Understanding
Psychological
Disorders

Enhanced 12th Edition

David Sue

Emeritus Professor of Psychology
Western Washington University

Derald Wing Sue

Department of Counseling and Clinical Psychology
Teachers College, Columbia University

Diane M. Sue

Private Practice

Stanley Sue

Emeritus Professor of Psychology
University of California, Davis
Palo Alto University

✳ Cengage

Australia • Brazil • Canada • Mexico • Singapore • United Kingdom • United States

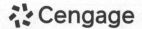

Understanding Psychological Disorders,
Enhanced 12th Edition
David Sue, Derald Wing Sue, Diane M. Sue,
Stanley Sue

SVP, Product: Cheryl Costantini

VP, Product: Thais Alencar

Portfolio Product Director: Laura Ross

Portfolio Product Manager: Marta Healey-Gerth

Product Assistant: Fantasia Mejia

Learning Designer: Kim Beuttler

Content Manager: Brett Rader

Digital Project Manager: Scott Diggins

Director, Product Marketing: Neena Bali

Product Marketing Manager: Chris Walz

Content Acquisition Analyst: Deanna Ettinger

Production Service: Lumina Datamatics Ltd.

Designer: Sara Greenwood

Cover Image Source: © iStockPhoto.com
/agsandrew

For product information and technology assistance, contact us at
Cengage Customer & Sales Support, 1-800-354-9706
or support.cengage.com.

For permission to use material from this text or product, submit all
requests online at **www.copyright.com**.

Library of Congress Control Number: 2023922187

ISBN: 979-8-214-13635-6

Cengage
5191 Natorp Boulevard
Mason, OH 45040
USA

Cengage is a leading provider of customized learning solutions.
Our employees reside in nearly 40 different countries and serve digital
learners in 165 countries around the world. Find your local representative at
www.cengage.com.

To learn more about Cengage platforms and services, register or access
your online learning solution, or purchase materials for your course,
visit **www.cengage.com**.

Printed at CLDPC, USA, 03-24

About the Authors

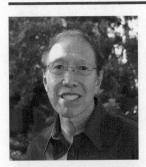

David Sue is Professor Emeritus of Psychology at Western Washington University, where he is an associate of the Center for Cross-Cultural Research. He has served as the director of both the Psychology Counseling Clinic and the Mental Health Counseling Program. He co-authored the books *Counseling and Psychotherapy in a Diverse Society* and *Counseling the Culturally Diverse: Theory and Practice*. He received his PhD in Clinical Psychology from Washington State University. His research interests revolve around multicultural issues in individual and group counseling. He enjoys hiking, snowshoeing, traveling, and spending time with his family.

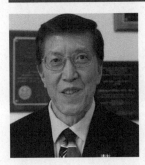

Derald Wing Sue is Professor of Psychology and Education in the Department of Counseling and Clinical Psychology at Teachers College, Columbia University. He has written extensively in the field of multicultural counseling/therapy, microaggression theory, and racial dialogue. He is author of *Counseling the Culturally Diverse: Theory and Practice*. Dr. Sue has served as president of the Society of Counseling Psychology and the Society for the Psychological Study of Ethnic Minority Issues and has received numerous awards for teaching and service. He received his doctorate from the University of Oregon and is married and the father of two children. Friends describe him as addicted to exercise and the Internet.

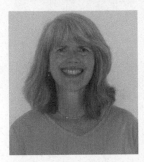

Diane M. Sue received her PhD from the University of Michigan, Ann Arbor. She has worked as a school psychologist and counselor as well as with adults needing specialized care for mental illness and neurocognitive disorders. Her areas of expertise include child and adolescent psychology, aging, and neuropsychology. She co-authored *Counseling and Psychotherapy in a Diverse Society* and is the author of *Remarkable Resilience: The Life and Legacy of Noémi Ban Beyond the Holocaust*. A former adjunct faculty member at Western Washington University, Dr. Sue received the Western Washington University College of Education Professional Excellence Award and the Washington State School Psychologist of the Year Award. She enjoys spending time with friends and family and is an advocate for climate justice.

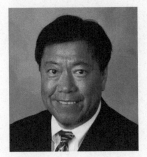

Stanley Sue is Emeritus Distinguished Professor of Psychology at University of California, Davis and at Palo Alto University. He was Assistant and Associate Professor of Psychology at the University of Washington (1971–1981); Professor of Psychology at University of California, Los Angeles (1981–1996); and Distinguished Professor of Psychology at University of California, Davis (1996–2010). He served as President of the Western Psychological Association in 2010; President of APA Division 45 (Society for the Psychological Study of Culture, Ethnicity, and Race) in 2015; and Science Editor for the U.S. Surgeon General's 2001 supplementary report for *Mental Health: Culture, Race, and Ethnicity*.

Brief Contents

Contents

Chapter 3 Assessment and Classification of Mental Disorders 85

Chapter 4 Research Methods for Studying Mental Disorders 117

Chapter 5 Anxiety and Obsessive-Compulsive and Related Disorders 147

Chapter 6 Trauma- and Stressor-Related Disorders 195

Chapter 7 Somatic Symptom and Dissociative Disorders **231**

Chapter 8 Depressive and Bipolar Disorders **267**

Chapter 9 Suicide 313

Chapter 10 Eating Disorders 353

Chapter 11 Substance-Related and Other Addictive Disorders   **391**

Chapter 12 Schizophrenia Spectrum Disorders   **433**

Chapter 15 Personality Psychopathology　　563

Chapter 16 Disorders of Childhood and Adolescence　　603

Chapter 17 Law and Ethical Clinical Practice 647

Features

■ Going Deeper

Focus on Resilience

Disorders Charts

Preface

We recognize that the times in which we are living are quite extraordinary and that the social conditions and societal disruptions sparked by political discord, the COVID-19 pandemic, and the climate crisis are unprecedented. The social inequities that became apparent early in the pandemic, coupled with the ongoing inequality and systemic racism spotlighted by the tragic killing of George Floyd, Breonna Taylor, and so many others, appeared to awaken many people to the issues of social injustice that have operated for centuries in the United States and throughout the world. Further, the tragic effects of extreme weather conditions, including changing patterns of global migration, have highlighted societal imbalance and the vulnerability of marginalized groups. These societal realities have brought attention to the enormous impact that social and sociocultural issues have on mental health. Stress, anxiety, and depression are affecting people throughout the United States and Canada but particularly those who have historically faced societal oppression. Although the disruptions related to current societal stressors have been quite challenging for people of all ages across the globe, the impact is particularly significant for those who are in college—a group on the threshold of integrating core values and discovering the contributions they will make to our changing society. Many students are facing this unprecedented and complicated period of history with full awareness of the challenges we need to address and the need for transformational societal changes with respect to social and climate justice. Many college students and youth are at the forefront in understanding how injustice, poverty, and economic inequality impact society as a whole. Awareness of the challenges we are confronting can certainly produce a degree of chronic stress, but it can also serve as a catalyst for choosing career paths or working with visionary organizations that will make the world a better place.

We realize that as you navigate these challenging and transformational times, many of you will be touched by mental health issues, either directly through your own emotional struggles or indirectly through friends or family. Recent events have both created and exacerbated social and economic challenges for many people, with resultant effects on emotional functioning and overall mental health. Given these realities, knowledge about symptoms, causes, and treatments associated with mental disorders and about methods for maintaining optimal mental health during challenging times is a highly relevant topic. It is our hope that this textbook will be personally meaningful to all who read it. For this reason, we look at the subject matter broadly and incorporate a variety of multicultural and contemporary examples to enhance the relevancy of our discussions.

In writing and revising this text, we have made great effort to update the content in an effort to engage students in the exciting process of understanding psychopathology and the techniques that mental health professionals employ when assessing and treating mental disorders. Four major objectives have guided our pursuit of this goal:

- to provide students with scholarship of the highest quality;
- to offer balanced coverage of abnormal psychology as both a scientific and a clinical endeavor, giving students the opportunity to explore topics thoroughly and responsibly;

- to expand awareness and empathy by focusing on the human face of mental illness, including an emphasis on both resilience and recovery; and

- to write a text that is inviting and stimulating to a wide range of students and that highlights meaningful topics that intersect with contemporary societal issues.

The enhanced 12th edition of *Understanding Abnormal Behavior*, now titled *Understanding Psychological Disorders*, has been revised to incorporate the text revision of the American Psychiatric Association's *Diagnostic and Statistical Manual of Mental Disorders, Fifth Edition* (DSM-5-TR), published in 2022, and some of the newest scientific, psychological, multicultural, and psychiatric research, as well as the continued controversies surrounding the classification and diagnosis of mental disorders. Although we have relied on the DSM-5 and the DSM-5-TR for much of our organizational framework and for the specific diagnostic characteristics of mental disorders, you will find that we do not follow the DSM in a mechanistic fashion. Instead, we remain committed to providing our readers with information from a variety of key organizations and from the multitude of medical and psychological publications that address mental health issues.

We feel a keen responsibility to keep our book fresh and to incorporate the burgeoning and immensely important research from the fields of neuroscience, psychology, and psychiatry. Thus, you will find many discussions of contemporary issues, controversies, and trends in these fields. In keeping with our commitment to the currency of the information presented, you will find that we have included many new references in this edition of the text. Most important, consistent with our goal of a balanced presentation, the references come from a wide variety of journals and other resources. Further, we have made every attempt to determine which research is most critical to a comprehensive understanding of each mental disorder and to present that information in an understandable, nontechnical manner. Although we strive to avoid overwhelming students with extensive data or too much theory, we are strong believers in sharing research-based information and evidence-based mental health practices. As with previous editions of this text, our goal is to include recent and cutting-edge research from a variety of resources in a manner that engages the reader.

We continue to receive very positive feedback about our multipath model of mental disorders, which is considered a highly effective visual and conceptual framework that helps students understand the multitude of factors that influence the development of various mental health conditions. In keeping with this model, we once again emphasize the importance of considering biological, psychological, social, and sociocultural factors and their interactions in the etiology of mental disorders. Our four-dimensional model ensures that instructors consistently consider sociocultural influences that are associated with specific disorders—an aspect made apparent by our current social unrest, yet often neglected by contemporary models of psychopathology. In this and previous editions of the text, we emphasize the importance of understanding multicultural influences on psychopathology, accentuating how marginalized populations, including women, people from underrepresented racial/ethnic groups and gender/racial minorities, are differentially affected by mental health issues. Readers will find that we take a balanced approach when discussing the etiology of mental disorders— emphasizing multicultural issues within the context of interactions between these cultural factors and biological, psychological, and social factors. In this edition of the text, we continue to connect the dots between societal oppression and the resultant effects on mental health. We highlight inherent societal factors, such as systemic racism, that influence both mental and physical health.

We are excited that the text continues to incorporate features that help students to organize the material and to consolidate their learning. For example, throughout the text, students will find Mental Disorders Charts that concisely describe symptoms and diagnostic criteria, prevalence, and gender data, as well as data on course and outcome for many of the disorders we cover. Students can easily compare and contrast the various disorders presented throughout the text by referring to these charts and the Multipath Model figures. We are pleased to continue our Focus on Resilience feature, introduced in the 10th edition. This feature encompasses contributions from the field of positive psychology and highlights key information relevant to both prevention and recovery from the symptoms associated with various disorders. This emphasis is particularly important given all of the recent data on neuroplasticity and the changes that are possible with prevention efforts and with evidence-based therapies that are able to successfully reduce or ameliorate the distressing symptoms of many disorders.

Overall, we believe readers will find the text more engaging and captivating than ever before. We have made a consistent effort to align the information presented from chapter to chapter in order to enhance students' understanding of more complex topics. We also connect our discussions with current events whenever possible and with issues of particular importance to college-age populations. We have concentrated on providing students with information that relates not only to the field of psychopathology but also to their day-to-day lives—material students will find valuable both now and in the future. In fact, we view this text as a meaningful tool that students can refer to when they encounter questions regarding mental health issues in their personal lives or with co-workers or clientele within the workforce.

We have also prioritized putting a human face on the various disorders and issues we discuss throughout the text. We have considered the fact that many students have direct experience with mental disorders, either because they are personally affected or because their friends or family members have experienced the distressing symptoms of a mental disorder. Many of the case studies we present highlight the perspective of individuals coping with the disorders discussed, which allows students to gain greater insight into the struggles involved in living with mental illness.

As illustrated by the new information added to each chapter, this edition of our book provides current and relevant information on a wide variety of topics in the field of psychopathology.

New and Updated Coverage of the Twelfth Edition and Enhanced Twelfth Edition

Our foremost objective in preparing the 12th edition and enhanced 12th edition was to thoroughly update the contents of the text to incorporate the DSM-5-TR and present the latest trends in research and clinical thinking. This has led to updated coverage of many topics throughout the text, including the following.

Chapter 1—Abnormal Behavior

- New statistics on the prevalence of mental disorders
- New discussions regarding the recovery movement; current stressors on mental health such as mass shootings, climate change, sexual harassment, and discrimination; overcoming stigma and stereotypes; the influence of social media on mental health; extreme risk protection orders; personnel shortages in the mental health field; and technological advances that enhance mental health research and treatment

Chapter 2—Understanding and Treating Mental Disorders

- Expanded multipath model coverage, including an enhanced discussion of epigenetics
- New discussion of the effects of systemic, structural, and internalized racism and social injustice on mental health
- Updated discussion of the social and sociocultural etiological dimensions, including further discussion of gender, poverty, and stress associated with immigration

Chapter 3—Assessment and Classification of Mental Disorders

- New discussion regarding the appropriateness of making a mental health diagnosis involving a public figure
- Expanded discussion of the dimensional approach to assessment incorporated into the DSM-5 and the DSM-5-TR
- Overview of the updated version of the Minnesota Multiphasic Personality Inventory
- Expanded coverage of cultural considerations in assessment and diagnosis

Chapter 4—Research Methods for Studying Mental Disorders

- New feature regarding the importance of critical thinking when evaluating the veracity of information presented in the media
- New discussion about the advantages and disadvantages of using large data sets gathered from the Internet and social media
- Updated information regarding the controversy about repressed memory

Chapter 5—Anxiety and Obsessive-Compulsive and Related Disorders

- New discussions of the impact of COVID-19 on anxiety symptoms and how acculturation conflicts, prejudice, and discrimination affect ethnic minority students
- Expanded discussion of treatment for anxiety disorders, including the use of virtual reality therapy, smartphone applications, and transdiagnostic treatment for disorders with similar emotional underpinnings
- Greater focus on how anxiety disorders manifest globally
- A new discussion comparing the minority stress model and the rejection sensitivity model as explanations for the higher incidence of mental and physical health challenges among marginalized populations

Chapter 6—Trauma- and Stressor-Related Disorders

- Discussion to deepen understanding of the stress associated with the COVID-19 pandemic
- Discussion of prolonged grief disorder, a disorder introduced in the DSM-5-TR
- Expanded discussion of epigenetic influences on stress disorders
- Discussion of stress, trauma, and health disparities associated with race-based discrimination and the concept of "skin-deep" resilience

- Research regarding the use of MDMA to treat posttraumatic stress disorder
- Discussion of the role of positive emotions in preventing stress disorders

Chapter 7—Somatic Symptom and Dissociative Disorders

- Updated discussion of the continuing controversy involving dissociative amnesia and repressed memory
- Enhanced analysis of issues surrounding the assessment and understanding of depersonalization
- Expanded discussion of dissociative identity disorder, including brain scan findings and the evolution of treatments for the disorder

Chapter 8—Depressive and Bipolar Disorders

- Updated data on the prevalence of depressive and bipolar disorders
- New discussion of functional brain alterations in depression and the effects of racism, discrimination, poverty, cannabis use, adverse childhood experiences, and prosocial characteristics on the development of depression and the relationship between stress and depression
- Updated discussion of depression treatments, including use of the anesthetic ketamine, probiotics, and brain stimulation and cognitive-behavioral therapies
- Information about personality traits associated with bipolar disorder and the role of cannabis in the development of bipolar disorder, as well as updates regarding treatment approaches used with bipolar disorder

Chapter 9—Suicide

- New data on the prevalence of suicide, including age and racial group differences
- New discussions regarding a proposed category of suicidal behavior disorder; moral, ethical, and legal issues surrounding suicide; psychological recovery after a suicide attempt; and innovative prevention and intervention strategies
- Updated discussion regarding the dramatic increase in youth suicides and the role that bullying, social media, drug and alcohol use, experiences with discrimination, and sleep difficulties play in suicidal behavior

Chapter 10—Eating Disorders

- Updated statistics on eating disorders and obesity
- New discussion of the role of genetic factors on metabolic dysfunction; the influence of social media and "fat shaming" on body dissatisfaction; and the role of emotional eating

Chapter 11—Substance-Related and Other Addictive Disorders

- Updated statistics and figures illustrating the prevalence of substance use and abuse, with a particular focus on alcohol
- Expanded discussion regarding the dangers of energy drinks and the abuse of illicit and prescription drugs, particularly opioids
- New discussion of the prevalence and risk of vaping
- Updated information on substance abuse treatment

Chapter 12—Schizophrenia Spectrum Disorders

- Updated research on schizophrenia and the DSM-5-TR diagnostic categories
- Expanded discussion of symptoms associated with schizophrenia spectrum disorders, including a focus on reasoning bias and on catatonia
- Updated discussion on attenuated psychosis syndrome
- New discussion about the role of machine learning in identifying spoken language unique to schizophrenia; the role of aberrant "pruning" of neural synapses as a cause of schizophrenia; and the success of integrated early intervention efforts with individuals at risk for psychotic disorders

Chapter 13—Neurocognitive and Sleep–Wake Disorders

- Presentation of new research on various neurocognitive disorders, particularly Alzheimer's disease
- Continued focus on neurocognitive disorders across the life span, with a strong emphasis on how modern lifestyle affects brain function and neurogenerative disorders
- Discussion of Robin Williams and Lewy bodies dementia
- Expanded discussion of traumatic brain injury and chronic traumatic encephalopathy in athletes and veterans
- New discussion on sleep deprivation in college students
- New table on sleep–wake disorders

Chapter 14—Sexual Dysfunctions, Gender Dysphoria, and Paraphilic Disorders

- Updated application of the multipath model to sexual disorders
- Discussion of new research on treatment for sexual dysfunctions, including new medications for low sexual desire in women
- New discussion regarding the relationship between Internet porn and sexual dysfunction
- Discussion of a sexual assault survey involving nearly 182,000 college students
- An expanded discussion of terminology related to gender expression and gender identity and the role of societal stressors and discrimination in the development of gender dysphoria

Chapter 15—Personality Psychopathology

- New case studies and expanded discussion of the 10 traditional personality categories, including updated research on the etiology and treatment of antisocial, borderline, and narcissistic personality disorders
- Expanded discussion of the six personality types and five personality trait domains included in the DSM-5 alternative model for diagnosing a personality disorder
- Critical discussion of the DSM-5 inclusion of two methods for diagnosing personality disorders and dimensional methods of personality assessment

Chapter 16—Disorders of Childhood and Adolescence

- Updated discussion of neurodevelopmental disorders, childhood anxiety, childhood posttraumatic stress disorder, reactive attachment disorder, tics and Tourette's syndrome, nonsuicidal self-injury (a category undergoing further study), disruptive mood dysregulation disorder, and disinhibited social engagement disorder
- Enhanced discussion regarding early prevention of lifelong mental illness and methods for enhancing resilience

Chapter 17—Law and Ethical Clinical Practice

- New discussion regarding the therapeutic and legal implications of confidentiality during mandatory therapy sessions for migrant children and with regard to violent behaviors; psychiatric advance directives for individuals with chronic, severe mental illness; extreme risk protection orders and red flag laws that allow a court to temporarily prohibit an individual from possessing or purchasing firearms; the lack of sufficient mental health resources; homelessness and incarceration among individuals living with chronic mental illness; Assertive Community Treatment programs; and conflicts between ethics and the law for psychologists working for the Veterans Administration

Our Approach

We take an eclectic, evidence- and research-based, multicultural approach to understanding psychological disorders, drawing on important contributions from various disciplines and theoretical perspectives. The text covers the major categories of disorders in the updated *Diagnostic and Statistical Manual of Mental Disorders* (DSM-5-TR), but it is not a mechanistic reiteration of the DSM. We believe that different combinations of life experiences and constitutional factors result in mental disorders, and we project this view throughout the text. This combination of influences is demonstrated in our multipath model, which was introduced in our 9th edition. There are several elements to our multipath model. First, possible contributors to mental disorders are divided into four dimensions: biological, psychological, social, and sociocultural. Second, factors in the four dimensions can interact and influence each other in any direction. Third, different combinations and interactions within the four dimensions can result in mental illness. Fourth, many disorders appear to be heterogeneous in nature; therefore, there may be different versions of a disorder or a spectrum of the disorder. Finally, distinctly different disorders (such as anxiety and depression) can be caused by similar factors.

Sociocultural influences, including cultural norms, values, and expectations, are given special attention in our multipath model. We are convinced that cross-cultural comparisons of psychological disorders and treatment methods can greatly enhance our understanding of disorders; cultural and gender influences are emphasized throughout the text. *Understanding Abnormal Behavior* was the first textbook on abnormal psychology to integrate and emphasize the role of multicultural factors. Although many texts have since followed our lead, the 12th edition and the enhanced 12th edition continue to provide the most extensive coverage and integration of multicultural models, explanations, and concepts available. Not only do we discuss how changing demographics increase the importance of multicultural psychology, we also introduce multicultural models of psychopathology in the opening chapters and address multicultural issues throughout the text whenever research findings and theoretical formulations allow. Such an approach adds richness to students' understanding of mental disorders.

As psychologists (and professors), we know that learning is enhanced whenever material is presented in a lively and engaging manner. We therefore provide case vignettes and clients' descriptions of their experiences to complement and illustrate symptoms of various disorders and research-based explanations. Our goal is to encourage students to think critically rather than to merely assimilate a collection of facts and theories. As a result, we hope that students will develop an appreciation of the study of psychological disorders.

Special Features

As previously noted, our multipath model provides a framework through which students can understand the origins of mental disorders. The model is introduced in Chapter 2 and applied throughout the book, with _multiple figures highlighting how biological, psychological, social, and sociocultural factors contribute to the development of various disorders. The 12th edition and enhanced 12th edition include a variety of features that were popular in earlier editions and that, in some cases, have been revised and enhanced. These features are aimed at helping students to organize and integrate the material in each chapter.

- *GOING DEEPER* boxes provide information and thought-provoking questions that raise key issues in research, examine widely held assumptions about mental illness, or challenge the student's understanding of the text material. These boxes stimulate critical thinking, evoke alternative views, provoke discussion, and allow students to better explore the wider meaning of psychological distress in our society.

- *Contemporary Trends and Future Directions* is a newer feature with which we conclude most of the chapters, providing a final look at current trends that are relevant to topics covered in each chapter.

- *Myth versus Reality* discussions challenge the many myths and false beliefs that have surrounded the field of psychopathology and help students realize that beliefs, some of which may appear to be "common sense," must be checked against scientific facts and knowledge.

- *Did You Know?* boxes found throughout the book provide fascinating, at-a-glance research-based tidbits that are linked to material covered in the main body of the text.

- *Learning Objectives* appearing in the first pages of every chapter provide a framework and stimulate active learning.

- *Chapter Summaries* provide students with a concise recap of the chapter's most important concepts via brief answers to the chapter's opening Focus Questions.

- *Case Studies* allow issues of mental health and mental disorders to "come to life" for students and instructors. Many cases are taken from journal articles and actual clinical files.

- *Disorder Charts* provide snapshots of disorders in an easy-to-read format.

- *Key Terms* are highlighted in the text and appear at the end of each chapter.

MindTap for Sue's *Understanding Psychological Disorders*

Today's leading online learning platform, MindTap for Sue's *Understanding Psychological Disorders*, gives you complete control of your course to craft a personalized, engaging learning experience that challenges students, builds confidence, and elevates performance.

MindTap introduces students to core concepts from the beginning of your course using a simplified learning path that progresses from understanding to application and delivers access to eTextbooks, study tools, interactive media, auto-graded assessments and performance analytics.

Use MindTap for Sue's *Understanding Psychological Disorders* as is or personalize it to meet your specific course needs. You can also easily integrate MindTap into your Learning Management System (LMS).

For students:

- MindTap delivers real-world relevance with activities and assignments that help students build critical-thinking and analytical skills that will transfer to other courses and their professional lives.

- MindTap helps students stay organized and efficient with a single destination that reflects what's important to the instructor, along with the tools students need to master the content.

- MindTap empowers and motivates students with information that shows where they stand at all times—both individually and compared to the highest performers in their class.

Additionally, for instructors, MindTap allows you to:

- Control what content students see and when they see it, with a learning path that can be used as is or aligned with your syllabus

- Create a unique learning path of relevant readings and multimedia activities that move students up the learning taxonomy from basic knowledge and comprehension to analysis, application, and critical thinking

- Integrate your own content into the MindTap Reader using your documents or pulling from sources such as RSS feeds, YouTube videos, Web sites, Google Docs, and more

- Use powerful analytics and reports that provide a snapshot of class progress, time in course, engagement, and completion

In addition to the benefits of the platform, MindTap for Sue's *Understanding Psychological Disorders* features:

- Videos from the Continuum Video Project
- Case studies to help students humanize psychological disorders and connect content to the real world

Learn more at https://www.cengage.com/mindtap.

Supplements

Continuum Video Project

The Continuum Video Project provides holistic, three-dimensional portraits of individuals dealing with psychopathologies. Videos show clients living their daily lives, interacting with family and friends, and displaying—rather than just describing—their symptoms. Before each video segment, students are asked to make observations about the individual's symptoms, emotions, and behaviors and then rate them on the spectrum from normal to severe. The Continuum Video Project allows students to connect with the disorder and the person on a human level; the videos also help students understand that mental illness can be viewed along a continuum.

Additional instructor resources for this product are available online. Instructor assets include an Instructor's Manual, Educator's Guide, PowerPoint® slides, and a test bank powered by Cognero®. Sign up or sign in at www.cengage.com to search for and access this product and its online resources.

Acknowledgments

We would like to thank the reviewers of the previous editions of *Understanding Abnormal Behavior* for sharing their valuable insights, opinions, and recommendations:

Sandra K. Arntz, Northern Illinois University

Julia C. Babcock, University of Houston

Jay Brown, Texas Wesleyan University

Jeffrey D. Burke, University of Pittsburgh

Catherine Chambliss, Ursinus College

Betty Clark, University of Mary-Hardin

Irvin Cohen, Hawaii Pacific University and Kapiolani Community College

Lorry Cology, Owens Community College

Bonnie J. Ekstrom, Bemidji State University

Joseph Falco, Rockland Community College

Greg A. R. Febbraro, Drake University

Kate Flory, University of South Carolina

David M. Fresco, Kent State University

Jerry L. Fryrear, University of Houston, Clear Lake

Michele Galietta, John Jay College of Criminal Justice

Alice L. Godbey, Daytona State College

Christina Gordon, Fox Valley Technical College

Robert Hoff, Mercyhurst College

Deborah Huerta, The University of Texas at Brownsville

George-Harold Jennings, Drew University

Kim L. Krinsky, Georgia Perimeter College

Arlene Lacombe, St. Joseph's University

Dawn Lin, Jackson State University

Katheryn Lovell, Thomas Nelson Community College

Brian E. Lozano, Virginia Polytechnic Institute and State University

Vicki Lucey, Las Positas College

Polly McMahon, Spokane Falls Community College

Jan Mohlman, Rutgers University

Sherry Davis Molock, George Washington University

Rebecca L. Motley, University of Toledo

Gilbert R. Parra, University of Memphis

Jeffrey J. Pedroza, Santa Ana College

Kimberly Renk, University of Central Florida

Tiffany Rich, East Los Angeles College

Mark Richardson, Boston University

Alan Roberts, Indiana University

Tom Schoeneman, Lewis and Clark College

Daniel L. Segal, University of Colorado at Colorado Springs

Michael D. Spiegler, Providence College

Sandra Terneus, Tennessee Technological University

Ma. Teresa G. Tuason, University of North Florida

Theresa A. Wadkins, University of Nebraska, Kearney

Susan Brooks Watson, Hawaii Pacific University

Fred Whitford, Montana State University

Jessica L. Yokley, University of Pittsburgh

We also wish to acknowledge the contributions of Marta Healy-Gerth, Associate Portfolio Product Manager; Brett Rader, Content Manager; Fantasia Mejia, Senior Product Assistant; and Sara Greenwood, Designer. We also thank the text designer and the text and photo researchers.

D. S.
D. W. S.
D. M. S.
S. S.

focus Questions

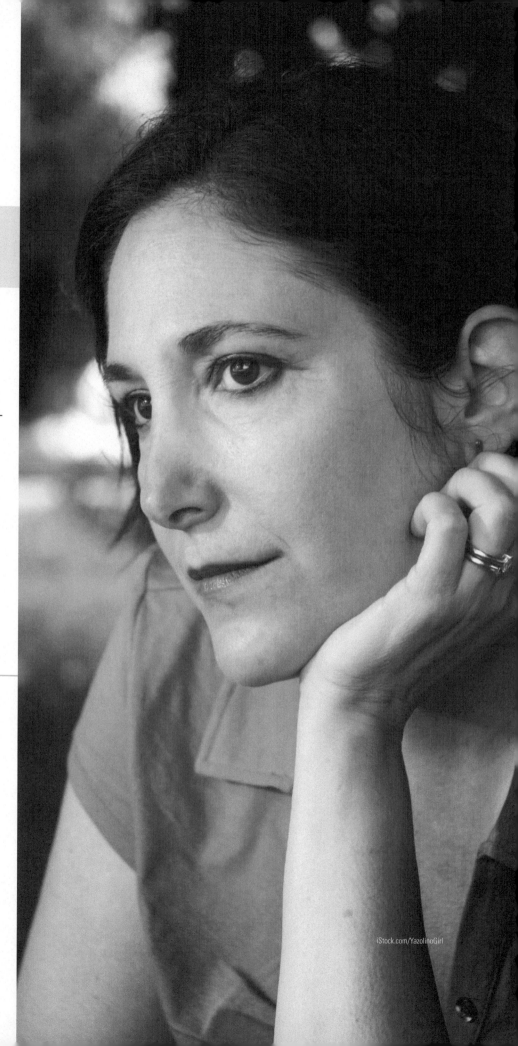

1

Understanding Psychopathology

Learning Objectives

After studying this chapter, you will be able to . . .

1-1 Define psychopathology.

1-2 Explain the various criteria used to determine psychopathology.

1-3 Summarize some of the data regarding the prevalence of mental disorders.

1-4 Discuss how sociopolitical experiences and cultural influences affect definitions of psychopathology.

1-5 Explain why it is important to confront the stigma and stereotyping associated with mental illness.

1-6 Discuss how explanations of psychopathology have changed over time.

1-7 Summarize early explanations regarding the causes of mental disorders.

1-8 Describe some contemporary trends in understanding psychopathology.

In the Early Morning Hours of January 8, 2011, 23-year-old Jared Lee Loughner posted a message on social media, prefaced with the word "Goodbye." The post continued: "Dear friends . . . Please don't be mad at me. The literacy rate is below 5%. I haven't talked to one person who is literate. I want to make it out alive. The longest war in the history of the United States. Goodbye. I'm saddened with the current currency and job employment. I had a bully at school. Thank you."

Hours later, Loughner took a taxi to a supermarket in Tucson, Arizona, where U.S. representative Gabrielle Giffords (D-AZ) was meeting with her constituents. Loughner approached the gathering and, using a semiautomatic handgun, opened fire on Giffords and bystanders, killing 6 people and injuring 13 others. Giffords, believed to have been Loughner's target, was shot in the head and left in critical condition (Cloud, 2011). After his arrest, Loughner was declared incompetent to stand trial due to his extensive mental confusion. However, 19 months after the shooting, his mental condition improved enough for him to participate in court proceedings. He pleaded guilty to all charges related to the shooting and received a life sentence without the possibility of parole. Fortunately, Giffords has demonstrated remarkable resilience and recovery from her brain injury. Although she resigned from her congressional seat in 2012, she has returned to public service as a well-respected advocate of gun control (Collins, 2019).

Untreated Mental Illness

This picture of Jared Lee Loughner was taken after his arrest for shooting Representative Gabrielle Giffords and killing numerous bystanders. It was not until after his arrest that he received a mental health evaluation and was diagnosed with paranoid schizophrenia.

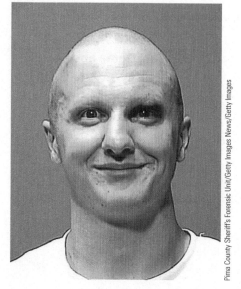

Pima County Sheriff's Forensic Unit/Getty Images News/Getty Images

As with other mass shootings, people around the country attempted to make sense of Loughner's irrational act, asking questions such as: What could have motivated him to take so many innocent lives? Was he a political extremist? Was he a callous, psychopathic killer? Was he suicidal? Was he high on drugs? What was Loughner like before the shooting? Did he have a **mental disorder**? Were there warning signs that he was so dangerous? Could therapy or medication have helped Loughner? Could *anything* have prevented this tragedy?

These questions are extremely difficult to answer for a number of reasons. First, understanding what might cause behavior and mental disturbance like Loughner's is not an easy task. We still do not know enough about the specific causes of psychopathology to arrive at a definitive answer. We do know, however, that **mental illness** does not generally result from a single cause but instead arises from an interaction of many factors, a fact that we discuss in the next chapter.

Second, trying to assess someone's state of mind can be extremely difficult. In the case of Loughner, his thinking and reasoning were so confused that he was unable to assist in his own defense for over 18 months. Given such mental confusion, any attempt to construct a portrait of Loughner's state of mind around the time of the shooting requires the use of secondary sources such as observations by family and acquaintances, school records, and other data such as Internet postings. Fortunately, unlike Loughner, many people recognize the need to seek help when they experience emotional distress or the behavioral, emotional, or physical symptoms of a mental disorder. Furthermore, the vast majority of those affected by mental illness display neither the violence nor the extreme mental confusion shown by Loughner (Lu & Temple, 2019).

As you can see, understanding mental disorders is a complex topic. The purpose of this book is to help you understand the signs, symptoms, and causes of mental illness. We also focus on research related to preventing mental disorders and successfully living with and recovering from mental illness. Before exploring mental health and mental illness, however, we discuss the study of psychopathology, including some of its history and emerging changes in the field. During our discussion, we will periodically refer to the Loughner case to highlight issues in the mental health field.

1-1 The Field of Psychopathology

The field of **psychopathology** focuses on the study of the symptoms and causes of mental distress as well as available treatments for behavioral and mental disorders. Our hope is that this textbook will help you understand how professionals in the field of psychopathology describe, explain, predict, and modify the behaviors, emotions, and thoughts associated with various mental conditions.

This book focuses on behavior that ranges from highly unusual to fairly common—from the very rare violent homicides and mental breakdowns that are widely reported by the news media to more prevalent concerns such as depression, anxiety, eating disturbances, and substance abuse. We also focus on methods for preventing and alleviating the distress and life disruption experienced by those with mental illness.

Describing Behavior

If you were undergoing emotional distress, you might decide to seek help from a **mental health professional**. If so, your therapist might begin by asking you some questions and observing your behavior and reactions while listening carefully to your concerns. The therapist would then use these observations paired with information you share about your background and symptoms as well as knowledge of societal circumstances to formulate a **psychodiagnosis**, an attempt to describe, assess, and understand your particular situation and the possibility that you might be experiencing a mental disorder. After gaining a better understanding of your situation, you and the professional would work together to develop a **treatment plan**, beginning with a focus on your most distressing symptoms.

Loughner never worked with a mental health professional before the shooting. However, he did undergo several psychiatric evaluations after his arrest. In addition to receiving a psychiatric diagnosis, Loughner was evaluated to assess his potential dangerousness, the degree to which he was in contact with reality, and whether he was mentally competent to assist in his own defense. Based on observations of Loughner and a review of available information, the examiners determined that Loughner had symptoms consistent with a diagnosis of schizophrenia (a serious mental disorder we discuss in Chapter 12).

Explaining Behavior

Identifying the **etiology**, or possible causes, for psychopathology is a high priority for mental health professionals. In the case of Loughner's actions, one popular explanation was that he was a right-wing political extremist who held positions diametrically opposed to those of Representative Giffords. However, Loughner's issues were much more complex. His Internet postings and YouTube videos highlighted his belief that the U.S. government was brainwashing people. Additionally, when attending a political event several years prior to the shooting, he asked Giffords, "What is government if words have no meaning?" Giffords declined to comment (probably because the question made no sense to her). Loughner apparently felt slighted and angered by her lack of response. This interaction reportedly fueled his rage and obsession with Giffords.

A closer look at Loughner's background reveals many other possible causes for his rampage:

- Friends noted that he seemed to undergo a personality transformation around the time he dropped out of high school. He again experienced academic difficulties when attending community college; he was suspended because of poor academic performance, disruptive behavior, and a YouTube posting in which he described the school as "one of the biggest scams in America." Could this pattern of academic failure have contributed to his downward spiral and resultant anger?

- Others noted that Loughner was devastated following a breakup with a high school girlfriend. The failed relationship reportedly triggered increasing use of marijuana, LSD, and other hallucinogens. When Loughner tried to enlist in the U.S. Army, he was deemed unqualified. Did the breakup, his drug use, or being rejected from military service play a role in his actions?

- Others have noted that biological factors may account for Loughner's mental breakdown. While incarcerated, he was diagnosed with schizophrenia. Research points to a biological basis for this disorder, with

Myth Mental illness causes people to become unstable and potentially dangerous.

Reality The vast majority of individuals who are mentally ill do not commit crimes, do not harm others, and do not get into trouble with the law. However, there is a slightly increased risk of violence among individuals with a history of mental illness, substance abuse, and prior victimization (Rozel & Mulvey, 2017).

It is very difficult to predict school violence. However, risk factors associated with increased potential for violence include male gender, access to weapons, threatening or violent communications, talking about plans to carry out an attack, feeling hopeless or suicidal, and having a history of being bullied or persecuted.

Source: Stubbe, 2019

vulnerability to schizophrenia exacerbated by marijuana use. Interestingly, Loughner's downward spiral in his early 20s is very consistent with the onset of schizophrenia, as are his paranoid beliefs and nonsensical speech. What role did biological factors play in his deteriorating mental condition?

These snippets from Loughner's life suggest many possible explanations for his actions, including **biological vulnerability** such as genetic susceptibility to mental illness, perhaps made worse by his use of marijuana, his belief in extremist political rhetoric, his academic and military failures, his anger about the breakup with his girlfriend, and his substance abuse. Some explanations may appear more valid than others. As you will learn in the next chapter, no single explanation adequately accounts for complex human behavior. Human behaviors occur along a continuum and result from interactions among various biological, psychological, social, and sociocultural factors.

Predicting Behavior

Many believe that there was sufficient evidence to predict that Loughner was a seriously disturbed and potentially dangerous young man. His parents, alarmed by his deteriorating behavior, encouraged him to seek professional help but were unsuccessful in their efforts. At Pima Community College, concerned staff and students contacted campus police regarding Loughner's disruptive conduct on at least five occasions. He posted hate-filled rants about the college on YouTube, and at least one teacher and one classmate expressed concern that he was capable of a school shooting.

To protect the campus, college administrators suspended Loughner, stipulating that he could return if (a) his behavior conformed to the codes of the college and (b) he received a mental health clearance confirming that his presence on campus would not constitute a danger to himself or others. In light of these reports, why was it that Loughner never received any type of psychological help or treatment? How could he purchase firearms during a period of obvious mental deterioration? If his parents and college officials were concerned that he was dangerous, why did mental health professionals or police officials not intervene?

There are several possible explanations for the lack of intervention. First, *civil commitment*, or involuntary confinement, represents an extreme decision that has major implications for an individual's civil liberties. Our legal system operates under the assumption that people are innocent until proven guilty. Locking someone up before they commit a dangerous act potentially violates that person's civil rights. In Loughner's case, there were concerns but no evidence that he presented an imminent threat. Second, because Loughner never agreed to mental health treatment, he was not in contact with a mental health professional who would have recognized the potential danger from his deteriorating mental condition. Even if Loughner had sought treatment, his therapy would have been confidential unless the therapist became aware of a clear and present danger to Loughner or to others. Regarding the purchase of firearms, Loughner met no criteria in Arizona that prevented him from purchasing weapons.

Further, even if someone had significant concerns about Loughner possessing a gun, Arizona

Intervening Through Therapy

Group therapy is a widely used form of treatment for many problems, especially those involving interpersonal relationships. In this group session, participants are learning to develop adaptive skills for coping with social problems rather than relying on alcohol or drugs to escape the stresses of life.

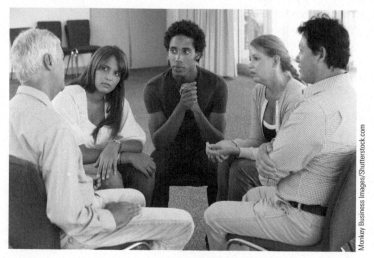

Monkey Business Images/Shutterstock.com

does not have a "red flag" law permitting police or family members to petition the court for an extreme risk protection order—a court order authorizing temporary removal of a firearm from someone who potentially poses a danger to themselves or others (a topic we discuss further in Chapter 17). Additionally, it is possible for someone with a deteriorating mental condition to appear relatively normal.

Modifying Behavior

Distressing symptoms can often be addressed and modified through **psychotherapy**, which involves systematic intervention designed to improve a person's behavioral, emotional, or cognitive state. Mental health professionals focus first on problematic symptoms and understanding the cause of a client's mental distress, taking into account any social or societal stressors. Next, they work with the client to plan treatment. Just as there are many ways to explain mental disorders, there are many therapies and many professional helpers offering their services. (Table 1.1 lists the qualifications and training of various mental health professionals.)

Among the mental health professionals, it is usually psychiatrists who prescribe medication. We are currently experiencing a national shortage of psychiatrists, which is exacerbated by retirements and insufficient numbers of psychiatrists-in-training (Merritt Hawkins, 2018). Other professionals

Table 1.1 The Mental Health Professions

Clinical psychologist	• Holds a PhD or a PsyD. • Coursework and internship focus on psychopathology, personality, psychological testing, diagnosis, therapy, and neuropsychology.
Counseling psychologist	• Academic and internship requirements are similar to those for a clinical psychologist, but with a focus on life adjustment problems rather than mental illness.
Mental health counselor; marriage/family therapist	• Holds a master's degree in counseling or psychology as well as supervised clinical experience.
Neuropsychologist	• Holds a PhD or a PsyD with specialization in brain–behavior relationships. • Coursework focuses on assessment, diagnosis, treatment planning, and research related to neurological, medical, developmental, or psychiatric conditions.
Psychiatrist	• Holds an MD degree; can prescribe medication. • Completes the 4 years of medical school required for an MD, and an additional 3 or 4 years of training in psychiatry.
Psychiatric nurse	• Holds an RN degree from a nursing program, plus specialized psychiatric training. • Performs assessment, diagnosis, and treatment of mental illness. • Some advanced practice registered nurses (APRNs) have completed master's or doctoral degrees and are allowed to prescribe medication.
Psychiatric social worker	• Holds a master's degree in social work. • Conducts assessment, screening, and therapy with high-need clients and facilitates outreach to other agencies.
School psychologist	• Holds a master's or a doctoral degree in school psychology. • Assesses and intervenes with the emotional and learning difficulties of students in educational settings.
Substance abuse counselor	• Professional training requirements vary; many practitioners have personal experience with addiction. • Works in agencies that specialize in the evaluation and treatment of drug and alcohol addiction.

with prescribing privileges—such as health advanced practice nurses (APRNs), physician assistants, and prescribing psychologists—are helping to fill this gap.

Many believe that if Loughner had received psychotherapy, his intense anger, disturbed thinking, and deteriorating mental condition would have been recognized as a serious concern and his violent rampage could have been prevented. Treatment might have included appropriate medications, anger management and social skills training, educating Loughner and his family about schizophrenia, and perhaps even temporary hospitalization to stabilize his mental situation.

1-2 Views of Psychopathology

Understanding and treating the distressing symptoms associated with mental illness is the main objective of those working in the mental health field. But how do mental health professionals evaluate symptoms and decide if a client is experiencing a mental disorder? *The Diagnostic and Statistical Manual of Mental Disorders* (5th ed., Text Revision DSM-5-TR; American Psychiatric Association [APA], 2022), the most widely used classification system of mental disorders, indicates that a mental disorder has the following components:

(a) involves a significant disturbance in thinking, emotional regulation, or behavior caused by a dysfunction in the basic psychological, biological, or developmental processes involved in normal development;

(b) causes significant distress or difficulty with day-to-day functioning; and

(c) is not merely a culturally expected response to common stressors or losses or a reflection of political or religious beliefs that conflict with societal norms.

This definition is quite broad and raises many questions. First, when are symptoms or patterns of behavior significant enough to have meaning? Second, is it possible to have a mental disorder without any signs of distress or discomfort? Third, what criteria do we use to decide if a behavior pattern is a reflection of an underlying psychological or biological dysfunction and not merely a normal variation or an expectable response to common stressors?

Complex definitions aside, most practitioners agree that mental disorders involve behavior or other distressing symptoms that depart from the norm and interfere with the individual's ability to adapt to life's demands. Nearly all definitions used in the field of psychopathology involve some form of comparative analysis to gauge deviations from normative standards. The four major factors involved in judging psychopathology are

- distress,
- deviance,
- dysfunction, and
- dangerousness.

Distress

Most people who seek the help of therapists are experiencing psychological distress that is affecting their social, emotional, or physical functioning. In the social sphere, an individual may become withdrawn and avoid

Societal Norms and Deviance

Societal norms often affect our definitions of expected behavior. When social norms begin to change, standards used to judge behaviors or roles also shift. Here we see a stay-at-home father cooking with his son. In the past, staying home to care for children was a role reserved for women.

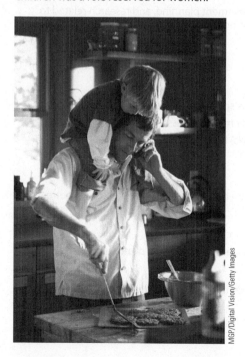

MGP/Digital Vision/Getty Images

interactions with others or, at the other extreme, may engage in inappropriate or dangerous social interactions. In the emotional realm, distress might involve crying, extreme agitation, or prolonged depression. Distress might also surface in the form of confused thinking or physical symptoms such as fatigue, pain, or heart palpitations. One disadvantage of assessing distress in determining psychopathology is that some individuals with severe mental illness experience **anosognosia**, an inability to recognize their own mental confusion.

Of course, we all have social, emotional, and physical ups and downs. We need to recognize that just as there is a continuum of human traits, such as height, there is a continuum associated with human emotions and behaviors. For example, you have probably felt temporarily depressed after experiencing a loss or a disappointment or felt anxious about situations involving friendships or school. The mere presence of a common symptom is not sufficient to warrant the diagnosis of a mental illness. Most professionals agree that many of us experience some of the symptoms associated with mental disorders. However, if your reaction is so intense or prolonged that it interferes with your ability to function adequately, the symptoms may reflect a mental disorder.

Deviance

Definitions of deviance rely on statistical standards (behaviors that occur infrequently), moral or religious beliefs (deviations from religious doctrine), or noncompliance with societal customs (departure from normative behavior). These methods of defining deviance are not mutually exclusive, and the importance of each may vary both within and between societies or cultural groups. Further, these standards are not fixed; they evolve or change over time. For example, "homosexuality" was considered a mental disorder until it was finally removed from the DSM in 1987. This decision was based on the many studies that demonstrate that gay men and lesbians are as well-adjusted as the heterosexual population. Public opinion has also evolved on sexual orientation. Although only 41 percent of the public supported same-sex marriage in 2004, approval rose to 70 percent in 2021 (McCarthy, 2021).

Certain behaviors are considered deviant in most situations. These behaviors include refusing to leave your house, sleeping for days because you are feeling depressed, fasting because you are terrified of gaining weight, forgetting your own identity, panicking at the sight of a spider, avoiding social contact because you fear people will judge you, believing that others can "hear" your thoughts, seeing aliens inside your home, collecting so many items that your health and safety are jeopardized, and intentionally making yourself sick with the goal of receiving attention. However, culture-related factors must be considered before labeling behaviors as symptomatic of a mental disorder. For instance, during some religious ceremonies, people display episodes of possession or loss of identity that are normative to the group and therefore would not be considered symptoms of a disorder (APA, 2022).

Personal Dysfunction

In everyday life, each of us fulfills a variety of social and occupational roles, such as friend, family member, student, or employee. Emotional problems sometimes interfere with our ability to adapt to life's demands and perform these roles. Therefore, role dysfunction is often considered when determining if someone has a mental disorder. One way to assess dysfunction

Did You Know?

During the Victorian era, women wore many layers of clothing to conceal their bodies from the neck down. Exposing an ankle was roughly equivalent to going topless at the beach today. Using words that might have a sexual connotation was also taboo. Victorians said *limb* instead of *leg* because the word *leg* was considered erotic; even pianos and tables were said to have limbs. People who did not adhere to these codes of conduct were considered immoral.

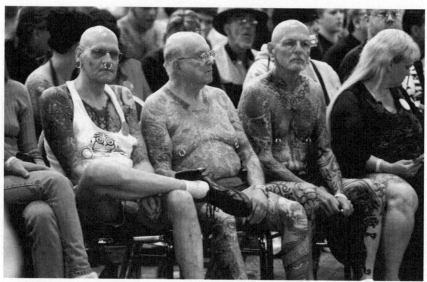

Behavioral Variation

By most people's standards, the full-body tattoos of these three men would be considered unusual. Yet these men openly and proudly display their body art at the National Tattoo Association Convention. These same individuals may be very typical in their work and personal lives. This leads to an important question: What constitutes psychopathological behavior, and how do we recognize it?

is to compare someone's performance with the requirements of a role. An employee who suddenly cannot concentrate sufficiently to fulfill job demands may be experiencing emotional difficulties. Dysfunction can also be assessed by comparing an individual's performance with their potential. For example, a sudden drop in academic performance may signal that a college student is experiencing anxiety, depression, or another common mental disorder.

Dangerousness

Even though it is rare for individuals who are living with a mental illness to commit violent crimes, media coverage of national tragedies has led the public to associate mental illness with violence. After mass shootings, we often hear the National Rifle Association and some politicians link gun violence to mental illness. Similarly, mass shootings often trigger an immediate increase in social media posts regarding mental illness (Budenz et al., 2019). Clearly, the public is inundated with messages that link mental illness and violence. In one study, over 60 percent of those surveyed believed that people with schizophrenia were dangerous, and 30 percent of the respondents indicated that people experiencing a major depression pose a danger to others (Pescosolido & Manago, 2019).

In reality, only a small minority of acts of violence involve someone with a serious mental disorder. Drug or alcohol abuse is much more likely to result in violent behavior (Friedman & Michels, 2013). Even though violence is rare, predicting the possibility that clients might be dangerous to themselves or to others has become an inescapable part of the role of mental health professionals. Therapists are required by law to take appropriate action when a client is potentially homicidal or suicidal. In the case of concern about harm to others, therapists have a duty to warn the intended victim or to contact officials who can provide protection, a topic we cover in Chapter 17. In the case of Loughner, although some community members believed he was dangerous, neither law enforcement nor mental health professionals were directly involved or in a position to intervene prior to the tragic shooting.

1-3 How Common Are Mental Disorders?

Many of us have direct experiences with mental disorders, either personally or through our involvement with family and friends. You may have wondered, "Just how many people are affected by a mental disorder?" To answer this question and to understand societal trends and factors that contribute to the occurrence of specific mental disorders, we turn to data from **psychiatric epidemiology**, the study of the frequency with which mental illness occurs in a society. Analyzing data from psychiatric epidemiology studies is critical because it can help guide us toward solutions that reduce the cost and distress associated with mental disorders. Epidemiological data allow public officials to determine how frequently or infrequently various conditions occur in the population. We can also use prevalence data to compare how disorders vary by ethnicity, gender, and age. Most importantly, monitoring changes in rates can inform decisions about whether current mental health practices are effective in preventing or treating various disorders.

The **prevalence** of a disorder is the percentage of people in a population who have the disorder during a given interval of time. For instance, the results from surveys conducted in 2021 by the U.S. Substance Abuse and Mental Health Services Administration (SAMHSA) revealed that 33.7 percent of the respondents ages 18 to 25 had experienced a mental disorder (not including a drug or alcohol use disorder) during the previous 12 months, with 11.4 percent facing a serious mental disorder such as schizophrenia. The annual prevalence of mental illness varies between adults in the major U.S. ethnic groups: Asian: 16.4 percent; Native Hawaiian/Pacific Islander: 18.1 percent; Hispanic: 20.7 percent; non-Hispanic Black: 21.4 percent; non-Hispanic White: 23.9 percent; American Indian/Alaska Native: 26.6 percent; and non-Hispanic mixed/multiracial: 34.9 percent. The annual prevalence of a mental disorder is highest (50.9 percent) among the demographic group that includes adults who are lesbian, gay, or bisexual (SAMHSA, 2023).

When looking at prevalence rates, it is important to consider the time interval involved. A **lifetime prevalence** rate refers to existence of the disorder during any part of a person's life, whereas the statistics just discussed involved a 12-month prevalence rate. In a study designed to determine if youth around the world are at high risk for mental disorders, Auerbach et al. (2018) and the World Health Organization compared the lifetime prevalence of various symptoms of mental illness among nearly 14,000 college students from eight countries: Australia, Belgium, Germany, Mexico, Northern Ireland, South Africa, Spain, and the United States. Over 35 percent of the students reported having experienced symptoms that would meet the criteria for at least one mental disorder (refer to Figure 1.1). Some students met the criteria for more than one disorder. Symptoms of the students' disorders usually began during early to middle adolescence and continued to the time of the

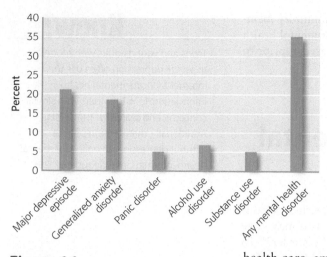

Figure 1.1

Lifetime Prevalence of Mental Disorders in College Students from Eight Countries

Over one third of a group of 14,000 college students who were surveyed in Australia, Belgium, Germany, Mexico, Northern Ireland, South Africa, Spain, and the United States reported having experienced a mental health disorder during their lifetime.

Source: Auerbach et al., 2018

survey. The authors of the study expressed concern that the large number of students who need mental health assistance may overwhelm college resources and suggested that therapeutic programs be made available to students via the Internet.

In addition to those who have a diagnosable mental health condition in a given year, many more people experience emotional or behavioral concerns that do not meet the exact criteria for a mental disorder. These problems may be equally distressing and debilitating unless adequately treated. The economic and social circumstances surrounding the COVID-19 pandemic took a toll on mental health and stretched already limited mental health resources. Further, **systemic racism** and the resultant racial and ethnic disparities in access to education, health care, employment, and housing remain an ongoing concern in the United States and in many countries throughout the world. Clearly, mental disturbance is widespread, and many people are coping with symptoms of mental distress. What is even more disconcerting is that in the United States fewer than one half of adults with a mental disorder are receiving treatment (SAMHSA, 2019).

1-4 Cultural and Sociopolitical Influences on Behavior

Considering the cultural and sociopolitical context of a person's behavior and emotional functioning is an essential aspect of determining if the person is experiencing significant mental health issues. Psychologists now recognize that all behaviors originate from a cultural context. **Culture** is the learned behavior that members of a group transmit to the next generation. Culture includes a group's shared values, beliefs, attitudes, and views about the world (Sue et al., 2022). **Cultural relativism** underscores the fact that our lifestyle, cultural values, and worldview affect our behavior and expression of emotions. According to cultural relativism, cultures vary in what they define as typical or expected behavior. Therefore, it's not surprising that one's cultural background can significantly influence one's understanding of mental illness. For this reason, it is essential to evaluate symptoms within a cultural framework, taking care to refrain from judging behavior based solely on our personal cultural perspective. For example, in some cultural groups, hallucinating (having false sensory impressions) is considered normal in some situations, particularly religious ceremonies. Yet within most cultural groups within the United States, hallucinating is typically viewed as a symptom of a psychological disorder.

Cultural universality, on the other hand, refers to the perspective that symptoms of mental disorders are the same in all cultures and societies. According to those who regard mental illness as a universal phenomenon, specific mental disorders have the same symptoms throughout the world. Which point of view is correct? Should the criteria used to determine psychopathology be based on cultural universality or cultural relativism? Few mental health professionals today embrace the extremes of either position, although most gravitate toward one or the other. Proponents of cultural universality focus on the symptoms of specific disorders and minimize cultural factors, while proponents of cultural relativism focus on the cultural context within which symptoms are manifested. Both views have some support. Many disorders have symptoms that are strikingly similar across cultures. In some cases, however, there are significant cultural differences in the definitions, descriptions, and understandings of mental illness.

Some scholars believe that we also need to consider behavior from a sociopolitical perspective—the social and political context within which a behavior occurs. The importance of considering the sociopolitical implications of defining mental illness was well-articulated by Thomas Szasz (1987). In a radical departure from conventional beliefs, he asserted that mental illness is a myth, a fictional creation that society uses to control and change people. According to Szasz, people may have "problems in living," but not "mental illness." His argument stems from three beliefs: (a) that societal characterization of a behavior as atypical does not necessarily mean that it is an illness; (b) that unusual beliefs are not necessarily incorrect; and (c) that unusual behavior or emotional distress is a reflection of something wrong with society rather than with the individual. Few mental health professionals would take the extreme position advocated by Szasz, but his arguments highlight an important area of concern. Therapists and other practitioners must be sensitive to the fact that personal bias, sociopolitical factors, or societal norms and values may influence decisions about diagnosis and treatment.

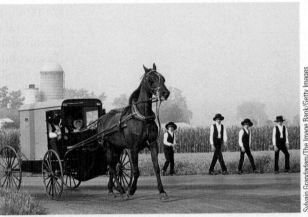

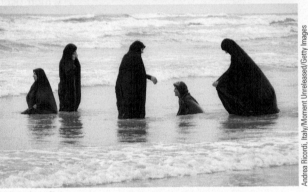

Sylvain Grandadam/The Image Bank/Getty Images

Andrea Ricordi, Italy/Moment Unreleased/Getty Images

Cultural Relativism

Cultural differences often lead to misunderstandings and misinterpretations. In a society that values technological conveniences and modern fashion, the lifestyles and cultural values of some groups may be perceived as strange. The Amish, for example, continue to rely on the horse and buggy for transportation. Women in both Amish and Islamic cultures wear simple, concealing clothing. According to the cultural norms of these communities, dressing in any other way would be considered deviant.

1-5 Overcoming Social Stigma and Stereotypes

Case Study "I have a mental illness. I cringe whenever I hear or read a story about a horrific tragedy committed by a person while in the deep throes of his or her own mental suffering. Time and again the story is told using the same damaging stereotypes. The story paints me and others living with a mental illness with the same brush without acknowledging that we are distinct individuals with our own histories. This one-dimensional story only reinforces the long-held belief that an individual with a mental illness is violent, unpredictable, dangerous, unreliable, irresponsible, and utterly incapable of managing all but very basic tasks." (Hughes, 2015)

The woman who wrote this, Stephanie Mitchell Hughes, is well aware of the **stereotypes** surrounding mental illness because she has lived with depression for over three decades. The distressing **social stigma** associated with mental illness and the resulting feelings of "shame" regarding her symptoms prevented Hughes from openly acknowledging her condition for many years. Research findings support her perceptions—that those with mental illness are often disapproved of, devalued, and set apart from others (Pescosolido & Manago, 2019). Sadly, although mental illness is found in many families and in all communities, negative stereotypes persist.

Individuals with mental illness often need to contend with two forms of stigma. First, they frequently must cope with the public stigma that is expressed through **prejudice** (belief in negative stereotypes) and **discrimination** (actions based on this prejudice). Prejudice and discrimination are sometimes more devastating than the illness itself. The effects of stigma can be particularly challenging for those who are simultaneously contending with other forms of discrimination based on factors such as race, ethnicity, gender, religion, or sexual orientation. Second, **self-stigma**, which occurs when individuals internalize negative beliefs or stereotypes regarding their group and accept the prejudice and discrimination directed toward them, can also be destructive to those living with mental illness. They come to accept negative societal stereotypes of being different, dangerous, unpredictable, or incompetent and then incorporate these negative beliefs into their self-image. As you might imagine, this negative self-image can lead to further distress and maladaptive reactions such as not socializing or not seeking work because of feelings of uselessness or incompetence (Mathison, 2019).

Unfortunately, self-stigma based on societal prejudices not only undermines feelings of self-worth and **self-efficacy** (belief in one's ability to succeed) but also can delay treatment and hinder recovery. For example, in a review of studies about postpartum depression, social stigma was found to be a primary reason why women failed to seek treatment despite distressing symptoms (Button et al., 2017). Further, individuals living with mental illness who are members of oppressed groups are faced with the additional challenge of contending with self-stigma involving internalized negative stereotypes based on societal factors such as systemic racism.

Can stigma be reduced by furnishing individuals living with mental illness with information about the causal factors associated with their disorder? Sixty individuals who had experienced psychosis (a period of losing touch with reality) were randomly exposed to varying explanations for their condition: (a) a psychosocial explanation attributing psychosis to difficult life circumstances such as abuse or bullying or (b) a biological explanation focused on dysfunctional brain development. Both interventions significantly reduced self-stigma—possibly through the mechanism of normalizing their experiences or increasing understanding of how their illness developed. However, only the psychosocial explanation reduced their belief in negative stereotypes associated with individuals who experience psychotic symptoms (Carter et al., 2019).

This leads to another question: Would stigma be reduced if the public better understood that mental illness results from a variety of factors, including biological vulnerability? The connection between (1) beliefs about the causes of severe mental disorders and (2) prejudice and discrimination toward the mentally ill was studied in 1996 and again in 2006 (Pescosolido et al., 2010). The researchers discovered a significant increase in public recognition of biological causes for mental illness and a shift away from blaming the individual or families. For instance, there was an increase in the number of people who cited biological reasons as the cause of major depression and schizophrenia.

Surprisingly, the researchers found that an improved understanding of biological causes did not lessen the desire for social distance from or perceived danger associated with individuals diagnosed with schizophrenia or major depression. Of the respondents, 62 percent reported they would not want to "work closely with" individuals with schizophrenia, and 60 percent believed individuals with schizophrenia are "violent to others." Similarly, 47 percent of respondents would be unwilling "to work closely with" colleagues with major depression, and 32 percent expressed concern that people coping with major depression would be "violent to others." Although understanding biological explanations may reduce the tendency to blame those with mental illness for their situation, it may have had the "unintended side effect" of increasing the perception of dangerousness and a desire for social distance (Kvaale et al., 2013).

Mental health advocates continue to work to counter inaccurate perceptions about mental illness and combat social stigma. National Alliance on Mental Illness (NAMI) and other organizations, such as Mental Health America, are strongly committed to the goal of educating the public about mental health issues and reducing the unfair stigma associated with mental illness. These organizations also highlight the challenges faced by individuals who contend with dual stigma, such as sexual and gender minorities or those subjected to societal stigma based on religion, race, or ethnicity. Their efforts have focused on increasing public awareness and providing accurate information about mental illness via media messages, such as those seen in the "You Are Not Alone" campaign launched by NAMI. Additionally, advocacy organizations are recognizing and commending those in the entertainment industry who are producing movies and television shows that humanize and present a more accurate portrayal of mental illness. Many hope that these educational efforts will reduce both public stigma and self-stigma and thereby improve the recovery of those living with mental illness.

Stigmatization is also reduced when well-known public personalities come forward to acknowledge and even openly discuss their own personal struggles with stress and various mental health symptoms. Such public disclosure and openness has come from well-known celebrities, including Adele, Miley Cyrus, Kendall Jenner, Dwayne Johnson, Demi Lovato, Zayn Malik, Nicki Minaj, Gina Rodriguez, and Emma Stone, and sports figures, including NFL wide receiver Brandon Marshall, gymnast and gold medal winner Simone Biles, professional basketball player Royce White, and tennis champions Naomi Osaka and Serena Williams. There is no doubt that the social stigma surrounding mental illness is reduced when the public is able to appreciate how talented people cope with and recover from distressing mental symptoms, rather than just hearing stories of untreated mental disturbance that end in violence or tragedy.

Professionals in the mental health field are encouraged by these attempts to reduce stigma, stereotyping, and common misconceptions about mental illness. Such efforts are important because social stigma can cause individuals and families to not only delay or avoid seeking treatment but also develop a "code of silence" regarding mental illness, especially when a family member has not "come out" regarding their situation. In countries where there is less discrimination and prejudice, people living with mental illness have less self-stigma and are more likely to see help. Additionally, they have a more positive quality of life and feel more optimistic about recovery. Personal **empowerment** through open discussion of mental illness is a first step in overcoming societal prejudice and discrimination.

A question we ask ourselves as we write this book is: If so many individuals are affected by mental illness in today's society, is it really unusual to have mental health challenges? When we look at the pervasiveness of anxiety, depression, eating disorders, and substance-use disorders, for example, it appears that dealing with trauma, stress, and mental health concerns is the new norm. The question then becomes: What can we do

Media Portrayals of Mental Illness

Many people learn about mental disorders from watching movies and television. Do media portrayals of mental illness, such as the severe depression experienced by Toby in the television series *This Is Us*, add to our understanding of mental illness or simply perpetuate stereotypes?

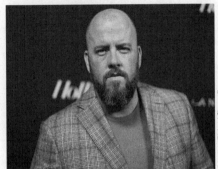

AP Images/Richard Shotwell

Famous people with mental disorders who have made important contributions to the world include Abraham Lincoln, Ernest Hemingway, and Vincent van Gogh, pictured here, as well as Michelangelo, Isaac Newton, and Ludwig van Beethoven, among many others.

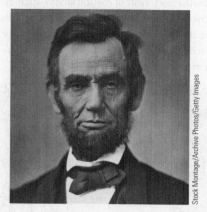
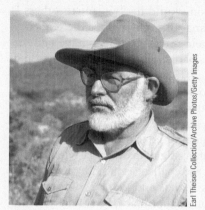
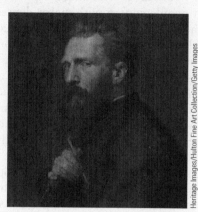

as a society to allow people to be open and honest about their mental health problems and to seek treatment without fear of being stigmatized? Someday soon the course you are now taking may have a more progressive title, such as "Promoting Mental Health and Overcoming Challenges in Living."

What can you do to help reduce stigmatization and stereotyping and assist those working to move mental illness out of the shadows? You can carefully consider your choice of words and avoid the many commonly used terms that perpetuate negative stereotypes about mental illness. For instance, stigmatizing attitudes can be reduced when we avoid noun-based labels such as calling someone "a schizophrenic" and instead refer to the person as "someone living with schizophrenia" (Krzyzanowski et al., 2019). You can also be respectful when discussing someone who is experiencing mental distress, and encourage friends or family who are experiencing emotional symptoms to seek help, perhaps letting them know that the sooner they receive treatment, the greater the likelihood of a full recovery. You can also be sensitive to the fact that many individuals are dealing with other forms of prejudice and everyday discrimination based on characteristics that are much more visible than mental illness (e.g., skin color, religious attire).

1-6 Historical Perspectives on Psychopathology

Definitions of psychopathology are firmly rooted in the system of beliefs that operates in a given society at a given time. This next section covering historical details is based on writings by Alexander and Selesnick (1966), Neugebauer (1979), Plante (2013), Spanos (1978), and Wallace and Gach (2008). We must be aware, however, that our discussion is strongly influenced by Western understandings of mental health and mental disorders. Other, non-Western societies have historical journeys and beliefs about atypical behavior that differ from those presented here.

Prehistoric and Ancient Beliefs

Prehistoric societies some half a million years ago did not distinguish between mental and physical disorders. According to historians, these ancient peoples attributed many forms of illness to demonic possession, sorcery, or retribution from an offended ancestral spirit. Certain symptoms and behaviors, from simple headaches to convulsions, were ascribed to evil spirits residing within a person's body. Within this system of belief, called *demonology,* people displaying symptoms were often held at least partly responsible for their misfortune.

It has been suggested that Stone Age cave dwellers may have treated behavioral and mental disorders with a surgical method called **trephining**, in which part of the skull was chipped away to provide an opening through which the evil spirits could escape, in hopes that the person would return to their normal state. Surprisingly, anthropologists have discovered some trephined skulls with evidence of healing, indicating that some individuals survived this extremely crude operation. Another treatment method used by the early Greeks, Chinese, Hebrews, and Egyptians was **exorcism**, during which elaborate prayers, noises, emetics (drugs that induce vomiting), and extreme measures such as flogging and starvation were used to cast evil spirits out of an afflicted person's body.

Naturalistic Explanations: Greco-Roman Thought

With the expansion of Greek civilization and its continuation into the era of Roman rule (500 B.C.–A.D. 500), naturalistic explanations gradually became distinct from supernatural ones. Early thinkers, such as Hippocrates (460–370 B.C.), a physician sometimes referred to as the father of Western medicine, actively questioned prevailing superstitious beliefs and proposed much more rational and scientific explanations for mental disorders. Hippocrates believed that, because the brain was the central organ of intellectual activity, deviant behavior was caused by **brain pathology**, that is, a dysfunction or disease of the brain. Hippocrates also considered heredity and the environment important factors in psychopathology. He classified mental illnesses into three categories—mania, melancholia (sadness or depression), and phrenitis (brain fever)—and provided detailed clinical descriptions of symptoms such as paranoia, alcoholic delirium, and epilepsy. Many of his descriptions of disorders are still used today, which is eloquent testimony to his keen powers of observation.

Other thinkers who contributed to the organic explanation of behavior were the philosopher Plato and the Greek physician Galen, who practiced in Rome. Plato (429–347 B.C.) carried on the thinking of Hippocrates; he insisted that people who were mentally disturbed were the responsibility of their families and that they should not be punished for their behavior. Galen (A.D. 129–199) made major contributions through his scientific examination of the nervous system and his explanation of the role of the brain and central nervous system in mental functioning. His greatest contribution may have been the coding and classification of all European medical knowledge from Hippocrates's time to his own.

Reversion to Supernatural Explanations: The Middle Ages

With the upheavals in society associated with the collapse of the Roman Empire, the rise of Christianity, and the devastating plagues sweeping

Trephining: Evidence of Therapy?

Anthropologists speculate that this human skull is evidence of trephining, the centuries-old practice of chipping a hole in the skull to release the evil spirits causing symptoms of mental disturbance.

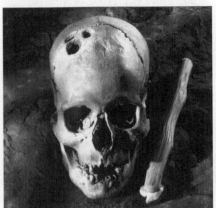

Paul Bevitt/Alamy Stock Photo

Did You Know?

Hippocrates believed that certain disorders in women (such as a sudden inability to speak or to walk) were due to the wandering of the woman's uterus in search of a child. The type of physical symptoms displayed depended upon where in the body the uterus was lodged. He often recommended marriage or more sexual activity to coax the uterus back to its proper place.

through Europe, rational and scientific thought gave way to a renewed emphasis on the supernatural. Religious dogma reinforced the idea that nature is a reflection of divine will and beyond human reason and that earthly life is a prelude to the "true" life experienced after death. Scientific inquiry—attempts to understand, classify, explain, and control nature—became less important than accepting nature as a manifestation of God's will. Religious truths were viewed as sacred, and those who challenged these ideas were denounced as heretics. Natural and supernatural explanations of illness were once again fused. Because of this atmosphere, rationalism and scholarly scientific works went underground for many years, preserved mainly by Arab scholars and European monks.

With people once again believing that many illnesses were the result of supernatural forces, treatment also shifted. In some cases, religious monks treated the mentally ill with compassion, allowing them to rest and receive prayer in monasteries and at shrines. In other cases, treatment was quite brutal, particularly when the illness was seen as resulting from God's wrath or possession by the devil. When the illness was perceived to be punishment for sin, the sick person was assumed to be guilty of wrongdoing; relief could only come through atonement or repentance. The humane treatment that Hippocrates had advocated centuries earlier was replaced by torturous exorcism procedures designed to combat Satan and eject him from the possessed person's body. Prayers, curses, obscene epithets, and the sprinkling of holy water—as well as such drastic and painful "therapies" as flogging, starving, and immersing in hot water—were used to drive out the devil. A time of trouble for everyone, the Middle Ages were especially bleak for the mentally ill.

Belief in the power of the supernatural became so prevalent and intense that psychological symptoms frequently affected whole populations. Beginning in Italy early in the 13th century, large numbers of people were affected by various forms of mass madness, or group **hysteria**, involving the sudden appearance of unusual symptoms that had no apparent physical cause. One of the better-known manifestations of this condition was **tarantism**, which was characterized by agitation and frenzied dancing. People would leap up, believing they had been bitten by a spider. They would then run out into the street or marketplace, jumping and dancing about, and be joined by others who also believed that they had been bitten. The mania soon spread throughout the rest of Europe, where it became known as *Saint Vitus's dance*.

How can these phenomena be explained? Outbreaks of mass hysteria are often associated with stress and fear. During the 13th century, for example, there was enormous social unrest. The bubonic plague had decimated one third of the population of Europe. War, famine, and pestilence were rampant, and the social order of the times was crumbling.

Witchcraft: The 15th Through 17th Centuries

During the 15th and 16th centuries, social and religious reformers increasingly challenged the authority of the Roman Catholic Church. Martin Luther attacked the corruption and abuses of the clergy, precipitating the Protestant Reformation of the 16th century. Church officials viewed such protests as insurrections that threatened their power. According to the church, Satan himself fostered the attacks on church practices. In effect, the church actively endorsed an already popular belief in demonic possession and witches.

During the Middle Ages, people with mental disorders were thought to be victims of demonic possession. The most prevalent form of treatment was exorcism, which was usually conducted by religious leaders. Here a televangelist and his daughters are participating in a modern-day exorcism.

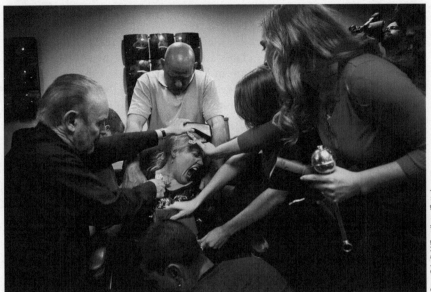

Steve Schofield/Contributor/Getty Images

To counter the satanic threat, Pope Innocent VIII issued a decree in 1484 calling on the clergy to identify and exterminate witches. This resulted in the 1486 publication of the *Malleus Maleficarum*, which officially confirmed the existence of witches, suggesting signs for detecting them (such as red spots on the skin and areas of anesthesia on the body) and methods to force confessions. Confession could be designated as "with" or "without" torture. The latter allowed "mild" bone crushing. The church initially recognized two forms of demonic possession: willing and unwilling. The willing person made a blood pact with the devil and had the power to create floods, pestilence, storms, crop failures, and impotence. Although those deemed unwilling victims of possession initially received more sympathetic treatment than those believed to have willingly conspired with the devil, this distinction soon evaporated.

Thousands of innocent men, women, and even children were beheaded, burned alive, or mutilated during the period of the witch hunts. It has been estimated that over 100,000 people (mainly women) were executed as witches from the middle of the 15th century to the end of the 17th century. Witch hunts also occurred in colonial America. The witchcraft trials of 1692 in Salem, Massachusetts, were infamous. Several hundred people were accused, many were imprisoned and tortured, and 20 were killed. Most psychiatric historians believe that many of those who were initially suspected of witchcraft were mentally ill. Additionally, the astonishingly high number of women who were accused and persecuted suggests that other sociological factors were involved, such as patriarchal (male-dominated) societal conditions (Reed, 2007). Although these events took place centuries ago, belief in witchcraft or supernatural causes for mental and physical disorders still exists today in the United States and other countries (Mariani, 2018). In fact, within the Catholic Church, there has been a significant revival in the belief in demonic possession and the practice of exorcism (Innamorati et al., 2019).

Did You Know?

The practice of casting out evil spirits still occurs among some Christian groups who believe that physical or psychological illnesses result from possession by demons. Many believe that such illnesses are due to sins committed by the individual or the person's ancestors.

Source: Mercer, 2013

The Rise of Humanism

A resurgence of rational and scientific inquiry during the 14th through 16th centuries led to great advances in science and **humanism**, a philosophical movement emphasizing human welfare and the worth and uniqueness of the individual. Prior to this time, most asylums were at best custodial centers in which people who were mentally disturbed were chained, caged, starved, whipped, and even exhibited to the public for a small fee, much like animals in a zoo (Dreher, 2013). For example, the term *bedlam*, which has become synonymous with chaos and disorder, was the shortened name of Bethlehem Hospital, an asylum in England that has come to symbolize the plight of people experiencing severe mental illness. Patients were bound by chains, left untreated, and exhibited to the public in the courtyard.

Johann Weyer (1515–1588), a German physician, published a revolutionary book that challenged the prevailing beliefs about witchcraft. He personally investigated many cases of demonic possession and asserted that many people who were tortured, imprisoned, and burned as witches were mentally disturbed, not possessed by demons (Metzger, 2013). Although both the church and the government severely criticized and banned his book, it helped pave the way for the humanistic perspective on mental illness. With the rise of humanism, a new way of thinking developed—if people were "mentally ill" and not possessed, they should be treated as though they were sick. A number of new treatment methods reflected this humanistic spirit.

The Moral Treatment Movement: The 18th and 19th Centuries

In France, Philippe Pinel (1745–1826), a physician, took charge of la Bicêtre, a hospital for mentally ill men in Paris. Pinel instituted what came to be known as the **moral treatment movement**—a shift to more humane care for people who were mentally disturbed. He removed patients' chains, replaced dungeons with sunny rooms, encouraged exercise outdoors on the hospital grounds, and treated patients with kindness and reason. Surprising many disbelievers, the freed patients did not become violent; instead, this humane treatment seemed to improve behavior and foster recovery. Pinel later instituted similar, equally successful, reforms at la Salpêtrière, a large mental hospital for women in Paris.

In England, William Tuke (1732–1822), a prominent Quaker tea merchant, established a retreat at York for the "moral treatment" of mental patients. At this pleasant country estate, the patients worked, prayed, rested, and talked out their problems—all in an atmosphere of kindness. This emphasis on moral treatment laid the groundwork for using psychological means to treat mental illness. Indeed, it resulted in much higher rates of "cure" than other treatments of that time (Charland, 2007).

In the United States, three individuals—Benjamin Rush, Dorothea Dix, and Clifford Beers—made important contributions to the moral treatment movement. Rush (1745–1813), widely acclaimed as the father of U.S. psychiatry, encouraged humane treatment of those residing in mental hospitals. He insisted that patients be treated with respect and dignity and that they be gainfully employed while hospitalized, an idea still evident in the modern concept of work therapy. Dorothea Dix (1802–1887), a New England schoolteacher, was a leader in 19th-century social reform in the United States. At the time, people who were mentally ill were often incarcerated in prisons and poorhouses. While teaching Sunday school to female prisoners, Dix was appalled to find jailed mental patients living

Dorothea Dix (1802–1887)

During a time when women were discouraged from political participation, Dorothea Dix, a New England schoolteacher, worked tirelessly as a social reformer to improve the deplorable conditions in which people who were mentally ill were forced to live.

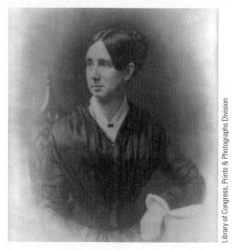

Library of Congress, Prints & Photographs Division

under deplorable conditions. For the next 40 years, she worked tirelessly on behalf of those experiencing mental disorders, campaigning for reform legislation and funds to establish suitable mental hospitals. Dix raised millions of dollars, established more than 30 mental hospitals, and greatly improved conditions in countless others. But the struggle for reform was far from over. Although the large hospitals that replaced jails and poorhouses had better physical facilities, the humanistic focus of the moral treatment movement was lacking.

The moral treatment movement was energized in 1908 with the publication of *A Mind That Found Itself*, a book by Clifford Beers (1876–1943) about his own mental collapse. His book describes the terrible treatment he and other patients experienced in three mental institutions, where they were beaten, choked, spat on, and restrained with straitjackets. His vivid account aroused public sympathy and attracted the interest and support of the psychiatric establishment, including such eminent figures as psychologist-philosopher William James. Beers founded the National Committee for Mental Hygiene (forerunner of the National Mental Health Association, now known as Mental Health America), an organization dedicated to educating the public about mental illness. This organization continues to advocate against ineffective or inappropriate treatment methods. Even the most severe critics of today's mental health system would acknowledge, however, that treatment for people who are mentally ill has improved over the years.

Did You Know?

Vincent van Gogh benefited from the moral treatment movement. He was admitted to Saint-Paul Asylum in 1889 after cutting off part of his ear. He received benevolent care and rehabilitation and was allowed short supervised walks and a studio for painting. During his 1-year stay, he produced 150 paintings.

Source: Harris, 2010

Going Deeper

What Role Should Spirituality and Religion Play in Mental Health Care?

Reluctance to incorporate religion into treatment may be understandable in light of the historical role played by the church in the oppression of people who are mentally ill. The role of demons, witches, and possession in explaining atypical behavior has been part and parcel of past religious teachings. Furthermore, psychology as a science stresses objectivity and naturalistic explanations of human behavior, an approach that is often at odds with religion as a belief system (Sue et al., 2022).

For many years, the mental health profession was largely silent about the influence of spirituality or religion on mental health. Apart from pastoral counselors, many therapists avoid discussing spiritual or religious issues with their clients, concerned they might appear to be proselytizing or usurping the role of the clergy. Further, therapists who are atheist or agnostic may feel inauthentic addressing the spiritual or religious aspects of a client's well-being.

Many people are open to medical and mental health care providers discussing spiritual and faith issues with them, including some individuals who do not participate in religious services. Additionally, for many members of racially and ethnically underrepresented groups, cultural identity is intimately linked with spirituality (Sue et al., 2022). More compelling are findings that reveal a positive association between spirituality or religion and optimal health outcomes; longevity; and lower levels of anxiety, depression, suicide, and substance abuse (Kasen et al., 2013; Portnoff et al., 2017). Similarly, higher levels of spirituality in gay and bisexual men are associated with psychological resilience and better mental health outcomes (Reist Gibbel et al., 2019).

Many mental health professionals are becoming increasingly open to the potential benefits of incorporating spirituality into treatment. As part of that process, psychologists are making distinctions between spirituality and religion. *Spirituality* is a broad term that includes finding meaning, purpose, and connection to a higher power or something larger within the universe, whereas *religion* involves a specific doctrine and particular system of beliefs. Spirituality can be pursued outside of a specific religion because it involves growth associated with self-discovery, faith, and deep connections. In many ways, spiritual growth can enhance the personal growth that occurs in therapy.

For Further Consideration

1. What thoughts do you have about the role of spirituality and religion in mental health and psychotherapy?

2. Should therapists avoid discussing religious or spiritual matters with clients?

3. If you were in therapy, how important would it be to discuss your religious or spiritual beliefs?

1-7 Causes of Mental Illness: Early Viewpoints

Paralleling the rise of humanistic treatment of mental illness was an inquiry into its causes. Two schools of thought emerged. The biological viewpoint holds that mental disorders are the result of physiological damage or disease. The psychological viewpoint stresses an emotional basis for mental illness. Elements of these positions were often combined.

The Biological Viewpoint

Hippocrates's suggestion of a biological explanation for mental illness was ignored during the Middle Ages but revived after the Renaissance. Not until the 19th century, however, did the **biological viewpoint**—the belief that mental disorders have a physical or physiological basis—flourish. The ideas of Wilhelm Griesinger (1817–1868), a German neurologist and psychiatrist who believed that all mental disorders had physiological causes, received considerable attention. Emil Kraepelin (1856–1926), a follower of Griesinger, observed that certain symptoms tend to occur regularly in clusters, called **syndromes**. Kraepelin believed that each cluster of symptoms represented a mental disorder with its own unique—and clearly specifiable—cause, course, and outcome. In his *Textbook of Psychiatry* (1883/1923), Kraepelin outlined a system for classifying mental illnesses based on their physiological causes. That system was the foundation for the diagnostic categories in the DSM, the classification system of the American Psychiatric Association that is still in use today.

The acceptance of organic or biological causes for mental disorders was enhanced by medical breakthroughs such as Louis Pasteur's (1822–1895) germ theory of disease. The biological viewpoint gained even greater strength with the discovery of the biological basis of *general paresis*, a degenerative physical and mental disorder associated with late-stage syphilis (a sexually transmitted infection). In 1897, Richard von Krafft-Ebing, a German neurologist, proved conclusively that the serious mental symptoms associated with general paresis resulted from syphilis bacteria invading the brain.

Finally, in 1905, a German zoologist, Fritz Schaudinn, isolated the microorganism that causes syphilis and develops into general paresis. These events strengthened the search for biological explanations for mental disorders. As medical breakthroughs in the study of the nervous system occurred, many scientists became hopeful that they would discover a biological basis for all mental disorders. As we discuss in the next chapter, the biological model, including the focus on genetic factors, brain structure, and biochemical processes, continues to generate considerable interest.

The Psychological Viewpoint

Some scientists noted, however, that certain emotional disorders do not appear to be associated with any obvious biological cause. Such observations led to the **psychological viewpoint**—the belief that mental disorders are caused by psychological and emotional factors. This view contends, for example, that personal challenges or interpersonal conflicts can lead to intense feelings of frustration, depression, and anger, which may consequently lead to deteriorating mental health. This perspective received support with the discovery that psychological interventions could both produce

Emil Kraepelin (1856–1926)

In an 1883 publication, psychiatrist Emil Kraepelin proposed that mental disorders could be directly linked to biologically based brain disorders and further proposed a diagnostic classification system for all disorders.

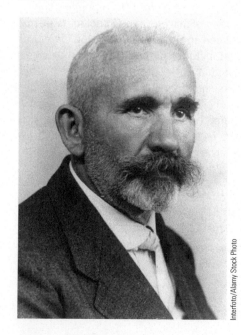

Interfoto/Alamy Stock Photo

and treat *hysteria*, a condition first identified in the Middle Ages involving physical symptoms that have a psychological rather than a physical cause.

Mesmerism and Hypnotism

The unique and exotic techniques to treat hysteria used by Friedrich Anton Mesmer (1734–1815), an Austrian physician who practiced in Paris, presented an early challenge to the biological viewpoint. Mesmer developed a theory of "animal magnetism," contending that disruptions in the flow of magnetic forces in the body could produce physical problems and that the use of magnetism could restore the flow to normal. Based on this theory, Mesmer developed a highly controversial treatment referred to as *mesmerism*, a technique that evolved into the modern practice of hypnotism. Mesmer performed his most miraculous cures by successfully treating hysteria, including symptoms of blindness, deafness, loss of bodily feeling, and paralysis. His system for curing hysteria involved inducing a sleeplike state, during which his patients became highly susceptible to suggestion and their symptoms often disappeared. Mesmer's dramatic and theatrical techniques earned him censure as well as fame. Although a committee of prominent thinkers, including Benjamin Franklin, investigated Mesmer and declared him a fraud, the theory of animal magnetism also became popular in some circles in the United States (Quinn, 2012).

Although Mesmer's theatrics and basic assumptions were discredited, he succeeded in demonstrating that the power of suggestion could treat hysteria. Following Mesmer, two physicians, Ambroise-Auguste Liébeault (1823–1904) and Hippolyte-Marie Bernheim (1840–1919), hypothesized that hysteria was a form of self-hypnosis. In treating hysterical patients using hypnosis, they were often able to cure symptoms of paralysis, deafness, and blindness. They were also able to produce these symptoms in healthy persons through hypnosis. Their work demonstrated that suggestion could cause certain symptoms of mental illness and that mental and physical disorders could have a psychological rather than a biological explanation. This conclusion represented a major breakthrough in the understanding of mental disorders.

Breuer and Freud

The idea that psychological processes could produce mental and physical dysfunction soon gained credence among physicians who were using hypnosis. Among them was the Viennese doctor Josef Breuer (1842–1925). He discovered that after one of his female patients spoke quite freely about her past traumatic experiences while in a trance, many of her physical symptoms disappeared. There was even greater improvement when the patient recalled and talked about previously forgotten memories of emotionally distressing events. This technique became known as the **cathartic method**, the therapeutic use of verbal expression to release pent-up emotional conflicts. It foreshadowed the practice of psychoanalysis initiated by Sigmund Freud (1856–1939), whose techniques have had a lasting influence and whose contributions we discuss in Chapter 2.

Behaviorism

Whereas psychoanalysis explained mental illness as an **intrapsychic** phenomenon involving psychological processes occurring within the mind, another viewpoint that emerged, behaviorism, was firmly rooted in laboratory science. The behavioristic perspective stressed the importance of directly observable behaviors and the conditions that produce and maintain symptoms of mental disorders. Behaviorism not only provided an alternative explanation regarding how symptoms of mental illness develop but also offered successful procedures for treating some psychological conditions.

Friedrich Anton Mesmer (1734–1815)

Mesmer's techniques were a forerunner of modern hypnotism. Although highly controversial and ultimately discredited, Mesmer's efforts stimulated inquiry into the possibility that psychological and emotional factors could cause mental disorders.

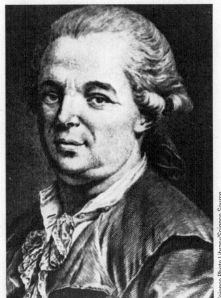

Science Photo Library/Science Source

Figure 1.2

2045 Census Projections: Racial and Ethnic Composition of the United States

Minorities now constitute an increasing proportion of the U.S. population, and new statistics project that the nation will become "minority White" by 2045. Mental health providers will increasingly encounter clients who differ from them in race, ethnicity, and culture.

Source: Frey, 2018

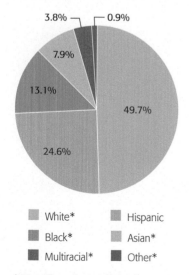

3.8% ⌐ 0.9%
7.9%
13.1%
49.7%
24.6%

■ White*   ■ Hispanic
■ Black*   ■ Asian*
■ Multiracial* ■ Other*

Non-Hispanic members of race

1-8 Contemporary Trends in Studying Psychopathology

Our understanding and treatment of mental disorders have changed significantly over the past 30 years. Views of mental illness continue to evolve as they incorporate the effects of several major trends in the field: (a) the influence of multicultural psychology; (b) the focus on resilience and positive psychology; (c) the recovery movement; and (d) changes in the therapeutic landscape such as psychiatric medications, managed health care and health care reform, evidence-based treatments, and the increased use of technology in treatment.

The Influence of Multicultural Psychology

The United States is quickly becoming a multicultural, multiracial, and multilingual society (Figure 1.2). Projections based on U.S. Census Bureau data indicate that in this decade fewer than 50 percent of children will be non-Hispanic White and that by 2045 the United States will have a "minority White" population (Frey, 2018). Additionally, the number of individuals identifying as having a biracial or multiracial background is steadily increasing. These changes are sometimes referred to as the diversification of the United States or, literally, the changing complexion of society.

Culture, ethnicity, and gender are recognized as powerful influences on many aspects of human development. Not surprisingly, the increasing diversity within the United States has had a major impact on the mental health profession, creating a field of study called **multicultural psychology**. Mental health professionals now recognize that it is essential to learn about the worldviews, lifestyles, and challenges faced by culturally diverse groups (including people with a multiracial or multicultural background) and to use culturally relevant approaches to therapy (Sue et al., 2022). The American Psychological Association (1990, 2017) guidelines related to work with diverse populations emphasize the importance of:

• understanding that culture and diversity play a significant role in the experiences and perspectives of members of diverse groups.

• using culturally sensitive assessment and carefully interpreting information provided by clients from diverse populations.

• helping clients determine if their presenting problem is a result of prejudice, discrimination, or systemic racism.

• recognizing that a therapist's own cultural background, values, and attitudes can influence his or her reactions to clients and the quality of services provided.

Understanding four key areas related to cultural diversity—social conditioning, cultural values and influences, sociopolitical influences, and bias in diagnosis—will help broaden your awareness of how cultural forces exert their influence.

Social Conditioning

How we are raised, the values we develop, and cultural expectations regarding our behavior can have a major effect on the types of symptoms we are most likely to experience. For instance, in U.S. culture, men are exposed to expectations regarding how to fulfill the masculine role—to be independent, assertive, courageous, unsentimental, and objective. Women, in contrast, are often raised to be helpful, conforming, and empathetic. As a result of this social conditioning, women are more likely to internalize their conflicts (resulting in anxiety and depression), whereas men are more likely to externalize and act out (resulting in impulsive behaviors or substance abuse). Although these gendered roles have begun to change and nonbinary expressions of gender are increasingly embraced, the effects of traditional gender stereotypes remain.

Cultural Values and Influences

Mental health professionals now recognize that mental disorders differ from country to country and that there are also variations within a country. For example, challenges faced by various racial and ethnic groups in the United States appear to influence overall health and susceptibility to emotional disorders. Culture can also influence the way in which emotional distress is expressed. For instance, among Latinx immigrants and Asian Americans, experiencing physical symptoms is a common and culturally accepted means of expressing psychological and emotional stress (Dunlop et al., 2020). Thus, mental health professionals working with members of these groups might hear complaints involving headaches, fatigue, restlessness, and disturbances of sleep and appetite rather than discussion of distressing emotions or situations. Within these cultural groups, many believe that physical problems cause emotional distress and that psychological symptoms will disappear as soon as the physical illness is treated. In addition, Asian groups view physical illness as acceptable, whereas mental illness may be a source of shame and disgrace (Dai et al., 2016).

Sociopolitical Influences

In response to the long history of prejudice, discrimination, and **racism** in the United States, many people of color have adopted various behaviors (e.g., distrusting members of the majority culture) that have proved important for their survival. Some people may define these actions as deviant, yet from an oppressed group's perspective, the behaviors function as healthy survival mechanisms. Early personality studies of African Americans concluded that, as a group, they appear more suspicious, mistrustful, and paranoid than their European American counterparts. But are African Americans inherently suspicious, as studies suggest, or are they making healthy, adaptive responses to societal conditions such as systemic racism? Many psychologists would argue that members of groups who have been targets of discrimination and oppression in a society not yet free of racism have good reason to be suspicious and distrustful of White society. Further, people from diverse populations are often exposed to **microaggressions**, the brief everyday statements or behaviors that slight or denigrate members of socially marginalized groups. Thus, a "paranoid orientation" may reflect not only survival skills but also an accurate depiction of reality. It is evident that we need to consider people's behaviors based on an understanding of the sociopolitical context in which they arise.

Diversity Is a Fact of Life

This group of students represents the increasing diversity of the United States.

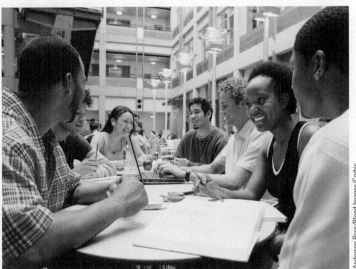

Anderson Ross/Blend Images/Corbis

Did You Know?

In 1851, the article "Diseases and Peculiarities of the Negro Race" described two forms of mental disorders found among enslaved African Americans: (a) Those who had an "unnatural desire for freedom" and ran away were considered to have *drapetomania*, and (b) those who resisted slavery, argued, and created disturbances were diagnosed with *dysaesthesia aethiopica*, also referred to as "rascality." In contrast, those who appeared interested in servitude and were faithful to their masters were considered "mentally healthy."

Source: Cartwright, 1851

Cultural and Ethnic Bias in Diagnosis

It is important to be aware of potential cultural biases inherent in diagnosis and the diagnostic system. For example, bias on the part of mental health professionals can affect their view of symptoms and their subsequent diagnosis. Mental health practitioners are not immune from inheriting the prejudicial attitudes and stereotypes of the larger society. It is possible for even the most enlightened and well-intentioned mental health professional to be influenced by ethnic, gender, and social class bias. One source of bias is the tendency to *overpathologize*—to exaggerate the severity of disorders—among clients from socioeconomic or ethnic groups whose cultural values or lifestyles differ markedly from the clinician's own. This overpathologizing of disorders has been found to occur in psychological evaluations of African Americans, Latinx Americans, women, and sexual and gender minorities (Sue et al., 2022).

Multicultural psychology is now incorporating studies from the growing field of cultural neuroscience in which researchers are using neuroimaging techniques to investigate the influence of gene–culture interactions on cultural variability in neural functioning (Pedraza, 2019). It appears that certain patterns of neural activity are associated with specific cultural practices. For example, individuals who meditate regularly show patterns of neural activity that are distinctly different from those who do not practice meditation (Craigmyle, 2013).

Positive Psychology

Positive psychology is a branch of the profession that seeks to add balance to our view of human functioning; its purpose is to study, develop, and achieve scientific understanding of the positive human qualities associated with thriving individuals, families, and communities. Positive psychologists argue against focusing primarily on deficits and pathology in human experiences and instead encourage an emphasis on human strengths (Seligman & Csikszentmihalyi, 2000). Positive psychology focuses on optimal human functioning in three domains: First, there is interest in the degree to which someone has feelings of well-being, contentment, and satisfaction regarding the past; hope and optimism for the future; and flow and happiness in the present. Second, research concentrates on positive personal traits such as resilience, courage, compassion, **spirituality**, and wisdom. Third, at the group level, positive psychology addresses civic virtues and the institutions that move us toward better citizenship and social responsibility.

What contributions has the field of positive psychology made to our understanding of mental health?

1. Consideration of a person's strengths and their capacity for growth and change has become increasingly important in therapeutic assessment and treatment. Therapists recognize that clients often have an unrealized potential for dealing with both personal and societal problems. Identifying strengths is a positive experience for clients and can assist with recovery. When therapists incorporate the positive qualities of human functioning and adaptive coping into treatment, clients increase their confidence in managing distressing emotional symptoms as well as day-to-day challenges. Taking into account diversity in life experiences, positive psychologists are also developing models of resilient functioning within members of racially and ethnically underrepresented groups (Perrin et al., 2020).

2. Positive psychologists also focus on prevention by addressing healthy methods for managing stress and increasing **psychological resilience**

by harnessing the power of positive emotions. The goal is to identify the strengths and assets of people, to arm them with adaptive coping skills, and to promote mental health—an approach that can vastly improve the functioning of individuals experiencing mental distress (Tse et al., 2016).

It is likely that you, and those around you, encounter stressful situations on a regular basis. Additionally, you may have also experienced a traumatic event or been subjected to violence, abuse, bullying, racism, or discrimination. What characteristics have helped you effectively cope with these kinds of stressors? Positive psychologists believe in teaching and promoting the qualities associated with effective coping and resilience—the same strategies that may have helped you cope during challenging times. These protective strategies help us effectively regulate our emotions; manage the challenges of life; and avoid developing depression, anxiety, or other mental health conditions.

Positive psychology has reawakened an interest in optimizing human functioning and presenting a more balanced picture of the human condition. In chapters throughout this text, you will find a section called *Focus on Resilience* that highlights psychological assets and strengths—information that relates to the prevention of or recovery from the various mental health conditions we discuss.

Recovery Movement

Historically, the public and some mental health professionals have held predominantly pessimistic views regarding the life prospects of those living with mental illness. Individuals with severe mental illness often were told that they would never recover or have a fulfilling future. In contrast to this pessimistic message, a reconceptualization of the possible outcomes for those with severe mental illness resulted in the **recovery movement**—the perspective that those with mental illness can recover and live satisfying, hopeful, and meaningful lives, even with limitations caused by illness. Recovery involves a continued focus on the meaning and purpose of one's life (Davidson, 2016).

Indeed, there is a move away from the view that severe mental disorders have an inevitably poor prognosis. Instead, with appropriate support and treatment, those with mental illness can look forward to a meaningful future. The recovery model, emphasizing optimism and collaborative support targeting each individual's potential for recovery, views severe mental disorders as chronic medical conditions, such as diabetes or heart disease—illnesses that may require treatment but that do not define the individual. The recovery model is based on the following assumptions (Dilks et al., 2010):

1. Recovery begins when a person realizes that positive change is possible.

2. Recovery is not a continual movement forward; occasional setbacks can be viewed as opportunities for new learning.

3. Healing involves separating one's identity from the illness and developing the ability to live and cope with psychiatric symptoms.

4. Self-acceptance and regaining belief in one's self are vital.

5. Recovery involves learning about personal capabilities, talents, and coping skills and using these strengths to engage in new life roles.

6. Self-direction allows one to learn to control and exercise choice on the journey to recovery and to participate in all decisions affecting one's life and well-being.

Psychology Is Also the Study of Strengths and Assets

Randy and Billy grew up in the same neighborhood, went to the same high school, joined the army together, and served two tours of duty in Iraq before leaving the service. In Iraq, they encountered threats of death, saw their comrades killed or wounded, and endured many hardships. While in the army, Billy frequently coped by using drugs and alcohol, especially after witnessing traumatic events. Although Randy went drinking with his friends, he never drank excessively.

Upon their return home, Randy and Billy both enrolled in a community college with the hopes of opening a car repair business. However, Billy's mental health deteriorated quickly. He was very anxious and had flashbacks about the war. Before long, he was heavily involved in drugs and dropped out of college. Randy finished his college program and opened a small, successful automobile repair shop with three employees. He has since married, and he and his wife are expecting their first child. In addition, he has become actively involved in helping other veterans at the local VA hospital.

After years of not seeing his friend Billy, Randy happened to run into him late one afternoon. Billy sat on a box on a street corner, talking to himself and occasionally swearing at people who walked by. He had an unkempt appearance and apparently had not bathed for days. He was begging for handouts and became verbally abusive to those who did not drop money into his hat. Billy did not seem to recognize Randy, even when addressed by name. He avoided eye contact, refused to speak, and simply pointed to his hat. Feeling sorry for his friend, Randy gave Billy all the cash he had.

Billy's mental state is understandable in light of his war trauma. Many soldiers returning from combat have experienced stress reactions, anxiety attacks, drug or alcohol abuse, and depression. The constant threat of death or bodily harm is a reality for soldiers serving in war zones, and the trauma they experience is often beyond human endurance. We know much about war trauma and the psychological harm that combat can produce. In many ways, we know more about pathology than about resilience and strength; we know more about mental illness than mental health, and thus we know more about Billy than we do about Randy.

It may sound strange to ask this question, but what *do* we know about Randy? He seems to have returned from Iraq unscathed; he completed his college education, started a successful business, married, and become an active member of his community. Didn't he go through the same war traumas as his friend Billy? Why didn't he show psychological symptoms? What helped him remain mentally healthy? How did he cope with and overcome the hardships of war?

There are benefits to addressing these questions and realizing that psychology is not just the study of pathology and damage but also the study of strength, character, and virtue. For example, even after experiencing significant combat trauma, Randy exhibits many positive traits—grit, perseverance, integrity, social responsibility, kindness, and compassion. This may be due to Randy's personal characteristics and coping skills, but it also may reflect other factors, such as his exposure to supportive social relationships before, during, and after his military service.

It is important for psychologists to study mental health as well as mental illness and to consider resilience, strengths, and **optimal human functioning.** Unfortunately, we often ignore these positive aspects of the human condition. By focusing on problems and symptoms, we inadvertently recognize a very narrow picture of human functioning. Thus, as we learn about psychopathology, it is important to focus on factors that can help people remain resilient, bounce back from adversity, and recover from mental disorders.

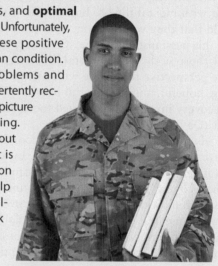

Straight 8 Photography/Shutterstock.com

7. Personal empowerment helps overcome the sense of dependence that results from traditional mental health care.

8. Establishing or strengthening social connections and helping others can facilitate healing.

9. Taking personal responsibility for the journey toward recovery begins with understanding one's experiences and identifying the most effective coping strategies and healing processes.

10. Understanding that barriers can be overcome allows one to confidently live, work, and participate in society.

Community and peer support resources that assist with recovery are increasingly available. For example, NAMI sponsors NAMI on Campus, a student-led group that not only supports students living with mental illness but also strives to educate campus communities regarding mental health, thereby increasing the chances that all students will have a positive college experience. The recovery model has also resulted in social justice actions such as identifying the impacts of stigmatization and discrimination on mental health; fighting policies that neglect the rights of individuals with mental illness; and promoting healing, growth, and respect for those affected by severe mental disorders.

A focus on recovery assists those living with mental illness to achieve their potential and live more meaningful and positive lives. Recognizing that many in the mental health field are still unfamiliar with or mistaken about what recovery encompasses, efforts have concentrated on providing recovery-focused training for community mental health professionals interested in providing recovery-oriented services.

Changes in the Therapeutic Landscape

The use of psychiatric medications combined with a focus on reducing health care costs, examining treatment effectiveness, and using technology in the treatment process have changed the therapeutic landscape of the mental health profession.

The Drug Revolution in Psychiatry

Many mental health professionals consider the introduction of **psychotropic medications** (psychiatric drugs) in the 1950s to be one of the great medical advances of the 20th century (Norfleet, 2002). First, lithium, a naturally occurring element, was discovered to radically calm some patients who had been psychiatrically hospitalized for years. Several years later, the drug chlorpromazine (brand name Thorazine) was found to be extremely effective in treating agitation in patients with schizophrenia. Before long, drugs were available to treat disorders such as depression, phobias, and anxiety. These drugs were revolutionary because they could sometimes rapidly and dramatically decrease or eliminate troublesome symptoms. As a result, confinement in mental hospitals was no longer necessary, and treatment became more cost-effective. The new drug therapies were credited with the depopulation of mental hospitals, a movement we discuss in Chapter 17. To handle the large number of patients returning to the community, outpatient treatment became the primary mode of service for those with severe symptoms. In addition to changing treatment, the introduction of psychiatric drugs revived interest in the role of biological influences on mental disorders. As we discuss later in the text, the burgeoning use of psychiatric medications has also led to many questions and concerns regarding the role of the medical industry and pharmaceutical lobby in influencing trends in diagnosis, treatment, and research.

The Development of Managed Health Care

Managed health care refers to the industrialization of health care, whereby insurance organizations in the private sector monitor and control the delivery of services. Traditionally, psychotherapy has been provided by individuals working independently or in small group practices. Health insurance companies allowed therapists and clients to determine the methods and duration of treatment. However, escalation of health expenditures and a need to control costs resulted in the implementation of managed health

I Have It, Too: The Medical Student Syndrome

To be human is to encounter difficulties and problems in life. A course in psychopathology dwells on human problems—many of them familiar. As a result, as you read this text, you may be prone to the medical student syndrome: Reading about a disorder may lead you to suspect that you have the disorder or that a friend or relative has the disorder. This reaction to the study of psychopathology is common and important for you to recognize. Similarly, medical students reading about physical disorders sometimes begin to imagine that they have the illnesses they are studying. "Distractibility? Fatigue? Trouble sleeping? That's me!" In this way, a cluster of symptoms—no matter how mild or how briefly experienced—can lead some people to suspect that they are ill.

Students who take a course that examines psychopathology are equally prone to believing that they have one or more of the mental disorders described in their text. The problem is compounded by easy access to the Internet, where brief research on mental disorders such as schizophrenia, depression, or anxiety can produce a multitude of descriptors that seem to fit them. It is possible, of course, that some students *do* have an undiagnosed psychological disorder and would benefit from counseling or therapy. Most, however, are merely experiencing an exaggerated sense of their vulnerability to disorders.

Two influences in particular may make us susceptible to imagining that we have a disorder. One is the universality of the human experience. All of us have experienced misfortunes in life. Depressed mood following the loss of a loved one or anxiety before giving a speech are perfectly normal reactions. We can all remember and relate to feelings of fear, apprehension, unhappiness, or euphoria. In most cases, however, these feelings are normal reactions to life situations, not symptoms of illness. Another influence is our tendency to compare our own functioning with our perceptions of how other people are functioning. The outward behaviors you observe your fellow students displaying may lead you to conclude that they experience few difficulties in life, are self-assured and confident, and are invulnerable to mental disturbance. If you were privy to their inner thoughts and feelings, however, you might be surprised to find that they share the same apprehensions and insecurities that you sometimes experience.

If you recognize yourself anywhere in the pages of this book, we hope you will take the time to discuss your feelings with a friend, a family member, one of your professors, or someone at the counseling center at your school. You may be responding to pressures that you have not encountered before—worries about friendships, your grades, or a heavy course load, for example—or may be experiencing other common difficulties associated with adjustment to college life. If you continue to suspect that you have a problem, we hope you will consider getting help from your campus counseling center or a mental health professional in your community. As you will read many times throughout this text, people who seek and receive treatment for mental health issues often find that their condition improves; by seeking help, they are able to prevent a downward spiral of increasing emotional distress.

care. This industrialization of health care brought about major changes in the mental health professions:

- Health insurers began to exert increasing control over psychotherapy by determining what mental conditions are eligible for treatment and the number of treatment sessions allowed.

- Many organizations, in an effort to reduce costs, began hiring therapists with master's degrees rather than those with doctoral degrees.

- Many insurance carriers only reimburse for evidence-based forms of treatment, so therapists must choose therapies that have strong research support.

Many mental health professionals have been frustrated by these trends, concerned that decisions are now made for business reasons rather than in the best interests of clients. On a positive note, in 2010, mental health advocates celebrated the enactment of groundbreaking legislation—the Affordable Health Care Act—which included provisions mandating that insurance companies offer mental health and substance use benefits with treatment limits that are equivalent to those offered for physical health conditions. This has resulted in an increased use of outpatient mental health services, particularly among individuals with employer-sponsored insurance (Mulvaney-Day et al., 2019). Additionally, provisions of the Affordable Health Care Act have allowed many people previously unable to purchase health insurance (due to high costs or preexisting conditions such as mental illness) to access both physical and mental health services.

An Increased Appreciation for Research

Breakthroughs in neuroscience combined with a focus on exploring evidence-based forms of psychotherapy have produced another contemporary trend: a heightened appreciation for the role of research in evaluating the effectiveness of treatments for mental disorders, with the goal of highlighting or even combining effective treatments for each mental disorder. Although the move toward evidence-based practice is important, it is not without controversy. Some claim that the call for empirically based treatments is biased against treatment connected with certain theoretical orientations. For instance, studies reveal that a large majority of treatments identified as effective are those based on cognitive-behavioral principles (Castelnuovo, 2010). Others assert that evidence-based practice is too restrictive and does not recognize clinical intuition and the dynamic basis of therapy. In addition, some question whether treatment research is applicable to members of racially and ethnically underrepresented groups without adaptations that take into account an individual's cultural background (Hall & Yee, 2014). Further, as noted earlier, some mental health professionals fear that managed care companies will use research data to place even more restrictions on the types of treatments they are willing to reimburse.

Technology-Assisted Therapy

Researchers and practitioners committed to treating mental disorders are making increasing use of technology to provide or supplement traditional therapies or as a stand-alone intervention. For example, telehealth services, involving the use of video communication platforms for both individual and group therapy, began to increase dramatically during the COVID pandemic and have since become an acceptable method of providing mental health support. In one survey of clinical psychologists, 76 percent provided "virtual" therapy to their clients and believed the video sessions were effective (Wallis, 2022). It appears that the use of telehealth will continue to remain an important means of providing psychotherapy.

Computer-assisted and online programs to treat psychological problems such as depression and anxiety are rapidly increasing. Many people seem open to these forms of "digital therapies" that depend on the use of apps and Web-based interventions. In general, computer-based programs that employ techniques paralleling those used in traditional therapy have shown the most success in reducing troublesome symptoms involving stress, anxiety, and depression (Heesacker et al., 2019). If you were depressed or stressed, would you consider using a computer program for treatment? One Web-based program (YOLO—"You only live once") succeeded in improving the mental health of college students. The YOLO program, based on a therapeutic approach that promotes self-acceptance, awareness of the present moment, and developing cognitive flexibility, was found to reduce depression, anxiety, and stress while simultaneously improving well-being, life satisfaction, self-compassion, and self-acceptance (Viskovich & Pakenham, 2019).

Therapists are also using technological devices in their work with clients. For example, virtual reality therapy, using helmets with computer screens that immerse the wearer into a realistic virtual world, has successfully treated phobias, stress disorders, and other problems (Fernández-Álvarez et al., 2020). We will go into more detail about this technology as we discuss treatments for anxiety in Chapter 5. Mobile apps have also helped clients track behaviors such as cravings, substance use, and the number and quality of social interactions (Weir, 2018). Another example involves the use of smartphones with a downloaded application that allows individuals with schizophrenia to monitor their symptoms; receive reminders to take medications; obtain suggestions on how to identify and avoid stressors; and, if their symptoms are intensifying, to access ideas for coping (Ben-Zeev et al., 2013). Many participants like using this technology, especially because support is readily available when needed. As these applications become more sophisticated, it is likely that the use of mobile devices for providing assistance to those in therapy will increase.

Social robots are another example of how technology is changing treatment options. In one example, researchers interested in treating depression in older adults developed a seal-like robot that reacts to sounds and voices by turning its head. Participants who interacted with the robot reported feeling less lonely, coping better when encountering stress, and increasing their participation in group activities—positive psychological and emotional changes similar to those obtained with animal-assisted therapies (Misselhorn et al., 2013). Similarly, children with severe social difficulties improved when an assistive robot helped model appropriate social skills, eye contact, and body posture while playing an interactive game (Rudovic et al., 2018). In Japan, scientists are developing robots that are more and more humanlike—robots that are improving the health of hospitalized patients (Akinaga, 2013). These amazing robots can mimic facial expressions and communicate with people, including answering questions in complete sentences. Do you think that robots have a future in assisting with therapy or reducing loneliness and depression in our aging population or in other socially isolated groups? Are there disadvantages to the idea of using social robots? What ethical issues may be involved? As you can see, technological advances are producing a surge of research into causes of and treatment for mental disorders, topics we cover extensively in Chapter 2.

Chapter Summary

1 What is psychopathology?

- The field of psychopathology involves the study of the symptoms and causes of behavioral and mental disorders; the objectives are to describe, explain, predict, and modify distressing emotions and behaviors.

2 How do we decide when behaviors are a significant concern?

- Four criteria have traditionally been used to determine and define psychopathology: distress, deviance, dysfunction, and dangerousness.

3 How common are mental disorders?

- Over the course of a year, approximately 34 percent of young adults in the United States experience a mental disorder.

- In a study of college students in eight countries, over one third of those surveyed met the criteria for a mental disorder at some point in their lives.

4 What societal factors affect definitions of psychopathology?

- Cultural context and sociopolitical factors can influence definitions of psychopathology. Criteria used to define psychopathology must be considered in light of community standards, changes over time, cultural values, and sociopolitical experiences.

5 Why is it important to confront the stigmatization and stereotyping associated with mental illness?

- Much of the stigma and stereotyping surrounding mental illness is based on inaccurate information, such as beliefs that those with mental illness are prone to violence or cannot make important social or career-related contributions. Unfortunately, some people living with mental illness come to believe this inaccurate information.

- Negative societal attitudes about mental illness and related discrimination produce additional barriers to recovery.

- A "code of silence" about mental illness allows inaccurate stereotypes to continue and may prevent people from seeking treatment.

6 How have explanations of psychopathology changed over time?

- Ancient peoples believed in demonology and attributed certain behaviors to evil spirits that inhabited the victim's body. Treatments consisted of trephining, exorcism, and bodily assaults.

- Rational and scientific explanations of mental illness emerged during the Greco-Roman era. Hippocrates believed that mental illness was due to biological causes, such as a dysfunction or disease of the brain. Treatment became more humane.

- With the collapse of the Roman Empire and the increased influence of the church, belief in the supernatural again flourished. During the Middle Ages, some of those killed in church-endorsed witch hunts were people with mental illness.

- The 14th through 16th centuries brought a return to rational and scientific inquiry, along with a heightened interest in humanistic methods of treating the mentally ill.

7 What were early explanations regarding the causes of mental disorders?

- In the 19th and 20th centuries, major medical breakthroughs reignited a belief in the biological roots of mental illness. An especially important discovery during this period was the microorganism that causes the symptoms of general paresis.

- The uncovering of a relationship between hypnosis and hysteria corroborated the belief that psychological processes could produce emotional difficulties.

8 What are some contemporary trends in the field of psychopathology?

- Multicultural psychology, positive psychology, the recovery movement, the drug revolution, managed care, evidence-based practice, and the use of technology have all influenced the field of psychopathology.

Chapter Glossary

anosognosia
a lack of awareness of or insight into one's own mental dysfunction

biological viewpoint
the belief that mental disorders have a physical or physiological basis

biological vulnerability
genetic or physiological susceptibility

brain pathology
a dysfunction or disease of the brain

cathartic method
a therapeutic use of verbal expression to release pent-up emotional conflicts

cultural relativism
the idea that a person's beliefs, values, and behaviors are affected by the culture within which that person lives

cultural universality
the assumption that a fixed set of mental disorders exists whose manifestations and symptoms are similar across cultures

culture
the configuration of shared values, beliefs, attitudes, and behaviors that is transmitted from one generation to another by members of a particular group

discrimination
unjust or prejudicial treatment toward a person based on the person's actual or perceived membership in a certain group

empowerment
increasing one's sense of personal strength and self-worth

etiology
the cause or causes for a condition

exorcism
a practice used to cast evil spirits out of an afflicted person's body

humanism
a philosophical movement that emphasizes human welfare and the worth and uniqueness of the individual

hysteria
an outdated term referring to excessive or uncontrollable emotion, sometimes resulting in somatic symptoms (such as blindness or paralysis) that have no apparent physical cause

intrapsychic
psychological processes occurring within the mind

lifetime prevalence
the percentage of people in the population who have had a disorder at some point in their lives

managed health care
the industrialization of health care, whereby large organizations in the private sector control the delivery of services

mental disorder
psychological symptoms or behavioral patterns that reflect an underlying psychobiological dysfunction; are associated with distress or disability; and are not merely an expectable response to common stressors or losses

mental health professional
health care practitioners (such as psychologists, psychiatrists, psychiatric nurses, social workers, and mental health counselors) whose services focus on improving mental health or treating mental illness

mental illness
a mental health condition that negatively affects a person's emotions, thinking, behavior, relationships with others, or overall functioning

microaggression
subtle comments or actions that intentionally or unintentionally insult or invalidate members of socially marginalized groups

moral treatment movement
a crusade to institute more humane treatment for people with mental illness

optimal human functioning
qualities such as subjective well-being, optimism, self-determinism, resilience, hope, courage, and ability to manage stress

positive psychology
the philosophical and scientific study of positive human functioning focused on the strengths and assets of individuals, families, and communities

prejudice
a biased, preconceived judgment about a person or group based on supposed characteristics of the group

prevalence
the percentage of individuals in a targeted population who have a particular disorder during a specific period of time

psychiatric epidemiology
the study of the prevalence of mental illness in a society

psychodiagnosis
assessment and description of an individual's psychological symptoms, including inferences about possible causes for the psychological distress

psychological resilience
the capacity to effectively adapt to and bounce back from stress, trauma, and other adversities

psychological viewpoint
the belief that mental disorders are caused by psychological and emotional factors rather than biological influences

psychopathology
the study of the symptoms, causes, and treatments of mental disorders

psychotherapy
a program of systematic intervention aimed at improving a client's behavioral, emotional, or cognitive symptoms

psychotropic medications
drugs used to treat or manage psychiatric symptoms by influencing brain activity associated with emotions and behavior

racism
subtle or direct prejudice, discrimination, or systemic oppression against an individual or group based on their race or ethnicity

recovery movement
the perspective that with appropriate treatment and support those with mental illness can improve and live satisfying lives despite any lingering symptoms of illness

self-efficacy
a belief in one's ability to succeed

self-stigma
acceptance of prejudice and discrimination based on internalized negative societal beliefs or stereotypes

social stigma
a negative societal belief about a group, including the view that the group is somehow different from other members of society

spirituality
the belief in an animating life force or energy beyond what we can perceive with our senses

stereotype
an oversimplified, often inaccurate, image or idea about a group of people

syndrome
certain symptoms that tend to occur regularly in clusters

systemic racism
deeply imbedded societal policies and structures that disadvantage certain racial groups

tarantism
a form of mass hysteria prevalent during the Middle Ages; characterized by wild raving, jumping, dancing, and convulsing

treatment plan
a proposed course of therapy, developed collaboratively by a therapist and client, that addresses the client's most distressing mental health symptoms

trephining
a surgical method from the Stone Age in which part of the skull was chipped away to provide an opening through which an evil spirit could escape

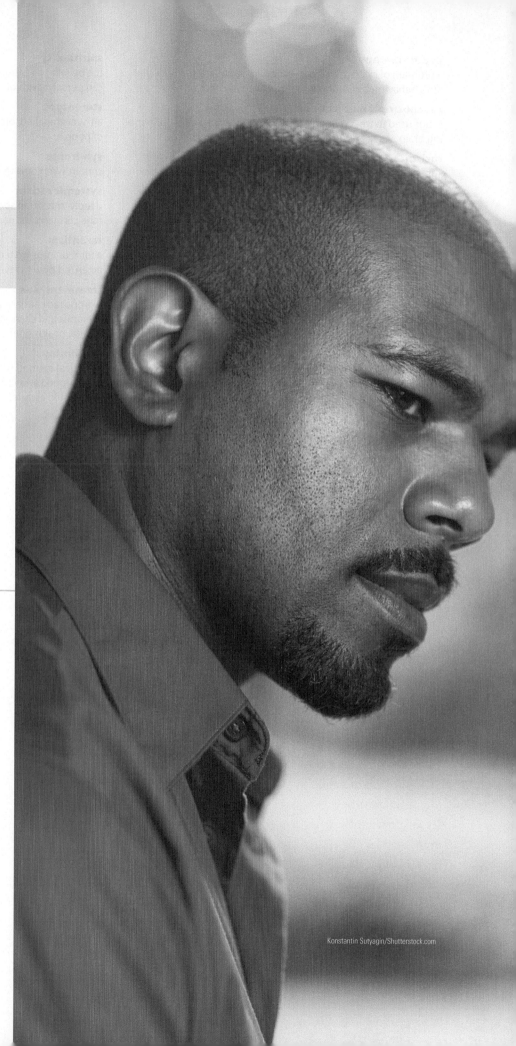

focus
Questions

2

Understanding and Treating Mental Disorders

Learning Objectives

After studying this chapter, you will be able to . . .

2-1   Identify and describe the models used to explain psychopathology.

2-2   Describe the multipath model of mental disorders.

2-3   Describe how biological factors contribute to mental illness.

2-4   Compare and contrast the psychological models that are used to explain the etiology of mental disorders.

2-5   Discuss the role social factors play in psychopathology.

2-6   Outline and describe some of the major sociocultural influences affecting mental illness.

2-7   Explain the importance of considering mental disorders from a multipath perspective.

Steve V., A 21-Year-Old College Student, has been struggling to cope with a debilitating bout of depression. He has a long psychiatric history, including two hospitalizations for severe depression and confused thinking.

Steve was born in a suburb of San Francisco, California, the only child of an extremely wealthy couple. His father is a prominent businessman who works long hours and travels frequently. On those rare occasions when he is home, Mr. V. is preoccupied with business and aloof toward his son. When they do interact, Mr. V. often criticizes and ridicules Steve, complaining that his son is timid and weak. Once, when 10-year-old Steve was bullied and beaten up by classmates, his father berated Steve for losing the fight.

Although Steve is extremely bright and earns good grades, Mr. V. feels that he lacks the "toughness" needed to survive and prosper in today's competitive world.

Although Mrs. V. experiences episodes of severe depression several times each year, she tries to remain active in civic and social affairs. She feels abandoned by Mr. V. and harbors a deep resentment toward him, which she is frightened to express. She sometimes treats Steve lovingly but spent little time with him as he was growing up and seldom defends Steve during Mr. V.'s insulting tirades. She also remains silent when Mr. V. complains that Steve inherited "bad genes" from her side of the family. In reality, Mrs. V. is quite lonely. When Steve was younger,

Mrs. V. often allowed Steve to sleep with her when her husband was away on business trips. This behavior continued until Steve was 12 and Mrs. V. caught Steve masturbating under her sheets one morning. She then abruptly refused to allow Steve into her bed.

Steve was raised by a series of full-time nannies. He had few playmates. His birthdays were celebrated with a cake and candles, but the only celebrants were Steve and his mother. By age 10, Steve occupied himself with "mind games," letting his imagination carry him off on flights of fancy. He frequently imagined himself as a powerful figure—Spiderman or Batman. His fantasies were often extremely violent, involving bloody battles with his enemies.

During high school, Steve became convinced that external forces were controlling his mind. After seeing a horror movie about exorcism, he was convinced that he was possessed by the devil. He also began to experience episodes of severe depression. On two occasions, suicide attempts led to his hospitalization. Steve initially did well in college. Recently, however, he has had little interest in attending classes or studying for exams.

S teve is certainly experiencing symptoms of a mental disorder. What do you think is going on with him? How do we explain his unusual thoughts and his deep depression? Is Steve correct in his belief that he is possessed by evil spirits? Is his father correct in suggesting that "bad genes" caused his disorder? What role did social isolation, constant criticism from his father, and confusing interactions with his mother play in the development of his problems? These complex questions lead us to a very important aspect of psychopathology: the **etiology**, or causes, of disorders. In this chapter, we propose an integrative *multipath model* for explaining symptoms associated with mental illness—a model that highlights how biological, psychological, social, and sociocultural factors affect the development of specific mental disorders. Before we begin, however, let's look at how traditional one-dimensional models might explain Steve's psychopathology.

2-1 One-Dimensional Models of Mental Disorders

Most contemporary explanations of mental disorders fall into four distinct camps: (a) biological views, including genetics and other physiological explanations; (b) psychological issues, rooted in the invisible complexities of the human mind; (c) dysfunctional social relationships, including stressful interactions with family members and peers; and (d) sociocultural influences, including the effects of discrimination and stressors related to race, gender, and poverty. Let's look at how each model might explain Steve's psychopathology.

- *Biological explanations*: Some form of biological dysfunction is causing Steve's difficulties. His problems are likely due to a genetic predisposition to depression and related abnormalities in brain functioning.

- *Psychological explanations*: Psychological explanations for Steve's behavior might focus on (a) early childhood experiences that created resentment and loneliness, (b) Steve's feelings of hostility toward his father and conflicted relationship with his mother, or (c) the role that irrational beliefs and distorted thinking played in Steve's mental confusion.

- *Social explanations*: From a social-relational perspective, a dysfunctional family system and pathological upbringing contributed to Steve's issues. Parental neglect, rejection, and psychological abuse may explain many of his symptoms. The constant bullying of Steve by his father and the confusing messages and lack of support from his mother are the primary culprits. Steve also led a very isolated life, with few opportunities to develop appropriate social skills and behaviors. Additionally, Steve lacks a network of supportive relationships.

- *Sociocultural explanations*: Societal and cultural context are important considerations in understanding Steve's difficulties. He is a European American man, born to a wealthy family. He was raised in a cultural context that values individual achievement, assertiveness, and competitiveness. Because Steve does not live up to his father's standards of masculinity, he is considered a failure not only by his father but also by himself.

These four explanations, perspectives, or viewpoints regarding psychopathology are referred to as *models* by psychologists. A **model** describes or attempts to explain a phenomenon or process that we cannot directly observe. The models used to explain the causes of mental disorders each embody a particular theoretical approach. Such models guide mental health professionals as they review relevant information, ask probing questions, make educated guesses about the causes of an individual's symptoms, and organize the accumulated information in a meaningful way. Theorists do not assume there is one definitive model that explains human behavior. They recognize the complexities involved in being human and realize that any model has limitations.

Models of psychopathology, whether biological, psychological, social, or sociocultural, help us to organize and make sense of what we know about mental illness. These models, however, can foster a one-dimensional and linear explanation of mental disorders, thus limiting our ability to consider other perspectives. If, for example, we use a psychological explanation of Steve's behavior and consider his problems to be rooted in unconscious sexual desire for his mother and competitiveness toward his father, we may unintentionally ignore research findings pointing to powerful biological, social, or sociocultural influences on his symptoms.

As you reviewed the one-dimensional explanations for Steve V.'s difficulties, it is likely that you concluded that each explanation contains kernels of truth, but that none of the explanations sufficiently addresses Steve's mental distress, including his unique physiology, experiences, and family background. You may have also concluded that it is more likely that a combination of biological, psychological, social, and sociocultural effects interacted and contributed to Steve's difficulties. If so, you are beginning to appreciate the complexities involved in understanding the etiology of mental disorders.

Scientists now recognize that one-dimensional perspectives are overly simplistic because they (a) set up a false "either–or" dichotomy between accepting one explanation or another (e.g., nature vs. nurture), (b) neglect the possibility that a variety of circumstances contribute to the development of mental disorders, and (c) fail to recognize the reciprocal interactions of the various contributing factors.

We will use our integrative and interacting *multipath model* to explain the mental disorders discussed throughout the text. The multipath model addresses the limitations associated with one-dimensional models and will help you conceptualize how various interacting forces can contribute to mental illness.

2-2 A Multipath Model of Mental Disorders

Research suggests that a variety of circumstances affect the development of a psychological disorder—influences that incorporate the perspectives of multiple theories. Some models do, in fact, consider multiple viewpoints. The **biopsychosocial model**, for example, suggests that interactions between biological, psychological, and social factors cause mental disorders. In Steve V.'s case, genetics and brain functioning (a biological perspective) may interact with ways of thinking (a psychological perspective) in a given family environment (a social perspective) to produce his symptoms. Although the biopsychosocial model highlights the fact that multiple circumstances can lead to the development of mental disorders, concerns remain: (a) there is limited focus on how elements interact to produce illness; (b) the model provides little guidance regarding how to treat the disorder; and (c) the model neglects the powerful forces of culture. Of particular concern is the relative neglect of **sociocultural influences** such as the effects of poverty or discrimination in explaining mental disorders.

What, then, is the "best" way to conceptualize the causes of mental disorders? Throughout this text, we will use the **multipath model**—an integration of biological, psychological, social, and sociocultural influences—as we consider the multitude of factors that researchers have confirmed are associated with each disorder we discuss. The multipath model is not a theory but a way of looking at the variety and complexity of contributors to mental disorders. It provides an organizational framework for understanding the numerous circumstances that increase risk for the development of a mental disorder, the complexity of potential interactions among these elements, and the need to view each disorder from a holistic perspective. The multipath model operates under several assumptions:

- No one theoretical perspective is adequate to explain the complexity of the human condition and the development of mental disorders.

- There are multiple pathways to and influences on the development of any single disorder. Explanations of behavior must consider biological, psychological, social, and sociocultural elements.

- Not all dimensions contribute equally to a disorder. In the case of some disorders, current research may suggest that certain etiological forces have the strongest effect on the development of that specific disorder. Additionally, our understanding of mental disorders often evolves as further investigation provides new insights into contributing factors.

- The multipath model is integrative and interactive. It acknowledges that factors may combine in complex and reciprocal ways so that people exposed to the same conditions may not develop the same disorder and that different individuals exposed to different circumstances may develop similar mental disorders.

- The biological and psychological strengths and assets of a person and positive aspects of the person's social and sociocultural environment can help protect against psychopathology, minimize symptoms, or facilitate recovery from mental illness.

As you can see, understanding the causes of various disorders is a complex process. Let's look at some of the details regarding how our multipath model conceptualizes the development of mental disorders. As we explain various disorders throughout the book, we will focus on these four dimensions.

- *Dimension One: Biological Factors*—Genetics, brain structure and physiology, central nervous system functioning, autonomic nervous system reactivity, and so forth
- *Dimension Two: Psychological Factors*—Personality, cognition, emotions, learning, coping skills, self-efficacy, values, and so forth
- *Dimension Three: Social Factors*—Family and other interpersonal relationships, social support, sense of belonging, community connections, and so forth
- *Dimension Four: Sociocultural Factors*—Race, gender, sexual orientation, spirituality or religion, socioeconomic status, ethnicity, culture, and so forth

As summarized in Figure 2.1, the etiology of mental disorders often involves the interaction of influences occurring within and between these dimensions. As we expand our discussion and dive deeper into the multipath model, keep in mind that the four dimensions have permeable boundaries with considerable overlap and various complexities. For example, it is important to be aware that:

1. Each dimension may include a variety of explanations for a disorder based on distinct theories; each theoretical perspective affects the explanations proposed and the research conducted. Let's take the psychological dimension as an example. Some psychological theories highlight the importance of unconscious impulses in the development of psychopathology, whereas other psychological perspectives emphasize learned patterns of thinking and behaving. Thus, there are considerable differences of opinion regarding the purported causes of a disorder even within a particular dimension.

2. Factors within each of the four dimensions can interact and influence each other in any direction. For example, let's consider the association

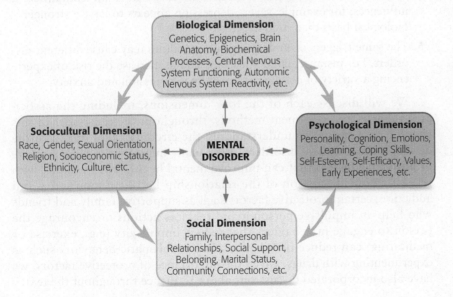

Figure 2.1

The Multipath Model

Each dimension of the multipath model considers factors found to be important in explaining mental disorders. Reciprocal interactions involving factors within and between any of these dimensions can also influence the development of psychopathology.

between **impulsivity** and addiction. Research suggests that certain patterns of brain functioning (a biological characteristic) are associated with impulsivity (a psychological characteristic). Additionally, if you are impulsive, it is quite possible that you have a parent or sibling who behaves impulsively; this might have affected your family relationships or your experiences growing up (a social factor). Also, if you have a tendency to make decisions without carefully considering the consequences, you might be more likely to hang around with friends who also engage in high-risk behaviors such as underage drinking or experimenting with drugs (a social factor) that result in additional biological influences (e.g., substance use affects brain regions associated with decision making).

Your impulsive behavior or substance use may also affect your ability to complete your education or keep a job. This makes you vulnerable to the influences of poverty or discrimination because of your inconsistent employment history (a sociocultural factor). These circumstances may increase your tendency to turn to drugs or alcohol; this pattern of substance use and addictive behavior may further affect your brain functioning, strain your relationships with family and friends, decrease your chances of stable employment, and so on. As you might imagine, other sociocultural factors such as being a woman, being a member of an underrepresented ethnic or religious group, or having a lesbian, gay, or bisexual orientation or transgender or nonbinary gender identity would add additional complexity to your situation.

3. A particular mental health condition may be caused by various combinations of influences within the four dimensions. For instance, let's look at the severe depression experienced by Steve V.'s mother. Her depression may be related to a single factor (e.g., an unhappy marriage) or may involve an interaction of elements in different dimensions (e.g., biological vulnerability to depression, child abuse occurring in early life, and stressors in adulthood). Although a single circumstance may trigger a disorder such as depression, it is more likely the result of a combination of factors.

4. Many disorders appear to be **heterogeneous** in nature. That is, there may be distinct versions of a specific disorder that result from different influences; for example, severe depression appears to have a stronger biological basis than mild depression.

5. The same triggers or underlying vulnerabilities may cause different disorders. For instance, child abuse appears to increase the risk of experiencing a variety of conditions, including depression and anxiety.

We will discuss each of the four dimensions, including the associated theories and treatment methods, throughout the remainder of this chapter. In addition to understanding the circumstances linked to the development of mental disorders, it is equally important to remain aware of **protective factors** that can improve mental health. For example, with respect to our discussion of the relationship between impulsivity and addiction, certain protective factors such as supportive family and friends who help an impulsive person avoid reckless actions or encourage the person to engage in behaviors that reduce impulsivity (e.g., exercise or meditating) can reduce the likelihood of problematic behaviors such as experimenting with drugs. Given the importance of protective factors, we have also incorporated discussions about resilience throughout the text.

Myth If one member of a family has a mental health condition, other members will probably develop the same disorder.

Reality The fact that mental health conditions run in certain families has caused undue anxiety for many people. Heredity plays a role in many mental disorders but does not guarantee that symptoms of mental illness will develop. Mental disorders result from interactions among a variety of influences. Fortunately, positive psychological, social, and cultural circumstances can help protect people from developing a disorder to which they are biologically predisposed.

A Multipath Model of Resilience

Most of us face various adversities during our lifetimes. How is it that some people bounce back quickly when affected by stressful circumstances? Just as biological, psychological, social, and sociocultural vulnerabilities contribute to mental disorders, these same factors influence our resilience—our ability to recover from stressful or challenging circumstances (refer to Figure 2.2). In other words, enhancing and using our strengths and relying on positive supports within our environment may decrease the likelihood that we develop a mental disorder. Similarly, if circumstances are such that we are coping with a mental health condition, these protective factors may decrease the duration or severity of our symptoms. Here are some examples of factors influencing resilience from a multipath perspective.

Biological Influences

Because adaptation is the key to our survival, our brains and bodies are primed for resilience. This biological ability to adapt and bounce back increases our chances of thriving even after we have faced challenging circumstances. Because some people appear to have high internal resilience, researchers are attempting to identify genes associated with this characteristic (Choi et al., 2019). Additionally, researchers have found that lifestyle factors such as healthy dietary choices, exercise, and sleep patterns can exert positive effects on our mental health (Zaman et al., 2019). Biological researchers interested in increasing resilience are also using neuroimaging procedures to investigate methods for optimizing emotional functioning (Bolsinger et al., 2018).

Psychological Influences

Psychological qualities such as mental flexibility, active coping, optimism, hope, self-efficacy, and adaptability allow people to tackle life challenges and increase resilience (Gallagher et al., 2020). In one study involving nurses working in a high-stress intensive care unit, characteristics such as these were associated with less burnout and fewer symptoms of anxiety or depression (Mealer et al., 2013). Additionally, our mindset—our views about our ability to make positive changes in our lives—can exert a powerful influence on our well-being; if we have positive expectations that sustained effort will influence outcome, we are less likely to succumb to distressing life circumstances (Schäfer et al., 2020).

Social Influences

Social support plays an important role in increasing our resilience. For instance, adolescents who reported high levels of peer support were less affected by stress compared to teens who reported average or low levels of support (Doane & Zeiders, 2013). Additionally, supportive family characteristics can help us cope with adversity (Mackin et al., 2017). Combining both psychological and social factors, the broaden-and-build theory of positive emotions posits that positive emotions increase our engagement in the world and thus enhance our resilience by building our coping skills and interpersonal resources (Fredrickson, 2013).

Sociocultural Influences

Cultural and community support can also increase our ability to deal with life's challenges. For example, ethnically underrepresented youth in Canada who remained involved in the culture and customs of their ethnic community showed good resilience (Ungar & Liebenberg, 2013). Presumably, cultural connections serve as a buffer to adverse situations. Similarly, adherence to traditional cultural values such as *familismo* (importance of family), respect, and ethnic identity were associated with strength in overcoming adversity among Mexican American college students (Morgan Consoli & Llamas, 2013). Latinx adolescents who possess a strong ethnic identity or bicultural identity have an increased likelihood of leading a lifestyle that promotes good mental health (Moise et al., 2019).

These are just a few of many possible examples demonstrating how biological, psychological, social, and sociocultural factors play a role in resilience. As you read about the risk factors associated with mental disorders, we hope you will remember that we all have personal and social strengths—positive life outlook, social support, coping skills, and social group identities—that we can rely on to help us bounce back when life is challenging. Additionally, just as we can improve our physical health, we also have the opportunity to engage in activities that improve our mental health and our resilience, even when presented with difficult personal circumstances. In fact, many mental health professionals are incorporating techniques from the resilience literature into their prevention efforts and therapeutic practices.

Figure 2.2

The Resilience Model

Strengths, assets, and protective factors help maximize mental health and allow individuals to bounce back from trauma and stressful life events.

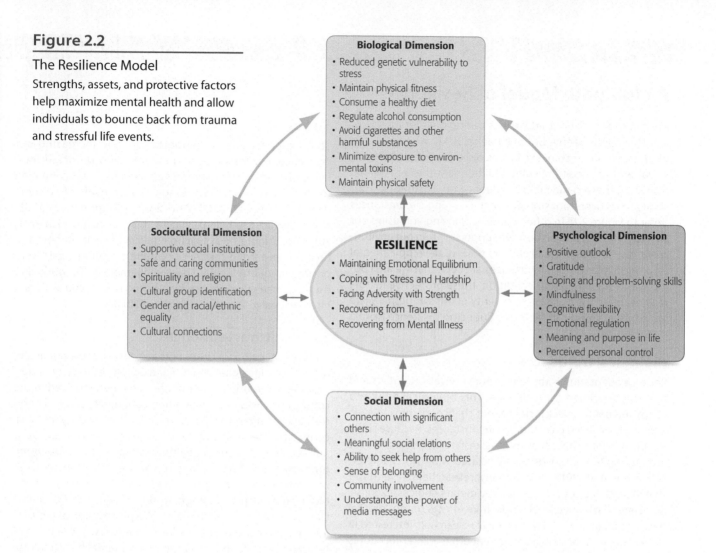

Biological Dimension
- Reduced genetic vulnerability to stress
- Maintain physical fitness
- Consume a healthy diet
- Regulate alcohol consumption
- Avoid cigarettes and other harmful substances
- Minimize exposure to environmental toxins
- Maintain physical safety

Sociocultural Dimension
- Supportive social institutions
- Safe and caring communities
- Spirituality and religion
- Cultural group identification
- Gender and racial/ethnic equality
- Cultural connections

RESILIENCE
- Maintaining Emotional Equilibrium
- Coping with Stress and Hardship
- Facing Adversity with Strength
- Recovering from Trauma
- Recovering from Mental Illness

Psychological Dimension
- Positive outlook
- Gratitude
- Coping and problem-solving skills
- Mindfulness
- Cognitive flexibility
- Emotional regulation
- Meaning and purpose in life
- Perceived personal control

Social Dimension
- Connection with significant others
- Meaningful social relations
- Ability to seek help from others
- Sense of belonging
- Community involvement
- Understanding the power of media messages

2-3 Dimension One: Biological Factors

Our understanding of the biological processes that play a role in mental disorders is expanding rapidly. Not only are research methods increasing in sophistication, scientists across the globe are also sharing and building on available research. Modern biological explanations of mental illness share certain assumptions:

1. Characteristics that make us who we are—our physical features, susceptibility to illness, and physiological response to stress, to name a few—are embedded in the genetic material of our cells. Additionally, many of our personal qualities result from complex interactions between our biological makeup and the environment.

2. Thoughts, emotions, and behaviors involve physiological activity occurring within the brain; changes in the way we think, feel, or behave affect these electrical and chemical processes and, over time, can change brain function and structure.

3. Many mental disorders are associated with inherited biological vulnerability and preexisting brain dysfunction.

4. Medications and other biological interventions used to treat mental disorders focus on modifying physiological processes within the brain and body.

We begin our discussion with an overview of brain structures and physiological processes associated with the development of mental disorders.

The Human Brain

The brain's role as the center of our thoughts, memories, and emotions is significant to psychopathology. The brain coordinates a variety of highly complex functions, including (a) regulating activities necessary for our survival (such as breathing and heartbeat), (b) receiving and interpreting sensory information (from both inside and outside our bodies), (c) transmitting information to our muscles and other organs, and (d) coordinating our responses to incoming stimuli.

Presented in cross section, the brain has three parts (refer to Figure 2.3):

- *the forebrain*—responsible for higher-level mental processes;
- *the midbrain*—involved with basic functions such as hearing and vision, motor movement, alertness and sleep–wake cycles, and temperature regulation; and
- *the hindbrain*—responsible for instinctive behavior related to self-preservation and survival as well as basic bodily functions involving physiological equilibrium such as heartbeat, respiration, and digestion.

Cerebrospinal fluid surrounds the entire brain. This fluid not only cushions and protects the delicate regions of the brain, but it also fills the cerebral ventricles—the linked system of open spaces found within the brain. A deep groove divides the outer layers of the brain and the deeper brain structures into virtually identical halves—the left and right hemispheres. These matching brain structures receive sensory input from and control muscle movement on the opposite side of the body. Each hemisphere has some specialized functions; the left hemisphere is associated with many language functions, whereas the right hemisphere is associated with visual-spatial abilities and has stronger connections to structures associated with emotion. Although some brain activities occur primarily in one hemisphere, most mental performance involves complex communication between brain regions. While all brain regions are critical for optimal functioning, some brain structures play a greater role in the development of mental disorders. Many of the structures relevant to psychopathology are in the forebrain.

The Forebrain

The forebrain contains brain structures associated with characteristics that make us human—thoughts, perceptions, intelligence, language, personality, imagination, planning, organization, and decision making. The forebrain includes the largest and most advanced part of the brain, the **cerebrum**. Another significant part of the forebrain is the **cerebral cortex**, which consists of layers of specialized nerve cells, called **neurons**, that transmit information to other nerve cells, muscles, and gland cells throughout the body.

The **prefrontal cortex**, the region of the cerebral cortex responsible for **executive functioning**, helps us manage our attention, behavior, and emotions, thus allowing us to accomplish short-term and long-term goals. Executive functioning involves a combination of emotional, social, and intellectual capacities. An important aspect of executive functioning—the

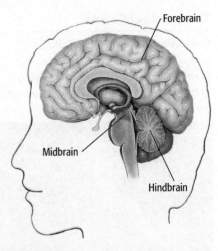

Figure 2.3

Three Major Divisions of the Brain
A cross-sectional view of the brain reveals the forebrain, midbrain, and hindbrain. Although the large size of the forebrain makes the other two divisions look trivial, the midbrain and hindbrain perform essential functions involving vision, hearing, breathing, movement, and maintaining balance.

The Cerebral Cortex

This section of the brain of an adult woman presents the cerebral cortex, with its extensive folding, and the underlying white matter—the connective networks of the brain.

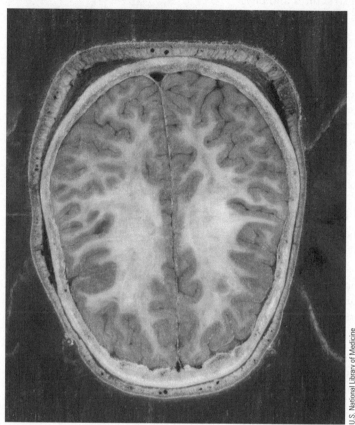

U.S. National Library of Medicine

ability to foresee the consequences of our actions—is guided by our assessment of present circumstances combined with memories of similar past experiences. When operating optimally, the prefrontal cortex helps inhibit many of the instinctual responses and reflexive actions that arise from the more primitive areas of the brain. In other words, the prefrontal cortex helps us exercise good judgment and keep our feelings and impulses in check. Unfortunately, many mental disorders involve dysfunction in the prefrontal cortex; when this occurs, a person may experience difficulty organizing and evaluating incoming information and planning appropriate responses.

The **limbic system** is a group of deep brain structures associated with emotions, decision making, and the formation of memories (Figure 2.4). The intricate connections in this system link our emotions and our recollections. One important structure in the limbic system, the **amygdala**, plays a key role by facilitating the recall of our emotional memories, thus guiding our response to potential threat. The amygdala activates in response to our thoughts or imagination, as well as real-world stimuli; this reactivity plays a key role in various mental disorders. Another structure in the limbic system is the **hippocampus**, which helps us form, organize, and store memory; this includes evaluating short-term memories and sending emotionally relevant memories to the cerebral cortex for long-term storage, as well as assisting with the recall of emotions associated with specific memories.

Emotional responses originating in the limbic system directly affect the **autonomic nervous system (ANS)**. The ANS coordinates basic functions such as digestion and respiration when we are at rest.

Figure 2.4

Structures in the Limbic System
The limbic system, comprised of an interconnected group of brain structures, controls emotional reactions and basic human drives. It is also involved in motivation, decision making, and the formation of memories.

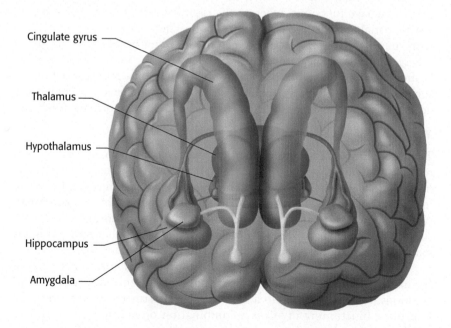

Cingulate gyrus

Thalamus

Hypothalamus

Hippocampus

Amygdala

It also regulates automatic physical responses associated with emotional reactions, most notably the "fight or flight" response that occurs when we perceive a situation as threatening. The **hypothalamus**, a structure that regulates our bodily drives—such as hunger, thirst, and sexual response—and body conditions—such as body temperature and circadian rhythms—plays a key role in our reactions via the **hypothalamic-pituitary-adrenal (HPA) axis**, a system activated under conditions of stress or emotional arousal. When stress or perceived threat triggers the HPA axis, the hypothalamus stimulates the **pituitary gland** to release **hormones** that produce a sequence of events (including stimulation of the **adrenal gland**) that prepare the body to respond to the potentially dangerous situation. Biochemical processes associated with the HPA axis can have a cascading effect throughout the brain and produce symptoms associated with various mental disorders.

Biochemical Processes Within the Brain and Body

Biochemical theories attempt to explain how irregularities in biochemical functioning trigger mental disorders. These theories focus on the critical role of biochemical actions in various physiological and mental processes, from sleeping and digestion to thinking and feeling. In order to understand the research investigating the link between biochemical dysfunction and psychopathology, it is important to understand the physiological processes underlying emotional functioning.

Optimal mental performance involves a variety of interconnected activities. Our brains are composed of billions of neurons and trillions of **glia**, cells that perform a variety of supportive roles, including shaping the brain's **neural circuits** or signal-relaying systems. Although neurons vary in the specific functions they perform, they all share certain characteristics. Each neuron has a cell body with the capacity to regulate the growth, metabolism, and repair of the neuron. On one end of the cell body are numerous **dendrites**, short, rootlike structures that receive chemical and electrical signals from other neurons (Figure 2.5). At the other end is an **axon**, a much longer extension that sends signals not only to other neurons but also to muscles and glands, often a considerable distance away. Incoming messages are received and transmitted to the cell body by a neuron's dendrites; the signal is then sent down the axon to bulblike swellings called axon terminals, usually located near dendrites of another neuron.

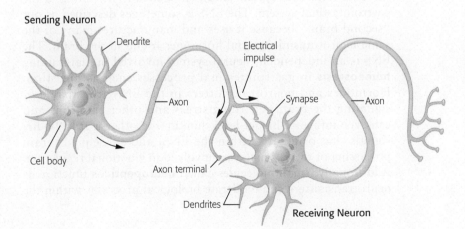

Figure 2.5

Synaptic Transmission
Electrical impulses travel along the axon, through the synapse, and to the dendrites of the next neuron. Neurotransmitters facilitate the transmission of the impulse across the synapse.

Thus, dendrites bring information *to* the body of the cell, and axons carry information *away* from the cell. Axons are covered with **myelin**, a fatty, insulating substance that forms a myelin sheath; **myelination** increases the efficiency of signal transmission and allows damaged nerve pathways to regenerate by providing tracks along which regrowth can occur. Some brain tissue (**white matter**) primarily consists of nerve pathways, myelinated axons, and the supportive glia cells that surround them, whereas other tissue (**gray matter**) consists of the cell bodies of neurons and glia (and the capillaries supplying them nutrients).

The functioning of the brain involves many continuous activities—neurons working in synchronization with processes occurring throughout the body. Effective communication between neurons relies on both electrical impulses and chemical signals. A variety of chemicals, called **neurotransmitters**, help relay messages by transmitting nerve impulses across the **synapse**, a tiny gap that exists between nerve cells. After crossing the synapse, the neurotransmitter binds to the correct receptor neuron on the other side, like a key fitting into a lock. Once neurotransmitters have performed their function, they are often reabsorbed by the axon that released them, a process called **reuptake**. If not reabsorbed, neurotransmitters are sometimes deactivated (neutralized) by enzymes in the synapse or removed by glial cells. (Refer to Table 2.1 for some of the neurotransmitters and hormones most frequently involved in mental disorders.)

Depending on the specific neurotransmitter and other physiological influences, the binding that occurs at the synapse (Figure 2.6) either excites the cell (stimulating continued transmission of the signal) or inhibits further signaling. Excitation causes electrical impulses to travel to other neurons, to muscles, or to gland cells that stimulate the release of hormones. Some neurotransmitters (such as gamma-aminobutyric acid [GABA] and serotonin) have inhibitory effects that decrease neural signaling, whereas others (such as epinephrine and norepinephrine) have excitatory effects that promote signal transmission. Some neurotransmitters, such as acetylcholine and dopamine, have the capacity to either increase or decrease the likelihood that neurons will fire depending on the type of receptors available. Additionally, some chemicals, such as epinephrine (also called adrenaline), can function both as a neurotransmitter and as a hormone.

Mental health researchers are paying increasing attention to the **enteric nervous system (ENS)**, embedded in the lining of the gastrointestinal system. The ENS is sometimes described as our "second brain" because it uses and manufactures many of the same neurotransmitters and hormones found in the brain. The ENS is an independent neural system involved in maintaining **homeostasis** in gastrointestinal processes such as digestion. Hormones and neurotransmitters in the ENS are capable of signaling the brain regarding stress and other emotions and can even influence higher-level thinking. In other words, bodily signals that originate within the ENS, and subsequent brain processing of these signals, are involved in emotional regulation. Additionally, small molecules called **neuropeptides** function as neurotransmitters and moderate biological processes within the

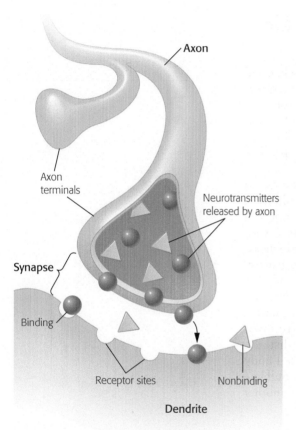

Figure 2.6

Neurotransmitter Binding

Neurotransmitters are released into the synapse and bind with receptor cells on the dendrites of the receiving neuron. Each neurotransmitter has a specific "shape" that corresponds to a receptor site. Like a jigsaw puzzle, binding occurs if the neurotransmitter fits into the receptor site.

Table 2.1 Major Neurotransmitters and Their Functions

Neurotransmitter	Function	Associated Disorders
Acetylcholine (ACh)	Influences attention and memory, dream and sleep states, and neuroplasticity; has excitatory and inhibitory effects	Alzheimer disease; schizophrenia; attention-deficit/hyperactivity disorder
Dopamine*	Influences motivation and reward-seeking behaviors; regulates movement, emotional responses, attention, and planning; has excitatory and inhibitory effects	Attention-deficit/hyperactivity disorder; autism spectrum disorder; depression; schizophrenia; substance use disorders; Parkinson disease
Epinephrine (adrenaline)* and norepinephrine (noradrenaline)*	Excitatory functions include regulation of attention, arousal and concentration, dreaming, and moods; as a hormone, influences physiological reactions related to stress response (attention, blood flow, heart rate, etc.)	Anxiety and stress disorders; sleep disorders
Glutamate	Major excitatory neurotransmitter involved in cognition, memory, and learning	Alzheimer disease; autism spectrum disorder; depression; obsessive-compulsive disorder; schizophrenia
Gamma-aminobutyric acid (GABA)	Major inhibitory neurotransmitter; calms the nerves; regulates mood and muscle tone	Anxiety disorders; attention-deficit/hyperactivity disorder; bipolar disorder; depression; schizophrenia
Serotonin	Inhibitory effects regulate temperature, mood, appetite, and sleep; reduced serotonin can increase impulsive behavior and aggression	Depression; suicide; obsessive-compulsive and anxiety disorders; posttraumatic stress disorder; eating disorders

Hormone	Function	Associated Disorders
Cortisol	Steroid hormone released in response to stress	Anorexia nervosa; depression; stress-related disorders
Ghrelin	Stimulates hunger and boosts the appeal of food	Eating disorders; obesity
Leptin	Suppresses appetite	Anorexia nervosa; schizophrenia
Melatonin	Regulates circadian sleep–wake cycles	Bipolar disorder; depression, particularly seasonal depression; schizophrenia; obsessive-compulsive disorder
Oxytocin	Neuropeptide hormone influencing lactation and complex social behavior (including nurturing and bonding)	Autism spectrum disorder; anxiety; schizophrenia

*These neurotransmitters also function as hormones.

ENS and the central nervous system; neuropeptides have the ability to both directly and indirectly affect a variety of hormones and neurotransmitters.

Neurotransmitters, hormones, neuropeptides, and related biochemical processes play an important role in our overall functioning, affecting our mood, behavior, coordination, communication, and higher-level thinking, as well as basic physiological activities occurring throughout our brains and bodies. Thus, dysfunction in biochemical transmission can produce symptoms seen in many mental disorders. Biochemical processes also play an important role in the adaptive structural changes that occur in the brain and central nervous system.

Neuroplasticity

The human brain evolves and adapts to ensure our survival. This process of frequent change, **neuroplasticity**, enables the brain to adjust to environmental conditions or to compensate for injury. Our brains respond to environmental circumstances by creating neural circuits as needed (e.g., to facilitate new learning or to cope with environmental stressors) and by pruning the neural pathways that are no longer used. Although neurons are long-lived cells that remain healthy over much of our lifetime, the synapses that connect neurons are constantly changing. Many factors influence these changes, including our interactions with people, places, and events; our thoughts and emotional reactions; and our health, nutritional intake, and exercise patterns.

You may have heard the saying "Neurons that fire together, wire together." This refers to another important concept related to neuroplasticity—nerve pathways that we use frequently become myelinated and thus become stronger and more efficient. Neural circuits are bolstered when we continually practice a new skill or a new way of reacting to a situation—the neural circuits become "hardwired" into the brain. This is true for healthy, productive thoughts and behaviors, as well as for the distressing or dysfunctional thoughts and behaviors associated with mental disorders.

Neuroplasticity also involves brain changes associated with the birth of new neurons (**neurogenesis**). We all have **neural stem cells**, uncommitted brain cells that can be stimulated to form new neurons and glia. This means we can alter brain functioning at any point in life by engaging in experiences that stimulate neurogenesis. Neural stem cells have the ongoing potential to generate neurons needed for new skills or experiences, as well as to compensate for brain damage or changes in the brain associated with illness or aging (Gelfo, 2019). Just as we know that conditions such as chronic stress can have negative effects on brain functioning, we also know that exercise, challenging mental activities, and some forms of psychotherapy can produce positive neuroplastic changes via neurogenesis (Levy et al., 2018).

Many mental disorders are associated with brain dysfunction. However, to fully understand the biological bases of psychopathology, we need to move beyond brain processes alone. Researchers across the globe are finding hundreds—perhaps even thousands—of pieces to add to the biological puzzle through the study of genetics and epigenetics.

Genetics and Heredity

Research strongly indicates that **heredity**—the genetic transmission of **traits**—plays an important role in the development of mental disorders. Genetics is a fascinating but incredibly complex field of study. Let's review some basic information associated with genetics and how traits are inherited. In the nucleus of each cell, most humans have 23 pairs of chromosomes that we inherit from our parents. Within each chromosome are **genes**; each gene contains specific information pertaining to the development of our cells, tissues, organs, and body systems, all coded as a DNA sequence. Scientists have been able to document that the entire human **genome** consists of approximately 20,000 to 25,000 protein-coding genes.

Our genetic makeup (the specific genes each of us inherits) is called our **genotype**. Our genotype and environmental circumstances interact and produce our **phenotype**, our observable physical and behavioral characteristics. Determining what exerts the most influence on our traits—our genotype or the environment—is sometimes difficult. For example, some characteristics, such as eye color, are determined solely by our genotype—by the coding in our genes. Other characteristics, such as height, are determined partly by our genes and partly by environmental factors. People who are malnourished in childhood, for instance, may not reach their genetically programmed height. Yet excellent nutrition does not produce growth beyond what our genes dictate.

Genetic characteristics can also result from **genetic mutations**. Throughout our lifetime, our bodies create new cells; each cell has a copy of our chromosomes and our DNA. Sometimes, errors occur in the cell duplication process, causing a spontaneous genetic mutation. Genetic mutations change the instructions within the gene and thus change the outcome of the genetic coding. Some mutations are helpful or have no noticeable outcome, whereas others result in biological dysfunction, including difficulties associated with mental illness. Toxins, viruses, or other environmental elements can produce genetic mutations. We can also inherit a genetic mutation. Additionally, some mental disorders are influenced by common genetic variations called **polymorphisms**; with polymorphic genes, people inherit various forms (**alleles**) of a particular gene. Any genetic variation—whether inherited or produced by cell division or environmental influences—can interact with environmental factors to produce varying phenotypes, including symptoms associated with mental disorders.

However, having a specific gene and encountering environmental stressors is not enough to increase the risk of developing a mental disorder. Rather, the configuration of the gene, the specific stressors, and the times at which stressors occur can all affect gene expression (Price et al., 2019). In particular, gene × environment interactions that occur during **critical periods**, such as early childhood, can set the stage for behavioral or physiological phenotypes that increase the likelihood of experiencing mental illness (Epel & Prather, 2018). This gene × environment interaction can affect cellular functioning in complex ways and exert a profound effect on the individual and on future generations through epigenetic processes.

Epigenetics

Epigenetics refers to the study of the complex biochemical processes that allow us to adapt to a changing environment. Although the DNA within our genes provides the foundation for and programs the sequence of human development, a variety of biochemical processes, triggered by the environment, shape the path that this development takes. In addition to the genetic information carried within our genes, chemical compounds outside of the genome control **gene expression** and thus determine whether or not specific genes are "turned on" or "turned off." Because each cell has a special function, only a small number of genes within a cell are expressed—the genes related to the function of that cell. The remaining genes in the cell stay inactive or dormant unless environmental circumstances trigger their activation. Further, environmental influences can result in the repression of genes that were previously activated. These epigenetic processes leave biological markers on the DNA responsible for regulating gene expression—markers that can produce traits different from those coded in our DNA. Thus, most genetically determined differences between people, including whether or not someone has an increased risk of developing a mental disorder, are due not only to variations in our genes but also to distinct epigenetic processes controlling which genes are expressed.

Genetic and Epigenetic Comparisons in Identical Twins

Identical twins Scott and Mark Kelly are the subjects of NASA's Twins Study. Scott (right) spent a year in space while Mark (left) stayed on Earth as a control subject. Researchers are looking at the effects of space travel on the human body, including genetic and epigenetic changes resulting from time spent in space.

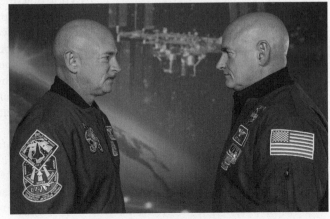

NASA

We are learning more about how environmental circumstances trigger processes that alter gene expression and allow for adaptive changes in cellular function based on various requirements of the internal and external environment. Epigenetic modifications appear to result from four primary categories of environmental influences: nutrition, behavior, exposure to stress, and contact with toxins (Faulk & Dolinoy, 2011). Even minor events that occur during certain critical periods of development can have significant epigenetic consequences. For example, environmental adversities such as poverty or stressful conditions within the home can produce epigenetic modifications, particularly when these events occur in very early childhood (Dunn et al., 2019). Epigenetic alterations in gene function are meant to serve an adaptive purpose—helping the person to respond to environmental circumstances and adversities. Interestingly, after 1 year in space, astronaut Scott Kelly had hundreds of epigenetic changes and even some different DNA patterns compared to his identical twin brother. Although many of the changes disappeared soon after his return to Earth, approximately 7 percent of the epigenetic changes (e.g., those related to immunity, DNA repair, and bone formation) remained (Carr, 2018).

There is mounting evidence that epigenetic changes, particularly those that occur early in life, may result in lifelong alterations in gene expression. Additionally, researchers have found that some epigenetic modifications in gene expression can be passed down from parent to child (via epigenetic markers in the egg or sperm), perhaps as a means of assisting our offspring to adapt to the same environmental variables that triggered the epigenetic alterations (Xavier et al., 2019). As with genetic mutations, not all epigenetic changes are positive. However, unlike genetic mutations, future changes in environmental influences (such as improved nutrition) can eliminate epigenetic markers and thus reverse the epigenetic processes that originally altered gene expression (Kane & Sinclair, 2019).

Biology-Based Treatment Techniques

Treatments based on biological principles aim to improve an individual's social and emotional functioning by producing changes in physiological functioning. Our increasing knowledge of human physiology and brain functioning has led to the development of a variety of biologically based therapies for mental disorders.

Psychopharmacology

Psychopharmacology is the study of how **psychotropic medications** affect psychiatric symptoms, including thoughts, emotions, and behavior. Ideally, psychotropic medications, widely used to treat a variety of mental health conditions, are prescribed only after careful diagnosis and analysis of symptoms. Many psychiatric medications correct physiological imbalances by normalizing biochemical processes (e.g., binding, reabsorption, or breakdown by enzymes) involving certain neurotransmitters, thereby increasing or decreasing the availability of the neurotransmitter. Some medications work by enhancing message transmission, while others block communication between neurons.

Classes of medication used to treat mental disorders include (a) *antianxiety drugs* (or minor tranquilizers), (b) *antipsychotics* (or major tranquilizers), (c) *antidepressants* (used for both depression and anxiety), and (d) *mood stabilizers* (sometimes called antimanic drugs). These powerful medications require careful monitoring because they all have the potential for producing side effects.

Antianxiety medications (minor tranquilizers) such as benzodiazepines (including Valium and Xanax) are used to calm people and to help them sleep. Benzodiazepines increase the activity of GABA, an inhibitory neurotransmitter, thereby reducing the transmission of nerve impulses, with a resultant reduction in symptoms of anxiety. Benzodiazepines are usually prescribed in low doses and on a short-term basis due to their addictive potential.

Antipsychotic medications (also referred to as *neuroleptics* or major tranquilizers) play a major role in treating the agitation, mental confusion, and loss of contact with reality associated with **psychotic symptoms**. In 1951, the first drug with antipsychotic properties (chlorpromazine; brand name Thorazine) was synthesized in France. Thorazine had the unexpected effect of significantly reducing agitation and mental confusion in severely ill psychiatric patients. Thorazine and the many other antipsychotic medications developed using Thorazine as a prototype (a group referred to as *typical antipsychotics*) exert their effect by binding tightly to and blocking dopamine receptors, thereby stopping nerve activity that relies on dopamine.

Unfortunately, the sizeable reduction in dopamine associated with these first-generation antipsychotics also produces a constellation of side effects, referred to as **extrapyramidal symptoms**—including involuntary muscle contractions that affect gait, movement, and posture. A newer generation of antipsychotics, referred to as *atypical antipsychotics*, has emerged; these medications produce biochemical changes with fewer extrapyramidal symptoms. Some atypical antipsychotics reduce dopamine transmission by loosely binding to dopamine receptors (creating a less drastic reduction in dopamine), whereas others influence other neurotransmitters.

Antidepressant medications are prescribed to help relieve symptoms of depression and anxiety. There are several well-known classes of antidepressants. Among the most popular medications for both depression and anxiety are the *selective serotonin reuptake inhibitors (SSRIs)*, which work by blocking the reabsorption of serotonin, allowing it to remain in the synapse and thus enhance neural-communication potential. The drugs Prozac (fluoxetine hydrochloride), Paxil (paroxetine), and Zoloft (sertraline) are SSRIs. Another class of antidepressants, the *tricyclic antidepressants*, increase the availability of both serotonin and norepinephrine. *Monoamine oxidase inhibitors (MAOIs)* are antidepressants that inhibit the action of monoamine oxidase, an enzyme that deactivates neurotransmitters after they are released into the synapse. There are other antidepressant medications with distinct biochemical properties, such as Wellbutrin (bupropion). The primary difference between SSRIs and other antidepressants is that SSRIs specifically target the neurotransmitter serotonin, whereas others target multiple neurotransmitters.

Mood-stabilizing medications are prescribed to treat the excitement associated with episodes of mania, as well as to help prevent future mood swings. Lithium, a naturally occurring chemical compound, is a well-known and frequently prescribed mood stabilizer. A variety of anticonvulsant (used to treat seizure disorders) and antipsychotic medications are also used for mood stabilization.

The use of psychotropic medication has improved the lives of many people with mental illness, especially those with severe symptoms. Many individuals using these medications report symptom improvement and are better able to participate in other forms of treatment, such as psychotherapy. In most cases, severe mental illness no longer requires long periods of hospitalization. Remember, however, that although symptoms improve, medications do not cure mental disorders; they just help alleviate symptoms.

Additionally, some people need to try many different medications before finding one that helps their symptoms. Further, some individuals are not helped by medication or are not able to tolerate the medication side effects.

Researchers hope to develop simple blood tests that will identify which medications work best for each person. A new field, *pharmacogenomics*, focuses on understanding the relationship between a person's genetic makeup and both positive and aversive responses to drug treatment (Cacabelos, 2020). Some prescribers now routinely order genetic testing to gain knowledge about how their patient's genetic makeup might interact with a particular medication. Also, given the communication occurring between the ENS and the brain, interventions aimed at modifying bacteria in the digestive tract, including the promotion of beneficial bacteria (probiotics), are now being used for some psychological disorders (Park et al., 2018).

Electroconvulsive Therapy

Electroconvulsive therapy (ECT) is a procedure that can change brain chemistry and reverse symptoms associated with some mental disorders. ECT, which is usually reserved for those who have not responded to other treatments, involves applying moderate electric voltage to the brain to induce a short convulsion (seizure). The person undergoing treatment receives a general anesthetic and muscle relaxant before the procedure. A related treatment currently being researched is magnetic seizure therapy, which involves the induction of seizures using magnetic stimulation instead of a direct electrical current (Fitzgerald et al., 2018).

Neurosurgical and Brain Stimulation Treatments

During the 1940s and 1950s, *psychosurgery*—performing brain surgery in an attempt to correct a severe mental disorder—became increasingly popular. The treatment, which involves destruction or removal of a small area of the brain, raised many scientific and ethical objections. As a result, psychosurgery is now very uncommon and has been replaced by neurosurgical techniques that focus on stimulation rather than destruction of brain tissue. These brain stimulation procedures, which aim to reduce symptoms by changing physiological processes within the brain, are used only with certain conditions, such as severe depression, and only when other treatments have not been effective.

A contemporary neurosurgical treatment, *deep brain stimulation (DBS)*, involves implanting electrodes that produce ongoing stimulation of specific areas of the brain. The brain region targeted for stimulation varies depending upon the specific disorder being treated. For many disorders, research continues regarding the optimal site for stimulation (Senova, Clair, et al., 2019). Another approach, *vagus nerve stimulation*, involves surgically implanting a pacemaker-like device under the skin on the chest; when activated, the device sends signals along a wire connected to the **vagus nerve** (the longest and most complex of the cranial nerves), which then sends signals to various regions of the brain.

An increasingly popular, noninvasive brain stimulation procedure—*repetitive transcranial magnetic stimulation (rTMS)*—involves

Repetitive Transcranial Magnetic Stimulation

Repetitive transcranial magnetic stimulation is used to treat a variety of disorders, including depression. This man has been undergoing the treatment for almost 2 years. He says he "walks in feeling one way and walks out feeling another."

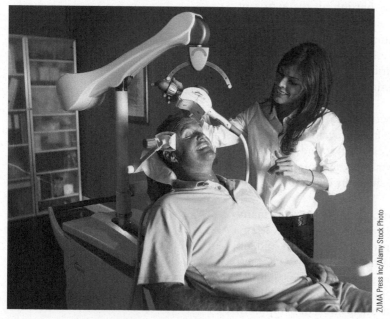

ZUMA Press Inc/Alamy Stock Photo

stimulation of the prefrontal cortex and regions of the brain involved with mood regulation; this is done by means of magnetic pulses emitted from an electromagnetic coil held against the forehead. Each rTMS treatment takes less than an hour and requires no sedation or anesthesia. Although some promising findings have been reported for treatment-resistant psychiatric disorders, the studies have involved small numbers of patients, conflicting results, and low-quality research (Guo et al., 2017).

Criticisms of Biological Models and Therapies

Biological models are criticized for their failure to consider an individual's unique life circumstances or psychological, social, or cultural influences on a person's symptoms. Although biological models have traditionally focused only on biological explanations, this has changed in recent years. For instance, most researchers now reject the simple linear explanation of genetic determinism; they no longer claim that mental disorders result primarily from "bad genes" or that there is "one gene for one disease" (Palk et al., 2019).

The majority of biological research comes from physicians and researchers whose worldview strongly supports the medical model and the use of medication to treat mental disorders. This is a particular concern given the rapid growth in the sale and marketing of psychotropic medications and the frequent use of these medications without first conducting a careful mental health evaluation (Alduhishy, 2018). There is also little discussion of where psychotherapy fits into treatment planning and at what point medication should be considered in the course of comprehensive treatment. All too often, medication is prescribed even when there are other effective treatment options available. In comparison to placebos, antidepressants and antipsychotic medications often offer only minimal or no greater effectiveness in treating disorders (Rief et al., 2016). Prescribing multiple medications has also become common, increasing the importance of watching for side effects and possible **drug–drug interactions**. Another concern is the limited focus on ethnic or gender group differences in physiological response to medication.

There is clearly a need for more discussion about how mental health professionals, health care providers, and clients can effectively collaborate in monitoring the effectiveness of medications and other biological interventions; however, it is equally important, particularly when making treatment decisions, that all involved consider psychological, social, and sociocultural factors that may be causing and maintaining symptoms.

2-4 Dimension Two: Psychological Factors

A number of psychological influences contribute to the etiology of mental disorders. The psychological dimension focuses on emotions, learned behavior, and cognitions. Interestingly, psychological explanations of mental illness vary considerably depending on the underlying theory. In this section, we describe four major psychological perspectives: psychodynamic, behavioral, cognitive, and humanistic-existential.

Sigmund Freud (1856–1939)

Freud began his career as a neurologist. He became increasingly intrigued with the relationship between illness and mental processes and ultimately developed psychoanalysis, a therapy in which unconscious conflicts are brought to the surface so they can be resolved.

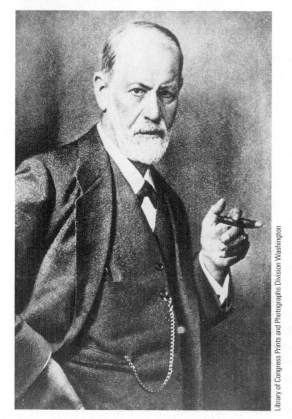

Library of Congress Prints and Photographs Division Washington

Psychodynamic Models

Psychodynamic models view mental disorders as the result of childhood experiences and unconscious conflicts. The early development of psychodynamic theory is credited to Sigmund Freud (1938, 1949). Freud originally characterized much of human behavior as attempts to express, gratify, or defend against sexual or aggressive impulses—instinctual drives that operate at an unconscious level, continually seeking expression. Psychological symptoms are associated with these sexual or aggressive impulses. Further, certain experiences or mental conflicts are too threatening to face, so we block them from consciousness. As a result, we sometimes experience emotional symptoms but do not understand their meaning. Freud believed that the therapist's role was to help individuals experiencing mental distress to achieve insight into these unconscious processes.

Personality Components

Freud developed a model suggesting that all behavior is a product of interactions between three personality components: the id, the ego, and the superego. The *id*, a key part of our unconscious psyche, is present at birth. The id operates from the **pleasure principle**—the impulsive, pleasure-seeking aspect of our being—and seeks immediate gratification of instinctual needs, regardless of moral or realistic concerns. In contrast, the *ego* represents the realistic and rational part of the mind. It is influenced by the **reality principle**—an awareness of the demands of the environment and of the need to adjust behavior to meet these demands. The ego's decisions are dictated by realistic considerations rather than by moral judgments. Moralistic considerations are the domain of the *superego*. The *conscience* is the part of the superego that instills guilt in us and helps prevent us from engaging in immoral or unethical behavior.

Psychosexual Stages

Human personality develops through a sequence of five **psychosexual stages**, each of which brings a unique challenge. If unfavorable circumstances prevail, the personality may be drastically affected. Because Freud stressed the importance of early childhood experiences, he saw the human personality as largely determined in the first 5 years of life—during the *oral* (first year of life), *anal* (around the second year of life), and *phallic* (beginning around the third or fourth year of life) stages. The last two psychosexual stages are the *latency* (approximately 6 to 12 years of age) and *genital* (beginning in puberty) periods. The importance of each psychosexual phase for later development lies in whether fixation occurs during that phase. *Fixation* halts emotional development at a particular psychosexual stage. Someone who is fixated at a particular stage may experience emotional disturbance resulting from the distinct conflicts associated with that period of development.

Defense Mechanisms

According to psychodynamic theory, we often use **defense mechanisms** to distance ourselves from uncomfortable feelings associated with unpleasant thoughts or other internal conflicts. Defense mechanisms are ways of thinking or behaving that operate unconsciously and protect us from anxiety, often by distorting reality. We all experience the self-deception associated with defense mechanisms from time to time. Defense mechanisms are considered

Table 2.2 Examples of Defense Mechanisms

Mechanism	Definition	Example
Repression	Preventing forbidden or dangerous thoughts or desires from entering one's consciousness	A soldier who witnesses the death of a friend in combat blocks the event from conscious thought.
Reaction formation	Acting in a manner opposite to one's unconscious wishes or feelings	A woman who gives birth to an unwanted child showers the child with superficial attention.
Projection	Distancing oneself from unwanted desires or thoughts by attributing them to others	A worker covers feelings of inadequacy by claiming fellow workers are incompetent.
Rationalization	Explaining one's behavior by giving socially acceptable reasons unrelated to one's true motives	A person justifies stealing a shirt from a store by saying that the store's prices are too high.
Displacement	Directing an emotion, such as hostility or anxiety, toward a substitute target	A clerk who is belittled by her boss yells at her husband.
Undoing	Attempting to right a wrong or negate an unconscious thought, impulse, or act	After making an insensitive comment to his daughter, a father makes amends by buying her a gift.
Regression	Retreating to an earlier developmental level that demands less mature responses and aspirations	A traumatized adult spends hours laying in a fetal position.

maladaptive, however, when they are overused—that is, if they become our predominant means of coping with stress and interfere with our ability to handle life's demands. Table 2.2 lists some common defense mechanisms.

Contemporary Psychodynamic Theories

As psychodynamic theory continued to evolve, theorists such as Adler (1929/1964) and Erickson (1968), unhappy with the prominence given to instinctual drives, suggested that the ego had adaptive abilities, including the capacity to function independently from the id. Other psychoanalytic theorists (Bowlby, 1969; Mahler, 1968) proposed that having our social needs met—the need to be loved, accepted, and emotionally supported—is of primary importance in early development and identity formation. Thus, children who do not receive emotional support from caregivers may experience difficulty achieving a healthy self-identity. Mental distress and problem behaviors occur when people seek interpersonal experiences lacking in childhood.

Therapies Based on the Psychodynamic Model

We begin with a brief overview of some of the techniques used by Freud and his approach to therapy. However, very few contemporary psychodynamic therapists rely only on these traditional methods. Instead, they emphasize interpersonal relationships and the ego's ability to cope with life challenges.

Traditional Psychodynamic Therapy Many of you have probably heard of psychoanalysis, but what is it? Psychoanalytic therapy, or **psychoanalysis**, aims to overcome a client's defenses so that material blocked from consciousness can be uncovered, allowing the client to gain insight into inner thoughts and unresolved childhood conflicts. If you were to undergo psychoanalysis, your therapist might use some of these methods:

- In **free association**, you say whatever comes to your mind, regardless of how illogical or embarrassing it may seem. The idea is that if you spontaneously express your thoughts, you will reveal the contents of your unconscious, including unrecognized worries and conflicts.

- **Dream analysis** is a technique focused on interpreting the hidden meanings in dreams. Psychoanalysts believe that when people sleep, ego defenses and inhibitions weaken so that unacceptable impulses or repressed anxieties are more likely to surface. Your therapist would help you understand the underlying meaning of your dreams.

- Your therapist would look for and attempt to analyze evidence of **resistance**—your unconscious attempts to impede therapy and prevent exposure of conflicts you are repressing. Your therapist would remain alert to see if you missed appointments, or suddenly changed the subject, lost your train of thought, or became silent during therapy. If you appear to be demonstrating resistance, the next step would be to uncover and analyze any unconscious conflicts your resistance might be trying to conceal.

- Psychoanalysts believe that client reactions such as anger, love, or disappointment directed toward the therapist are signs of other relationship issues; they refer to this process as **transference**. If your therapist noticed you displaying frustration or anger during therapy, you would be encouraged to work through the true meanings of your reactions.

Because psychoanalysts believe that unconscious impulses and instinctual drives cause psychological symptoms, they focus almost exclusively on the internal world of clients and work to allow unconscious conflicts to surface. Psychoanalysts assume that healthy behavior patterns will develop once clients understand and resolve their unconscious issues.

Therapy Based on Later Psychodynamic Theories Contemporary psychodynamic therapists view experiences with early attachment figures as having powerful effects on current interpersonal difficulties. Therefore, therapy focuses on existing social and interpersonal relationships rather than on unconscious conflicts. Some psychodynamic therapists look for recurring themes in problematic relationships and use the client–therapist relationship to work through conflicts that develop (Barsness, 2020). One contemporary therapy, short-term psychodynamic psychotherapy, addresses past relationship issues and the role they play in current emotional and relationship experiences (Ho & Adcock, 2017). Another approach, interpersonal psychotherapy, identifies the link between childhood experiences and current problematic relational patterns. Therapists using interpersonal psychotherapy focus on improving interpersonal relationships, decreasing social distress, and helping clients learn ways of interacting that are more effective than maladaptive patterns acquired during childhood (Ravitz et al., 2019).

Criticisms of Psychodynamic Models and Therapies

Psychodynamic theory strongly influenced the emerging field of psychology but is now treated with more skepticism. First, Freud relied heavily on case studies and on his own self-analysis as a basis for his theory. Second, his patients represented a very narrow spectrum of society—relatively affluent Victorian-era Austrian women. Thus, traditional psychoanalysis fails to address external issues such as racial or gender inequality. A third criticism is that traditional psychoanalysis has minimal therapeutic value with people who are less talkative, less psychologically minded, or more severely disturbed.

Psychodynamic theories are difficult to investigate in a scientific manner because the processes and outcomes are dynamic rather than specific. Therefore, there are far fewer outcome studies evaluating psychodynamic therapies compared to the large number of studies conducted on other contemporary treatment techniques (although short-term psychodynamic and interpersonal psychotherapy are accruing a research base). Research is further complicated because there are many different approaches to psychodynamic therapy.

Behavioral Models

The **behavioral models** of psychopathology are concerned with the role of learning in the development of mental disorders and are based on experimental research. The differences among the models lie in their explanations of how learning occurs. The three learning paradigms are *classical conditioning*, *operant conditioning*, and *observational learning*.

The Classical Conditioning Paradigm

Early in the 20th century, Ivan Pavlov (1849–1936), a Russian physiologist, discovered that automatic responses (such as salivation) can be learned through association. Pavlov was measuring dogs' salivation as part of a study of their digestive processes when he noticed that the dogs began to salivate at the sight of an assistant carrying their food. This response led to his formulation of the theory of **classical conditioning**, sometimes referred to as *respondent conditioning*. Pavlov reasoned that food is an **unconditioned stimulus (UCS)** that automatically elicits salivation; this salivation is an unlearned or **unconditioned response (UCR)** to the food.

Pavlov then presented a previously *neutral* stimulus (the sound of a bell) to the dogs just before feeding them. Initially, no salivation occurred with just the bell alone. However, after several repetitions of the bell combined with food powder in the mouth, the dogs began to salivate when hearing the bell. The bell had become a **conditioned stimulus (CS)**; that is, the sound induced salivation due to its previous pairings with the food (UCS). The salivation elicited by the bell is a **conditioned response (CR)**—a learned response to a previously neutral stimulus. Each time a CS (the bell) is paired with a UCS (food powder), the CR (salivation) is reinforced, or strengthened. Pavlov also discovered that if he kept presenting the bell (CS) without following it with the food powder (UCS), **extinction** would occur; eventually, the bell no longer produced salivation. Figure 2.7 presents Pavlov's conditioning process.

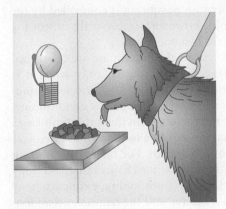
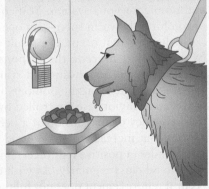
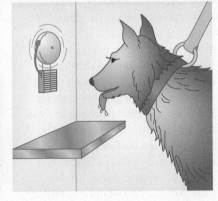

Stimulus:	UCS (food)	UCS & CS (food and bell)	CS (bell alone)
Response:	UCR (salivation)	UCR (salivation)	CR (conditioned salivation)

Figure 2.7

A Basic Classical Conditioning Process

Dogs normally salivate when food is provided (left). With his laboratory dogs, Ivan Pavlov paired the ringing of a bell with the presentation of food (middle). Eventually, the dogs would salivate to the ringing of the bell alone, when no food was near (right).

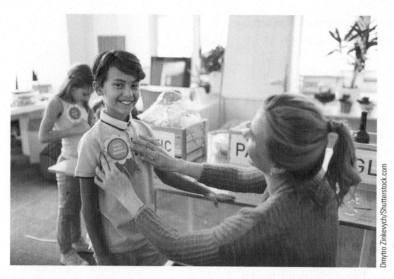

Operant Conditioning in the Classroom

In operant conditioning, positive consequences increase the likelihood and frequency of a desired response. Young children often learn that appropriate behavior will be rewarded and that inappropriate behavior will be punished. Here a student proudly receives a reward from his teacher.

Did You Know?

A 54-year-old woman in a mental institution carried a broom with her everywhere. What accounted for this behavior? Behavioral psychologists had shaped her actions using operant conditioning. They gave her a reward first when she approached the broom, then when she touched or picked up the broom, and finally when she carried the broom. Later, the researchers asked two psychodynamic psychiatrists to explain the woman's behavior; the psychiatrists hypothesized that the broom represented a "loving child," a "phallic symbol," or a "magical scepter." Does our theoretical orientation influence how we view behaviors? Are there ethical issues with this study?

Source: Ayllon et al., 1965

John B. Watson (1878–1958) is credited with recognizing how classical conditioning can help explain emotional distress. In a classic experiment, Watson and Rosalie Rayner (1920) demonstrated how classical conditioning experiences can create *phobias* (an extreme fear of particular objects or situations). In an investigation that most people would now consider highly inappropriate, they performed experiments with an 8-month-old infant, Albert, in an attempt to determine if there might be "simple methods" by which emotional responses develop. Could little Albert learn to fear objects through classical conditioning? They presented Albert with a number of objects, including a white rat. None of the items produced a fear response. Then they again showed Albert the white rat, immediately followed by a loud bang from a hammer striking a steel bar. Albert was startled and began crying. After several pairings of the rat and the loud sound, Albert showed a fear response when presented with the rat alone. This finding has helped us understand the etiology of anxiety and fear responses. The passive nature of classical conditioning limits its usefulness, however, as an explanatory and treatment tool.

The Operant Conditioning Paradigm

Operant conditioning was first formulated by Edward Thorndike (1874–1949) and further elaborated by B. F. Skinner (1904–1990). Their operant models are based on observations that behaviors are sometimes influenced by events that follow them. Rather than the involuntary physiological reactions (e.g., sweating, salivating, and fear responses) involved in classical conditioning, **operant conditioning** involves voluntary behaviors. An **operant behavior** is a controllable behavior, such as walking or talking, that "operates" on an individual's environment. In an extremely warm room, for example, you would have difficulty consciously controlling your sweating (an involuntary response) because perspiring is controlled by the autonomic nervous system. You could, however, simply walk out of the uncomfortably warm room—an operant behavior.

Behaviors that occur as a result of *classical* conditioning are controlled by events that *precede* the response: Salivation occurs only when it is preceded by an unconditioned stimulus (food) or a conditioned stimulus (the thought of sizzling onions, for example). In *operant* conditioning, however, behaviors are controlled by **reinforcers**—anything that influences the frequency or magnitude of a behavior. **Positive reinforcement** involves actions that increase the likelihood of a behavior. For instance, receiving good grades (a positive reinforcer) might increase the chances that you study and attend class regularly. As with classical conditioning, extinction may occur if reinforcement does not follow a behavior: If the reinforcer is no longer present, the behavior will eventually diminish. For example, you might have noticed that class attendance decreases if an instructor does not consider class participation when assigning grades. Studies have demonstrated a relationship between environmental reinforcers and certain abnormal behaviors. Self-injurious behavior, such as head banging, is a dramatic form of psychopathology that occurs in some individuals. If caregivers give attention and show concern whenever self-injurious behavior occurs, they may unwittingly be providing positive reinforcement for these behaviors.

Although positive reinforcement can account for some undesirable behaviors, other variables also influence behavior. For instance, **negative reinforcement**—when behavior is reinforced because something aversive has been removed—can increase the likelihood of certain actions. For example, you may spend time reviewing your class notes because studying removes the anxiety associated with upcoming exams. Notice that the focus is on the *effect* of the reinforcer. Negative reinforcement can also strengthen and maintain maladaptive behaviors. Imagine you are in a class in which the instructor requires oral reports. The thought of doing an oral presentation in front of the class terrifies you. If you decide to transfer to another class where the instructor does not require oral presentations, you will escape the aversive feelings. Thus, you would negatively reinforce your avoidance behavior; this could lead to similar escape tactics the next time you face an anxiety-provoking situation.

The Observational Learning Paradigm

The traditional behavioral theories of learning—classical conditioning and operant conditioning—require that the individual be directly involved in the learning process. In contrast, **observational learning theory** suggests that we can acquire new behaviors and emotional reactions simply by watching other people perform or experience them (Bandura, 1997). The process of learning by observing models (and later imitating them) is called *vicarious conditioning* or **modeling**. Reinforcement for imitation of the model is not necessary for learning to occur. Watching someone respond fearfully to a stimulus can cause a fear reaction to develop. For example, Bandura and Rosenthal (1966) found that individuals who watched someone receive a shock when a buzzer sounded also began to react to the buzzer.

Voluntary behaviors are also learned through observation (Bandura, 1997). In a series of experiments, children exposed to models displaying "unique" behaviors later demonstrated the very same behaviors themselves. Thus, observation of another individual can result in new behavior, including socially undesirable behaviors. Similarly, we sometimes inhibit a behavior if we see others punished for the behavior; for example, you may have reduced your driving speed after seeing someone receive a traffic ticket.

Social learning theory greatly expanded our understanding of the ways in which behaviors are learned. Bandura (1982) further developed his social learning theory to encompass *self-efficacy*, individuals' belief in their ability to make changes in their environment. His work introduced the idea that humans are not merely the "subjects" of conditioning—we are quite capable of mastering situations and producing positive outcomes. Bandura's research also reinforced the idea that we learn to persevere when we observe others succeeding through sustained effort.

In explaining psychopathology, social learning theory posits that exposure to disturbed models is likely to produce disturbed behaviors. For instance, when children watch their parents respond with fear, they may learn to respond in a similar manner. Similarly, if we are exposed to models who display impulsivity, helplessness, or aggression, we are more likely to acquire these characteristics.

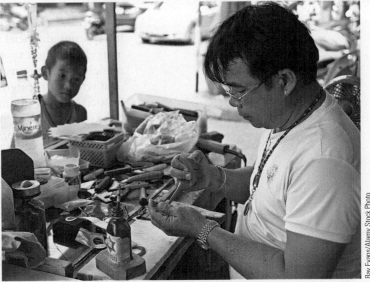

Ray Evans/Alamy Stock Photo

Learning by Observing

Observational learning is based on the theory that behavior can be learned by observing it. Although much has been made of the relationship between violence and aggression viewed on television and in movies and violent behavior in real life, observational learning can have positive benefits as well.

Behavioral Therapies

Classical conditioning and the concept of extinction are the basis for therapies that involve having clients directly face their fears. **Exposure therapy**, also known as *extinction therapy*, can involve *graduated exposure*, which involves gradually introducing a person to feared objects or situations, or *flooding*, which involves rapid exposure to produce high levels of anxiety. For example, if you had a spider phobia, the therapist might ask you to imagine seeing a spider 10 feet away (a first step in graduated exposure) or might hand you a jar containing a live spider (flooding). Therapists often prefer to use the graduated approach because flooding creates extreme discomfort. Similarly, extinction therapy can also involve virtual reality procedures using computer-generated images that immerse clients in a realistic setting. For example, a therapist might treat your spider phobia by having you use a virtual reality helmet to view spiders in a variety of situations.

Another effective behavioral technique, **systematic desensitization**, developed by Joseph Wolpe (1958), involves having the extinction process occur while the client is in a competing physiological state, such as relaxation. If you were undergoing systematic desensitization to decrease your fear of public speaking, you would first learn to relax, and then imagine yourself engaged in a hierarchy of behaviors related to giving a speech (perhaps beginning with imagining yourself practicing the talk at home and ending with giving the speech to a large audience). Combining exposure with relaxation appears to be an efficient method of facilitating extinction of fear responses (Keller et al., 2020).

Social skills training, which involves the teaching of specific skills needed for appropriate social interactions, is an effective behavioral intervention for individuals who experience social difficulties. Social skills training includes modeling and the use of role-play activities to practice behaviors associated with appropriate social interactions. *Assertiveness training* is a form of social skills training that teaches individuals (especially those who tend to be overly timid or overly aggressive) the difference between nonassertive, aggressive, and assertive responses. This training offers participants an opportunity to consider challenging, real-life situations and then practice how they might confidently convey their message, with attention to clear verbal communication and confident body posture, voice intonation, and facial expression. Culturally appropriate assertiveness programs have been developed to take into account the social norms of specific cultural groups (Omura et al., 2019).

Criticisms of the Behavioral Models and Therapies

Although behavioral approaches to psychopathology have provided considerable insight into the etiology and treatment of mental disorders, critics point out that behaviorism neglects—or places minimal emphasis on—factors such as inner determinants of behavior or the sociocultural context in which the behavior occurs. They also criticize behaviorists' use of results obtained from animal studies to solve human problems. Some also charge that the behaviorist perspective is mechanistic, viewing people as "empty organisms." These theories, like many others, also tend to view behavioral symptoms in a linear and one-dimensional fashion.

Cognitive-Behavioral Models

Cognitive theorists, such as Aaron Beck (1921–2021) and Albert Ellis (1913–2007), were among the first to break away from traditional behavioral approaches. They both theorized that the manner in which we interpret situations can profoundly affect our emotional reactions and behaviors. Further, their theories link psychopathology with irrational and maladaptive assumptions and thoughts. In other words, emotional responses such as anger, depression, fear, and anxiety result from our *thoughts* about events rather than from the events themselves.

The *A-B-C theory of emotional disturbance*, developed by Albert Ellis (1997, 2008), describes how we develop irrational thoughts. *A* is an event, a fact, or someone's behavior or attitude. *C* is our emotional or behavioral reaction. The activating event *A* never causes the emotional or behavioral consequence *C*. Instead, *B*, our beliefs about *A*, causes *C*. Let's imagine you were interviewed for a job you really wanted, and then you learned someone else was hired for the job (activating event *A*). If your reaction was "How awful to be rejected! I'll never get a good job" (irrational belief *B*), and you continued thinking this way, you might become depressed and withdrawn (emotional and behavioral consequence *C*). Imagine instead that when you learned you didn't get the job (activating event *A*), you responded by thinking, "I really wanted that job, so it's hard being rejected. Maybe next time I'll be considered the best match for the job" (rational belief *B*), and you continued looking for another job (healthy consequence *C*).

Thus, if you interpret the rejection as "awful and catastrophic," you are more likely to become distressed and postpone your job search efforts. If, on the other hand, you don't take the rejection personally and you recognize that many people experience rejection during a job search, your motivation and self-esteem will remain intact and you will continue seeking employment, thereby increasing your chances of finding a job. Figure 2.8 presents the A-B-C relationship and explains how a cognitive therapist might work with a client who is depressed over the loss of a job.

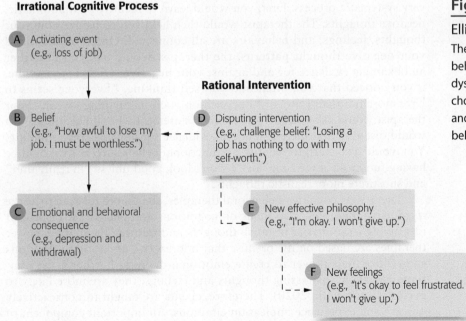

Irrational Cognitive Process

A Activating event (e.g., loss of job)

B Belief (e.g., "How awful to lose my job. I must be worthless.")

C Emotional and behavioral consequence (e.g., depression and withdrawal)

Rational Intervention

D Disputing intervention (e.g., challenge belief: "Losing a job has nothing to do with my self-worth.")

E New effective philosophy (e.g., "I'm okay. I won't give up.")

F New feelings (e.g., "It's okay to feel frustrated. I won't give up.")

Figure 2.8

Ellis's A-B-C Theory of Personality
The development of emotional and behavioral problems is often linked to dysfunctional thinking. Cognitive psychologists assist their clients to identify and modify irrational thoughts and beliefs.

Cognitive-Behavioral Approaches to Therapy

Cognitive-behavioral therapy (CBT) is rapidly becoming the treatment of choice for many disorders. Cognitive approaches to psychotherapy help clients recognize patterns of illogical thinking and replace them with more realistic and helpful thoughts (Chand et al., 2020). Although these therapies emphasize cognitions (patterns of thinking), they are called cognitive-behavioral therapies because they also incorporate changes in social skills and other behaviors. Cognitive-behavioral therapists encourage clients to become actively involved in their treatment outside of therapy sessions by assigning homework that includes practicing skills learned during therapy.

Albert Ellis and Aaron Beck developed distinct varieties of therapy based on their views regarding the connection between thought processes and emotional reactions and behaviors. Rational emotive behavior therapy (REBT) has a strong focus on challenging illogical thinking (Ellis, 1997). Ellis believed that mental distress occurs when someone takes a reasonable desire such as "I'd like to perform well and be approved by others" and changes it into an illogical expectation such as "I *must* perform well and be approved" (Ellis referred to this pattern of problematic thinking as "musturbation"). Ellis often confronted clients about their irrational thinking patterns and encouraged them to change "*musts*," or irrational demands, into more rational "preferences."

Beck's approach to cognitive therapy, which has strong research support for treating depression and other conditions, focuses on mental **schema**—the framework from which we automatically organize and give meaning to information. We develop cognitive schemas so we can process information more efficiently. In effect, a schema is the lens through which we view the world and ourselves. Because dysfunctional schemas such as "I'm stupid," "I'm helpless," or "people are dangerous" result in emotional distress, Beck's therapy helps clients recognize their dysfunctional attitudes and belief systems. Clients eventually learn to replace automatic negative thinking with more adaptive thoughts.

If you worked with a cognitive therapist, you would go through a very systematic process. First, you would learn to identify your automatic, negative thoughts. The therapist would then help you recognize how your thoughts, feelings, and behaviors are all connected. Once you identified your negative thought patterns, the therapist would ask you to gather and examine evidence for and against your negative views. For example, if you noticed that you often find yourself thinking, "Everyone seems to have more fun than I do" or "I never look good in anything I wear," your therapist would ask you to "prove" your statements. In all likelihood, you would discover that there is minimal evidence for your negative thinking. You would also learn to identify dysfunctional beliefs such as "I should be having fun most of the time" or "I won't look good unless I'm really thin" and substitute more realistic thoughts.

The newest cognitive-behavioral therapies, sometimes referred to as the *third wave therapies*, also focus on cognitions and behaviors. Instead of identifying irrational or negative thoughts and refuting them, these newer therapies are based on the premise that nonreactive attention to emotions can reduce their power to create emotional distress. Further, if we continuously avoid distressing thoughts and feelings, they are more likely to persist (Garey et al., 2020). Therefore, clients are taught to nonreactively observe and experience unpleasant emotions. An important component of third wave therapies is **mindfulness**, maintaining conscious attention to the present, including negative emotions or thoughts, with an open, accepting, and nonjudgmental attitude. Mindfulness allows us to experience stressful emotional states without undue distress or physiological arousal. *Mindfulness-based stress reduction* is an 8-week evidence-based program that teaches mindfulness meditation as a means of coping with stress and reducing emotional reactivity (Janssen et al., 2018).

Dialectical behavior therapy (DBT) is a supportive and collaborative therapy involving cognitive-behavioral techniques and therapist–client teamwork. This therapy, developed by psychologist Marsha Linehan, uses an empathetic and validating environment to help clients learn to mindfully experience and regulate their emotions, cope with stress, and improve interpersonal skills and social relationships (Linehan, 2020). Therapists actively reinforce positive actions while avoiding the reinforcement of maladaptive behaviors, including behaviors that interfere with therapy. Components of Eastern spiritual philosophy (Zen) are also part of the therapy—specifically, mindfulness and the acceptance of things that cannot be changed. DBT differs from traditional cognitive therapies due to the emphasis on the therapist–client relationship and the priority given to accepting and validating the client.

DBT is very structured and relies on four interrelated modules:

- *Mindfulness*—Learning to tolerate and accept your emotions by observing them objectively and nonjudgmentally
- *Distress tolerance*—Viewing yourself and your circumstances in an objective and dispassionate manner so that you can take productive actions rather than responding emotionally
- *Emotional regulation*—Identifying and labeling your emotions rather than being emotionally reactive; learning to change your negative thoughts and increase your positive emotions
- *Interpersonal effectiveness*—Improving your skills in dealing with difficult interpersonal situations such as learning to make requests assertively and to say "no" when appropriate

Using a similar approach, *acceptance and commitment therapy (ACT)* encourages noticing, accepting, and even embracing unpleasant feelings and emotions rather than avoiding them. Therapists who use ACT also help their clients develop **psychological flexibility**, the ability to adapt to situational demands. They also help clients make a commitment to take action toward achieving valued goals. Studies have found that ACT is effective for psychological disorders and for physical symptoms such as chronic pain (Kuba & Weißflog, 2017).

Criticisms of the Cognitive-Behavioral Models and Therapies

Some behaviorists remain quite skeptical of the **cognitive models** and therapies. Just before his death, B. F. Skinner (1990) warned that cognitions are not observable phenomena and cannot form the foundations of empiricism. In this context, he echoed the beliefs of John B. Watson, who stated that the science of psychology was about observable behaviors, not "mentalistic concepts." Cognitive-behavioral theories are also criticized for failing to acknowledge that human behavior involves more than thoughts and beliefs. Others question the role of the therapist as teacher, expert, and authority figure and the cross-cultural applicability of cognitive behavioral approaches. In response, culturally adapted CBT has been developed for diverse populations (Pan et al., 2020).

The Universal Shamanic Tradition

Since the beginning of human existence, all societies and cultural groups have developed their own explanations of symptoms associated with mental distress and their own culture-specific ways of dealing with human suffering (Redvers & Blondin, 2020). In recent decades there has been a revival of interest in non-Western Indigenous explanations of physical and mental disorders and their treatments. Much of this is due to our changing demographics, including an influx of immigrants who hold non-Western beliefs regarding illness, wellness, and healing.

Western science focuses on what we can observe and measure through the five senses. However, many indigenous people believe that the nature of reality transcends the senses. The **universal shamanic tradition** incorporates a belief in special healers who are blessed with powers to gain insight from nature and call forth healing energies. Shamans treat mental and physical disorders using rituals, prayers, and sacred symbols that summon spiritual forces. They are admired for their ability to enter altered states of consciousness, journey to an existence beyond the physical world, and contact and communicate with a deeper consciousness.

Universal shamanic traditions view illness, distress, and problematic behaviors as the result of an imbalance in human relationships; a disharmony between the person and the group; or a lack of synchrony among mind, body, spirit, and nature. Many cultures believe that accessing higher states of consciousness can enhance perceptual sensitivity, clarity, concentration, and emotional well-being. Interestingly, meditation and yoga are the most widely practiced forms of therapy in the world today. These ancient practices can help with anxiety, phobias, substance abuse, chronic pain, and high blood pressure, as well as enhance self-confidence (Sue et al., 2022).

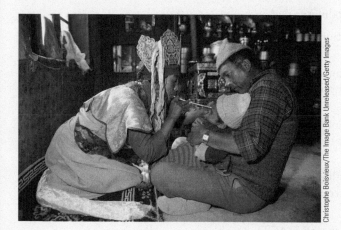

Christophe Boisvieux/The Image Bank Unreleased/Getty Images

For Further Consideration

1. Can you identify commonalities between what therapists and shamans do?

2. What can we learn from indigenous beliefs and forms of healing?

3. Are there dangers or downsides to shamanism as a belief system or form of treatment?

Humanistic-Existential Models

The humanistic-existential models include a group of theories that emphasize the whole person rather than looking at parts of the personality such as the id, ego, and superego (psychoanalysis) or specific behavior patterns (behavioral theories). In fact, the humanistic-existential approaches evolved in reaction to the failure of these early models of psychopathology to acknowledge the role of free will. Although each of the humanistic theories has a different emphasis, they all have a belief in the innate goodness of humanity, in our uniqueness and individuality, and in our capacity to choose our life direction. Humanistic approaches are philosophical in nature. They deal with values, decry the use of diagnostic labels, and prefer a holistic view of the person.

The humanistic-existential perspectives represent many schools of thought, but they share a set of assumptions that distinguishes them from other approaches. The first is that what we see as "reality" is a product of our unique experiences and perceptions of the world. Our subjective universe—how we construe events—is more important than the events themselves. Therefore, to understand a person's behavior, it is important to understand the person's perspective on the world. Second, humanistic theorists assume that we have the ability to make free choices and are responsible for our own decisions. Third, they believe in the wholeness or integrity of the person and assume that we will lead lives that are best suited to who we are.

The Humanistic Perspective

The best known of the humanistic psychologists is Carl Rogers (1902–1987). His theory of personality (Rogers, 1959, 1961) reflects his concern with human welfare and his deep conviction that humans are basically good, forward moving, and trustworthy. This **humanistic perspective** is based on the idea that people are motivated not only to satisfy their biological needs (e.g., for food, warmth, and sex) but also to cultivate, maintain, and enhance the self. Related to this view is Abraham Maslow's concept of **self-actualization**—our inherent tendency to strive toward the realization of our full potential.

Humanistic Views on the Development of Psychopathology Humanistic approaches were not developed to explain psychopathology. Instead of concentrating on problems, the humanistic approach focuses on bettering the state of humanity and helping people *actualize* their potential. Rogers believed that when allowed to grow and develop freely, unencumbered by societal restrictions, people will thrive. Anxiety, depression, and other problems occur when society blocks this innate tendency for growth by imposing conditions on whether we have personal value and we begin to believe we have worth only when we have the approval of others. This belief can prevent us from developing optimally and can result in mental distress. According to Rogers, when circumstances allow us to reach our full potential, we avoid mental illness.

The Existential Perspective

The **existential approach** is not a systematized school of thought but a set of attitudes. It shares with humanistic psychology an emphasis on our individual uniqueness, our quest for freedom and for meaning in life, and a belief that we all have positive attributes that we express unless environmental factors interfere. In contrast to humanists, existentialists focus on the irrationality, difficulties, and suffering all humans encounter in life and believe we must be viewed within the context of the human condition. As members of the human race, we have responsibility not only to ourselves but also to others. Existentialists maintain that human unhappiness and psychopathology stem from the avoidance of important life challenges, resulting in a life that is directionless and without meaning. Thus, we are responsible for our own unhappiness if we ignore choices available to us or "unconsciously" choose an unfulfilling path.

Humanistic and Existential Therapies

Within the humanistic tradition, the relationship between the client and therapist (the therapeutic alliance) is viewed as the key to successful psychotherapy. For therapists, this means fostering conditions that allow clients to grow and fulfill their potential, an approach known as *person-centered therapy*. Rogers emphasized that therapists' attitudes and ability to communicate respect, understanding, and acceptance are more important than specific counseling techniques. He believed that an accepting therapeutic environment encourages clients to reactivate their potential for self-actualization. With unconditional positive regard, clients can make constructive changes and learn to accept themselves, including

Did You Know?

Humanistic psychologists believe that promoting a person's inner resources results in self-actualization. This approach—focusing on a person's assets and strengths rather than weaknesses and deficits—was a forerunner to contemporary positive psychology.

any imperfections. This self-growth allows clients to cope with present and future problems. The person-centered therapeutic focus on developing a strong therapist–client relationship is increasingly incorporated into contemporary psychological therapies (Rockwell, 2019).

Existential therapy is rooted in an understanding of the universal challenges of existence faced by all humans. As with other humanistic therapies, the therapist–client relationship is important. It is through this relationship that a client can acknowledge or deal with universal challenges. Existential therapists work to have their clients consider ways in which their freedom is impaired so they can remove obstacles to autonomy and increase their opportunities for choice. They also look for underlying meaning in what clients say, and challenge clients to examine their lives. When clients become aware of choices they have made, they are more able to select a new direction. The goal is to help people become intentional in directing their lives. Consistent with humanistic traditions, therapists who have studied transpersonal psychology (based on the works of Carl Jung, William James, and Abraham Maslow) focus on deeper aspects of the human experience and healing the whole person; thus, they emphasize spiritual, physical, and creative well-being as well as emotional growth.

Criticisms of the Humanistic and Existential Models and Therapies

Critics of the humanistic-existential approaches point to their imprecise nature, lack of scientific grounding, and reliance on people's unique, subjective experiences. Others question the power of the self-actualizing tendency and whether the therapist–client relationship in and of itself is sufficient to promote change. Although these approaches have been extremely creative in describing the human condition, they have been less successful in constructing treatment strategies. Moreover, they are not suited to scientific or experimental investigation. It is difficult, for example, to verify the humanistic concept of people as rational, inherently good, and moving toward self-fulfillment.

Another major criticism leveled at the humanistic-existential approaches is that they do not explain many mental disorders, nor do they address cultural diversity or acknowledge social factors such as poverty, discrimination, and prejudice. They seem to be most effective with well-educated individuals experiencing mild distress or adjustment difficulties. These limitations have hindered the application of these perspectives to the treatment of mental illness. Nevertheless, the humanistic and existential concepts of freedom, choice, and responsibility have had a profound influence on third wave therapies and on contemporary thought beyond the field of psychology.

2-5 Dimension Three: Social Factors

The theories of psychopathology discussed so far focus primarily on the individual rather than on the social environment. They are relatively silent when it comes to addressing important aspects of our lives such as how social interactions affect the expression of mental distress. It is clear that we are social beings and that our relationships can influence the development, manifestation, and amelioration of mental disorders.

Social-Relational Models

Social-relational models consider a variety of interpersonal relationships, including those involving intimate partners, nuclear or extended family, and connections within the community. Studies show that social isolation and lack of emotional support and intimacy are associated with a variety of symptoms of mental illness and difficulty coping with stress. Social-relational explanations of mental distress make several important assumptions (Johnson & Johnson, 2003; Santini et al., 2015):

1. Healthy relationships are important for optimal human development and functioning.

2. Social relationships provide many intangible benefits (emotional support, love, compassion, trust, sense of belonging, etc.).

3. When relationships prove dysfunctional or are absent, the individual may be vulnerable to mental distress.

Family, Couples, and Group Perspectives

In contrast to traditional psychological models, social-relational models emphasize how other people, especially significant others, influence our behavior and emotional well-being. For instance, the **family systems model** assumes that the behavior of one family member directly affects the entire family system. According to this model, our behavior can be shaped by both healthy and unhealthy family circumstances. There are three distinct beliefs underlying the family systems approach (Corey, 2017). First, our personality development is strongly influenced by our family's characteristics, especially the way our parents interacted with us and other family members. Second, mental illness in an individual often reflects unhealthy family dynamics, especially poor communication among family members. Thus, the cause of mental disorders resides within the family system, not within the individual. Third, therapy must focus on the family system, rather than the individual; treatment may be ineffective unless the entire family is involved.

Social-Relational Treatment Approaches

The family systems model has spawned a number of treatment approaches. One method, the *conjoint family therapeutic approach*, developed by Virginia Satir (1967), stresses the importance of clear and direct communication and teaches message-sending and message-receiving skills to family members. Like other family therapists, Satir believed that a family member experiencing mental distress or behavioral difficulties (referred to as the "identified patient") is a reflection of dysfunction in the family system. *Strategic family approaches* (Haley, 1963, 1987) consider power struggles within the family and attend to developing a healthier power distribution. *Structural family approaches* (Minuchin, 1974) attempt to reorganize family relationships based on the assumption that family dysfunction occurs when family members have too much or too little involvement with one another. All of these approaches emphasize communication, equalizing power within the family, and restructuring the troubled family system.

Another social-relational approach, **couples therapy**, targets marital relationships and intimate relationships between unmarried partners.

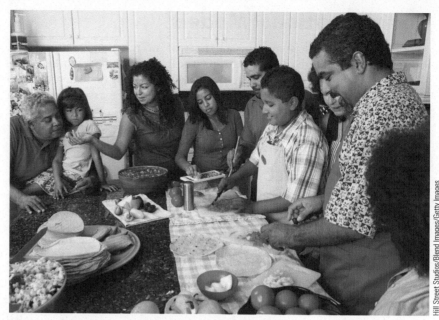

Family Dynamics and Positive Self-Image

Family interaction patterns can exert tremendous influence on a child's personality development, determining the child's sense of self-worth and the acquisition of appropriate social skills. This picture shows a Latinx family preparing dinner together. Notice how the family members are actively involved in working together and how the children are experiencing family cohesion and belonging.

Treatment helps couples to improve their communications and to understand and clarify role relationships, unfulfilled needs, and unrealistic or unmet expectations. Couples therapy has become an increasingly popular treatment for those who find that the quality of their relationship needs improvement (Gurman et al., 2015).

Another form of social-relational treatment is **group therapy**. Unlike couples and family therapy, participants in group therapy are often initially strangers. However, group members may share certain characteristics, such as experiencing a similar life stressor (e.g., chronic illness, domestic violence, divorce, or death of a family member) or having similar mental disorders or similar therapeutic goals. Most group therapies focus on a specific topic or on interactions among members. Despite their wide diversity, successful group therapies share several features that promote change in clients (Corey, 2017; Yalom, 2005). For example, the group experience:

- allows participants to become involved in a social situation and to see how their behavior affects others;
- permits the therapist to see how clients actually respond in a real-life social and interpersonal context;
- provides group members an opportunity to develop new communication skills, social skills, and insights;
- allows group members to feel less isolated and less fearful about their problems; and
- provides participants with strong social and emotional support.

The feelings of intimacy, belonging, protection, and trust (which participants may not be able to experience outside the group) can provide powerful motivation for group members to confront their emotions and to overcome personal difficulties.

Criticisms of Social-Relational Models

There is no denying that we are social beings, and that the social-relational models provide important insight into our understandings of psychopathology. However, social-relational research studies are generally not rigorous in design and have often lacked control groups, solid outcome measures, or adequate sample sizes (Jiménez et al., 2019). Critics have also voiced concern that family approaches to therapy can result in negative consequences. For example, family therapists who believe that behavioral problems in children result from maladaptive family communication patterns may not consider other possible influences and may unfairly blame parents for factors beyond the parents' control. For this reason, many contemporary family therapists prefer to use an educational model where family members are viewed as partners in developing more effective interaction skills (McFarlane, 2016). Further, traditional couples and family therapies often do not consider cultural diversity and may fail to recognize the hierarchical structure that guides interactions in familial and intimate relationships within many cultural groups—a significant difference from the relationship equality and freedom of expression that is accepted in most Western cultures.

2-6 Dimension Four: Sociocultural Factors

Sociocultural perspectives emphasize the importance of considering ethnicity, gender, sexual orientation, religious preference, socioeconomic influences, and other such factors in explaining mental disorders. The importance of the sociocultural dimension is evident in the *Diagnostic and Statistical Manual of Mental Disorders* (DSM), which lists disorders that are limited to a specific society or cultural group. For instance, *maladi moun* is the term that Haitians use to refer to certain mental and physical illnesses they believe are "sent" by an envious enemy who wishes to cause harm. Similarly, *khyal cap* is a condition that occurs among Cambodians, involving symptoms such as shortness of breath, asphyxia, dizziness, and tinnitus; this "wind attack" is believed to result from a windlike substance that arises in the body and blood. It is clear that people's cultural experiences play an important role in their beliefs about mental health. Further, the cultural groups to which we belong may expose us to unique stressors or may affect how we express mental distress. We briefly discuss four major sociocultural influences to explain their importance in understanding psychopathology: gender, socioeconomic class, acculturative stress, and race and ethnicity.

Gender Factors

The importance of gender in understanding psychopathology becomes evident when we consider research which consistently concludes that women have a higher prevalence of many mental health conditions. (It should be noted that most research continues to address gender from a binary perspective.) There are many influences in U.S. society that help explain this disparity in mental health between men and women. For example, girls and women are subjected to ongoing socialization processes regarding the importance of physical appearance and stereotyped standards of beauty. The related objectification and sexualization of women that is evident in advertising, social media, television, music, and movies can affect the mental health of girls and women. These sociocultural standards not only influence body dissatisfaction but can also lead to anxiety, depression, and eating disorders (APA, 2018).

Women are also subjected to more stress than their male counterparts. They are often placed in the unenviable position of needing to fulfill expectations associated with a variety of socially defined feminine social roles. Even when employed full-time outside of the home, women have more responsibility for domestic chores and child care (APA, 2018). During the COVID-19 pandemic, women around the world were more likely than men to give up their employment, be engaged in unpaid household duties, and assume responsibility for caring for children and other family members as well as providing home-schooling (Savage, 2020). A report by the United Nations raised concerns that the pandemic may have caused a setback in equality for women. In addition, the report indicated that gender-based violence increased during the pandemic, particularly among women who were isolated at home with their abusers (United Nations, 2020).

Throughout their life span, girls and women have an increased risk of physical and sexual victimization. Approximately 8 percent of girls experience childhood sexual abuse, which is associated with disorders such as posttraumatic stress disorder (PTSD), major depressive disorder, and other psychiatric diagnoses (Pérez-Fuentes et al., 2013). Additionally, exposure to sexual harassment often begins during the middle school years, with effects on both psychological well-being and learning (Eom et al., 2015). Sexual violence is also a particular concern for women. In one report that studied college women, 28 percent reported experiencing some form of sexual assault that ranged from unwanted sexual touching to rape (Mellins et al., 2017). Gender challenges are often accentuated for women of color. For instance, some African American women feel the need to adopt a "strong woman" role by projecting an image of strength and success while simultaneously helping others. Such a role can produce chronic "wear and tear" on their physiological and psychological systems (Allen et al., 2019). These are just a few of the many findings documenting stressors that have a major effect on the mental health of girls and women.

Socioeconomic Class

Social class and poverty are frequently overlooked sociocultural influences on mental health. Lower socioeconomic class is associated with a limited sense of personal control, poorer physical health, and higher incidence of depression. Increasingly, psychologists are recognizing the degree to which poverty exposes people to multiple stressors. Life in poverty is associated with low wages, unemployment or underemployment, housing insecurity, food insufficiency, limited access to health care, and lack of savings. Meeting even the most basic needs of food and shelter becomes a major challenge. In such circumstances, people are likely to experience feelings of hopelessness, helplessness, dependence, and inferiority (Sue et al., 2022).

Circumstances associated with the social, economic, and physical environment experienced by those living in poverty have a strong effect on both mental and physical health. For this reason, interventions are necessary not only at the individual level (e.g., nutrition, health care) but also at the community level (e.g., safer neighborhoods, access to healthy food and affordable housing) and nationwide level (e.g., reduction of poverty and discrimination, increased educational and employment opportunities). Multilevel interventions such as this are necessary to reduce the chronic environmental stressors that affect the well-being of individuals living in poverty (Wahlbeck et al., 2017).

Immigration and Acculturative Stress

Many immigrants face **acculturative stress**, the psychological, physical, and social pressures associated with a move to a new country. Not only do immigrants face the challenge of adjusting and adapting to new cultural customs, but they also sometimes receive a hostile reception from both the government and the public. Placed in unfamiliar settings and missing their accustomed social support from the communities they left behind, severe culture shock may occur. Feelings of isolation, loneliness, helplessness, anxiety, and depression are common. Many immigrants face additional challenges as they negotiate the educational system, learn a new language, and seek employment. Men who immigrate often experience a loss of status and develop a sense of powerlessness. Problems of gender inequity and spousal abuse can increase under these conditions (Sabri et al., 2018). Acculturation conflicts are common, especially among first-generation immigrants and their children. The children may experience difficulty fitting in with their peers, yet may be considered "too Americanized" by their parents. Racism and discrimination can compound these already stressful circumstances (Sue et al., 2022).

Immigrants without legal status are especially vulnerable to chronic stress. One group of undocumented students attending community college reported high levels of fear, anxiety, and depression over concerns about possible deportation for themselves, family members, or friends. They felt socially isolated and, although they were engulfed with fear, they did not feel it was safe to discuss their situation with their college teachers or classmates (Alif et al., 2020). Further, U.S. immigration policies that focused on separating immigrating children from their families at the U.S.–Mexico border were a source of "toxic stress" that seriously influenced the developing brains of children affected by these actions as well as youth within the United States who were aware of the separations. For those seeking asylum, being housed in prison-like detention centers with the threat or reality of family separation compounded the already frightening experience of fleeing violence in their countries of origin and intensified their fear—an emotion that reverberated throughout immigrant communities across the United States (Linton, 2019). The emotional shock of separation not only led directly to stress, anxiety, and depression among those involved but also may manifest at a later time in a variety of physical and emotional symptoms (Aleaziz, 2020).

Race and Ethnicity

Early attempts to explain differences between various underrepresented groups and their counterparts in the majority culture tended to adopt one of two models. The first, the **inferiority model**, was based on the overtly racist premise that underrepresented racial and ethnic groups are inferior to the majority population. For example, those with this perspective have suggested that the reduced academic achievement and higher unemployment among African Americans and Latinx Americans are due to biological differences such as low motivation or limited intelligence. The second model—the deprivation or **deficit model**—explained differences as the result of "cultural deprivation." This perspective was promoted by Euro-American men, a group attempting to maintain the power and authority they achieved during colonization. Those who subscribe to this perspective believe that underrepresented groups lack the "right" culture, and do not believe there is value in diversity of traditions or beliefs. A tragic example of this attitude is the long-standing U.S. policy that forced Native American children to be separated from their families and placed in Indian Residential Schools—with the goal of eliminating their native language and cultural traditions. Both models are criticized as being inaccurate, racially biased, and unsupported by scientific research.

During the late 1980s and early 1990s, a new and conceptually different perspective, the **multicultural model**, emerged in the literature. The multicultural approach emphasizes that being culturally different does not mean that someone is deviant, pathological, or inferior; instead, it is important to recognize that each culture has strengths and limitations. The multicultural model also points out that all theories of human development and psychopathology arise from a particular cultural context. Thus, many traditional models of psychopathology operate from a European American worldview that is not experienced or shared by other cultural groups. For instance, individualism and autonomy are valued in the United States; children are encouraged to become increasingly independent, to make their own decisions, and to "stand on their own two feet." In contrast, many cultural groups within the United States embrace collective, interdependent relationships; thus, the psychosocial unit of importance is the family or community rather than the individual. Whereas European Americans fear the loss of individuality, members of collectivist cultural groups fear the loss of belonging and group membership (Sue et al., 2022).

According to the multicultural model, all behavior should be considered from a cultural perspective. Cultural understanding is particularly crucial when assessing a person's mental health. Therapists who lack awareness of cultural variations in experiences or values may make inaccurate assumptions about clients who come from a different background. For instance, a mental health professional who does not understand that Asian Americans and Latinx Americans typically value a collectivistic identity might see clients with interdependent family relationships as overly dependent, immature, or unable to make decisions on their own. Further, behavior considered disordered in one context—seeing a vision of a dead relative, for example—might be considered acceptable within a cultural context in which **hallucinations** such as this are viewed as positive spiritual events, particularly during bereavement or religious ceremonies.

The multicultural model emphasizes that mental health difficulties are sometimes due to sociocultural stressors residing in the social system rather than conflicts within the person. Economic hardships, overt discrimination, and **implicit bias** associated with systemic racism are just a few of the realities faced by members of ethnic minorities and other marginalized groups. In some cases, **internalized racism** develops in which members of oppressed groups begin to believe the negative societal stereotypes directed at their own group. Given these detrimental societal influences, it is often more productive to focus on ameliorating oppressive or harmful social conditions rather than attempting therapy aimed at changing the individual. Supportive individual therapy may be beneficial, however, if it allows clients to discuss their experiences and possible strategies for coping with societal stressors.

Did You Know?

We all learn societal stereotypes, biases, and prejudices. On a conscious level, most of us believe we would never intentionally discriminate against others. However, implicit bias studies demonstrate that unconscious discrimination is common because many of our stereotypes operate outside the level of conscious awareness.

Source: Schnierle et al., 2019

Does Social Injustice Influence Mental Health?

The COVID-19 pandemic that began early in 2020 brought to light the significant racial and ethnic disparities that exist in the United States with respect to health and access to health care. And on May 25, 2020, the widely publicized police killing of George Floyd in Minneapolis, Minnesota, reignited the Black Lives Matter movement and the focus on police violence and societal oppression directed toward communities of color. The synchronicity of these two events led to a deepened understanding of the need to address issues of social and racial injustice and how various societal systems have contributed to these disparities.

These events also heightened our awareness of the many faces of *systemic racism*, the deeply embedded societal policies that have disadvantaged certain racial groups over multiple generations. The general public suddenly appeared more open to learning about the history of racism and the repercussions of a system in which a dominant group (i.e., White people) organizes society into categories (i.e., "races") and then both explicitly and implicitly deems members of the nondominant groups as inferior.

More people began to understand that these artificial divisions, created and perpetuated for the comfort and profit of the dominant group, have resulted in societal systems that provide fewer opportunities for members of oppressed groups. In other words, our society is set up in a way that prevents certain people from having equal access to resources, paving the way for the dominant group to gain wealth and power while simultaneously limiting opportunities for the groups they have disadvantaged. Systemic racism such as this occurs on multiple levels.

- *Structural racism* (also known as institutional racism) refers to the societal systems that advantage one group over another. Structural racism perpetuates discrimination toward disadvantaged groups via actions and policies within a variety of systems, including education and employment, policing and judicial treatment, banking and access to credit, housing, and health care. For example, discrimination in housing opportunities leads to segregated neighborhoods and segregated school systems, which subsequently affect access to higher education and well-compensated employment.

- *Cultural racism* involves the societal acceptance and internalization of stereotyped portrayals that perpetuate inaccurate beliefs about the supposed inferiority of certain groups. This negative imagery, often reinforced by the media, can take the form of prevailing norms or implicit assumptions and accepted discriminatory language pertaining to these groups. This socialization is so pervasive that members of oppressed groups sometimes develop internalized racism and begin to believe in these negative stereotypes regarding their own group.

- *Individual racism* occurs when members of a society engage in racial discrimination—the unequal treatment of certain people based on their race or ethnicity. Discriminatory events are usually sudden, negative, and beyond the control of the individual subjected to the racist action. Discrimination can produce hurt and trauma, whether it is overt and intentional (e.g., name-calling or direct harassment) or subtle and unintentional (e.g., differential treatment based on implicit bias).

All forms of racism directly and indirectly affect the mental and physical health and life span of people of color (Williams et al., 2019). As you will see throughout the text, the pervasiveness of racism not only affects physical health but also creates significant emotional distress. Racism is a significant etiological influence in the development of many of the disorders covered in this text. The sudden and uncontrollable aspects of racist actions are not only traumatic for those affected but can also result in those targeted feeling chronic stress and a need for constant vigilance in order to avoid future racist events. Knowledge of actions that have threatened the safety of members of one's own racial group (such as police violence against African Americans) can be equally traumatizing.

Although most of us would never choose to engage in racist actions, inequitable policies and practices are deeply interwoven in the economic, social, and political systems that surround us. Thus, we are all inadvertently involved in racism. Recognition is the first step in ensuring that we transform our racialized systems and replace them with policies and actions that allow for true racial equity and a humane society where power and opportunity are equalized.

For Further Consideration

1. Have you ever considered ways in which your race or ethnicity has served as an advantage or disadvantage for you?

2. Why do you think the Black Lives Matter movement was reignited across the globe following the tragic killing of George Floyd? Do you believe this would have occurred if we were not in the midst of a global pandemic?

3. Do you believe that your school or home community is ready to embrace social justice reform?

4. What ideas do you have for encouraging people to work together to bring about needed societal reforms?

Multicultural Perspectives and Behavior

Multicultural models of human behavior regard race, culture, and ethnicity as central to the understanding of problematic emotions and behaviors. In China, children are taught to value group harmony over individual competitiveness. In contrast, in the United States, individual efforts and privacy are valued. These values are evident in the common use of cubicles in work settings to separate people from one another.

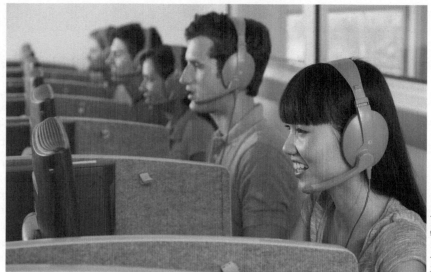

Tetra Images/Getty Images

Sociocultural Considerations in Treatment

Multicultural counseling has been called the "fourth force" in the field of psychotherapy, following the other major schools of psychoanalytic, cognitive-behavioral, and humanistic-existential therapies. Multicultural counseling is assuming greater importance as our population becomes more diverse. Therapists who use a multicultural approach take care to show respect for clients' cultural background and to incorporate cultural and societal themes for disadvantaged groups into traditional psychotherapeutic techniques. Problems are not assumed to reside only in the individual—the possible etiological influences of the community and society are also considered. The effects of discrimination, marginalization, and environmental adversities on the mental and physical health of specific populations are also evaluated (Sue & Sue, 2008).

Because mainstream counseling therapies are based on Western values and perspectives, they often do not meet the needs of clients from diverse ethnic and racial groups. Not surprisingly, compared to White clients, people from diverse ethnic and racial groups are more likely to terminate therapy after one session (Kilmer et al., 2019). Additionally, traditional therapies often do not consider the importance of other diversity issues, such as gender, disability, or sexual orientation, nor societal issues such as poverty, racism, or discrimination. Cultural influences, such as family experiences and degree of assimilation, are also essential to consider in assessment and treatment. At the same time, therapists need to be careful not to assume that all clients who are a member of a particular group necessarily identify with or share the cultural values of that group.

Criticisms of the Multicultural Model and Related Therapeutic Techniques

Critics of the multicultural model argue that a disorder is a disorder, regardless of the cultural context in which it occurs. For instance, they would contend that someone who is hallucinating lacks contact with reality. This behavior would represent a dysfunction, according to this viewpoint, even if the person considers the hallucination desirable. Another criticism leveled at the multicultural model is that it relies heavily on case studies and ethnographic analyses and that formal research has not yet validated many of the concepts associated with the model. However, culturally adapted therapies do seem to address the shortcoming of Western-based interventions for diverse populations and have proven to be more effective than non-adapted therapies with a variety of cultural groups (Cachelin et al., 2019; Parra-Cardona et al., 2017).

Applying the Models of Psychopathology

A useful learning exercise to evaluate your mastery of the various models is to apply them to a case study. We invite you to try your hand at explaining the behavior of Nikeesha, a hypothetical client, from the perspective of some of the models we have discussed. Afterward, we invite you to attempt a more integrated multipath approach to explaining Nikeesha's difficulties.

Nikeesha, a 27-year-old African American woman and recent law school graduate, decided to seek counseling due to her increasing anxiety and sleep difficulties as well as recent panic attacks. Nikeesha found it was easy to open up to her therapist, an older African American woman. She shared how she often felt close to tears, but did everything possible not to cry because "showing weakness is not an option," especially at the law firm where she was recently hired. When asked about her family, Nikeesha described how her mother, Betty, raised her as a single mom and taught her the importance of being self-sufficient, independent, and able to stand up for herself. Nikeesha admired her mother's self-reliance and ability to support the two of them on the wages she earned working at the local grocery store; although Betty occasionally experienced episodes of severe anxiety, she never missed a day of work.

When asked to describe her early experiences in school, Nikeesha smiled as she recalled that during elementary and middle school, she often took a leadership role and was voted president of her eighth-grade class. Her priorities were to do well in school and "not get into trouble." Nikeesha's hard work and academic success resulted in an opportunity for her to attend a highly rated high school in another area of the city. Leaving her friends and adjusting to an unfamiliar school environment where there were few students of color was challenging for Nikeesha, particularly when she overheard some of her new classmates making overtly racist comments about her. Further, when Nikeesha voiced her opinions in class, fellow students called her "pushy" and "aggressive." Despite her discomfort at being one of the only Black students at the school, Nikeesha was excited by the academic challenges and continued to receive good grades and positive support from many of her teachers. However, instead of having a close group of friends like she did in middle school, Nikeesha felt isolated from other students. She also became very anxious and began to have difficulty sleeping. Nikeesha coped by suppressing her emotions, putting on invisible "armor," and working even harder to succeed. However, after returning home from school, she often burst into tears.

During college and law school, Nikeesha continued to succeed academically but felt even more socially isolated. Although she was hired by a prestigious law firm, her life did not feel rewarding. She started to have more anxiety and feelings of depression. Nikeesha's stress had recently increased after her mother, who was only 60 years old, experienced a debilitating stroke. Although Betty was slowly recovering, Nikeesha was now her mother's primary caregiver. Nikeesha had recently missed several days of work taking her mother to medical appointments—a decision that Nikeesha believed the managing partners in the law firm did not understand or support. When appearing in court to argue a recent case, Nikeesha felt her heart pounding and had to ask for a brief recess to prevent a panic attack—an event that prompted her to seek therapy.

Table 2.3 summarizes the various models to review as you begin this exercise.

- Consider what each theory would propose as the basis of Nikeesha's stress, anxiety, sleep issues, and panic attacks. Consider the type of information that each perspective would consider most important.

- Compare and contrast the views of several of the models.

- As you attempt to explain Nikeesha's mental and physical distress, notice how your adoption of a particular framework influences the type of data you consider important. Is it possible that all the models hold some semblance of truth? Are their positions necessarily contradictory? How would you explain Nikeesha's difficulties if you integrated all of the background information into a unified explanation using the multipath model?

Table 2.3 Comparison of the Most Influential Models of Psychopathology

Model	Motivation for Behavior	Theoretical Foundation	Source of Symptoms	Treatment
Biological	State of biological integrity and health	Animal and human research, case studies, neuroimaging	Genetics, epigenetics, brain anatomy, and physiology; autonomic overreactivity	Medications; ECT; rTMS; DBS; vagus nerve stimulation
Psychodynamic	Unconscious influences	Case studies, correlational methods	Early childhood experiences	Psychoanalysis; uncovering unconscious conflict; dream analysis; free association
Behavioral	External influences	Animal research, case studies, experimental methods	Learning maladaptive responses, not acquiring appropriate responses	Directly modifying behavior; analyzing and changing the environmental factors controlling behavior
Cognitive	External and cognitive influences	Human research, case studies, experimental methods	Learned patterns of irrational or negative thoughts or self-statements	Understanding the relationship between thoughts and problem behavior; modifying internal dialogue
Humanistic	Self-actualization	Case studies, correlational methods	Incongruence between self and experiences	Nondirective reflection; unconditional positive regard
Existential	Capacity for self-awareness; freedom to decide one's fate	A philosophical approach to understanding the human condition	Failure to actualize human potential, avoidance of choice and responsibility	Providing conditions for maximizing self-awareness and growth and concern for others
Family systems	Interaction with significant others	Case studies, social psychological studies, experimental methods	Faulty family interactions and inconsistent communication patterns	Treating the entire family, not just the identified patient
Multicultural	Cultural values and norms	Data about cultural groups from various disciplines	Culture conflicts, discrimination, and oppression	Adapting therapy to consider both individual and cultural factors

2-7 Contemporary Trends and Future Directions

A truly comprehensive model of human behavior must address the likelihood that biological, psychological, social, and sociocultural factors are all involved. We hope it is now clear why it is important to consider mental disorders from a multipath perspective, and to embrace integration of the various theories and treatment approaches. Fortunately, our evidence-based understanding of mental disorders has evolved in recent decades. Let's take biological explanations as an example. Researchers have increasingly come to reject a simple linear explanation of biological effects on mental health. Instead, the majority of scientists now view mental disorders as resulting from complex interactive and oftentimes reciprocal processes (Alam et al., 2017).

Further, epigenetic research is revealing how reciprocal gene × environment interactions modify gene expression. Additionally, we are learning how behavioral traits associated with certain genes or gene combinations can lead to stressful personal or environmental circumstances. For example, genetic factors may predispose a person to seek out situations (such as using drugs or alcohol or selecting unstable friends or romantic partners) that increase the risk of experiencing stressors that trigger depression. Accumulating evidence demonstrates that biochemistry, brain activity, and even brain structures and neural circuitry can change in response to a variety of psychological, social, cultural, and other environmental influences (Tozzi et al., 2018).

Regardless of which etiological pathways have created a specific person's mental health condition, we know that a variety of therapeutic strategies can change many of the dysregulated physiological processes occurring within that person's brain and body. We know, for example, that fear can cause the secretion of adrenaline and noradrenalin. Through brain imaging studies, we also know that psychotherapeutic interventions can "normalize" brain circuitry in people experiencing symptoms of various mental disorders (Lazaridou et al., 2017). Thus, although biology may affect the development of mental disorders, the environment can exert an equally powerful effect on recovery from mental distress.

Sociocultural factors are increasingly recognized as playing an important role in the etiology of mental health conditions, particularly among diverse populations. Over the past few decades, major research universities have been focusing on *cultural neuroscience*—the study of how biology shapes culture and culture shapes biology (Pedraza, 2019). Fortunately, mental health professionals are learning more about the importance of using therapeutic practices that consider clients' diverse cultural backgrounds, their culturally based experiences, and their views regarding the causes of their difficulties and their opinions regarding treatment goals. In fact, we are seeing much more individualization of both psychologically and biologically based treatment approaches. As our understandings of the complex causes of mental disorders increase, there is an increased focus on earlier diagnosis, preventive interventions, and evidence-based treatments that are guided by a comprehensive understanding of a client's biological, psychological, social, and sociocultural characteristics.

Chapter Summary

1 What models of psychopathology have been used to explain symptoms of mental illness?

- A variety of one-dimensional models have traditionally been used to explain emotional and behavioral symptoms. They are inadequate because mental disorders are multidimensional.

2 What is the multipath model of mental disorders?

- The multipath model provides a framework for understanding biological, psychological, social, and sociocultural influences on mental disorders; the complexity of their interacting components; and the need to view disorders from a holistic framework.

3 How is biology involved in mental disorders?

- Genetics, brain anatomy, biochemical imbalances, central nervous system functioning, and autonomic nervous system reactivity are often involved in mental disorders. Neurotransmitters seem to play a significant role in emotions and behavior, and genetic inheritance and epigenetic factors are associated with many psychopathologies.

4 How do psychological models explain mental disorders?

- Psychodynamic models emphasize childhood experiences and the role of the unconscious in determining adult behavior.
- Behavioral models focus on the role of learning in symptoms of mental disorders. Behaviors are acquired through association (classical conditioning), reinforcement (operant conditioning), or modeling (observational learning).

- Cognitive models are based on the assumption that mental disorders are due to irrational beliefs or distorted cognitive processes.
- The humanistic-existential models view an individual's reality as a product of personal perception and experience, see people as capable of making free choices and fulfilling their potential, and emphasize the whole person.

5 What role do social factors play in psychopathology?

- Poor-quality or absent social relationships are associated with increased susceptibility to mental disorders.
- Family systems approaches view mental distress as the result of distorted or faulty communication or unbalanced relationships within the family.

6 What sociocultural factors influence mental health?

- Proponents of the sociocultural approach believe that race, culture, ethnicity, gender, sexual orientation, religious preference, socioeconomic status, and other societal variables are powerful influences on the development and manifestation of mental disorders.

7 Why is it important to consider mental disorders from a multipath perspective?

- Focusing on only one theoretical perspective can overlook important aspects of the individual.
- The majority of mental disorders result from complex and reciprocal interactions among biological, psychological, social, and sociocultural factors.

Chapter Glossary

acculturative stress
the psychological, physical, and social pressures experienced by individuals who are adapting to a new culture

adrenal gland
a gland that releases sex hormones and other hormones, such as cortisol, in response to stress

allele
each of two or more alternative forms of a gene responsible for a specific trait

amygdala
the brain structure involved with physiological reactivity and emotional memories

autonomic nervous system (ANS)
a system that coordinates basic physiological functions and regulates physical responses associated with emotional reactions

axon
an extension on the neuron cell body that sends signals to other neurons, muscles, and glands

behavioral models
models of psychopathology concerned with the role of learning in the development of behavior

biopsychosocial model
the perspective suggesting that interactions between biological, psychological, and social factors cause mental disorders

cerebral cortex
the outermost layers of brain tissue; covers the cerebrum

cerebrum
the largest part of the brain, consisting of the right and left hemisphere

classical conditioning
a process in which responses to new stimuli are learned through association

cognitive models
explanations based on the assumption that thoughts mediate an individual's emotional state or behavior in response to a stimulus

conditioned response (CR)
in classical conditioning, a learned response to a previously neutral stimulus that has acquired some of the properties of another stimulus with which it has been paired

conditioned stimulus (CS)
in classical conditioning, a previously neutral stimulus that has acquired some of the properties of another stimulus with which it has been paired

couples therapy
a treatment aimed at helping couples understand and clarify their communications, role relationships, unfulfilled needs, and unrealistic or unmet expectations

critical periods
a specific time in early development during which there is heightened sensitivity to environmental influences or experiences

defense mechanism
in psychoanalytic theory, an ego-protection strategy that shelters the individual from anxiety, operates unconsciously, and distorts reality

deficit model
an early attempt to explain differences in minority groups that contended differences are the result of "cultural deprivation"

dendrite
a short, rootlike structure on the neuron cell body that receives signals from other neurons

dream analysis
a psychoanalytic technique focused on interpreting the hidden meanings of dreams

drug–drug interactions
when the effect of a medication is changed, enhanced, or diminished when taken with another drug, including herbal substances

enteric nervous system (ENS)
an independent neural system involved with digestion; capable of signaling the brain regarding stress and other emotions

epigenetics
a field of biological research focused on understanding how environmental factors influence gene expression

etiology
the cause or origin of a disorder

executive functioning
mental processes that involve the planning, organizing, and attention required to meet short-term and long-term goals

existential approach
a set of philosophical attitudes that focus on human alienation, the individual in the context of the human condition, and personal responsibility to others as well as to oneself

exposure therapy
a treatment approach based on extinction principles that involves gradual or rapid exposure to feared objects or situations

extinction
the decrease or cessation of a behavior due to the gradual weakening of a classically or operantly conditioned response

extrapyramidal symptoms
side effects of antipsychotic medications that can affect a person's gait, movement, or posture

family systems model
an explanation that assumes that the family is an interdependent system and that mental disorders reflect processes occurring within the family system

free association
a psychoanalytic therapeutic technique in which clients are asked to say whatever comes to mind for the purpose of revealing their unconscious thoughts

gene expression
the process by which heritable information in a gene is translated into a specialized function within a cell; although the DNA within the cell does not change, epigenetic changes can be passed on to new cells during cell division and can be inherited

genes
segments of DNA coded with information needed for the biological inheritance of various traits

genetic mutation
an alteration in a gene that changes the instructions within the gene; some mutations result in biological dysfunction

genome
the complete set of DNA in a cell; the human genome consists of approximately 30,000 genes located in the nucleus of every cell

genotype
a person's genetic makeup

glia
the cells that support and protect neurons

gray matter
brain tissue comprised of the cell bodies of neurons and glia

group therapy
a form of therapy that involves the simultaneous treatment of two or more clients and may involve more than one therapist

hallucination
a sensory experience (such as an image, sound, smell, or taste) that seems real but that does not exist outside of the mind

heredity
the genetic transmission of personal characteristics

heterogeneous
different or diverse

hippocampus
the brain structure involved with the formation, organization, and storing of emotionally relevant memories

homeostasis
the ability to maintain internal equilibrium by adjusting physiological processes

hormones
regulatory chemicals that influence various physiological activities, such as metabolism, digestion, growth, and mood

humanistic perspective
the optimistic viewpoint that people are born with the ability to fulfill their potential and that mental distress results from disharmony between a person's potential and self-concept

hypothalamic-pituitary-adrenal (HPA) axis
a system activated under conditions of stress or emotional arousal

hypothalamus
the brain structure that regulates bodily drives, such as hunger, thirst, and sexual response, and body conditions, such as body temperature and circadian rhythms

implicit bias
unconscious assumptions about or stereotyping of members of a specific group

impulsivity
a tendency to act quickly without careful thought

inferiority model
an early attempt to explain differences in minority groups that contended racial and ethnic minorities are somehow inferior to the majority population

internalized racism
unconscious belief and acceptance of the dominant culture's negative portrayal of one's own racial group

limbic system
a group of deep brain structures associated with emotions, decision making, and memory formation

mindfulness
nonjudgmental awareness of thoughts, feelings, physical sensations, and the environment

model
an analogy used by scientists, usually to describe or explain a phenomenon or process they cannot directly observe

modeling
the process of learning by observing models and later imitating them

multicultural model
a contemporary view that emphasizes the importance of considering a person's cultural background and related experiences

multipath model
a model that provides an organizational framework for understanding the numerous influences on the development of mental disorders, the complexity of their interacting components, and the need to view disorders from a holistic framework

myelin
white, fatty material that surrounds and insulates axons

myelination
the process by which myelin sheaths increase the efficiency of signal transmission between nerve cells

negative reinforcement
increasing the frequency or magnitude of a behavior by removing something aversive

neural circuits
a signal-relaying network of interconnected neurons

neural stem cells
uncommitted cells that can be stimulated to form new neurons and glia

neurogenesis
the birth and growth of new neurons

neuron
a nerve cell that transmits messages throughout the body

neuropeptides
small molecules that can directly and indirectly influence a variety of hormones and neurotransmitters

neuroplasticity
the process by which the brain changes to compensate for injury or to adapt to environmental changes

neurotransmitter
any of a group of chemicals that help transmit messages between neurons

observational learning theory
the theory that suggests an individual can acquire new behaviors by watching other people perform them

operant behavior
voluntary and controllable behavior, such as walking or thinking, that "operates" on an individual's environment

operant conditioning
the theory of learning that holds that behaviors are controlled by the consequences that follow them

phenotype
observable physical and behavioral characteristics resulting from the interaction between the genotype and the environment

pituitary gland
the gland that stimulates hormones associated with growth, sexual and reproductive development, metabolism, and stress responses

pleasure principle
the impulsive, pleasure-seeking aspect of our being, from which the id operates

polymorphism
a common DNA mutation or variation of a gene

positive reinforcement
desirable actions or rewards that increase the likelihood that a particular behavior will occur

prefrontal cortex
the outer layer of the prefrontal lobe responsible for inhibiting instinctive responses and performing complex cognitive behavior such as managing attention, behavior, and emotions

protective factors
conditions or attributes that lessen or eliminate the risk of a negative psychological or social outcome

psychoanalysis
therapy aimed at helping clients uncover repressed material, achieve insight into inner motivations and desires, and resolve childhood conflicts that affect current relationships

psychodynamic model
a model of psychopathology concerned with unconscious conflicts

psychological flexibility
the ability to mentally and emotionally adapt to situational demands

psychopharmacology
the study of the effects of medications on thoughts, emotions, and behaviors

psychosexual stages
in psychodynamic theory, the sequence of stages—oral, anal, phallic, latency, and genital—through which human personality develops

psychotic symptoms
the loss of contact with reality that may involve disorganized thinking, false beliefs, or seeing or hearing things that are not there

psychotropic medications
drugs that treat or manage psychiatric symptoms by influencing brain activity associated with emotions and behavior

reality principle
an awareness of the demands of the environment and of the need to adjust behavior to meet these demands, from which the ego operates

reinforcer
anything that increases the frequency or magnitude of a behavior

resilience
the ability to recover from stress or adversity

resistance
during psychoanalysis, a process in which the client unconsciously attempts to impede the analysis by preventing the exposure of repressed material

reuptake
the reabsorption of a neurotransmitter after an impulse has been transmitted across the synapse

schema
a mental framework for organizing and interpreting information

self-actualization
an inherent tendency to strive toward the realization of one's full potential

sociocultural influences
factors such as gender, sexual orientation, spirituality, religion, socioeconomic status, race/ethnicity, and culture that can exert an effect on mental health

synapse
a tiny gap that exists between the axon of the sending neuron and the dendrites of the receiving neuron

systematic desensitization
a treatment technique involving repeated exposure to a feared stimulus while a client is in a competing emotional or physiological state such as relaxation

trait
a distinguishing quality or characteristic

transference
the process by which a client undergoing psychoanalysis reenacts early conflicts by applying to the analyst feelings and attitudes that the person has toward significant others

unconditioned response (UCR)
in classical conditioning, the unlearned response made to an unconditioned stimulus

unconditioned stimulus (UCS)
in classical conditioning, the stimulus that elicits an unconditioned response

universal shamanic tradition
the set of beliefs and practices from non-Western Indigenous traditions that assume that special healers are blessed with powers to act as messengers between the human and spirit worlds

vagus nerve
a nerve that creates a mind–body pathway from the brain through the digestive tract to the abdomen; regulates autonomic nervous system processes and body reactivity

white matter
brain tissue comprised of myelinated nerve pathways

focus
Questions

1 How do we know if psychological tests and evaluation procedures are accurate?

2 How do mental health professionals evaluate a client's mental health?

3 How do professionals make a psychiatric diagnosis?

4 What changes are occurring in the field of psychological assessment?

Assessment and Classification of Mental Disorders

Learning Objectives

After studying this chapter, you will be able to . . .

3-1 Explain how psychological tests and assessment procedures are evaluated for accuracy.

3-2 Describe the kinds of tools that clinicians employ in evaluating a client's mental health.

3-3 Explain how professionals make a psychiatric diagnosis.

3-4 Discuss current trends in the field of psychopathology and their impact on assessment.

Police Were Called when Ms. Y. became physically aggressive, breaking several windows, biting and spitting at her boyfriend, and leaving her home in disarray. Because Ms. Y. was too confused to be interviewed, her boyfriend provided background information. He reported that Ms. Y. had previously been hospitalized on three occasions: earlier in the year when she was hearing voices and claiming she was God, and twice when she experienced hallucinations after experimenting with drugs as a teenager. Ms. Y.'s family history includes an aunt diagnosed with schizophrenia (Lavakumar et al., 2011).

ifferent conditions can cause the symptoms Ms. Y. exhibited. To determine the exact cause, a thorough assessment must be performed. In the case of Ms. Y., a drug screen ruled out alcohol and illicit drugs as causal factors. There was also no evidence of infections or other medical conditions that might produce her symptoms. However, when asked about the use of medications, Ms. Y. volunteered that she had been taking an over-the-counter weight-loss supplement containing the amino acid L-carnitine. In fact, eager to lose weight, Ms. Y. had been taking twice the recommended levels of the supplement. In addition, she had been drinking energy drinks containing L-carnitine as one of the main ingredients. The mental health team concluded that her mental confusion was due to carnitine intoxication.

When dealing with psychiatric symptoms, assessment is critical. Mental health professionals collect and organize information about a person's current condition and past history using observations, interviews, psychological tests, and neurological tests, as well as input from relatives and friends. Information gathered from a variety of sources allows for a more thorough understanding of a client's symptoms and mental state, especially because findings from different sources often diverge from one another and must be integrated in order to obtain an optimal understanding of what is occurring (Bottini et al., 2019). Further, it is important to rule out physical causes for psychological symptoms (e.g., anemia, medication reactions, thyroid, or cardiac irregularities), particularly when there is a sudden onset of symptoms for no apparent reason. In the case of Ms. Y., the therapists relied on observations, laboratory tests, and interviews to arrive at their diagnosis. Knowledge about Ms. Y.'s excessive use of L-carnitine was an important piece of the puzzle regarding the sudden changes in her behavior. As we noted in Chapter 1, evaluation of a client's concerns, pattern of symptoms, and background information leads to a *psychodiagnosis*, a description of the individual's psychological state and judgments about possible causes of the psychological distress. Psychodiagnosis is usually the first step in the treatment process.

In this chapter, we examine assessment methods and tools used to make a psychodiagnosis. We also discuss the most widely used diagnostic classification system, as well as criticisms regarding labeling and classification. We begin with a discussion of methods for ensuring the accuracy of assessment tools.

3-1 Reliability and Validity

There are many tests and procedures that professionals can use to evaluate clients who are seeking help. The best assessment tools for accurately diagnosing psychological disorders are both reliable and valid.

Reliability is the degree to which a procedure, test, or classification system yields the same results repeatedly under the same circumstances. There are many types of reliability, including the following:

- *Test-retest reliability* determines whether a measure yields the same results when given at two different points in time. For example, if you take a personality test in the morning and then retake the test later in the day, the test is reliable if the results are consistent from one point in time to another. If the test results vary, we would say the test has poor reliability.

- *Internal consistency reliability* requires that various parts of a test yield similar or consistent results. For example, on a test assessing anxiety, each test item should reliably measure characteristics related to anxiety.

- *Interrater reliability* refers to how consistent (or inconsistent) test results are when scored by different test administrators. For instance, imagine that two clinicians trained to diagnose individuals according to a certain classification system are given the same list of symptoms to review and are asked to formulate a psychodiagnosis. If one clinician diagnoses an anxiety disorder and the other diagnoses depression, there would be poor interrater reliability.

It is also important to consider **validity**, the extent to which a test or procedure actually performs the function it was designed to perform. If a measure intended to assess depression actually measures motivation, the measure is an invalid measure of depression. Common forms of validity considered in assessment are predictive, construct, and content validity.

- *Predictive validity* is how well a test or measure predicts or forecasts a person's behavior, response, or performance. Colleges and universities often use applicants' SAT or ACT scores to predict future college grades. If the tests have good predictive validity, they should be able to differentiate students who will perform well in college from those who will perform poorly.

- *Construct validity* is how well a test or measure relates to the characteristics or disorder in question. For example, a test to measure social anxiety should be constructed to match other measures of social anxiety, including questions about physical symptoms seen in people who are socially anxious, such as muscle tension, sweating, or startle responses.

- *Content validity* is how well a test measures what it is intended to measure. For instance, we know that depression involves cognitive, emotional, behavioral, and physiological symptoms. If a self-report measure of depression contains items that assess only cognitive characteristics, such as difficulty concentrating, the measure has poor content validity because it fails to assess the other areas we know are associated with depression.

Let's look at the reliability and validity of a measure developed to assess the unusual thinking patterns and impaired sense of reality seen in **psychosis**. The test creators (Cicero et al., 2010) wanted to determine if the instrument they developed was a valid and reliable measure of the likelihood of developing psychosis. The items for the test were based on descriptions of psychosis, including characteristics observed during the early stages of schizophrenia (a disorder involving symptoms of psychosis), and interviews with people diagnosed with schizophrenia. The test's internal consistency reliability—the consistency among the items—was high (.89).

To determine the construct validity—how well the measure actually assesses the likelihood of developing psychosis—the inventory was compared to other scales that measure psychosis. It was highly correlated to other measures of psychosis, thus demonstrating good construct validity and increasing confidence in the measure. Because the inventory assesses the likelihood of developing psychosis, you would also expect that individuals with a history of psychosis would score higher on this test compared to individuals with other mental disorders. This was also found. Thus, the researchers concluded that their inventory is a useful measure of susceptibility to psychosis.

Test accuracy is also influenced by the conditions under which tests are administered. **Standardization**, or standard administration, requires professionals administering a test to follow common rules or procedures. If an examiner creates a tense or hostile environment for some individuals who are taking a test, for example, the test scores may vary simply due to differences in

Did You Know?

The TSA behavioral checklist for identifying possible terrorists at airports includes "arriving late for a flight," "exaggerated yawning," "trembling," "avoids eye contact," and "appears to be in disguise." Those who exceed a certain threshold of stress-related or deceptive signs are interrogated. This program, which cost nearly $1 billion, has been found to be inaccurate and based on invalid evidence such as newspaper articles and opinion pieces.

Source: U.S. Government Accountability Office, 2017

the testing situation. An additional concern is the **standardization sample**—the group of people who originally took the measure and whose performance is used as the basis for comparison. Clinicians use the standardization sample to compare and interpret test results. For test scores to be valid, test takers should be similar to the original group or sample. For instance, would comparing the test score of a 20-year-old African American woman with a standardization sample consisting of middle-aged European American men provide accurate information? Most would agree that the standardization group is too different to allow for a valid interpretation of the results.

3-2 Assessment and Classification of Mental Disorders

Psychological assessment involves gathering information and drawing conclusions about the traits, skills, abilities, emotional functioning, and psychological problems of an individual. Clinicians use four main methods of assessment: interviews, observations, psychological tests and inventories, and neuropsychological measures. Using several different assessment methods can provide a more accurate view of the client and increase diagnostic accuracy.

Interviews

The clinical interview is a time-honored means of psychological assessment that allows the mental health professional to get to know their client. Observation of verbal and nonverbal behaviors, as well as any specific information the client shares, provides important information to assist with psychodiagnosis and treatment planning. Client interviews can also explore social and sociocultural factors that may affect mental health. For example, the therapist can determine whether issues such as religion, sexual orientation, age, gender, social class, or disability may be playing a role in the difficulties a client is experiencing.

Interviews can vary in their degree of structure and formality. The most structured interview is the formal standardized interview, which often includes a standard series of questions or the use of standardized rating scales. Generally, standardized measures involve yes/no responses or ratings (e.g., Never = 1; Occasionally = 2; Fairly often = 3; Frequently = 4) in response to specific questions such as "Have you been told by others that you have done or said things that you do not remember?" Unstructured interviews involve open-ended questions and queries such as "What problems have you experienced when you attempt to limit your consumption of alcohol?" With an unstructured interview, the clinician has the opportunity to initiate follow-up discussion to gain further understanding of any issues that seem pertinent to diagnosis and treatment.

Although structured interviews limit conversation and in-depth probing of responses, they have the advantage of collecting consistent and comprehensive information, are less subject to interviewers' biases, and tend to produce higher levels of reliability and validity when compared to semi- or nonstructured methods (Groth-Marnat & Wright, 2016; Shankman et al., 2018).

Observations

> **Case Study** [A] 9-year-old boy . . . was referred to a neurologist for treatment of "hysterical paralysis." . . . Medical tests indicated no apparent neurological damage . . . He reported that his legs simply did not work no matter how he tried. As the child was describing his difficulties, we noted that he would shift his feet and legs in his wheelchair so his legs could swing freely . . . When we asked him to describe his paralysis, he would look at his feet and . . . his leg movements would diminish. However, when we asked him to discuss other topics (e.g., school, friends), he would look up, become engaged in the interview, and his feet would swing. (O'Brien & Carhart, 2011, p. 14)

Both formal and informal behavioral observations can provide key information. In the case of this 9-year-old boy, observations provided critically important data—he seemed to be able to move his legs under some circumstances. Sometimes observations are highly structured and specific. For example, a school psychologist observing a child in a classroom may count episodes of off-task behavior and the circumstances under which the off-task behaviors occur. On other occasions, observations may be less formal and more subjective, such as when the school psychologist observes a child interacting with peers on the playground. Informal observations such as this tend to be more subjective and less reliable or valid than structured observations (Bergold et al., 2019).

Mental health professionals informally observe behavior when they interview or work with clients. Often, behavioral clues have diagnostic significance, as seen in the following case.

> **Case Study** Margaret was a 37-year-old woman treated by one of the authors for symptoms of severe depression. It was obvious from a casual glance that Margaret had not taken care of herself for weeks. Her face, hands, and hair were dirty. Her beat-up tennis shoes were only halfway on her sockless feet. Her disheveled appearance and stooped body posture made her appear much older than she was.
>
> Throughout the interview, Margaret sat as though she lacked the strength to straighten her body. She avoided eye contact and stared at the floor. When asked questions, she responded in short phrases: "Yes," "No," "I don't know," "I don't care." There were long pauses between the questions and her answers.

Although Margaret did not have the energy for much conversation, her lack of grooming and low energy levels helped confirm her family's concern that she was in the midst of a deep depression.

Naturalistic Observations

Naturalistic observations are made in naturally occurring environments. In this photo, a female researcher is observing children as they interact with their teacher in a preschool classroom.

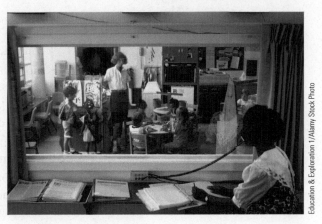

Education & Exploration 1/Alamy Stock Photo

Mental Status Examination

A widely used semi-structured clinical assessment is the mental status examination. This examination uses questions, observations, and tasks to briefly evaluate a client's cognitive, psychological, and behavioral functioning. As the exam is administered using a combination of specific, structured questions and open-ended inquiries, the clinician considers the

Should Strengths Be Assessed?

A 25-year-old woman reported extreme anxiety, frequent crying spells, difficulty sleeping, and a lack of happiness in her life. Although she had always been anxious, a recent breakup with her partner made her feel that she was going to "fall apart." Instead of focusing primarily on her problems, the therapist began to help the client identify her strengths and to generate positive emotions. When the client described herself as "quirky," explaining how she liked science fiction movies, "weird dancing," and "strange poetry," she began to smile and became more engaged in the session. She also described experiences that made her happy, such as being in the sun, listening to music, and breathing fresh morning air. These areas were further explored, and strengths such as intelligence, self-reflection, and empathy were identified. These positive characteristics were discussed as the therapist worked with the client to increase her self-compassion, acceptance of difficult emotions, and ability to maintain healthy interpersonal boundaries. At the end of therapy, the client expressed that she liked herself more, understood more about the person she would like to be, and felt capable of handling feelings of depression and establishing healthy relationships (Hawley et al., 2020).

Although the identification of strengths, positive qualities, and supportive relationships is important in creating hope and motivation (Lopez et al., 2018), it is much more common for deficits, symptoms, problem behaviors, and emotional difficulties to be the focus of psychological assessments and classification systems such as the DSM. The negative picture this emphasis creates can affect a client's self-concept as well as the therapist's view of the client. In contrast, assessing strengths can provide a more balanced picture for both the mental health professional and the client. Recognizing the importance of acknowledging personal assets, Peterson and Seligman (2005) developed a classification system involving character strengths and virtues to complement the DSM; their system focuses on six overarching virtues (wisdom, courage, humanity, justice, temperance, and transcendence), characteristics that are important to assess and consider when working with anyone experiencing emotional distress.

Fortunately, as we saw in the case study, therapists are also recognizing the importance of focusing not only on clients' problems but also on their strengths—their positive personal characteristics, accomplishments, and prior successes in dealing with adversities and stress. This goal-focused positive therapy not only reduces symptoms but also increases resilience and improves quality of life (Conoley & Scheel, 2018).

What do you think are the advantages of assessing client strengths? If you were a client, would you want the therapist to concentrate on your strengths as well as your concerns?

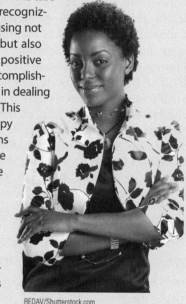

REDAV/Shutterstock.com

appropriateness and quality of the client's responses and then attempts to render an initial, tentative opinion regarding diagnosis and treatment needs (Voss & Das, 2020). A mental status report on Margaret (described in the previous case study) might indicate the following:

- *Appearance*: Poor self-care in grooming; disheveled appearance; shoes halfway off her feet; stooped body posture; avoidance of eye contact.

- *Mood*: Appears severely depressed. Margaret verified that she has felt "depressed," "exhausted," "hopeless," and "worthless" for months.

- *Affect*: Margaret demonstrates minimal emotional responsiveness. Her overall demeanor is suggestive of depression.

- *Speech*: Margaret speaks and responds slowly, with short replies. She frequently stated, "I don't know" and "I don't care."

- *Thought process*: Margaret's lack of responsiveness made it difficult to assess her thought processes. There was no evidence of racing thoughts or confused thinking.

- *Thought content*: Margaret denies experiencing hallucinations or delusions (false beliefs). She reports thinking about suicide almost daily but denies having a suicide plan or thoughts of hurting someone else. She reports constantly worrying about what others think of her.

- *Memory*: Margaret seems to have good recall of family details, past events, jobs, and educational background. However, she had difficulty with short-term memory—she was able to recall only one out of three words after a 5-minute delay.

- *Abstract thought*: Margaret was slow to respond but was able to explain the proverbs "A rolling stone gathers no moss" and "People in glass houses should not throw stones."

- *General knowledge*: Margaret was able to name the last four presidents but gave up before determining the number of nickels in $1.35, explaining that she "just can't concentrate."

The mental status examination is a useful diagnostic tool that helps clinicians assess areas that are not included in most clinical interviews. However, many aspects of the exam are subjective, and one's cultural background can influence the assessment. As Goldberg (2009) points out, "There is a major distinction between 'different' and 'abnormal.' A 'failure' to provide a correct interpretation of a proverb, for instance, may have nothing to do with an individual's cognitive functioning but rather may simply reflect a different upbringing or background. Similarly, tests of memory which require the subject to recite past presidents may not be an appropriate measuring tool depending on a person's country of origin, language skills, educational level, etc." (p. 3).

A client's eye contact and body posture may also reflect cultural factors. Individuals from diverse cultural backgrounds may display patterns of eye contact, dress, and body postures that appear atypical but are consistent with the client's culture and upbringing (Sue et al., 2022).

Psychological Tests and Inventories

Psychological tests and inventories are standardized tools that measure characteristics such as personality, social skills, intellectual abilities, or vocational interests. Tests differ in structure, degree of objectivity, content, and method of delivery (e.g., some tests are administered individually and others in groups). To demonstrate some of these differences, we examine several types of personality measures (projective and self-report inventories), tests of intelligence and cognitive impairment, and neuropsychological and neurological assessment procedures. Keep in mind that the psychometric properties of tests may vary for different cultural groups.

Projective Personality Tests

If you were to take a **projective personality test**, the examiner would present you with ambiguous stimuli, such as inkblots, pictures, or incomplete sentences, and ask you to respond to them in some way. The stimuli would be unfamiliar and you would be unaware of the true purpose of the test, which might involve revealing attitudes, unconscious conflicts, or personality characteristics. Projective tests presumably tap into a person's unconscious needs and motivations.

The Rorschach test, created by Swiss psychiatrist Hermann Rorschach, consists of 10 cards that display

The Rorschach Technique

Devised by Swiss psychiatrist Hermann Rorschach in 1921, the Rorschach technique uses a number of cards, each containing a symmetrical inkblot design similar to the one included here. The earlier cards in the set are in black and white; the later cards are more colorful. A client's responses to the inkblots are interpreted according to assessment guidelines and can be compared with responses of individuals diagnosed with various disorders.

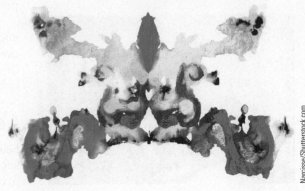

Narcisse/Shutterstock.com

symmetrical inkblot designs. Inkblots are considered appropriate stimuli because they are ambiguous, nonthreatening, and unfamiliar, so learned responses are unlikely. If you were taking the Rorschach test, the examiner would show you the cards one at a time and ask you to describe what you see in the blots. The examiner would then analyze your responses, paying close attention to how you describe the blots, whether you attend to large areas or to details, whether you respond to color, and whether your perceptions suggest movement—all of these factors are assumed to be symbolic of inner promptings, motivations, and conflicts (Masuda, 2019; Woods & Nashat, 2012).

You may have correctly guessed that the Rorschach test and the interpretation of responses rely on psychoanalytic theory and an assumption that certain answers are associated with particular unconscious conflicts. For example, seeing eyes or buttocks may imply paranoid tendencies; seeing fierce animals may imply aggressive tendencies; seeing blood may imply strong uncontrolled emotions; and seeing food may imply dependency needs (Klopfer & Davidson, 1962). Although intriguing, research has found that interpretation of these "signs" is unreliable and highly subject to clinician bias. Although there are many questions about the validity and reliability of the Rorschach test, over half of the practicing psychologists who responded to a national survey reported including the Rorschach in their assessments (Wright et al., 2017).

The Thematic Apperception Test (TAT), another projective personality test, was developed in 1935 (Murray & Morgan, 1938). It consists of 30 picture cards, most depicting two human figures. Their poses and actions are vague and ambiguous enough to be open to different interpretations. If you were to take the TAT, the examiner would ask you to tell a story about what is going on in each of the 20 TAT cards, what led up to it, and what the outcome will be. As with the Rorschach technique, your responses to the TAT items would be analyzed to provide information about your personality and your unconscious conflicts, worries, or motives (Miller, 2015).

Other types of projective tests include sentence-completion and draw-a-person tests. In the *sentence-completion test*, you would be given a list of partial sentences and asked to finish each sentence. You might be presented with partial sentences such as "My ambition . . .," "My mother was always . . .," and "I can remember . . . ." The examiner would try to interpret the meaning of your responses. In *draw-a-person tests*, such as the Machover D-A-P (Machover, 1949), you would be asked to draw a person. The examiner would analyze characteristics of your drawing, such as the size, position, and details you included, assuming that the drawing would provide clues about you. Well-controlled studies cast doubt on such diagnostic interpretations (Imuta et al., 2013). Because of the lack of research support of projective tests, fewer academic programs are including instruction on these techniques in their clinical and professional courses (Piotrowski, 2015).

Projective tests do not meet reliability and validity standards, and, therefore, are subject to error and wide variation in interpretation. The low reliability, low validity, and limited cultural relevance of these instruments suggest that they should be used with caution and only in conjunction with other assessment measures (Butcher, 2010).

Self-Report Inventories

Self-report inventories are used to assess personality or symptoms such as depression, anxiety, or emotional reactivity. Self-report inventories may involve completing open-ended questions or

The Thematic Apperception Test

In the Thematic Apperception Test, the person being assessed is asked to tell a story about each of a series of pictures. These pictures—often depicting one, two, or three people doing something—are less ambiguous than Rorschach inkblots.

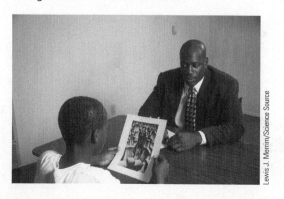

Lewis J. Merrim/Science Source

Wikipedia and the Rorschach Test

In 2009, editors of the online encyclopedia Wikipedia decided to publish the entire set of Rorschach inkblot plates, the most common responses for each inkblot, and the characteristics each inkblot is purported to measure. One of the inkblots, for instance, represents a "father figure." Responses to this card are supposed to reveal one's attitude toward males and authority figures.

Although the reliability and validity of the inkblot test are questionable, many clinicians still use this assessment tool. As Bruce Smith, president of the International Society of Rorschach and Projective Methods, states, "The more test materials are promulgated widely, the more possibility there is to game the test" (Cohen, 2009, p. 1). In other words, knowing the typical answers may change the responses of individuals taking the test and invalidate the results.

In defense of their decision to publish the inkblot information, editors at Wikipedia argue that the Rorschach test is in the public domain because intellectual property rights have expired, and it does not have copyright protection. Did Wikipedia go too far in publishing the entire Rorschach inkblot test?

---

responding to a list of self-descriptive phrases. For example, you might be asked to indicate the extent of your agreement with a list of statements. The inventory would be scored by comparing your responses to a standardization sample or to responses from individuals with specific mental disorders.

The *Minnesota Multiphasic Personality Inventory*, or *MMPI*, is a self-report personality inventory that is frequently used by practicing psychologists (Wright et al., 2017). The aim of the MMPI is to describe an individual's personality as clearly as possible. The most recent revision, the Minnesota Multiphasic Personality Inventory-3 (MMPI-3), published in 2020, incorporates contemporary views of personality by considering each person's distinct personality characteristics along a continuum. The developers of the MMPI-3 addressed concerns regarding validity by incorporating a large and diverse normative sample and by including a Spanish-language version of the test. Approximately 24,000 participants were involved in developing the norms and in field testing the MMPI-3 in mental health, medical, and forensic settings (Sellbom, 2019).

Unlike the MMPI, which assesses different personality characteristics, some self-report inventories or questionnaires focus only on certain traits or emotional problems, such as impulsivity, depression, or anxiety. For example, the *Beck Depression Inventory-II (BDI-II)* is composed of 21 items that measure various aspects of depression, such as mood, appetite, functioning at work, suicidal thinking, and sleeping patterns (Beck et al., 1996).

Though widely used, self-report inventories have limitations (Sollman et al., 2010), including the following:

1. The fixed number of answer choices can make it difficult for individuals to answer in a manner that clearly describes them. For instance, if asked to answer "true" or "false" to the statement "I am suspicious of people," you would not have an opportunity to explain your answer. You might mark "yes" because you have had personal experiences to which suspiciousness is a logical reaction.

2. Respondents often have a unique response style or response set (i.e., a tendency to respond to test items in a certain way regardless of content) that may affect the test results. For example, if you have a tendency to present yourself in a favorable light (which many people do), your answers might be socially acceptable but might not accurately reflect your true mental state.

Did You Know?

In a study involving therapy outcomes, clients undergoing treatment for depression defined a positive outcome with descriptors not typically measured by traditional assessment tools such as depression scales. They defined *success* as feeling empowered and confident, making one's own choices, having personal boundaries, and being able to manage their lives independently. Do you believe measures of therapeutic success should include outcomes such as these?
Source: De Smet et al., 2020

3. Interpretations of the responses of people from different cultural groups may be inaccurate if test norms for these groups are lacking (Laher & Cockcroft, 2017).

4. Cultural factors may shape the way a trait or characteristic is viewed. For example, although Asian Americans tend to score higher on measures of social anxiety, their scores may reflect cultural values of modesty and self-restraint rather than a sign of psychopathology; similarly, African Americans demonstrate a unique pattern of responding to measures of social anxiety (Melka et al., 2010).

5. Scores on inventories may not accurately reflect the client's perspective. For example, approximately half of a sample of 274 outpatients with major depressive disorder who demonstrated "good" improvement according to the Hamilton Rating Scale for Depression (a questionnaire that measures the severity of depression) did not consider their symptoms to have lessened or resolved. As the researchers noted, the findings call into question the clinical usefulness of the scale, as well as the validity of studies that rely exclusively on questionnaire scores to document symptom improvement (Zimmerman et al., 2012).

Despite these potential problems, many self-report inventories have good reliability and validity and are widely used.

Intelligence Tests

Intelligence testing, intended to obtain an estimate of a person's current level of cognitive functioning, results in a score called the *intelligence quotient (IQ)*. An IQ score indicates an individual's level of performance relative to that of other people of the same age (refer to Figure 3.1). Through statistical procedures, IQ test results are converted into numbers, with 100 representing the mean, or average, score. An IQ score is an important aid in predicting school performance or detecting intellectual disability, a topic we discuss in Chapter 16.

The two most widely used intelligence tests are the Wechsler scales (Wechsler, 1981) and the Stanford-Binet scales (Terman & Merrill, 1960;

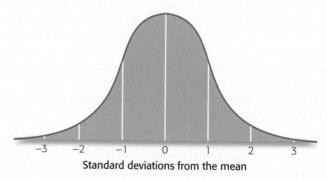

Standard deviations from the mean

Figure 3.1

A Bell Curve

The distribution of certain traits in a population resembles the shape of a bell, with most scores hovering over the mean and fewer scores falling in the outlying areas of the distribution. IQ scores are generally distributed in this manner. The mean for IQ scores is 100. One standard deviation from the mean (about 15 IQ points above or below the mean, or IQ scores between 85 and 115) encompasses about 68 percent of the scores.

Should We Assess the Assessor?

A foreign-born psychiatric resident attempted to find out what precipitated a client's problem by asking, in poor and halting English, "How brought you to the hospital?" The patient responded, "I came by car" (Chambliss, 2000, p. 186). Later, during the case conference, the resident argued that the patient's response reflected concrete thinking, a quality that is sometimes displayed by people with schizophrenia. The rest of the treatment team, however, believed the response was due to a poorly worded question.

Researchers have found that errors can occur in assessment due to attributes, beliefs, or personal values of the assessor. For instance, the biases or personal perspectives of mental health professionals have been found to influence IQ scores (McDermott et al., 2013), cross-cultural assessment results (Alcantara & Gone, 2014), responses to clinical cases involving African American clients (Santee et al., 2022), and the diagnosis of attention-deficit/hyperactivity disorder (Kazda et al., 2021). In one study, psychotherapists provided clinical ratings based on a fictitious intake report regarding a male client whose sexual orientation was identified as heterosexual, gay, or bisexual. Although heterosexual or gay sexual orientation had little impact on clinical ratings, the bisexual male was rated as more disturbed despite the fact that all of the other case information provided was identical. The researchers concluded that the difference was due to the stereotype of bisexual men being "confused and conflicted" (Mohr et al., 2009).

Despite their subjectivity, professional judgments can have profound consequences, including decisions regarding who is eligible for capital punishment. The U.S. Supreme Court has generally supported the concept that executing individuals with significant intellectual disability (someone with an IQ score below a certain threshold) is unacceptable because it violates the standard of "cruel and unusual punishment." To work around this prohibition, some prosecutors have contended and some courts have accepted the use of "cultural adjustment"—the argument that the IQ scores of defendants from ethnically underrepresented groups should be adjusted upward because IQ tests unfairly underestimate the intelligence of individuals from diverse or impoverished backgrounds. In other words, they use professional judgment about the need for "cultural adjustment" of an IQ score to help ensure that certain culturally diverse defendants with low IQ scores remain eligible for capital punishment. In fact, several defendants have been executed with adjusted IQ scores based solely on professional judgement and not on empirical studies (Shapiro et al., 2019).

For Further Consideration

1. It is clear that the characteristics, attitudes, and beliefs of mental health professionals can influence the assessment process. Given this reality, what can be done to ensure accuracy in the assessment?

2. Should state agencies responsible for the licensing of mental health professionals include screening for potential biases in applicants?

3. In what situations would you consider cultural adjustments on intellectual measures to be harmful or helpful?

Thorndike et al., 1986). The fourth edition of the *Wechsler Adult Intelligence Scale* is administered to individuals age 16 and older. Using a combination of questions and specific tasks, this intelligence test assesses four areas: verbal comprehension, perceptual organization, working memory, and processing speed. Other versions of the Weschler scales are available for use with children. The fifth edition of the *Stanford-Binet Intelligence Scale* assesses intelligence in individuals ages 2 to 85. If you were to take the Stanford-Binet, the examiner would first establish a basal age (the level where you pass all subtests) and a ceiling age (the level where you fail all subtests) as part of the process of calculating your IQ score. Although somewhat complicated to administer and score, the Stanford-Binet is the standard to which other tests are compared because of its long history, careful revision, and periodic updating (Kline, 2005).

There are various critiques regarding IQ tests. First, some psychologists believe that IQ tests largely reflect cultural and social factors rather than innate intelligence. The issue of racial differences in innate intelligence has a long history of debate. Publication of the controversial book *The Bell Curve* (Herrnstein & Murray, 1994) refocused attention on this issue when the book's authors proposed that racial differences in IQ scores are

Testing for Intellectual Functioning

Intelligence tests can provide valuable information about intellectual functioning and help psychologists assess intellectual disability and deterioration. Although criticized for being culturally biased, if used with care, they can be beneficial tools. Here a second-grade student is working with a school psychologist who is administering a subtest of the Wechsler Intelligence Scale for Children.

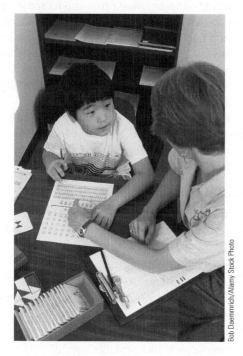

Bob Daemmrich/Alamy Stock Photo

genetically determined; they further argued that there is little that can be done to overcome the social and status differences between racial groups because of these inherent IQ differences. Richwine (2009) made a similar claim about Hispanic immigrants, arguing that their IQ is "substantially lower than that of the White native populations" and that their children and grandchildren will continue to have low IQs. Politically charged assertions such as these fail to consider other important influences such as English language proficiency, culture, poverty, discrimination, and oppression (Nisbett et al., 2012).

Tests for Cognitive Impairment

Clinical psychologists, especially those working in medical settings, are concerned with detecting and assessing cognitive impairment resulting from brain damage, a topic we address in our discussion of neurocognitive disorders in Chapter 13. Brain dysfunction can have profound effects on physical skills, such as motor coordination, as well as on cognitive skills, such as memory, attention, and learning. A common method of screening for cognitive impairment is the *Bender-Gestalt Visual-Motor Test* (Bender, 1938; Brannigan et al., 2004), displayed in Figure 3.2. Nine geometric designs, each drawn in black on a piece of white cardboard, are presented one at a time to the test taker, who is asked to copy them on a piece of paper. Certain drawing errors are characteristic of neurological impairment. Among these are rotation of figures, perseveration (unusual continuation of a pattern), and inability to copy angles.

Comprehensive neuropsychological tests are also used to assess cognitive impairment. In fact, they are far more accurate in documenting cognitive deficits than are interviews or informal observations (Malik, 2013). For example, the *Halstead-Reitan Neuropsychological Test Battery* successfully differentiates patients with brain damage from those without brain damage and can provide valuable information about the type and location of the damage (Goldstein & Beers, 2004). The full battery consists of a series of tasks that assess sensorimotor, cognitive, and perceptual functioning, including abstract concept formation, memory, and attention.

Figure 3.2

The Nine Bender Designs

The figures presented to participants are on the left. The distorted figures drawn by an individual with suspected brain damage are on the right.

Source: Bender, 1938

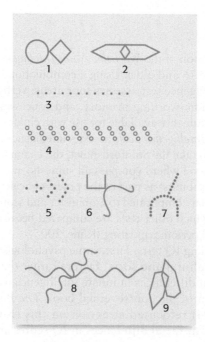

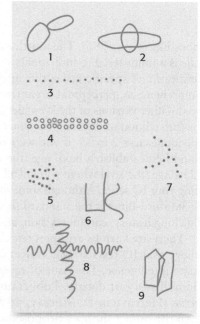

Neurological Tests

Various neurological tests are used to research and diagnose impairment associated with psychiatric and neurocognitive disorders. Neuroimaging techniques allow medical professionals and researchers to noninvasively visualize brain structures (**structural imaging**), as well as monitor the physiological processes occurring within the brain (**functional imaging**). We begin by discussing structural imaging procedures (refer to Table 3.1); the anatomical views of the brain obtained through these procedures can help detect brain tumors, bleeding within the brain, or significant changes in brain tissue associated with substance abuse and disorders such as schizophrenia, depression, and Alzheimer disease.

A well-known and widely available structural imaging procedure is the computerized axial tomography (CT) scan. CT scans combine multiple X-rays to produce three-dimensional, cross-sectional brain structure images. Although CT scans are useful for diagnosis, excess radiation exposure may increase cancer risk, especially in children, so efforts are made to keep radiation doses as low as possible (Meulepas et al., 2019).

Magnetic resonance imaging (MRI) is another structural imaging procedure. Radio waves within a magnetic field create images by scanning one layer at a time to produce an amazingly clear cross-sectional "picture" of the brain and its tissues; these images look remarkably similar to postmortem brain slices. Unlike CT scans, MRIs do not involve radiation exposure and cancer risk. MRIs provide highly detailed pictures but are more expensive and less widely available than CT scans. Although MRIs have been used to examine brain changes associated with psychiatric symptoms, their use in routine care is severely limited because of their high cost (Baroud et al., 2019).

Functional imaging methods (refer to Table 3.2) allow doctors and researchers to study physiological and biochemical processes in the brain. One of the most basic functional techniques is the *electroencephalograph (EEG)*. During an EEG, electrodes attached to the scalp record electrical activity (brain wave patterns); an EEG can detect even brief episodes of irregular electrical activity associated with seizures or other brain conditions. A newer procedure, *magnetoencephalography (MEG)*, uses electrodes within a helmet to measure electrical activity in the magnetic field close to the surface of the brain; the MEG process is even more precise in localizing brain dysfunction. Unfortunately, these techniques do not measure electrical activity occurring deep within the brain.

CT Scan Revealing Brain Atrophy

Cerebral CT scans, which involve multiple, cross-sectional X-rays of the brain, are able to document changes in brain tissue and brain structures. This CT scan of the brain of a 94-year-old woman reveals enlarged ventricles and atrophy indicative of a loss of neurons in some brain regions.

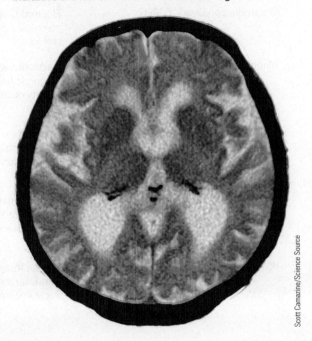

Scott Camazine/Science Source

Table 3.1 Structural Imaging Techniques

Structural imaging techniques allow noninvasive study of major brain structures and the detection of injury or disease, including skull fractures, brain tumors, bleeding within the brain, and changes in brain tissue associated with substance abuse and many mental disorders.

Structural Imaging Technique	Description	What Is Detected?
Computerized axial tomography (CT)	Uses multiple cross-sectional X-rays to rapidly produce brain images	Brain deterioration or major abnormality, including swelling, bleeding, skull fractures, or tumors
Magnetic resonance imaging (MRI)	Uses a constant magnetic field and radio waves to produce detailed images of the brain and its tissues	White matter and gray matter abnormalities seen in many psychiatric disorders

Table 3.2 Functional Imaging Techniques

Functional imaging techniques allow for direct visualization of brain activation patterns, including the physiological and biochemical processes associated with specific mental activities (such as thinking; feeling; or reacting to visual, auditory, or tactile stimuli) and symptoms of various mental disorders.

Functional Imaging Techniques	Description	What Is Detected?
Electroencephalograph (EEG)	Electrodes attached to the scalp detect electrical activity from neurons firing in the cortex	Confirms coma or brain death; detects seizures
Magnetoencephalography (MEG)	Electrodes within a helmet measure the magnetic field generated from electrical activity occurring close to the brain's surface	Provides even more precise localization and measurement of surface electrical activity than the EEG
Functional magnetic resonance imaging (fMRI)	Constant magnetic field and radio waves measure changes in blood flow and oxygenation	Can detect location and patterns of brain activation associated with different mental processes and reduced blood flow associated with clots
Diffusion tensor imaging (DTI)	An MRI variation that uses a magnetic field and radio waves to track diffusion of water molecules throughout the brain	Provides data regarding axons, nerve fibers, and connections, including how white matter injury relates to cognitive or motor symptoms
Positron emission tomography (PET)	Nuclear imaging technique using computer monitoring of a radioactive tracer injected into the bloodstream	Can detect neuronal damage and neurochemical changes, including gene expression and activity of some neurotransmitters, as well as other brain activity
Single photon emission computed tomography (SPECT)	Less expensive and less detailed nuclear imaging technique	Provides basic information about metabolism and blood flow for a longer time period than a PET scan

Electroencephalograph (EEG)

This woman is undergoing an electroencephalograph (EEG). Electrodes placed on her skull are measuring and recording her brain waves.

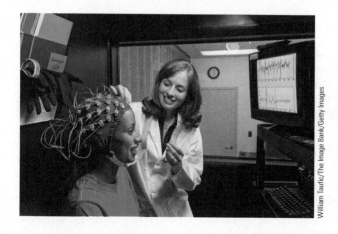

William Taufic/The Image Bank/Getty Images

Other forms of functional imaging can measure metabolic processes on the brain's surface and much deeper. Rather than a static image of the brain's anatomy, it is possible to evaluate the brain in action. In fact, functional imaging demonstrates which brain regions are active during the resting state and the changes that occur during various mental activities or emotional states. For example, nuclear imaging procedures such as *positron emission tomography (PET)* reveal brain processes using small quantities of radioactive substances and special cameras that detect radioactivity. If you were to have a PET scan, you would be given an intravenous injection of glucose (sugar) combined with a radioactive (positron-emitting) tracer; the scanner then follows the tracer to evaluate how your brain is metabolizing the glucose. Brain activity and subtle metabolic changes measured during PET imaging can indicate active disease or malignant tumors. Researchers also use PET scans to compare the outcomes of psychotherapy and medications by observing brain activity changes in regions of the brain associated with the disorder being treated (McGrath et al., 2013; Yuan et al., 2022).

Although most neuroimaging techniques cannot elucidate biochemical changes occurring within the brain, the radioactive tracers used in PET provide unique information regarding the release, uptake, and transport of neurotransmitters and gene expression (Potter et al., 2013). Unfortunately, the tracers used in PET technology are short-lived, requiring close proximity to expensive generators (cyclotrons) equipped to produce radioactive substances. *Single photon emission computed tomography (SPECT)* imaging is a less expensive nuclear imaging technique that uses a longer-lived radioactive substance to produce images of metabolic activity and blood flow similar to those obtained through PET scans, but with less detail.

Functional magnetic resonance imaging (fMRI) provides images of brain structures combined with physiological activity in different brain regions. It is a newer, noninvasive procedure that does not involve radioactivity. fMRI reveals details such as where blood is flowing and which nerve cells are actively using oxygen. Medical professionals also use a multimodal neuroimaging technique in which EEG and fMRI data are recorded simultaneously in order to study the association between electrical brain activity and blood circulation within the brain. Another variation of MRI technology is *diffusion tensor imaging (DTI)*, which tracks the diffusion (movement) of water molecules throughout the brain; this imaging provides pictures of axons and the networks of nerve fibers (white matter) that connect different brain areas.

These techniques, either individually or in combination, allow the study of brain abnormalities and distinct metabolic patterns of people diagnosed with a mental disorder. Each of the neuroimaging techniques has strengths and weaknesses in terms of costs, benefits, and possible side effects. Evaluating the risks and benefits helps determine which tools to use for research, diagnosis, treatment, and monitoring of disease progression. Because of these techniques, our knowledge of brain structure and function associated with a variety of mental disorders has increased significantly. Combining these procedures with other assessments helps us learn even more about how physiological processes relate to psychological processes. Some researchers predict that these techniques will eventually allow clinicians to make more rapid and more specific diagnoses and provide information that helps guide treatment.

PET Scan

These PET scans illustrate the difference in brain activity between someone with normal brain functioning (left) and someone with neurological dysfunction in which brain activity is significantly reduced (right).

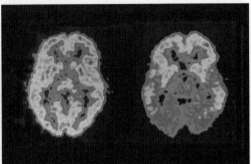

Mediscan/Alamy Stock Photo

3-3 Diagnosing Mental Disorders

After gathering assessment data, clinicians formulate diagnoses using a psychiatric classification system. These classification systems use various indicators of atypical behavior, thought processes, and emotional disturbance to make a determination regarding which distinct category is the closest match to the client's symptoms. Psychiatric classification systems are like a catalog: A detailed description accompanies each mental disorder. Thus, the pattern of behavior and symptomology associated with each diagnosis is distinctly different. For example, the concerns associated with social anxiety disorder are different from the symptoms that define schizophrenia. At the same time, each category also accommodates symptom variations. For instance, the exact symptoms, symptom severity, and length of depressive episodes vary among people who receive the diagnosis of major depressive disorder.

Structural MRI (left) and functional MRI (right) scans reveal that some violent individuals have structural and metabolic abnormalities in the anterior cingulate cortex, a brain region associated with the regulation of impulses (blue area in the front part of the brain at the left and corresponding yellow area in brain at the right). The two types of MRI scans reveal differences in brain volume (structural MRI) and brain activity (functional MRI).

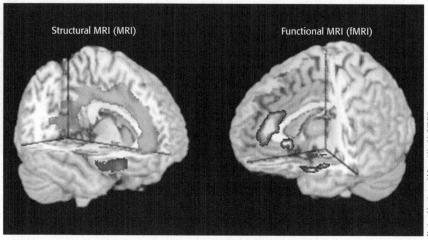

Structural MRI (MRI)   Functional MRI (fMRI)

National Institute of Mental Health (NIMH)

The *Diagnostic and Statistical Manual of Mental Disorders*

The *Diagnostic and Statistical Manual of Mental Disorders* (DSM) is a widely used classification system for psychiatric disorders. The DSM lists all officially designated mental disorders and the characteristics or symptoms needed to confirm a diagnosis. Diagnostic criteria include the physical, behavioral, and emotional characteristics associated with each disorder. For all disorders, the symptoms must cause significant distress or impairment in social, occupational, or other important areas of functioning (APA, 2022).

The DSM is based on the classification philosophy developed by Emil Kraepelin in the mid-19th century. Kraepelin believed that mental disorders were like physical disorders, each with a specific set of symptoms. Thus, the DSM has traditionally been a categorical system, listing disorders and the various characteristics, course, and outcome associated with each. As with physical illnesses, the diagnostic process involves deciding whether a person meets the specific criteria for a particular condition. The process of diagnosing mental disorders, however, is complex because disorders often have overlapping symptoms, making it difficult to distinguish one from another. For example, depressive and anxiety disorders share some of the same symptoms and have common neurobiological underpinnings and responsiveness to antidepressant medications (Grisanzio et al., 2018).

To add to the complexity, the number of identified psychological disorders has increased dramatically over time. In 1840, the U.S. census had only two categories of mental disorders—idiocy or insanity (Cloud, 2010). Since then, the number of disorders acknowledged by the American Psychiatric Association, the organization that publishes the DSM, has increased:

- DSM, 1952: 106 mental disorders
- DSM-II, 1968: 182 mental disorders
- DSM-III, 1980: 265 mental disorders

- DSM-III-R, 1987: 292 mental disorders
- DSM-IV, 1994: 297 mental disorders

The most recent revisions of the diagnostic manual, DSM-5 (APA, 2013) and DSM-5-TR (APA, 2022), did not significantly increase the number of diagnostic categories but did include changes in some diagnostic criteria as well as the addition of several new disorders. The areas that received the most extensive updating included prevalence, prognostic signs, sex- and gender-related diagnostic issues, cultural-related factors, and symptom codes for suicidal and self-injurious behavior. Table 3.3 lists the DSM-5/DSM-5-TR categories of mental disorders, most of which are discussed in this book. Although the DSM-5-TR and the previous DSM-5 are touted as an improvement over previous editions of the manual, they are not without their own set of controversies.

Table 3.3 DSM-5/DSM-5-TR Disorders

Categories of Disorders	Features
Neurodevelopmental Disorders	Cognitive, learning, and language disabilities evident early in life
Neurocognitive Disorders	Psychological or behavioral abnormalities associated with dysfunction of the brain
Substance-Related and Addictive Disorders	Excessive use of alcohol, illicit drugs, or prescription medications that results in impaired functioning; behavioral addictions such as gambling
Schizophrenia Spectrum and Other Psychotic Disorders	Disorders marked by severe impairment in thinking and perception; often involving delusions, hallucinations, and inappropriate affect
Bipolar and Related Disorders	Disorders characterized by episodes of mania or hypomania, alternating with periods of normal and/or depressed mood
Depressive Disorders	Disorders involve feelings of sadness, emptiness, and social withdrawal
Anxiety Disorders	Disorders characterized by excessive or irrational anxiety or fear, often accompanied by avoidance behaviors and fearful cognitions or worry
Obsessive-Compulsive and Related Disorders	Disorders characterized by obsessions (recurrent thoughts) and/or compulsions (repetitive behaviors) and other compulsive behavior such as hoarding
Trauma and Stressor-Related Disorders	Disorders associated with chronic or acute reactions to trauma and stress
Somatic Symptom and Related Disorders	Disorders involving physical symptoms that cause distress and disability, including high levels of health anxiety and disproportionate concern over bodily dysfunctions
Dissociative Disorders	Disturbance or alteration in memory, identity, or consciousness, including amnesia, having two or more distinct personalities, or experiencing feelings of depersonalization
Sexual Dysfunctions	Disorders involving the disruption of any stage of a normal sexual response cycle, including desire, arousal, or orgasm
Gender Dysphoria	Significant distress associated with conflict between biological sex and gender assigned at birth
Paraphilias	Recurrent, intense sexual fantasies or urges involving nonhuman objects, pain, humiliation, or children
Eating Disorders	Disturbed eating patterns and body dissatisfaction, involving bingeing, purging, and excessive dieting
Sleep-Wake Disorders	Problems in initiating/maintaining sleep, excessive sleepiness, sleep disruptions, sleepwalking, or repeated awakening associated with nightmares
Personality Disorders	Disorders involving stable personality traits that are inflexible and maladaptive and notably impair functioning or cause subjective distress

Each revision of the DSM has attempted to correct or reduce problems in previous editions and improve the reliability and validity of the diagnostic system. Testing the reliability and validity of a diagnostic category involves having clinicians independently interview and formulate diagnoses for the same client, based on DSM criteria. Agreement between the clinicians (interrater reliability) is then measured. Studies conducted with prior editions of the DSM found poor agreement (poor interrater reliability) in diagnosis based on the same information; one clinician reviewing case information on an individual might diagnose an anxiety disorder, whereas another clinician reviewing the same information might diagnose depression. Although the reliability and validity of many of the DSM diagnoses have been problematic over the years, there has been improvement with each successive edition, with the exception of the DSM-5. With the DSM-5, some, but not all, diagnostic categories achieved adequate validity and reliability (refer to Figure 3.3). What is especially problematic is the "questionable" reliability of some of the most common diagnoses—major depressive disorder and generalized anxiety disorder. Both of these diagnoses now have lower reliability compared to the two previous editions of the DSM (Stetka et al., 2013).

Dimensional Perspective

The DSM employs a categorical model—it provides a category or label for each disorder. Many researchers and mental health professionals believe that a categorical diagnostic system such as the DSM is problematic because individuals with a specific diagnosis often display a range of symptoms. Additionally, as we previously discussed, some diagnostic categories have overlapping symptoms. For example, in addition to the overlap in characteristics associated with depression and anxiety disorders, similarities in symptom patterns have been found between major depressive disorder, panic disorders, and posttraumatic stress disorder (Grisanzio et al., 2018) and between obsessive-compulsive disorder and generalized anxiety disorder (Gillan et al., 2019).

Comorbidity refers to the presence of two or more disorders in the same person. The fact that certain disorders often co-occur (are comorbid) is another complication of a categorical system. Along the same lines, some medications are effective across diagnostic categories, a finding that brings into question whether the diagnostic categories are truly distinct (Gillan et al., 2019). For instance, depression is often accompanied by an anxiety disorder (comorbidity), and certain antidepressants have demonstrated effectiveness with both conditions. Because of these problems, clinicians and researchers involved in revising the DSM discussed the possibility of changing the DSM to a dimensional classification system. However, this perspective was rejected—the categorical system was deemed to be of greater use in clinical practice.

In a dimensional model of mental disorders, disorders are seen to occur on a continuum, with "normality" appearing at one end of the continuum and severe forms of a disorder at the opposite end. From a dimensional perspective, anxiety, depression, and even psychotic-like experiences would not constitute an "either–or" phenomenon; instead, clinicians would rate the degree to which a person demonstrates characteristics of a particular condition (Komasi et al., 2022). Such an approach would allow characteristics that occur across different disorders to be identified and specifically studied.

Research targeting specific symptoms that occur across different disorders might enhance our understanding of causal factors and improve treatment. Using a dimensional approach to diagnosis would also address

Did You Know?

Learning one's genetic risk for obesity may cause physical and psychological changes that are independent of actual genetic risk. A group of adults diagnosed with obesity were genotyped for genetic risk of obesity and assessed on measures of satiety, exercise capacity, and cardiovascular response to exercise. They were then randomly assigned to receive "information" that they were at either high or low genetic risk of obesity. Regardless of their actual genotype, the genetic "feedback" they received influenced subsequent measures of their satiety, cardiorespiratory responses, and exercise endurance levels (Turnwald et al., 2019).

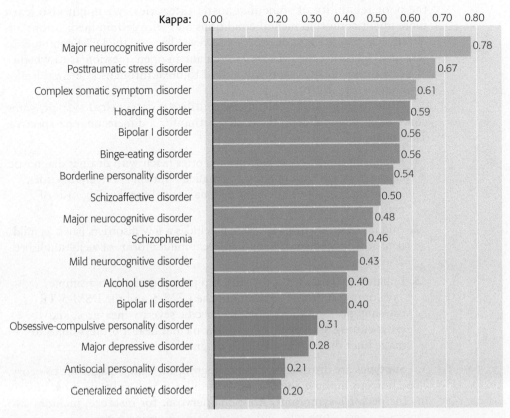

Adult Diagnoses

	Kappa
Major neurocognitive disorder	0.78
Posttraumatic stress disorder	0.67
Complex somatic symptom disorder	0.61
Hoarding disorder	0.59
Bipolar I disorder	0.56
Binge-eating disorder	0.56
Borderline personality disorder	0.54
Schizoaffective disorder	0.50
Major neurocognitive disorder	0.48
Schizophrenia	0.46
Mild neurocognitive disorder	0.43
Alcohol use disorder	0.40
Bipolar II disorder	0.40
Obsessive-compulsive personality disorder	0.31
Major depressive disorder	0.28
Antisocial personality disorder	0.21
Generalized anxiety disorder	0.20

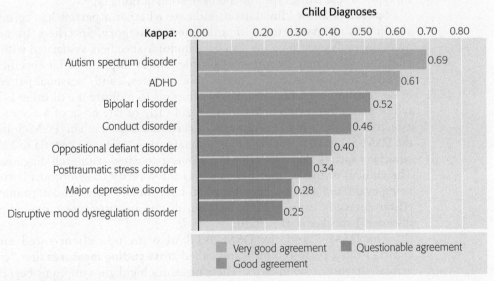

Child Diagnoses

	Kappa
Autism spectrum disorder	0.69
ADHD	0.61
Bipolar I disorder	0.52
Conduct disorder	0.46
Oppositional defiant disorder	0.40
Posttraumatic stress disorder	0.34
Major depressive disorder	0.28
Disruptive mood dysregulation disorder	0.25

Very good agreement   Questionable agreement
Good agreement

Figure 3.3

Interrater Reliability of DSM-5 Diagnostic Categories*

During the DSM-5 field trials, individuals undergoing diagnostic evaluation were assessed by two clinicians; each clinician interviewed the person and made a diagnosis. Kappa scores from the field trials (which take into account diagnostic agreement between clinicians and data regarding the frequency of a diagnosis) varied significantly for both adult and child/adolescent diagnostic categories.

Source: Modified from Freedman et al., 2013

*Interrater reliability for the diagnostic categories was not updated for the DSM-5-TR.

some of the shortcomings of a categorical classification system, including the poor reliability of some diagnostic categories. We might also learn more about comorbid mental conditions and why certain medications are effective across different disorders. However, because the DSM continues to rely on diagnostic categories, it will remain an open question as to whether or not a dimensional system would lead to breakthroughs in mental health research and treatment.

Although the DSM continues to utilize a categorical system, some concessions were made to those advocating for a dimensional perspective. They include:

1. Replacing the different autism categories (each with distinct diagnostic characteristics) with one disorder called "autism spectrum disorder," and adding an alternative dimensional model for the diagnosis of personality disorders.

2. Adding "risk syndromes," which includes a few disorders (such as mild neurocognitive disorder) that represent milder forms of well-established disorders.

3. Enhancing assessment procedures to permit more than a simple "yes-or-no" option. For example, the DSM-5 and the DSM-5-TR use subtypes, specifiers, disorder-specific severity measures, and cross-cutting assessments that allow mental health professionals to make finer distinctions within a diagnosis.

Subtypes are distinctly different subgroups within a diagnostic category. The clinician making the diagnosis decides which subtype most closely fits the person's symptoms. Anorexia nervosa, for instance, includes two subtypes: a restricting type and a binge-eating/purging type.

Specifiers allow clinicians to indicate whether a person has certain characteristics associated with a diagnostic category. Specifiers are not mutually exclusive, so people can have multiple specifiers associated with a diagnosis. With major depressive disorder, for example, possible specifiers include "anxious distress," "melancholic features," and "seasonal pattern of depression." Specifiers also allow clinicians to indicate if a disorder is in full or partial **remission** or if someone had early or late onset of a disorder, a factor that affects the **prognosis** of certain disorders. The DSM-5 and the DSM-5-TR also provide a dimensional rating scale with criteria to help clinicians specify the severity of symptoms associated with each diagnosis. The clinical utility of specifiers such as the severity of symptoms is still being evaluated and has been found to have limited value in determining effectiveness of treatment for at least one diagnostic category—binge-eating disorder (Lydecker et al., 2020).

The DSM-5 and the DSM-5-TR also include client-rated and clinician-rated symptom measures called **cross-cutting measures** that "cut across" diagnostic boundaries. These measures highlight symptoms beyond those associated with a diagnosed disorder. Clinicians first use a brief screening questionnaire involving symptoms that frequently occur in individuals coping with a mental disorder, such as suicidal tendencies. A follow-up questionnaire is then used to further assess areas that emerge as a possible concern. These questionnaires identify and address key symptoms that may affect prognosis and treatment. Additionally, they help clinicians track the severity of symptoms and monitor changes throughout treatment. They also help clinicians determine if a person has a comorbid disorder.

In addition to assessment and diagnosis, clinicians also identify factors that may affect a client's prognosis. For example, therapists consider the causes of diagnosed disorders to help plan treatment. The DSM, therefore, includes a focus on "other conditions that may be a focus of clinical attention." Let's look at an example of a comprehensive diagnostic evaluation based on the DSM-5-TR.

Case Study Mark is a 50-year-old machine operator referred for treatment by his work supervisor due to concerns about his frequent absenteeism and difficulty getting along with others. Coworkers complain that Mark distrusts others and overreacts with anger to any perceived criticism. The supervisor suspects that Mark drinks alcohol during work hours. The supervisor is unaware that Mark recently received a diagnosis of cirrhosis of the liver due to his heavy drinking. In his assessment interview, Mark acknowledged that he consumes a large quantity of alcohol daily. He also shared that his wife recently left him, claiming she could no longer tolerate his drinking, his emotional withdrawal, his extreme jealousy, and his accusations of infidelity. Mark indicated he has no close friends, although he does hang out with "regulars" at a local bar.

During interviews with the therapist, Mark revealed that he began drinking in his early teens to help him "get through the day." He admitted drinking on the job but claimed it was "no big deal." He blames his parents and his wife for his drinking problems. Mark eventually shared that his father is an alcoholic who physically and verbally abused Mark and his siblings. Mark believes that his mother has stayed with his father only because of the family's Catholic religion.

Mark's pattern of heavy alcohol use is clearly interfering with his social and occupational functioning, and he continues drinking despite the loss of his marriage and risk of losing his job. This pattern is consistent with a diagnosis of alcohol use disorder with severe symptoms. Mark's distrust, suspiciousness, and hostility toward others have interfered with relationships since childhood and suggest a comorbid paranoid personality disorder.

Upon completing the DSM-5-TR cross-cutting screening measure, Mark's therapist noted problems with depression, sleep, memory, and excessive use of prescription medications as additional concerns. Further assessment revealed that Mark met the diagnostic criteria for a major depressive disorder with mild severity. His depressive symptoms have been evident since childhood and preceded his alcohol use. Assessments conducted by the therapist also revealed that Mark has some mild cognitive deficits, presumably resulting from his heavy alcohol consumption. Cirrhosis of the liver is a significant medical condition. The clinician noted Mark's pending divorce, work difficulties, and poor relationships with coworkers when assessing psychosocial functioning. Mark's diagnosis included:

- Alcohol use disorder; with a specifier of "severe"
- Paranoid personality disorder
- Major depressive disorder; with a specifier of "mild"
- Physical disorder: cirrhosis of the liver
- The clinician also addressed additional factors associated with Mark's diagnosis:

1. *Biological/genetic*—There is a family history of alcohol abuse. The early onset of Mark's heavy drinking may be related to genetic vulnerability to alcohol abuse or depression.

2. *Environmental*—Mark is in jeopardy of losing his job and is facing financial stress due to his upcoming divorce.

3. *Developmental*—Mark's father exhibited paranoia and drank heavily. Mark endured physical and psychological abuse throughout childhood. Mark began drinking in early adolescence to cope with feelings of worthlessness; early substance use appears to have affected emotional maturation and social development.

4. *Social*—There is limited family support. Mark's wife is seeking a divorce. Mark has very few friends other than a few "drinking buddies."

5. *Cultural*—Due to his Catholic upbringing, Mark is very concerned about family reactions to his upcoming divorce.

6. *Behavioral*—Mark tends to blame others and reacts with anger to perceived criticism. Mark has a strong tendency to be suspicious of others, a characteristic that has consistently interfered with social relationships. Mark has a long history of withdrawing and using alcohol to cope at home and at work.

Mark also completed the *World Health Organization Disability Schedule*—an instrument used to assess overall level of impairment and disability. His total score of 72 suggests moderately severe impairment; he has severe problems understanding, communicating, and getting along with other people and participating in society, and mild to moderate disability in getting around, self-care, and life activities. The therapist will use all of the information obtained from Mark's diagnostic assessment to develop a plan of treatment.

Cultural Factors in Assessment

Case Study David Henderson, an associate professor of psychiatry at Harvard Medical School, worked as a psychiatrist in Cambodia. While working in Cambodia, he found that every patient he interviewed reported hearing voices. He wondered why so many Cambodians had this symptom. When he later asked his Cambodian colleagues whether they had ever heard voices, they all answered affirmatively and observed, "It looks as if Dr. Henderson is the only one among us who has not been in touch with his ancestors." (Treichel, 2011)

Dr. Henderson's story is an excellent example of how our culture affects our worldview, including our view of psychological "symptoms." The influence of culture is also evident in the results of a study in which psychiatrists from either the United States or India ranked which symptoms they considered most important when making a variety of diagnoses. For most disorders, there was concurrence on the four most critical diagnostic symptoms. However, the psychiatrists diverged when diagnosing depression—with psychiatrists from India placing much more emphasis on somatic symptoms such as pain, sleep, and changes in appetite (Biswas et al., 2016).

Beyond understanding each client's cultural background, clinicians must also recognize how the presentation of mental illness varies across cultures. They must be able to determine whether a behavior is consistent with cultural norms or is evidence of mental illness. Culture not only affects diagnosis but also influences a person's willingness to seek help; it can also affect treatment variables such as how medication is metabolized (Lin, 2022).

Unfortunately, mental health assessment and diagnosis often fail to adequately consider racial or cultural factors. This issue needs to be addressed, given the projection that people from ethnically underrepresented groups will constitute over half of the U.S. population by the year 2045 (Frey, 2018). Although some progress has been made, advocates of culturally competent practice are concerned that more effort is needed to ensure that all clinicians understand the degree to which culture and ethnicity can influence assessment, diagnosis, and treatment (Sue et al., 2022).

The DSM affirms that cultural factors can impact how a person's symptoms are expressed and thus encourages consideration of cultural influences when making a diagnosis. To support increased consideration of culture, diagnostic characteristics for each DSM disorder now includes culture-related and gender-related diagnostic issues and risk factors such as discrimination and racism. Additionally, to improve the assessment and diagnosis of mental disorders among ethnically and culturally underrepresented populations, the DSM now includes a list of topics to explore with culturally diverse clients. This list includes factors such as the degree to which clients identify with their ethnic background, the presence of acculturation conflicts or stressors within their social network, and whether factors such as experiences with racism or discrimination might influence interactions during assessment and treatment or hamper the therapeutic relationship.

The DSM-5 and the DSM-5-TR also include an in-depth guide for conducting a cultural assessment interview that lists 16 questions to help determine the possible impact of culture on a client's symptoms. Here are some sample questions:

- "What do you think is causing your problem?" This question helps the therapist to understand the client's perception of the factors involved, including interpersonal, social, and cultural influences.

- "Why is this happening to you?" This question taps into the issue of causality and possible spiritual or cultural explanations for the problem.

- "What have you done to cope with or treat this condition?" This question can lead to a discussion of previous interventions, the possible use of spiritual remedies, and the client's evaluation of the usefulness of these treatments.

- "Your cultural identity or background can be a source of strength or can contribute to problems. How is it affecting your problem?" In answering this question, the client can discuss the positive aspects of cultural identity and the effects of factors such as discrimination and acculturation conflicts.

- "How has this condition affected your life?" This question helps identify individual, interpersonal, health, and social issues related to the concern.

In addition, there are queries regarding current stressors and supports, as well as perceived barriers to seeking help. The use of this clinical formulation interview combined with a brief training focused on improving a clinician's skill in working with culturally diverse populations appears to help therapists elicit their clients' perspectives regarding the concerns discussed, improve clinician–client rapport, and increase the clinician's understanding of the social and cultural context of the client's symptoms (Jarvis et al., 2020).

Did You Know?

People from ethnically underrepresented groups are now the majority in five states and in the District of Columbia.

Hawaii	78.2 percent
Washington, DC	63.5 percent
California	63.0 percent
New Mexico	62.6 percent
Texas	58.1 percent
Nevada	51.2 percent

Source: U.S. Census Bureau, 2018

Evaluation of the DSM-5/DSM-5-TR Classification System

The DSM-5 and the DSM-5-TR have received criticism regarding their construction, the lack of dimensional considerations, changes in diagnostic criteria for disorders, and the addition of new disorders. Along with the lower reliability for many diagnostic categories compared with previous DSM editions, other concerns include the following:

1. Viewing autistic and personality disorders along a continuum may have the unexpected consequence of broadening diagnostic boundaries to encompass people with less severe symptoms (Frances, 2013; Zeidan et al., 2022).

2. Criteria for certain disorders have changed and may increase the number of individuals receiving a diagnosis. For example, a review of 12 studies found that the DSM-5 criteria increased the prevalence of alcohol use disorder (Bartoli et al., 2015).

3. Decisions regarding the DSM-5 diagnostic categories may have been unduly influenced by outside pressure. For instance, 70 percent of the professionals who developed the DSM-5 had direct ties to pharmaceutical companies. This raises the concern that there may have been subtle pressure to broaden diagnostic categories, thereby increasing access to medication as a form of treatment (Cosgrove & Krimsky, 2012).

4. "Addictive" disorders now include gambling disorder, which opens the possibility that other "behavioral addictions" (e.g., Internet, video games, shopping, eating) may eventually be included in this category. In fact, Internet gaming disorder is currently under review for inclusion in the DSM.

5. A new diagnosis in DSM-5-TR, prolonged grief disorder, has the potential of turning intense grief into a pathological condition. For children and adolescents, the diagnosis can be given if the grief over the loss of a loved one lasts more than 6 months. The diagnosis has not been field tested, and little is known about its reliability or validity (Cacciatore & Frances, 2022).

6. Premenstrual dysphoric disorder, a diagnosis added during the DSM-5 revision, has been the subject of heated discussion. Critics of this category contend that symptoms associated with hormonal changes during menses should be treated as a physiological or gynecological disorder and that it is stigmatizing to women to label severe premenstrual mood swings as a psychiatric disorder. Pharmaceutical companies strongly supported this diagnosis (Schroll & Lauritsen, 2022).

7. Although the DSM has strengthened cultural considerations in diagnosis, the cross-cultural applicability of the system is still questioned. The prevalence of some disorders differs across the globe. It may be that some descriptions of disorders developed in Western countries simply do not fit other cultures.

Although there are many valid criticisms of the DSM, it is the most frequently used diagnostic and classification system in the United States and some other countries. Classification systems, like the DSM, not only facilitate diagnosing disorders, but they also help diagnosticians differentiate one disorder from another. Classification systems also facilitate communication between mental health professionals and provide diagnostic consistency for researchers who study the etiology and treatment of mental disorders. Without a classification system to identify, differentiate, and group disorders, it would be difficult to accomplish the above goals.

Although the DSM is widely used in the United States, another important classification system is the 11th edition of the International Classification of Disease (ICD), which took effect in 2022. The World Health Organization oversees the ICD system, which covers all health conditions, including mental disorders. Although there are significant differences between the DSM and the ICD diagnostic systems, the DSM diagnostic definitions increasingly align with the ICD classification of mental disorders. Both the DSM and the ICD affect consumers, health care providers, insurance companies, and the pharmaceutical industry.

Objections to Classification and Labeling

Although classification systems such as the DSM and the ICD are essential for diagnosing disorders, communicating information about disorders, and conducting research, they are also subject to criticism because of the negative consequences that sometimes result from classification and labeling.

1. *Labeling a person as having a mental disorder can result in overgeneralization, stigma, and stereotypes.* Stereotypes about certain mental disorders can lead to inaccurate generalizations about individuals and assumptions that may result in discriminatory behavior. When we respond to someone according to stereotypes, we are less likely to appreciate the person's strengths and unique qualities.

2. *A label may lead those who are labeled to believe that they do indeed possess characteristics associated with the label or may cause them to behave in accordance with the label.* When people are told that they have particular characteristics, they may come to believe what they are told; this may lead to cognitive and behavioral changes. Labels and stereotypes can influence individuals not only to act out the stereotypes but also to devalue their personal status. Internalized self-stigma can have a profound effect on a person's self-image (Drapalski et al., 2021).

3. *Although health care organizations often require labels, a mental health diagnosis does not necessarily provide useful information.* Despite health care systems' reliance on diagnoses for making decisions about treatment and health care reimbursement, a diagnosis itself does not provide information about treatment needs. The assessment of an individual's functioning at work, home, school, and elsewhere is often of much greater utility in treatment planning than is a particular clinical diagnosis.

Should Presidential Candidates Undergo Psychiatric Assessment?

During the 2016 presidential election campaign, Fox News requested that their medical team analyze videos of Hillary Clinton in which she displayed unsteady movements, coughing episodes, and uncharacteristic laughter. These medical professionals concluded that Clinton might be displaying signs of a postconcussion syndrome resulting from a head injury incurred in 2012 (Higbee, 2016). Dr. Drew, a celebrity physician, similarly claimed that Clinton was exhibiting signs of brain damage (Allen, 2016).

During the same election cycle, several psychologists were asked to give a diagnosis of Donald Trump for *Vanity Fair* magazine. Behaviors such as an exaggerated sense of self-importance, lack of empathy for others, inflation of achievements, denigration of others, and a constant need to prove himself resulted in agreement that Donald Trump met the criteria for a narcissistic personality disorder (Kilgore, 2015). Other psychiatrists volunteered to testify about President Trump's "dangerous and fragile" mental state during his first impeachment hearing (Feinberg, 2019).

Should mental health professionals and physicians give their opinion regarding a diagnosis involving politicians or celebrities? Although most physicians and mental health professionals are not bound by professional constraints against sharing their views, psychiatrists are ethically prohibited from expressing their opinion about an individual who is in the public eye unless that person has disclosed personal information through public media. In such circumstances, a psychiatrist may share opinions about psychiatric issues in general. However, a psychiatrist may not offer a professional opinion about someone without having conducted an examination and being granted authorization for making a public statement about the evaluation (Ghaemi, 2016).

This ethical standard, popularly known as the "Goldwater rule," was adopted in 1973 as a result of a magazine survey of psychiatrists regarding the mental status of U.S. presidential candidate Barry Goldwater. Of the psychiatrists who responded to the survey, almost 1,200 believed Goldwater was mentally unfit to serve as president. Some saw him as paranoid, schizophrenic, or having a personality disorder. The American Psychiatric Association was aghast that these diagnostic opinions were given without a personal evaluation and without Mr. Goldwater's consent. Dr. Maria Oquendo, past president of the American Psychiatric Association, agreed that psychoanalyzing presidential candidates is not only unethical but also irresponsible (Oquendo, 2016).

Not everyone agrees with the Goldwater rule. Nassir Ghaemi, a psychiatrist, believes that a personal evaluation is not necessary if "sufficient documentation" of the individual's mental status is available. In addition, he believes that there are times when psychiatrists have a duty to report a diagnosis about political leaders even if consent has not been obtained, for example, if not knowing the diagnosis would lead to "serious political and social circumstances." Ghaemi refers to Adolph Hitler as an example where information regarding a diagnosis would have had significant societal importance. To avoid this ethical dilemma, Ghaemi believes that all political candidates should undergo not only a physical examination but also a psychiatric evaluation (Ghaemi, 2016).

For Further Consideration

1. What are the advantages and disadvantages of the Goldwater rule?

2. Should this ethical restriction also apply to physicians and other mental health professionals?

3. Under what circumstances might a professional have sufficient documentation to make an accurate diagnosis of a political figure?

4. How can we be certain that biases on the part of the assessor are not influencing the process of sharing public opinions about a politician's mental health?

3-4 Contemporary Trends and Future Directions

Two trends in assessment and classification, with somewhat opposing perspectives, have emerged: (1) increased reliance on the biological model to provide guidance in assessing and diagnosing mental disorders and (2) increased and more careful consideration of psychological, social, and sociocultural factors along with a focus on comprehensive, multifaceted assessment.

Let's first consider the biological perspective and the view that the DSM is an inadequate categorical diagnostic system based only on clusters of symptoms that have insufficient validity for guiding treatment and research. Because of these concerns, there has been an increased interest in a neuroscientific or "precision medicine" approach to mental illness focused on identifying and grouping psychiatric symptoms based on biological markers such as genes, brain structure, and physiological functioning. This alternative framework known as RDoC (Research Domain Criteria) is directed toward the classification of patients based on neurobiological measures such as genetic profiles, imaging results, or physiological traits (Alonso et al., 2019). In addition to identifying biomarkers associated with psychiatric disorders, some researchers are using noninvasive imaging such as transcranial magnetic stimulation (TMS) to both examine cortical functioning patterns in psychiatric patients and to treat symptoms by modulating neural dysfunctions (Ferrarelli & Phillips, 2021). Although there is no immediate plan for the RDoC framework to replace the DSM diagnostic system, some researchers expect that this evidence-based system of biological research into how physiological processes affect behaviors and mental functioning will ultimately yield novel diagnostic approaches that will improve treatment.

Although it is hoped that simple biomarkers will be able to inexpensively and reliably predict an individual client's response to treatment, researchers have not yet located biomarkers that reliably assist with the identification of causes, outcome, or treatment of mental illnesses (Lozupone et al., 2017). Despite this reality, many biological researchers characterize mental disorders as disorders of neural patterns or brain circuits (Cao et al., 2021). Kupfer (2013), a leader in the development of the DSM-5, calls the search for biological and genetic markers a welcome effort but believes success in the quest to locate such biomarkers remains "disappointingly distant."

Other researchers believe that viewing mental disorders as biomedical illnesses similar to cancer or diabetes is a mistake. They argue that current models of neuroscience are insufficiently developed to take a predominant role in the development of diagnostic systems (Paris & Kirmayer, 2016). They contend that it is impossible to learn all that we need to know about a client by studying genetics, brain structure, and brain circuits and that we cannot afford to ignore the influence of factors such as cultural and social stressors, discrimination, abuse, trauma, and poverty on the development and course of mental illness (Kim et al., 2018). Additionally, there is no doubt that psychological processes, such as maladaptive thinking patterns, play a role in the development of some mental disorders. It is significant that certain psychotherapies, such as cognitive-behavioral therapy, have proven to be more effective than medication for some mental illnesses (Öst et al., 2015).

Although biological research and neuroscience continue to provide new insight into the study of mental disorders, many hope that we do not abandon research into the many psychological, social, and sociocultural influences associated with mental illness. Interestingly, the increased focus on appropriate assessment practices for those from diverse backgrounds has highlighted the importance of ensuring that all clinicians understand how social and cultural factors can influence the development of mental disorders as well as the assessment process.

There is a growing consensus that mental health professionals are not merely objective observers, and that accurate diagnosis and treatment of mental disorders are dependent upon the characteristics, values, and worldview of both the clinician and the client (APA Presidential Task Force on Evidence-Based Practice, 2006; Marquine & Jimenez, 2020).

Thus, it is increasingly recognized that self-assessment is a necessary step when clinicians work with clients whose backgrounds differ from their own. For example, assumptions a clinician holds regarding aging, gender roles, sexual orientation, social class, or political philosophy may influence the diagnostic process. Careful self-assessment allows clinicians to identify and counteract any biases, errors in thinking, or stereotypes that may be influencing their work.

In the areas of diagnosis and assessment, we will continue to benefit from advances based on biological research as well as acknowledging the importance of psychological, social, and sociocultural factors in the development of psychopathology. We believe that an integrative assessment framework, such as the multipath model, that emphasizes consideration of the multitude of factors that can affect both mental health and mental illness, is essential if we want to effectively assess, diagnose, and treat mental disorders.

Chapter Summary

1 **How do we know if psychological tests and evaluation procedures are accurate?**

- In developing assessment tools and classification systems, it is important to consider reliability (the degree to which a procedure or test yields consistent results) and validity (the extent to which a test or procedure actually performs the function it was designed to perform).

2 **How do mental health professionals evaluate a client's mental health?**

- Clinicians primarily use four methods of assessment: observations, interviews, psychological tests and inventories, and neurological tests.

- Interviews involve a face-to-face conversation, after which the interviewer reviews and interprets information obtained from the interviewee.

- Observations of behaviors and personal characteristics can have diagnostic significance.

- The mental status examination is frequently used as an interview tool during assessment.

- Psychological tests and inventories provide a more formalized means of obtaining information.

- Neurological assessments, including X-rays, CT and PET scans, EEG, and MRI, have added highly important and sophisticated means to detect brain abnormalities.

3 **How do professionals make a psychiatric diagnosis?**

- Professionals consider all available information and evaluate the pattern of symptoms to determine if there is a mental disorder. The DSM, used by the majority of mental health professionals, contains detailed diagnostic criteria.

- The DSM-5 and the DSM-5-TR primarily use categorical assessment but include some dimensional measures, symptom rating systems, and culturally relevant interviews that enhance assessment.

4 **What changes are occurring in the field of psychological assessment?**

- Neuroscientists are advocating for assessment systems that rely on biologically based data.

- Other groups advocate for the use of comprehensive assessment models that include psychological, social, and sociocultural as well as biological factors; the importance of considering the worldview and potential biases of those conducting the assessment is also emphasized.

Chapter Glossary

comorbidity
co-occurrence of two or more disorders in the same person

cross-cutting measure
assesses common symptoms that are not specific to one disorder

functional imaging
procedures that provide data regarding physiological and biochemical processes occurring within the brain

prognosis
prediction of the probable outcome of a disorder, including the chances of full recovery

projective personality test
testing involving responses to ambiguous stimuli, such as inkblots, pictures, or incomplete sentences

psychological assessment
the process of gathering information and drawing conclusions about an individual's traits, skills, abilities, and emotional functioning

psychosis
a condition involving loss of contact with or a distorted view of reality, including disorganized thinking, false beliefs, or seeing or hearing things that are not there

reliability
the degree to which a procedure or test yields consistent results

remission
a significant improvement in the symptoms of a disorder

specifier
specific features associated with a diagnostic category

standardization
the use of identical procedures in the administration of tests

standardization sample
the comparison group on which test norms are based

structural imaging
procedures that allow for visualization of brain anatomy

subtype
mutually exclusive subgrouping within a diagnosis

validity
the extent to which a test or procedure actually measures what it was designed to measure

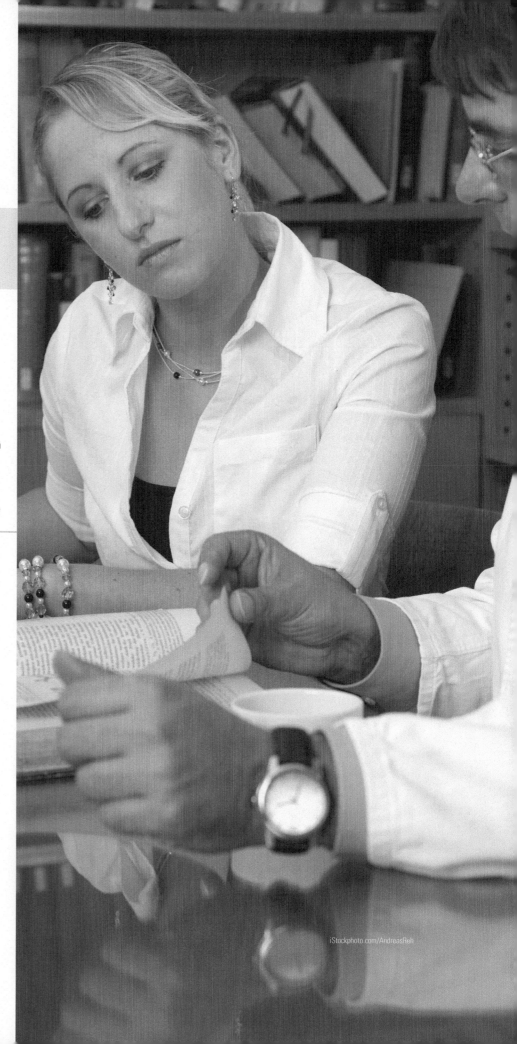

focus
Questions

1 What methods do researchers use to study the causes of and treatments for psychopathology?

2 How does biological research help us understand the causes of psychopathological behavior?

3 Why is epidemiological research important in understanding mental illness?

4 What are current trends in research into psychopathology?

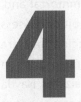

Research Methods for Studying Mental Disorders

Learning Objectives

After studying this chapter, you will be able to . . .

4-1 Outline the methods that researchers use to study the causes of and treatments for psychopathology.

4-2 Explain how biological research can help us to understand the causes of psychopathological behavior.

4-3 Describe why epidemiological research is important in understanding mental illness.

4-4 Discuss current trends in research into psychopathology.

A 24-Year-Old Married Woman from Puerto Rico, Nayda, reported that she was in "utter anguish" and incapacitated by "epileptic fits." A strong headache usually preceded her seizures, which involved convulsions and a loss of consciousness. A neurologist diagnosed her condition as intractable (difficult-to-treat) epilepsy. Nayda's psychotherapist, however, believed that some of Nayda's symptoms were inconsistent with those seen in epilepsy. First, when regaining consciousness, Nayda sometimes did not recognize her husband or children. Second, during her seizures, she appeared fearful and would beg an invisible presence to have mercy and not to kill her. Third, during these episodes, Nayda often hit herself and burned

items in the house. Her most recent seizures included hallucinations involving blood and an attempt to strangle herself with a rope.

Because Nayda's symptoms were not consistent with those commonly seen in epilepsy, the therapist wanted to determine if the seizures were psychogenic (generated from psychological causes). She asked Nayda if she had suffered any significant trauma in her life. Nayda told of an event that had occurred when she was 17 years old—2 years before the seizures began. She tearfully related that one night at about 2 a.m., she was awakened by the smell of something burning. She was shocked to find her grandmother's house in flames (her grandmother lived in a small house in the backyard). Strangely, she decided to go back to sleep and repeatedly told herself, "Tomorrow I will tell my parents of the fire" (Martinez-Taboas, 2005, p. 8). A few minutes later, the smoke awakened the rest of the family. Their attempts to rescue the grandmother failed. It was later determined that the grandmother had set the fire to take her own life. When asked about her feelings regarding the incident, Nayda cried profusely, saying she was responsible for her grandmother's death.

The therapist concluded that it was highly probable that this traumatic event was causing the seizure episodes. She also wanted to investigate the possibility that cultural influences were contributing to Nayda's symptoms. In many Latin American countries, there is a belief in *espiritismo*—that the soul is immortal and, under certain circumstances, able to inhabit or possess a living person. Auditory or visual hallucinations are common among those experiencing espiritismo. When asked what she believed was causing her seizures, Nayda explained that the spirit of her grandmother was not at peace and was causing her seizures and other problems. She believed that her failure to help her grandmother resulted in a disturbed and vengeful spirit. Using the case study method to understand Nayda's psychological distress and then employing a therapeutic approach that combined cognitive therapy with Nayda's cultural beliefs, the therapist succeeded in eliminating Nayda's distressing seizure episodes.

Science and research inform the study of psychopathological behavior. Nayda's story demonstrates several important points regarding clinical research. First, professionals tend to interpret events from a perspective that is consistent with their own background and field of study. For example, proponents of the biological model may focus on physical causes for symptoms, with little attention to psychological or environmental factors. In the case of Nayda, the neurologist believed that the seizures were due to epilepsy and prescribed an antiseizure medication to treat her condition. Conversely, psychological theorists tend to view disorders primarily from a psychological framework, placing less emphasis on biological, social, or sociocultural explanations. For instance, a psychologist with a cognitive-behavioral perspective might focus on Nayda's irrational thoughts and intervene by challenging her illogical beliefs. Fortunately, in Nayda's case, the therapist viewed the symptoms from both a psychological and a sociocultural perspective; this broader perspective acknowledged both the distress associated with Nayda's intense self-blame and important aspects of Nayda's cultural belief system.

Similarly, researchers frequently design studies based on their personal perspectives about possible causes of psychopathology. When you review research, remembering this fact will help you keep an open mind and avoid inaccurate assumptions. Instead of concluding that a single factor is responsible for a condition, you can consider how a particular study intersects with other research and how various contributing factors may interact. For example, shortly after the discovery of a gene associated with obesity made headlines, media attention focused on another study that reported an increased likelihood of obesity among those who socialize with people who are overweight. After reading such divergent explanations, you might wonder: Is obesity due to genetic influences, or is it related to our social relationships? To answer questions such as this, it is important to evaluate the perspectives of the researchers and the quality of the research and to consider whether other researchers are coming to similar conclusions.

We now know that the majority of mental health disorders are the result of a convergence of biological, psychological, social, and sociocultural risk factors. Thus, when you come across mental health research, it is essential to remember that mental disorders are complex and, therefore, best understood from an integrative perspective. Researchers and mental health practitioners must open-mindedly investigate all possible causes and consider alternative explanations for behavior, the approach taken by Nayda's therapist. Additionally, as you will discover in this chapter, understanding different research designs and their shortcomings will help you evaluate reported findings about psychopathology.

4-1 Research Methods Used to Study Mental Disorders

Mental health practitioners rely on scientifically verified information to guide both diagnosis and treatment. Thus, they rely on data generated using the **scientific method**—a process of inquiry that incorporates systematic collection of data, controlled observation, and the testing of hypotheses. A **hypothesis** is a tentative explanation for certain facts or observations— an idea that can be tested by further investigation. Examples of hypotheses investigated by researchers include "Seasonal forms of depression are due to decreases in light," "Exposure to certain food dyes causes hyperactivity," and "Eating disorders develop due to exposure to models and celebrities who are extremely thin." A **theory**—a group of principles and hypotheses that together explain some aspect of a particular area of inquiry—is much broader than a hypothesis.

Recalling the large number of theories developed to explain psychopathology that we covered in Chapter 2, you probably would not be surprised to learn that researchers generate many different hypotheses when studying mental disorders. For example, hypothesized explanations for eating disorders include genetic vulnerability, fear of sexual maturity, societal demands for thinness in women, and unhealthy family relationships. Each of these hypotheses comes from a different theoretical perspective. Researchers in the field of psychopathology design studies to test hypotheses about the causes of and treatments for mental disorders.

Scientists are often described as skeptics. Rather than accept the conclusions from a single study, scientists demand that other researchers replicate (repeat) the results. As Nosek observed, "Learning new things is hard, and a single study is not enough to establish new knowledge" (Samarrai, 2013). Replicating research reduces the chance that findings are due to experimenter bias, methodological flaws, or unusual characteristics of the group studied. Let's consider research findings that were initially reported as "conclusive" in the mass media. As you can see, some of the conclusions changed after further investigation:

- *Childhood vaccines may cause autism.* Due to media reports suggesting that childhood vaccines caused autism, many parents reported concerns about vaccine safety and side effects. The percentage of parents who felt vaccines were important dropped from 94 percent in 2001 to 84 percent in 2019 (Reinhart, 2019).

Brain Mapping

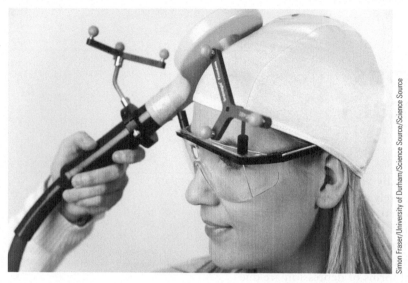

This woman is participating in an image-guided transcranial magnetic stimulation (TMS) brain mapping study, a technique that has advanced our understanding of brain physiology and psychiatric disorders.

Simon Fraser/University of Durham/Science Source/Science Source

Status: Research does not support a link between vaccines and autism, even among vaccinated high-risk children whose older sibling has a diagnosis of autism (DeStefano & Shimabukuro, 2020). In fact, the World Health Organization listed the antivaccination movement as one of the top risks to global health in 2019 (Trimble, 2019).

- *Antidepressants raise suicide risk in children and adolescents.* In 2004, there was considerable public reaction when the Food and Drug Administration (FDA) made the decision to require manufacturers of certain antidepressants to include a warning about increased risk of suicidal symptoms in children and adolescents.

  Status: This finding needs further research. Although some studies concluded that use of certain antidepressants is associated with an increase in suicide attempts in youth taking these antidepressants (Spielmans et al., 2013), others have found no such relationship (Strawn et al., 2015). In a meta-analysis of 34 studies involving 14 antidepressants prescribed to treat major depression in children and adolescents, only one antidepressant was linked to an increased risk of suicidal thoughts and attempts (Cipriani et al., 2016). However, the researchers concluded that the vast majority of antidepressants worked no better than a placebo—at least with children and adolescents diagnosed with major depression.

- *Cannabis use leads to the development of psychosis.* Drug prevention efforts nationwide cite this concern regarding marijuana use.

  Status: A number of well-designed studies support an association between marijuana use during adolescence and an increased risk of developing psychosis, particularly among those with a preexisting genetic vulnerability (Hill et al., 2022; Hjorthøj et al., 2023).

- *The majority of children who have experienced sexual abuse exhibit signs of trauma that can be reliably detected by experts in the field of child sexual abuse.* Many believe certain behaviors in children—including masturbating or mimicking movements of sexual activity, sleep disturbances, acting out behaviors, and regression to an earlier stage of life—are signs of sexual abuse.

  Status: There are no signs or symptoms that characterize the majority of children who have experienced sexual abuse. Although one should be alert to behavioral changes and indicators of stress, the signs above are nonspecific, and most children who have experienced abuse have no identifiable psychological symptoms (Pataki & Johnson, 2016).

As you can see, the search for "truth" is often a long journey. Reports regarding the causes of psychopathology come and go, and questions sometimes remain unanswered, as the following example demonstrates.

A mysterious illness involving uncontrolled bodily tics and verbal outbursts was reported in 15 teenagers (14 girls and 1 boy) in upstate New York. One girl spent most of her time in a wheelchair due to the severity of her symptoms. All of those affected attended Le Roy High School when these behavioral changes began (Graham, 2012). The New York Department of Health and local physicians found no medical or environmental explanations for the symptoms (Moisse & Davis, 2012).

Clinical phenomena such as the behaviors displayed by these teenagers need to be assessed and evaluated. Quality clinical research requires the development of specific hypotheses and decisions about which variables to investigate. Examples of hypotheses regarding the cause of the mysterious illness in New York have included suggestions that the symptoms may have resulted from (1) an environmental toxin, (2) an infection or other medical condition, or (3) psychological stressors. Researchers used the scientific method as they evaluated these hypotheses and other possible causes of the behaviors displayed by the teens. Specialists assessed the background and personal characteristics of each teen. Many of the girls had family issues that could cause psychological symptoms; for instance, one was assaulted by her father, and one witnessed her father's suicide (Porter, 2012). Doctors also looked for common medical conditions or environmental exposures that might explain the symptoms but found nothing.

Unfortunately, this situation remains unsolved. Some professionals are convinced that the symptoms are due to psychological factors, whereas others remain adamant that the teens' distressing symptoms resulted from unidentified environmental influences and that more inquiry is needed. Concern has been raised that the investigation into environmental toxins was prematurely terminated in favor of psychological explanations, thus resulting in a biased inquiry (Goldstein & Hall, 2015).

In evaluating research, we must consider the adequacy of the design used. Case studies (used with Nayda and the teens in New York), correlational approaches, and experimental designs are tools used in the field of psychopathology to study the characteristics, causes, and appropriate treatment for mental disorders. As Hunsley (2007) observed, "not all evidence is created equal" (p. 114). Some types of studies provide stronger evidence (more accuracy, reliability, and generalizability) because of their methodological or conceptual soundness (refer to Table 4.1).

If we were to construct an evidence hierarchy based on **internal validity** considerations (i.e., confidence that one thing causes another),

Table 4.1 Levels of Evidence

Randomized experimental designs are considered the gold standard in research because they can provide information regarding cause and effect relationships. Correlational and case studies furnish other important information, including ideas for hypotheses that can be tested using an experimental design.

Level 1: Randomized, controlled studies
Level 2: Observational studies and single-subject research design
Level 3: Case studies and clinical judgments or opinions

Adapted from Ghaemi (2010)

expert opinion and case studies would be placed on the lowest level of the hierarchy. Group research designs (such as correlational studies) and single-participant experimental designs generally provide stronger evidence and thus appear in the middle. Randomized controlled designs that involve random assignment of participants to experimental and control conditions provide the most reliable evidence and are thus the "gold standard" in research (Hariton & Locascio, 2018).

Each kind of study has its own strengths and weaknesses. In general, scientists view evidence from higher levels of the hierarchy as most valid, although higher levels do not guarantee certainty without replication (Ghaemi, 2010). Even when randomized controlled designs are used to compare different forms of therapy, for example, researcher bias (such as the belief that a certain therapy is superior) can influence the outcome of studies (Buetow & Zawaly, 2022). It is particularly important for practitioners to choose treatment methods based on solid scientific evidence, as you will read about in the following case.

> **Case Study** A 10-year-old girl named Candace was diagnosed with a reactive attachment disorder, a condition that interferes with the formation of trusting relationships. In an attempt to help Candace bond with her adoptive mother, her therapist decided to use "rebirthing therapy." Candace was wrapped in a blanket and surrounded by four adults pressing pillows against her, in a process intended to simulate birth. During the 70-minute session, Candace complained that she was unable to breathe. After being unwrapped, Candace had no pulse—the "treatment" caused her to die from suffocation (Kohler, 2001). Because of this case, laws prohibiting rebirthing therapy have been passed in Colorado and in North Carolina, where Candace was born. Bans have also been proposed in California, Florida, Utah, and New Jersey (Watson, 2019).

This heartbreaking story is an example of the importance of using scientifically verified approaches to treating mental illness. The research literature is replete with studies designed to evaluate the effectiveness of various treatment methods in alleviating symptoms of mental disorders. Some treatment outcome studies, designed to investigate conditions associated with treatment effectiveness, analyze the therapy process itself—how therapists, clients, or situational factors influence one another during the course of treatment. You are probably wondering if therapists actually use the scientific method to determine the effectiveness of the approaches they choose when treating mental disorders. Fortunately, many practitioners choose therapies based on data from rigorous experimental studies that have proven that the treatments are effective for specific disorders. However, some proponents of **evidence-based therapies**—treatments that have the highest level of research support—are concerned that many psychotherapists value their own experience and judgment over that of research (Lee & Hunsley, 2015).

Characteristics of Clinical Research

Clinical research relies on various characteristics of the scientific method, including the potential for self-correction, the development of hypotheses about relationships, the use of operational definitions, consideration of reliability and validity, the acknowledgment of base

Attacks on Scientific Integrity

- Examination of a cohort of 105 studies conducted to evaluate the effectiveness of various antidepressant medications found that 98 percent of the studies published supported the use of medication. However, up to half of the randomized controlled studies that did not support antidepressants were never submitted for publication. In addition, some studies with negative or questionable results were written as if the drugs were effective (De Vries et al., 2018).

- Approximately 40 percent of the opioid overdose deaths in the United States are due to prescribed medications. During one 2-year period, pharmaceutical companies spent nearly $40 million marketing opioids to physicians using advertisements and financial incentives (e.g., speaking and consulting fees, meals, travel expenses). Physicians receiving the incentives were more likely to prescribe opioids (Hadland et al., 2019).

- Approximately 80 percent of the marketing budget of some drug companies goes to purchasing meals for physicians and other prescribers. Comparisons in prescribing patterns of medical professionals who received a pharmaceutical-sponsored meal versus those who did not reveal that free meals were associated with increased prescribing of the marketed brand-name drug over the generic drug counterpart (DeJong et al., 2016).

The scientific method requires a commitment from researchers to search for the truth and to remain objective. When personal beliefs, values, political position, or conflicts of interest are allowed to influence the interpretation or dissemination of data, scientific integrity is threatened. We rely on scientists to maintain high ethical standards so we can make informed decisions based on valid research. There is suspicion that many findings unfavorable to "interested parties" such as drug developers or pharmaceutical manufacturers are not published. In some cases, the publication of any data resulting from a company-sponsored study is subject to the approval of the company. Additionally, some have expressed concern because over two thirds of the mental health professionals who assisted in developing the DSM-5 worked for pharmaceutical companies as consultants, researchers, or promoters of certain medications (Cosgrove & Krimsky, 2012). Unfortunately, when financial considerations intersect with science, research can become a tool of interested parties rather than a mechanism to promote the welfare of society.

For Further Consideration

1. Can the interests of consumers be promoted and scientific integrity be maintained when researchers and key decision makers receive funding from pharmaceutical companies?

2. Should individuals be excluded from conducting research or promoting products in which they have a financial conflict of interest?

3. Should pharmaceutical companies be prohibited from offering financial incentives to psychiatrists and other physicians?

rates, and the evaluation of research findings based on their statistical significance. These characteristics allow us to understand exactly what researchers are studying and how much confidence we can place in research findings.

Potential for Self-Correction

One of the unique characteristics of the scientific method is the potential for self-correction. Under ideal conditions, research data and conclusions are freely exchanged and experiments are replicable (reproducible). Clinical research is most easily replicated when hypotheses are explicitly stated and when the variables of concern are clearly defined and easily measurable. The use of open discussion, testing, and verification of research minimizes influence from scientists' personal beliefs, perceptions, biases, and values.

Operational Definitions

Operational definitions are concrete definitions of the variables that researchers are studying. Operational definitions are important because they encourage researchers to be very explicit about what they are measuring.

Did You Know?

The Center for Open Science promotes the reproduction of scientific research. In their latest test of reproducibility, they were able to replicate only 13 of the 21 psychological studies published in one journal. In some cases, failure to replicate occurred because the researchers provided insufficient details about their research and data collection process. This project ignited considerable discussion and anger from the researchers whose work was not replicated.
Source: Camerer et al., 2018

Additionally, researchers choose participants or assessment measures based on the operational definitions they use. For example, researchers studying treatments for depression have the option of defining depression in a variety of ways, including (1) a specific pattern of responses to a self-report depression inventory, (2) a rating assigned by an observer using a depression checklist, or (3) a specific pattern of neuroimaging results associated with depression. This specificity allows others to agree or disagree with the definition used.

When operational definitions of a phenomenon differ, comparing research is problematic, and conclusions can be faulty. Let's consider the definition of *child sexual abuse*, a stressor associated with a number of negative effects such as anxiety, eating disorders, depression, and substance abuse (Hailes et al., 2019). Unfortunately, studies exploring this important topic vary in the definitions used. For example, Mathews and Collin-Vézina (2019) found that definitions of *child sexual abuse* varied on a number of dimensions, including:

- the degree of sexual contact ranged from penetrative acts to "unwanted acts" to "sexual things"; and
- the age difference between victim and perpetrator ranged from "no mention of age" to "adult perpetrators only" to a range of 3 to 5 years age difference between victim and perpetrator.

Consider a few other operational definitions of *child sexual abuse* used in the research literature:

- "A child or adolescent under the age of 16 being involved in sexual activities they do not and cannot fully comprehend and to which they do not fully consent"
- "Any sexual contact between a child of 13 years or younger with another person who was at least 5 years older or a family member who was at least 2 years older"

The use of so many different definitions of *child sexual abuse* make it difficult to compare studies, evaluate the research, and reach conclusions. Operational definitions need to be clear, precise, and consistent.

Reliability and Validity of Measures and Observations

The scientific method requires that measures provide accurate results. **Reliability** refers to the degree to which a measure or procedure yields the same results repeatedly. Consider, for example, an individual who has been diagnosed, by means of a questionnaire, as having a personality disorder. If the questionnaire is reliable, the individual should receive the same diagnosis after filling out the questionnaire on another occasion. Results must be consistent if we are to have any faith in them. Even if consistent results are obtained, questions can arise over the **validity** of a measure. Does the testing instrument really measure what it was developed to measure? For instance, if our research uses a test to determine the severity of anxiety, we must demonstrate that the test has good validity and can accomplish this task.

Base Rates

A **base rate** is the rate of natural occurrence of a phenomenon in the population studied. Knowledge of the base rate of specific behaviors or circumstances can help us avoid jumping to inaccurate conclusions.

Further, data on the base rates of variables being studied help ensure that we do not misinterpret research findings. For example, both unwanted sexual events and eating problems are reported by a high percentage of women. As a result, clinicians may find that many of their clients with disordered eating report a history of sexual abuse. In some cases, the relationship may be causal. That is, it is *possible* that emotional responses to sexual abuse *may* result in an eating disorder. However, knowing that both of these conditions occur with high frequency (have high base rates) ensures that we do not mistakenly assume that one causes the other.

The importance of base rates is also evident in clinical research related to psychosis. We need to know how frequently psychotic symptoms (the unusual thoughts or reactions seen in individuals with schizophrenia) occur in the general population. Depending on the study, psychotic-like symptoms are reported by between 5 percent and 35 percent of children and adolescents; however, only a small percentage of these individuals go on to develop a psychotic disorder (Rembert, 2017). Similarly, Johns et al. (2004) found that 66 percent of a control group of adults endorsed having one or more psychotic symptoms (Figure 4.1).

Base rates may also differ between populations. One cross-cultural study found significant differences in reports of psychotic symptoms between countries. For instance, the prevalence of hallucinations ranged from 0.1 percent in Vietnam to 31.0 percent in Nepal; these data suggest that clinicians and researchers should take base rates from a client's country of origin into account when interpreting psychotic symptoms. The researchers did find, however, that the more symptoms reported, the greater the likelihood the individual had a mental illness (Nuevo et al., 2012).

Statistical Versus Clinical Significance

The scientific method also requires that research findings be evaluated in terms of their **statistical significance**—the statistical probability that the findings are not due to chance alone. Even a statistically significant finding may have little practical significance in a clinical setting, as demonstrated in the following studies:

- Wearing compression socks significantly reduced the number of episodes of sleep apnea (cessation of breathing) from 48 to 31 episodes per hour, a highly significant finding from a statistical perspective. However, the results were not clinically significant, since the number of apnea episodes remained in the severe range (Redolfi et al., 2011).

- A study with a large sample size found that an expensive new blood pressure medication reduces systolic blood pressure readings by 2 mm Hg more than a proven less expensive medication. Although the change of 2 mm Hg is statistically significant, it does not represent a clinically significant reduction in blood pressure (Yueh, 2020).

When evaluating research, we must always keep in mind whether the statistical significance reported is truly "clinically" significant. This problem—a finding being statistically significant but not necessarily meaningful—is most likely to occur in studies with large sample sizes.

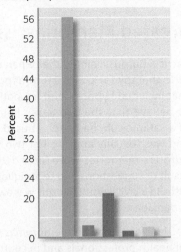

Percent reporting this over the past year

- ■ Feeling very happy without a break for days on end
- ■ Thoughts being interfered with or controlled by some outside force or person
- ■ Felt that people were against you
- ■ Heard voices or saw things that other people could not
- ■ Felt like something strange was going on

Figure 4.1

Base Rate Responses to Psychosis Screening Questionnaire

It is important to know the base rate of responses when interpreting questionnaire data. This figure presents the percentage of "normal" individuals endorsing items on a questionnaire used to identify psychotic thinking and beliefs. Based on these data, do you think this questionnaire is a valid measure of psychotic thinking?

Source: Data from Johns et al., 2004

Repressed Memories: Issues and Questions

Patricia Burgus claimed that when undergoing psychiatric therapy for postpartum depression—treatment that included hypnosis and hypnotic drugs—she came to believe that she had eaten human flesh, was part of a satanic cult, had been abused by numerous men, and was sexually abusing her two sons (Ewing, 1998). Burgus's memories were later determined to be the result of suggestions and techniques used by her therapists. In a civil lawsuit, Burgus was awarded $10.6 million in damages.

The battle over repressed memory has taken place among mental health professionals and in courts of law—a dispute characterized as a "memory war" between those who believe and those who do not believe that repressed memory is a genuine phenomenon. This debate intensified during the 1990s when therapists increased their use of treatment methods designed to retrieve "repressed" memories of childhood abuse in their clients. Even today, some clinicians raise the possibility that certain clients have repressed memories (Otgaar et al., 2019). Although psychoanalysts and hypnotherapists are the most likely to believe that traumatic memories are repressed and can be retrieved, this belief is also held by college undergraduates and the general public (Otgaar et al., 2021).

On the other hand, based on their knowledge of how memory works, memory experts and research-oriented clinicians are highly skeptical of the validity of repressed memories. Elizabeth Loftus argues that there is little scientific evidence that a memory, however painful, can be banned from consciousness and return years later (Loftus et al., 2008). Further, studies have found that it is not difficult to convince research subjects that a suggested childhood event (i.e., an implanted memory) actually occurred (Scoboria et al., 2017). Thus, "repressed" memories can arise by means of therapist suggestion or through techniques such as hypnosis, guided imagery, or age regression (Otgaar et al., 2022; Ulatowska & Sawicka, 2017).

Similarly, Pope and Hudson (2007) believe that repressed memory is not a scientifically valid phenomenon but rather a condition "manufactured" after the 1800s. In fact, they offered a $1,000 reward to anyone who could produce a published case of the phenomenon in fiction or nonfiction before 1800. They argue that if "repressed memory" were genuine, it would have been the subject of writings in the past. After reviewing over 100 submissions, they did find that one character (Nina, from a 1786 opera) met their criteria, and they awarded the money. However, they still maintain that genuine psychological phenomena such as depression, anxiety, and hallucinations are abundantly represented in historical works, unlike repressed memories (Pope et al., 2009).

For Further Consideration

1. Do you believe repressed memories are real? What research approach would you take to determine if it is a genuine phenomenon?

2. Why are research psychologists more likely than clinicians to have doubts regarding the existence of repressed memories?

3. Why do you think undergraduates and the general public are more likely to believe that repressed memories occur? How might they have formed that opinion?

Experiments

The **experiment** is perhaps the best tool for testing cause and effect relationships. In contrast to case study and correlational methods, experiments allow researchers to investigate causal relationships. When researchers manipulate (change) experimental variables, they can draw conclusions about the effects of the manipulated variables on other variables. In its simplest form, an experiment involves the following:

1. An **experimental hypothesis**, which is a prediction concerning how an independent variable will affect a dependent variable

2. An **independent variable** (the possible cause), which the experimenter manipulates to determine its effect on a dependent variable

3. A **dependent variable**, which is expected to change as a result of changes in the independent variable

Let's clarify these concepts by examining an actual research study.

Research conducted by Thom et al. (2000) seemed to provide some direction. In their study of individuals with dental phobia, 50 patients who needed dental surgery were assigned to one of three groups: psychological treatment, medication, or no treatment. The psychological treatment consisted of one stress management training session (relaxation exercises, visualization of dental work, use of coping thoughts) followed by 1 week of practicing these techniques at home. Those in the medication group took an antianxiety pill 30 minutes before the dental procedure. All participants (including those in the no-treatment control group) were told that their surgeon specialized in patients with dental anxiety and would treat them carefully.

The Experimental Group

An experimental group is a group exposed to an independent variable. In their study, Thom and her colleagues created two experimental groups: One group received a single session of stress management training plus 1 week of daily, home-based stress reduction activities. The other experimental group received antianxiety medication. Because the investigators were interested in how treatment affects levels of anxiety and reports of panic, their dependent variables included pretreatment and posttreatment self-reports of dental fear and ratings of pain during the procedure. The investigators also tabulated how many of the patients completed dental treatment with further appointments. Thus, the dependent variables were self-reports of fear, ratings of pain when undergoing dental surgery, and participation in further dental care.

The Control Group

If the participants in the two experimental groups in the study by Thom and her colleagues demonstrated a reduction in dental fear between pretesting and posttesting measures, could the researchers conclude that the treatments were effective forms of therapy? The answer would be no, because participants may have reported less anxiety about dental procedures merely due to the passage of time or as a function of completing the assessment measures. The use of a control group enables researchers to eliminate such possibilities. A control group is a group that is similar in every way to the experimental group except they are not exposed to the independent variable. In the study by Thom and her colleagues, the control group also took the pretest measures, received reassurance about their surgeon, underwent dental surgery, and took the posttest measures. However, those in the control group did not receive medication or stress management training, the treatments being investigated. Because of this, we can be more certain that any differences found between the control and experimental groups were due to the independent variable (i.e., the treatment received).

Did You Know?

Many research findings in the leading psychology journals are based on undergraduate students, particularly those majoring in psychology. Because of the reliance on college students as subjects in Western countries, the term *WEIRD* (Westernized, Educated, from Industrialized, Rich Democracies) has been used to describe this population. Psychology research is supposed to reveal information about human nature. How generalizable is research based on college students?
Source: Grohol, 2018

Myth Building more controls into an experiment always results in greater generalizability of the findings.

Reality Although a tightly controlled study increases internal validity, problems can occur with external validity—that is, the findings may not be generalizable to other populations because the conditions existing in an experimental setting may not resemble those found in real-life situations. Both internal validity and external validity have to be considered when designing a study.

Double-Blind Design

When researching the effects of a drug, researchers often use a double-blind design to ensure that neither participants nor experimenters are aware of the experimental conditions. Here a physician is holding a bottle containing either medication or placebo pills. Neither she nor the participants in the study will know the type of pill received. This design is used to control for expectancy effects.

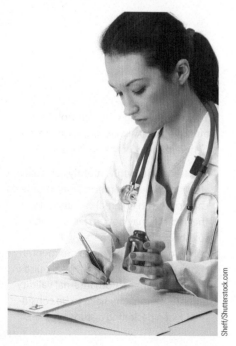

Sheff/Shutterstock.com

The findings revealed that the groups who received stress management training or antianxiety medication reported significantly less fear and pain when undergoing surgery than the control group. However, those treated with medication continued to display dental phobia following their surgery, whereas those who received stress management training demonstrated sustained improvement and continued their dental treatment. Of those who completed additional dental procedures, 70 percent had been in the psychological intervention group, 20 percent in the medication group, and 10 percent in the control group. Given these findings, the therapist told River that both treatments could help during their dental appointment but that psychological intervention was more likely to produce long-term effects.

The Placebo Group

Some researchers have found that if participants have an expectation that they will improve from treatment, it may be this expectancy—referred to as the **placebo effect**—rather than specific treatment that accounts for improvement. In fact, studies developed to test the effectiveness of medications often use a **placebo**—an inactive substance—for the purpose of making a comparison. Interestingly, placebos can actually produce meaningful symptom reduction and physiological changes. For example, one group of chronic pain patients who responded to a placebo demonstrated biological changes in the amygdala, hippocampus, and nucleus accumbens, areas of the brain associated with emotion and reward. Interestingly, those who responded to the placebo tended to possess characteristics such as being emotionally aware and attuned to their bodily sensations (Vachon-Presseau et al., 2018).

To control for placebo effects, researchers often design their experiments to include a placebo control group. For instance, Thom and her colleagues could have given another group a medication capsule containing a placebo or designed a presumably ineffective single-session intervention such as a therapist reading an informational pamphlet and asking the client to review the pamphlet daily for 1 week. If the experimental groups (i.e., medication or psychological treatment) improved more than the placebo control groups, the researchers could be even more confident that the treatment, rather than expectancy, was responsible for the results.

Additional Controls in Experimental Research

Because experimenter and participant expectations can also influence the outcome of a study, researchers sometimes use a **single-blind design**, in which participants in an experiment are unaware of the purpose of the research. The single-blind study can be problematic because clinicians who know the experimental condition have been found to exhibit subtle changes in facial expressions or behaviors that are picked up by patients during their clinical interactions. These cues may then affect the response of subjects to the treatment being studied (Chen, Cheong, et al., 2019).

To control for this possibility, researchers often use a **double-blind design**, in which the impact of both experimenter and participant expectations is reduced. In the double-blind procedure, neither the individual working directly with the participant (such as a therapist or physician) nor the participant is aware of the experimental conditions. The effectiveness of this design is dependent on whether participants are truly "blind" to the intervention, which may not always be the case. For example, in medication studies, over 75 percent of subjects may correctly guess their treatment assignment due to either the presence or absence of physical symptoms or other side effects (Perlis et al., 2010). Physicians are also able to distinguish between placebos and actual medications based on patient reactions.

Ethical Considerations—Risk/Benefit Versus Social Value

Randomized controlled experiments that include components such as placebo trials and random assignment represent the "gold standard" of research designs. However, all experiments must consider the risk/benefit ratio to the participants and the social value of the data obtained. Consider the following experiment and decide if you have concerns with the study.

Romanian officials asked researchers to conduct a study regarding the effects of institutional care. One hundred thirty-six young children living in a Romanian orphanage were randomly assigned either to continued institutional care or to placement in foster care (Zeanah et al., 2009). These Romanian orphans received mental health assessments (1) before the random assignment and (2) after they were 54 months of age. Noninstitutionalized Romanian children served as a comparison group. The findings revealed that children assigned to foster care had fewer psychiatric problems than those who remained in the orphanage. It was concluded that placement in foster care can ameliorate some of the effects of early institutionalization. The children were reexamined at 12 years of age. Those who had been placed in institutions were more like to show psychological symptoms compared to the children who had never been institutionalized (Humphreys et al., 2015).

For Further Consideration

1. What is your reaction to this study?
2. What are the potential risks or benefits of this study?
3. Are there other research designs that might furnish the same information?

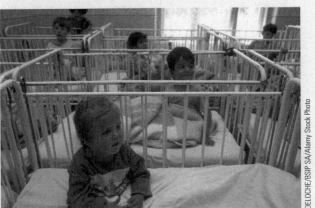

DELOCHE/BSIP SA/Alamy Stock Photo

Although experimental studies have the greatest credibility with respect to cause and effect relationships, shortcomings also exist. Questions are sometimes raised about the generalizability of the results of experimental studies. For instance, some wonder if findings generated in clinics or research settings apply to other environments. The tight control of variables that might influence the outcome of a study may not resemble the real world where this kind of control does not exist.

Additionally, some variables cannot be manipulated. For example, for ethical reasons, we cannot conduct an experiment to investigate if child abuse increases the risk of depression. Investigating this hypothesis using an experimental design would require randomly assigning children to conditions of child abuse or no child abuse to determine if those in the abuse condition are more likely to develop depression. In this case, a correlational study (described next) analyzing the association between child abuse and depression would be the most appropriate research approach.

Correlational Studies

Correlational studies allow researchers to look at data from a large group to determine if variations in one variable are accompanied by increases or decreases in a second variable. If we wanted to investigate a possible link between child abuse and depression, we would operationally define both variables (child abuse and depression), find a large sample where we had access to data on these variables, and then perform a statistical analysis to determine if degree of exposure to child abuse was associated with increases in symptoms of depression. The statistical analysis would tell us if there was a **correlation**—a relationship between the variables.

For instance, in a correlational study involving 3,000 children who were 5 years old, greater consumption of soft drinks was associated with increased frequency of aggressive behavior (Suglia et al., 2013). This study demonstrates a *positive correlation* in which an increase in one variable (soft drink consumption) was accompanied by an increase in the other (aggressive behavior). A *negative correlation* involves an increase in one variable accompanied by a decrease in the other variable. The greater the value of correlation, positive or negative, the stronger the relationship between the variables. Refer to Figure 4.2 for examples of correlations. Correlational studies are very important to scientific inquiry because they allow analysis of variables that cannot be controlled—variables such as age, annual income, or frequency of exposure to traumatic experiences.

Although correlational studies provide data regarding the degree to which two variables are related, they do not explain the reason for the relationship. Thus, correlational studies cannot be used to demonstrate cause and effect. For instance, eating highly processed foods (e.g., sweets, fried food, refined grains, high-fat dairy) is correlated with an increased likelihood of depression and anxiety symptoms (Lane et al., 2022). However, because these data come from correlational studies, it is possible that the relationship between dietary patterns and depression is due to variables other than those studied. In other words, we cannot conclude that consuming processed foods causes depression; it is possible that depressed individuals are more prone to eating unhealthy foods or that a third variable affects both dietary habits and depression. Similar issues arise when you consider the previously mentioned

Figure 4.2

Possible Correlation Between Two Variables

The more closely the data points approximate a straight line, the greater the magnitude of the correlation. The slope of the regression line rising from left to right in example (a) indicates a perfect positive correlation between two variables, whereas example (b) reveals a perfect negative correlation. Example (c) demonstrates a lower positive correlation. Example (d) involves no correlation whatsoever.

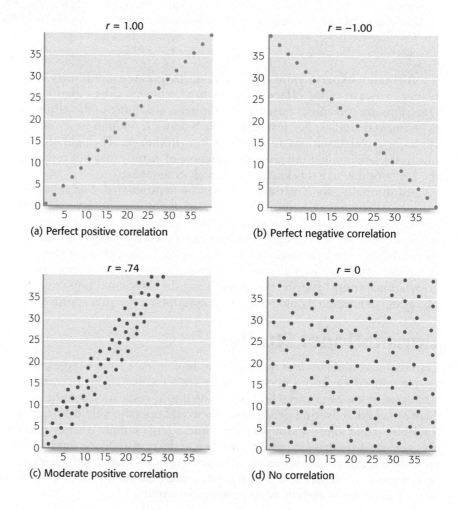

(a) Perfect positive correlation $r = 1.00$

(b) Perfect negative correlation $r = -1.00$

(c) Moderate positive correlation $r = .74$

(d) No correlation $r = 0$

study that reported a positive correlation between the consumption of soft drinks and aggressive behavior in young children.

Let's consider another study assessing the relationship between the amount of exposure to violence in television programs and films and aggressive behaviors in a sample of 1,990 adolescents. The researchers found a significant correlation between the variables studied; higher rates of exposure to media violence were associated with higher levels of aggression. This correlation was evident even when the researchers took into consideration other risk variables such as family conflict, impulsivity, and sensation-seeking (Khurana et al., 2019). However, even though possible confounding risk variables were considered, an inference of causality cannot be made due to the possibility that another, unstudied variable was responsible for the relationship between exposure to media violence and aggression.

There are numerous ways that a third variable might affect a correlation. Consider the following observations. What third-variable explanations can you suggest?

- There is a positive correlation between the number of churches in a city and the number of individuals living in the city who have been diagnosed with depression.
- There is a positive correlation between the number of mental health professionals working in a community and the number of violent crimes committed in the region.

When interpreting correlational data, it is always important to remember that "correlation does not mean causation" and to consider alternative possibilities. Some of the misinformation regarding immunizations causing autism, mentioned earlier in the chapter, occurred, in part, because the age of onset of autism is correlated with the timing of childhood vaccines; this association resulted in the widespread but inaccurate assumption that childhood vaccines cause autism—a conclusion that has since been dispelled by many studies.

In summary, correlational studies are a very important method of scientific inquiry. Because sample sizes are large and the research can be replicated, this method of investigation has a strong scientific foundation. However, interpreting the outcome of correlational studies can be problematic. Even when variables are causally related, the direction of causality may be unclear. It is also possible that variables that are highly correlated are, in fact, causally unrelated or influenced by an additional, not-yet-identified variable.

Analogue Studies

As we have noted, ethical, moral, or legal standards may prevent researchers from devising certain studies. Additionally, studying real-life situations is often not feasible because it is difficult to control all possible variables. Sometimes researchers resort to an **analogue study**—an investigation that attempts to replicate or simulate, under controlled conditions, a situation that occurs in real life. Here are some examples of analogue studies:

- To study the possible effects of a new treatment for anxiety disorders, the researcher experiments with students who have test anxiety rather than individuals diagnosed with an anxiety disorder.
- To test the hypothesis that human depression is caused by continual encounters with events that one cannot control, the researcher exposes rats to uncontrollable aversive stimuli and looks for depressive-like behaviors (such as lack of motivation, inability to learn, and general apathy) or changes in chemical activity in the brains of the animals.

Many individuals who are involved in or witness a disaster experience severe emotional and physical trauma. Disasters provide a unique, though unwelcome, opportunity to observe events and reactions of individuals in the natural environment. Can social scientists remain detached and objective when recording a tragedy?

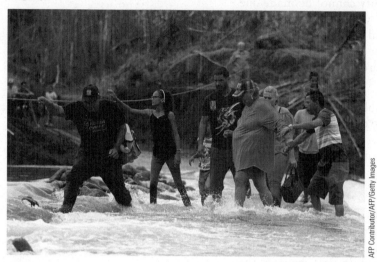

AFP Contributor/AFP/Getty Images

- To test the hypothesis that sexual sadism is influenced by watching sexually violent media, an experimenter exposes college fraternity members to either violent or nonviolent sexual videos. The students then complete a questionnaire assessing their attitudes toward women and their likelihood of engaging in sexually violent behaviors.

Obviously, each example is only an approximation of real life. Students with test anxiety may not be equivalent to individuals with an anxiety disorder. Findings based on rats may not be applicable to human beings. And exposure to one violent sexual film and the use of a questionnaire may not be sufficient to allow a researcher to draw the conclusion that sexual sadism is caused by long-term exposure to such films. However, analogue studies can give researchers insight into the processes that might be involved in the development of a mental disorder and can facilitate the search for effective treatment.

Field Studies

In some cases, it may be too difficult to develop an analogue study that accurately reflects a real-life situation. Investigators may then resort to a **field study**, in which they observe and record behaviors and events in their natural environment. Field studies examine behavior after events of major consequence such as wars, floods, and earthquakes, or explore reactions to personal crises such as major surgery or terminal disease. Field studies sometimes employ data collection techniques, such as questionnaires, interviews, and analysis of existing records, but the primary technique is observation. Observers must be highly trained and have enough self-discipline to avoid disrupting or modifying the behavioral processes they are observing and recording.

Although field studies offer a more realistic investigative environment than other types of research, they suffer from certain limitations. First, as with other nonexperimental research, field work does not provide information about causality. Second, so many factors affect real-life situations that it is impossible to control—and sometimes even distinguish—all possible variables. As a result, the findings may be difficult to interpret. Third, observers can never be absolutely certain that their presence did not influence the interactions they observed.

Single-Participant Studies

Most researchers believe we learn the most when a study includes large numbers—the more people studied, the easier it is to uncover the basic principles governing behavior. This approach, called the *nomothetic orientation*, is concerned with formulating general laws or principles while deemphasizing individual variations or differences. Experiments and correlational studies are nomothetic. Other scientists advocate the in-depth study of one person, exemplified by the single-participant study. This approach is called the *idiographic orientation*. There is much debate regarding which method is more fruitful in studying psychopathology.

Although the idiographic method of studying a single participant has many limitations, especially lack of generalizability, it has proven very valuable in applied clinical work. Furthermore, it is not productive to argue about which method is more helpful because both approaches provide important insight into psychopathological behavior. The nomothetic approach seems appropriate for researchers, whereas the idiographic approach seems appropriate for psychotherapists, who regularly face the challenge of providing effective treatment.

There are two types of single-participant studies: the **case study** and the **single-participant experiment**. Both techniques may be used to examine a rare or an unusual phenomenon, demonstrate a novel diagnostic or treatment procedure, test an assumption, generate future hypotheses on which to base controlled research, or analyze comprehensive information to better understand an individual. Only the single-participant experiment, however, can determine cause and effect relationships. Nevertheless, case studies often provide crucial information.

The Case Study

In psychology, a case study is an in-depth look at data about an individual, including observations, medical and psychological tests, and historical and biographical information. Clinicians using the case study method, such as the therapist working with Nayda, develop a strong therapeutic relationship with the client and make every effort to understand the client's background, symptoms, and distress. The therapist can then formulate hypotheses regarding possible causes of the client's behavior or distress and test out different therapeutic strategies. Innovative methods of assessment or treatment often arise from case studies—strategies that can be evaluated with further research (Piccirillo et al., 2019). In Nayda's case, the therapist adapted a therapeutic approach to incorporate Nayda's cultural beliefs. In addition to facilitating new therapeutic or diagnostic techniques, case studies are also used to study rare psychological phenomena such as the mysterious physical symptoms experienced by the teenagers in New York described at the beginning of this chapter. A case study is exemplified in the following example.

Case Study Rosa is a 63-year-old woman who was born on a Spanish-speaking island in the Caribbean. Her parents brought her to the United States when she was 3 years old. She is divorced and has one adult son. Throughout her childhood, her family life was full of conflict. Rosa was particularly traumatized from witnessing her father's frequent drunken outbursts and physical abuse of her mother. Although she tried to develop a close relationship with her mother by acceding to all her wishes, Rosa faced constant rejection. She became the scapegoat of the family and was continually criticized and shamed because she had the darkest skin color in her family. Despite these early problems, Rosa had a successful career as a school counselor. However, since retiring, Rosa has made few friends and feels isolated. She decided to seek therapy because she was feeling depressed and anxious.

In analyzing the case, it was evident that Rosa's current problems stemmed from her early history of abuse and trauma, a topic she tried to avoid. She was clearly reluctant to talk about her traumatic past and tried to change the discussion to focus on problems with her son. The therapy chosen by the therapist addressed attachment difficulties and focused on enhancing Rosa's capacity to address difficult emotions. A breakthrough occurred when the therapist shared that she also spoke Spanish. This produced a positive emotional response from Rosa, who started to language switch—using Spanish to explore the emotion-laden events from her childhood. After 23 sessions, Rosa reported marked improvement in her symptoms. She also felt empowered and was able to set boundaries with her son (Fosha, 2018).

This case study provides information regarding how early life trauma can lead to depression and anxiety. It also explores the damaging effects of intrafamilial colorism (discrimination based on the darkness of one's skin color). Also of interest is that Rosa was better able to explore difficult topics in her native language. A case study such as this provides in-depth information about the development and experience of a disorder, as well as insight into possible treatments.

However, case studies have limitations. First, because the study involves a single individual or specific situation, questions arise about whether the findings are applicable to other individuals with similar problems. Second, the data gathered in case studies often reflect the theoretical perspective or bias of the investigator. The clinician may operate from a biological, psychological, sociocultural, or other perspective and ignore other viewpoints. Third, case studies do not generally provide scientifically reliable information about causes. Because of these problems, group designs such as correlational and experimental studies that allow for replication and larger sample sizes provide a more solid research foundation for investigating mental disorders. In summary, case studies provide detailed information regarding the development and features of psychopathology in a specific individual but lack the control and objectivity of many other methods.

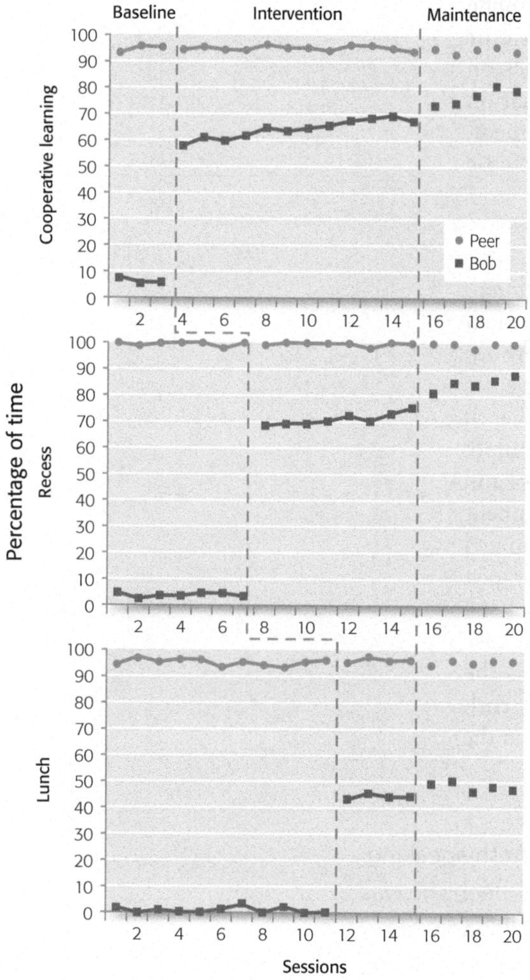

The Single-Participant Experiment

The single-participant experiment involves research on one person; the person's current behavior is used as a control or baseline for comparison with future behaviors (Kazdin, 2019). To determine the effectiveness of a treatment, for example, the experimenter first determines the frequency of a behavior before intervention. The treatment occurs, and the person's behavior is again observed. Once behavior change occurs, the treatment is withdrawn. If, after the withdrawal of treatment, the person's behavior again resembles behavior observed during the baseline condition, we can be fairly certain that the treatment was responsible for the behavior changes observed earlier. In the final step, the treatment is reinstated.

A **multiple-baseline study** is a single-participant experimental design in which baselines on two or more behaviors or the same behavior in two or more settings are obtained prior to intervention. An intervention is first introduced for one behavior or setting, its effects are observed, and then the intervention is applied to the next behavior or setting. If the behaviors change only with the intervention, confidence is increased that the intervention caused the behavior change.

Bock (2007) used a multiple-baseline approach to determine the effectiveness of a training program for four children diagnosed with autism who were experiencing significant difficulty developing peer relationships and understanding social customs. Baseline information for each child's behaviors was obtained during (1) cooperative learning activities, (2) recess, and (3) lunch with peers. Prior to the intervention, the four children used very few appropriate social behaviors in any of these settings. The intervention program, called SODA, taught each child how to attend to social cues and to respond appropriately. The children were prompted to use the SODA strategies in different settings—first in the cooperative learning situation, then during recess, and finally when eating lunch in the school cafeteria. Figure 4.3 demonstrates how one of the students, Bob, increased appropriate behaviors in each of the three conditions after the intervention. (The other three students demonstrated similar improvement.)

Figure 4.3

A Multiple-Baseline Study

The figures summarize the percentage of time Bob and a classmate spent behaving appropriately during cooperative learning, recess, and lunch. During baseline, Bob displayed appropriate behaviors in cooperative learning, recess, and lunch less than 10 percent of the time. With the SODA intervention, the percentage increased to about 70 percent during cooperative learning and recess and to more than 40 percent during lunch. At a 5-month follow-up, Bob maintained his gains in appropriate behaviors.

Source: From Bock, 2007 (p. 92)

How Can We Enhance Critical-Thinking Skills?

False news stories are rampant and, despite their inaccuracies, they take hold and spread rapidly. Untrue stories are retweeted more often and spread faster than accurate news stories, creating an unjustified sense of support and consensus for falsified information. Further, automated social bots have the capacity to dramatically increase the number of posts or tweets on a particular theme. Russian bots, targeting the United States and other Western democracies, have attempted to stoke public division over race relationships and create societal conflict on controversial issues. For example, bots have spread antivaccine messages such as claiming that there is a secret government database of vaccine-damaged children (Broniatowski et al., 2018; Broniatowski et al., 2020).

Many people take what they read or see on the Internet at face value without pausing to critically reflect on the veracity of the data. Unfortunately, even a single exposure to a false headline can increase the believability of the story, with the belief strengthening with each subsequent exposure (Giotakos, 2022; Ross et al., 2019). In a study to determine if high school students could determine the veracity of information displayed on the Internet, Breakstone et al. (2019) analyzed online survey responses from 3,446 students with the following results:

- When presented with a grainy video that claimed to expose the stuffing of ballot boxes during the 2016 Democratic primaries, 52 percent of the students rated the video as "strong evidence" of voter fraud within the United States. Although the video was actually produced in Russia and an Internet search would have quickly indicated that

the video was a hoax, only three students attempted to find the source for the video.

- When presented with actual news reports and "sponsored" articles, the students deemed them equally reliable sources of information and made no attempt to identify the source of sponsored articles.

- After exposure to Web site information on climate change produced by the fossil fuel industry, many of the students did not understand why the source of the data might influence the credibility of the information.

Some suggestions for combating fake news include (1) carefully considering the source and remaining aware that some illegitimate actors attempt to mimic legitimate sources, (2) researching the background and affiliation of the writer, (3) checking the date to ensure that the information is current, (4) keeping in mind your own biases before deciding to either accept or reject the information, (5) reading beyond the topic line to understand the substance of the story, and (6) using reliable sources to fact check the details (Kiely & Robertson, 2016).

For Further Consideration

1. How can we encourage people to look at social media and Internet content more critically?

2. Why is it difficult for people to use critical-thinking skills when exposed to information via social media?

3. What influences your decisions to share or retweet information you encounter online?

Single-participant designs can provide valuable information but are seldom used because researchers often rely on research designs that involve group comparisons. Because only one participant is observed at a time in a single-participant design, questions are raised about **external validity**, or the generalizability of the findings, even when the approach is applied to several children as in the evaluation of the SODA intervention.

4-2 Biological Research Strategies

Researchers in the field of psychopathology often rely on biological research to enhance their understanding of factors influencing the development of mental disorders and to guide research on effective treatment. Researchers study biological processes involved in mental illness from many directions, including endophenotypes; twin comparisons; genetic studies; and, more recently, the study of epigenetic processes.

Twin Studies

Identical twins are often used in studies to determine the influence of genetic factors. They tend to demonstrate greater behavioral similarities than do fraternal twins or siblings. This similarity is attributed to genetic factors.

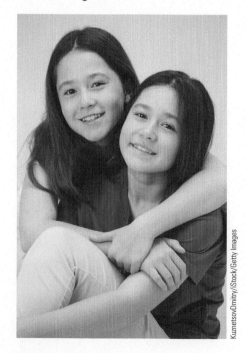

KuznetsovDmitry/iStock/Getty Images

The Endophenotype Concept

Endophenotypes are measurable characteristics, such as atypical cognitive functioning or anatomical or chemical differences in the brain—traits that indicate the genetic pathways involved in a disorder. To be considered an endophenotype, the characteristic must be heritable (can be inherited), seen in family members who do not have the disorder, and occur more frequently in affected families than in the general population. For example, as many as 80 percent of individuals diagnosed with schizophrenia (a severe mental illness we will discuss in Chapter 12) and 45 percent of their close relatives demonstrate irregularities in the way they track objects with their eyes. In families without schizophrenia, only 10 percent have this trait (Gottesman & Gould, 2003).

This irregularity thus qualifies as an endophenotype: It is inherited, is seen in families with a particular disorder (schizophrenia), and occurs more often in those families than in the general population. Although the majority of **asymptomatic** relatives never develop the disorder, identifying endophenotypes associated with a disorder can guide prevention and early treatment efforts (Braff & Tamminga, 2017). Despite strong interest in the use of endophenotypes, progress has been slow. As we learned in Chapter 2, there are many possible pathways leading to the development of a disorder, not just those involving genetics. Additionally, the search for clear-cut indicators of risk for specific disorders is complicated because the symptoms and severity of symptoms can vary significantly even for those given the same diagnosis.

Twin Studies

Ongoing developments in the field of genetic research are contributing to our understanding of psychopathology. Researchers often study monozygotic (MZ) twins, commonly called identical twins, because they originate from the same egg. MZ twins not only share the same DNA but also experience similar environmental influences prenatally and during childhood. Fraternal, or dizygotic (DZ), twins also provide important information; although they originate from two eggs and thus have no more genetic similarity than non-twin siblings (sharing approximately half of inherited traits), fraternal twins do share similar prenatal and childhood environments. Researchers often make comparisons between identical and fraternal twins to evaluate hereditary and environmental influences on development. In rare cases, twins are raised apart; when this occurs, researchers have even more opportunity to investigate the influence of genetic and environmental factors.

Genetic Linkage Studies

The goal of a **genetic linkage study** is to determine whether a disorder follows a genetic pattern. With genetically linked disorders, individuals closely related to the person with the disorder (who is called the *proband*) are more likely to display that disorder or a related disorder.

Genetic studies of psychiatric disorders often employ the following procedure (Iorfino et al., 2021):

1. The proband and their family members are identified.
2. The proband may be asked about the psychiatric history of family members.

3. Family members are contacted and given some type of assessment, such as psychological tests, brain scans, or neuropsychological examinations, to determine whether they have the same or a related disorder.

This research strategy depends on the accurate diagnosis of both the proband and the relatives. Caution must be used in employing the family history method in genetic linkage studies. Variables such as psychiatric status ("ill" or "well") may influence the accuracy of a person's assessment of the mental health of relatives. Researchers often reduce this bias by using multiple informants or assessing family members directly. In one comprehensive study looking at psychological disorders in more than 11,000 twins, researchers increased the reliability of their findings by interviewing each twin and co-twin at least twice and at different points of time; they also relied on independent assessments of the psychiatric status of family members to increase the accuracy of their research (Kendler & Prescot, 2006).

Genetic research is also complicated by the fact that genes vary in their penetrance. **Penetrance** refers to the proportion of individuals with a particular genotype (carrying a specific gene) who manifest the phenotype (observable characteristics) associated with the gene. Complete penetrance occurs when a carrier *always* manifests the characteristic associated with the gene. In mental disorders, incomplete penetrance is the rule—many people carry the genotype but do not display the trait. Even in cases of schizophrenia (a disorder with high heritability), only about half of the identical twins of a proband develop the disorder. When genes have lower penetrance, it is particularly difficult to differentiate between genetic and environmental influences. Additionally, epigenetic effects (discussed in the next section) can influence whether or not a gene is expressed and thus affect gene penetrance. Not surprisingly, epigenetics has become a major focus of research.

Epigenetic Research

Epigenetic researchers focus on the role of epigenetic influences on gene expression. In particular, they consider environmental factors that may influence whether or not a gene is expressed; the manner in which epigenetic changes regulate how and when genes are turned on or turned off; and how epigenetic modifications influence an individual's risk of developing a mental disorder. These researchers have found that trauma and other adversities (such as unsafe neighborhoods or financial stress within the home) have the greatest impact during the sensitive period of brain development that occurs prior to 3 years of age (Dunn et al., 2019).

Children's experiences early in life not only affect their own development but also may influence traits inherited by their descendants (Bošković & Rando, 2018). This occurs when epigenetic changes leave an *imprint* (a genetic marker) on eggs or sperm, a marker that influences whether specific genetic characteristics appear in future generations. Epigenetic researchers conduct laboratory studies to learn more about the molecular and chemical processes involved with epigenetic regulation of genes. They also research genome-wide distribution of epigenetic changes, sometimes using human epidemiological studies to look for changes that may have affected large numbers of people in a population.

The Human Genome Project

The Human Genome Project, a massive undertaking that involved deciphering, mapping, and identifying DNA sequencing patterns and variations in approximately 30,000 human genes, has resulted in a variety of significant scientific and medical benefits. Pictured here is a sample of DNA and a sequencing chromatograph revealing the DNA sequence associated with the sample.

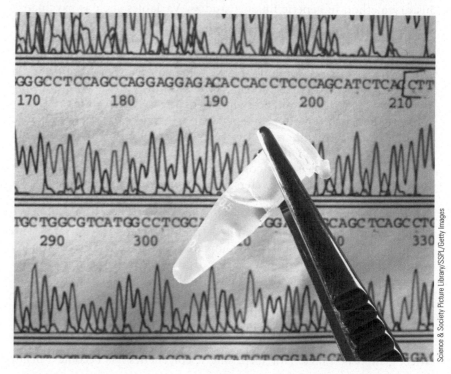

Science & Society Picture Library/SSPL/Getty Images

Using Animals in Biological Research

The use of *animal models*, relying on animals as surrogates for humans in research, is a frequent practice in biological research, particularly in genetic and epigenetic studies. Such experiments allow for considerable control over the variables studied and analysis across multiple generations. Animal studies also permit experimental procedures that would not be practical to use with humans.

For instance, animal studies have been used extensively in an effort to better understand and treat posttraumatic stress disorder (PTSD), an often-debilitating disorder that results from exposure to an extreme stressor. Exposing animals to traumatic circumstances allows researchers to determine how the disorder develops, which brain systems and neurochemicals are involved, and what medications might be useful for treatment (Lowery-Gionta et al., 2019). Alcohol abuse has also been studied by training rats to binge drink; the animals then develop an "addiction" to alcohol and experience withdrawal symptoms when alcohol is no longer available. Alcohol is also given to pregnant rats in order to study the effects of alcohol on a developing fetus, something that cannot be studied experimentally in humans (Crowley et al., 2019). Of course, opponents point to ethical concerns with animal research.

Animal Observations

Research on animals can provide clues to the development of emotions in humans. In this photo, the scientist is looking carefully at the rat's emotional response to an experiment.

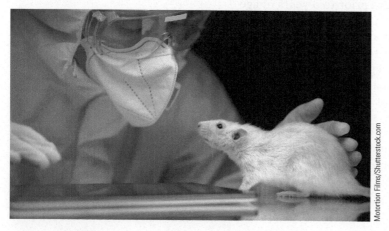

Motortion Films/Shutterstock.com

4-3 Epidemiological Research

Epidemiological research examines the frequency and distribution of mental disorders in a population. This important type of research is used to determine both the extent of mental disturbance found in a targeted population and the factors that influence the rate of mental illness. Two terms, *prevalence* and *incidence*, are used to describe the frequency with which mental disorders occur. As noted in Chapter 1, prevalence tells us the percentage of individuals in a targeted population who have a particular disorder during a specific period of time. For example, we might be interested in how many school-age children had a spider phobia during the previous 6 months (6-month prevalence), during the previous year (1-year prevalence), or at any time during their lives (lifetime prevalence). In general, shorter time periods have lower prevalence rates. Determining the prevalence rate is vital for planning treatment services because mental health workers need to know the base rates and the percentage of people who are affected by particular disorders.

Epidemiological studies also provide information regarding **incidence**—the number of new cases of a disorder that appear in an identified population within a specified time period. The incidence rate is lower than the prevalence rate because incidence involves only new cases, whereas prevalence includes both new and existing cases. Incidence rates are important for examining hypotheses about the causes or origins of a disorder. For instance, if we find an increased incidence of a disorder (i.e., more new cases) in a population exposed to a particular stressor compared with another population not exposed to the stressor, we can hypothesize that the stressor contributed to the development of the disorder. Epidemiological research, then, is important not only in describing the frequency and distribution of disorders but also in determining possible causal factors.

Surveys, which involve collecting data from all or part of a population to assess the relative prevalence, distribution, and interrelationships of different phenomena, are frequently used in epidemiological research. For instance, survey researchers often collect data and then correlate certain variables, such as family income and frequency of psychiatric hospitalization, to discover whether they are related. Surveys are also used in **longitudinal research**, a methodology that involves observing, assessing, and evaluating people's behaviors over a long period. In fact, researchers often combine elements of different methods in their research. For example, an investigator conducting treatment outcome studies may use both surveys and longitudinal studies.

Myth We can accurately predict the outcome of treatment.

Reality Treatment sometimes produces unexpected results.
Iatrogenic effects are the unintended effects of therapy—such as an unintended change in behavior resulting from a medication prescribed or a psychological technique employed by a therapist. For example, some medications can produce unanticipated side effects or interact negatively with other drugs (Fava & Rafanelli, 2019). When this occurs, additional medication is sometimes required to counteract the iatrogenic effects of the original medication.

4-4 Contemporary Trends and Future Directions

Clinical practice continues to be guided by research. Therefore, mental health professionals must be able to easily sort through and evaluate research data. Several contemporary trends are facilitating this effort. For example, meta-analysis has simplified the process of comparing research results from the many studies published each year. **Meta-analysis** is a statistical method in which researchers combine and analyze the results from numerous studies focused on the same or similar phenomena. The aim is to increase the precision of the results. In general, the studies included in a meta-analysis meet particular criteria, such as having a certain sample size or research design. However, unless studies chosen for inclusion in the systematic review are well designed and use meaningful operational definitions, the outcome may be suspect. Additionally, a meta-analysis is only as good as the information going into it—or, as some say, "garbage in, garbage out."

In the fields of psychology and psychiatry, there is also increasing emphasis on **evidence-based practice**. Evidence-based practice is based on the principle that treatment decisions must incorporate three components: (1) high-quality research such as randomized controlled studies; (2) clinician judgment and experience; and (3) client culture, values, needs, and perspectives (Morales & Norcross, 2010). Following this trend, the American Psychological Association and other organizations maintain a list of evidence-based therapies that are effective for specific mental disorders. The use of evidence-based therapies for members of underrepresented groups has become more available as multicultural counselors increasingly conduct research using evidence-based practices with various ethnic groups. For example, culturally modified, evidence-based treatments have been developed for Latinx immigrants (Parra-Cardona et al., 2017) and for other diverse populations (Hall et al., 2016). However, the implementation of evidence-based practices in community agencies is not yet widespread, since some therapists and organizations believe the approach does not consider therapists' therapeutic preferences, requires specialized training, and imposes a standardized approach to each client (Munson et al., 2022).

Another area of rapid growth has been the use of large data sets. Researchers can now access data sets of unimaginable sizes from online surveys or social media posts. These data can be collected on a worldwide basis. For instance, Bleidorn et al. (2016) collected over 985,000 online surveys from adults (ages 16 to 45) in 48 countries in their investigation of the relationship between age, gender, and self-esteem. The results of studies based on online survey and social media data are likely to be deemed more valid than research based on college students because findings based on people of different educational or income levels, ethnicities, religions, and political perspectives are more reflective of the real world.

However, problems also exist with online surveys. The quality of input from online respondents is likely to be variable, depending on each person's commitment to and interest in responding—ranging from those who are deeply interested in the study to those simply looking for a distraction. Additionally, some participants might answer dishonestly in an effort to skew the results. The honesty of responses may be especially problematic for researchers studying a rare phenomenon with fewer respondents and, thus, a smaller sample size. In such cases, low-quality or fraudulent responses could exert a much stronger effect on the results (Chandler et al., 2020).

Ethical standards may have to be changed for the digital age. For example, a Facebook researcher and a professor from Cornell University collaborated on a study investigating emotional contagion; specifically, they wanted to know if our emotions are affected by the postings of our Facebook friends. The design of the study involved altering the emotional content of the newsfeed of over 600,000 Facebook users (without their knowledge or consent) and then monitoring the emotional content of those users' subsequent posts (Kramer et al., 2014). While many criticized the study as unethical, some argued that the study was appropriate because it yielded useful information (Ross, 2014). Many Facebook users are unaware that much of their data on social media is publicly available for research or how it is being used (Lathan et al., 2023). In the absence of strict ethical guidelines, if you use social media, you might wish to carefully review the terms of agreement, especially if you would prefer not to unknowingly become a research subject.

Another contemporary trend is the concerted effort to reduce bias and misconduct in research. Retractions of articles due to fraud, plagiarism, and duplication of previously published data have been increasing, especially in the last few decades (Chen et al., 2022). As we mentioned earlier, many pharmaceutical companies avoid publishing studies that fail to support their products. Further, clinical trials of some medications have been found to include falsified data. In one study where falsified data (involving one specific medication) were removed from a meta-analysis, the results no longer favored that drug (Garmendia et al., 2019).

There is an ongoing need to continually monitor and address these issues of publication fraud and bias through actions such as:

- increasing the transparency of research by having researchers register their studies, including their hypotheses and statistical methods;
- facilitating access to both published and unpublished studies regarding specific medications or treatments;
- reducing conflicts of interest by identifying pharmaceutical or other financial ties for all researchers;
- congressional action such as the Physician Payments Sunshine Act, passed in 2010, which compels pharmaceutical companies to publicly report payments they make to medical researchers or mental health professionals; and
- encouraging all researchers to demand openness in research.

Finally, biological researchers are continuing to focus on locating biomarkers and endophenotypes for particular disorders. Locating specific neurochemical, neuroanatomical, cognitive, or neuropsychological traits associated with specific disorders will provide important information regarding possible genetic pathways and physiological processes involved in their etiology. If we know who is at greatest risk to develop a particular disorder, it is then possible to focus efforts on prevention or on rapid diagnosis and treatment if symptoms develop.

Chapter Summary

1 What methods do researchers use to study the causes of and treatments for psychopathology?

- The scientific method is a method of inquiry involving the systematic collection of data, controlled observation, and the testing of hypotheses.

- Characteristics such as the potential for self-correction, the development of hypotheses, the use of operational definitions, the consideration of reliability and validity, an acknowledgment of base rates, and the evaluation of the statistical significance of the results enable us to have greater faith in research findings.

- The experiment is the most powerful research tool we have for determining and testing cause and effect relationships. In its simplest form, an experiment involves an experimental hypothesis, an independent variable, and a dependent variable.

- Correlational studies measure the degree to which two variables are related to each other. Correlational techniques provide less precision, control, and generality than experiments provide, and they do not answer questions about cause and effect relationships.

- Analogue studies are used to create a situation as close to real life as possible. They permit the study of phenomena under controlled conditions when such study might otherwise be ethically, morally, legally, or practically impossible.

- Field studies rely on naturalistic observations in real-life situations; events are observed as they naturally occur. However, a field study cannot determine causality, and it may be difficult to sort out all the variables involved.

- A case study is an intensive study of one individual that relies on clinical data, such as observations, psychological tests, and historical and biographical information.

- Single-participant experiments differ from case studies in that cause-and-effect relationships can be determined. A multiple-baseline study is a type of single-participant experimental design in which baselines on two or more behaviors or the same behavior in two or more settings are obtained prior to intervention.

2 How does biological research help us better understand the causes of psychopathological behavior?

- Biological research strategies allow us to search for genetic and epigenetic factors involved in psychological disorders and to identify biological indicators of a disorder.

- Biological researchers study biological processes involved in mental illness from many directions, including endophenotypes, the measurable and heritable traits that give clues regarding the genetic pathways involved in a disorder.

- Researchers often make comparisons between identical, or monozygotic (MZ), twins and fraternal, or dizygotic (DZ), twins to evaluate hereditary and environmental influences on development.

- Genetic linkage studies allow researchers to determine whether a disorder follows a genetic pattern by assessing individuals who have a mental disorder and their close relatives.

- Epigenetic researchers seek to determine which environmental factors influence whether or not a gene is expressed and how gene expression is associated with the development of mental disorders.

- Researchers frequently use animals as surrogates for humans, particularly in genetic and epigenetic studies.

3 What is epidemiological research and what does it tell us about mental illness?

- Epidemiological research examines the rate and distribution of mental disorders in a population. It can also provide insight into what groups are at risk for mental disturbance and what factors may influence the development of mental disorders.

- There is often confusion between prevalence rates and incidence rates. Prevalence rates include both new and existing cases during a specified time period. Incidence rates involve only new cases.

4 What are current trends in research into psychopathology?

- Meta-analytic research combines and analyzes the results from numerous studies focused on the same or similar phenomena.
- The recent focus on evidence-based practice helps ensure that therapies for mental disorders are based on solid research.

- Professionals are concerned about reducing bias and misconduct in research.
- Biological researchers continue to focus on locating biomarkers for particular disorders with the goal of preventing or intervening early to treat mental disorders.

Chapter Glossary

analogue study
an investigation that attempts to replicate or simulate, under controlled conditions, a situation that occurs in real life

asymptomatic
without symptoms

base rate
the rate of natural occurrence of a phenomenon in the population studied

case study
an intensive study of one individual that relies on clinical data, such as observations, psychological tests, and historical and biographical information

correlation
the extent to which variations in one variable are accompanied by increases or decreases in a second variable

dependent variable
a variable that is expected to change when an independent variable is manipulated in a psychological experiment

double-blind design
an experimental design in which neither those helping with the experiment nor the participants are aware of experimental conditions

endophenotypes
measurable characteristics (neurochemical, endocrinological, neuroanatomical, cognitive, or neuropsychological) that can give clues regarding the specific genes involved in disorders

epidemiological research
the study of the prevalence and distribution of mental disorders in a population

evidence-based practice
treatment decisions based on best current research combined with clinician judgment and client characteristics and needs

evidence-based therapies
treatment techniques that have strong research support

experiment
a technique of scientific inquiry in which a prediction is made about two variables; the independent variable is then manipulated in a controlled situation, and changes in the dependent variable are measured

experimental hypothesis
a prediction concerning how an independent variable will affect a dependent variable in an experiment

external validity
the degree to which findings of a particular study can be generalized to other groups or conditions

field study
an investigative technique in which behaviors and events are observed and recorded in their natural environment

genetic linkage studies
studies that attempt to determine whether a disorder follows a genetic pattern

hypothesis
a tentative explanation for certain facts or observations

iatrogenic effects
unintended effects of an intervention—such as an unintended change in behavior resulting from a medication or a psychological technique used in treatment

incidence
the number of new cases of a disorder that appear in an identified population within a specified time period

independent variable
a variable or condition that an experimenter manipulates to determine its effect on a dependent variable

internal validity
the degree to which changes in the dependent variable are due solely to the effect of changes in the independent variable

longitudinal research
a research method that involves observing, assessing, or evaluating a group of people over a long period of time

meta-analysis
a statistical method in which researchers combine and analyze the results from numerous studies focused on the same or similar phenomena

multiple-baseline study
a single-participant experimental design in which baselines on two or more behaviors or the same behavior in two or more settings are obtained prior to intervention

operational definition
a concrete description of the variables that are being studied

penetrance
the proportion of individuals carrying a specific variant of a gene (allele or genotype) who also express the associated trait (phenotype)

placebo
an ineffectual or sham treatment, such as an inactive substance, used as a control in an experimental study

placebo effect
improvement produced by expectations of a positive treatment outcome

reliability
the degree to which a measure or procedure yields the same results repeatedly

scientific method
a method of inquiry that provides for the systematic collection of data, controlled observation, and the testing of hypotheses

single-blind design
an experimental design in which only the participants are unaware of the purpose of the research

single-participant experiment
an experiment performed on a single individual in which some aspect of the person's behavior is used as a control or baseline for comparison with future behaviors

statistical significance
the likelihood that a research finding is not due to chance alone

theory
a group of principles and hypotheses that together explain some aspect of a particular area of inquiry

validity
the degree to which an instrument measures what it was developed to measure

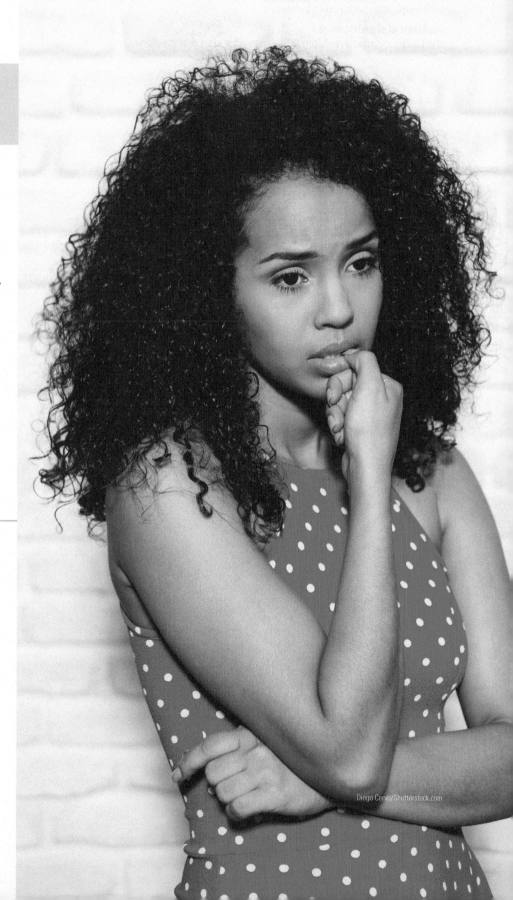

focus
Questions

5

Anxiety and Obsessive-Compulsive and Related Disorders

Learning Objectives

After studying this chapter, you will be able to . . .

5-1 Discuss how biological, psychological, social, and sociocultural factors are involved in the development of anxiety disorders, and why the multipath model is important.

5-2 Discuss phobias, what contributes to their development, and how they are treated.

5-3 Describe panic disorder, what produces it, and how it is treated.

5-4 Describe generalized anxiety disorder, its causes, and how it is treated.

5-5 Describe the characteristics of obsessive-compulsive and related disorders, their causes, and how they are treated.

"I've Frozen, Mortifyingly, Onstage at public lectures and presentations, and on several occasions I have been compelled to bolt from the stage . . . I've abandoned dates, walked out of exams, and had breakdowns during job interviews, plane flights, train trips, and car rides, and simply walking down the street. My anxiety can be intolerable" (Stossel, 2014).

Scott Stossel, a Harvard graduate, is the editor of *Atlantic* magazine and author of several best-selling books. He has lived with anxiety since childhood, when he was often terrified by worries that his parents might die. Anxiety has also been an ongoing issue throughout his adult years. While making his wedding vows, he leaned on his bride so that he would not collapse from anxiety; during the birth of his child, the nurses had to stop attending to his wife so they could help him as he turned pale and keeled over. Even today, Stossel drinks a small quantity of alcohol and takes several antianxiety medications to cope with the strong physiological reactions he experiences before making a public presentation.

A nxiety takes many forms. People vary in how they express anxiety and what triggers their anxiety. People also differ in the severity of their anxiety reactions. Why do so many of us, like Scott Stossel, feel our hearts race, our muscles tense, and our bodies tremble during public speaking or other social situations when no actual danger exists? Why do some people have extreme fears of clowns, spiders, flying, or enclosed places; experience constant worry; or feel compelled to perform rituals?

In this chapter, we answer these questions and discuss various conditions involving extreme anxiety—*phobias*, *panic disorder*, and *generalized anxiety disorder*. We also cover obsessive-compulsive and related disorders (*obsessive-compulsive disorder*, *body dysmorphic disorder*, *hair-pulling disorder*, and *skin-picking disorder*) in this chapter because of their strong association with anxiety. We begin our discussion with the multipath model outlined in Chapter 2 to explain some of the etiological factors associated with anxiety disorders.

5-1 Understanding Anxiety Disorders from a Multipath Perspective

We have all experienced the uneasiness or apprehension associated with anxiety. **Anxiety** often produces tension, worry, and physiological reactivity. Anxiety is frequently an anticipatory emotion—a sense of unease about a dreaded event or situation that has not yet occurred. What causes so many of us to experience anxiety? From an evolutionary perspective, anxiety may be adaptive, producing bodily reactions that prepare us for "fight or flight." Thus, mild or moderate anxiety prevents us from ignoring danger and allows us to cope with potentially hazardous circumstances. **Fear** is a more intense emotion experienced in response to a threatening situation. In some cases, as we saw with Scott Stossel's reactions to various events in the opening vignette, fear and anxiety occur even when no danger is present. Unfounded fear or anxiety that interferes with day-to-day functioning and produces clinically significant distress or life impairment is a sign of an **anxiety disorder**.

Those who are affected by anxiety have plenty of company. Anxiety disorders are the most common mental health condition in the United States and affect about 19.1 percent of adults—63 million people—in a given year. Based on nationwide surveys before the COVID-19 pandemic, past-year prevalence for anxiety disorders in the United States was 23 percent for women and 14.3 percent for men. Among adolescents, 31.9 percent had experienced an anxiety disorder (lifetime prevalence), with 8.3 percent experiencing severe impairment (National Institute of Mental Health [NIMH], 2017b). Among 18- to 26-year-old students, the percentage experiencing anxiety disorders doubled between 2008 and 2018 from 10 to 20 percent. Anxiety disorders disproportionately affect Latinx, African American, and transgender people, groups who traditionally experience the stress of everyday discrimination (Kane, 2019). The reported rates of specific anxiety disorders for adults and children can be seen in Figure 5.1.

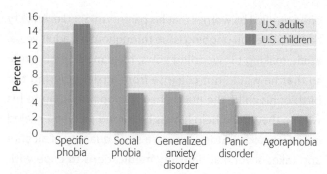

Figure 5.1

Reported Rates of Anxiety Disorders in Adults and Children in the United States

Source: Matthews, 2017

Anxiety disorders are responsible for a great deal of distress and dysfunction, especially because they are often accompanied by depression or substance abuse (Penninx et al., 2021). Anxiety reactions, such as a *phobia*, can significantly interfere with a person's quality of life, as you will read in the following case of a young person who developed a fear of dogs.

> **Case Study** Emily was hiking with her dog when another dog attacked her and bit her wrist. She was terrified. The wound became badly infected and very painful, requiring medical treatment. On another occasion, her sister, Marian, was walking in the fields when three large, growling dogs chased her. The owner heard the commotion and intervened before she was physically injured. Marian developed a fear of dogs; she now avoids visiting friends who have dogs or participating in leisure activities where dogs might be present. In contrast, Emily, who experienced painful injuries, did not develop a fear of dogs. What could account for these differences in reactions between the sisters? (Mineka & Zinbarg, 2006)

Emily experienced a traumatic dog attack, but it was her sister, Marian, who developed a phobia. What might be some factors that increased Marian's vulnerability to experiencing anxiety and fear around dogs and what might have protected Emily from developing a phobia? In general, single **etiological models**, whether biological, psychological, social, or sociocultural, do not adequately explain why people vary in their enduring responses to fearful situations.

A number of factors play a role in the acquisition of disorders involving anxiety and fear, including biological influences such as genetically based vulnerabilities and psychological factors such as personality characteristics. In addition, social stressors and cultural rules or norms can influence the development and expression of anxiety. You can appreciate the variety of contributors that can potentially influence the development of an anxiety disorder in the multipath model presented in Figure 5.2. We begin our etiological discussion with a focus on the biological underpinnings of anxiety.

Biological Dimension

For phobias and all anxiety disorders, it is important to rule out possible medical or physical causes of anxiety symptoms, such as medication side effects, excessive caffeine intake, hyperthyroidism (overactive thyroid), cardiac arrhythmias, or withdrawal from alcohol (Bhat et al., 2019). Beyond these physiological causes of anxiety symptoms, two main biological factors influence the development of anxiety disorders: fear circuitry in the brain and genetics.

Fear Circuitry in the Brain

A variety of limbic system structures and processes are involved in fear and anxiety responses. The amygdala plays a central role in triggering a state of fear or anxiety. As you may recall from Chapter 2, the amygdala is involved in our recollection of intense emotions, particularly memories associated with danger. But how is the amygdala involved in producing fear or anxiety reactions? When we encounter a situation that may affect our safety and security, two separate neural pathways are activated. In the first, when we come across a possible threat, the potentially dangerous stimulus rapidly activates the amygdala, triggering the hypothalamic-pituitary-adrenal (HPA)

Did You Know?

Neuroimaging studies of a woman who was unable to experience fear or recognize life-threatening situations revealed bilateral damage to her amygdala. It is likely that this brain abnormality was the reason for her absence of fear.

Source: Feinstein et al., 2011

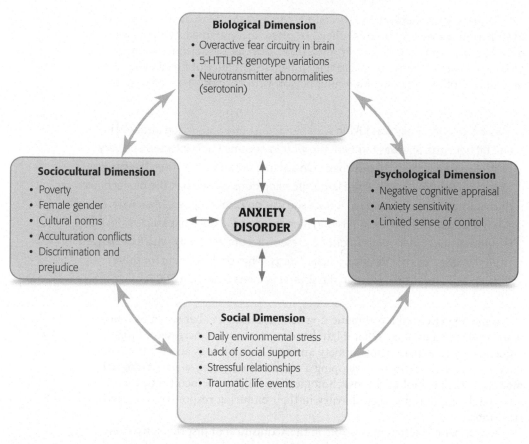

Figure 5.2

Multipath Model of Anxiety Disorders

The dimensions interact with one another and combine in different ways to result in a specific anxiety disorder. The importance and influence of each dimension vary from individual to individual.

axis to prepare for immediate action—the "fight or flight" response. The ensuing chemical cascade prepares us to defend ourselves or to flee. In some cases, fear results in a "freeze" response. Our emotional reaction may be so strong that our perceptions are narrowed and primitive survival responses take over, interfering with rational thinking and productive action (Marek et al., 2019).

Fortunately, a potentially threatening stimulus simultaneously activates the second and slower pathway in which sensory signals travel to the **hippocampus** and prefrontal cortex. These structures process the sensory input and evaluate any potential danger associated with the situation. If this secondary fear circuit determines that no threat exists, signals are sent to the amygdala to curtail the HPA axis activity, thus overriding the initial fear response. For example, if you were on an airplane, sudden turbulence might activate your amygdala and produce an immediate fear response. However, more precise mental processing of the event involving your hippocampus and prefrontal cortex—putting the turbulence in context perhaps by activating memories of prior air travel where you remained safe despite turbulence—would provide reassurance, inhibit your fear, and reduce your anxiety. But if you misinterpret or magnify the significance of the environmental signals—such as concluding that turbulence must be dangerous or questioning the competence of the pilot—you might react with undue anxiety.

Once the HPA axis activity is activated, the reaction continues until higher-level mental processing terminates the response; because our initial fear responses are turned on or off rather than regulated like a thermostat, we are not able to curtail our initial, reactive responses without this higher-order mental processing. As you might expect, when the HPA axis is activated frequently, the neural connections associated with environmental triggers are strengthened ("neurons that fire together, wire together"), paving the way for increased emotional reactivity, including heightened or more frequent anxiety. Neuroimaging techniques such as positron emission tomography (PET) scans and magnetic resonance imaging (MRI) have confirmed this increased reactivity in the amygdala when individuals with anxiety disorders are exposed to emotional stimuli (Hattingh et al., 2013).

In some individuals this overactivity in the fear network appears to be associated with insufficient availability of certain neurotransmitters that inhibit neural activity. For instance, some studies have linked anxiety and fear with a reduction in **GABA** (gamma-aminobutyric acid) activity in the hippocampus and amygdala (Delaney et al., 2018). As you may recall, GABA is an inhibitory neurotransmitter that reduces neural communication; thus, with less GABA activity, there is potentially less inhibition of fear responses.

Our understanding of the biological aspects of anxiety also comes from studies that monitor changes that occur in individuals who have received treatment for an anxiety disorder. For example, neuroimaging techniques suggest that certain medications and certain therapies (e.g., cognitive-behavioral therapy) produce a reduction in limbic activity that results in symptom improvement (Gorka et al., 2019). Medication appears to directly decrease activity in the amygdala and thus "normalize" anxiety reactions, whereas therapy appears to reduce physiological arousal by strengthening distress tolerance and the ability of the prefrontal cortex to inhibit fear responses (refer to Figure 5.3). Interestingly, some psychotherapies appear to enhance amygdala–prefrontal cortex connectivity, which suggests that the neurological mechanisms that inhibit fear responses have been strengthened (Hölzel et al., 2013).

Genetic Influences

Genes modestly contribute to anxiety disorders; genetic effects are most pronounced when genetic factors interact with stressful environmental influences (Sharma et al., 2016). Researchers are now trying to identify how genes influence the development of anxiety disorders. As you learned in Chapter 2, neurotransmitters are chemicals that help transmit messages in the brain. One specific neurotransmitter, **serotonin**, is strongly associated with anxiety disorders. Consequently, a variation in the serotonin transporter gene (5-HTTLPR) has been the focus of considerable research.

In the case of the 5-HTTLPR genotype, a **polymorphic variation** (a common DNA mutation) affects the length of one region of the associated **alleles** (the gene pair responsible for specific traits); it is possible to inherit two short alleles, two long alleles, or one short and one long allele. Researchers have found that short alleles of the 5-HTTLPR gene are associated with both a reduction in serotonin activity and increased fear- and anxiety-related behaviors. This means that carriers of the short allele are more likely to show reactivity of the amygdala when exposed to threatening stimuli. In contrast, long alleles of the 5-HTTLPR gene appear to protect against negative effects from exposure to distressing circumstances, particularly early childhood stressors (Nestor et al., 2019).

It is likely that numerous genes affect vulnerability to anxiety disorders. Additionally, identified genes only influence an individual's **predisposition**

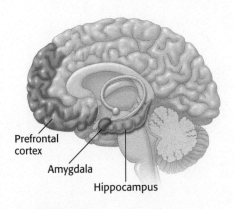

Prefrontal cortex

Amygdala

Hippocampus

Figure 5.3

Neuroanatomical Basis for Panic and Other Anxiety Disorders

The fear network in the brain is centered in the amygdala, which interacts with the hippocampus and areas of the prefrontal cortex. Antianxiety medications appear to desensitize the fear network. Some psychotherapies also affect brain processes associated with anxiety.

to develop an anxiety disorder. For example, although the presence of certain alleles increases the chances that a characteristic such as anxiety is expressed, actual expression of the gene depends on interactions between the genotype and the environment.

Interactions Between Biological and Environmental Influences

How do environmental variables influence the expression of genes related to anxiety? Researchers were initially puzzled by conflicting findings regarding carriers of the short allele of the 5-HTTLPR gene and **behavioral inhibition**. If the short allele of the 5-HTTLPR genotype is associated with anxiety, why do only some children who are carriers of this allele demonstrate persistent behavioral inhibition or significant shyness?

N. A. Fox and colleagues (Nichols & Schwartz, 2005) hypothesized that behavioral inhibition occurs when certain environmental factors such as parental behaviors interact with a child's genetic predisposition. Using a longitudinal design, researchers observed and rated characteristics of behavioral inhibition in 153 children at age 14 months and again at 7 years. They also rated the mothers' nurturing behaviors and tendency to provide social support to their children. Based on DNA genotyping, they divided the children into two groups: those with and those without a short 5-HTTLPR allele. The researchers found that children with the short allele showed behavioral inhibition only when they were raised in a stressful environment with low levels of maternal social support. As Fox observed:

> If you have two short alleles of this serotonin gene, but your mom is not stressed, you will be no more shy than your peers as a school age child. . . . But . . . if you are raised in a stressful environment, and you inherit the short form of the gene, there is a higher likelihood that you will be fearful, anxious or depressed. (Association for Psychological Science, 2007)

Further research suggests that the presence of the short allele of 5-HTTLPR increases neuroplasticity in response to environmental influences. Thus, social and cultural influences such as positive family or community support can reduce or eliminate the behavioral inhibition associated with the short variant of 5-HTTLPR (Johnson et al., 2016). Interestingly, a study conducted in China—a culture that tends to nurture inhibited behavior in young children—found that Chinese children with two short alleles had more confidence interacting with peers and with a stranger than their peers with other allele combinations. While behavioral inhibition in young children in Western cultures is often viewed as a concern, this does not occur in China, where parents traditionally regard the ability to inhibit impulsive behavior as a sign of social maturity. This finding supports the role of sociocultural environment on genetic expression (Chen et al., 2014).

Psychological Dimension

Psychological characteristics can also interact with biological predispositions to produce anxiety symptoms. People who have **anxiety sensitivity**—a tendency to interpret physiological changes in the body as signs of danger—are particularly vulnerable to developing anxiety symptoms. This pattern of anxiety sensitivity has been found to increase anxious arousal among Latinx college students adjusting to college life (Jardin et al., 2018).

Did You Know?

Having chronic anxiety can affect your physical well-being. Disorders involving fear and anxiety have been linked to the shortening of telomeres (the end part of chromosomes) and poorer physical health.

Source: Malouff & Schutte, 2017

Reducing Risk of Lifelong Anxiety

Some infants and toddlers demonstrate high levels of behavioral inhibition characterized by distress and emotional reactivity to environmental changes. Inhibited children tend to be cautious, shy, and wary of unfamiliar situations or people. New experiences are difficult because children with these characteristics show negative emotional reactions to novelty and attempt to avoid or escape from uncomfortable social situations. Such behavioral inhibition is thought to result from biological predispositions involving heightened fear responses (Fox et al., 2005). However, less than half of children who are biologically predisposed to anxiety continue to be inhibited in middle childhood (Degnan & Fox, 2007).

What protective factors enhance the resilience of these children? Nurturing behaviors on the part of parents and other caretakers play a key role in reducing symptoms of inhibition. A supportive parenting style can foster prosocial behaviors through modeling and reduce anxiety by building a child's self-confidence; sense of security; and feelings of mastery, including the belief that it is possible to control anxiety (Eisenberg et al., 2019).

Other helpful parental behaviors include encouraging the child to explore

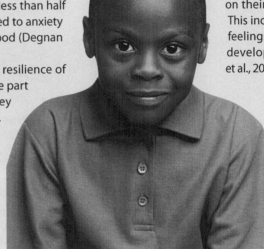

Kevin Peterson/Photodisc/Getty Images

new situations by reinforcing independent behaviors, supporting the child's attempts to approach situations that evoke anxiety, and giving comfort when needed. Such exposure allows children to develop the skills needed to develop prosocial behaviors and regulate their emotional reactivity (Eisenberg et al., 2015). As inhibited children increasingly engage with anxiety-evoking situations, they begin to focus on positive aspects of the situation rather than solely on their anxiety and vigilance to threats. This increase in emotional regulation and feelings of mastery decreases the risk of developing an anxiety disorder (White et al., 2011).

Thus, the behaviors of parents or other caretakers can produce adaptive emotional regulation skills in young children and help them overcome their biological predisposition toward behavioral inhibition; in fact, such support can reduce the innate physiological reactivity and emotional overarousal associated with anxiety disorders.

In general, those of us who engage in **negative appraisal**—interpreting events, even ambiguous ones, as threatening—have an increased likelihood of developing an anxiety disorder. In contrast, individuals who practice adaptive forms of emotional regulation such as using the skill of **reappraisal**—minimizing negative responses by looking at a situation from various perspectives—demonstrate fewer anxiety symptoms (Goldin et al., 2021).

One's sense of control may also be a factor in the development of an anxiety disorder. Young monkeys reared in environments in which they could control access to water and food showed less fear when exposed to anxiety-provoking situations compared to monkeys without this control. Having a sense of self-control and mastery also appears to reduce susceptibility to anxiety in humans (Gallagher et al., 2014). Thus, a number of psychological characteristics can affect individual vulnerability to anxiety disorders.

Social and Sociocultural Dimensions

Any etiological theory of anxiety disorders must consider the influence of social and sociocultural factors and stressors. Daily stress can produce anxiety, especially in individuals who have biological or psychological

Did You Know?

Concerns regarding risk of infection, shortages of protective equipment, isolation from families, fear of infecting family members, working long hours, and compassion fatigue created high levels of anxiety among health care workers who were dealing with the COVID-19 outbreak.

Source: Kang et al., 2020

Self-Control and Mastery Decrease Anxiety

Children who develop a sense of control and mastery are less susceptible to anxiety disorders. In this case, the child is allowed to choose her dinner from an assortment of healthy foods and to serve herself.

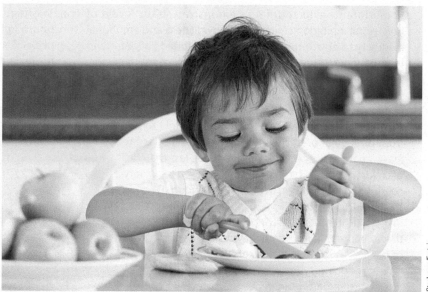

iStock.com/Fertnig

vulnerabilities. For instance, experiencing financial strain due to a low income is associated with higher rates of anxiety disorders. Young adults from families that have problems paying bills are nearly three times as likely to have problems with anxiety compared to those whose families do not face financial difficulty (Kane, 2019). Environmental conditions such as experiencing poverty, an unsafe environment, or adverse working conditions can lead to or exacerbate anxiety (Yatham, Sivathasan, et al., 2018). Further, events such as terrorist attacks, school shootings, and natural disasters are also associated with increased rates of anxiety disorders (Vandentorren et al., 2018). Perceptions of having limited social support from family, friends, and peers can exacerbate these anxiety reactions, especially among those genetically predisposed to anxiety sensitivity (Reinelt et al., 2014).

The emergence of the COVID-19 illness significantly increased anxiety throughout the world. For instance, in the United States, during the first month of the pandemic (February 16, 2020 through March 15, 2020), prescriptions for antianxiety medications increased by 34 percent—a striking upturn after a 5-year decline in antianxiety prescription rates. Given the large number of individuals affected either directly or indirectly by the pandemic, there is concern about the potential for a marked increase in anxiety disorders in the coming years (Stettin, 2020).

Gender plays a role in the development of anxiety disorders. Women are more frequently diagnosed with anxiety disorders compared to men. Is the reason biological, social, or a combination of the two? Women are more likely to be diagnosed with emotional disorders due to their lack of power and status, as well as stressors associated with poverty, lack of respect, and limited choices, according to researchers (World Health Organization, 2020b). These social factors may increase the production of stress hormones that increase vulnerability to both depression and anxiety. Thus, interactions between psychological, social, and biological factors may help explain why women are more likely to develop anxiety disorders. Similarly, combinations of these factors may account for the varied age of onset for the various anxiety disorders (refer to Figure 5.4).

Exposure to discrimination and prejudice can increase the anxiety of people who are members of ethnically underrepresented or marginalized groups, such as gender and sexual minorities or individuals with disabilities. For example, discrimination, expectations of rejection, and the perceived need for identity concealment in LGBT populations have been connected not only with increased anxiety but also with other mental health conditions linked to anxiety (MacIntyre et al., 2023; Valentine & Shipherd, 2018). The roots of this anxiety may develop at an early age, particularly among those who experience ongoing rejection. One longitudinal study found that discrimination experienced by Mexican-born 5th graders living in the United States was associated with anxiety symptoms in the 12th grade, particularly among the students who continued to experience racism during their middle school and early high school years (Stein et al., 2019).

Internalization of societal and cultural prejudices and attitudes toward one's own group, either consciously or subconsciously, has also been linked to increases in anxiety symptoms (Cénat et al., 2023). Among one group of Black college students attending a predominately White university, both moderate and high levels of internalized racism were linked to anxiety and distress in the college environment (Sosoo et al., 2020). Similarly, the presence of covert and overt racism on a predominantly White campus combined with a perception that their values and beliefs were not a "good fit" with the university environment contributed to high levels of academic and social anxiety for one group of Native American students (Chee et al., 2019). Further, fear over raids, discovery, or deportations has resulted in traumatic stress and anxiety for undocumented immigrants as well as their families and friends (Sanchez, 2019).

Cultural factors such as acculturation conflicts also contribute to anxiety disorders among ethnically underrepresented groups. For example, Asian American undergraduate students report higher levels of anxiety related to academic achievement and parental expectations compared to their European American counterparts (Saw et al., 2013). Culture can also influence how anxiety is expressed. For instance, in the United States and other Western countries, social anxiety involves fear of embarrassing oneself, whereas in some Asian countries, social anxiety involves worries about being offensive to others (Nakagami et al., 2017). Awareness of cultural manifestations of anxiety in different groups is essential for clinicians working with clients from diverse backgrounds.

You now have some ideas about some of the factors associated with anxiety—the emotion underlying the disorders we discuss in this chapter. Keep these influences in mind as we turn our attention to the specific anxiety disorders, beginning with phobias (refer to Table 5.1).

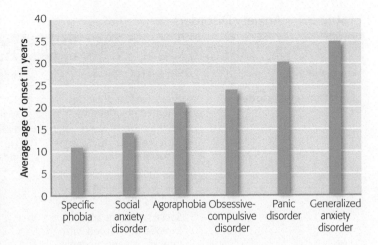

Figure 5.4

Age of Onset for Anxiety Disorders

This graph, based on a compilation of data from multiple studies, demonstrates the mean age of onset for specific phobia, social anxiety disorder, agoraphobia, obsessive-compulsive disorder, panic disorder, and generalized anxiety disorder.

Source: Adapted from Lijster et al., 2017

Table 5.1 Anxiety Disorders

Disorders Chart			
Disorder	**DSM-5-TR Criteria**	**Prevalence**	**Age of Onset**
Social anxiety disorder	• Excessive fear of being watched or judged by others • Extreme self-consciousness in social situations • Fear that anxiety symptoms will be humiliating or offend others • Social situations are avoided or endured with intense fear and anxiety	• 12-month prevalence of 7% to 8% • Twice as common in women and adolescent girls	• Mid-teens
Specific phobia	• Excessive fear of specific objects or situations • Intense fear or panic attacks produced by exposure • Object or situation avoided or endured with great anxiety	• 12-month prevalence from 8% to 12% • Some phobias twice as common in women and girls	• Childhood or early adolescence (depends on type of phobia)
Agoraphobia	• Anxiety or panic in situations where escape is difficult or embarrassing • Situations nearly always produce panic and are avoided	• 12-month prevalence of up to 1.7% • Twice as common in women	• Usually late adolescence, with two thirds before age 35 • Onset sometimes occurs late in life
Panic disorder	• Recurrent and unexpected intense attacks of fear or terror • Worry about future panic attacks • Can occur with or without agoraphobia	• 12-month prevalence of 2.7% • Twice as common in women	• Early adulthood
Generalized anxiety disorder	• Excessive anxiety and worry over life circumstances (e.g., money, family, or school) • Difficulty in controlling worry • Vigilance, muscle tension, restlessness, edginess, and difficulty concentrating	• 12-month prevalence ranges from .9% in adolescents to 2.9% for adults • At least twice as prevalent in women	• Median age of diagnosis is about 35, but symptom onset is often earlier

Source: American Psychiatric Association, 2022

5-2 Phobias

The word *phobia* comes from the Greek word for "fear." A **phobia** is a strong, persistent, and unwarranted fear of some specific object or situation (refer to Table 5.2). Phobias are the most common mental disorder in the United States. Individuals with a phobia often experience extreme anxiety or panic when encountering the phobic stimulus. Adults with phobias usually realize that their fear is excessive, although children may not.

There are three categories of phobias: social anxiety disorder, specific phobias, and agoraphobia. The diagnosis of these disorders requires that symptoms are present for at least 6 months.

Social Anxiety Disorder

> **Case Study** In any social situation, I felt fear. I would be anxious before I even left the house, and it would escalate as I got closer to a college class, a party, or whatever. When I would walk into a room full of people, I'd turn red, and it would feel like everybody's eyes were on me. I was embarrassed to stand off in a corner by myself, but I couldn't think of anything to say.... It was humiliating.... I couldn't wait to get out. (NIMH, 2016b, p. 9)

A **social anxiety disorder (SAD)**, sometimes referred to as a social phobia, involves an intense fear of being scrutinized or of doing something embarrassing or humiliating in the presence of others. According to DSM-5-TR, the fear is out of proportion to the circumstances and results in avoidance of the situation or experiencing intense fear or anxiety when enduring the situation. Individuals with SAD are so self-conscious that they literally feel sick with fear at the prospect of public activities. SAD often involves high levels of anxiety in most social situations, although some people experience anxiety only in situations in which they must speak or perform in public (*performance only type*). The most common forms of SAD involve public speaking and meeting new people (APA, 2022).

SAD affects from 7 to 8 percent of adults in a given year; women are 2 times as likely as men to have this disorder. More than 48 percent of those with SAD rate the severity of their symptoms as "mild." However, SAD can be chronic and disabling, especially for those who develop the disorder early in life (Bhat et al., 2019). In a 5-year naturalistic follow-up study, only 40 percent of those with SAD recovered (Beard et al., 2010). The 2-year recovery rate is much lower for African Americans and Latinx Americans, with less than 1 percent reporting a significant reduction in SAD symptoms (Bjornsson et al., 2014; Sibrava et al., 2013). The chronic nature of SAD within oppressed groups may be explained by the ongoing nature of everyday experiences of discrimination in social settings. SAD is often **comorbid** with (i.e., often occurs with) depressive disorders, substance-use disorders, and suicidal thoughts or attempts (Bhat et al., 2019).

Individuals with high social anxiety tend to believe that others are evaluating them or viewing them negatively. Thus, they remain alert for "threat" cues such as signs of disapproval or criticism. They avoid drawing attention to themselves by engaging in "safety behaviors" such as avoiding eye contact, talking less, sitting alone, holding a glass tightly to prevent tremors, or wearing makeup to hide blushing (Cougle et al., 2020). Those with SAD also tend to be socially submissive in an effort to avoid conflicts with others (Zaffar & Arshad, 2020).

Not surprisingly, individuals with SAD often report stressful interpersonal relationships. In an exploration of communication patterns among romantic couples, partners with high levels of social anxiety attended more to negative information, showed less interest in and support for their partners when communicating, and made fewer supportive comments in

Table 5.2 Examples of Phobias

Phobia	Object of Phobia
Acrophobia	Heights
Ailurophobia	Cats
Algophobia	Pain
Astrapophobia	Storms, thunder, lightning
Dementophobia	Insanity
Genophobia	Fear of sexual relations
Hematophobia	Blood
Microphobia	Germs
Monophobia	Being alone
Mysophobia	Contamination/germs
Nyctophobia	Dark
Pathophobia	Disease
Trypophobia	Holes, irregular clusters of holes
Phobophobia	Phobias
Pyrophobia	Fire
Xenophobia	Strangers

Did You Know?

Men with social anxiety disorder often report feeling fearful in dating situations and using alcohol and illicit drugs to cope with their anxiety. Women have a wider variety of social fears and are more likely to be treated with medications.

Source: Xu et al., 2012

response to shared positive events; not surprisingly, these couples were more likely to have ended their relationship 6 months later (Kashdan et al., 2013).

Specific Phobias

A **specific phobia** is an extreme fear of a specific object or situation. Exposure to the stimulus nearly always produces intense panic or anxiety that is out of proportion to the actual danger represented by the object or situation (APA, 2022). The primary types of specific phobias are:

- living creatures (e.g., spiders, insects, dogs, snakes),
- natural environmental (e.g., heights, earthquakes, thunder, water),
- blood/injections or injury (e.g., needles, dental treatment, invasive medical procedures), and
- situational (e.g., enclosed places, flying, driving, being alone, the dark, traveling in tunnels or over bridges).

The following case study demonstrates a common specific phobia exhibited by a 26-year-old public relations executive.

> **Case Study** If I see a spider in my house, I get out! I start shaking, and I feel like I'm going to throw up. I get so scared, I have to bolt across the street to drag my neighbor over to get rid of the spider. Even after I know it's gone, I obsess for hours. I check between my sheets 10 times before getting in bed, and I'm so creeped out that I won't get up and go to the bathroom at night, even if my bladder feels like it's about to burst. (Kusek, 2001, p. 183)

This case reveals how phobias can be extremely distressing and how they can interfere with daily life, especially if it is difficult to avoid the feared object or situation. It is not unusual for an individual to have more than one phobia. Scott Stossel, introduced at the beginning of the chapter, has not only social anxiety disorder but also phobias involving germs, vomiting, enclosed spaces, heights, flying, and cheese.

Specific phobias affect approximately 30 million adults in a given year in the United States (approximately 9.1 percent of the population) and are twice as common in women as in men (NIMH, 2017f). Specific phobias are less common in Asian and Latinx Americans than in African and non-Latinx European Americans and less common in older individuals (APA, 2022).

Specific phobias often begin during childhood. Animal phobias tend to have the earliest onset (age 7), followed by blood phobia (age 9), dental phobia (age 12), and claustrophobia (age 20) (Öst, 1992). Excessive fears are common in young children and most **remit**, or disappear, without treatment (APA, 2022; Reynolds et al., 2014).

Approximately 4 percent of the U.S. population has experienced a phobic reaction to the sight of blood. Blood phobia differs from other phobias because it is associated with a unique physiological response: fainting in the phobic situation. Fainting appears to result from an initial increase in physiological arousal followed by a sudden drop in blood pressure and heart rate. Nearly 70 percent of those with a blood phobia report a history of fainting in medical situations; many avoid medical examinations or are unable to care for injured family members if there is blood involved (Meuret et al., 2017). Blood-injection-injury phobias appear to activate disgust as well as fear responses (Mason et al., 2022).

Phobias

Coulrophobia, a fear of clowns, may result from their painted eyes and smiles and never-changing expressions. Musician Sean "P. Diddy" Combs is reportedly so fearful of clowns that he demands a "no-clown clause" in his performance contracts.

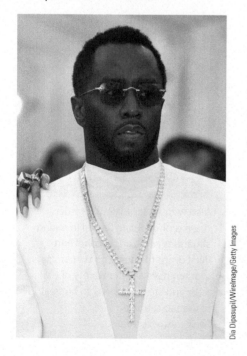

Dia Dipasupil/WireImage/Getty Images

Agoraphobia

Agoraphobia is an intense fear of at least two of the following situations: (a) being outside of the home alone, (b) traveling via public transportation, (c) being in open spaces (e.g., a parking lot or playground), (d) being in stores or theaters, or (e) standing in line or being in a crowd. These situations are feared because escape or help may not be readily available. The fears are out of proportion to actual dangers and result in avoidance of the situation or intense fear or anxiety when enduring the situation (APA, 2022).

People coping with agoraphobia have a fear that they might become incapacitated or severely embarrassed by fainting, losing control over bodily functions, or displaying excessive fear in public. In some cases, people refuse to leave their homes due to concern they might have a **panic attack**, which is an episode of intense fear accompanied by uncomfortable physiological symptoms. Individuals who have agoraphobia often have *anxiety sensitivity*, which is the tendency to misinterpret and overreact to normal physiological changes. This precipitates anxiety, which further increases bodily sensations (e.g., sweating or heart palpitations), resulting in a vicious cycle that can culminate in a panic attack (Jurin & Biglbauer, 2018).

Agoraphobia is relatively uncommon (affecting about 1 percent of U.S. adults in a given year). However, 41 percent of those affected rate their symptoms as serious. This phobia occurs about 2 times more in women compared to men, and is nearly 2.5 times more common in adolescent girls compared to adolescent boys (NIMH, 2017a). Agoraphobia sometimes develops in older adults, with about 11 percent experiencing their first episode at age 65 or older. Risk factors for late-onset agoraphobia include severe depression or a prior tendency to be anxious (Ritchie et al., 2013).

Etiology of Phobias

How do such strong and "irrational" fears develop? In most cases, predisposing genetic factors interact with psychological, social, and socio-cultural influences, as discussed earlier. Scott Stossel, for example, has a family history of anxiety that traces back to his great grandfather. His mother, an attorney, has panic attacks and many of the same phobias that Scott experiences. In addition to these biological factors, Scott observed his mother's fear reactions and panic episodes throughout his childhood. Scott also suspects that the unhappy relationship between his mother and father as well as their divorce may have played a role in his phobias. Although his parents' child-rearing practices were well intentioned and loving, Scott believes that he had few opportunities to develop "autonomy and a sense of self-efficacy." So, are Scott's phobias a result of genetics, psychological influences, social experiences, or their combination? In this section, we examine the factors related to the etiology of phobias, as presented in Figure 5.5.

Biological Dimension

All phobia subtypes involve a moderate genetic contribution. The highest rate of heritability is for animal and blood–injury–injection phobias, according to studies of twin pairs (Van Houtem et al., 2013). Some individuals with phobias appear to have an innate tendency to be anxious and experience strong emotional responses. This exaggerated responsiveness of the amygdala and other areas of the brain associated with fear may make an individual more susceptible to developing a phobia. Neuroimaging studies have confirmed that individuals with phobias show increased

Figure 5.5

Multipath Model of Phobias
The dimensions interact with one another and combine in different ways to result in a phobia.

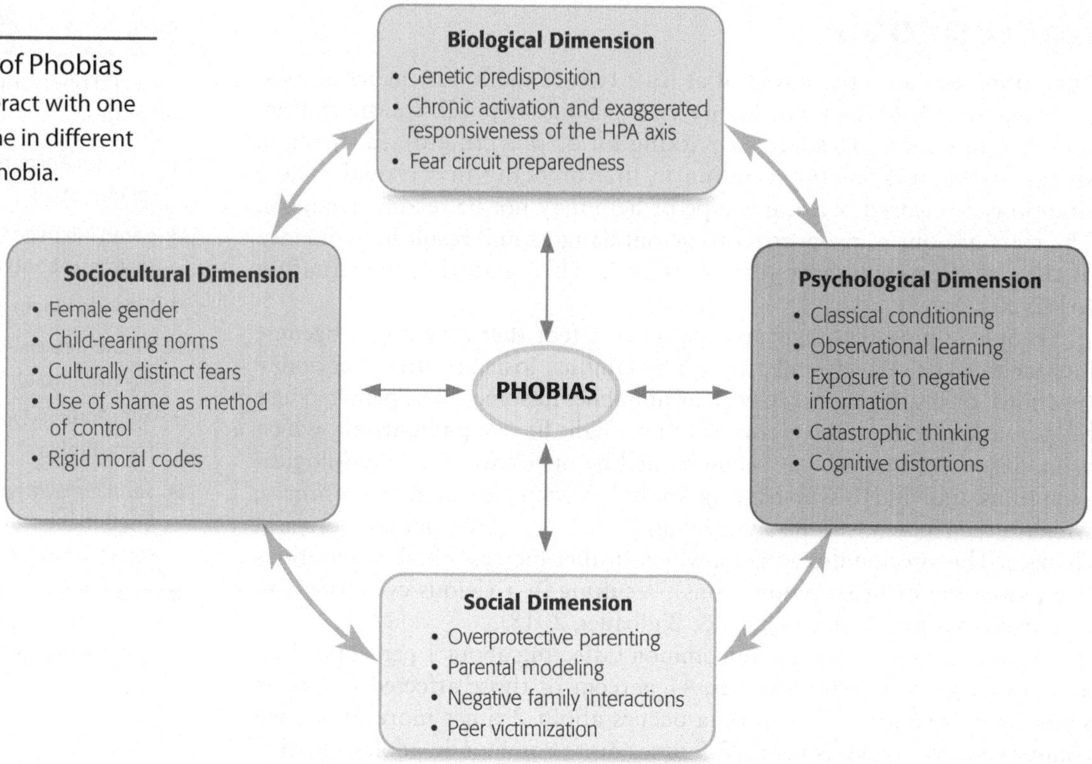

Biological Dimension
- Genetic predisposition
- Chronic activation and exaggerated responsiveness of the HPA axis
- Fear circuit preparedness

Sociocultural Dimension
- Female gender
- Child-rearing norms
- Culturally distinct fears
- Use of shame as method of control
- Rigid moral codes

PHOBIAS

Psychological Dimension
- Classical conditioning
- Observational learning
- Exposure to negative information
- Catastrophic thinking
- Cognitive distortions

Social Dimension
- Overprotective parenting
- Parental modeling
- Negative family interactions
- Peer victimization

Did You Know?

- Nearly half of all U.S. Americans have experienced a severe phobic reaction regarding an injection.

- Up to 50 percent of adolescents and between 20 and 30 percent of young adults in the United States have a fear of injections.

- Fifty percent of individuals who use medications that require self-injections are unable to perform the injections.

- Those with an injection phobia fear pain or have unrealistic thoughts such as "the needle might break off."

Source: Huff, 2021; Mohr et al., 2005

physiological fear responses in reaction to phobic-related stimuli (Kovner et al., 2019). Interestingly, when a man underwent brain surgery designed to eliminate seizures by removing part of his left amygdala (an area associated with the storage and retrieval of frightening stimuli), he lost his intense fear of spiders. He now views them with interest, can observe them closely, and can even touch them. However, his fear of public speaking remains—suggesting that this fear may be processed in a different part of the amygdala (Franco, 2014).

A different biological view of the development of fear reactions is that of *preparedness*. Proponents of this position argue that fears do not develop randomly. They believe that it is easier for humans to develop fears to which we are physiologically predisposed, such as a fear of heights or snakes. Such quickly aroused (or "prepared") fears may have been necessary to human survival. In fact, evolutionarily prepared fears (e.g., fear of fire or deep water) occur even without exposure to traumatic conditioning experiences (Muhlberger et al., 2006). Although preparedness is an interesting theory, it is hard to believe that most phobias stem from prepared fears. Many simply do not fit into the prepared-fear model. It would be difficult, for example, to explain the survival value of social anxiety disorder, as well as many of the other specific phobias. In addition, phobias involving snakes and spiders (prepared fears) are usually not difficult to eliminate with exposure therapy (Luck et al., 2020). In one review of numerous fear-conditioning studies involving snakes and spiders, only 31 percent supported predictions based on preparedness theory (Åhs et al., 2018).

Psychological Dimension

There are multiple psychological pathways that can lead to the development of phobias: (a) direct conditioning of a fear response, (b) observational learning or modeling, (c) receiving negative or threatening information, and (d) cognitive distortions such as overestimating potential danger.

Is It Fear or Disgust?

Do phobias such as fears of spiders and rats result from feelings of disgust rather than from a threat of physical danger? Some researchers have pointed out that spiders and rats are, in general, harmless. These researchers believe that phobias result from an inborn or "prepared" fear of disease or contamination, rather than a threat of physical danger. Others feel that the emotion of disgust underlies certain phobias. For instance, a tendency to be easily disgusted appears to be a precursor to the development of phobias involving spiders, blood, injections, and injury (Olatunji et al., 2019). In an experiment to determine whether disgust is involved in spider phobia, Mulkens, de Jong, and Merckelbach (1996) asked women with and without spider phobias to indicate their willingness to eat a cookie that a "medium-sized" spider had walked across. The researchers reasoned that if disgust was a factor, those with a spider phobia should be more reluctant to eat the "contaminated" cookie. Results supported this idea: Only 25 percent of women with spider phobia eventually ate some of the cookie, compared with 70 percent of the control-group participants.

For Further Consideration

1. Does the avoidance of spiders, snakes, or blood stem from fear, disgust, or both?

2. Since insects such as cockroaches, maggots, and slugs also elicit disgust, why do they not result in phobias?

Classical Conditioning Perspective   The view that phobias are conditioned fear responses evolved from psychologist John B. Watson's classic conditioning experiment with an infant, Little Albert. Watson caused Little Albert to develop a fear of white rats by pairing a white rat with a loud sound (Watson & Rayner, 1920), demonstrating that fears can result through an association process. Similarly, classical conditioning occurred when eight lions at a preserve were given beef laced with a deworming medication that made them temporarily nauseous. After repeated pairings with this medicated meat, seven of the lions refused to eat any beef and the eighth lion temporarily refused all food (Platt, 2011).

Observational Learning Perspective   Fears can develop through observational learning. For example, after being told that they would participate in a similar experiment, participants in a study watched a video in which a man received an uncomfortable shock in response to a stimulus. After viewing the video, they were exposed to the stimulus that was associated with the shock. Not surprisingly, the participants responded with fear. Their fear response was documented by neuroimaging scans that showed activation of the amygdala (Olsson et al., 2007). Observational fear learning not only results in avoidance but also has been found to affect physiological responses such as heart rate (Reynolds et al., 2014).

Children can develop fear responses by observing others displaying fear in real life or in the media. In one study, parents of children ages 8 to 12 were trained to act anxiously or in a relaxed manner before their child took a spelling test (Burstein & Ginsburg, 2010). Children exposed to an anxious-acting parent reported higher anxiety levels, more anxious thoughts, and a greater avoidance of the spelling test than did those in the relaxed parent condition. In another study, watching peers who showed either calm or anxious behaviors when interacting with a novel animal influenced how much fear children displayed when asked to interact with the animal (Broeren et al., 2011). Similarly, children who watched adults display an expression of genuine pain while performing a pain-inducing task with their hands immersed in colored water developed a fear response to the color of water associated with the painful look on the adult's face; this fear reaction did not generalize to water of a different color (Van Lierde et al., 2020).

Scary or Cute?

Fears can be induced through negative information. Children's reactions to the cuscus depended on the descriptions furnished to their parents about the unfamiliar animal.

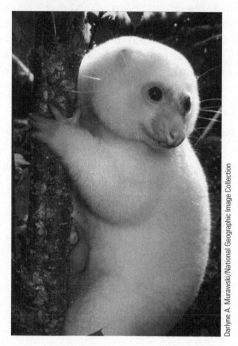

Darlyne A. Murawski/National Geographic Image Collection

Negative Information Perspective   Can information cause someone to fear an object or situation? To determine this, parents were given descriptions regarding an unfamiliar animal (a cuscus) and were asked to use the information to tell their children how the cuscus might behave in certain situations. Parents received one of three descriptions: (a) negative (has sharp claws and long teeth, can jump at your throat); (b) ambiguous (has white teeth, can jump, likes to drink all sorts of things); or (c) positive (has nice tiny teeth, eats tasty strawberries, likes to play with other animals). Children whose parents received the negative description reacted with more fear to the cuscus than those whose parents received positive or ambiguous information (Muris et al., 2010). Interestingly, one group of college students reported that exposure to negative information was responsible for their fears involving academic failure or becoming a victim of crime or violence, but that classical conditioning events most likely explained their acquisition of specific phobias (Loxton et al., 2018).

Cognitive-Behavioral Perspective   Why do individuals with spider phobia react with such terror at the sight of a spider? Some researchers believe that catastrophic thoughts and cognitive distortions (including overestimating possible threat) may cause strong fears to develop. For example, compared with people with a low fear of spiders, those who are highly fearful overestimate the size of spiders and report thinking that the spider "will attack" or "will take revenge" (Leibovich et al., 2016; Mulkens et al., 1996). Similarly, individuals with social anxiety believe the people around them are watching and judging them (NIMH, 2016b).

Social Dimension

Parental behaviors and family interaction patterns can also influence the development of phobias and social anxiety. Overprotection of socially withdrawn children and lack of support for their independence can increase their sense of insecurity and decrease opportunities for them to practice approaching novel situations. The children are thus prevented from developing emotional regulation and coping skills—and social anxiety is more likely to continue (Clarke et al., 2013).

Children with high levels of behavioral inhibition (shyness) appear to be more vulnerable to the effects of poor parenting (Ryan & Ollendick, 2018). In one study, behavioral inhibition and family interactions were measured in a sample of 242 boys and girls at age 3 and again 4 years later. Negative family interactions at age 3 and family stress in middle childhood were both associated with social anxiety symptoms (Volbrecht & Goldsmith, 2010). Additionally, a punitive maternal parenting style (based on child report) was linked with an increased tendency to have fearful beliefs (Field et al., 2007).

Victimization by peers during childhood is an unequivocal risk factor for the development of social anxiety. Further, ongoing ostracism and bullying maintain and exacerbate social anxiety symptoms, especially when those who have been victimized feel a need to avoid situations in which they may encounter the peers responsible for the harassment (Pontillo et al., 2019).

Sociocultural Dimension

Women and girls are more likely to have phobias, with the gender difference showing up as early as 9 years of age. However, this difference mainly involves fear of creatures that elicit a disgust response, such as snakes, rather than animals such as dogs. Some of the gender differences in phobias may occur because women show a stronger disgust

Minority Stress or Rejection Sensitivity?

Alma, a 10-year-old African American girl, was accused of shoplifting a button. She insisted she was innocent and showed her empty pockets. To get out of the stressful situation, she gave the cashier one dollar. After this episode, she developed unwanted and intrusive thoughts of slapping the woman who had accused her. She also became hypervigilant regarding "dangerous situations" and developed a compulsion to lock and unlock her door repeatedly.

Vincent, a gay African Latino adolescent, was rejected by his father because of his sexual orientation. Vincent faced additional homophobia and abuse from his siblings and was forced to undergo conversion therapy. He was also subject to racist behavior while in the community. At a restaurant, someone threw an object at him. Another person shouted, "Go back to Africa!" In school, he was rejected both for his sexual orientation and his race. He became very fearful in social situations and actively avoided social interactions (MacIntyre et al., 2023).

Both of these cases demonstrate how prejudice and discrimination toward individuals who are members of stigmatized groups can impact mental and physical health. How does this happen? According to the *minority stress model* (Meyer, 2020):

1. External stressors (e.g., prejudice, microaggression, aggression) directed toward individuals of stigmatized groups increase their level of psychological and physiological burden.

2. Vulnerability increases for those who internalize the social stigma and/or expect rejection.

3. Resilience resources such as positive group identification, coping skills, community involvement and social support from family or friends can help mitigate the distress caused by external pressures.

4. The interaction of these factors influences the mental and physical well-being of the individual.

Instead of focusing on external stressors, Feinstein (2020) has proposed a *rejection sensitivity model* which suggests that internal cognitive processes involving "rejection sensitivity" and a tendency to expect rejection contribute greatly to the stress of many members of oppressed groups. This "oversensitivity" to experiencing rejection is viewed as maladaptive when it becomes automatically activated in response to minimal threat. Thus, it is the expectation of stigma-related experiences that can result in emotional reactions such as anxiety.

For Further Consideration

1. Analyze the cases above using the minority stress and the rejection sensitivity models.

2. What are the implications of selecting one model over the other?

3. Can the two perspectives be combined?

response than men and because some phobic objects produce feelings of both fear and disgust (Olatunji et al., 2019). Fewer gender differences exist for social fears, fears of bodily injury, and fears of enclosed spaces. Gender differences may be due to a combination of biological and temperamental factors, as well as social norms and socialization experiences (Christiansen, 2016).

Social anxiety appears to be more common in collectivistic cultures in which individual behaviors are seen to reflect on the entire family or group. Because social interdependence is more important than independence in collectivistic cultures, social actions can result in higher anxiety, since they not only implicate the individual, but even more importantly, they are perceived as a reflection on the family or cultural group (Krieg & Xu, 2018). Furthermore, parents who are highly concerned about the opinions of others tend to use shame as a method of control (Bruch & Heimberg, 1994). These are common child-rearing practices among some cultural groups, including Asians; not surprisingly, fear of negative evaluation by others is more common in Asian children and adolescents than in Western comparison groups (Khambaty & Parikh, 2017). The higher levels of social anxiety found in people of Asian heritage may result, in part, from discrepancies between traditional cultural behavioral norms and social expectations of the mainstream culture (Hsu et al., 2012).

Social anxiety disorder is also common among Arab college students, with a prevalence rate between 12 percent and 13 percent. These high rates of social anxiety may be due not only to collectivism but also to other cultural factors, such as a strong sense of personal responsibility for social behaviors, a perceived need to follow a set of rigid moral codes and rituals, and the threat of being ostracized for deviations from social norms (Iancu et al., 2011). Prejudice and discrimination from the mainstream culture may also explain their tendency to feel anxious in social situations.

It is important to note that social fears may be expressed differently in different cultures. *Taijin kyofusho*, for instance, is a culturally distinctive phobia found in Japan that is similar to a social anxiety disorder. However, instead of a fear involving social or performance situations, *taijin kyofusho* is a fear of offending or embarrassing others, a concept that is consistent with the Japanese cultural emphasis on maintaining interpersonal harmony (Nakagami et al., 2017). Individuals with this disorder are fearful that their appearance, facial expression, eye contact, body parts, or body odor might be offensive to others.

Treatment of Phobias

Phobias are successfully treated by both pharmacological and cognitive-behavioral methods.

Biochemical Treatments

In treating phobias, a number of medications demonstrate some effectiveness, although symptoms often recur when the medication is discontinued. The SSRI antidepressants are considered the first-line treatment for chronic conditions such agoraphobia and social anxiety disorder. The serotonin-norepinephrine reuptake inhibitors (SNRIs) and older tricyclic and monoamine oxidase inhibitors (MAOIs) also have some efficacy in treating these disorders. Although these medications begin to alter brain chemistry after the very first dose, they require about 4 to 6 weeks before they begin to reduce symptoms. Beta-blockers, medications used to treat high blood pressure and heart conditions, can also reduce the physical symptoms that accompany certain anxiety disorders, particularly social anxiety disorder. When a feared situation is anticipated (such as taking an exam), physicians sometimes prescribe a beta-blocker to keep physical symptoms of anxiety under control (Butt et al., 2017).

Benzodiazepines (a class of antianxiety medication) have been found to have some effectiveness for anxiety disorders. You may recall that benzodiazepines reduce symptoms of anxiety by increasing the activity of the inhibitory neurotransmitter GABA. Short-acting benzodiazepines, such as lorazepam (Ativan) and alprazolam (Xanax), are used in short-term situations such as a traveler with a fear of flying, whereas long-acting benzodiazepines, such as diazepam (Valium), are used for longer-term treatment needs. As with most medications, side effects can occur; best practice guidelines suggest prescribing benzodiazepines only for a limited period to avoid drug dependency or misuse (Ströhle et al., 2018). Caution in prescribing benzodiazepines is particularly important with older adults, due to the additional concerns of precipitating cognitive deterioration or fall-related injury (Luta et al., 2020).

Cognitive-Behavioral Treatments

Phobias are also successfully treated with a variety of cognitive-behavioral approaches. These approaches include:

- *Exposure therapy*: Gradually introducing the individual to the feared situation or object until the fear dissipates
- *Systematic desensitization*: Exposure to the feared situation or object combined with a competing response, such as relaxation
- *Cognitive restructuring*: Identifying and changing irrational or anxiety-arousing thoughts associated with the phobia
- *Modeling therapy*: Viewing another person's successful interactions with the feared object or situation

Exposure Therapy   In **exposure therapy**, treatment involves gradual and increasingly difficult encounters with a feared situation. For instance, when treating a client with agoraphobia, a therapist may first ask the client to visualize or imagine opening the door and leaving their residence. Eventually, the client might walk outside with the therapist and then remain outside alone. A modified exposure technique using a smartphone app allowed one therapist to help a client extinguish agoraphobic fears involving traveling on a train, attending a concert, and standing on a bridge. After the client identified specific goals, the therapist used a Web-based viewer to determine the time the client spent at each predetermined location. In this manner, the client achieved gradual exposure to each of the feared situations until he was able to perform the most challenging actions, such as boarding a train (Miralles et al., 2020).

A variant of exposure therapy has been successful for the treatment of blood and injection phobia, at least for individuals who show the physiological pattern of a sudden drop in blood pressure (Ritz et al., 2013). A procedure known as *applied tension* (described in the following case study) is combined with exposure techniques.

Case Study   Mr. A. reported feeling faint when exposed to any stimuli involving blood, injections, injury, or surgery. Even hearing an instructor discuss the physiology of the heart caused Mr. A. to feel sweaty and faint. Mr. A. was taught to recognize the first signs of a drop in blood pressure and then to combat this autonomic response by tensing the muscles of his arms, chest, and legs until his face felt warm. He was then taught to stop the tension for about 15 to 20 seconds and then to reapply the tension, repeating the procedure about five times (the rise in blood pressure that follows this process prevents fainting, and the fear becomes extinguished). After going through this process, Mr. A. was able to watch a video of thoracic surgery, watch blood being drawn, listen to a talk about cardiovascular disease, and read an anatomy book—stimuli that in the past would have caused him to faint. (Anderson et al., 1996)

Virtual reality therapy—replacing real-life exposure with an immersive virtual environment—is now viewed as an effective alternative to conventional exposure therapy in reducing or eliminating certain phobias such as a fear of heights (Donker et al., 2019). In fact, devices such as virtual reality screens can enhance the effects of exposure-based psychotherapy. For instance, after successful behavioral treatment, phobias sometimes recur if the person encounters the feared object in a context that is different from the one used in treatment. In an effort to determine if virtual reality exposure to multiple contexts reduces the likelihood of symptom recurrence, 30 individuals with a spider phobia were each exposed to a virtual spider either in a single context (e.g., the spider was pictured on a chair) or in multiple contexts. Each of four successive exposures produced a reduction in various physiological and behavioral measures of fear. However, those exposed to the spider in a single context later displayed phobic reactions when the spider was presented in a novel context, whereas those who had been exposed to multiple contexts did not. Thus, the virtual reality technique involving multiple contexts improved treatment outcome by reducing the chances that the phobic response would reappear (Shiban et al., 2013).

Systematic Desensitization   **Systematic desensitization** uses muscle relaxation to reduce the anxiety associated with phobias. Wolpe (1958, 1973), who developed the treatment, first taught clients to relax their muscles. Then he had them visualize feared stimuli (arranged from least to most anxiety provoking) while in the relaxed state. This continued until clients reported little or no anxiety with the stimuli. This procedure was adapted for a man who had a fear of urinating in restrooms when others were present. He was trained in muscle relaxation and, while relaxed, learned to urinate under the

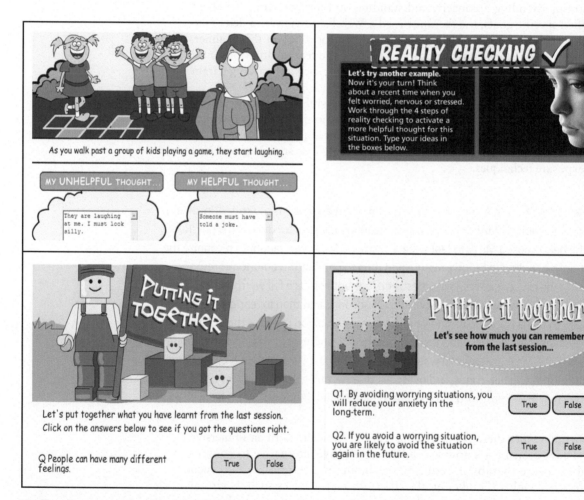

Source: Reprinted with permission of the authors from Spence, S. H., Donovan, C. L., March, S., Gamble, A., Anderson, R., Prosser, S. Kercher, A. & Kenardy, J. (2008). Online CBT in the treatment of child and adolescent anxiety disorders: Issues in the development of BRAVE-ONLINE and two case illustrations. *Behavioural and Cognitive Psychotherapy, 36*, 411–430.

Online Program for Social Anxiety

Pictured are sample items from a computerized treatment program dealing with social anxiety disorder in children and adolescents.

following conditions: no one in the bathroom, therapist in the stall, therapist washing hands, therapist at adjacent urinal, therapist waiting behind client. The easier items were practiced first until anxiety was sufficiently reduced (McCracken & Larkin, 1991).

Cognitive Restructuring In **cognitive restructuring**, unrealistic thoughts believed to be responsible for phobias are altered. Individuals with social phobias, for example, tend to be intensely self-focused and fearful that others will perceive them as anxious, incompetent, or weak. Their own self-criticism maintains their phobia. Therapists use cognitive strategies to help clients "normalize" social anxiety by encouraging them to question their negative thoughts, generate alternative views, and create new rational and positive thoughts regarding the situation (Norton & Abbott, 2016).

Modeling Therapy In **modeling therapy**, the individual with the phobia observes a model (either on a video or in person) coping with or responding appropriately to the fear-producing situation. The individual with the phobia may be asked to replicate the model's interactions with the phobic object. In one study testing this process, 99 children saw a video in which a peer interacted positively with an unfamiliar animal. After watching positive peer modeling, the children's fear toward the animal decreased significantly (Broeren et al., 2011).

Modeling

Watching a fear-producing act being performed successfully can help people overcome their fear. In this photo, a friend exposes a reluctant teen (on the right) to a python. Why do you think modeling works?

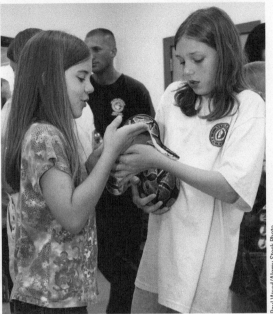

Paul Wood/Alamy Stock Photo

5-3 Panic Disorder

Case Study During final exams, I would be terrified . . . My hands would sweat, making the exam paper so wet that I could hardly write on it. . . . I felt physically sick and I thought I was going crazy. . . the teacher had to call my parents as I could not breathe and I thought I was going to die . . . . The fear of having a panic attack made me avoid . . . public transport, highways, enclosed spaces, escalators, and cinemas. (Rossiter, 2018)

According to the DSM-5-TR, a diagnosis of **panic disorder** involves recurrent unexpected panic attacks in combination with (a) apprehension over having another attack or worry about the consequences of an attack or (b) changes in behavior or activities designed to avoid another panic attack. These reactions must be present for a period of 1 month or more. As you can determine from the preceding case description, the attacks are extremely distressing because they often involve strong physiological reactions and occur without warning. There are some cultural variations in the manner in which symptoms are expressed. People of European ancestry generally report cardiac and respiratory symptoms, whereas Cambodian refugees may have somatic symptoms involving the head, neck, and gastrointestinal areas; African Americans may experience numbing sensations in their extremities and fears of dying; and Native Americans may report a pounding heart, dizziness, and altered perceptions of time (Sawchuk et al., 2017).

The past-year prevalence of panic disorder in U.S. adults is about 2.7 percent, with the disorder about twice as common in women than men. The lifetime prevalence is approximately 4.7 percent. Nearly 45 percent of those with a panic disorder rate the degree of impairment to be severe (NIMH, 2017e). Lower prevalence rates are reported among Latinx, African and Asian Americans compared to European Americans (APA, 2022). Many individuals diagnosed with a panic disorder also develop agoraphobia; this occurs because they fear having a panic episode in a public place (Locke et al., 2015).

Although panic disorder is diagnosed in only a small percentage of individuals, panic attacks are fairly common. Panic episodes often begin in late adolescence or early adulthood. In a cross-national study, the average lifetime prevalence of panic attacks was 13.2 percent, with about two thirds having recurrent episodes. Panic attacks are more prevalent in high-income as compared to low-income countries (de Jonge et al., 2016).

Etiology of Panic Disorder

As with the other disorders we have discussed so far, biological, psychological, social, and sociocultural factors and their interactions play a role in the etiology of panic disorder, as presented in Figure 5.6.

Biological Dimension

Higher **concordance rates** (i.e., percentages of relatives sharing the same disorder) for panic disorder have been found in monozygotic (identical) twins compared to dizygotic (fraternal) twins. Heritability is estimated to be between 30 percent and 40 percent, which is considered a modest contribution (Forstner et al., 2021; Na et al., 2011). As we mentioned

Figure 5.6

Multipath Model of Panic Disorder
The dimensions interact with one another and combine in different ways to result in panic disorder.

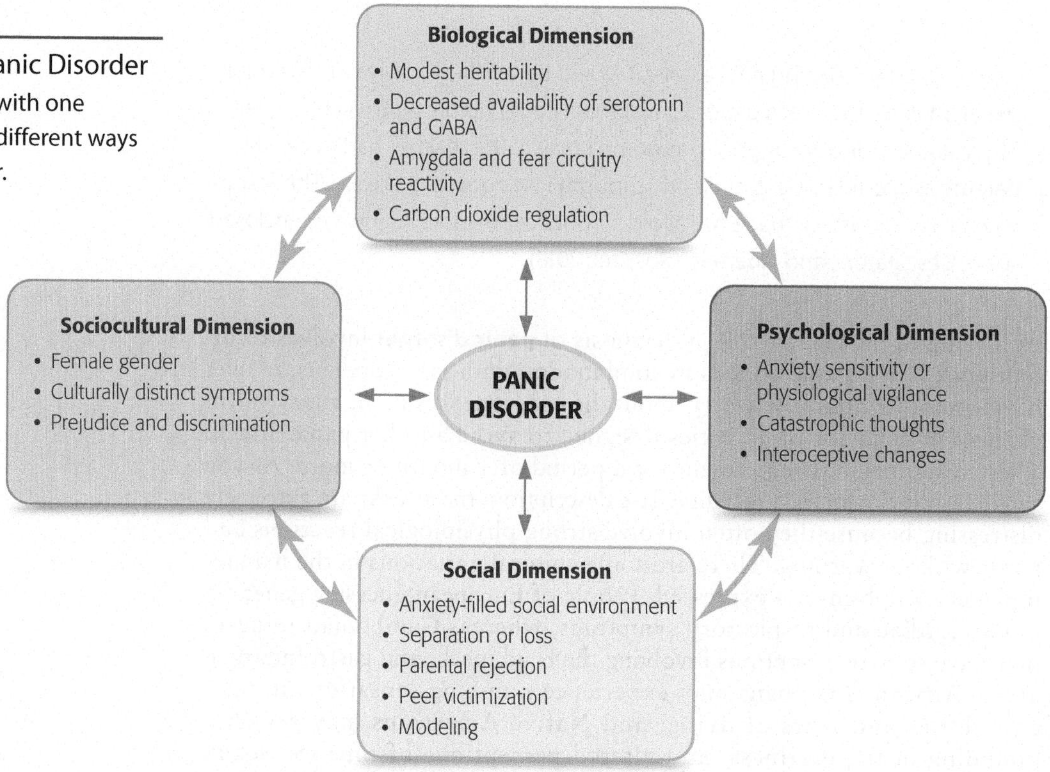

Biological Dimension
- Modest heritability
- Decreased availability of serotonin and GABA
- Amygdala and fear circuitry reactivity
- Carbon dioxide regulation

Sociocultural Dimension
- Female gender
- Culturally distinct symptoms
- Prejudice and discrimination

PANIC DISORDER

Psychological Dimension
- Anxiety sensitivity or physiological vigilance
- Catastrophic thoughts
- Interoceptive changes

Social Dimension
- Anxiety-filled social environment
- Separation or loss
- Parental rejection
- Peer victimization
- Modeling

earlier, the brain fear network involving the amygdala, hippocampus, and prefrontal cortex is implicated in anxiety disorders, including panic disorder.

The exact physiological processes that produce panic episodes are unclear, but research has focused on neurotransmitter abnormalities involving GABA and serotonin, both of which play an important role in emotions such as fear. GABA and serotonin both inhibit nerve impulses and thereby regulate neuronal excitability. One theory suggests that the hyperarousal associated with panic episodes may occur in individuals who have decreased availability of these essential neurotransmitters. Support for this hypothesis comes from neuroimaging studies, which have revealed that individuals with panic disorder have reduced expression of genes associated with serotonin receptors, thus decreasing the availability of serotonin (Bighelli et al., 2018). It is also interesting to note that SSRIs, antidepressant medications designed to increase levels of serotonin, are effective in treating panic disorders, as well as other anxiety disorders (Adigun et al., 2015). Others believe that panic disorder is associated with hypersensitivity in the neural network associated with respiratory and carbon dioxide regulation; this hypothesis is supported by research showing that increases in carbon dioxide levels produce panic attacks in many people with panic disorder (Zulfarina et al., 2019).

Psychological Dimension

Certain psychological characteristics have been associated with panic disorder. Individuals with this disorder score high on anxiety sensitivity measures and show heightened fear responses to bodily sensations; they display hypervigilance over changes in their heart rate, blood pressure, and respiration (refer to Figure 5.7). When these physiological changes are detected, anxiety increases, resulting in even more physical symptoms and more anxiety; this cycle often culminates in a panic attack (Woud et al., 2014). Anxiety sensitivity has been found to be such an important vulnerability for the development of panic disorder that the presence of this characteristic is predictive of the onset of panic symptoms several years into the future (Jurin & Biglbauer, 2018).

Cognitive-Behavioral Perspective The cognitive-behavioral model proposes that panic attacks occur when unpleasant bodily sensations are misinterpreted as indicators of an impending disaster. These inaccurate cognitions and somatic symptoms create a feedback loop that results

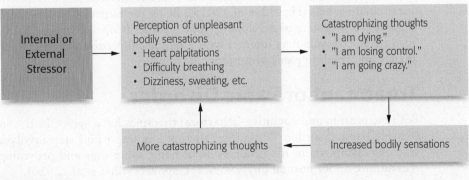

Figure 5.7

Role of Cognitions in Panic Attacks

A positive feedback loop between cognitions and somatic symptoms leads to panic attacks.

Source: Roy-Byrne et al., 2006, p. 1027

Table 5.3 Examples of Catastrophic Thoughts in Panic Disorder

Physical	Mental	Social
"I will die"	"I will go crazy"	"People will think I'm crazy or weird"
"I will have a heart attack"	"I will become hysterical"	"People will laugh at me"
"I will suffocate"	"I will uncontrollably try to escape"	"People will stare at me"

Source: Hicks et al., 2005

in increasing anxiety (refer to Table 5.3). Thus, the following pattern is associated with the development of a panic disorder (Van Diest, 2019):

1. A physiological change occurs (e.g., faster breathing or increased heart rate) due to factors such as exercise, excitement, or stress.

2. Catastrophic thoughts develop, such as "Something is wrong," "I'm having a heart attack," or "I'm going to die."

3. These thoughts bring about increased apprehension and fear, resulting in even more physiological changes.

4. A circular pattern develops as the amplified bodily changes now result in even more fearful thoughts.

5. This pairing of changes in internal bodily sensations with fear results in **interoceptive conditioning**—a classical conditioning process in which fear is associated with the perception of bodily changes. As this association strengthens, somatic changes can automatically produce panic attacks.

Research support for the cognitive-behavioral hypothesis includes the finding that a decrease in panic-related cognitions and anxiety sensitivity is associated with a subsequent reduction in panic symptoms (Pompoli et al., 2016).

Social and Sociocultural Dimensions

Anxiety sensitivity and a tendency to display panic symptoms may be acquired via modeling—by watching family or friends express fears about physical sensations or use avoidance to cope with fear-producing situations (Lindner et al., 2014). Not surprisingly, many individuals with panic disorder report a stressful childhood involving separation anxiety, family conflicts, school problems, or loss of a loved one (Klauke et al., 2010). Exposure to racial or ethnic-based discrimination is also associated with panic attacks, especially among those exposed to the greatest number of discriminatory acts (Hearld et al., 2015). Being the target of bullying also increases vulnerability to developing panic disorder (Copeland et al., 2013). Such social stressors may interact with a biological predisposition toward anxiety and result in panic symptoms.

Treatment of Panic Disorder

Both medication and cognitive-behavioral therapies have been effective in treating panic disorder. With either therapy, an important step involves teaching clients about the progression of panic symptoms and providing reassurance about normal physiological responses (Imai et al., 2016).

Biochemical Treatment

Different classes of medications have been used to treat panic disorder. As with phobias, SSRI antidepressants are considered the first choice for psychopharmacological treatment, although these medications take between 4 and 6 weeks to become fully effective. Tricyclic antidepressants are also

Did You Know?

The word *panic* originates from Greek mythology. Pan, a Greek demigod who lived in isolated forests, amused himself by making noises while following travelers through the woods. He would continue to frighten them until they bolted in panic.

prescribed for panic disorder. Benzodiazepines (antianxiety medications) can help reduce the frequency of panic attacks, but long-term use is problematic because of dependency issues, sedation effects, and cognitive impairment. Up to 45 percent of individuals with panic disorder are not responsive to medication, and among those who report improvement, one fourth to one half find that their symptoms return when their medication is discontinued. Thus, researchers continue to search for new and more effective medications for panic disorder (Zulfarina et al., 2019).

Cognitive-Behavioral Treatment

Cognitive-behavioral treatment is successful in producing long-term decreases in panic symptoms. In general, cognitive-behavioral treatment for panic disorder involves the following steps (Pompoli et al., 2018; Strauss et al., 2019):

1. Educating the client about panic disorder and correcting misconceptions regarding the symptoms

2. Identifying and correcting catastrophic thinking—for example, the therapist might comment, "Maybe you are overreacting to what is going on in your body" or "A panic attack will not stop your breathing"

3. Teaching the client to self-induce physiological symptoms associated with panic (such as hyperventilating or breathing through a straw) in order to extinguish the interoceptive bodily cues

4. Instructing the client on breathing techniques that will prevent hyperventilating during a panic attack

5. Encouraging the client to emotionally face rather than resist the symptoms, both within the session and in the outside world, using statements such as "Allow your body to have its reactions and let the reactions pass"

6. Reviewing the skills acquired and making a plan to prevent relapse

Going Deeper

Panic Disorder Treatment: Should We Focus on Self-Efficacy?

Imagine you are standing in a busy mall when your heart suddenly starts to pound and you begin to sweat. You may not realize it, but you are experiencing a panic attack. Soon you feel nauseated and disoriented, and can barely breathe. You fear you are going to either pass out or die. What is happening to you? What brought on this terrifying experience? Will it happen again? When you regain your composure, you think about what has just happened. You decide to explore treatment options. What treatment techniques will you choose? Consider the following studies.

Abraham Bakker et al. (2002) compared two groups of individuals with panic disorder. One group was treated with cognitive-behavioral therapy (CBT)—a therapy that encouraged clients to accept personal control over their panic reactions. The other group was treated with antidepressant medications without psychotherapy. Clients in the CBT group had lower relapse rates than those treated pharmacologically, perhaps because those in the CBT group learned to view their gains as the result of their own efforts rather than due to medication.

A number of studies using CBT have found that developing skills to combat catastrophic thoughts and frightening bodily symptoms is not only therapeutic but also enhances *panic self-efficacy*—confidence in coping with or controlling panic attacks. In fact, self-efficacy has been found to be a mediator of change for those who undergo cognitive-behavioral treatment for panic disorder (Schønning & Nordgreen, 2021). Individuals who believe (or come to believe) that successful control of panic symptoms is up to them are significantly more likely to reduce panic symptoms than are those who attribute their improvement to external factors, such as medication.

For Further Consideration

1. CBT does not typically emphasize self-efficacy. Do you believe that including this as a therapeutic goal would strengthen the effectiveness of CBT and reduce relapse?

2. How might therapists help their clients increase self-efficacy?

This method of cognitive-behavioral intervention extinguishes the fear associated with both internal bodily sensations (e.g., heart rate, sweating, dizziness, breathlessness) and fear-producing environmental situations. With this treatment approach, clients increasingly develop confidence in their ability to recognize and successfully deal with panic symptoms.

5-4 Generalized Anxiety Disorder

Case Study Jake, a 6-year-old boy, had a pattern of excessive worry and apprehension. Some of his recurring worries involved injuring his friend by accidentally brushing against him; leaving a favorite toy in the car, causing it to melt; a bird flying through a window and injuring itself; lying on a hammock and then experiencing the hammock collapse; and being attacked by bullies. Jake's worries resulted in constant anxiety, sleep difficulties, feelings of exhaustion, and the need to frequently seek reassurance from his parents. (Michael et al., 2012)

Many of us have had specific concerns and worries, but when is this worry considered a significant problem? **Generalized anxiety disorder (GAD)** is characterized by persistent, high levels of anxiety and excessive and difficult-to-control worry over life circumstances; these feelings are accompanied by physical symptoms such as feeling restless or tense. For a DSM-5-TR diagnosis of GAD, the symptoms must be present on the majority of days for at least 6 months and cause significant distress or impairment in life activities. As we saw with Jake, the pervasive worry and anxiety associated with GAD can significantly interfere with optimal functioning. Worry appears to be the defining characteristic of GAD, and some believe a better term for this disorder would be *pathological worry behavior* (Songco et al., 2020).

In any given year, about .9 percent of adolescents and 2.9 percent of the U.S. adult population is affected by GAD, with over 32 percent describing their degree of impairment as "serious." In epidemiological studies, women are at least twice as likely to have this condition as men. Individuals of Asian or African descent are less likely to meet the criteria for this disorder than those of European descent (APA, 2022; NIMH, 2017c).

Etiology of Generalized Anxiety Disorder

GAD results from predisposing biological variables combined with psychosocial stressors, as presented in Figure 5.8. Let's take a look at each of the factors that may contribute to the etiology of GAD.

Biological Dimension

Genetic contributions appear to play a small but significant role in the development of GAD, with familial and twin studies suggesting heritability of 31 percent (Gottschalk & Domschke, 2017). Genes associated with

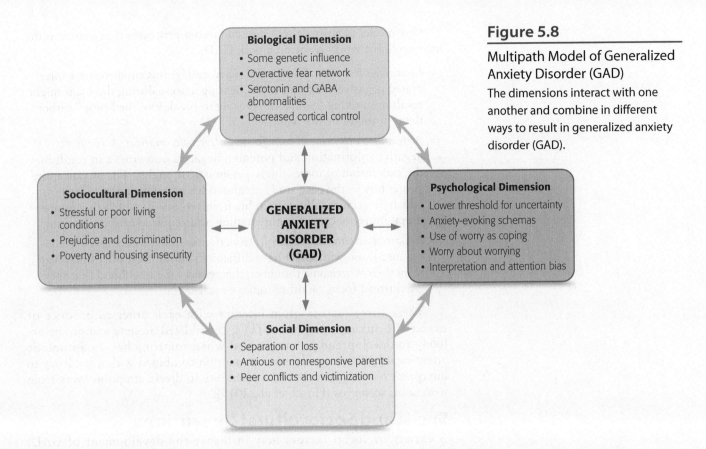

Figure 5.8

Multipath Model of Generalized Anxiety Disorder (GAD)

The dimensions interact with one another and combine in different ways to result in generalized anxiety disorder (GAD).

Biological Dimension
- Some genetic influence
- Overactive fear network
- Serotonin and GABA abnormalities
- Decreased cortical control

Sociocultural Dimension
- Stressful or poor living conditions
- Prejudice and discrimination
- Poverty and housing insecurity

GENERALIZED ANXIETY DISORDER (GAD)

Psychological Dimension
- Lower threshold for uncertainty
- Anxiety-evoking schemas
- Use of worry as coping
- Worry about worrying
- Interpretation and attention bias

Social Dimension
- Separation or loss
- Anxious or nonresponsive parents
- Peer conflicts and victimization

anxiety are often expressed in terms of serotonin or GABA abnormalities or overactivity of the HPA axis. As with phobias and panic disorder, the neuro-correlates of GAD involve irregularities within the limbic system and prefrontal cortex—excessive physiological reactivity combined with failure of the prefrontal cortex to dampen the emotional centers of the brain. As mentioned earlier, our prefrontal cortex modulates our responses to threatening situations; therefore, as an individual attempts to regulate the anxiety aroused by ongoing worries, there is increased activation in this region. Further, in GAD, a fleeting concern can lead to a cascade of fearful thoughts; without any brakes on the system, worries become magnified and anxiety continues unabated (Goossen et al., 2019). Supporting this perspective is the finding that successful cognitive-behavioral therapy for GAD reduces amygdala activity and increases activity of the prefrontal regulatory systems (Klumpp et al., 2014).

Psychological Dimension

Cognitive theories of GAD emphasize the role of dysfunctional thinking and beliefs. Individuals with this disorder have a lower threshold for uncertainty, which leads to worrying and a focus on bodily changes (Wauthia et al., 2019). Some researchers believe that the roots of GAD lie in beliefs regarding the function of worrying (Wells, 2005, 2009). In this model, there are two types of worry. The first involves the frequent use of worry to cope with stressful events or situations that might occur. However, the stress of constantly generating solutions to "what if" scenarios eventually results in a belief that worry is uncontrollable, harmful, and dangerous. GAD develops when the second type of worry ("worrying about worry") occurs. This dynamic (worrying about worry) leads to increased anxiety (Ellis & Hudson, 2010).

Did You Know?

A 2-year study of adolescents with either GAD or social anxiety disorder revealed the following:

- GAD (but not social anxiety disorder) was associated with increased frequency of underage drinking.
- Adolescents with social anxiety disorder used less alcohol and cannabis than those with GAD or no anxiety disorder.

Source: Frojd et al., 2011

One model identifies three interconnected processes that maintain the uncontrollable worry associated with GAD:

- *Interpretation bias.* This occurs when ambiguous situations are interpreted negatively. For example, hearing a noise during the night might result in thinking "Someone is trying to break into the house" rather than "It might be the wind."
- *Automatic attentional bias for negative information.* A focus on negative information and potential negative outcomes can result in the generation of increasingly pessimistic thoughts. For instance, the young boy in the case study escalated his worry from a scenario in which he accidentally injured his friend to one in which the unintentional injury became life-threatening and required hospitalization.
- *Impaired attentional control.* Anxiety-provoking thoughts continue because those with GAD have difficulty shifting their attention away from their worrisome thoughts; this reduces the likelihood that they will instead focus on other topics or tasks.

These three factors often interact with each other to produce or exacerbate anxiety symptoms. Thus, generalized anxiety symptoms are likely to develop and be maintained when someone has an automatic attentional bias for worrisome information combined with a tendency to interpret events negatively and an inability to divert attention away from worrisome scenarios (Hirsch et al., 2019).

Social and Sociocultural Dimensions

A variety of social factors may influence the development of GAD. Mothers who themselves have anxiety symptoms may be less responsive and engaged with their infants than mothers who are not anxious. These behaviors appear to increase the likelihood that the child will develop GAD (Stein et al., 2012). Conflict in peer relationships, including being the target of bullying, can increase the chances of developing GAD (Copeland et al., 2013). Stressful conditions such as poverty and poor housing also contribute to GAD. The disorder is twice as prevalent among those with low income (Kessler et al., 2005). It is also seen more frequently in individuals who are separated, divorced, or widowed (Wittchen & Hoyer, 2001).

Treatment of Generalized Anxiety Disorder

Benzodiazepines are often used in treating GAD; however, because GAD is a chronic condition, drug dependence is a concern. If medication is necessary, antidepressants are usually preferred because they do not have the potential for the physiological dependence seen with benzodiazepines (NIMH, 2017c).

Cognitive-behavioral therapy (CBT) is an effective psychological treatment for GAD. A meta-analysis found CBT to be successful in reducing pathological worry, with nearly 60 percent of those treated with CBT demonstrating significant improvement that continued 12 months after treatment (Hanrahan et al., 2013). CBT has been specifically adapted to treat the dysfunctional cognitive processes that maintain the cycle of worry associated with GAD (Hirsch et al., 2019). In this approach, the therapist encourages the client to:

- View worrisome thoughts as "mental magnets" that result from a "thinking habit" involving a selective focus on negative concerns and to use attentional control to replace this unhelpful practice with more useful habits—shifting the spotlight from worries to other tasks at hand

Myth Because brain activity associated with anxiety disorders can be "normalized" with medication, biological therapies provide the best alternatives for treatment.

Reality Psychotherapy is highly effective with anxiety disorders and can also normalize brain functioning. Medications appear to influence the fear network at the level of the amygdala, whereas cognitive-behavioral therapy leads to fear inhibition mediated by the prefrontal cortex and hippocampus.

- Keep a record of all worries and then consider evidence for and against each of the worries, determining whether a negative outcome actually occurred in any of the worrisome situations
- Develop habits of mental self-control, including monitoring and challenging irrational thinking and substituting more positive, coping thoughts
- Create "worry-free zones" by deliberately moving attention away from worry to the task at hand, practicing this shifting of attentional control until it becomes a strong habit
- Use muscle relaxation to deal with any physiological anxiety symptoms
- Keep a positive data log of situations in which the use of adaptive skills has resulted in reduced anxiety

Mindfulness practices can enhance the effectiveness of CBT in the treatment of GAD (Hofmann & Gómez, 2017). The process involves teaching a client to remain nonjudgmental in the presence of anxiety—accepting any emotions and bodily sensations that arise and allowing the experience to occur without reacting. Practicing mindfulness allows the individual to discover that uncomfortable emotions and bodily sensations are temporary and to understand that reactive thinking exacerbates anxiety symptoms.

We now discuss another set of disorders characterized by persistent troublesome thoughts and underlying anxiety: obsessive-compulsive and related disorders.

5-5 Obsessive-Compulsive and Related Disorders

Case Study   Mrs. A. is a 32-year-old married mother of two who spends at least 4 hours each day cleaning and making sure everything in her house is in its perfect place. If Mrs. A. sees or hears words pertaining to death, she immediately begins to repeat the Lord's Prayer in her mind 100 times. She believes that failure to perform this ritual will lead to the untimely death of her children. (Greenberg, 2010)

Obsessive and compulsive symptoms such as those experienced by Mrs. A. can be extremely distressing and debilitating. In this section, we will learn more about obsessive-compulsive and related disorders, including obsessive-compulsive disorder, hoarding disorder, body dysmorphic disorder, hair-pulling disorder (trichotillomania), and excoriation (skin-picking) disorder (Table 5.4). These disorders are grouped together because they have similar symptoms, such as repetitive disturbing thoughts and irresistible urges, and are believed to have similar neurobiological causes. Not surprisingly, disorders involving obsessive and compulsive symptoms are comorbid with a number of other disorders, including depression, anxiety disorders, and schizophrenia spectrum disorders (Rowe et al., 2022).

Obsessive-Compulsive Disorder

The primary symptoms in **obsessive-compulsive disorder (OCD)** are **obsessions**, which are persistent, anxiety-producing thoughts or images (e.g., Mrs. A.'s concern that her children might die), and **compulsions**,

Table 5.4 Obsessive-Compulsive Spectrum Disorders

Disorders Chart			
Disorder	**DSM-5-TR Criteria**	**Gender and Cultural Factors**	**Age of Onset**
Obsessive-compulsive disorder	• Repeated disturbing and intrusive thoughts or impulses • Inability to control or suppress the thoughts or behaviors • Brief relief after performing the behaviors	• 12-month prevalence rate about 1.2% • Slightly more common in women • Cultural factors or racial stereotypes may influence content of obsessions and type of compulsions	• Usually evident by age 20 • Onset after age 35 is unusual • 25% of cases begin by age 14
Body dysmorphic disorder	• Distressing and impairing preoccupation with imagined or slight defects in appearance	• Prevalence rate of 2.4%; up to 13% in those seen by dermatologists • Slightly more common in women and girls, especially during adolescence and early adulthood	• Usually early adolescence to early adulthood • Disorder tends to be chronic
Hair-pulling disorder (trichotillomania)	• Repeated pulling out of hair, resulting in hair loss	• 12-month prevalence rate of 1% to 2% • Lifetime prevalence up to 4%; 2 to 10 times more common in women and girls	• Usually before age 17 • Symptoms may disappear and reappear
Excoriation (skin-picking) disorder	• Repeated picking at the skin, resulting in lesions	• Lifetime prevalence rate of 3.1% • 75% of those diagnosed are women or girls	• Usually begins in adolescence, although can occur at any age
Hoarding disorder	• Difficulty discarding items because of perceived need, resulting in cluttered living areas	• From 2% to 6% at any given time • Women more prevalent in clinical samples • 3 times more prevalent in older adults	• Usually begins by age 16 and produces clinically significant impairment by the thirties

Source: Based on American Psychiatric Association, 2022

which involve an overwhelming need to engage in activities or mental acts to counteract anxiety or prevent the occurrence of a dreaded event (e.g., Mrs. A.'s mental repetition of the Lord's Prayer). The obsessions and compulsions consume at least 1 hour of time per day and cause significant distress or impairment in life activities. You can probably imagine how upsetting it must feel to be unable to control disturbing thoughts or refrain from performing ritualistic acts. The obsessions are often accompanied by sensory experiences. For example, Mrs. A. had the visual sensation of seeing her children dying, whereas individuals obsessed with a fear of contamination might have the tactile feeling of dirt on their skin. These sensory experiences significantly increase the intensity of the anxiety linked with the obsession (Moritz et al., 2018).

People who experience the intrusive and often irrational thoughts or images associated with obsessions find it difficult to control their thinking. Although they may try to ignore the obsession or push it from their minds, the thoughts persist. Common themes associated with obsessions include:

• contamination, including concern about dirt, germs, body wastes, or secretions and fear of being polluted by contact with items, places, or people considered to be unclean or harmful;

- errors of uncertainty, including obsessing over decisions or anxiety regarding daily behaviors such as locking the door or turning off appliances;
- unwanted impulses, such as thoughts of sexual acts or harming oneself or others; and
- orderliness, including striving for perfect order or symmetry.

Compulsions often involve repetitive, observable behaviors such as hand washing, checking, or ordering objects. They can also involve mental acts such as praying, counting, or repeating words silently. Compulsions are usually connected to the recurring thoughts or distressing images associated with an obsession. Distress or anxiety occurs if the behavior is not performed or if it is not done "correctly." Recent studies indicate that just prior to performing a compulsive action, up to 60 percent of individuals with OCD experience feelings of incompleteness or a sense that something is "just not right" (Simpson et al., 2020).

Although obsessions and compulsions sometimes occur separately, they frequently occur together; in fact, only 25 percent of those with OCD report distressing obsessions without compulsive behaviors (Markarian et al., 2010). Compulsions are frequently performed to neutralize or counteract a specific obsession. For instance, individuals with an obsession about contamination may compulsively wash their hands. Table 5.5 contains additional examples of obsessions and compulsions.

Individuals with OCD often describe their obsessive or compulsive thoughts and actions as being out of character for them and not under their voluntary control. Most recognize that their thoughts and impulses are senseless, yet they feel unable to use willpower to stop these unwanted thoughts or actions. If they try to avoid engaging in their rituals, they feel more and more anxious. As one individual noted, "The reason I do these kinds of rituals and obsessing is that I have a fear that someone is going

Did You Know?

OCD may be underdiagnosed. If it is suspected, screening questions such as these are asked:

- Do you have unwanted ideas, images, or impulses that seem silly, nasty, or horrible?
- Are you constantly worried that something bad will happen because you forgot something important, like locking the door or turning off appliances?
- Are there things you feel you must do excessively or thoughts you must think repeatedly in order to feel comfortable or ease anxiety?
- Do you wash yourself or things around you excessively?
- Do you have to check things over and over or repeat actions many times to be sure they are done properly?
- Do you feel a very strong need to perform certain rituals repeatedly and feel like you have no control over what you are doing?

Source: Anxiety and Depression Association of America, 2020

Table 5.5 Clinical Examples of Obsessions and Compulsions

Client Age	Gender	Duration of Obsession in Years	Content of Obsession or Compulsion
21	M	6	Teeth are decaying, particles between teeth
55	F	35	Fetuses lying in the street, people buried alive
29	M	14	Shoes dirtied by dog excrement
32	F	7	Contracting AIDS
42	F	17	Hand washing triggered by touching surfaces touched by other people
21	M	2	Intense fear of contamination after touching money
9	M	4	Going back and forth through doorways 500 times

Source: Based on Greenberg, 2010; Jenike, 2001; Kraus & Nicholson, 1996; Rachman et al., 1973; Zerdzinski, 2008

Obsessive-Compulsive and Related Disorders | **177**

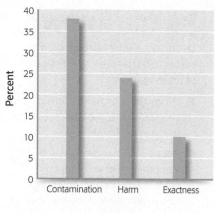

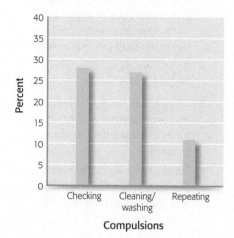

Figure 5.9

Common Obsessions and Compulsions

Many individuals with OCD report both obsessions and compulsions, including the symptoms demonstrated by individuals in this clinical sample.

Source: Based on Foa & Kozak, 1995

to die. This is not rational thinking to me. I know I can't prevent somebody from dying by putting 5 ice cubes in a glass instead of 4" (Jenike, 2001, p. 2122). Refer to Figure 5.9 for some clinical examples of disabling obsessions and compulsions.

In a given year, about 1 percent of the U.S. adult population experience OCD symptoms significant enough to constitute a disorder. Over half of those affected report the severity of the disorder as "serious." OCD is slightly more common among boys in childhood but is somewhat more common in women than men during adulthood. Onset is usually by age 20 with about 25 percent of the cases occurring by age 14. Men have an earlier age of onset than women. Sociocultural factors can influence the content or form of obsession and compulsions (APA, 2022; Mathes, Morabito, & Schmidt, 2019). Many people with this disorder are depressed and may abuse substances, possibly because of the emotional distress associated with their symptoms (Canavera et al., 2010).

How common are intrusive, unacceptable thoughts and impulses? Many people report experiencing occasional intrusive ideas or impulses to behave in an uncharacteristic manner (e.g., shouting during a religious service, injuring a family member). In fact, between 9 percent and 25 percent of the general population report having obsessive-compulsive symptoms, but without the severity required to meet the diagnostic criteria for OCD (Fullana et al., 2009; Jaisoorya et al., 2017). Additionally, the content of obsessions reported by individuals with OCD overlaps considerably with intrusive thoughts reported by those with less severe symptoms. However, with OCD, the obsessions last longer, are more intense, are more upsetting, produce more discomfort, and are more difficult to dismiss (Radomsky et al., 2014). For all of us, intrusive thoughts are more likely to occur during times of stress. For instance, over two thirds of new mothers report unwanted intrusive worries such as concern that their baby might stop breathing, be dropped, or be injured by accident. In fact, about half of mothers have had distressing thoughts of intentionally harming their infant (Collardeau et al., 2019).

Compulsions are also common in the general population (Barzilay et al., 2019). A continuum appears to exist between "normal" rituals and "pathological" compulsions. Mild compulsions include superstitions such as refusing to walk under a ladder, throwing salt over one's shoulder, or knocking on wood. In individuals with OCD, the compulsions are much more frequent and intense, and they produce discomfort. Additionally, the behaviors are repetitive and are often conducted in a mechanistic fashion; if compulsive acts are not performed in a certain manner or a specific number of times, the individual is flooded with anxiety.

Hoarding Disorder

Case Study Rose, a 39-year-old woman with two children, came into treatment for compulsive hoarding. Over 75 percent of her house was inaccessible because of piles of boxes, small appliances, food items, cans, and clothes. The dining room was unusable because the chairs, tables, and floor were covered with objects and boxes. She could not use her stove because of all of the items piled on top of it. Even a portion of her bed was covered with clothes and boxes. She was unable to discard items because she thought, "Maybe I will need this item in the future" and "If I throw it away, I will regret it." (St-Pierre-Delorme et al., 2011)

According to the DSM-5-TR, **hoarding disorder** is diagnosed when there is (a) an inability to discard items regardless of their value, (b) a perceived need for items and distress over the thought of giving or throwing them away, and (c) an accumulation of items that produces congestion and clutter in the living area. The hoarding results in distress or impairment in life activities or interferes with safety within the home. For example, Rose was unable to perform daily activities because a vast majority of her house was inaccessible, and the accumulated objects posed a fire hazard. She also avoided inviting friends and family to her house because of the clutter and because she believed that they might try to convince her to give away, sell, or junk some of her belongings. Social pressure to discard possessions or cease hoarding is distressing for individuals with hoarding disorder because of their irrational emotional attachment to the items (Kalogeraki & Michopoulos, 2017).

The prevalence of hoarding disorder ranges from 2 percent to 6 percent of adults and typically begins by late adolescence. It is more common among women in clinical samples and is most prevalent in older adults (APA, 2022); up to 25 percent of individuals with anxiety disorders report significant hoarding symptoms (Zaboski et al., 2019). People with hoarding disorder respond similarly to those with OCD on most neuropsychological measures. However, they tend to have more difficulties with attention and memory, which has led to the hypothesis that individuals with hoarding disorder may cling to their possessions in order to avoid forgetting (Tolin et al., 2018).

Hoarding

Individuals with hoarding disorder believe that the items collected are valuable and resist having them removed, even when the possessions are worthless, are unsanitary, or create a fire danger.

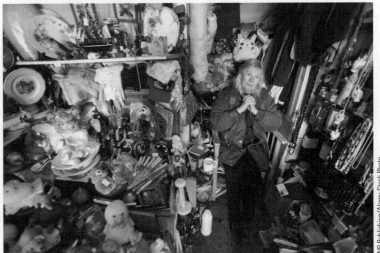

WR Publishing/Alamy Stock Photo

Body Dysmorphic Disorder

Case Study A 14-year-old girl complained of dark circles under her eyes and too-large eyebrows, which, she said, made her "look dead" or "punched in both eyes." She was also concerned about her uneven skin tone and blemishes. She spent between 5 and 9 hours a day tweezing her eyebrows and applying makeup to cover her perceived defects. To be able to get to school on time, she had to get up at 1 a.m. to begin this routine and refused to leave her home unless she felt that her "defects" were adequately covered. (Burrows et al., 2013)

The DSM-5-TR criteria for **body dysmorphic disorder (BDD)** include (a) preoccupation with a perceived physical defect in a normal-appearing person or excessive concern over a slight physical defect; (b) repetitive behaviors such as checking one's appearance in mirrors, applying makeup to mask "flaws," and comparing one's appearance to those of others; and (c) significant distress or impairment in life activities due to these symptoms. Concern commonly focuses on bodily features such as excessive hair; lack of hair; or the size or shape of the nose, face, or eyes (refer to Figure 5.10). This disorder may be underdiagnosed because individuals feel embarrassed or ashamed about bringing attention to their "problem" (Krebs et al., 2017).

Did You Know?

Many people have some preoccupation with physical characteristics. Questions such as these are used to screen for body dysmorphic disorder:

- Do you believe that there is a defect in your appearance or in a part of your body?
- Do you spend considerable time checking this defect?
- Do you attempt to hide or cover up this defect, or remedy it by exercising, dieting, or seeking surgery?
- Does this belief cause you significant distress, embarrassment, or torment?
- Does the defect interfere with your ability to function at school, at social events, or at work?
- Do friends or family members tell you that there is nothing wrong or that the defect is minor?

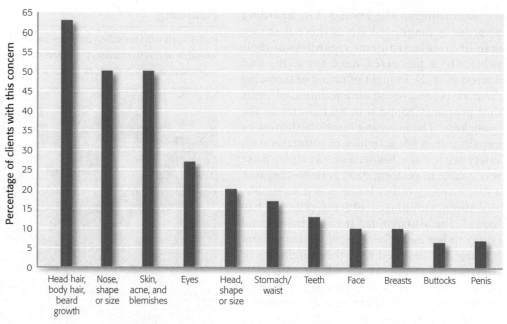

Figure 5.10

Imagined Defects in Patients with Body Dysmorphic Disorder

This graph presents the percentage of 30 patients who targeted different areas of their body as having "defects." Many of the patients selected more than one body region.

Source: Phillips, 2005

Although some individuals with BDD recognize that their beliefs are untrue, up to half maintain strong **delusions** (false beliefs) about their bodies (Phillips et al., 2014). Individuals with BDD regard their "defect" with embarrassment and loathing and are concerned that others may be looking at or thinking about the defect. They are ashamed to be seen and are detached in intimate relationships, believing themselves to be "flawed" (Stechler & Henton, 2022). Up to 60 percent of individuals with BDD undergo unnecessary cosmetic surgeries. As a group, they tend to be dissatisfied with the results and are more likely than other patients to sue the doctor. Unfortunately, few plastic surgeons screen individuals for BDD (Joseph et al., 2017).

The prevalence of BDD ranges from 0.7 percent to 2.4 percent in community samples, but has been found to be as high as 13 percent among individuals undergoing psychiatric hospitalization. Sixty percent of individuals with BDD have experienced an anxiety disorder, including 38 percent who have social anxiety (Mufaddel et al., 2013). It is slightly more common in women especially during adolescence and early adulthood (APA, 2022).

BDD tends to be chronic and difficult to treat due to comorbidity with depression and substance abuse. About 70 percent of individuals with BDD have poor insight into their condition, which makes attempts to change their delusional beliefs very challenging. Cognitive-behavioral therapy to address perceptions of perceived flaws has met with some success, especially among those who demonstrate readiness for change and have positive expectations for treatment (Greenberg et al., 2019).

Muscle dysmorphia, the belief that one's body is too small or insufficiently muscular, is a specific type of BDD. Some bodybuilders show a pathological preoccupation with their muscularity; these individuals have high body dissatisfaction and show negative biases and emotions even when observing parts of their body that are large and very muscular (Waldorf et al., 2019).

Hair-Pulling Disorder (Trichotillomania)

Trichotillomania involves recurrent and compulsive hair pulling despite repeated attempts to stop the behavior. Trichotillomania results in hair loss and significant distress. The most common areas for hair pulling are the scalp, eyebrows, and pubic region. The behavior may occur sporadically throughout the day or continue for hours at a time. Trichotillomania may be precipitated by boredom, stress, or anxiety. In some, the hair pulling relieves tension or is pleasurable. Although the hair pulling may occur with some consciousness, it is often an automatic act. For instance, one woman became aware that she had pulled her hair only after she snapped out of her "daze" and saw a pile of her hair on her desk (Grant & Chamberlain, 2016).

Trichotillomania has a 12-month prevalence rate between 1 percent and 2 percent and a lifetime prevalence of 4 percent, with women having a fourfold to tenfold increased likelihood of developing the disorder (APA, 2022). Although hair pulling is not uncommon before age 17, many younger children outgrow the behavior. Nevertheless, up to 11 percent of college-age individuals continue to pull their hair occasionally (Woods & Houghton, 2014). Trichotillomania is often comorbid with major depressive disorder and excoriation disorder (Titus-Lay et al., 2020).

Excoriation (Skin-Picking) Disorder

Case Study A woman sought therapy due to her 3-year history of skin picking resulting in lesions around her lips, cheeks, chin, and nose. The urge to pick occurred many times during the day and was followed by feelings of relief as soon as she engaged in the behavior. This activity was frequent, lasting for hours and preceded by emotional stress. Attempts to resist the urge were highly distressing. (Luca et al., 2012)

Excoriation (skin-picking) disorder involves repetitive and recurrent picking of the skin. Individuals with excoriation disorder spend 1 hour or more per day thinking about, resisting, or actually picking the skin. Episodes are preceded by rising tension; picking results in feelings of relief or pleasure (Lochner et al., 2017). According to the DSM-5-TR, a diagnosis of excoriation disorder occurs only when the behavior causes skin lesions and clinically significant distress or impairment and when there are repeated unsuccessful attempts to decrease or stop the behavior.

The lifetime prevalence of excoriation disorder is approximately 3.1 percent in adults and is most prevalent during early adolescence, although the onset for some individuals is during middle age. Those with a later onset tend to have less severe symptoms compared to those whose skin-picking behavior begins in adolescence. About three quarters of individuals with this disorder are women or girls (APA, 2022). It is often comorbid with depression, OCD, anxiety disorders, BDD, or trichotillomania (Stargell et al., 2016). As with trichotillomania, individuals with excoriation disorder report psychosocial impairment and an impaired quality of life (Ricketts et al., 2018).

Did You Know?

- More than half of plastic surgeons report seeing patients who want to improve their appearance for selfies: many of these patients report using photo-editing apps like Facetune, which allow people to make their skin look smoother, their eyes seem larger, and their teeth appear whiter—alterations that were previously available only to celebrities. Is pervasive photo editing changing the standards of beauty for ordinary people and creating body dissatisfaction?

Source: Beos et al., 2021; Rajanala et al., 2018

Etiology of Obsessive-Compulsive and Related Disorders

In this section, we examine the biological, psychological, social, and sociocultural factors associated with obsessive-compulsive and related disorders (refer to Figure 5.11). The causes of these disorders remain speculative. OCD itself may involve distinct disorders with different triggers and etiologies.

Biological Dimensions

Biological explanations for obsessive-compulsive and related disorders are based on findings from genetic and neurological studies. Genetic research suggests that although heredity is involved in OCD, with the greatest risk of OCD occurring in first-degree relatives, nonshared environmental influences are equally important (Purty et al., 2019). Genetic factors are also involved in body dysmorphic disorder (Ahmed et al., 2014), compulsive hoarding (Lervolino et al., 2009), and skin-picking disorder (Monzani et al., 2012), although environmental factors play a greater role in their etiology compared with OCD.

Environmentally based biological factors associated with an increased risk for OCD include maternal smoking during pregnancy, cesarean section delivery, preterm birth, unusually low or high weight at birth, and breech presentation at labor. If the mother smoked 10 cigarettes or more a day during her pregnancy, the OCD risk for the child increases by 27 percent. These conditions may adversely alter brain development in the fetus (Brander et al., 2016).

Figure 5.11

Multipath Model of Obsessive-Compulsive Disorder

The dimensions interact with one another and combine in different ways to result in obsessive-compulsive disorder.

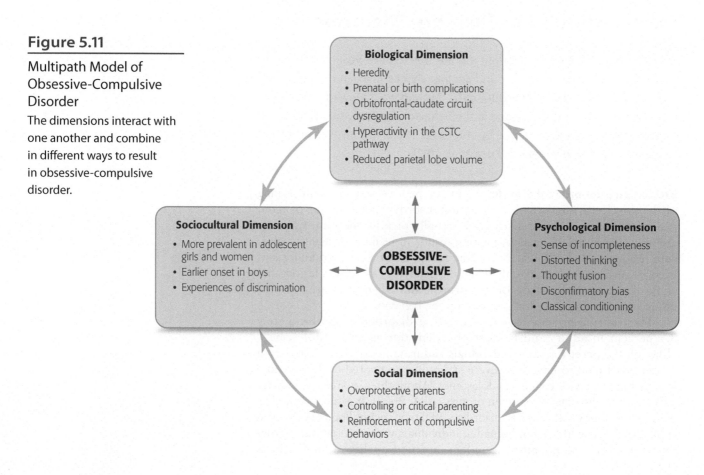

Biological Dimension
- Heredity
- Prenatal or birth complications
- Orbitofrontal-caudate circuit dysregulation
- Hyperactivity in the CSTC pathway
- Reduced parietal lobe volume

Sociocultural Dimension
- More prevalent in adolescent girls and women
- Earlier onset in boys
- Experiences of discrimination

OBSESSIVE-COMPULSIVE DISORDER

Psychological Dimension
- Sense of incompleteness
- Distorted thinking
- Thought fusion
- Disconfirmatory bias
- Classical conditioning

Social Dimension
- Overprotective parents
- Controlling or critical parenting
- Reinforcement of compulsive behaviors

As we have discussed, OCD affects cognitive functions associated with executive functioning, resulting in (1) impaired planning and decision making and (2) difficulty inhibiting or shifting attention away from intrusive thoughts or compulsive behaviors. Not surprisingly, researchers have focused their efforts on the brain circuits and structures that help mediate planning, movement, habitual behavior, and behavioral reactions to strong emotions. Neuroimaging studies confirm that OCD involves alterations in brain structures and neural networks associated with these cognitive areas as well as atypical and complex patterns of interactions between separate areas of the brain (Moreira et al., 2017). First-degree relatives of individuals with OCD show impairment in decision making, planning, and mental flexibility, so these cognitive characteristics may represent an **endophenotype** for the disorder (Cavedini et al., 2010). OCD is also associated with less volume in certain regions of the prefrontal cortex, most notably the parietal lobe (a brain structure associated with attention, planning, and response inhibition). Thus, impairment in the executive functions associated with this region may explain the inability to inhibit the recurring thoughts and behaviors associated with OCD (van den Heuvel et al., 2020).

Symptoms of OCD are also consistent with dysregulation of the orbitofrontal-caudate circuit, sometimes referred to as the orbitofrontal-striatal circuit. Supporting this perspective, brain studies have revealed that some people with OCD show increased metabolic activity within the **orbitofrontal cortex** and deep brain networks within the basal ganglia, particularly the **caudate nuclei** located within the **striatum** (refer to Figure 5.12). It is hypothesized that dysfunctional brain circuitry in this area can influence OCD symptoms due to their association with movement, emotion, and memory (Carmi et al., 2018). The orbitofrontal cortex alerts the rest of the brain when something is wrong. Thus, the amygdala and the HPA axis become activated, creating feelings of anxiety. When this system becomes hyperactive, the feeling that something is not right can lead to the sensation that something is "deadly wrong" and needs to be corrected. The caudate nuclei, which process information based on memories of

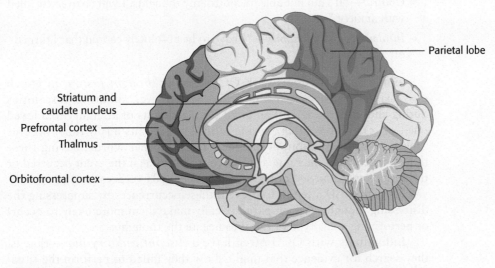

Parietal lobe

Striatum and caudate nucleus

Prefrontal cortex

Thalmus

Orbitofrontal cortex

Figure 5.12

Neuroanatomical Basis for Obsessive-Compulsive Disorder

Symptoms of obsessive-compulsive disorder involve increased metabolic activity within the orbitofrontal cortex and deep brain networks within the basal ganglia, particularly the caudate nucleus located within the striatum.

prior experiences, may then become overwhelmed and unable to flexibly shift to other activities; the network thus becomes stuck in an obsessive-compulsive loop, and the individual's ability to regulate behavior is compromised. Scientists have documented structural changes in the amygdala in individuals with OCD, which may be related to the atypical fear conditioning that occurs in this disorder (Zhang et al., 2020). Other recent research that extends the orbitofrontal-striatal model of OCD includes the finding that those with the disorder have excessive neural connectivity within the cortico-striatal-thalamo-cortical (CSTC) pathway—a looping brain network (connecting the cortex, striatum, and thalamus) that is associated with movement and habit formation (Katz et al., 2022).

Psychological Dimension

Some researchers maintain that obsessive-compulsive behaviors develop because they reduce anxiety. Classical conditioning theory provides a possible explanation for this connection. If certain thoughts or behaviors become associated with an unpleasant event, they can become a conditioned stimulus. Because these actions or thoughts are unpleasant, individuals may develop behaviors that help them avoid the initial unpleasant event. These avoidance behaviors reduce anxiety and are thus reinforcing. During the COVID pandemic, concerns over getting infected produced an increase in contamination obsessions and handwashing symptoms (Linde et al., 2022). If this type of behavior reduces anxiety over health concerns and the pairing occurs frequently, a compulsive behavior could develop.

Psychologists have also studied cognitive factors that lead to the severe anxiety and doubts associated with obsessive-compulsive behavior. As we have discussed, individuals with OCD believe that if they do not act in a certain way, negative consequences will occur. Individuals with OCD show certain cognitive characteristics, including distorted thinking in the following areas (Pozza et al., 2019):

- *Exaggerated estimates regarding the probability of harm*—"If the door isn't locked, I'll be killed by an intruder."
- *Control*—"If I am not able to control my thoughts, I will be overwhelmed with anxiety."
- *Intolerance of uncertainty*—"I have to be absolutely certain that I turned off the computer."

Similarly, individuals with OCD display *thought fusion*, in which distressing thoughts regarding (a) an action (e.g., shouting obscenities during church services), (b) an event (e.g., thoughts of an injury to a loved one), or (c) an object (e.g., seeing a black cat means misfortune) become "fused" with the action, event, or object. In other words, having these thoughts produces the same distressing emotions as if the event occurred or the actions were carried out (Myers & Wells, 2013). Because of this, individuals with OCD attempt to prevent these occurrences by suppressing the distressing thoughts (which paradoxically make them more likely to occur) or performing some type of ritual to negate the thoughts.

Individuals with OCD often have a *disconfirmatory bias*—that is, they search for evidence that might show they failed to perform the ritual correctly. Compulsions occur because they are unable to trust their own memories or judgment and feel a need to determine whether they actually performed the behavior or performed it "correctly." Further, they may need to repeat the ritual multiple times until it is "just right." Thus, individuals with a compulsive need to check things may repeatedly lock their doors (even though they have seen and heard the lock engage) because they are unable to convince themselves that the door is indeed locked. Those with OCD often experience an inner sense of uneasiness that an act is somehow "incomplete" or "incorrect" and attempt to resolve this discomfort by repeating actions or by focusing on symmetry when arranging objects in their environment (Mathes, Kennedy, et al., 2019).

Cognitive influences or beliefs also play an important role in hoarding disorder. Individuals with this disorder appear to have the conviction that objects they collected have some type of intrinsic, instrumental, or sentimental value. They feel a sense of responsibility toward the items and have feelings of guilt at the thought of discarding them. Individuals who hoard believe "I might need this someday." These beliefs are sometimes reinforced when a retained item is, in fact, useful. The cognitive explanatory model of hoarding disorder also notes that those who hoard often have difficulties with information processing, attention, memory, and decision making that may influence their tendency to retain possessions (Kalogeraki & Michopoulos, 2017).

Social and Sociocultural Dimensions

Family variables such as a controlling, overly critical style of parenting; minimal parental warmth; and discouragement of autonomy are associated with the development of OCD symptoms (Blanco-Vieira et al., 2021). Individuals raised by overprotective parents with rigid rules may develop maladaptive beliefs relating to personal responsibility; they may overestimate threats and believe it is up to them to prevent harm to themselves or others (Collins & Coles, 2018). Individuals with OCD who perceive their relatives to be critical or hostile tend to have more severe symptoms (Van Noppen & Steketee, 2009).

Although we tend to think about OCD as an individual problem, it often develops within an interpersonal context. Friends, roommates, and family members also have to deal with OCD symptoms, as seen in the following case.

Case Study As soon as I'd go into the bathroom, they'd be banging on the door. "How long are you going to be in there?" . . . I'd have to lock myself in the bathroom . . . and I'd shake a third of this thing of Ajax in the toilet, a third in the sink and a third in the bath and I'd be there about an hour scrubbing everything up until it was pristine." (Murphy & Perera-Delcourt, 2014, p. 118)

Understandably, the long wait to use the bathroom was frustrating for family members; however, such negative reactions to OCD symptoms can increase symptom severity. Interestingly, symptoms also increase when loved ones provide assistance (e.g., helping someone clean or check doors and locks) or reassurance regarding the rituals. Although this might temporarily reduce distress, such assistance may actually reinforce or prolong the symptoms and contribute to poorer treatment outcome (Boeding et al., 2013). On rare occasions, living with a partner or family member with OCD can produce a shared psychopathology in which two individuals develop the same OCD symptoms. One woman who engaged in frequent cleaning in an attempt to help her husband with his obsession with cleanliness eventually developed her own severe cleaning compulsion that persisted even after her husband's symptoms improved (Benatti et al., 2019).

Stressful environmental conditions can also affect the prevalence of OCD. During the COVID pandemic, obsessive and compulsive-like symptoms increased in the general population and worsened the condition of those with contamination-related obsessive-compulsive disorder (Guzik et al., 2021). Similar results were found in children and adolescents with OCD. However, instead of increases in cleaning or washing rituals, symptom increases involved obsessions over the possible death of their parents, grandparents, or caregivers (Nissen et al., 2020).

Sociocultural factors and experiences can influence the form, content, and severity of obsessions and compulsions. For example, men are more likely to have symptoms associated with forbidden thoughts and symmetry, while women are more likely to experience thoughts or actions related to cleaning (APA, 2022). Environmental experiences or negative racial stereotypes may be responsible for the finding that African and Asian Americans report more contamination themes in OCD than European Americans (Wheaton et al., 2013). In addition, exposure to racism and discrimination by African Americans with OCD has been associated with an increased severity of OCD symptoms (Williams, 2020).

Treatment of Obsessive-Compulsive and Related Disorders

The primary methods of treatment for obsessive-compulsive and related disorders are either biological or cognitive-behavioral in nature. Behavioral therapies have been used successfully for many years, but treatment with medication is becoming more common.

Biological Treatments

Antidepressant medications that increase serotonin availability (SSRIs) are often used to treat OCD and related disorders. Unfortunately, only about 60 percent of people with OCD respond to SSRIs, and often the relief is only partial. In one group of individuals with moderate OCD symptoms treated with SSRIs, many had significantly reduced symptoms after 2 years. However, about one third experienced a recurrence of symptoms during a 5-year follow-up period; the likelihood of relapse was lowest for those who had a full remission of symptoms (Cherian et al., 2014). Alternative medications such as antipsychotics are sometimes used for those who do not improve with SSRIs.

More recently, deep brain stimulation has become an approved treatment for individuals with treatment-resistant OCD; research continues regarding the optimal brain regions for stimulation and whether an individual's specific symptoms should guide such decisions (Senova, Clair, et al., 2019).

Behavioral Treatments

The treatment of choice for OCD is a combination of the behavioral techniques of exposure and response prevention. This approach has been proven effective in reducing the symptoms of OCD and has a lower relapse rate compared to treatment by medications (Richter & Ramos, 2018). In treating OCD, exposure therapy involves actual or imagined exposure to an anxiety-arousing situation; it can involve gradual exposure to a distressing stimulus or **flooding**, which is the immediate presentation of whatever stimulus is most likely to trigger the urge to engage in a compulsive behavior. **Response prevention** involves not allowing the individual with OCD to perform the compulsive behavior after the urge is activated. The steps in exposure therapy with response prevention generally include (Ojalehto et al., 2020):

1. psychoeducation about OCD and the rationale for exposure and response prevention;
2. development of an exposure hierarchy (from somewhat fearful to most-feared situations);

3. exposure to feared situations (such as contact with the restroom floor) until anxiety has diminished;

4. prevention of the performance of compulsive rituals such as hand washing after exposure to the cues that trigger the compulsion;

5. repeated exposure to a variety of triggering situations without performing compulsive rituals; and

6. review of relapse prevention strategies.

CBT that focuses on correcting dysfunctional beliefs can also assist with OCD symptoms; unfortunately, up to 30 percent of those treated with CBT for OCD do not achieve symptom relief (Murphy & Perera-Delcourt, 2014). Interestingly, SSRI medications reduce OCD symptoms by targeting overactive neural connections (Cheng et al., 2013), whereas cognitive-behavioral treatments appear to induce neuroplasticity that results in more functional connectivity—retraining the brain so that the fear circuitry no longer activates when a cue for obsessions or compulsions is present (Ressler & Rothbaum, 2012).

CBT has been modified to treat the specific features of hoarding disorder (Tolin et al., 2015). This approach includes:

- motivational interviewing to increase readiness for change;
- graded exposure involving opportunities to resist the urge to acquire items;
- identification and correction of maladaptive beliefs about the need for specific possessions;
- practice in sorting and discarding items; and
- placement of retained items in appropriate places in the home to encourage continued decluttering.

CBT for the treatment of skin-picking and trichotillomania includes (1) training in awareness of and self-monitoring for the undesirable behavior and (2) habit-reversal training, which involves practicing a competing and incompatible response (such as fist clenching) when the hair-pulling or skin-picking urge occurs (Jones et al., 2018).

CBT has also produced promising results in the treatment of body dysmorphic disorder (BDD). Wilhelm et al. (2014) developed a modified CBT-BDD program that focused on the "core" components of the disorder. Along with psychoeducation regarding BDD, the approach involves:

- motivational enhancement to address ambivalence about complying with treatment;
- cognitive restructuring focused specifically on negative thoughts about personal appearance;
- exposure and response prevention focused on eliminating mirror checking, seeking reassurance, and the camouflaging of imagined defects; and
- mindfulness training focused on learning to observe and describe one's body without judgment.

In addition, participants learn to move away from self-focus, to pay attention to others and to their environment, and to base their self-esteem on qualities such as being a good friend rather than physical attractiveness. The success of this program has prompted the development of modified CBT treatments for other difficult-to-treat disorders (Wilhelm et al., 2019).

5-6 Contemporary Trends and Future Directions

> **Case Study** I have, since the age of 10 ... tried in various ways to overcome my anxiety ... individual psychotherapy (three decades of it), family therapy, group therapy, cognitive-behavioral therapy, rational emotive behavior therapy, acceptance and commitment therapy, hypnosis, meditation, role-playing, interoceptive exposure therapy, in vivo exposure therapy, self-help workbooks, massage therapy, prayer, acupuncture, yoga, Stoic philosophy, and audiotapes. ... Lots of medication. (Stossel, 2014)

Although there have been many advancements in treating the disorders covered in this chapter, many of those affected continue to experience distressing symptoms even after receiving treatment, as is the case for Scott Stossel. Cognitive-behavioral therapies are considered to be the most effective treatments for anxiety and obsessive-compulsive and related disorders. Yet, even among those who show improvement, the distressing symptoms often return.

Three areas receiving attention in the field of cognitive-behavioral therapies are (a) specialized therapy programs that target specific disorders, (b) identifying neurobiological measures that accurately predict who might be responsive to treatment, and (c) using a unified protocol for treatment that is effective across disorders. We will consider examples of research in these areas.

Specialized Therapy Programs

Specialized treatment approaches are being developed that are very specific to the needs of those with anxiety and obsessive-compulsive disorders, particularly those who refuse treatment or have not benefited from traditional methods of treatment. For example, a new treatment for hoarding disorder focuses on innovative methods for engaging clients who are reluctant to initiate therapy because of their inability to tolerate separating from their collected items (Francalanza., Raila, & Rodriguez, 2021). The treatment incorporates a less threatening approach involving imaginal exposure, a therapeutic technique that involves having the client repeatedly imagine feared scenarios and experiencing the evoked emotions. This strategy aims to allow those with hoarding disorder to "acclimate" to the idea of discarding their possessions. Participants in the study spent 20 minutes each day writing and thinking about worst-case scenarios involving the discarding of a possession. In their pilot study with eight patients with hoarding disorder, the intervention was found to be "acceptable and tolerable."

Use of Technology to Predict Response to Therapy

Researchers, aware that many individuals with anxiety disorders do not improve with traditional biological or psychological therapies, are interested in determining if there are physiological, demographic, or clinical characteristics that can be used to predict responsiveness to therapy. Frick et al. (2020) studied a group of 47 individuals with social anxiety disorder who were treated either with CBT plus SSRIs or with CBT plus placebo. Areas of the cortex and the amygdala anterior were scanned (using fMRI imaging) during a cognitive interference task conducted prior to treatment. The researchers used a machine-learning algorithm to analyze this neuroimaging data combined with demographic and clinical data (such as the severity of symptoms) to determine which data had the highest level of accuracy in differentiating between participants who responded or did not respond to each type of intervention. Surprisingly, only one variable—reactivity of the anterior cingulate cortex during the cognitive interference task—predicted treatment response, with 83 percent accuracy. Similar findings were reported by Feurer et al. (2022). It is hoped that additional research using machine-learning algorithms will assist in identifying predictors of treatment responsiveness for other disorders.

Treatment Protocols for Multiple Disorders

Paradoxically, not only is there interest in improving treatment outcomes by modifying CBT for specific anxiety disorders, but there is also interest in developing CBT interventions that can be used across a wide variety of psychological disorders. This approach makes sense for many of the anxiety and obsessive-compulsive disorders because, as you have seen in this chapter, they share etiological pathways and respond to similar biological and psychological treatments.

Farchione et al. (2012) argued against the "proliferation of diagnosis-specific treatment manuals, many of which have only minor and somewhat trivial variations in treatment procedures" (p. 519). They wondered: Is there a unifying factor that is common across different anxiety disorders and, if so, can we develop a treatment package that adheres to a "single set of therapeutic principles"? Thus, they developed the Unified Protocol for Transdiagnostic Treatment of Emotional Disorders, which is a CBT program that is applicable to all anxiety and depressive disorders. Based on the theory that emotional dysregulation underlies these disorders, the treatment protocol targets aspects of emotional processing and regulation and consists of five modules focusing on (1) increasing present emotional awareness, (2) increasing cognitive flexibility, (3) identifying and preventing patterns of emotion avoidance, (4) increasing awareness and tolerance of emotion-related physical sensations, and (5) exposing the individual to physiological and emotional triggers.

In an early randomized clinical trial of individuals with panic disorder, generalized anxiety disorder, obsessive-compulsive disorder, and social anxiety disorder, the effectiveness of single disorder protocols (SDPs) designed for the specific disorders were compared to those treated with unified protocol (UP) therapy. At the end of the study, 64 percent of those in the UP condition no longer met the diagnostic criteria for the disorders as compared to 57 percent of those in the SDPs condition. At a 6-month follow-up, the percentages increased to 71 percent for the UP condition and 63 percent for the SDPs condition (Barlow et al., 2017). In a review of studies utilizing UP therapy, the results were described as "encouraging" (Osma et al., 2021).

Other studies have also found the UP to be efficacious in treating body dysmorphic disorder (Mohajerin, Bakhtiyar, et al., 2019) and mood disorders with comorbid anxiety symptoms (Ellard et al., 2017; Sauer-Zavala et al., 2019). These results are promising and will help simplify treatments for emotional disorders. However, specialized treatments may still be necessary for individuals who are not responsive to Unified Protocol therapy.

Chapter Summary

1 According to the multipath model, how are biological, psychological, social, and sociocultural factors involved in the development of anxiety disorders?

- The multipath model stresses the importance of considering the contribution of and *interaction* between biological, psychological, social, and sociocultural factors in the etiology of anxiety disorders.

- For instance, genetically predisposed individuals (e.g., those with inherited overactivity of the fear circuitry in the brain) who grow up in a supportive family or social environment may not develop an anxiety disorder. Similarly, although sociocultural factors (e.g., discrimination, poverty) can increase the risk of anxiety disorders, personality variables (such as a sense of control and mastery) can help mitigate the impact of stressors.

2 What are phobias, what are their causes, and how are they treated?

- Phobias are strong, irrational fears. Social anxiety disorder involves anxiety over situations in which others can observe the person. Agoraphobia is an intense fear of being in public places where escape or help may not be possible. Specific phobias include a variety of irrational fears involving objects and situations.

- Biological explanations are based on studies of the influence of genetic, biochemical, and neurological factors and on the idea that humans are predisposed to develop certain fears. Psychological explanations include classical conditioning, observational learning, and distorted cognitions.

- The most effective treatments for phobias include medications (especially antidepressants) and cognitive-behavioral therapies (exposure, systematic desensitization, modeling, and graduated exposure).

3 What is panic disorder, what causes it, and what interventions decrease panic symptoms?

- Panic disorder is marked by unexpected episodes of extreme anxiety and feelings of impending doom. There are cultural variations in the presentation of symptoms.

- The causes of panic disorder include biological factors (genetics, neural structures, and neurotransmitters), psychological factors (catastrophic thoughts regarding bodily sensations), and social and sociocultural factors (peer victimization, an anxiety-filled social environment, prejudice, and discrimination).

- Treatments for panic disorder include medications (benzodiazepines and antidepressants) and behavioral treatments (identifying catastrophic thoughts, correcting them, and substituting more realistic ones).

4 What is generalized anxiety disorder, what are its causes, and how is it treated?

- Generalized anxiety disorder (GAD) involves chronically high levels of anxiety and excessive worry.

- There appears to be less support for the role of genetics in GAD than in other anxiety disorders, although overactivity of the anxiety circuitry in the brain is implicated. Cognitive-behavioral theorists emphasize erroneous beliefs regarding the purpose of worry or the existence of attentional bias, interpretation bias, and impaired attentional control. Social and sociocultural factors such as poverty and discrimination can also contribute to GAD.

- Antidepressant medications and cognitive-behavioral therapies are used for treatment.

5 What are obsessive-compulsive and related disorders, what causes these disorders, and how are they treated?

- Obsessive-compulsive disorder (OCD) and related disorders involve thoughts or actions that are involuntary, intrusive, repetitive, and uncontrollable.

- OCD is associated with increased metabolic activity in the orbitofrontal cortex and excessive neural connectivity involving the prefrontal cortex. According to the anxiety-reduction hypothesis, obsessions and compulsions develop because they reduce anxiety. Cognitive-behavioral theorists have focused on cognitive factors such as an intolerance of uncertainty or overestimating the probability of harm.

- Body dysmorphic disorder involves excessive concern or preoccupation with a perceived body defect.

- Hair-pulling disorder (trichotillomania) involves the compulsive pulling out of one's hair, resulting in noticeable hair loss.

- Excoriation (skin-picking) disorder involves the repetitive picking of one's skin, resulting in the development of lesions.

- Hoarding disorder involves accumulating possessions and having difficulty discarding items, including items that appear to have little or no value.

- Antidepressant medications and cognitive-behavioral therapies are used to treat these disorders.

Chapter Glossary

agoraphobia
an intense fear of being in public places where escape or help may not be readily available

alleles
the gene pair responsible for a specific trait

anxiety
an anticipatory emotion that produces bodily reactions that prepare us for "fight or flight"

anxiety disorder
fear or anxiety symptoms that interfere with an individual's day-to-day functioning

anxiety sensitivity
a trait involving fear of physiological changes within the body

behavioral inhibition
shyness

body dysmorphic disorder (BDD)
a condition involving a preoccupation with a perceived physical defect or excessive concern over a slight physical defect

caudate nuclei
the deep brain structure that stores and processes memories and signals when something is amiss

cognitive restructuring
a cognitive strategy that attempts to alter unrealistic thoughts that are believed to be responsible for fears and anxiety

comorbid
existing simultaneously with another condition

compulsion
the need to perform acts or mental tasks to reduce anxiety

concordance rate
the degree of similarity between twins or family members with respect to a trait or disorder

delusion
a firmly held false belief

endophenotype
measurable characteristics that can give clues regarding the specific genetic pathways involved in a disorder

etiological model
model developed to explain the cause of a disorder

excoriation (skin-picking) disorder
distressing and recurrent compulsive picking of the skin resulting in skin lesions

exposure therapy
treatment that involves introducing the client to increasingly difficult encounters with a feared situation

fear
an intense emotion experienced in response to a threatening situation

flooding
a technique that involves inducing a high anxiety level through continued actual or imagined exposure to a fear-arousing situation

GABA
gamma-aminobutyric acid, an inhibitory neurotransmitter involved in inducing sleep and relaxation

generalized anxiety disorder (GAD)
a condition characterized by persistent, high levels of anxiety and excessive worry over many life circumstances

hippocampus
the part of the brain involved in forming, organizing, and storing memories

hoarding disorder
a condition involving congested living conditions due to the accumulation of possessions and distress over the thought of discarding them

interoceptive conditioning
when internal bodily sensations of fear and anxiety that have preceded panic attacks serve as signals for new panic attacks

modeling therapy
a treatment procedure involving observation of an unfearful individual successfully interacting with a phobic object or situation

muscle dysmorphia
a belief that one's body is too small or insufficiently muscular

negative appraisal
interpreting events as threatening

obsession
an intrusive, repetitive thought or image that produces anxiety

obsessive-compulsive disorder (OCD)
a condition characterized by intrusive, repetitive anxiety-producing thoughts or a strong need to perform acts or dwell on thoughts to reduce anxiety

orbitofrontal cortex
the brain region associated with planning and decision making

panic attack
an episode of intense fear accompanied by symptoms such as a pounding heart, trembling, shortness of breath, and fear of losing control or dying

panic disorder
a condition involving recurrent, unexpected panic attacks with apprehension over future attacks or behavioral changes to avoid attacks

phobia
a strong, persistent, and exaggerated fear of a specific object or situation

polymorphic variation
a common DNA mutation of a gene

predisposition
a susceptibility to certain symptoms or disorders

reappraisal
minimizing negative responses by looking at a situation from various perspectives

remit
diminish or disappear

response prevention
a treatment in which an individual is prevented from performing a compulsive behavior

serotonin
a neurotransmitter associated with mood, sleep, appetite, and impulsive behavior

social anxiety disorder (SAD)
an intense fear of being scrutinized in social or performance situations

specific phobia
an extreme fear of a specific object (such as snakes) or situation (such as being in an enclosed place)

striatum
the region within the basal ganglia associated with movement planning, goal-directed action, memory, and decision making

systematic desensitization
a treatment technique involving repeated exposure to a feared stimulus while a client is in a competing emotional or physiological state such as relaxation

trichotillomania
recurrent and compulsive hair pulling that results in hair loss and causes significant distress

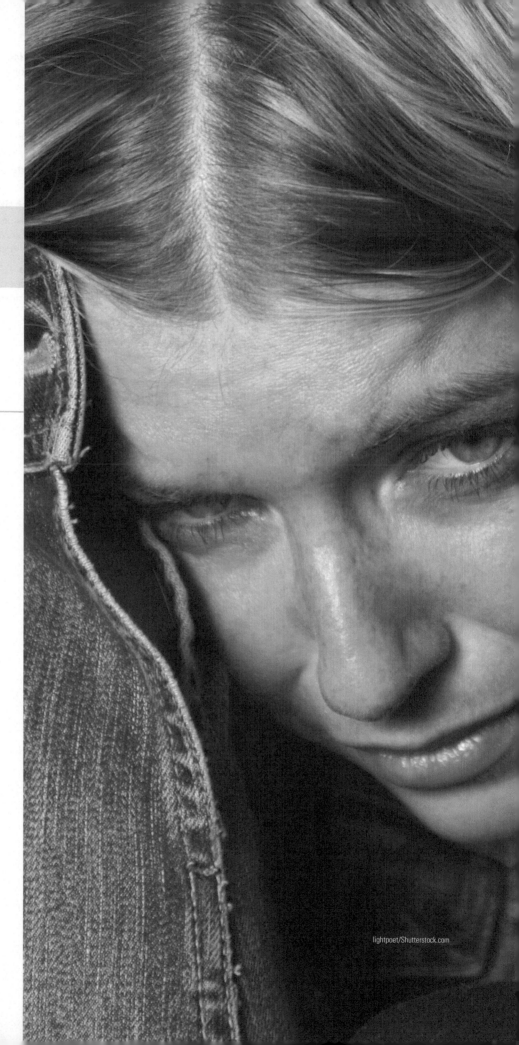

focus
Questions

1 What do we know about disorders caused by exposure to stressors or traumatic events?

2 In what ways can stress affect our physical health?

6

Trauma- and Stressor-Related Disorders

Learning Objectives

After studying this chapter, you will be able to . . .

6-1 Compare and contrast prolonged grief disorder, adjustment disorder, acute stress disorder, and posttraumatic stress disorder, and explain how trauma-related disorders develop and are treated.

6-2 Describe various medical conditions affected by stress (coronary heart disease, hypertension, headaches, and asthma) and discuss the etiological influences and treatments associated with psychophysiological disorders.

Grisham, an Army Veteran, experienced a number of traumatic events while serving in Iraq, including shooting a person being used as a human shield and helping a distressed Iraqi family recover a dead loved one from a burned-out car. He had flashbacks and nightmares about these events. Even after returning to the United States, he remained extremely vigilant and fearful of crowded situations; he searched for exits before entering any building and always sat with his back against the wall so he could observe people approaching him (Tucker, 2012).

S tress can affect our mental and physical health in a variety of ways. **Stressors** are external events or situations, such as challenging or difficult life circumstances, that place physical or psychological demands on us. We all encounter numerous stressors throughout our lives—ranging from daily situations that may result in irritation or frustration to life-changing, traumatic events such as those experienced by Grisham, the army veteran in the introductory vignette.

Stress is our internal psychological or physiological response to a stressor. Most of us understand that traumatic events can affect us physically and psychologically. However, exposure to worrisome but less traumatic events can also significantly influence our health and well-being. Unfortunately, most of us experience stress on a regular basis. During the early months of the COVID-19 pandemic, approximately two thirds of U.S. adults reported experiencing significant stress due to the weakened economy and the ineffective governmental response to the crisis. Over one third of the adults surveyed were exhibiting signs of anxiety or depression (or both), and 20 percent reported having a physical reaction when thinking about the pandemic (Beheshti, 2020).

Everyday stress can negatively influence our health and lead to the development of both psychological and physical conditions. Additionally, long-term exposure to adversities can suppress our immune system and subsequently increase the risk of illness (Strain, 2018). And exposure to traumatic stressors can result in the distressing symptoms associated with trauma-related disorders. But how does this occur? And why are some people who are exposed to stressors, even traumatic ones, able to adjust without too much difficulty, whereas others develop intense, long-lasting psychological or physical symptoms? As you will see, the answers are complex, involving interactions among a variety of biological, psychological, social, sociocultural, and resiliency factors. In this chapter, we focus on trauma- and stressor-related disorders as well as stress-related physical conditions.

6-1 Trauma- and Stressor-Related Disorders

The DSM-5-TR includes a variety of disorders involving intense reactions to traumatic or stressful events. We will discuss four of these trauma- and stressor-related disorders: *prolonged grief disorder*, *adjustment disorder*, *acute stress disorder*, and *posttraumatic stress disorder*. The remaining trauma- and stressor-related disorders, *reactive attachment disorder* and *disinhibited social engagement disorder*, result from childhood trauma and are covered in our discussion of childhood disorders in Chapter 16. Understanding trauma reactions is important because trauma, especially early childhood trauma, appears to underlie many psychological disorders.

Did You Know?

The most common stressors for adults in the United States involve concern about:

- mass shootings (71 percent)
- health care (69 percent)
- acts of terrorism (60 percent)
- climate change (56 percent)
- immigration (48 percent)
- sexual harassment (45 percent)

Reports of discrimination have risen significantly and are now a source of stress for 25 percent of U.S. Americans. Generation Z adults report the highest stress levels, while the lowest levels are reported by older adults.

Source: American Psychological Association, 2019b

Prolonged Grief Disorder

Case Study Alice, age 78, and her younger brother, Charles, age 69, were very close and enjoyed spending time together. They often talked for hours on the phone, and he regularly drove a significant distance to visit her. Alice knew Charles had some health problems, but was surprised to learn that he had been hospitalized for COVID and was on a ventilator. Alice was not able to visit her brother in the hospital and was not with him when he died. Alice is filled with remorse, feeling that she abandoned her brother. She has extreme sadness and guilt feelings, is unable to sleep, and has lost weight. She yearns to be with her brother and is unable to believe that he is actually gone. (Goveas & Shear, 2020)

According to the DSM-5-TR, the diagnosis of prolonged grief disorder includes:

1. A persistent grief reaction to the loss of a loved one that lasts for at least 1 year (for children and adolescents for at least 6 months)

2. Intense yearning and/or preoccupation with thoughts of the person

3. Three or more clinically significant symptoms such as a disruption of identity, a disbelief of the death, avoiding memories of the person's death, intense emotional pain, difficulty engaging in past relationships and activities, emotional numbness, feelings that life is meaningless, and intense loneliness

In general, bereaved individuals with moderate or high levels of grief are able to adjust and integrate the loss into their lives. Most do not need psychotherapy or other interventions. However, up to 10 percent of bereaved individuals show persistent grief, especially those with other psychological conditions (Szuhany et al., 2021).

The exact prevalence of prolonged grief disorder is unclear, since it is a new disorder and past studies have used different definitions for prolonged grief. During the COVID pandemic, rates of prolonged grief may have been higher because of social isolation, the inability to be with loved ones during their illness, guilt over the possibility of having infected them, and not being able to go through the normal grieving rituals for a death (Eisma & Tamminga, 2022). For example, clinically significant symptoms of trauma (34 percent) and intense grief (55 percent) were reported among a group of adolescents who lost a loved one to COVID-19 (Murata et al., 2021).

Prolonged grief disorder continues to be a controversial diagnosis, since it is difficult to delineate what constitutes normal grief. Should it be defined by a certain time period without regard for the specific circumstances of the death? Should children only be afforded 6 months of intense grief before they are considered to have prolonged grief disorder? Because of these and other concerns, some clinicians and researchers are worried that this new diagnostic category will result in normal grief being labeled a pathological condition (Cacciatore & Frances, 2022).

Adjustment Disorder

An **adjustment disorder** (AD) occurs when someone has difficulty coping with or adjusting to a specific life stressor—the reactions to the stressor are disproportionate to the severity or intensity of the event or situation. Common stressors such as interpersonal or family problems, divorce, academic failure, harassment or bullying, loss of a job, or financial problems may lead to an AD. According to the DSM-5-TR, the following is necessary for a diagnosis of AD:

1. Exposure to an identifiable stressor that results in the onset of significant emotional or behavioral symptoms that occur within 3 months of the event

2. Emotional distress and behavioral symptoms that are out of proportion to the severity of the stressor (normal bereavement is excluded from the AD diagnosis) and result in significant impairment in social, academic, or work-related functioning, or other life activities

3. These symptoms last no longer than 6 months after the stressor or consequences of the stressor have ended

AD is a common diagnosis among people seeking help from medical or mental health professionals. The prevalence ranges from 5 percent to 20 percent in mental health clinics and is up to 50 percent higher in certain groups, such as the recently bereaved and unemployed (APA, 2022). AD can be acute, occurring immediately after a specific one-time stressor, or chronic, involving multiple or repeated stressors. Although AD is considered a time-limited disorder that often resolves without treatment, the symptoms sometimes remain months after the traumatic event, such as when someone experiences a major injury (O'Donnell et al., 2019). Individuals who experience repeated distressing stressors may qualify for a diagnosis of AD for up to 6 months after each stressor. They may also qualify for an alternative diagnosis if distressing symptoms associated with a stressor persist for more than 6 months.

Adjustment disorders often involve mood or behavioral changes, including symptoms of anxiety or depression. It is not always easy to distinguish between normal adaptive stress, adjustment disorders, and depressive and anxiety disorders. The main differentiating factor is that a specific stressor precedes the symptoms experienced in AD and that the person experiences an unusually intense reaction to the stressor. To increase diagnostic accuracy and to rule out preexisting mental health conditions, clinicians also consider a person's emotional functioning prior to encountering the stressor (Zelviene & Kazlauskas, 2018).

As with prolonged grief disorder, there is concern that the AD diagnostic category may be pathologizing normative responses to stressors. Determining whether someone's reaction to a stressful situation is "out of proportion" can be difficult. Is a young adult who is overwhelmed with feelings of depression 3 weeks after being diagnosed with cancer demonstrating an AD, a normal adaptive emotional reaction, or the onset of a depressive disorder? In fact, symptoms of an AD are quite common among those who have received a worrisome medical diagnosis; for instance, up to one third of those receiving treatment for cancer meet the criteria for an AD diagnosis, a finding that highlights the difficulty of determining when a mental health diagnosis is appropriate (Strain, 2019). As you will read about in the next section, in contrast to the broad range of possible life events and stressors associated with an AD diagnosis, the other trauma-related disorders we will be discussing (acute and posttraumatic stress disorders) require the presence of specific traumatic stressors (refer to Table 6.1).

Trauma-Related Disorders

Case Study I was raped when I was 25 years old. For a long time, I spoke about the rape as though it was something that happened to someone else. I was very aware that it had happened to me, but there was just no feeling. Then I started having flashbacks. They kind of came over me like a splash of water. I would be terrified. Suddenly I was reliving the rape. Every instant was startling. I wasn't aware of anything around me. I was in a bubble, just kind of floating. And it was scary. (National Institute of Mental Health, 2009, p. 7)

Table 6.1 Trauma- and Stressor-Related Disorders

	Disorders Chart			
Disorder	**DSM-5-TR Criteria[a]**	**Prevalence**	**Gender and Cultural Factors**	**Course**

Prolonged grief disorder	• Persistent grief reaction lasting for at least 1 year (at least 6 months for children and adolescents)
	• Intense yearning and/or preoccupation with thoughts of the deceased person
	• Clinically significant symptoms (3 or more)
	  • Disruption of identity
	  • Disbelief of the death
	  • Avoidance of memories involving the person's death
	  • Intense emotional pain
	  • Difficulty engaging in past relationships and activities
	  • Emotional numbness
	  • Feelings that life is meaningless
	  • Intense loneliness
		• Up to 10% in adults and 18% in youth	• No significant gender disparity
			• Symptoms vary across cultures
				• Prolonged grief for death of a child
				• More chronic for traumatic death or suicide

Adjustment disorder	• Exposure to a stressor of any type or severity • Symptoms begin within 3 months of exposure to the stressor • Lasts no longer than 6 months after termination of the stressor or consequences from the stressor	• About 5% to 20% in mental health clinics • Up to 50% in medical and psychiatric samples, recently bereaved, and unemployed	• More common in women and those with disadvantaged life circumstances	• Most adults recover • Adolescents may be at risk for other disorders

Acute stress disorder	• Direct or indirect exposure to a traumatic stressor involving actual or threatened death, serious injury, or sexual violence
	• Nine or more symptoms involving:
	  • intrusive memories
	  • avoidance of reminders of event
	  • negative thoughts or emotions
	  • heightened arousal
	  • dissociation or inability to remember details
	• Disturbance persists from 3 days to 1 month after exposure to trauma
		• Up to 20% for most traumatic events; higher rates for those involving interpersonal situations
		• Varies according to the type, intensity, and personal meaning of the traumatic stressor
			• More prevalent in women, possibly due to more interpersonal trauma
			• Symptoms may vary cross-culturally
				• About one half will later receive a PTSD diagnosis; the remainder will remit within 30 days

Posttraumatic stress disorder[b]	• Direct or indirect exposure to a traumatic stressor involving actual or threatened death, serious injury, or sexual violence
	• One or two symptoms involving each of the following:
	  • Intrusive memories
	  • Avoidance of reminders of the event
	  • Negative thoughts or emotions
	  • Heightened arousal and hypervigilance
	• Symptoms present for at least 1 month
		• Lifetime prevalence for U.S. adults is up to 8.3%
		• 12-month prevalence is 4.7%
		• Varies according to the traumatic stressor and population involved; higher rates for rape, military combat, and emergency responders
			• Twice as prevalent in women
			• Adolescent girls have higher prevalence (6.6%) compared to adolescent boys (1.6%)
			• Low prevalence in Asian Americans
			• Higher prevalence in Latinx and African Americans
			• Symptoms may vary cross-culturally
				• Symptoms fluctuate
				• About 50% recover within the first 3 months
				• In some cases, PTSD is a chronic condition

[a]Symptoms produce significant distress or impairment in social interactions, ability to work, or other areas of functioning.
[b]Applies to those over 7 years of age.
Source: APA, 2022; O'Donnell et al., 2019; Szuhany et al., 2021

Unfortunately, exposure to trauma, such as the terrifying sexual assault described in this case, is not uncommon. In fact, as many as 85 percent of undergraduate students have experienced a traumatic event sometime in their lives (Table 6.2). After exposure to traumatic incidents, there are four common outcomes or trajectories (Bryant, 2013):

1. *Resilience*—Relatively stable functioning and few symptoms resulting from the trauma

2. *Recovery*—Initial distress with a reduction in symptoms over time

3. *Delayed symptoms*—Few initial symptoms followed by increasing symptoms over time

4. *Chronic symptoms*—Consistently high trauma-related symptoms that begin soon after the event

The trauma-related disorders we will discuss—**acute stress disorder (ASD)** and **posttraumatic stress disorder (PTSD)**—both begin with normal adaptive responses to extremely upsetting circumstances. However, individuals who develop these disorders find that their anxiety and reactivity to cues associated with the traumatic circumstances do not fade away. As you will learn from our discussion, the risk of developing

Going Deeper

Understanding Intergenerational Trauma

Intergenerational trauma refers to the concept of collective historic trauma that is passed down from generation to generation. Thus, unresolved emotional distress based on prior traumatic occurrences exerts an undue influence on the well-being of future generations. This occurs through mechanisms such as pervasive stress, difficulties with trust, or maladaptive coping behavior—conditions that lead to social and emotional disconnection within families and communities. This type of intergenerational trauma has affected Native Americans (beginning with colonization), African Americans (originating with slavery), and Mexican Americans in the southwestern United States (following both Spanish and Anglo colonialism), as well as the survivors of modern-day genocide, including the Holocaust. In many cases, those affected by historic trauma are further traumatized by ongoing displacement, segregation, and oppression. This generational transmission of trauma not only has significant implications for emotional and spiritual well-being but also can directly and indirectly jeopardize physical health (DeAngelis, 2019).

Researchers have begun to examine the biological pathways through which historical trauma has the potential to influence health by examining the role of epigenetic modifications in the generational transmission of psychophysiological illness. They argue that the physical condition of future generations is affected when disease-associated epigenetic changes occur (Youssef, 2022). This can happen when an individual in a historically traumatized population:

1. is personally exposed to stressors or traumatic events (e.g., incidents related to behavior patterns associated

with multigenerational trauma such as substance abuse or domestic violence) or

2. has inherited epigenetic changes from their parents and grandparents—transmissible genetic modifications that were produced by a prior generation's direct exposure to the traumatic event or circumstances.

As you can see, there are a multitude of ways in which historical trauma can have adverse health outcomes in contemporary generations. The Black Lives Matter movement has made it abundantly clear that in order to heal historical wounds, we need to engage in a concerted effort to genuinely acknowledge, examine, and account for the events of the past and their effects in the present. This is true not only for African Americans but also for other groups (particularly Native Americans) for whom the cultural wounds from genocide, war, displacement, and colonization have not yet been adequately addressed or healed.

For Further Consideration

1. What can be done to assist with reconciliation and healing for members of cultural groups who have been oppressed and historically affected by subjugation through colonization or slavery?

2. Do you believe that the concept of intergenerational trauma should also apply to families in which there is no specific historic precipitant but there is a history of trauma-producing behavior within the family (e.g., substance abuse or domestic violence)?

Table 6.2 Undergraduates' Lifetime Exposure to Traumatic Events

Natural disaster (e.g., tornado, hurricane, earthquake)	57.5%
Unexpected death of someone close to you	26.7%
Witnessing a serious accident (e.g., car, fire, explosion)	24.4%
Target of violent crime (e.g., rape, robbery, assault)	13.9%
Relationship physical abuse	13.0%
Danger of losing your life or being seriously injured	11.9%
Experience of physical or sexual abuse as a child	11.7%
Traumatic experiences that you feel you can't tell anyone	7.9%
Unwanted sexual experiences with threat or force as adult	6.6%
Other very traumatic events (surgery, divorce, illness)	32.8%

Source: Yeung et al., 2016

either ASD or PTSD depends on a number of variables, including the type of trauma and degree of perceived threat, the magnitude of the event, the extent of exposure to the stressor, and risk and protective factors specific to the individual. People who face severe psychological or physical trauma such as military combat, sexual assault, or other life-threatening situations are particularly vulnerable to ongoing psychological or physical reactions.

Diagnosis of Acute and Posttraumatic Stress Disorders

Trauma-related disorders begin with direct or indirect exposure to specific traumatizing stressors, including actual or threatened death, serious injury, or sexual violence. The initial stress reactions that occur shortly after a traumatic event are normative responses to an overwhelming and threatening stimulus. Fortunately, most individuals recover from traumatic events and demonstrate a marked lessening of symptoms as time passes (McDonald et al., 2019). For some people, however, the response to a traumatic experience lasts for more than several days and results in the heightened reactivity and ongoing fear, alarm, and distress that are characteristic of ASD or PTSD. The trauma may be so overwhelming that the person finds it difficult to process or make sense of the event. Indirect exposure to trauma such as witnessing a traumatic event involving others, learning of a traumatic event involving loved ones, or repeated contact with aversive details of a traumatic event (such as professionals frequently exposed to details of violence or abuse) can also result in ASD or PTSD (Bradford & de Amorim Levin, 2020).

A diagnosis of ASD or PTSD requires direct or indirect exposure to the traumatic event, as well as symptoms from these major symptom clusters (American Psychiatric Association [APA], 2022):

- Intrusion symptoms: *Intrusive thoughts, including distressing recollections, nightmares, or flashbacks of the trauma; psychological distress triggered by external or internal reminders of the trauma; physical symptoms such as increased heart rate or sweating.* Carmen, a 19-year-old college student, was raped by her best friend's father when she was 13 years old. The release of the perpetrator when

Keeping Hope Alive

On May 6, 2013, Amanda Berry (front) and Gina DeJesus, who were abducted in their teens and held captive for almost a decade, finally escaped from their sadistic kidnapper. These courageous women collaborated on a book, *Hope: A Memoir of Survival in Cleveland*, in which they describe the role of hope in surviving and recovering from their ordeal.

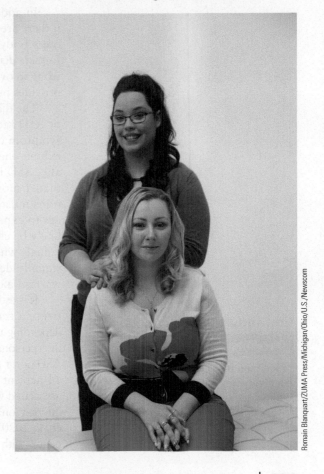

Romain Blanquart/ZUMA Press/Michigan/Ohio/U.S./Newscom

she was in college increased her PTSD symptoms. Flashbacks of the assault began to occur, sometimes triggered by her boyfriend touching her or older men looking at her (Frye & Spates, 2012).

- Avoidance: *Avoidance of thoughts, feelings, or physical reminders associated with the trauma, as well as places, events, or objects that trigger distressing memories of the experience.* One Iraq War veteran avoided social events and cookouts; even grilling hamburgers reminded him of the burning flesh he encountered during combat in Iraq (Keltner & Dowben, 2007).

- Negative alterations in mood or cognition: *Difficulty remembering details of the event; persistent negative views about oneself or the world; distorted cognitions leading to self-blame or blaming others; frequent negative emotions; limited interest in important activities; feeling emotionally numb, detached, or estranged from others; persistent inability to experience positive emotions.* The woman in the vignette presented earlier poignantly described her experience of numbness and detachment resulting from her rape. "I spoke about the rape as though it was something that happened to someone else. I was very aware that it had happened to me, but there was just no feeling. . . . I was in a bubble, just kind of floating."

- Arousal and changes in reactivity: *Feelings of irritability that may result in verbal or physical aggression, engaging in reckless or self-destructive behaviors,* **hypervigilance** *involving constantly remaining alert for danger, heightened physiological reactivity such as exaggerated startle response, difficulty concentrating, and sleep disturbance.* War veterans can become "unglued" at the sound of a door slamming, a nail gun being used, or a camera clicking (Lyke, 2004).

In addition to the symptoms already described, clinicians also specify if there are recurrent symptoms of *depersonalization* (feeling detached from one's body or thoughts) or *derealization* (a persistent sense of unreality). In fact, **dissociation**, a protective reaction involving mental disconnection from an overwhelming situation, is commonly associated with trauma, as it provides psychological distance from the traumatic event.

The diagnostic criteria for ASD and PTSD are very similar. A diagnosis of ASD requires the presence of at least nine symptoms from any of the symptom clusters, whereas a PTSD diagnosis requires that the individual exhibit one or two symptoms from each of the symptom clusters. Additionally, ASD involves symptoms that persist for at least 3 days but no longer than 1 month after the traumatic event; for a PTSD diagnosis, the symptoms must be present for at least 1 month. If someone with ASD continues to experience distressing symptoms after 30 days, the diagnosis would likely be changed to PTSD. This sequence occurs in up to half of the individuals who have received an ASD diagnosis. Expression of PTSD is occasionally delayed—symptoms are not evident or sufficiently distressing to warrant a diagnosis until 6 months or more after the trauma (APA, 2022).

It is estimated that between 12 percent and 26 percent of adults who experience a traumatic event develop ASD, with the risk of ongoing symptoms depending upon the specific trauma (Ophuis et al., 2018). If the event involved interpersonal trauma such as assault or rape, higher rates (up to 50 percent) of ASD occur (APA, 2022). In one sample of traumatized children and adolescents, 14 percent met the criteria for ASD 2 weeks after the trauma. Risk factors associated with developing ASD were younger age, female gender, exposure to interpersonal violence, and severity of initial reaction to the trauma (Lenferink et al., 2020). The prevalence of ASD is most likely underestimated, since many people with short-term symptoms do not seek treatment.

Continuum Video Project

Darwin: **PTSD**

"I led men into combat. And sometimes when I made decisions, people died."

Access the Continuum Video Project in MindTap.

A significant number of people experience prolonged reactions to trauma. In the United States, it is estimated that the lifetime prevalence of PTSD for women is between 8 to 11 percent and from 4 to 5 percent in men. Higher prevalence rates are reported among those occupationally subjected to traumatic situations such as firefighters, police, and emergency workers. Approximately half of those exposed to interpersonal violence such as rape, combat, or captivity develop PTSD. The prevalence varies across cultural groups and may reflect differential exposure to traumatic stressors, cultural differences in response to trauma, or differences in vulnerability. The lifetime prevalence of PTSD is highest among African Americans, Hispanic Americans, and Native Americans (APA, 2022).

Having the symptoms of PTSD can be quite distressing. Intrusive memories of the traumatic event via nightmares or flashbacks often occur unexpectedly and can be extremely upsetting both physically and psychologically. Trauma can shatter one's sense of safety and security, and lead to feelings of disillusionment or helplessness. Irritability and verbal or physical reactivity or feelings of numbness, dissociation, and disconnection from others can strain friendships and other close relationships. Avoiding cues associated with the trauma can become a priority and further interfere with normal functioning. It is not surprising that up to half of individuals with PTSD develop depression (Barbano et al., 2019). PTSD has a variable course; it may remit after several months or last for years (Santiago et al., 2013).

Etiology of Trauma- and Stressor-Related Disorders

Only a relatively small percentage of those exposed to a life-threatening trauma develop a trauma disorder. What factors increase risk? Certain stressors such as severe physical injuries or personalized trauma are more likely to result in PTSD (refer to Table 6.3). For example:

- Individuals who have serious injuries to the head or extremities have increased risk of developing PTSD (Haagsma et al., 2012).

- Approximately one third of individuals hospitalized with major burn injuries demonstrated PTSD symptoms after their trauma (McKibben et al., 2008).

- Over two thirds of women who are raped or sexually assaulted develop PTSD (Dworkin et al., 2023).

PTSD symptoms are more likely among those exposed to intentional trauma (e.g., assaults) than nonintentional trauma (e.g., car accidents) and when the perpetrator of an interpersonal trauma such as sexual assault is someone with whom the person has a close relationship (Martin et al., 2013). Factors such as a person's cognitive style, childhood history, genetic vulnerability, and availability of social support also influence the impact of a traumatic event (Lindstrom et al., 2013). In this section, we use the multipath model to consider biological, psychological, social, and sociocultural factors associated with the development of trauma-related disorders (refer to Figure 6.1). Although we refer to PTSD throughout the discussion, the information also pertains to the acute reactions to trauma that occur in those diagnosed with ASD.

Impact of Natural Catastrophes

Acute stress disorder is often observed among people who experience natural disasters. Leona Watts sits in a chair amid wreckage caused by a hurricane/tornado. Returning to look for some of her belongings, she was overwhelmed by the extent of the damage.

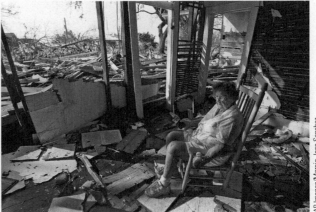

AP Images/Marcio Jose Sanchez

Did You Know?

In 2009, the Department of Defense ruled that veterans whose primary wartime injury is PTSD will not be awarded the Purple Heart, the honor given to wounded veterans. In part, this decision was made because physical wounds can be objectively identified, whereas "mental wounds" are subjective.

Source: Beresin, 2019

Table 6.3 Lifetime Prevalence of Exposure to Stressors by Gender and PTSD Risk

Trauma	Lifetime Prevalence (%)		PTSD Risk (%)	
	Men	**Women**	**Men**	**Women**
Life-threatening accident	25.0	13.8	6.3	8.8
Natural disaster	18.9	15.2	3.7	5.4
Threat with weapon	19.0	6.8	1.9	32.6
Physical attack	11.1	6.9	1.8	21.3
Rape	0.7	9.2	65.0	45.9

Some traumas are more likely to result in PTSD than others. Significant gender differences were found in reactions to "being threatened with a weapon" and "physical attack." What accounts for the differences in risk for developing PTSD among the specific traumas and for the two genders?

Source: Ballenger et al., 2000

Biological Dimension

Many individuals who develop trauma-related disorders have a nervous system that is more reactive to fear and stress when compared to people who are exposed to trauma but do not develop a disorder. Although our biological systems are designed for rapid recovery from traumatic events and for homeostasis (physiological balance), some people are more prone to the physiological reactivity associated with trauma-related disorders.

The normal response to a fear-producing stimulus is quite rapid, occurring in milliseconds, and involves the amygdala, the part of the brain that activates following threat detection and is the major interface between events occurring in the environment and physiological fear responses. The amygdala has multiple connections to regions of the prefrontal cortex that are concerned with attention, managing emotional reactions, and anticipating events. In response to a potentially dangerous situation, the amygdala sends out a signal to the prefrontal cortex and the **sympathetic nervous system**, preparing the body for action (i.e., to fight or to flee). The hypothalamic-pituitary-adrenal (HPA) axis (the system involved in stress

Figure 6.1

Multipath Model for Posttraumatic Stress Disorder
The dimensions interact with one another and combine in different ways to result in posttraumatic stress disorder (PTSD).

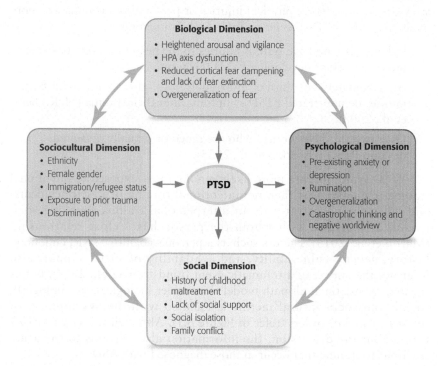

Biological Dimension
• Heightened arousal and vigilance
• HPA axis dysfunction
• Reduced cortical fear dampening and lack of fear extinction
• Overgeneralization of fear

Psychological Dimension
• Pre-existing anxiety or depression
• Rumination
• Overgeneralization
• Catastrophic thinking and negative worldview

Social Dimension
• History of childhood maltreatment
• Lack of social support
• Social isolation
• Family conflict

Sociocultural Dimension
• Ethnicity
• Female gender
• Immigration/refugee status
• Exposure to prior trauma
• Discrimination

PTSD

and trauma reactions) then releases hormones, including **epinephrine** and **cortisol**. These hormones prepare the body for "fight or flight" by raising blood pressure, blood sugar levels, and heart rate; the body is thus prepared to react to the potentially dangerous situation. Homeostasis returns once it becomes evident that the danger has passed and the "fight or flight" response is dampened.

Individuals with PTSD, however, continue to demonstrate an enhanced startle response and exaggerated physiological sensitivity to stimuli associated with the traumatic event (Schmidt et al., 2013). These physiological stress reactions persist even when the stressor is no longer present. For example, neuroimaging studies of individuals with PTSD demonstrate heightened amygdala reactivity in response to a broad range of stimuli that "resemble" the original traumatic event. This overgeneralization and expansion of "threatening" cues results in hyperarousal and increased vigilance. Brain scans using functional magnetic resonance imaging have documented that the degree of neurological activity associated with this overgeneralization is associated with the severity of PTSD symptoms (Berg et al., 2020).

Because many people with PTSD exhibit minimal **fear extinction**, their trauma-related fear responses do not decline with the passage of time. This impaired fear inhibition and difficulty discriminating safe situations is a hallmark of PTSD. In one study involving the neurological testing of soldiers before they were deployed, participants who displayed the least fear extinction before deployment (i.e., more prolonged reactivity to a fearful stimulus) were the most likely to exhibit PTSD after returning home. The researchers believe that deficiencies in fear extinction occur when the medial prefrontal cortex is unable to adequately inhibit fear responses. Unfortunately, even after fear reactions to the specific traumatic event finally subside (i.e., fear extinction occurs), various trauma-related cues may continue to trigger fear reactions (Lommen et al., 2013).

Why this reactivity occurs in the first place (i.e., why homeostasis is not restored soon after the trauma) is unclear. It is possible that the chronic release of stress hormones such as cortisol alters brain structures associated with stress regulation. Disruptions caused by excess cortisol can lead to neuronal loss and affect brain structure in the hippocampus, amygdala, and cerebral cortex (Gerson & Rappaport, 2013). Further, the heightened physiological arousal and cortisol production associated with PTSD have been associated with oxidative stress and inflammation throughout the brain and body (Miller et al., 2018). The brain is particularly vulnerable to the effects of cortisol during childhood, a time when the brain is still developing. Many individuals who develop trauma-related disorders in adulthood have experienced childhood trauma. This pattern of heightened amygdala reactivity has been documented in children exposed to child abuse and domestic violence (McLaughlin et al., 2019).

Stress-related alterations in connectivity within the orbitofrontal cortex may also help explain the vigilance and cognitive rigidity associated with PTSD (McEwen, 2017). Additionally, individuals with PTSD exhibit altered structural and functional connectivity between the amygdala and the ventromedial prefrontal cortex—neurological changes that appear to strengthen reactivity and hypersensitivity to threat. Lower glutamate levels in these regions may be responsible for these atypical patterns of connectivity (Ousdal et al., 2019).

Genetic differences are also implicated in vulnerability to trauma-related disorders. In twin studies, the heredity of PTSD is about 30 percent. Epigenetic alterations associated with environmental stressors such as poverty or early childhood abuse can influence how genes are expressed or regulated. The genes believed to be involved in trauma-related disorders are those related to

Social Support Following a Disaster

The city of El Paso, Texas, organized a prayer vigil after a racially motivated killing in which a heavily armed man walked into a crowded Walmart on August 3, 2019, and began shooting, an event that left 23 people dead and 23 injured. Local citizens, such as the woman pictured here, found support by gathering as they tried to make sense of the violent rampage and mourned those who lost their lives.

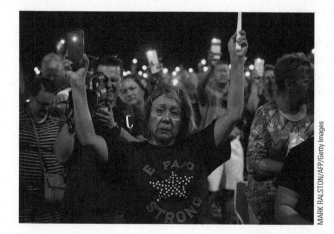

MARK RALSTON/AFP/Getty Images

the HPA axis and glucocorticoid receptors (Daskalakis et al., 2018). Genetic research has also focused on individuals with two short alleles (SS genotype) of the serotonin transporter gene (5-HTTLPR). Those with this genotype appear to have increased stress sensitivity and are more prone to heightened anxiety reactions when subjected to severe trauma (Gressier et al., 2013).

Psychological Dimension

What psychological factors contribute to the development of a trauma-related disorder? Preexisting conditions such as anxiety and depression as well as depleting emotions such as hostility and anger are risk factors for the development of PTSD (Schweizer et al., 2017). Individuals with higher anxiety or depleting emotions may react more intensely to a traumatic event because they ruminate about the event or overestimate the probability that additional aversive events will follow (Sadeh et al., 2015). A tendency to generalize trauma-related stimuli to other situations and to avoid circumstances associated with the trauma (e.g., a rape survivor avoiding contact with anyone similar to the perpetrator) can maintain the fear response because the person is not able to learn that such situations are not dangerous; in other words, there is less opportunity for fear extinction.

As with anxiety disorders, individuals with specific cognitive styles or dysfunctional thoughts about themselves (e.g., "I am inadequate") or the environment (e.g., "The world is a dangerous place") are more likely to develop PTSD (Harned et al., 2018). They may interpret stressors in a catastrophic manner and thereby increase the psychological impact of trauma. Negative thoughts such as these may produce sustained and heightened physiological reactivity, making the development of PTSD more likely (Iyadurai et al., 2018). People with ASD or PTSD who also have a negative worldview may have difficulty envisioning a positive future. These negative appraisals sustain hyperarousal, the trauma-related symptoms, and avoidance behavior (Kimble et al., 2018).

On the other hand, a cognitive style that results in active problem solving, reframing traumatic events in a more positive light, and optimistic thinking can increase resilience and reduce the risk of PTSD (Gil & Weinberg, 2015). Recovery from PTSD symptoms is also more likely with individuals who possess psychological flexibility, practice mindfulness, and demonstrate self-compassion (Meyer et al., 2019). In therapy, helping trauma survivors decrease dysfunctional trauma-related appraisals is effective in reducing PTSD symptoms (Kleim et al., 2013).

Social Dimension

Case Study Ebaugh was traumatized when she was abducted and raped by a man with a knife. She begged him to release her, but instead he handcuffed her and threw her from a bridge four stories above the water. She managed to reach the shore by swimming on her back and survived. This terrifying ordeal resulted in PTSD. (Hughes, 2012)

Ebaugh recovered from this trauma and was eventually free of PTSD symptoms. She attributes her resilience to support from caring people. The truck driver who found her took her to a nearby store and gave her a cup of tea, the police were very sympathetic when questioning her, the physician at the hospital treated her like a daughter, and a close friend took her in. In addition, her family was supportive. Social support can prevent or diminish PTSD symptoms by affecting brain processes (such as the release of endorphins) that reduce stress and anxiety (Hughes, 2012). Social support may also dampen the anxiety associated with trauma or prevent negative cognitions from occurring. Among U.S. service members and veterans, social support, especially from nonmilitary sources, is a strong protective factor against PTSD symptom severity (Blais et al., 2021). In contrast, individuals who are socially isolated and lacking in support systems appear to be more vulnerable to PTSD after encountering a traumatic event. For example, women who receive negative reactions from others after disclosing sexual abuse experience higher levels of distress and depression (Hakimi et al., 2018)

Additionally, less-than-optimal social support during childhood or exposure to childhood traumas such as physical or sexual abuse or severe bullying can increase the risk of developing trauma-related disorders. Preexisting family conflict or overprotective family interactions may also increase the impact of stress following exposure to a traumatic event (Bokszczanin, 2008). Social factors can affect our physiological and psychological reactions. For instance, conflicts or abuse in our family of origin may increase anxiety, lead to a pessimistic cognitive style, alter stress-related physiological activity and HPA axis functioning, or "trigger" a genetic predisposition toward greater physiological reactivity, and thus increase the risk of developing PTSD (Keding et al., 2021; McGowan, 2013).

Sociocultural Dimension

Ethnic differences have been found in the prevalence of PTSD. In a survey of 1,008 New York City residents following the terrorist attacks of September 11, 2001, symptoms consistent with PTSD were reported by 3.2 percent of Asian Americans, 6.5 percent of European Americans, 9.3 percent of African Americans, and 13.4 percent of Hispanic Americans (Galea et al., 2002). Among workers at the World Trade Center exposed to the horrific circumstances following the attacks (toxic fumes, human remains, and dangerous working conditions), PTSD was highest for Latinx (40 percent), followed by Black (27 percent) and White (26 percent) responders. Factors associated with vulnerability to PTSD include gender, educational and income levels, exposure to additional stressful life events, minimal social support at work, and prior psychiatric history (Whealin et al., 2022).

Race-based discrimination can produce psychological trauma and result in trauma symptoms (Polanco-Roman et al., 2016). In a study of PTSD among African American and Latinx adults, exposure to racism and discrimination accounted for up to 38 percent of the variance in PTSD diagnostic status. Discriminatory experiences such as "being called names or insulted," "witnessing friends of your ethnic group treated unfairly," and "being treated as not as smart because of your ethnic group" were predictive of PTSD status. For African Americans, the most frequent reported discriminatory experiences included "being disliked or treated unfairly because of your ethnicity" and "being treated unfairly in restaurants and stores at least once a week." These experiences not only increase the risk of disorders like PTSD but may be responsible

Posttraumatic Stress Disorder

A woman speaks about the ongoing distress she has experienced since a sexual assault that occurred during her freshman year of college. Women who are survivors of sexual assault experience high rates of PTSD.

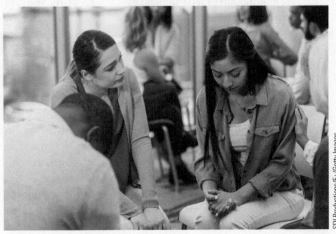

SDI Productions/E+/Getty Images

for the finding that the vast majority of participants in this sample remained chronically ill during a 5-year follow-up period (Sibrava et al., 2019). Ethnic group differences may also result from preexisting variables such as differential exposure to previous trauma or cultural differences in responding to stress.

Women are twice as likely as men to be diagnosed with a trauma-related disorder (Christiansen & Berke, 2020). This may result from physiological differences or because women have greater risk of exposure to stressors that are likely to result in PTSD. In analyzing the data from the National Violence Against Women Survey, Cortina and Kubiak (2006) concluded that the greater prevalence of trauma-related disorders in women was due, in part, to more frequent exposure to violent interpersonal situations.

Women who become police officers face greater assaultive violence than civilian women, yet they are less likely to have symptoms of PTSD (Lilly et al., 2009). Similarly, female veterans deployed to Iraq and Afghanistan appear to be as resilient as men to combat-related stress (Maguen et al., 2012; Vogt et al., 2011). What accounts for the difference in PTSD prevalence among civilian women and women who join the police force or the military? Women who choose these career paths may differ biologically from civilian women, may engage in emotional suppression to cope with the challenges of their work, or may conform to male norms (Lilly et al., 2009). It is also possible that training for combat or police duties increases resilience.

Treatment of Trauma-Related Disorders

In our discussion of treatment of trauma-related disorders, we will focus on methods for ameliorating the distressing symptoms found in those with ASD and PTSD. We have not extended our discussion to prolonged grief disorder and adjustment disorders because there is limited research on those conditions. Many individuals with prolonged grief disorder exhibit diminished grief over time without intervention. For individuals who seek treatment, cognitive-behavioral therapy specifically tailored to deal with severe grief has been successful in reducing the severity of symptoms (Reitsma et al., 2023). In general, therapists working with clients who have an adjustment disorder use brief forms of therapy that focus on removing or modifying the stressor or developing strategies for coping with the stressor.

Medication Treatment for Trauma-Related Disorders

Certain antidepressant medications (SSRIs) are moderately effective in treating individuals with ASD and PTSD. These medications appear to help by altering serotonin levels, decreasing reactivity of the amygdala, and desensitizing the fear network (Kaysen et al., 2019). However, they are effective in less than 60 percent of people with PTSD; additionally, only about 20 percent to 30 percent of those who respond to antidepressants report a full recovery (Berger et al., 2009).

Several other medications to treat PTSD symptoms have had variable success. In clinical trials, the medication D-cycloserine appears to act on the brain to boost fear extinction processes (Inslicht et al., 2022) and has demonstrated a small augmentative effect on improving the outcome of cognitive-behavioral therapy for PTSD (Mataix-Cols et al., 2017). Prazosin, a hypertension medication sometimes prescribed to reduce nightmares associated with PTSD, has not demonstrated substantial effectiveness in reducing distressing dreams or improving sleep quality (Skeie-Larsen et al., 2022).

Myth A PTSD diagnosis is a successful legal defense against criminal charges.

Reality Although PTSD is sometimes used as a legal defense, it is rarely successful. Among one group of defendants who attempted this defense, 86 percent were charged with a violent crime, including 40 percent who faced charges of homicide. The PTSD defense worked in only 7 percent of these cases—with the desired verdict of "not guilty by reason of insanity." Forty percent of the defendants were found guilty on the original charge, and 23 percent were sentenced after entering a guilty plea to a lesser charge (Cohen & Appelbaum, 2016).

Is There a Silver Lining to Adverse Life Events?

Stressful and traumatic life events are common. Although some people develop trauma- or stress-related disorders, many individuals appear to be resilient to stressors—that is, they are able to rebound after exposure to adversity. In fact, many who encounter significant stressors not only recover but also display "posttraumatic growth" and a greater capacity for future resilience (Whealin et al., 2020). One group of college students who experienced posttraumatic growth following trauma possessed a variety of characteristics. They perceived negative events as opportunities for transformation and had learned to embrace change. They also used positive reframing and active coping strategies to deal with stressors. These qualities, including the ability to recognize that difficult circumstances often lead to personal growth, may have helped increase their resilience when encountering stressful or fear-producing events or circumstances (Yeung et al., 2016).

In a study to determine the accuracy of these perspectives, Seery et al. (2010) assessed the cumulative lifetime exposure to 37 negative events (e.g., death of family members, serious illness or injury, divorce, physical or sexual assaults, and exposure to natural disasters) experienced by several thousand respondents. Participants completed measures of mental health and well-being that involved life satisfaction; overall psychological stress; distress during the previous week; and PTSD symptoms, including impairment in day-to-day functioning. For the next 2 years, respondents completed periodic questionnaires regarding stressors encountered and current mental health. The researchers

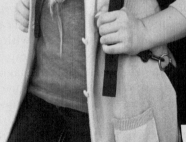

Take A Pix Media/Shutterstock.com

found an interesting relationship between adversity and mental health: Those who reported experiencing moderate amounts of prior adverse events demonstrated better mental health (higher life satisfaction, lower global distress, fewer PTSD symptoms) than those who had either minimal or high levels of prior adversity. In addition, those with moderate exposure to adversity appeared to be more resilient to the adversities encountered within the 2-year follow-up period.

Thus, it does appear that moderate amounts of adversity can generate resiliency to future stressors. This may be because individuals who encounter adversities learn that challenges can be overcome, thereby increasing a sense of mastery and control. These qualities may buffer the impact of future stressors and reduce physiological stress reactions. Individuals with very limited exposure to adversity may not have had the opportunity to develop the skills necessary for overcoming challenges. Conversely, individuals confronted by multiple adverse events may feel overwhelmed and develop feelings of hopelessness and helplessness. Along these lines, one study of disaster survivors in Chile found that the greater the number of previous stressors faced by a survivor, the more likely it was that the survivor would go on to develop PTSD or major depressive disorder (Fernandez et al., 2020). More research is needed to determine if certain stressors or traumas are more toxic than others and which kinds of prior stressors are most likely to "inoculate" against future traumatic events.

The drug MDMA has demonstrated effectiveness when combined with exposure-based therapy for PTSD. It works by suppressing the emotional memory circuits involved with intrusive memories, thus permitting the use of exposure therapy (i.e., revisiting the traumatic event) without creating a situation where the client is overwhelmed by fear. MDMA-assisted therapy was found to be effective in reducing severe PTSD symptoms (Lewis et al., 2023). In early 2023, Australia became the first country to approve the use of MDMA for the treatment of PTSD. In the United States, the FDA has given the drug an "expanded access status," allowing its use as an adjunct with psychotherapy for very severe cases of PTSD while continuing to review the data in preparation for granting full approval for its use in the treatment of PTSD (Mitchell, 2022).

Psychotherapy for Trauma-Related Disorders

Case Study When Castellanos arrived at the hospital for treatment, he checked the bathroom's stalls for bombs or hidden insurgent fighters. In the therapy area, he was handed an unloaded M16 rifle and a virtual reality headset. During 13 weeks of therapy, he regularly spent time in a virtual world, riding in a convoy in Iraq with a Blackhawk helicopter flying overhead. After he witnessed images of an explosion and felt a puff of air against his neck, his heart rate accelerated and he began sweating profusely. After each virtual session, he was asked to describe in detail the trauma he had witnessed. He cried throughout many of the sessions, but gradually the scene had less and less impact. After treatment, Castellanos no longer showed a physiological response to the previously traumatic virtual scene and described himself as a completely changed person. (Parkin, 2017)

Treatment strategies focus on extinguishing the fear of trauma-related stimuli and correcting dysfunctional cognitions. Efficacious therapies including prolonged exposure therapy (PE), cognitive-behavioral therapy (CBT), trauma-focused cognitive-behavioral therapy (TF-CBT), and eye movement desensitization and reprocessing (EMDR) have proven to be beneficial in treating PTSD (Schrader & Ross, 2021). In general, when compared to the use of medication, these treatments are not only more successful but also preferred by clients (Simiola et al., 2015).

Prolonged exposure therapy involves imaginary and real-life exposure to trauma-related cues. Extended exposure to avoided thoughts, places, or people can help individuals with PTSD realize that these situations do not pose a danger. As we saw with Castellanos as he underwent virtual exposure therapy, fear extinction can be facilitated through the use of visual immersion helmets equipped with realistic combat scenes (Parkin, 2017). More commonly, exposure therapy involves asking participants to re-create the traumatic event in their imagination. For example, trauma survivors may be asked to repeatedly imagine and describe the event "as if it were happening now," verbalizing not only details but also their thoughts and emotions regarding the incident. This repetitive process results in extinction of fear reactions (Foa et al., 2013). Prolonged exposure therapy is a preferred treatment modality among military personnel and is used in both individual and group sessions (Rauch et al., 2019). Although reduced depression is not a direct treatment goal, exposure therapy has also decreased depressive symptoms among veterans (Eftekhari et al., 2013).

Cognitive-behavioral therapy (CBT) and **trauma-focused cognitive-behavioral therapy (TF-CBT),** which uses a combination of CBT techniques and trauma-sensitive principles, focus on helping clients identify and challenge dysfunctional cognitions about the traumatic event and current beliefs about themselves and others. These therapies address underlying dysfunctional thinking or pervasive concerns about safety. For example, survivors of domestic abuse with PTSD often have thoughts associated with guilt or self-blame. Cognitions such as "I could have prevented it" or "I'm so stupid" can maintain PTSD symptoms. Therapy may include education about PTSD, developing a solution-oriented focus, reducing negative self-talk, and receiving therapeutic exposure to fear triggers such as photos of their abusive partner or movies involving domestic violence (Samuelson et al., 2017). Mindfulness training, which involves paying attention to emotions and thoughts on a nonjudgmental basis without reacting to symptoms, also demonstrates promise as an intervention for PTSD (Boyd et al., 2018).

Eye movement desensitization and reprocessing (EMDR) is a nontraditional therapy used to treat PTSD. The aim is to decrease physiological reactivity and weaken the impact of negative emotions. In this unique approach, clients visualize their traumatic experience while engaged in an activity involving both sides of the body, such as visually following a therapist's fingers moving from side to side. The therapist prompts the client to substitute positive cognitions (e.g., "I am in control") for negative cognitions associated with the experience (e.g., "I am helpless"). Processing the trauma in a relaxed state allows the client to detach from negative emotions and replace them with more adaptive appraisals of the trauma. EMDR incorporates aspects of prolonged exposure, since visualization of the trauma allows desensitization and fear extinction to occur. EMDR also employs many of the cognitive reappraisal strategies used in CBT. After a series of EMDR sessions, many individuals with PTSD report significant reductions in hyperarousal and other trauma-related symptoms (Gainer et al., 2020).

Psychiatric Service Dogs

Trained service dogs can mitigate PTSD symptoms in veterans by checking out anxiety-evoking environments before the veteran enters and reducing panic symptoms by giving the veteran a friendly nudge. Here, a medically retired Special Operations Army Ranger stands with his service dog, who served beside him in Iraq. This veteran and his loyal companion are helping each other recover from combat trauma and symptoms of PTSD.

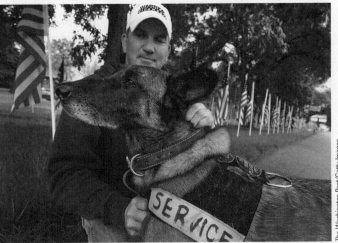

The Washington Post/Getty Images

6-2 Psychological Factors Affecting Medical Conditions

Case Study   Data from 200 patients who happened to have cardiac defibrillators implanted prior to the World Trade Center attack on September 11, 2001, provided interesting information regarding the physiological impact of the stressful event. The defibrillators, which record and respond to serious heart arrhythmias, revealed a doubling of life-threatening arrhythmias during the month following the terrorist attacks. (Steinberg et al., 2004)

Stress causes a multitude of physiological, psychological, and social changes that influence health conditions. Unfortunately, stress is pervasive. Among a national sample of U.S. college students, 15.9 percent of the men, 24.2 percent of the women, and 45.7 percent of transgender and gender nonconforming students reported "serious psychological distress" during the previous 12 months (American College Health Association, 2021). The American Psychological Association (2020b) conducted a survey that was focused on stressors during the early days of the COVID-19 pandemic; the results revealed high levels of stress, particularly among parents. Specific stressors included concerns about oneself or family members getting coronavirus (74 percent),

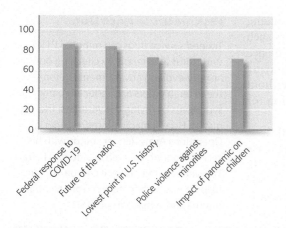

Figure 6.2

Five Leading Causes of Stress in America

The Stress in America survey, documenting high levels of stress among U.S. adults, highlights how the COVID-19 pandemic took a toll on the well-being of adults in the United States.

Source: American Psychological Association, 2020c

disrupted routines (74 percent), managing online learning for children (71 percent), and access to basic needs such as food and housing (70 percent). People of color reported the highest levels of stress. (Refer to Figure 6.2 for other major causes of stress.)

Although stress can have beneficial functions such as alerting us to the need to deal with a challenging situation or energizing us to accomplish important goals, most researchers acknowledge that excessive stress can negatively affect our physical well-being. In the past, *psychosomatic* was the term applied to physical disorders—such as asthma, hypertension, and headaches—made worse by psychological influences. This term attempted to distinguish between physical disorders affected by psychological factors and medical conditions considered strictly physical in nature. Now, however, medical and mental health professionals recognize the complexity of mind–body connections and that psychological factors influence many medical conditions.

In the DSM-5-TR, the diagnostic category "Psychological Factors Affecting Other Medical Conditions" refers to situations where psychological or behavioral factors adversely influence the course or treatment of a medical disorder, constitute an additional risk factor for the medical condition, or make the illness worse. Emotional states, patterns of interpersonal interaction, and coping styles are just a few examples of how psychological factors can affect physical illness. For the sake of brevity in discussing this topic, we sometimes substitute the term **psychophysiological disorder**—which references any physical disorder that has a strong psychological basis or component—instead of "psychological factors affecting other medical conditions." We begin by discussing how stress and other psychological factors or behaviors influence the development of and exacerbate symptoms of a variety of medical conditions. We will conclude with a discussion of etiological factors influencing various psychophysiological disorders.

Medical Conditions Influenced by Psychological Factors

Case Study Cyndy Bizon was under a great deal of stress. Her husband, Joe, suffered a heart attack while in recovery from routine surgery. Cyndy became increasingly stressed over her husband's condition and camped out in the hospital. Two days after his heart attack, she walked up to the nurses' station, felt faint, and dropped to the floor. A rush of stress hormones (e.g., adrenalin) had stunned her heart muscle. The hospital staffers were able to revive her and get her heart back to its normal rhythm. She had been experiencing "broken heart" syndrome. (Naggiar, 2012)

Broken heart syndrome, a reversible cardiac condition, occurs when severe stress results in the release of high levels of norepinephrine (i.e., noradrenaline) and a sudden reduction in heart function. As occurred with Cyndy, any strong emotional reaction can produce this physiological response (Matta & Carrie, 2023). In one study, researchers described 19 adults who developed severe cardiac symptoms after exposure to a highly emotional event (e.g., car accident, news of a death, surprise birthday party, armed robbery, court appearance). The emotional stress resulted in the cardiac changes associated with broken heart syndrome (Wittstein et al., 2005).

Symptoms and test results associated with broken heart syndrome are very similar to those of a heart attack. However, there is no evidence of blocked heart arteries or other cardiac abnormalities. For some unknown reason, this condition, which has been on the increase, is 7.5 times more likely to occur in women, particularly those between the ages of 65 and 70. In general, the cardiac abnormalities resolve in hours or weeks (Y-Hassan & Tornvall, 2018).

Medical conditions influenced by psychological factors can involve actual tissue damage (e.g., coronary heart disease), a disease process (e.g., impairment of the immune system), or physiological dysfunction (e.g., asthma, migraine headaches). Both medical treatment and psychotherapy may be required. The relative contributions of physical and psychological factors to a physical disorder can vary greatly. In some cases, the repeated association between a stressor and symptoms of the disorder provides important clues regarding psychological influences that may be involved.

In this section, we discuss several of the more prevalent psychophysiological disorders—coronary heart disease, hypertension (high blood pressure), headaches, and asthma. We also review research identifying biological, psychological, social, and sociocultural influences on specific psychophysiological disorders.

Coronary Heart Disease

Coronary vascular disease (CVD) involves the narrowing of cardiac arteries due to **atherosclerosis** (hardening of the arterial walls), resulting in complete or partial blockage of the flow of blood and oxygen to the heart, as presented in Figure 6.3. When coronary arteries are narrowed or blocked, less oxygen-rich blood reaches the heart muscle. This can result in angina (chest pain) or, if blood flow to the heart is completely blocked, a heart attack.

Heart disease is the leading cause of death in the United States. Someone dies of CVD every 40 seconds. Each year, about 605,000 people in the United States have an initial heart attack and almost 200,000 have a recurrent attack. A variety of psychological and behavioral factors increase risk and affect prognosis with CVD, including unhealthy eating habits, hypertension, cigarette smoking, diabetes, cholesterol, obesity, and lack of physical activity (Centers for Disease Control and Prevention [CDC], 2022). Psychosocial factors such as depression, perceived stress, and difficult life events can increase CVD risk as much as smoking, which is a well-known risk factor for CVD (Gianaros & Jennings, 2018).

Stress can also affect our heart rhythm. This occurs when a stressor causes the release of hormones that activate the sympathetic nervous system, which can lead to heart rhythm changes such as *ventricular fibrillation* (rapid, ineffective contractions of the heart), *bradycardia* (slowing of the heartbeat), *tachycardia* (speeding up of the heartbeat), or *arrhythmia* (irregular heartbeat). In fact, studies of heart recordings have demonstrated that mental stress can trigger potentially fatal ventricular tachycardias (Lampert, 2016). Figure 6.4 presents an example of ventricular fibrillation, a potentially fatal heart condition, that can be influenced by stress.

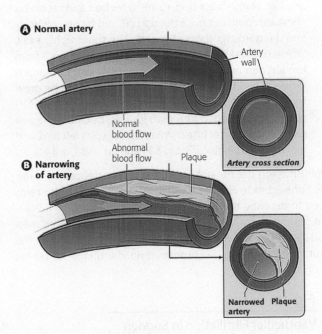

Ⓐ Normal artery

Artery wall

Normal blood flow

Abnormal blood flow

Plaque

Artery cross section

Ⓑ Narrowing of artery

Narrowed artery   Plaque

Figure 6.3

Atherosclerosis

Atherosclerosis occurs when fat, cholesterol, and other substances build up in arteries and form a hard structure called *plaque*. The buildup of plaque and resultant narrowing of the arteries can result in arteriosclerosis, or hardening of the arteries, a condition that can reduce or even stop blood flow to tissues and major organs.

Hmong Sudden Death Syndrome

Vang Xiong is a Southeast Asian immigrant who left dangerous conditions in Laos and resettled in Chicago in 1980. City life in a new country was a significant change from the familiar farm life and rural surroundings of his native Hmong village. Vang had experienced the trauma of seeing people killed prior to his escape from Laos, and expressed feelings of guilt about leaving his brothers and sisters behind. His physical difficulties began soon after his move to Chicago.

[He] could not sleep the first night in the apartment, nor the second, nor the third. After three nights of sleeping very little, Vang went to see his resettlement worker, a bilingual Hmong man named Moua Lee. Vang told Moua that the first night he woke suddenly, short of breath, from a dream in which a cat was sitting on his chest. The second night, the room suddenly grew darker, and a figure, like a large black dog, came to his bed and sat on his chest. He could not push the dog off, and he grew quickly and dangerously short of breath. The third night, a tall, White-skinned female spirit came into his bedroom from the kitchen and lay on top of him. Her weight made it increasingly difficult for him to breathe, and as he grew frantic and tried to call out he could manage but a whisper. He attempted to turn onto his side, but found he was pinned down. After fifteen minutes, the spirit left him, and he awoke, screaming. (Tobin & Friedman, 1983, p. 440)

The terrifying dream-state symptoms experienced by Vang are connected to *Hmong sudden death syndrome*—the term used to describe hundreds of cases of sudden death involving Southeast Asian refugees. Almost all cases involved men and most occurred within their first 2 years of residence in the United States. Autopsies produced no identifiable cause for the deaths. All of the reports were the same: People in apparently good health died in their sleep. Many family members reported that their deceased loved ones displayed labored breathing, screams, and frantic movements just before death. Some consider the deaths to represent an extreme and very specific example of the impact of psychological stress on physical health (refer to Figure 6.4). Similar cases of sudden unexplained death have been reported in Asian countries. Interestingly, as the refugees settled in, the incidence of cases of sudden death among Southeast Asian refugees residing in the United States decreased from 59 per 100,000 in 1981 to 1 per 100,000 in 1987. One hypothesis is that the stressors involved in the immediate aftermath of fleeing one's country, being a refugee, and living in a foreign country (perhaps in combination with some kind of underlying cardiac abnormality) produced the ventricular arrhythmia associated with Hmong sudden death syndrome (Zheng et al., 2018).

Vang was one of the lucky people with the syndrome—he survived. In many non-Western cultures, physical or mental problems are attributed to supernatural forces such as witchcraft or evil spirits. For this reason, Vang sought treatment from a Hmong woman, a highly respected shaman in Chicago's Hmong community. She believed unhappy spirits were causing his problem and performed ceremonies to release them. After this spiritual treatment, Vang reported no more physical problems or nightmares during sleep.

For Further Consideration

1. How would a doctor practicing Western medicine interpret Vang's symptoms?

2. What do you think accounted for the shaman's success in treating Vang?

Figure 6.4

Ventricular Fibrillation in Sudden Unexplained Death

A Thai man fitted with a defibrillator exhibited ventricular episodes (rapid spikes on the graph) when asleep. Part A represents a transient episode that resolved itself. Part B depicts a sustained ventricular episode accompanied by labored breathing. Part C demonstrates that his defibrillator was set off, which normalized the heart rate. Is this the explanation for sudden unexplained death syndrome?

Source: Nademanee et al., 1997

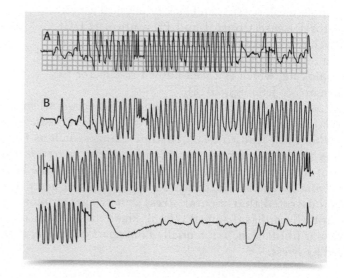

Hypertension

Case Study   On October 19, 1987, the stock market drastically dropped 508 points. By chance, a 48-year-old stockbroker was wearing a device measuring stress in the work environment on that day. The instrument measured his pulse every 15 minutes. At the beginning of the day, his pulse was 64 beats per minute and his blood pressure was 132 over 87. As stock prices fell dramatically, the man's physiological system surged in the other direction. His heart rate increased to 84 beats per minute and his blood pressure hit a dangerous 181 over 105. His pulse was "pumping adrenaline, flooding his arteries, and maybe slowly killing him in the process." (Tierney, 1988)

Undiagnosed Hypertension

David Thomas was buying groceries and decided to get a blood pressure check at a clinic located in the store. He found that he had high blood pressure and was a prime candidate for a stroke.

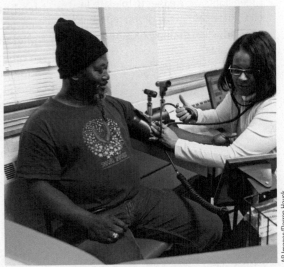

AP Images/Darren Hauck

The stockbroker's reaction in the case study demonstrates the impact of a stressor on **blood pressure**, the measurement of the force of blood against the walls of the arteries. **Normal blood pressure** is considered a **systolic pressure** (force when the heart contracts) lower than 120 mm Hg and a **diastolic pressure** (the arterial pressure that occurs when the heart is relaxed after a contraction) lower than 80 mm Hg. We all experience transient physiological responses to stressors, but some people develop a chronic condition called **hypertension**, in which the systolic blood pressure equals or exceeds 130 mm Hg or the diastolic pressure is 80 mm Hg or higher. **Elevated blood pressure** refers to a borderline level of blood pressure (systolic pressure between 120 and 129 mm Hg and diastolic pressure less than 80 mm Hg) that is believed to be a precursor to hypertension, stroke, and heart disease (Riley et al., 2018).

About 116 million (45 percent) of U.S. adults have high blood pressure requiring treatment. Unfortunately, about 74 percent of adults with hypertension do not have their condition under control. The highest rates of hypertension are found in adults age 65 and older (77 percent) and in African American adults (56 percent). (Figure 6.5 presents age, gender, and ethnic comparisons of hypertension among U.S. adults.) Chronic hypertension leads to *arteriosclerosis* (hardening of the arteries) and to increased risk of stroke and heart attack. In 2020, more than 670,000 fatalities involved hypertension as a primary or contributing causal factor. In about 90 percent of the cases of hypertension, the exact cause is not known, but both psychological and behavioral factors can play a role (CDC, 2023).

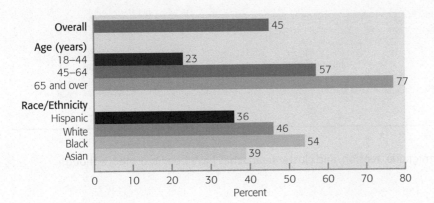

Figure 6.5

Age, Gender, and Ethnic Differences in Hypertension Among Adults in the United States

Source: CDC, 2021

Migraine, Tension, and Cluster Headaches

Headaches are among the most common stress-related psychophysiological complaints. Nearly everyone has a headache occasionally, and about one half of adults in the world had a headache during the last year; 1 in 20 people have a headache every or nearly every day. The intensity of headaches can vary from dull and annoying to excruciating. For some people, debilitating headaches decrease quality of life and impair family, social, and occupational functioning. In addition to the most common headaches (migraine, tension, and cluster headaches), medication-overuse headache is a common secondary headache disorder that affects up to 7 percent of some population groups. Ironically, this condition, which is especially prevalent among women, results from rebound headache effects associated with excessive use of headache medication (Kulkarni et al., 2021). Although we cover each category of headaches separately, the same person can be susceptible to more than one variety of headache. (Figure 6.6 presents some differences between the headaches.)

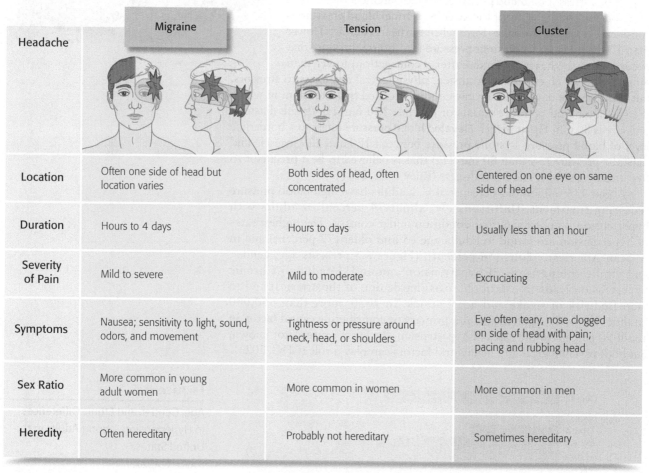

Headache	Migraine	Tension	Cluster
Location	Often one side of head but location varies	Both sides of head, often concentrated	Centered on one eye on same side of head
Duration	Hours to 4 days	Hours to days	Usually less than an hour
Severity of Pain	Mild to severe	Mild to moderate	Excruciating
Symptoms	Nausea; sensitivity to light, sound, odors, and movement	Tightness or pressure around neck, head, or shoulders	Eye often teary, nose clogged on side of head with pain; pacing and rubbing head
Sex Ratio	More common in young adult women	More common in women	More common in men
Heredity	Often hereditary	Probably not hereditary	Sometimes hereditary

Figure 6.6

Three Types of Headaches

Some differences in the characteristics of migraine, tension, and cluster headaches have been reported, although similarities between them also exist.

Source: Data adapted from Harvard Health, 2019

> **Case Study** A 31-year-old woman, the marketing director of a large business, became increasingly stressed when confronted with multiple upcoming projects. She began to experience severe throbbing headaches on the right side of her forehead that were accompanied by nausea and dizziness. Sunlight from the window or staring at her computer screen worsened her headaches. Sleeping for an hour or two usually resolved the pain. (Physiopedia, 2019)

Migraine headaches involve neurologically based head pain accompanied by symptoms such as nausea, vomiting, and hypersensitivity to environmental stimuli. Migraine episodes may last from a few hours to several days, with discomfort that ranges from mild to severe. Up to one third of individuals with migraines experience an **aura** prior to the headache—involving unusual physical sensations or visual symptoms such as flashes of light, unusual visual patterns, or blind spots (Harvard Health, 2019). Migraine headaches, especially those with an aura, are associated with an increased risk of cardiovascular events such as strokes and heart attack (Kurth et al., 2016). Migraines are associated with modifiable risk factors such as high levels of caffeine consumption, overeating, and poor sleep quality (Torres-Ferrús et al., 2020).

Migraine headaches affect about 20 percent of the U.S. population and are three to four times more common in women compared to men. The prevalence of severe migraines is highest in Native Americans (17.7 percent), followed by European Americans (15.5 percent), Hispanic Americans (14.5 percent), African Americans (14.5 percent), and Asian Americans (9.2 percent). Severe migraines are more prevalent in women than men across all ethnic groups (Najib et al., 2019). About 10.2 percent of college students surveyed reported being diagnosed with or receiving treatment for migraine headaches in the previous 12 months. The highest rate (16.2 percent) was reported by transgender and gender nonconforming students (American College Health Association, 2021).

Most people with migraines report having them up to 3 times per month; 19 percent have them 4 to 7 times per month, 11 percent have them 8 to 14 times per month, and 12 percent have them more than 15 times per month. Up to 26 percent report experiencing "severe disability" during the migraines, and 24 percent sought treatment at an emergency department (Lipton et al., 2022). Migraine headaches are the second leading cause of disability in the world and the first among young women (Steiner et al., 2020).

Between 80 percent and 90 percent of those who have migraines report sensitivity to light and/or sound during the migraine episode. Brain scans of people with migraines reveal hypersensitivity in the visual cortex, which may explain their light sensitivity. Further, increased connectivity within other brain regions (the audio cortices, anterior insula, and thalamus) might explain the intense pain and increased sensitivity to sound experienced by people who experience migraines (Pearl et al., 2020). Brain imaging of individuals with severe migraine headaches also reveals altered neuronal activity and structural changes in the brain, including white matter anomalies (Straube & Andreou, 2019).

Tension Headaches **Tension headaches** are produced when stress creates prolonged contraction of the scalp and neck muscles, resulting in vascular constriction and steady pain. With tension headaches, the most common form of headache, the pain often disappears once the stress is reduced.

Did You Know?

In one study of Norwegian neurologists, 26 percent of those surveyed reported experiencing migraines—twice the prevalence found in the Norwegian adult population.
Source: Alstadhaug et al., 2012

The pain is usually described as dull and pressing—as if there were a tight band around the head. Tension headaches are generally not as severe as migraine headaches but still can be debilitating (Ashina et al., 2021). Individuals with chronic tension headaches who frequently turn to aspirin or other analgesics for pain relief are at risk of developing medication overuse headaches (Scripter, 2018).

Tension headaches typically begin to occur during the teenage years and are more prevalent in women and girls. Approximately 70 percent of adolescents and adults experience tension headaches each year (World Health Organization [WHO], 2016).

Cluster Headaches

> **Case Study** A patient seeking help for excruciating headaches described the pain in the following manner: "It feels like someone walked up to me, took a screwdriver and jammed it up in my right eye and kept digging it around for 20 minutes" (Linn, 2004, p. A1).

Cluster headaches involve the rapid onset of an excruciating stabbing or burning sensation located in the eye or cheek. These recurring, painful attacks usually focus in or around one eye, often causing tears and redness of the eye, and sometimes resulting in drooping of the eyelid and nasal congestion on the affected side. They are referred to as "suicide headaches" because the symptoms are so severe that affected individuals report suicidal thoughts during episodes (Rimmele et al., 2023).

Cluster headaches are relatively uncommon, affecting about 1 in 1,000 adults; they generally develop during adulthood and are six times more prevalent in men (WHO, 2016). Cluster headaches occur in cycles, with incapacitating episodes that may arise several times a day. Each attack may last from 15 minutes to 3 hours before ending abruptly. Headache cycles may continue over a period of a few days to several months, followed by pain-free periods. Only about 10 percent to 20 percent of cluster headaches are chronic, with no periods of respite. In about 25 percent of cases, cluster headaches are preceded by migraine-like symptoms such as nausea and sensitivity to light and noise (Song et al., 2019).

Asthma

Asthma, a chronic inflammatory disease of the lungs, can be aggravated by stress or anxiety. During asthma episodes, various environmental influences trigger excessive mucus secretion as well as spasms and swelling of the airways; these physiological changes reduce the amount of air that can be inhaled (Figure 6.7). Asthma symptoms range from mild and infrequent wheezing or coughing to severe respiratory distress requiring emergency care. People with asthma often underestimate the magnitude of airflow obstruction during an asthma attack and, therefore, may neglect to self-administer medication or seek needed treatment. Additionally, ongoing psychological or economic stressors can interfere with adherence to protocols for the use of preventative medications or rescue inhalers (Barsky et al., 2018). Unfortunately, when there is a delay in seeking emergency assistance for a severe asthma attack, death can result.

In the United States, the prevalence of asthma has increased dramatically since the 1980s. It affects up to 7.8 percent of the U.S. population (over 25 million individuals) and is more prevalent among women, those living in poverty, American Indian/Alaska Natives, and African Americans. The highest prevalence rate (10.3 percent) occurs among

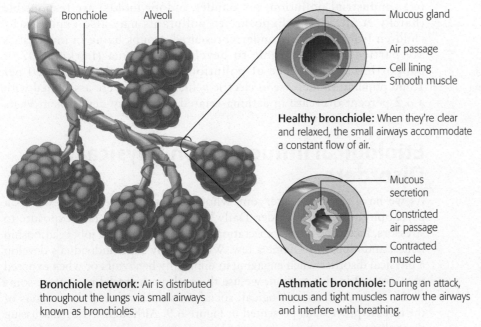

Healthy bronchiole: When they're clear and relaxed, the small airways accommodate a constant flow of air.

Bronchiole network: Air is distributed throughout the lungs via small airways known as bronchioles.

Asthmatic bronchiole: During an attack, mucus and tight muscles narrow the airways and interfere with breathing.

Figure 6.7

Physiological Mechanisms Underlying an Asthma Attack
Asthma attacks and deaths have increased dramatically since the 1980s.

Source: Cowley & Underwood, 1997, p. 61

young adults between the ages of 20 and 24 (CDC, 2022). (Figure 6.8 presents asthma prevalence among different groups.)

The increase in the number of asthma cases in the United States is puzzling. Some researchers suspect that, in addition to increasingly stressful life circumstances, a variety of environmentally based triggers

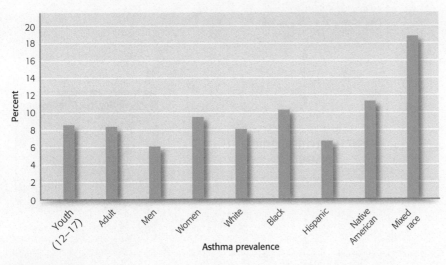

Figure 6.8

Asthma Prevalence
This figure indicates the prevalence of asthma among adults and children, men and women, and members of different ethnic groups.

Source: CDC, 2022

(e.g., industrial pollution, pet dander, indoor molds) are responsible (Barsky et al., 2018). Exposure to pollutants may also explain why children from ethnically underrepresented groups living in inner cities are particularly vulnerable to developing asthma (Larkin, 2023). Supporting the influence of pollution, zip codes that had a 20 per 1,000 population increase in electric vehicles (EVs) were associated with a 3.2 percent decrease in asthma-related emergency department visits (Garcia et al., 2023).

Etiological Influences on Physical Disorders

As we have seen, not everyone who faces stressful events develops a psychophysiological disorder. Daily living involves constant exposure to stressors, including work expectations at school or on the job, relationship issues, and illness—to name a few. Why do only some individuals develop a physical disorder when engaging in unhealthy behaviors or when exposed to stressors? In this section, we use the multipath model to explore some of the biological, psychological, social, and sociocultural dimensions of the disease process, as presented in Figure 6.9. Although we are discussing these dimensions separately, many interactions can occur among factors within and between dimensions.

Biological Dimension

Stressors, especially chronic ones, can dysregulate physiological processes occurring throughout the brain and body. When a stressor activates the HPA axis and the sympathetic nervous system, a cascade of hormones

Figure 6.9

Multipath Model of Psychophysiological Disorders
The dimensions interact with one another and combine in different ways to result in a specific psychophysiological disorder.

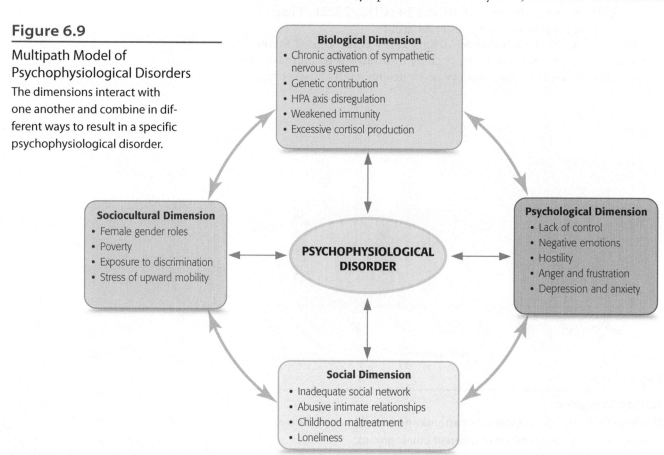

Biological Dimension
- Chronic activation of sympathetic nervous system
- Genetic contribution
- HPA axis disregulation
- Weakened immunity
- Excessive cortisol production

Sociocultural Dimension
- Female gender roles
- Poverty
- Exposure to discrimination
- Stress of upward mobility

PSYCHOPHYSIOLOGICAL DISORDER

Psychological Dimension
- Lack of control
- Negative emotions
- Hostility
- Anger and frustration
- Depression and anxiety

Social Dimension
- Inadequate social network
- Abusive intimate relationships
- Childhood maltreatment
- Loneliness

is released, including epinephrine, norepinephrine, and cortisol. These hormones assist the sympathetic nervous system to prepare the body for emergency action by increasing heart rate, respiration, and alertness. This preparation helps us respond quickly to a crisis situation. However, when such activation occurs over an extended period of time (i.e., there are chronic stressors), a psychophysiological disorder can develop.

Research supports the view that while brief exposure to stressors enhances immune functioning, long-lasting stress can impair immune response (Shan et al., 2020). Heightened or ongoing preparedness to face stress results in increased cortisol production, which can have a detrimental effect on physiological processes. For example, excess cortisol has been linked with coronary artery calcification, a contributor to coronary heart disease (Iob & Steptoe, 2019). Further, when excessive production of cortisol suppresses the immune system, white blood cells, responsible for destroying pathogens such as bacteria, viruses, fungi, and tumors, may be less able to multiply and we are therefore less capable of fighting infection. If natural defenses are weakened, illness is more likely to compromise the health of individuals with underlying psychophysiological conditions (Straub & Cutolo, 2018). Table 6.4 compares short-term adaptive responses to stress with symptoms that can result from chronic stress.

Additionally, genetic influences contribute to psychophysiological disorders. For instance, cardiovascular stress reactivity, as measured by blood pressure, is more similar among identical twins than among fraternal twins (De Geus et al., 2007). Genetic factors also appear to play a role in asthma. Among African American men, having a higher percentage of African ancestry increases the risk of developing severe asthma (Grossman et al., 2019). Further, twin studies have estimated the heritability of asthma to be around 35 percent. Asthma has been associated with genes that regulate immune response to environmental allergens (Reséndiz-Hernández & Falfán-Valencia, 2018). Migraine headaches appear to involve a biological predisposition that affects the reactivity of sensory neurons that stimulate the cerebral blood vessels and the sensitization of pain receptors (Zhao et al., 2020). A genetic predisposition for cluster headaches was found in a genome-wide association study (O'Connor et al., 2021).

Table 6.4 Adaptive and Maladaptive Responses to Stress

Adaptive Responses (Short-Term Stress)	Maladaptive Responses (Chronic Stress)
Increased glucose	Hyperglycemia (diabetes)
Increased blood pressure	Hypertension, breakage of plaque in arteries
Increased immunity	Impaired immune response to illnesses
Increased vigilance	Hypervigilance
Diminished interest in sex	Global loss of interest in sex
Improved cognition and memory	Increased focus on traumatic events, lack of attention to current environment
Faster blood clotting	Increased thickness of coronary artery walls (coronary vascular disease, strokes)

Source: Keltner & Dowben, 2007; Lee et al., 2015

Early environmental influences, such as traumatic childhood experiences, interacting with the alleles of certain genes may produce lasting changes in stress-responsive neurobiological systems, resulting in increased vulnerability to the development of a psychophysiological disorder through epigenetic mechanisms (McEwen, 2017). For example, one group of mothers who smoked during pregnancy increased the risk of asthma in their offspring by influencing the genes involved in lung development. Having a father who smoked before the age of 15 appears to be an independent risk factor for asthma, possibly through transmittable epigenetic changes in sperm cells. This epigenetic vulnerability may be passed across generations; for instance, a grandmother's smoking may increase asthma risk among grandchildren, even when the mother of the children does not smoke (Accordini et al., 2018).

Psychological Dimension

Psychological and personality characteristics can influence health status. Positive emotions, such as optimism, happiness, joy, and contentment, can help regulate heart rate, blood pressure, and other physiological stress reactions, whereas negative emotions accentuate the stress response. High levels of well-being and life satisfaction are associated with an increased likelihood of disease-free living and six more years of life compared to low levels of well-being (Zaninotto & Steptoe, 2019). In a comprehensive study involving nearly 10,000 women studied for 8 years, those who scored high on optimism ("In unclear times, I usually expect the best") had a 9 percent lower risk of developing heart disease and a 14 percent lower risk of dying. In contrast, women who had hostile thoughts about others were 16 percent more likely to die during the same time period (Tindle et al., 2009).

Control and the perception of control over the environment and its stressors (i.e., the ability to apply effective coping strategies when undergoing stress) can mitigate the negative effects of stress (Koffer et al., 2019). One group of older adults agreed to keep a daily journal describing stressful situations and their perceptions of perceived control over life events. Individuals who reported greater daily stress and lower control were more likely to have thickening of the lining of the carotid artery, a marker of atherosclerosis (Kamarck et al., 2007). Similarly, women with demanding jobs involving little personal control had nearly double the chance of having a heart attack compared to women with more personal control over stressful jobs (Albert et al., 2010). Among older adults with physical health problems, those who vowed to take charge of their health by engaging in health-improving behavior demonstrated less biological decline and had a decreased likelihood of cardiovascular illness despite risk factors for heart disease (Yanek et al., 2013).

In contrast to the health-promoting aspects of positive emotions, negative emotional states such as depression, hostility, anxiety, and cynicism increase the risk for psychophysiological disorders. In a 10-year follow-up study, pessimism was a substantial risk factor for CVD among men (Pankalainen et al., 2015). Depression and anxiety can influence both physiological functioning and behaviors that affect health. Individuals with high levels of these emotions exhibit irregularities in the autonomic nervous system (e.g., elevated levels of the adrenal hormones epinephrine and norepinephrine) that suggest exaggerated cardiovascular responses to stressors (Lambiase et al., 2014). In addition, depression may result in behaviors—such as excessive sleep, reduced exercise, consumption of unhealthy food, or increased use of alcohol or cigarettes—that increase susceptibility to illness.

Can Humor Influence the Course of a Physical Illness?

Can humor influence the course of a physical illness? Author Norman Cousins wrote a book that described how laughter improved his life after he was diagnosed with a degenerative condition involving chronic inflammation. He claimed that 10 minutes of laughter would provide 2 hours of pain relief (Cousins, 1979). The Association for Applied and Therapeutic Humor, a nonprofit organization dedicated to the study and application of humor, maintains a searchable database that includes academic research articles focused on the applied use of humor and laughter to achieve a variety of outcomes, including managing or preventing physical illness. Over 700 organizations provide "clown therapy" in hospitals across the world to reduce anxiety and promote healing (Catapan et al., 2019; Fusetti et al., 2022).

How might humor influence the disease process? Several routes are possible:

1. Humor may directly affect immune functioning.

2. Humor may serve as a psychological buffer to stress, thus reducing the impact of stressors on physical health.

3. Humor may increase social connections and enhance social support from friends and family, thus exerting an indirect positive influence on health.

Over the years, research has demonstrated that laughing or watching humorous videos can reduce stress as well as improve immune system and heart function. In fact, daily or frequent laughter in adults age 65 and older was associated with a lower prevalence of cardiovascular disease compared to elders who never or almost never laughed (Hayashi et al., 2016). Further, a longitudinal study involving Japanese adults (age 40 and older) revealed that those who laughed frequently had a lower risk of cardiovascular disease and all-cause mortality compared to individuals who seldom laughed (Sakurada et al., 2020). Perhaps what Norman Cousins said is true: "Each patient carries his own doctor inside him."

For Further Consideration

1. Do you believe humor can reduce a person's stress levels and improve health outcomes? How would you go about testing this proposition?

Hostility is associated with several psychophysiological disorders, particularly CVD (Jennings et al., 2017). The association between hostility and CVD may exist because negative emotions such as hostility can increase cardiovascular reactivity, subsequently increasing the risk of developing CVD. Further, anger produces pathophysiological reactions such as coronary vascular constriction and the formation of plaques (Aghaei et al., 2015). One group of healthy young men who responded to unfair treatment with anger or frustration displayed elevated cholesterol levels, a factor associated with increased risk of developing CVD (Richards et al., 2000). Among African American and European American adolescents, those who scored high on anger or hostility measures had increased abdominal fat and greater arterial stiffness (hardening of the arteries); these associations were particularly strong for the African American participants (Midei & Matthews, 2009).

Social Dimension

Social stressors can influence immunological functioning and produce undesired health outcomes. The acute and chronic stress associated with the physical or emotional abuse that occurs in intimate partner relationship violence can result in a wide range of health conditions (Sugg, 2015). For example, adversities such as physical, emotional, or sexual abuse in pregnant women increase the likelihood of headaches and hypertension (Gelaye et al., 2016; Kidd et al., 2011). We also know that asthma symptoms increase in response to social stress (Landeo-Gutierrez, Marsland, Acosta-Pérez, et al., 2020). Another case in point is the generational effect of interpersonal maltreatment on the development of asthma. In one study, the sons of Hispanic American and African American women who were exposed to violence during pregnancy had twice the risk of experiencing wheezing at age 2 and asthma at age 6 (Landeo-Gutierrez, Forno, Miller, et al., 2020).

Did You Know?

For both men and women, a romantic relationship with a happy partner is independently related to happiness in oneself and leads to a healthier life. This may be due to stronger immune functioning, less vulnerability to stress, or an increased likelihood of adopting a healthy lifestyle.
Source: Chopik & O'Brien, 2017

A lack of social support can lead to immune system dysregulation with less natural killer cell activity and elevated inflammation. In contrast, having social support (i.e., feelings of being loved, valued, and cared for) is associated with positive health (Leschak & Eisenberger, 2019). In fact, good relationships may moderate the link between hostility and poor health. In one study, hostile individuals in high-quality relationships displayed reduced physiological reactivity to stress compared to those with similar personality characteristics who lacked positive social relationships (Guyll et al., 2010).

Given the importance of social relationships for most women, social isolation is more likely to negatively affect the health of women. In a longitudinal study of men and women, high loneliness in women (discrepancy between actual and desired social relationships) was associated with a nearly 80 percent increase in CVD; this association was not found in men (Thurston & Kubzansky, 2009). Social support may exert an indirect influence on health. For instance, individuals with supportive family relationships or with a large social network may receive encouragement for healthy eating habits, exercise, and other health-promoting activities, thus increasing resistance to disease.

Sociocultural Dimension

Sociocultural factors associated with gender, race, or ethnicity can have a major impact on health. For example, women have an increased likelihood of exposure to stressors associated with their role as caregivers for children, partners, and parents (Versey, 2017). Additionally, women are more likely to live in poverty and experience the sociocultural stressors and chronic disparities associated with having limited economic resources. Women are not only more likely to experience high levels of stress, but they are also more likely to report physical or emotional reactions to stress, not getting enough sleep, and using food as a way of dealing with stress. Further, women who are married are more likely to experience headaches or emotions such as fatigue, irritability, anger, or feeling as if they are on the verge of tears (American Psychological Association, 2020a).

A variety of stressful experiences associated with race and ethnicity affect the health of people who are socially oppressed. Although genetic and other biological factors may perhaps partially explain the high rate of hypertension in African Americans, another line of research supports a sociocultural explanation: Exposure to discrimination has been found to heighten stress responses and elevate blood pressure and heart rate among African Americans—conditions that increase risk for chronic hypertension and CVD (Hill et al., 2017). Additionally, African Americans have a much higher risk of sudden cardiac death compared to European Americans; this risk is particularly pronounced for African American women. The incidence of sudden cardiac arrest for African Americans was up to 80 percent greater in low socioeconomic neighborhoods compared to the neighborhoods with the highest income levels. This may be due to the stressors of living in poverty and having limited access to medical care (Zhao et al., 2019).

African Americans who come from severely disadvantaged backgrounds, but who excel in school, succeed at work, and achieve

Maintaining Tradition and Reducing Risk

Japanese Americans who maintain traditional lifestyles have a lower rate of coronary heart disease than those who have acculturated to mainstream U.S. culture.

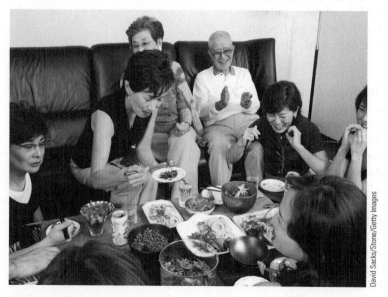

David Sacks/Stone/Getty Images

upward mobility have been found to be at increased risk for adverse health consequences. Despite "skin-deep resilience" and outward accomplishments, individuals in this situation have greater cellular aging and increased likelihood of experiencing diabetes, asthma, respiratory infection, and weakened immunological functioning. Researchers believe that this paradox may be due to the physiological stress that occurs because their upward mobility exposes them to a nondiverse (i.e., White) sociocultural environment with an increased likelihood of social isolation and experiences of racism and discrimination (Brody et al., 2020). Supporting this hypothesis, young Latinx and African American adults exhibited increases in cortisol levels on days they were exposed to discriminatory microaggressions—findings that link the impact of subtle racism to increases in HPA axis activity (Zeiders et al., 2018). Social support may be an important means of counteracting the physiological toll of racism. Among one group of African American women exposed to racist behavior, those with limited social support experienced the greatest increases in blood pressure, whereas those who frequently reached out for social support did not display this tendency (Clark, 2006).

Treatment of Psychophysiological Disorders

Treatment for psychophysiological disorders usually involves medical treatment for the physical symptoms and psychotherapy to eliminate stress and anxiety. Successful psychological approaches for stress management include relaxation training, biofeedback, or cognitive-behavioral therapy (Perlini et al., 2020). A nontraditional approach, acupuncture, is a promising treatment for chronic tension headaches (Zheng et al., 2022).

Relaxation Training

Relaxation training is a therapeutic technique in which a person acquires the ability to relax the muscles of the body under almost any circumstance. Imagine that you are a client who is beginning relaxation training. You are instructed to concentrate on one set of muscles at a time—first tensing and then relaxing them. You might tightly clench your fists for approximately 10 seconds, then release the tension. As your tightened muscles relax, you are asked to focus on the sensation of warmth and looseness in your hands. You practice this tightening and relaxing cycle several times before proceeding to the next muscle group, perhaps in your lower arms. After you have practiced tensing and relaxing various muscle groups, you might be asked to tighten and then relax your entire body.

The emphasis throughout the procedure is on the contrast between the feelings produced during tensing and those produced during relaxing. For a novice, the entire exercise lasts about 30 minutes. Progressive muscle relaxation has been effective in reducing physiological arousal and mitigating the physiological impact of stressors (Meyer et al., 2018). Individuals who learn stress reduction techniques such as this experience decreases in stress hormones and autonomic reactivity, and report less pain, less anxiety, improved sleep, and a higher quality of life (Blume et al., 2012).

Biofeedback Training

Biofeedback is a self-regulation technique that allows people to alter physiological processes in order to improve physical or mental health (Blase et al., 2021). If you were undergoing **biofeedback training**, your therapist would teach you to voluntarily control a physiological function, such as heart rate or blood pressure. During training, you would receive

Controlling Physiological Responses

Meditation is associated with a deeply relaxed bodily state produced by minimizing distractions and focusing internally or on a positive image, mantra, or word. Meditation can help regulate emotions and decrease stress hormones.

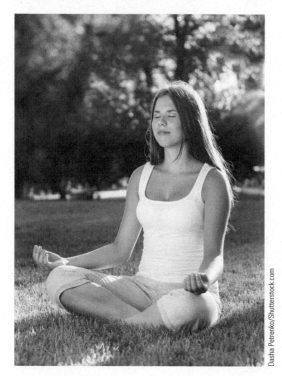

Dasha Petrenko/Shutterstock.com

second-by-second information (feedback) regarding a specific physiological activity. If you were trying to lower blood pressure, for example, you would receive feedback on your blood pressure, presented visually on a screen or via auditory signals. After repeated training sessions, you would be able to maintain your blood pressure in the desired range. The goal of biofeedback training is to continue the improvement in physiological responses outside of the training setting.

Biofeedback works because the visual and auditory feedback reinforces relaxation responses. It has been used to help people lower their heart rates and decrease their blood pressure during stressful situations (Peira et al., 2014), treat migraine and tension headaches (Kondo et al., 2019), and reduce stress-induced airway constriction (Taghizadeh et al., 2019).

Cognitive-Behavioral Therapy

Cognitive strategies designed to enhance coping skills and stress management can improve physiological functioning and psychological distress in individuals with chronic illness. For instance, cognitive-behavioral therapy has proven effective in controlling asthma symptoms, reducing anxiety levels, and enhancing the quality of life for those living with illness (McGovern et al., 2019). Mindfulness strategies have proven effective in improving emotional regulation and reducing symptoms of stress. Mindfulness-based stress reduction programs, designed to help foster nonjudgmental awareness of sensations and feelings, have been successful in producing significant decreases in stress, anxiety, depression, and physiological markers associated with stress (Green & Kinchen, 2021). Strategies taught in these programs include sitting and walking meditation (being aware of one's experiences while sitting or mindfully walking), mindful movement (awareness during yoga-like movement and poses), and body scan techniques (attention to sensations in different parts of the body). Mindfulness training has also significantly reduced physiological signs of distress in college students (Voss et al., 2020).

Another cognitive-behavioral approach, acceptance and commitment therapy, focuses on helping clients accept life difficulties and commit to behaviors that are consistent with their personal values. This intervention has also helped improve the well-being of individuals experiencing stress associated with serious health conditions (Kuba & Weißflog, 2017).

6-3 Contemporary Trends and Future Directions

Many questions remain about the biological underpinnings of trauma-related disorders and psychophysiological illness. For example, can psychotherapy or preventive interventions alter someone's biological predisposition to fear reactivity? Is it possible to reverse the epigenetic changes or the alterations in brain functioning or other physiological processes that result from trauma or stress? Neurophysiological, epigenetic, and psychological studies are currently underway to provide answers to these questions.

There are also continuing questions regarding the influence of psychological factors on individual responses to stress or trauma. As we have discussed, negative emotions amplify the consequences of trauma or stressful events, whereas cognitive characteristics such as perceived control, optimism, and self-efficacy appear to moderate the impact of stressors. Research continues to address how positive emotions affect stress responses and influence the risk of infection or disease. Do positive psychological states directly influence the biochemical processes occurring throughout the brain and body, or do positive emotions promote resilience more indirectly? Future research will provide more clarification about the role that psychological factors play in the etiology of serious diseases, as well as the prevention of psychophysiological conditions.

Given the role that social and sociocultural factors play in producing stress and physiological reactions to stress, researchers are continuing to explore how gender, race, and ethnicity intersect to influence the development and expression of trauma- and stressor-related symptoms. Are gender and racial/ethnic differences primarily the result of biological, social, or culture-related factors? Psychological, sociological, and medical research is continuing to explore the ways in which systemwide stressors and societal inequalities such as poverty, inadequate education, limited access to health care, racism, and discrimination are linked to the disorders discussed in this chapter. There is little doubt that these kinds of systemic stressors constitute a major public health problem, especially for marginalized groups. Unfortunately, most of our treatment and intervention strategies deal with problems at the individual level rather than addressing the root causes that occur at the social and sociocultural level.

The COVID-19 pandemic placed a spotlight on racial and ethnic disparities in our health care systems and on the higher prevalence of serious health conditions within communities of color. It is all too clear that we need to address these issues at the societal level. The elimination of racial and socioeconomic inequities can be accomplished by developing "communities of opportunity" that include high-quality child care and early childhood education programs, policies aimed at reducing poverty by providing work and income support, and ensuring safe and secure neighborhood conditions. Public health practitioners also emphasize the need for people of color to be invited to actively participate in health care reform and be offered the opportunity to share ideas for expanding preventive health care and ensuring access to high-quality health care (Hilliard-Boone et al., 2022). Advocates also stress the need to provide more educational opportunities for members of oppressed communities so they can become part of an increasingly diversified medical workforce. Elimination of stereotyping, implicit bias, microaggressions, and direct discrimination within the health care system is also an essential component of health care reform. Actions such as these would certainly be a step forward in eliminating health disparities and improving the health of marginalized populations (Williams & Cooper, 2019).

Chapter Summary

1 What do we know about disorders caused by exposure to specific stressors or traumatic experiences?

- Prolonged grief disorder involves clinically significant grief symptoms such as intense yearning, persistent thoughts about the deceased person, and disbelief over their death that last for at least 1 year in adults or 6 months in children and adolescents.

- Adjustment disorder involves clinically significant emotional distress and impairment in daily functioning that begins within 3 months after exposure to a stressor. An adjustment disorder persists no longer than 6 months after the end of the stressor or consequences from the stressor.

- Acute and posttraumatic stress disorders involve direct or indirect exposure to a life-threatening or violent event, resulting in intrusive memories of the occurrence, attempts to forget or repress the memories, emotional withdrawal, and increased arousal.

- In acute stress disorder, symptoms last up to 1 month; posttraumatic stress disorder (PTSD) is diagnosed when symptoms continue for more than 1 month after the traumatic event.

- Many factors are associated with the risk of developing a trauma-related disorder. Possible biological factors involve stress hormones and a sensitized autonomic nervous system. Psychological factors include anxiety, depression, and maladaptive cognitions. Maltreatment during childhood and inadequate social support are risk factors, as are various sociocultural factors, such as experiences with discrimination or racism.

- Certain medications are somewhat effective in treating trauma and stressor-related disorders. Prolonged exposure therapy, cognitive-behavioral therapies, and eye movement desensitization and reprocessing (EMDR) are often effective with these disorders.

2 What role does stress play in our physical health?

- External events that place a physical or psychological demand on a person can serve as stressors and affect physical health.

- A psychophysiological disorder is any physical disorder that has a strong psychological component. Psychophysiological disorders can involve actual tissue damage, a disease process, or physiological dysfunction.

- Not everyone develops an illness when exposed to the same stressor or traumatic event. Individuals may react to the same stressor in very different ways.

- Biological explanations for stress-related physical conditions include chronic activation of the sympathetic nervous system and continual release of stress hormones, as well as genetic influences.

- Psychological contributors include characteristics such as cynicism, pessimism, and hostility, as well as feelings of depression or anxiety.

- Social contributors include having an inadequate social network, abusive intimate partner interactions, and childhood maltreatment.

- Sociocultural factors such as gender, racial, and ethnic background increase the risk of some psychophysiological disorders. Stressful environments associated with poverty, discrimination, and racism increase risk of psychophysiological illness.

- Psychophysiological disorders are treated with interventions aimed at reducing stress and physiological reactivity combined with medical treatment for associated physical symptoms.

Chapter Glossary

acute stress disorder (ASD)
a condition characterized by flashbacks, hypervigilance, and avoidance symptoms that last up to 1 month after exposure to a traumatic stressor

adjustment disorder
a condition involving reactions to life stressors that are disproportionate to the severity or intensity of the event or situation

asthma
a chronic inflammatory disease of the airways in the lungs

atherosclerosis
a condition involving the progressive thickening and hardening of the walls of arteries due to an accumulation of fats and cholesterol along their inner lining

aura
a visual or physical sensation (e.g., tingling of an extremity or flashes of light) that precedes a migraine headache

biofeedback training
a physiological and behavioral approach in which an individual receives information regarding particular autonomic functions and is rewarded for influencing those functions in a desired direction

blood pressure
the measurement of the force of blood against the walls of the arteries

cluster headache
excruciating stabbing or burning sensations located in the eye or cheek

coronary vascular disease (CVD)
a disease process involving the narrowing of cardiac arteries, resulting in the restriction or partial blockage of the flow of blood and oxygen to the heart

cortisol
a hormone released by the adrenal glands in response to stress

diastolic pressure
the arterial force exerted when the heart is relaxed and the ventricles of the heart are filling with blood

dissociation
a psychological coping mechanism characterized by a sense of disconnection from traumatic circumstances

elevated blood pressure
a condition believed to be a precursor to hypertension, stroke, and heart disease, characterized by systolic blood pressure of 120 to 129 mm Hg and diastolic pressure less than 80 mm Hg

epinephrine
a hormone released by the adrenal glands in response to physical or mental stress; also known as *adrenaline*

eye movement desensitization and reprocessing
a therapy for PTSD involving visualization of the traumatic experience combined with rapid, rhythmic eye movements

fear extinction
the elimination of conditioned fear responses associated with a trauma

hypertension
a chronic condition characterized by a systolic blood pressure of 130 mm Hg or higher or a diastolic pressure of 80 mm Hg or higher

hypervigilance
a state of ongoing anxiety in which the person is constantly tense and alert for threats

migraine headache
moderate to severe head pain resulting from abnormal brain activity affecting the cranial blood vessels and nerves

normal blood pressure
the normal amount of force exerted by blood against the artery walls; systolic pressure is less than 120 mm Hg and diastolic pressure is less than 80 mm Hg

posttraumatic stress disorder (PTSD)
a condition characterized by flashbacks, hypervigilance, avoidance, and other symptoms that last for more than 1 month and that occur as a result of exposure to extreme trauma

prolonged exposure therapy
an approach incorporating sustained imaginary and real-life exposure to trauma-related cues

prolonged grief disorder
clinically significant grief symptoms over the loss of a loved one that last more than a year for adults and more than 6 months for children and adolescents

psychophysiological disorder
any physical disorder that has a strong psychological basis or component

relaxation training
a therapeutic technique in which a person acquires the ability to relax the muscles of the body in almost any circumstance

stress
the internal psychological or physiological response to a stressor

stressor
a difficult life circumstance or event that places a physical or psychological demand on a person

sympathetic nervous system
the part of the nervous system that automatically performs functions such as increasing heart rate, constricting blood vessels, and raising blood pressure

systolic pressure
the force on blood vessels when the heart contracts

tension headache
head pain produced by prolonged contraction of the scalp and neck muscles, resulting in constriction of the blood vessels and steady pain

trauma-focused cognitive-behavioral therapy
a therapeutic approach that helps clients identify and challenge dysfunctional cognitions about a traumatic event

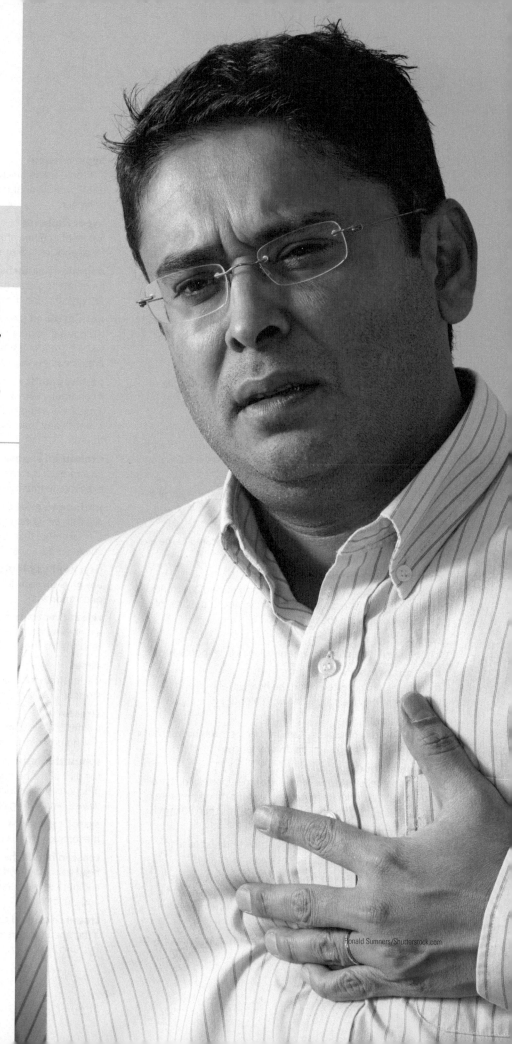

focus
Questions

1 What are the somatic symptom and related disorders, and what do they have in common? What causes these conditions, and how are they treated?

2 What are dissociations? Why do they occur, and how are they treated?

7

Somatic Symptom and Dissociative Disorders

Learning Objectives

After studying this chapter, you will be able to . . .

7-1 Compare the somatic symptom and related disorders and describe the causes and treatments of these conditions.

7-2 Compare and contrast the dissociative disorders and describe treatments for these disorders.

7-3 Describe possible explanations regarding why dissociation occurs and debate the controversies surrounding dissociative identity disorder.

A Boy Who Was 12 Years Old Was Referred for Evaluation because he suddenly began to walk in an unusual staggering manner. A comprehensive clinical examination showed no neurological abnormality. Shortly before his symptoms developed, he had been promoted to an academically rigorous secondary school. He was unable to meet the high scholastic expectations, and the teacher who taught his favorite subject humiliated him by rejecting classwork he had done and throwing his workbook on the floor (Leary, 2003, p. 436).

Joe Bieger, a Beloved Husband, Father, Grandfather, and High School Assistant Athletic Director, walked out of his front door one morning with his two dogs. Minutes later, his identity was seemingly wiped from his brain's hard drive. For the next 25 days, he wandered the streets of Dallas, unable to remember what his name was, what he did for a living, or where he lived. Finally, a contractor he worked with happened to recognize him and notified his family (Associated Press, 2007).

In this chapter, we discuss (a) somatic symptom disorder and related disorders, including conditions that involve highly distressing thoughts related to bodily symptoms, and (b) dissociative disorders, which involve alterations in memory, consciousness, or identity. These disorders, and the distress they cause, are associated with underlying biological, psychological, social, and cultural factors. We discuss somatic symptom and dissociative disorders together because research finds they have common etiological roots (Perez et al., 2018). Those with somatic symptom disorders often express stress through physical symptoms, while dissociative disorders involve psychological mechanisms for coping with overwhelming stress. We begin with a discussion of somatic symptom and related disorders.

7-1 Somatic Symptom and Related Disorders

Somatic symptom and related disorders are a disparate group of disorders that include *somatic symptom disorder*, *illness anxiety disorder*, *functional neurological symptom disorder*, and *factitious disorder*. The DSM-5-TR groups these disorders together because they all have prominent **somatic symptoms** (physical or bodily symptoms) that are associated with significant impairment or distress (refer to Table 7.1). Actual physical illnesses may or may not be present. However, these diagnoses emphasize the presence of "distressing somatic symptoms plus abnormal thoughts, feelings and behaviors in response to these symptoms" (American Psychiatric Association [APA], 2022, p. 349). Characteristics of the somatic symptom and related disorders are presented in Table 7.2. We begin with a discussion of somatic symptom disorder.

Somatic Symptom Disorder

Case Study A married man of South Asian descent complained of losing weight because of gastrointestinal symptoms such as bloating and retching. He reported that he had difficulty swallowing and retaining food. He appeared very frail, and was very concerned about his condition. Medical professionals conducted numerous examinations, including endoscopies; CT scans; and X-rays of his esophagus, stomach, and small bowel, but could find no organic cause for his symptoms (Lau et al., 2021).

Table 7.1 Comparison of DSM-5-TR Somatic Symptom and Related Disorders

Disorder	Identifiable Medical Condition?	Voluntarily Produced?	Cognitive Distortions Regarding Illness?
Psychophysiological disorders*	Yes	No	No
Somatic symptom disorder	Sometimes	No	Yes
Illness anxiety disorder	Sometimes	No	Yes
Functional neurological symptom disorder	No, but involves physical symptoms	No	No
Factitious disorder	Possibly, but self-induced	Yes	No

*Covered in Chapter 6

Table 7.2 Somatic Symptom and Related Disorders

	Disorders Chart		
Disorder	**DSM-5-TR Criteria**	**Prevalence**	**Course**
Somatic symptom disorder	At least one distressing somatic symptom and one of the following: a. Persistent thoughts about symptoms b. High anxiety c. Excessive time devoted to symptoms	• Ranges from 6.7% to 17.4% in population-based studies • Somewhat more prevalent in women	• Tends to be chronic and comorbid with depression and anxiety
Illness anxiety disorder	• Preoccupation with health and excessive worry about serious illness • No somatic symptoms or very mild symptoms • Excessive health anxiety • Repeated checking for signs of illness or avoiding medical contact for fear that illness will be confirmed	• Ranges from 1.3% to 10% • Similar prevalence in men and women	• Begins in adulthood • Tends to be chronic chronic
Functional neurological symptom disorder	• Motor or sensory disturbances • Symptoms incompatible with medical findings	• 5% to 15% in neurology clinics; up to 25% in hospital settings • More common in women and girls	• May be transient or chronic • Prognosis better for children
Factitious disorder, imposed on self or others	• Physical or mental symptoms fabricated or induced in oneself or others • Presents self or other as ill or injured • Absence of external rewards for illness	• About 1% in hospital settings • Diagnosed twice as often in women	• Varies from single episode to intermittent; persistent less common

Source: APA, 2022; Lowe et al., 2022

Individuals diagnosed with **somatic symptom disorder (SSD)** have a pattern of reporting and reacting to pain or other distressing physical or bodily symptoms. This pattern continues for at least 6 months and also involves persistent thoughts or high anxiety regarding the symptoms and associated health concerns. Thus, SSD involves not only excessive focus on somatic symptoms but also catastrophic thoughts related to these symptoms (Mewes, 2022). Refer to Table 7.3 for examples of somatic complaints reported by individuals with SSD.

People with SSD report a variety of physical complaints that involve discomfort in different parts of the body: gastrointestinal symptoms such as nausea, diarrhea, and bloating; sexual symptoms such as sexual indifference, irregular menses, or erectile dysfunction; and pseudoneurological symptoms such as difficulties speaking or breathing (Yates, 2014). Diagnostic tests that rule out disease or other physical conditions do little to reassure individuals with SSD or reduce their anxiety. They remain convinced they have a serious disease. In some cases, it may be true. Up to 9 percent of symptoms that are initially considered to be psychologically based are later discovered to be the first signs of a disease or medical condition (Yao et al., 2018).

Using estimates from questionnaires, the prevalence of SSD ranges from 6.7 percent to 17.4 percent in adolescent and adult samples (APA 2022). In general, higher prevalence rates are reported among women, African Americans, individuals with less than a high school education, and those with lower incomes (Kim et al., 2019; Noyes et al., 2006). The SSD diagnosis is most common in hospital settings, involving as many as 50 percent of the cases in which psychiatric consultations are requested (Yates, 2014). Medical patients with conditions such as cancer, cardiovascular disease, diabetes, and kidney disease sometimes display the high levels of

Table 7.3 Symptoms Reported by Patients with Somatic Symptom Disorder

Gastrointestinal Symptoms	Pseudoneurological Symptoms
Vomiting	Amnesia
Abdominal pain	Difficulty swallowing or talking
Nausea	Seizures
Bloating and excessive gas	Impaired mobility
Pain Symptoms	**Reproductive Organ Symptoms**
Diffuse pain	Burning sensation in sex organs
Pain in extremities	Pain during intercourse
Joint pain	Irregular menstrual cycles
Headaches	Excessive menstrual bleeding
Cardiopulmonary Symptoms	**Other Symptoms**
Shortness of breath at rest	Vague food allergies
Palpitations	Hypoglycemia
Chest pain	Chronic fatigue
Dizziness	Chemical sensitivity

Source: So, 2008

somatic anxiety, overutilization of health resources, functional impairment, and work disability associated with SSD (Norbye et al., 2022).

For many, SSD is a chronic condition. When SSD is diagnosed in adolescents, there is an increased likelihood that the adolescent will experience a serious mental illness later in life. In a 15-year longitudinal study, adolescents with somatic symptoms had an increased risk of developing depression and other mental disorders during adulthood. Those with the most severe somatic symptoms during adolescence were also most likely to attempt suicide later in life (Bohman et al., 2012); these findings reinforce the importance of early identification and intensive treatment for adolescents with SSD. In one study involving adolescent psychiatric patients hospitalized with a diagnosis of SSD, 49 percent showed complete remission. Another 32 percent showed improvement, and 19 percent showed no change. This compares with a remission rate of only 18 percent among adult outpatients (Löwe et al., 2022).

Many people undergo unnecessary surgical or assessment procedures and could potentially meet the diagnostic criteria for SSD due to the high levels of distress associated with their symptoms. Although medical professionals sometimes believe that those with SSD are faking their symptoms, mental health professionals do not agree. They do not believe that SSD involves feigning (faking) or exaggerating symptoms. Rather, they understand that for those with SSD, the symptoms are very real and extremely distressing.

Somatic Symptom Disorder with Predominant Pain

Case Study Ms. J. is a 37-year-old woman who came to the emergency department due to abdominal pain. She reported that she has lived with chronic pain since her adolescence. She has a history of multiple abdominal surgeries; the most recent was for pain due to scar tissue from her previous surgeries. These operations have failed to reduce her complaints of pain. Eventually, the medical professionals working with her began to focus on helping her identify sources of stress and practice healthy coping mechanisms (Yates, 2014).

When pain is the primary complaint expressed by someone with a SSD (as we saw with Ms. J.), the diagnosis becomes **somatic symptom disorder with predominant pain**. According to the DSM-5-TR, those with this pattern experience persistently high levels of distress over pain along with an excessive amount of time and energy devoted to the pain symptoms. Although pain complaints result in frequent medical appointments, diagnostic tests often cannot identify specific causes for the chronic pain. As you can imagine, those with SSD who are experiencing pain often feel angry and frustrated, particularly if they believe that medical staff are questioning their reports of pain (Henningsen, 2018).

Deciding if someone meets the diagnostic criteria for SSD with predominant pain can be problematic because chronic pain is relatively common, affecting about 20 percent of U.S. adults (National Center for Health Statistics, 2023). Pain symptoms are most prevalent among women, older adults, and those living in poverty or in rural areas (Dahlhamer et al., 2018). Although there is no overall difference in the prevalence of chronic pain between European Americans, African Americans, and Hispanic Americans, the latter two groups report greater pain severity (Meints et al., 2019). African Americans, in particular, disproportionately experience debilitating consequences from chronic pain. These differences may arise from differential exposure to psychosocial factors such as adverse childhood experiences, racial discrimination, and socioeconomic stressors, all of which have been associated with chronic pain (Aroke et al., 2019).

Illness Anxiety Disorder

Case Study   When she was a teenager, her cousin died suddenly in his 30s, presumably because of an undiagnosed heart problem. She began to have nearly constant fear that she had undiagnosed cardiac disease … [with] frequent sensations of heart palpitations and light headedness. … As she grew older, concerns expanded to include fear that she had appendicitis (based on mild gastrointestinal sensations) and diabetes (based on feeling tired and sore after exercise). Multiple worrisome bodily sensations led to extensive researching of conditions on the internet and repeatedly calling her parents for reassurance (Scarella et al., 2019, p. 398).

This woman's distress is associated with an **illness anxiety disorder**. This condition occurs in individuals who have minimal or no somatic symptoms but who report a chronic pattern (at least 6 months) of preoccupation with having or contracting a serious illness. The prevalence of illness anxiety disorder depends upon the specific definition used and how it is measured. Estimates range from 2.1 percent to 13.1 percent of the population (Kosic et al., 2020). This condition is found equally in men and women (APA, 2022).

People with illness anxiety disorder are very apprehensive and easily alarmed about their health. They show three characteristics: (1) disease conviction—their belief in having a serious illness cannot be dissuaded by negative lab results; (2) disease fear—great concern about the possibility of developing an illness; and (3) body preoccupation—obsessive attention to bodily signs or changes as warning signs of an illness (Scarella et al., 2019). This anxiety may result in excessive health-related behaviors such as continual checking of one's body for signs of illness, or avoidance behaviors (e.g., refusing to go to the doctor) due to extreme fear of possible illness.

A Physical or Psychological Disorder?

Somatic symptom disorder with pain is most frequently diagnosed in women, in members of underrepresented groups, and in people living in poverty. How can we determine if the cause of the pain is psychological, physical, or both?

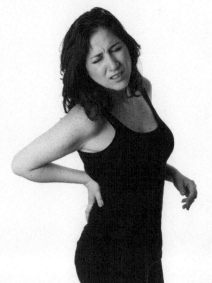

Paul Hakmata Photography/Shutterstock.com

Table 7.4 Percentage of Adults with Illness Anxiety Disorder Who Endorse Selected Fears Related to Health

Item	Much Agree or Very Much Agree (%)
When I notice my heart beating rapidly, I worry I might have a heart attack.	51
When I get aches or pains, I worry that there is something wrong with my health.	75
It scares me when I feel "shaky" (trembling).	47
It scares me when I feel tingling or prickling sensations in my hands.	50
When I feel a strong pain in my stomach, I worry it might be cancer.	62

Source: Walker & Furer, 2008

Some people with illness anxiety disorder have an actual medical condition or a high risk of developing a medical condition (perhaps due to a strong family history of a disease); in these cases, illness anxiety disorder is diagnosed when there is impairment due to excessive or disproportionate worry about this situation (APA, 2022). Illness anxiety disorder is much more likely to be present in those with existing physical conditions than those without (Bobevski et al., 2016). Refer to Table 7.4 for examples of the fears related to health found in individuals with illness anxiety disorder.

Illness anxiety disorder is strongly associated with a person's cognitions; that is, the individual misinterprets bodily variations or sensations as indications of a serious illness or undetected disease and becomes distressed. If unpleasant or "unusual" symptoms are detected, the bodily focus produces feelings of extreme distress and alarm (Scarella et al., 2019). For example, because of concerns over COVID-19 during the pandemic, some individuals with illness anxiety disorder experienced heightened alarm if they experienced a cough or muscle aches, fearing they had been infected with the virus (Asmundson & Taylor, 2020).

Individuals with illness anxiety disorder frequently check for signs of illness or disease, seek reassurance from others, continuously research and gather information on diseases on the Internet, and avoid activities or circumstances they believe might result in an illness. The term *cyberchondria* was coined to describe the maladaptive use of technology to continually check for information regarding physical disorders (Mathes et al., 2018). Paradoxically, these behaviors only serve to increase health anxiety.

Functional Neurological Symptom Disorder (FNSD)

Case Study A previously healthy 11-year-old girl came to the hospital after experiencing two weeks of debilitating "dizziness." She became unsteady when she stood up or sat up, but felt better when lying flat. The results of lab tests and physical examinations were within normal limits. During her 4-day hospital stay, the physiotherapy service provided daily strengthening exercises and she gradually recovered all functioning. It is believed that the interventions succeeded because they "validated her symptoms" (Caulley et al., 2018).

A boy, age 10, was first believed to have a case of juvenile myasthenia gravis (a physical disorder involving weakening of the voluntary muscles). For 5 weeks, he had been unable to open his eyes and could not attend school because of his "blindness." On examination, nothing was found that could explain his inability to see. On the hospital ward, it was noted that he did not walk into furniture and appeared to be able to follow football games on TV when alone. Just before his difficulties began, the boy, a sport's star within his village's youth league, had been blamed for his team's defeat during an important match (Leary, 2003).

Functional neurological symptom disorder (FNSD) involves motor, sensory, or seizure-like symptoms that are inconsistent with any recognized neurological or medical disorder and that result in significant distress or impairment in life activities. As these two cases demonstrate, symptoms such as muscle weakness or paralysis, unusual movements, swallowing difficulties, speech problems, dizziness, seizures, or loss of sensation may be involved (APA, 2022). Other suggestive clinical features include sudden onset, symptoms that disappear with distraction, and variability in symptom severity. The most common functional neurological symptoms found in neurological clinics involve **psychogenic** movement disorders, such as disturbances of stance and walking; sensory symptoms, such as blindness, loss of voice, or dizziness; abnormal movements; difficulty swallowing; tremors; and psychogenic seizures (Pourkalbassi et al., 2019). Although an FNSD diagnosis is relatively rare, up to one quarter of patients in general hospital settings may be experiencing functional neurological symptoms. It is estimated that from 5 percent to 15 percent of patients in neurological clinics have FNSD. These disorders are more prevalent in women (APA, 2022; Butz et al., 2019).

Diagnosis is confirmed when the symptoms an individual is displaying are incompatible with neurological findings. For instance, one woman had seizure-like attacks that were preceded by seeing white spots, followed by twitching of her upper and lower extremities involving one or sometimes both sides of her body and lasting for about 20 minutes. Electroencephalograph (EEG) monitoring during the episodes revealed no abnormalities that would suggest any form of epilepsy (Baslet & Hill, 2011). In some cases, the presenting symptoms—such as glove anesthesia (Figure 7.1), which involves a loss of feeling in the hand ending in a straight line at the wrist, or an inability to talk or whisper combined with the ability to cough—are easily diagnosed as symptoms of FNSD. The diagnosis is not complicated because coughing indicates intact vocal cord function, and in glove anesthesia, the area of sensory loss does not correspond to the distribution of nerves in the body.

In general, individuals with FNSD disorder are not physically damaged by the symptoms. For example, a person with psychogenic paralysis of the legs rarely shows the atrophy of the lower limbs that occurs when there is paralysis due to an underlying biological cause. In some persistent cases, however, long-term disuse of muscles can result in atrophy (Schonfeldt-Lecuona et al., 2003).

Discriminating between FNSD and actual medical conditions can be difficult, because there are no specific tests to confirm the diagnosis. For this reason, neurologists and other physicians are reluctant to conclude there is an FNSD unless they are absolutely certain that the condition is psychologically based. In many cases, medical providers order extensive neurological and physical examinations to rule out a true medical disorder before diagnosing an FNSD (Espay et al., 2018).

Individuals with FNSD are not consciously faking symptoms. In other words, they are not **malingering** (feigning illness for an external purpose

Figure 7.1

Glove Anesthesia

In glove anesthesia, the lack of feeling covers the hand in a glovelike shape. It does not correspond to the distribution of nerve pathways. This discrepancy leads to a diagnosis of functional neurological symptom disorder.

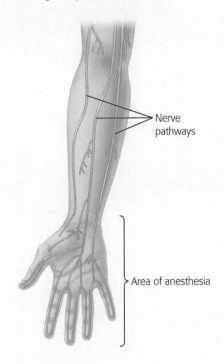

Nerve pathways

Area of anesthesia

such as getting out of work duties). People with this disorder believe that the problem is genuine and not under their control, and they are distressed by their symptoms. Most individuals with the disorder report that their symptoms developed soon after experiencing a distressing life event. The following cases of FNSD demonstrate how functional neurological symptoms are related to trauma or stressors (Becker et al., 2013; Gillig, 2013):

- Development of seizures by a college honors student after he failed an introductory biology exam
- Motor weakness and frequent falling in a man whose wife abruptly left him for someone else
- Bilateral vision loss after a 25-year-old man discovered that his childhood friend had accidentally died due to autoerotic asphyxiation

What is the prognosis for individuals with FNSD? In a review of long-term outcomes studies, about 39 percent of individuals with this disorder reported that their symptoms remained the same or became worse. A sudden onset of symptoms, early diagnosis, shorter duration of symptoms, and good premorbid (before the illness) functioning increase the likelihood of a positive outcome (Gelauff et al., 2014). The prognosis may be better for children and adolescents. In a sample of 204 youth between the ages of 7 and 15 with FNSD, a 12-month follow-up showed that all had improvement in their symptoms (Ani et al., 2013).

Factitious Disorder and Factitious Disorder Imposed on Another

Factitious disorders are mental disorders in which a person deliberately induces or simulates symptoms of physical or mental illnesses with no apparent incentive other than attention from medical personnel or others. The DSM-5-TR includes **factitious disorder imposed on self**, which involves inducing or simulating illness in oneself, and **factitious disorder imposed on another**, which involves inducing or falsifying illness in someone else.

Before we discuss the factitious disorders, we should note that these disorders are completely different from malingering—where the specific goal is usually evident, and the individual can "turn off" the symptoms whenever they are no longer useful. In factitious disorders, the purpose of the simulated or induced illness is much less apparent. Complex psychological variables are involved, and those with a factitious disorder are usually unaware of the motivation for their behavior. Simulation of illness is often done almost compulsively.

Factitious Disorder Imposed on Self

Case Study   Mandy was not hesitant to discuss how she was diagnosed with leukemia at age 37, right after her husband left her. She shared how chemotherapy damaged her immune system, liver, and heart, resulting in a stroke and weeks in a coma. She posted her story and updates online, and the virtual community rallied to support her as she shared details of additional surgeries and bouts of life-threatening infections. It was later discovered that Mandy was not sick and had made up the entire story (Kleeman, 2011).

Factitious disorder imposed on self is characterized by the presentation of oneself to others as ill or impaired through the recurrent falsification or induction of physical or psychological symptoms. This is done without any obvious external rewards. However, the symptoms do provide attention, support, and social relationships that the individual may not have otherwise obtained (Jafferany et al., 2018).

In the past, this condition was referred to as *hospital addiction* or *professional patient syndrome*. In 1951, it was given the name Munchausen syndrome after an 18th-century German nobleman who was noted for making up fanciful stories (Tatu et al., 2018). Although most of the cases involve physical symptoms, psychoactive drugs are sometimes used to simulate mental disorders or, instead of using substances, an individual might falsely report having delusions, hallucinations, or confusion in thinking (Sousa Filho et al., 2017).

In some situations, as in the case of Mandy, the individual obtains attention and social support as a result of completely fabricated stories of "illness." In other situations, people engage in behaviors that produce actual physical problems. One young woman, for example, requested medical attention for pain and infection in her limbs. It was discovered that she was inserting thin wires into different parts of her body to produce injury and infection (Sinha-Deb et al., 2013). In another case, a 27-year-old woman went to the emergency department complaining of abdominal pain and bleeding from her rectum. Comprehensive tests, including computed tomography (CT) scans, upper gastrointestinal endoscopy, colonoscopy, and biopsies, came out negative. Later, a nurse found the patient in a bathroom inserting a toothbrush into her rectum, producing the bleeding she had been complaining of (IsHak et al., 2010).

Signs of factitious disorder may include multiple lingering, unexplained illnesses that require numerous surgeries or complex treatments; "remarkable willingness" to undergo painful or dangerous treatments; a tendency to become angry if the illness is questioned; and the involvement of multiple doctors (Yates & Feldman, 2016). People with this condition appear to have a pathological need for attention and care (Dickerman & Jiménez, 2023).

Because of underdiagnosis and misdiagnosis, the prevalence of factitious disorder imposed on self is not known, although it is estimated to be less than 1 percent of the population (Schrader et al., 2019). The availability of virtual support groups and the opportunity for online attention may be increasing the prevalence of factitious disorders (Lancaster, 2021). In a large study of 455 cases of factitious disorder, 66.2 percent of the patients were women with a mean age of 34.2. Comorbid mental disorders were common; 42 percent had a current or past diagnosis of depression, 16.5 percent had a personality disorder, and 15 percent had a substance use or an anxiety disorder. Nearly 60 percent of the group self-induced their symptoms, while 40 percent either simulated or falsely reported symptoms. About 57 percent had worked or were working in the health care system or in a medical laboratory (Yates & Feldman, 2016). Factitious disorder is most often diagnosed in women, but the more chronic forms of the disorder tend to be found in middle-aged men (Elwyn et al., 2019).

Factitious Disorder Imposed on Another

Case Study   During the first 7 years of his life, Christopher's mother took him to the hospital or to see a medical professional 323 times for various physical ailments. He underwent 13 major surgeries, and was fitted with a feeding tube that was directly attached to his small intestine due to his mother's complaint that Christopher was unable to hold down any food. His mother also reported that he had severe seizures, placed him on a lung transplant waiting list, and enrolled him in hospice. When concerned medical professionals finally contacted Child Protective Services, Christopher was removed from his mother's care and placed in a hospital, where he ate regularly without a problem and did not experience any seizures, even when all medications were removed (Boyd, 2017).

If an individual deliberately feigns or induces physical or psychological symptoms in another person (or even a pet) in the absence of any obvious external rewards, the diagnosis is *factitious disorder imposed on another* (DSM-5-TR); this condition is sometimes referred to as *Munchausen syndrome by proxy*. In fact, parents sometimes produce symptoms in their own children with no apparent motive other than the attention they receive due to the child's "illness," as demonstrated in the case of Christopher and as presented in these examples (Truesdell, 2020):

- A hidden camera at a children's hospital captured the image of a mother injecting fecal material into the IV line of her 5-month-old son while the infant was undergoing treatment for repeated bouts of bacterial infection.

- A mother documented her 5-year-old son's battle with a "mysterious" illness on social media as she was feeding him the large quantities of salt that led to his death.

Little information is available on prevalence, age of onset, or familial patterns with this diagnostic category. In the vast majority of cases, the individual is a mother (often married) who appears to be loving and attentive toward her infant or young child while simultaneously sabotaging the child's health. It is not unusual for those with this behavior to be employed in health care or a related profession (Yates & Bass, 2017). Medical providers begin to suspect this disorder when a parent insists on unnecessary medical tests and invasive physical procedures or when the symptoms occur only when the parent is around. A mortality rate of up to 12 percent of the targeted children has been reported—either from the abuse itself or from unnecessary, invasive medical procedures. Of the data available on perpetrators, after the abuse was discovered, 37 percent were separated from the child, 14 percent were imprisoned, 10 percent received therapy, 4 percent continued living with their victim, and 1 percent committed suicide. When the child stayed with the offender, the probability of recurrence of the behavior was quite high (Abdurrachid & Gama Marques, 2022).

Diagnosis of this condition is difficult, and some believe that the diagnosis is so unclear, unreliable, and subject to misdiagnosis that it should be eliminated as a psychiatric diagnosis. They cite cases of possible false accusations of child endangerment made against parents purported to have this disorder (Siemaszko, 2019). Others argue, however, that investigation is essential whenever there is a possibility that the health of a child may be in danger due to deliberate acts on the part of a parent or caregiver.

Factitious Disorder Imposed on Another

Lacey Spears was found guilty of murdering her 5-year-old son, Garrett, who died from salt poisoning. For years prior to his death, Spears had gained attention and sympathy by posting about Garrett's frequent episodes of illness on social media and on a personal blog.

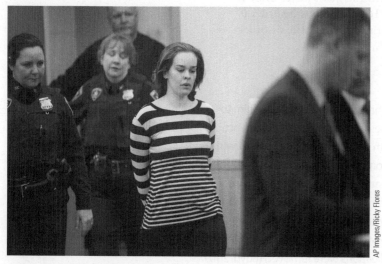

AP Images/Ricky Flores

Etiology of Somatic Symptom and Related Disorders

A variety of biological, psychological, social, and sociocultural factors may contribute to the development of somatic symptom, illness anxiety, functional neurological symptom, and factitious disorders (see Figure 7.2).

Biological Dimension

Genetic factors only modestly contribute to the development of SSD and related disorders, according to twin and family studies However, genetic factors may influence the

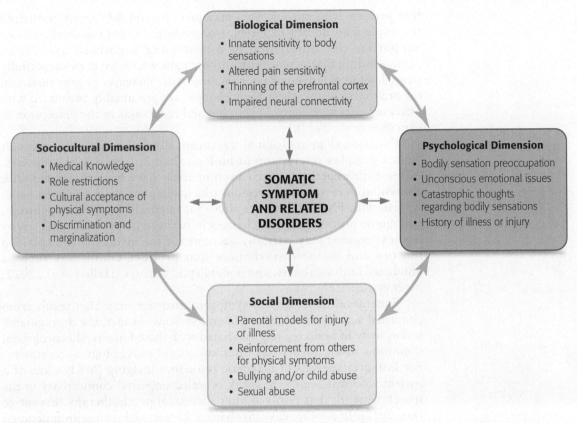

Figure 7.2

Multipath Model of Somatic Symptom and Related Disorders

The dimensions interact with one another and combine in different ways to result in a somatic symptom or related disorder.

development of somatic symptoms and health anxiety by means of biological vulnerabilities, such as heightened sensitivity to pain and somatic cues, particularly among individuals who have experienced childhood adversities (Henningsen, 2018).

Psychological, social, and sociocultural influences can produce alterations in brain function and structure that affect pain sensitivity. For example, a study comparing woman with chronic pelvic pain with matched control subjects found that the pain patients were three times more likely to have experienced childhood adversities such as abuse or exposure to domestic violence (Krantz et al., 2019). It is possible that repetitive activation of the sympathetic nervous system due to chronic exposure to stressors increases sensitivity of the nerves associated with pain and subsequently heightens pain sensation (Löffler et al., 2022). The finding that war veterans with combat exposure are more likely to report high levels of somatic symptoms compared to veterans without exposure to trauma also supports this hypothesis (Ginzburg & Solomon, 2010).

People who have experienced episodes of verifiable pain sometimes develop chronic, unexplained pain due to a process of *central sensitization* in which the pain modulating systems in the central nervous system become hyperexcitable and, therefore, hypersensitive to pain (den Boer et al., 2019). Consistent with this perspective, researchers have found differences in cortical thickness in areas of the sensorimotor cortex and temporal lobe when comparing individuals with chronic pain and people without a history of frequent pain. The thinning cortex in these regions suggests that patients with chronic pain may process pain differently compared to people who do not experience ongoing pain (Magon et al., 2018). Supporting this differential pain processing hypothesis are studies demonstrating that people with chronic pain who have been successfully treated with cognitive-behavior therapy show increases in gray matter in the prefrontal cortex; these brain changes are presumably associated with increased cognitive control over pain and reductions in the perception of pain (Bao et al., 2022).

Functional neurological symptom disorder appears to result from a complex interaction of biological and psychosocial processes. Adverse life experiences such as child abuse have been associated with alterations in certain brain regions (the insular and cingulate cortices) in women with FNSD. These are sites that integrate emotions, cognition, and motor processes. Thus, changes in brain structure and connectivity in these regions may partially account for the medically unexplained sensory and motor disturbances that produce conditions such as blindness, limb weakness, and nonepileptic seizures (Hallett et al., 2022; Perez et al., 2017).

Functional neurological symptom disorder may also result from abnormal actions of inhibitory neural systems. In fact, the dysregulated connectivity in brain regions associated with these functional neurological symptoms often normalizes after successful psychological treatment. For instance, analysis of magnetic resonance imaging (MRI) scans of a patient who was unable to speak revealed impaired connectivity in the speech network that resolved after successful psychotherapy (Bryant & Das, 2012). In another case involving a 25-year-old man with functional visual blindness, his initial MRI showed overreactivity in the frontoparietal regions of the brain along with suppressed responses in interconnected visual areas (indicating that visual cues were being suppressed); however, these abnormalities disappeared when his condition improved (Becker et al., 2013).

Psychological Dimension

Psychological theoretical explanations for somatic symptom and related disorders have focused on psychodynamic and cognitive-behavioral perspectives. Certain psychological characteristics have also been associated with these disorders.

Psychodynamic Perspective In psychodynamic theory, somatic symptoms serve the purpose of keeping unconscious emotional issues at a distance. Freud believed that "hysterical reactions" (biological complaints of pain, illness, or loss of physical function) were caused by the repression of some type of conflict, usually sexual in nature. To protect the individual from intense anxiety, this conflict is converted into a physical symptom (Breuer & Freud, 1895/1957). The psychodynamic view suggests that two mechanisms produce and then sustain somatic symptoms. The first involves a *primary gain* because the physical symptoms provide psychological protection from the anxiety associated with unacceptable desires or conflicts. This focus on the body keeps the person from becoming aware of the underlying conflict. Then a *secondary gain* accrues when the person's dependency needs are fulfilled through the attention and sympathy received in response to the physical symptoms.

Cognitive-Behavioral Perspective Reinforcement, modeling, maladaptive cognitions, or a combination of these influences are important in the development of SSD, according to cognitive-behavioral researchers.

Did You Know?

A 58-year-old African American woman reported that she had been experiencing morning sickness, abdominal cramps, abdominal distension, and backache while her daughter was pregnant. She then experienced labor pain when her daughter was in delivery. The woman was diagnosed with pseudocyesis, a rare somatic symptom disorder also known as sympathetic pregnancy.

Source: Thippaiah et al., 2018

Some contend that people with SSD, FNSD, and factitious disorder assume the "sick role" because it is reinforcing and allows them to escape unpleasant circumstances or to avoid responsibilities. Not surprisingly, many individuals with SSD and related disorders have experiences associated with convalescence, including serious illness, physical injury, and depression (Burton et al., 2010); in fact, these situations are all associated with an increased risk of developing SSD.

Catastrophic misinterpretations of bodily sensations or changes in bodily functions appear to be important in the etiology of SSD and illness anxiety disorder. Health anxiety arises because symptoms are interpreted as life-threatening conditions that could result in disability or death. Individuals' preoccupation with disease and inordinately high anxiety levels are fueled by intrusive imagery such as "visualizing the doctor telling me that I have cancer" or "I'm lying on my death bed with my children and partner crying" (Muse et al., 2010).

According to this perspective, catastrophic cognitions related to somatic symptoms are more likely to develop in individuals who are biologically or psychologically predisposed to having these thoughts—people who have somatic sensitivity, a low pain threshold, a history of illness, or who have received parental attention for somatic symptoms (Mewes, 2022). It is hypothesized that distressing cognitions develop in the following manner (Walker & Furer, 2008):

1. External triggers (traumatic or anxiety-evoking stressors) or internal triggers (anxiety-producing thoughts such as "My father died of cancer at age 47") result in physiological arousal.

2. The individual notices bodily changes associated with these triggers (e.g., increased heart or respiration rate).

3. Thoughts and worries about possible disease begin in response to these physical sensations.

4. These thoughts amplify bodily sensations, causing further physical reactions and concern.

5. Catastrophic thoughts increase in response to the magnified bodily sensations, creating a circular feedback pattern.

Consistent with this perspective, individuals with SSD tend to misinterpret and overestimate the dangerousness of bodily symptoms (Shi et al., 2022). One group of individuals with SSD involving chest pain in the absence of cardiac pathology were highly attuned to cardiac-related symptoms and exhibited anxiety reactions in response to heart palpitations and chest discomfort (White et al., 2010). Similarly, individuals with health anxiety interpreted nine common bodily sensations as indications of disease, whereas healthy controls were more likely to use normalizing explanations and view the symptoms as insignificant (Neng & Weck, 2014).

Social Dimension

A variety of social factors appear to influence somatic symptom and related disorders. Workplace bullying has been found to produce not only emotional distress and trauma but also musculoskeletal pain and cardiovascular complaints, especially among those with a genetic variant in the serotonin transporter gene (Jacobsen et al., 2018). Some individuals with SSD report being rejected or abused by family members and feeling unloved (Tunks et al., 2008). A history of childhood or sexual abuse has been associated with chronic pelvic pain in women (Krantz et al., 2019). Similarly, childhood trauma is reported by over 70 percent of patients with FNSD (Van der Feltz-Cornelis et al., 2020). More than 50 percent of a sample of individuals with somatic symptom, illness anxiety, or FNSD had experienced a serious physical illness in the preceding 12 months (Smith et al., 2000).

Degree of social support is also important. Individuals with high levels of health anxiety often report having few or no close friends that they can talk with or get support from (Norbye et al., 2022). Contact with medical staff may serve as a source of attention or comfort among those with limited social support. Social isolation and increased social media use during the COVID-19 pandemic appear to have contributed to an increase in the prevalence of cyberchondria—a type of illness anxiety involving an incessant search for health-related information about vulnerability to medical conditions, such as COVID-19 (Yalcin et al., 2022).

Individuals with SSD frequently have parents or family members with chronic physical illnesses (Schulte & Petermann, 2011). One group of mothers with high illness anxiety expressed significant health-related concerns for their child, displayed highly protective behaviors when their child was not feeling well, and reported they were less satisfied with pediatrician visits. This type of overprotection may reinforce illness complaints and increase a child's attention to bodily symptoms. Modeling also occurs when the child observes the mother expressing anxiety over her own health (Thorgaard et al., 2017).

Sociocultural Dimension

There is a long history of sociocultural explanations for some somatic disorders. FNSD, initially called *hysteria*, was originally viewed as a problem that afflicted only women; in fact, it derived its name from *hystera*, the ancient Greek word for uterus. Hippocrates believed that a shift or movement of the uterus resulted in complaints of breathing difficulties, paralysis, and seizures. He presumed that the movement was due to the uterus "wanting a child." However, others have argued that hysteria was more prevalent in women because restrictive social mores did not provide them with appropriate channels for emotional or sexual expression (Satow, 1979).

Around 1880, Anna O., a 21-year-old woman, developed a variety of symptoms, including muscle rigidity and insensitivity to touch. Her physician, Josef Breuer, later coauthored a book with Sigmund Freud, in which they proposed that hysterical symptoms such as those experienced by Anna O. result from intrapsychic conflicts. They made no mention of the possible impact of social role restrictions on psychogenic symptoms. According to Hollender (1980), Anna O. was highly intelligent, but her educational and intellectual opportunities were severely restricted because she was a woman.

As Hollender pointed out, "Not only was Anna O., as a female, relegated to an inferior position in her family with future prospects limited to that of becoming a wife and mother, but at the age of twenty-one she was suddenly called on to assume the onerous chore of nursing her father" (Hollender, 1980, p. 798). It is possible that many of her physical symptoms resulted from her resentment of this duty. The symptoms also allowed her to maintain the intellectually stimulating contact with Breuer. Later in her life, Anna O. made significant contributions to the field of social work and became recognized as a feminist leader.

Cultural factors can influence the frequency, expression, and interpretation of somatic complaints. Among Asian populations, physical complaints often occur in reaction to stress (Sue et al., 2022). Cultural differences such as this may account for the finding that nearly 34 percent of outpatients in a community hospital in China met the diagnostic

Severely Disturbed?

Anna O., whose real name was Bertha Pappenheim, was diagnosed as being severely disturbed, even though her later years were extremely productive. Were the paralysis and other physical disturbances she experienced products of societal restrictions on the role of women in the late 1800s? Or was it something totally different?

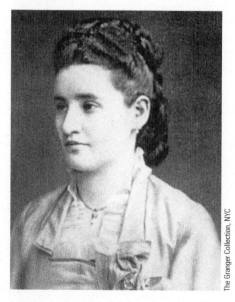

The Granger Collection, NYC

Culture and Somatic Symptom and Dissociative Disorders

- A 56-year-old Brazilian man requested an evaluation and treatment due to an ongoing somatic complaint. He had the firm belief that his penis was retracting and entering his abdomen, and he was reacting with a great deal of anxiety. He attempted to pull on his penis to prevent the retraction, a strategy he felt had been effective with a previous episode that occurred when he was 19 (Hallak et al., 2000).

- Dibuk ak Suut, a Malaysian woman, goes into a trancelike state in which she startles easily, blithely follows commands, blurts out offensive phrases, and mimics the actions of people around her. She displays profuse sweating and increased heart rate, but claims to have no memory of what she says or does. The episodes occur if she is suddenly frightened (Osbourne, 2001).

The symptoms of the first case fit the description of *koro*, a cultural syndrome that is found primarily in Southeast Asia, although cases have also been reported in West Africa and South America (Strong et al., 2023). Symptoms of koro involve an intense fear that the penis—or, in a woman, the labia, nipples, or breasts—is receding into the body. Episodes of koro are usually brief and responsive to positive reassurances. In the second case study, Dibuk is displaying symptoms related to *latah*, a condition found in Malaysia and many other parts of the world that involves dissociation or a trancelike state associated with a hyperstartle response, mimicking the behavior of others, and automatic obedience (Lanska, 2018). Other cultural syndromes related to either somatic symptom or dissociative disorders include the following:

- *Brain fag.* Found primarily in West Africa, this condition affects high school and college students who report somatic symptoms involving a fatigued brain, neck or head pain, or blurring of vision associated with difficult course work or classes.

- *Dhat syndrome.* This is a term used in India to describe severe anxiety over the discharge of semen. The condition produces feelings of weakness or exhaustion.

- *Ataque de nervios.* Commonly found in Latinx people residing in the United States and Latin America, the somatic and dissociative symptoms of this condition can include brain aches, stomach disturbances, anxiety symptoms, and trancelike states.

- *Piblokto.* Generally found in Inuit communities, this condition involves dissociative-type episodes accompanied by extreme excitement that are sometimes followed by convulsions and coma. The individual may perform aggressive and dangerous acts and report amnesia after the episode.

- *Zar.* This condition, found in Middle Eastern and North African societies, involves the experience of being possessed by a spirit. Individuals in a dissociative state may engage in bizarre behaviors, including shouting or hitting their head against a wall.

Cultural syndromes are interesting because they point to the existence of a pattern of symptoms that are associated primarily with specific societies or groups. These "disorders" do not fit easily into the DSM-5 classification system or into many of the biological and psychological models used to explain dissociative and somatic symptom disorders. What does it mean when unusual behavioral patterns are discovered that do not fit into Western-developed classification systems?

criteria for SSD (Cao et al., 2020). Some African cultural groups express somatic complaints, such as feelings of heat, crawling sensations, and numbness, that differ from those expressed in Western cultures (Brown & Lewis-Fernández, 2011). Latinx American college students are more likely to report pain symptoms, perhaps due to the cultural acceptance of physical problems as an expression of distress. Pain-related anxiety is associated with greater bodily vigilance, worry, and anxious arousal (Zvolensky et al., 2020). Other factors associated with SSD and related disorders include lower educational levels and immigrant status (Noyes et al., 2006).

Discrimination and marginalization because of social conditions is an important etiological factor in chronic pain. Marginalized populations that are subject to discrimination, trauma, and poor living conditions (such as members of racially underrepresented or sexual and gender minority groups, recent immigrants, and refugees) have higher rates of chronic pain (Craig et al., 2020). Discrimination has been found to directly impact the physical health of African Americans, resulting in increases in psychological and physiological stress responses that are associated with somatic symptoms such as pain (Seaton & Zeiders, 2020).

There are also different cultural views of the relationship between mind and body. The dominant view in Western culture is the *psychosomatic* perspective—that psychological conflicts are sometimes expressed via physical symptoms. But many other cultures have a *somatopsychic* perspective—that physical problems produce psychological and emotional symptoms. Although many of us believe that our psychosomatic view is the correct one, the somatopsychic view is the dominant perspective in numerous cultures.

Treatment of Somatic Symptom and Related Disorders

Case Study Mr. X., a 68-year-old Chinese man, reported sleep disturbance, loss of appetite, dizziness, and a sensation of tightness around his chest. Several episodes of chest pain led to admission and medical evaluation at the local hospital. All results, including tests for heart disease, were normal. He was referred for psychiatric consultation. Because traditional Chinese views of medicine recognize an interconnection between mind and body, the psychiatrist accepted and showed interest in the somatic concerns, such as their onset, duration, and factors that relieved or increased the symptoms. Arguments between Mr. X. and his wife appeared to be a significant stressor. The psychiatrist shared strategies for improving communication with Mrs. X., which led to a decrease in physical complaints (Yeung & Deguang, 2002).

Although somatic symptom and related disorders are considered difficult to treat, newer psychological approaches are showing some success. Treatment for SSD and related disorders is enhanced when the clinician understands the problem from the client's perspective. Therapists now realize that it is necessary to focus on mind–body connections, understand clients' perspectives regarding their somatic symptoms, and acknowledge the role of stressors in the development of physical complaints, as occurred in the case study of Mr. X. Individuals with somatic symptom, illness anxiety, and functional neurological symptom disorders are often frustrated, disappointed, and angry following years of encounters with the medical profession. They believe that treatment strategies have been ineffective and resent the implication that they are "fakers" or "problem patients." Medical personnel do, in fact, show negative reactions when interacting with individuals with these disorders (Howman et al., 2016). Because of these attitudes, it may be difficult for patients to establish a positive therapeutic relationship with medical personnel.

A compassionate approach to treating SSD and illness anxiety disorder involves demonstrating empathy regarding the physical complaints, accepting them as genuine, and providing information about stress-related symptoms. For instance, medical professionals can enhance their working relationship with a patient and reduce anxiety by eliciting the patient's views regarding the symptoms prior to providing psychoeducation regarding the relationship between stress, somatic symptoms, and emotional states. They might reassure the patient that certain physiological symptoms are quite common and that due to the absence of any concerning medical findings, they are confident that the symptoms will subside (Marshall et al., 2013).

In another approach, SSD is viewed within a social context—somatic complaints are regarded as reflecting unsatisfying social relationships. Individuals who assume a "sick role" may control others through bodily complaints or receive reinforcement for their condition by receiving attention or escaping responsibility. Therapy is directed toward developing and improving the individual's social network and adaptive coping skills. A therapist may say something such as: "There is treatment available that may be helpful to you, if you would like to participate. This involves learning new ways of understanding and coping with stresses, other than going to the nearest emergency room. Treatment will also involve learning more about yourself and finding out what gets in the way of developing more fulfilling relationships" (Gregory & Jindal, 2006, p. 34).

Cognitive-behavioral approaches focused on correcting misinterpretations and cognitive distortions, such as a conviction that they are especially vulnerable to disease, have benefited clients with health anxiety. In one program, individuals with illness anxiety disorder who feared having cancer, heart disease, or other fatal illnesses were educated about the relationship between misinterpretations of bodily sensations and selective attention to the topic of illness. Researchers taught the participants to monitor and challenge anxiety-producing, illness-related thoughts. After completing the program, most participants showed considerable improvement, and the gains were maintained at a 6-month follow-up (Hiller et al., 2002).

Similar cognitive-behavioral programs that add exposure and habituation also produce marked reductions in somatic symptoms and illness concerns in individuals with SSD (Saer & Witthöft, 2022). Because individuals with SSD often show a fear of internal bodily sensations, cognitive-behavioral therapists include *interoceptive exposure* (exposure to bodily sensations) during treatment. Therapists ask clients to perform activities that typically trigger physical sensations associated with anxiety (e.g., light-headedness, chest discomfort, or increased heart rate) by visiting hospitals, performing physical activities, and deliberately imagining anxiety-arousing situations. These activities are repeated until the client's bodily sensations no longer produce anxiety or fear (Axelsson et al., 2020).

Mindfulness-based cognitive therapy is another approach that can improve the functioning of people coping with chronic pain. Therapists teach their clients to experience and observe their problematic thoughts and symptoms without judgment or emotion. Instead of reacting with fear or anxiety, the individual merely observes and reflects on what they are experiencing, including their thoughts and physical symptoms. This process weakens the connection between emotional arousal, physical experiences, and distressing thoughts; thus, the individual is more able to cope with pain (Holmes et al., 2019).

Therapists who use acceptance and commitment therapy combine the teaching of mindfulness practices with a focus on helping the client embrace the possibility of leading a meaningful life, even when experiencing pain. The therapist also helps the client understand that it may not be necessary to reduce pain before focusing on important goals, performing meaningful tasks, and strengthening social networks. As the client increases engagement in valued activities, the perception of pain often diminishes (Vowles et al., 2019). Another promising approach involves the use of an immersive virtual reality experience to provide a distraction from chronic pain. Combining this technique with the use of deep breathing and relaxation techniques has proven to be an effective treatment (Castaneda, 2019).

7-2 Dissociative Disorders

Case Study A 29-year-old woman visiting China for an academic trip was found unconscious in the hotel bathroom. She was unable to remember her identity or any information about her life. Examinations showed no neurological abnormalities or evidence of substance use. She remained in an amnesiac state for 10 months, until blood on her fingers triggered memories of witnessing a murder in China and, because of her fear, being unable to help the person who had been attacked. Once this memory surfaced, she began to remember other aspects of her life (Reinhold & Markowitsch, 2009).

The **dissociative disorders**—dissociative amnesia (localized, generalized, and fugue), depersonalization/derealization disorder, and dissociative identity disorder—are summarized in Table 7.5. These disorders involve some sort of dissociation, or separation, of a part of the person's consciousness, memory, or identity. Although some dissociative disorders have been highly publicized and sensationalized, they are considered rare.

Table 7.5 Dissociative Disorders

Disorders Chart				
Disorder	**DSM-5-TR Criteria**	**Prevalence**	**Age of Onset**	**Course**
Dissociative amnesia	• Sudden inability to recall information of specific events or of one's identity or life history—results from stress or a traumatic event	• 1.8% in a community sample with 1% for men and 2.6% for women • 3.6% in college students	• Any age group	• Acute forms may remit spontaneously, although may become chronic
Dissociative amnesia, with dissociative fugue	• Sudden amnesia that may include wandering to a new area with inability to recall one's past and confusion about personal identity	• 0.2%; may increase during natural disasters or wartime	• Usually adulthood	• Related to stress or trauma; recovery is generally rapid
Depersonalization/ derealization disorder	• Persistent changes in perception and detachment from one's own thoughts and body • May feel things are unreal or a sense of being in a dreamlike state • Intact reality testing	• About 2%; up to 20% in outpatient clinics; 50% of adults may experience brief episodes of stress-related depersonalization	• Adolescence or childhood; less than 20% after 20 years of age; onset after age 40 is rare	• May be short-term or chronic
Dissociative identity disorder	• Identity disrupted by two or more distinct personality states or by the experience of possession (self-reported or observed) • Altered behavior, mood, sense of self, memories, emotions, cognitions, and perceptions • Frequent gaps in memory of everyday events or inability to recall important personal information	• Sharp rise in reported cases since the 1980s • Up to 9 times more frequent in women in clinic settings • 1.5% in a community sample, with slightly higher prevalence in men	• Any age group	• Fluctuating; tends to be chronic and recurrent • Impairment can be minimal or profound

Source: APA, 2022; Gill et al., 2023; Johnson et al., 2006; Yang et al., 2023

In contrast, **dissociation** (disconnection from one's emotions, thoughts, or surroundings) is a fairly common coping strategy, especially among survivors of trauma. In fact, a variety of stressors such as kidnapping, rape, sexual abuse, combat, or other life-threatening events are associated with dissociation (Granieri et al., 2018).

Dissociative Amnesia

According to the DSM-5-TR, **dissociative amnesia** occurs when a traumatic event or stressful circumstances result in a sudden partial or total loss of important personal information or memory of a specific event. An affected individual may be unable to recall information such as their name, address, or names of relatives, yet remember the necessities of daily life—how to read, write, and drive. You can probably imagine how distressing it would be to discover lapses in your memory. Fortunately, unlike amnesia associated with strokes, substance abuse, or other medical conditions, dissociative amnesia results from psychological factors or stressors, so the memory is potentially retrievable. In one study, comparing patients with neurologically based memory impairment and those with dissociative amnesia, loss of personal identity was found only in the patients with dissociative amnesia. Those with dissociative amnesia also reported significantly higher rates of prior head injury (an unexpected finding), depression, PTSD symptoms, and family and financial problems when compared to patients with neurological impairment (Harrison et al., 2017).

Dissociative amnesia may be more common in college students compared to the general population. In a meta-analysis involving college students, 3.6 percent of the students were experiencing dissociative amnesia at the time they were interviewed, a figure higher than previous studies of the disorder in the general population (Kate et al., 2020). In a community sample in New York, the 12-month prevalence was 1.8 percent, with over twice as many women experiencing symptoms of the disorder (Johnson et al., 2006).

Localized Amnesia

Case Study An 18-year-old woman who survived a dramatic fire claimed not to remember the event nor the death of her child and husband in the fire. She claimed her relatives were lying about the fire. She became extremely agitated and emotional several hours later, when her memory abruptly returned.

The most common form of dissociative amnesia, **localized amnesia**, involves an inability to recall events that happened in a specific period, often centered on some highly painful or disturbing event. As this case of the young woman demonstrates, localized amnesia often begins and ends very abruptly, particularly when it is in response to an overwhelming traumatic event (Harrison et al., 2017). People vary in the degree and type of memory that is lost in localized amnesia. Some individuals display **systematized amnesia**, which involves the loss of memory for certain categories of information. Individuals may be unable to recall memories of their families or of a particular person. In one case, shortly after the sudden death of her only daughter, an elderly woman appeared to have no recall of having had a daughter, but other memories were unaffected.

Some people display **selective amnesia**, an inability to remember certain details of an incident. For example, a parent remembered having an automobile accident but could not recall that their child had died in the crash. Selective amnesia is claimed by approximately 20 percent to

Hypnosis as Therapy

Some practitioners continue to use hypnosis to assess and treat dissociative disorders, based on the belief that these disorders may be inadvertently induced by self-hypnosis.

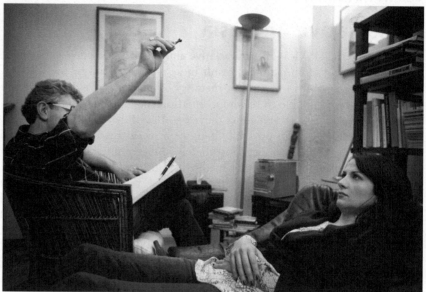

Amelie-Benoist/BSIP SA/Alamy Stock Photo

30 percent of people accused of violent criminal offenses; many murderers report that they remember arguments but do not remember killing anyone. In a limited number of cases, this may be true, since extreme emotion can prevent the encoding of a traumatic memory (Jelicic, 2018). However, because the diagnosis of dissociative amnesia depends primarily on self-report, faking to escape responsibility for criminal behavior is all too common. For this reason, criminal investigators have developed a variety of procedures to assist in the detection of feigned amnesia (Zago et al., 2019).

In some cases of localized amnesia, the amnesia comes to light only after the individual begins to recall the previously lost details of a traumatic event—repressed memories. Cases of **repressed memory** are believed to result from exposure to trauma that is so overwhelming or threatening that the individual represses the event, often for a sustained period of time, as in the following case study.

Case Study   A 21-year-old woman with severe fibromyalgia was being treated with hyperbaric oxygen therapy. While in the chamber, she suddenly experienced shortness of breath, overwhelming fear, and a loss of control. This was followed by flashbacks of fragmented memories of being raped by several classmates at the age of 14, an event that she had not previously remembered (Efrati et al., 2018).

Not all researchers believe in the validity of repressed memory or the hypothesis that certain threatening memories can be pushed out of consciousness. Otgaar et al. (2019) point out the complexities involved in interpreting reports of repressed memories:

- Suggestive techniques such as hypnosis and guided imagery have been used to "retrieve" false memories.

- Many abuse survivors with recovered memories claim that they had forgotten their traumatic abuse, but studies show that traumatic events are typically remembered in heightened detail.
- Memory is malleable; details can change over time, and false memories can be planted, intentionally or unintentionally.
- Just because a memory report is detailed and confidently expressed with significant emotion does not mean that it reflects a true experience; false memories can have these same features.

Some experts further argue that family members or therapists can unintentionally plant or strengthen implausible memories. At this point, it is not clear how many cases of genuine repressed memory exist, or whether the phenomenon exists at all. Belief in repressed memory is still high among undergraduates and many clinicians. Those least likely to believe that the phenomenon is real are experimental psychologists and memory experts (Patihis et al., 2014).

Dissociative Amnesia with Fugue

> **Case Study** A 26-year-old male was . . . found by police . . . wandering around a central London park. He reported that he did not know where he was, why he was there, or what he was doing. The police found an address in his bag and took him home, where he did not recognize his family . . . he had become depressed before the onset of his fugue: he described anxiety about finances, falling behind in rental payments, and caring for a sick mother (Harrison et al., 2017).

Dissociative Amnesia with Fugue

Jeff Ingram was on his way to visit a terminally ill friend in Alberta and woke up 4 days later in Denver without any memory of his life. He was without his car or any personal identification. Ingram now wears a necklace flash drive and a bracelet that contains his personal information.

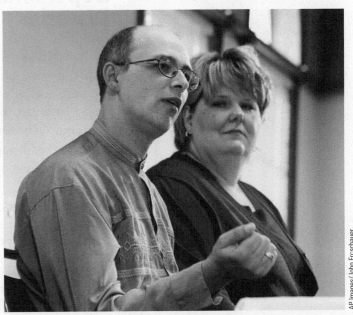

AP Images/John Froschauer

Another form of dissociative amnesia is **dissociative amnesia with fugue**, which involves bewildered wandering or purposeless travel accompanied by amnesia for one's identity and life history. The incidence of this disorder in the general population is rare and estimated to be 0.2 percent (Gill et al., 2023). The case study of the young man in London is an example of the extensive loss of personal identity that occurs during a dissociative fugue state. Similar to others who experience a fugue state, the man ended up in a new location, with no recall of his identity. As with localized amnesia, recovery from a fugue state is often abrupt and complete, although the gradual return of bits of information may also occur (Harrison et al., 2017). In some circumstances, however, a fugue state may last for an extended period and may recur, as found in the following case.

> **Case Study** Mr. A., a 74-year-old man, was brought to the hospital emergency room after awakening on a park bench not knowing who or where he was. He reported having no memory of how he got to the park, nor did he know his name or where he was from. Mr. A. was treated with an antianxiety medication and recovered his memory. His family was contacted, and his sister reported that Mr. A. had disappeared on two other occasions when under stress (Ballew et al., 2003, p. 347).

Some individuals who, like Mr. A., have experienced several fugue episodes, wear personal identification in the event of a future occurrence. Because of the complete loss of memory associated with dissociative fugue states, law enforcement agencies or hospitals often become involved. However, some individuals act completely normal during a fugue episode and slowly begin to take on a new identity, until bits of information about the past begin to return or someone recognizes them.

Depersonalization/Derealization Disorder

Case Study   A 35-year-old woman began to experience dissociative symptoms in high school and described feeling like her surroundings were "unreal" or "off." These symptoms worsened after the death of a family member. She reported feeling as though she was "inside her head . . . was watching herself . . . unable to distinguish dreams from real life." She told her therapist, "Looking at you right now, I feel like I'm in a movie" and then added, "I can live like this, but I don't enjoy it" (Weber, 2020).

Depersonalization/derealization disorder (DDD) is the most common dissociative disorder. It is present in up to 2 percent of the general population, in 5 percent to 20 percent of clients engaging in therapy on an outpatient basis and in 17.5 percent to 42 percent of psychiatric inpatients (Yang et al., 2023). It typically begins during later childhood and adolescence; DDD rarely has an onset after the age of 40 (APA, 2022).

According to DSM-5-TR, DDD is characterized by recurrent or persistent symptoms of *depersonalization* (feelings of unreality, detachment, or being an outside observer of one's own thoughts, feelings, or behaviors) and/or *derealization* (sense of unreality or dreamlike detachment from one's environment) that cause significant impairment or distress. During depersonalization/derealization episodes, the person remains in contact with reality. Episodes of depersonalization can be chronic and can produce great anxiety, as was true for the woman in the case study.

A diagnosis of DDD occurs only when the feelings of unreality and detachment, disembodiment, and emotional numbing cause major impairment in social or occupational functioning. This disorder is often accompanied by mood and anxiety disorders (Choi et al., 2017). Depersonalization episodes are sometimes brief, or they may last for decades—depending on individual circumstances. Transient depersonalization symptoms are common. For instance, fleeting experiences of depersonalization are reported by up to 70 percent of college students and 23 percent of the general population (Sierra, 2012). In one population-based study of health in Germany, 8.7 percent of the 13,182 participants were bothered by symptoms of depersonalization. Those who expressed depersonalization concerns had an increased risk of anxiety and depressive symptoms when assessed during the 2.5-year follow-up (Schlax et al., 2020).

The prevalence of this disorder has been questioned because the assessments used, such as the Dissociation Experiences Scale (DES), can conflate nonpathological experiences with symptoms of DDD. For example, the DES asks about experiences such as "driving a car and not realizing what happened during part of the trip," "feeling that things around you are unreal," "listening to a conversation and not hearing parts of it," and "sometimes feeling as though you were two different people."

In studies of the general population, 83 percent endorsed "missing part of a conversation" and 50 percent endorsed "feeling as though I was two different people," suggesting that this assessment instrument may indeed be pathologizing normal experiences (Canan & North, 2019).

Dissociative Identity Disorder

> **Case Study** "Little Judy" is a young child who laughs and giggles. "Gravelly Voice" is a man who speaks with a raspy voice. "The one who walks in darkness" is blind and trips over furniture. "Big Judy" is articulate, competent, and funny. These are 4 of the 44 personalities that existed within Judy Castelli. She was initially diagnosed with schizophrenia, but was later told that dissociative identity disorder was the appropriate diagnosis. She is a singer, a musician, an inventor, and an artist who has also become a lay expert on mental health issues (Castelli, 2009).

Dissociative identity disorder (DID), formerly known as *multiple-personality disorder*, is a disruption of identity as evidenced by two or more distinct personality states. According to the DSM-5-TR, those with DID have a disturbed sense of self and show alterations in behaviors, attitudes, and emotions when these alternate personality states occur. In most cases, the switches in states of consciousness and identity are subtle. Only a minority of cases involve distinct personality identities with different names, clothing, and speech, such as the changes experienced by Judy Castelli. Recurrent gaps in memory for personal information or for everyday or traumatic events are also evident. These symptoms (which may be self-reported or observed by others) cause significant distress and impairment in functioning. DID can also involve an experience of **possession**, in which the person's sense of personal identity is replaced by a supernatural presence. Possession was added to the DID definition in the DSM-5-TR to include cultural symptoms of dissociation (APA, 2022).

The estimated 12-month prevalence of DID in one community sample was about 1.5 percent, with the rate being slightly higher in men than women (Johnson et al., 2006). In a meta-analysis of studies involving diagnostic interviews with college students, the prevalence of DID was 3.7 percent (Kate et al., 2020). Many individuals with DID report depressive disorders, substance use disorders, nonsuicidal self-injury, and suicide attempts, as well as symptoms of functional neurological symptom disorder and posttraumatic stress disorder (Brand et al., 2019).

The process of dissociation and switching to an alternate personality state usually occurs during highly stressful situations and may be preceded by trancelike behavior, blinking, rolling of the eyes, or changes in posture (Gentile et al., 2013). Only one personality is evident at any moment. However, one or more personalities may be aware of the existence of the others. The personality states usually differ from one another and sometimes are direct opposites, as we saw in the case of Judy Castelli. In many cases, the role of the alternate personality (the alter) is to protect the emotional well-being of the main personality from stress or trauma.

Former NFL Star, Heisman Trophy Winner, and Senatorial Candidate Herschel Walker

Herschel Walker wrote about his ongoing struggle with dissociative identity disorder and his efforts to integrate his 12 alters in his recent book, *Breaking Free: My Struggle with Dissociative Identity Disorder*. He describes his alters as including "The Warrior," who appeared as he played football, and "The Hero," who had the role of making public appearances.

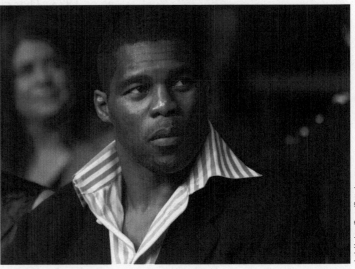

Josh Hedges/Forza/Getty Images

Figure 7.3

Comparison of Characteristics of Reported Cases of Dissociative Identity Disorder

This graph depicts characteristics of dissociative identity disorder (DID) cases reported in the 1980s versus those reported between 1800 and 1965. What could account for these differences?

Source: Based on Goff & Simms, 1993

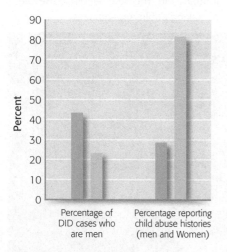

Between 1800 and 1965
1980s

Gaps in memories similar to symptoms of dissociative amnesia and fugue are present in individuals with DID. For instance, one 28-year-old woman mentioned receiving messages from people she did not know saying that they had a "great time" with her. Her phone contained phone numbers that she did not recognize, and she had a feeling she might have been sexually involved with a man but had no memory of it (Gentile et al., 2013). Many individuals with DID also report finding themselves at unusual locations without knowing how they got there.

Complex legal debate arises regarding acts performed when an individual with DID is purportedly in a dissociated state. The following examples offer a glimpse into this controversy:

- A therapist claimed that it was one of her client's 24 personalities who kidnapped and sexually assaulted her and that the main personality was not responsible (Haley, 2003).

- A man was convicted of sexual assault after a woman with DID claimed that two of her 21 personalities did not consent to the sexual activity—one was a 20-year-old woman who had just appeared and another was a 6-year-old child. The conviction was overturned because the defense psychiatrist had not been allowed to interview the woman before trial (Grimminck, 2015).

- A woman with DID claimed it was one of her alternate personalities who killed four of her relatives (Collins, 2013).

Cases such as these raise questions regarding dissociative disorders and responsibility. Does a diagnosis of DID constitute mitigating circumstances? Are people with DID responsible for the behaviors and actions of their alternate personalities?

Diagnostic Controversy Involving Dissociative Identity Disorder

DID is both complex and intriguing, especially because the characteristics associated with DID have changed over time. Goff and Simms (1993) compared professional and historical case reports from the years 1800 to 1965 with those from the 1980s. The earlier cases involved an average of 3 personality states (versus 12 in the more recent cases), a later age of onset of first dissociation (age 20, as opposed to age 11 in the 1980s), a greater proportion of men, and a much lower prevalence of child abuse (Figure 7.3).

There had been fewer than 200 reported cases of DID worldwide as of 1973. That changed when a book based on the life story of Sybil (a pseudonym) became a bestseller and the story was further popularized in a two-part television movie. The movie poignantly portrayed the story of how Sybil had coped with severe physical abuse perpetrated by her mother by developing 16 different personalities. Following this introduction of DID into popular culture in the 1970s, many new cases of DID were reported and continue to be reported each year. The DID diagnosis has become a source of controversy between clinicians and researchers in the field. Some clinicians contend that DID is relatively common, but that it is often not recognized and diagnosed (Brand et al., 2019). Others in the mental health field believe that DID is extremely rare and that the increase in numbers may be due to clinician bias, invalid assessment procedures, or the use of therapeutic techniques that increase the likelihood of a DID diagnosis (Ulatowska & Sawicka, 2017).

Temporary dissociation involving symptoms such as alterations in memory, thoughts, and perceptions or a sense of depersonalization (feeling detached or numb) is fairly common during periods of stress. Some clinicians may mistakenly interpret these symptoms as evidence of DID.

Additionally, the use of hypnosis or suggestion appears to increase the likelihood that a client is viewed as having a dissociative disorder involving multiple personality states. Whether the increase in diagnosis of DID is the result of more accurate diagnosis, false positives, hypnosis, or an actual increase in the incidence of the disorder is still being debated.

Etiology of Dissociative Disorders

The possible causes of dissociative disorders are subject to much conjecture. Because diagnosis depends heavily on self-report, faking is always a possibility. Fabricated amnesia, dissociative fugue, or DID can be produced by individuals who are attempting to avoid the social, legal, or financial consequences of their behaviors. However, true cases of these disorders may also result from these types of stressors. Differentiating between genuine cases of dissociative disorders and situations where the disorder is feigned can be difficult. In addition, the evidence for dissociative disorders tends to be weak and is based primarily on cases studies (Mangiulli et al., 2022).

In this section, we consider possible etiological explanations for the dissociative disorders (Figure 7.4). Although two models—the psychologically based *posttraumatic model* and the *sociocognitive model*—are the most influential etiological perspectives, neither is sufficient to explain why only some individuals develop these disorders. It is likely that biological, psychological, social, and sociocultural vulnerabilities all play a role.

Biological Dimension

Biological explanations for dissociative disorders have focused on disruptions in encoding of memories due to acute stress and the inability to retrieve autobiographical material due to the release of hormones such as glucocorticoid, which may impede the recall of traumatic events. Atypical functioning in brain structures associated with memory encoding and retrieval has been documented in various dissociative disorders. For example, diffusion tensor imaging of the brains of individuals with depersonalization/derealization disorder has revealed abnormalities in the structural connectivity between the frontolimbic brain regions, areas associated with the integration and regulation of emotions. This finding may help explain the emotional detachment that occurs with this disorder (Sierk et al., 2018).

Brain alterations also occur with dissociative amnesia. One woman with ongoing amnesia underwent an fMRI scan while being presented with photographs of friends, family, and strangers; although she said she did not recognize any of the photos, her brain wave patterns differed when she was presented with photos of the people she knew before the amnesia versus strangers. Thus, recognition did occur at a subconscious level. The scan also revealed decreased activation of the hippocampus, suggesting an alteration in this memory-sensitive part of the brain (Chechko et al., 2018). Further, positron emission tomography (PET) scans of people with dissociative amnesia show reduced metabolism in an area of the prefrontal cortex that is involved in the retrieval of autobiographical memories (Brand et al., 2009).

Neuroimaging of the brain structure of individuals with DID and healthy controls also reveals structural differences between the two groups. Researchers are hoping that these biomarkers will be useful in the early detection of DID, because

Myth Dissociative identity disorder is relatively easy to diagnose, and most mental health professionals accept the category.

Reality There are no objective measures for diagnosing DID. Those who question the category suggest that symptoms of the disorder are inadvertently produced through suggestion or techniques such as hypnosis.

Cross-Cultural Factors and Dissociation

Dissociative trance states are part of certain cultural or religious practices, as demonstrated by these Haitian women participating in a voodoo ceremony.

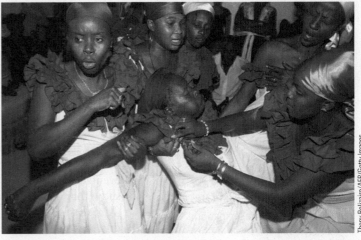

Thony Belizaire/AFP/Getty Images

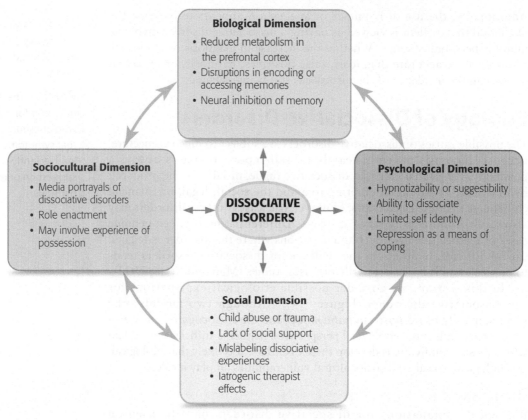

Figure 7.4

Multipath Model of Dissociative Disorders

The dimensions interact with one another and combine in different ways to result in a dissociative disorder.

individuals with DID often receive an average of four mistaken diagnoses before a diagnosis of DID occurs (Reinders et al., 2019). Overall, these neurological findings are difficult to interpret because it is unclear what causes them and what specific role they play, if any, in dissociative disorders.

Psychological Dimension

The primary psychological explanations for the dissociative disorders come from psychodynamic theory, although individual vulnerabilities such as hypnotizability or suggestibility are also thought to play an important role. According to psychodynamic theory, dissociative disorders are caused by an individual's use of repression to block unpleasant or traumatic events from consciousness; this provides emotional protection from painful memories or conflicts (Loewenstein, 2018). In dissociative amnesia and fugue, for instance, memories of specific events or large parts of the individual's personal identity are no longer available to conscious awareness. Dissociation is carried to an extreme in DID. There, the splits in mental processes become so persistent that independent identities are formed, each with a unique set of memories. Interestingly, although individuals with DID often report *interidentity amnesia* (i.e., an inability to recall the events experienced by an altered personality), objective psychological tests show that memory functioning is intact and comparable to healthy controls (Marsh et al., 2018). It is hypothesized that people who believe they have different personalities may consider certain memories unavailable and thus make no effort to retrieve those memories.

Did You Know?

Many individuals diagnosed with DID report hearing voices before the age of 18. They hear two or more voices (often child and adult) and also report tactile and visual hallucinations.

Source: Dorahy et al., 2009

Contemporary psychodynamic theorists propose a posttraumatic model of DID that focuses on the role of severe childhood abuse, parental neglect or abandonment, or other early traumatic events (Dalenberg et al., 2012; Loewenstein, 2018). According to this model, the factors necessary for the development of DID include:

- being exposed to overwhelming childhood stress, such as traumatic physical or sexual abuse;
- genetic or biological predisposition including the capacity to dissociate; and
- environmental circumstances that prevent a child from developing a strong sense of self, resulting in multiple, disconnected selves.

According to the posttraumatic model, DID develops when there are traumatic early experiences combined with an inability to escape them, an absence of emotional support, and the use of dissociation or self-hypnosis as a means of coping (refer to Figure 7.5). From this psychodynamic perspective, a child who is exposed to chronic and severe abuse uses dissociation as a protective mechanism to form different personality structures containing traumatic memories that are walled off from one another. In the case of Sybil, who reportedly experienced severe physical abuse by her mother, Dr. Wilbur—Sybil's psychiatrist—speculated that Sybil escaped "an intolerable and dangerous reality" by dividing into different personalities (Schreiber, 1973). Consistent with this perspective, most individuals diagnosed with DID do report a history of physical or sexual abuse during childhood. In fact, individuals with DID have the highest rate of childhood psychological trauma compared to people with other psychiatric disorders (Loewenstein et al., 2017). The psychodynamic explanation of DID further requires that the individual have the capacity to dissociate—or separate—certain memories or mental processes in response to traumatic events. In fact, people who have DID are very susceptible to hypnotic suggestion. Additionally, women with DID report various experiences involving alterations in consciousness, including trance states and sleepwalking (APA, 2022).

As with most psychodynamic conceptualizations, it is difficult to formulate and test hypotheses. In addition, the posttraumatic model presupposes dissociation in response to childhood trauma, yet few studies have directly examined the relationship between childhood trauma and dissociation and, as was mentioned earlier, many measures used to assess for dissociation have questionable validity (Canan & North, 2019). In most studies, information on child abuse is based on self-reports, is not independently corroborated, and involves varying definitions and degrees of abuse (Gharaibeh, 2009).

Social and Sociocultural Dimension

The sociocognitive model of DID focuses on social and sociocultural factors as the primary explanation for DID, proclaiming that DID is not a valid mental health condition, but rather a diagnosis created by psychiatrists and the media. This perspective describes DID as:

displays of multiple role enactments that have been created, legitimized, and maintained by social reinforcement. Patients with DID synthesize these role enactments by drawing on a wide variety of sources of information, including the print and broadcast media, cues provided by therapists, personal experiences, and observations of individuals who have enacted multiple identities. (Lilienfeld et al., 1999, p. 507)

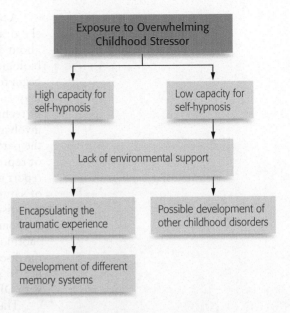

Figure 7.5

The Posttraumatic Model of Dissociative Identity Disorder
Note the importance of each of the factors in the development of dissociative identity disorder.
Source: Adapted from Kluft, 1987; Loewenstein, 1994

According to this model, developed by Spanos (1994) and further elaborated by Lilienfeld et al. (1999), individuals with the disorder learn about DID and its characteristics through the mass media. Those with biological or social vulnerabilities, such as exposure to childhood trauma, begin to act out these roles (Lynn et al., 2014). These susceptible individuals may enact certain behaviors when therapists inadvertently use questions or techniques that evoke dissociative descriptions by clients. In one study involving 2,326 U.S. adults who had undergone psychotherapy, 9 percent of the participants indicated that their therapist had brought up the possibility of repressed memories. People in this group were 20 times more likely to report recovered memories of abuse (including two cases involving memories of satanic ritual abuse) compared with individuals whose therapists had not discussed the issue of repressed memories (Canan & North, 2019). Proponents of the sociocognitive model support their perspective by citing the enormous increase in DID cases that occurred after mass media portrayals of the disorder. For example, after the 1973 publication of *Sybil*, which detailed her 16 personalities, the mean number of personalities for those diagnosed with DID rose from 3 to 12 (Goff & Simms, 1993).

Therapists exposed to mass media portrayals of DID may inadvertently look for and encourage reports of DID from clients. Thus, DID could be an **iatrogenic disorder**—a condition unintentionally produced by a therapist through mechanisms such as selective attention, suggestion, reinforcement, and expectations that are placed on the client. Across studies reviewed, techniques such as guided imagery, dream analysis, and hypnosis or the use of leading questions or comments induced false beliefs or memories in between 20 percent and 50 percent of participants (Muschalla & Schönborn, 2021). In a criminal case in Italy, the court ruled that a therapist implanted false memories of abuse in a young girl using highly suggestive questions that implied the father had abused her. Before treatment, she had no recollection of any abuse by her father (Otgaar et al., 2022). Could some or even most cases of dissociative identity disorder be iatrogenic? A number of researchers and clinicians say yes. They believe that many of the cases of DID and dissociative amnesia have unwittingly been produced by therapists, self-help books, and the mass media (Ulatowska & Sawicka, 2017). Clients most sensitive to these influences may have certain predisposing characteristics. For example, individuals who report dissociation score high on fantasy proneness and fantasy susceptibility (Giesbrecht et al., 2008). Similarly, maltreated children had higher levels of spontaneous negative false memories during an experimental procedure than non-maltreated children (Otgaar et al., 2017).

The authenticity of the well-known story of Sybil and her multiple personalities has also been seriously challenged. Herbert Spiegel, a hypnotist who used Sybil to demonstrate hypnotic phenomena, described her as an "hypnotic virtuoso" because she was so easy to hypnotize. When working with Spiegel, Sybil told him that her psychiatrist, Cornelia Wilbur, had wanted her to be "Helen," a name she gave to a feeling she expressed during therapy; this may have facilitated the conversion of different memories or emotions into "personalities." Tapes of sessions between Wilbur and Sybil further suggest that Wilbur may have described various personalities for Sybil during their therapy

A Famous Case of Dissociative Identity Disorder

Chris Sizemore, whose experiences with dissociative identity disorder inspired the book and movie *The Three Faces of Eve*, was photographed in 2008 at her home in Florida.

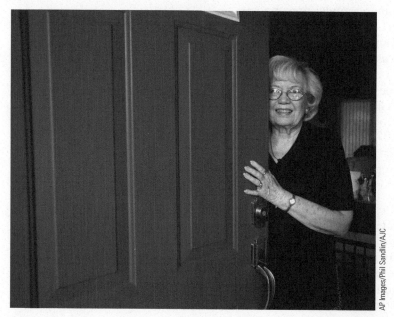

AP Images/Phil Sandlin/AJC

sessions (Rieber, 2006). In her recent book, *Sybil Exposed: The Extraordinary Story behind the Famous Multiple Personality Case*, journalist Debbie Nathan conducted extensive research into the case and concluded that the multiple personality and abuse story emerged from a combination of manipulation by Dr. Wilbur and fabrication by the real-life Sybil (Carey, 2017).

Although iatrogenic influences can occur in any disorder, such effects may be more common with dissociative disorders, because of the high levels of hypnotizability and suggestibility, as well as the number of comorbid mental disorders found in individuals with these conditions, including a high prevalence of borderline personality disorder (Foote & Van Orden, 2016). As Goff has stated, it is "no coincidence that the field of [multiple-personality disorder] studies in the United States largely originated among practitioners of hypnosis" (1993, p. 604). Hypnosis and other memory-retrieval methods may *create* rather than uncover personalities in suggestible clients. Although some cases of DID may be influenced by therapeutic techniques, many cases do not appear to be a result of the therapy process.

Treatment of Dissociative Disorders

A variety of treatments for the dissociative disorders have been developed, including supportive counseling, the use of hypnosis and personality reconstruction, and trauma therapy. Currently, there are no specific medications for the dissociative disorders. However, medications are sometimes prescribed to treat comorbid conditions.

Going Deeper

"Suspect" Techniques Used to Treat Dissociative Identity Disorder

Bennett Braun, who founded the International Society for the Study of Multiple Personality and Dissociation and trained many therapists to work with clients with dissociative identity disorder, was brought up on charges by the Illinois Department of Financial and Professional Regulation. A former patient, Patricia Burgus, claimed that Braun inappropriately used hypnotic drugs, hypnosis, and leather strap restraints to stimulate abuse memories. While undergoing this "repressed-memory therapy," Burgus became convinced that she possessed 300 personalities, was a high priestess in a satanic cult, ate meatloaf made of human flesh, and sexually abused her children. Burgus later began to question these "memories." In November 1997, she won a $10.6 million lawsuit, alleging inappropriate treatment and emotional harm (Associated Press, 1998). Braun lost his license to practice for 2 years and was placed on probation for an additional 5 years.

Another former patient, Elizabeth Gale, also won a $7 million settlement against Braun and other staff at the hospital where he worked. She had been convinced she was raised as a "breeder" to produce babies who would be subjected to sexual abuse. She has since sought to reestablish relationships with family members whom she accused of being part of a cult (Dardick, 2004). Braun moved to Montana, where he was again able to obtain a license to practice and was sued by a woman who went to him for treatment for anxiety and postconcussive syndrome. She claimed he prescribed her antipsychotic medications that resulted in various physical symptoms associated with tardive dyskinesia. Because the dosage was so high, her neurologist is convinced that her physical condition is permanent (Dunlap, 2019).

Although the cases against Braun appear to be warranted, such lawsuits create a quandary for mental health practitioners. Many feel intimidated by the threat of legal action if they attempt to treat adult survivors of childhood sexual abuse, especially cases involving recovered memories. However, discounting the memories of clients could result in further trauma. Especially worrisome is the use of techniques such as hypnosis, trance work, body memories, and age regression, because they may produce inaccurate "memories" (Patihis & Pendergrast, 2018).

For Further Consideration

1. In the case of repressed memories, should clients be told that some techniques may produce inaccurate information?

2. Under what conditions, if any, should a therapist express doubt about information remembered by a client?

3. Given the high prevalence of child sexual abuse and the indefinite nature of repressed memories, how should clinicians proceed if a client discusses early memories of abuse?

Kim Noble, a mother, artist, and author, first began painting during the art therapy she received as part of her treatment for dissociative identity disorder. Kim and each of her alters have their own distinctive painting style.

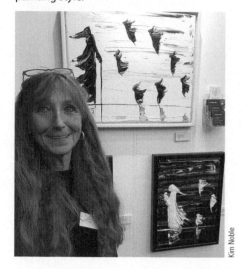

Kim Noble

Treating Dissociative Amnesia and Dissociative Amnesia with Fugue

The symptoms of dissociative amnesia and dissociative amnesia with fugue tend to disappear over time, with dissociative fugue having faster recovery (Harrison et al., 2017). It has been noted that depression, conflictual family relationships, and legal issues, as well as financial- and employment-related concerns, are often associated with these dissociative disorders. A reasonable therapeutic approach is to treat dissociative amnesia by using antidepressants, cognitive-behavioral therapy, and stress management techniques to alleviate the depression and environmental stressors that may underlie the dissociative symptoms (Gill et al., 2023).

Treating Depersonalization/Derealization Disorder

Depersonalization/derealization disorder is also subject to spontaneous remission, but at a much slower rate than typically occurs with dissociative amnesia. Treatment generally concentrates on alleviating underlying feelings of anxiety or depression or the fear associated with the symptoms of detachment. Because catastrophic attributions and appraisals sometimes play a role in the development of depersonalization/derealization symptoms, some therapists focus on "normalizing" minor dissociative reactions and thoughts in response to stressful situations (Hunter et al., 2014). Mindfulness techniques in which the individual focuses on the breathing process itself, with awareness of sensations in different parts of the body combined with acceptance of thoughts and feelings, including nonjudgmentally observing dissociative sensations, can help reduce the fear and anxiety associated with DDD (Mishra et al., 2022).

Treating Dissociative Identity Disorder

The mental health literature contains more information on treating DID than on all of the other dissociative disorders combined. Trauma-focused therapy for DID is often used to help the individual develop healthier ways of dealing with stressors and to assist the different self-states to become aware of one another, consider each other as a legitimate part of the individual, and resolve their differences. Each of the personalities is validated for helping the main personality cope with stressors and traumatic events. The desired outcome is an integration or harmony among the different selves and a final fusion of the personality states. In other words, the goal is for the selves to be completely integrated, merged, and assimilated into one personality.

A hierarchical treatment approach to achieve this integrated functioning involves the following steps (Brand et al., 2019):

Phase 1—Working on safety issues, emotional stabilization, and the reduction of symptoms using psychoeducation and cognitive-behavioral strategies focused on reducing cognitive distortions, managing emotional dysregulation, and coping with current stressors

Phase 2—Identifying and working though any traumatic memories underlying the disorder, while remaining attentive to safety and stability as the memories are addressed and processed

Phase 3—Focusing on personality integration by assisting all alter personalities to view themselves as a legitimate part of the self

Full remission of DID is difficult to achieve and is particularly challenging when an alter personality does not wish to become integrated. Treatment generally involves 3 or more years of therapy. In a 30-month follow-up involving 119 individuals with DID who underwent comprehensive treatment, it was concluded that therapy resulted in fewer symptoms of dissociation and PTSD. Further, many of the participants increased adaptive behaviors such as socializing, attending school, working, or volunteering. However, these individuals were not "cured"; they still experienced dissociative and other stress symptoms (Brand et al., 2012).

Treatments for DID continue to evolve, with most of the newer treatments emphasizing the importance of developing emotional regulation skills to deal with traumatic memories and everyday stressors rather than on integration of personalities. One group of 111 individuals with DID completed an online psychoeducational program in collaboration with their therapists. This therapeutic program—focused on improving emotional regulation skills; managing safety issues; and decreasing symptoms of PTSD, dissociation, and nonsuicidal self-injury—produced large improvements in emotional self-management and significantly reduced self-injurious behaviors (Brand et al., 2019). This intervention used many techniques that are included in dialectical behavior therapy (originally developed for borderline personality disorder), another approach that has been found to be effective in treating DID (Foote & Van Orden, 2016).

Cognitive-behavioral therapy was used to treat five women with DID. The therapy began with a focus on adaptive emotional regulation skills, including cognitive reappraisal, emotional awareness, and tolerance of distressing emotions. After these skills were achieved, the participants slowly began to work through traumatic memories. After 15 to 22 sessions of treatment (one individual required 42 sessions due to acute suicidal ideation), all participants showed increased emotional self-regulation and significant reductions in dissociation, anxiety, and depression. After treatment, the participants no longer met the criteria for a diagnosis for DID or for any other disorder; these gains were maintained at a 6-month follow-up (Mohajerin et al., 2019).

One group of researchers is investigating the use of schema therapy to treat DID (Huntjens et al., 2019). Their approach combines cognitive-behavioral therapy with interpersonal therapy, which has a strong focus on the therapeutic relationship as a catalyst for changing the emotional dysfunction caused by childhood neglect or abuse. Instead of accepting the idea of different alters that are walled off from one another, this approach reframes the alters as modes of behavior and feelings that are present in everyone. The alters that develop in DID are recast as extreme examples of dysfunctional methods of coping. This approach validates the feeling that people with DID have of alternating "identities" while simultaneously helping them learn how to modify dysfunctional methods of coping with stressful conditions or emotions.

Continuum Video Project

Lani and Jan: Dissociative Identity Disorder

"It's like living with 13 roommates . . . and your responsibility is to make sure everyone's needs get met."

Access the Continuum Video Project in MindTap.

7-3 Contemporary Trends and Future Directions

With each edition of the DSM, the criteria for certain disorders are amended. Sometimes these modifications are improvements, but some diagnostic changes create controversy. The change in criteria for somatization disorder in the DSM-IV to somatic symptom disorder (SSD) as described in the DSM-5 and DSM-5-TR was quite dramatic; the former required a more extensive history of physical complaints, many more somatic symptoms, and documentation that the symptoms were "medically unexplained." Some researchers and clinicians believed that the previous criteria were too restrictive and were especially concerned with the "medically unexplained" aspect of the criteria because it is difficult for medical professionals to verify that there is no physical basis for someone's somatic complaints. This situation often created an adversarial relationship between health care professionals and patients, particularly if patients concluded that the doctor believed their symptoms were "imaginary." Due to these concerns, the SSD diagnosis no longer emphasizes the "medically unexplained" nature of the symptoms and focuses instead on the degree of distress and impairment caused by the physical symptoms.

However, there is concern that the removal of "medically unexplained" has produced its own set of problems. Further, the diagnosis of SSD requires the presence of only one problematic physical symptom. The clinician then decides if the individual has persistent, distressing thoughts about the symptom; has high levels of anxiety about the symptom; or devotes excessive time and energy to the symptom, thereby confirming the diagnosis. Further, because actual illnesses are not excluded, many individuals with physical conditions now meet the criteria for SSD. For example, up to 26 percent of individuals who reported long-lasting post-COVID-19 symptoms such as impaired concentration and fatigue and who experienced excessive concern over their symptoms met the criteria for SSD (Schneider et al., 2023). In another study, nearly two thirds of people with long-lasting neurological symptoms post-COVID-19 met the criteria for SSD (Kachaner et al., 2022). Other studies have found that 26 percent of the individuals with irritable bowel syndrome or fibromyalgia and 15 percent of those with cancer or heart disease would meet the criteria for SSD due to their persistent concern and distress about their medical condition (Frances, 2013). This is also true in 26 percent of those with asthma or arthritis (Löwe et al., 2022). These statistics suggest that it will be difficult to decide if people with a chronic or potentially life-threatening illness have "too much" anxiety over their condition, spend an "inordinate" amount of time or energy on their symptoms, or have "excessive" thoughts regarding the seriousness of their illness.

In removing the "medically unexplained" aspect from SSD, are we now in danger of giving a psychiatric diagnosis to individuals with legitimate concerns about a diagnosed physical condition? Who is to say whether a person with an illness such as heart disease or cancer or long-COVID is devoting "excessive time or energy" or showing "too much" anxiety in response to their condition? The criteria for this disorder remain controversial. Time will tell if the changes are beneficial or have instead created a new set of concerns that will require further revisions in future editions of the DSM.

Controversy also exists with the repressed memory concept associated with the dissociative disorders. While many health care professionals, psychologists, and psychiatrists believe that memories of traumatic events can be repressed, most memory researchers and experimental psychologists reject the validity of this phenomenon (Otgaar et al., 2021; Pathis et al., 2021). This conflict has been called the memory war. The central issue is whether a memory that has formed can be repressed, or pushed out of consciousness, and later retrieved. A resolution to this debate is important, since the lives of abuse survivors, therapists, and accused perpetrators are at stake.

Chapter Summary

1 What are the somatic symptom and related disorders, and what do they have in common? What causes these conditions, and how are they treated?

- Somatic symptom and related disorders involve prominent somatic complaints that cause significant distress or impairment in the life of the individual and include somatic symptom, illness anxiety, conversion, and factitious disorders.

- Somatic symptom disorder (SSD) is characterized by at least one physical complaint accompanied by excessive anxiety, thoughts, or behaviors associated with health concerns.

- Illness anxiety disorder is characterized by a belief that one has a serious and undetected illness or physical problem. In contrast to somatic symptom disorder, somatic symptoms are not a major feature of this disorder.

- Functional neurological symptom disorder (FNSD) involves neurological-like symptoms that are incompatible with a medical condition.

- Factitious disorders involve self-induced or feigned physical complaints, or symptoms induced in others.

- Biological explanations have suggested that there is increased vulnerability to somatic symptom disorders when individuals have high sensitivity to bodily sensations, a lower pain threshold, or a history of illness or injury.

- Psychological factors include high anxiety or stress, and catastrophic thoughts regarding bodily sensations.

- Social explanations suggest that the role of "being sick" is reinforcing. External stressors such as sexual abuse, bullying, or role models who attend to illness can also be influential.

- From a sociocultural perspective, somatic symptom disorders result from societal restrictions placed on women, who are affected by these disorders to a much greater degree than are men. Additionally, marginalization, social class, limited knowledge about medical concepts, and cultural acceptance of physical symptoms can play a role.

- Treatment involves psychoeducation about physical complaints, altering distorted cognitions, and strategies for tolerating changes in bodily sensations.

2 What are dissociations? Why do they occur, and how are they treated?

- Dissociation involves a disruption in consciousness, memory, identity, or perception, and may be transient or chronic.

- Dissociative amnesia, including localized amnesia and dissociative amnesia with fugue, involves a selective form of forgetting in which the person cannot remember information that is of personal significance.

- Depersonalization/derealization disorder (DDD) is characterized by feelings of unreality—distorted perceptions of oneself and one's environment.

- Dissociative identity disorder (DID) involves the presence of two or more personality states in one individual, or an experience of possession.

- Biological explanations for DID have included atypical neurological connectivity, disruptions in encoding memories, and atypical neural activity that may indicate an inhibition of brain areas associated with memory. Some researchers believe that childhood trauma and chronic stress can result in permanent structural changes within the brain.

- Psychoanalytic perspectives attribute these disorders to the use of repression to block unpleasant or traumatic events from consciousness.

- Social explanations include childhood abuse, subtle reinforcement, mislabeling of dissociative experiences, and responding to the expectations of a therapist.

- Sociocultural explanations for dissociation include exposure to media portrayals of dissociation and role enactment by vulnerable individuals.

- Dissociative amnesia, dissociative amnesia with fugue, and DDD tend to remit spontaneously; cognitive-behavioral therapy and stress management techniques can be beneficial in preventing symptom recurrence. DID is often treated with trauma-focused cognitive therapy that addresses safety concerns and the integration of the personality states. Therapy incorporates strategies for eliminating cognitive distortions and dealing with current stressors. Newer approaches reframe the perception of alter personalities as modifiable methods of coping with stress or trauma.

Chapter Glossary

depersonalization/derealization disorder (DDD)
a dissociative condition characterized by feelings of unreality concerning the self and the environment

dissociation
a mild to extreme lack of connection with one's surroundings or emotions in reaction to stressful or traumatic circumstances

dissociative amnesia
a psychologically based sudden loss of important personal information or recall of events

dissociative amnesia with fugue
an episode involving complete loss of memory of one's life and identity, unexpected travel to a new location, or assumption of a new identity

dissociative disorders
a group of disorders, including dissociative amnesia, dissociative identity disorder, and depersonalization/derealization disorder, all of which involve some sort of dissociation, or separation, of a part of the person's consciousness, memory, or identity

dissociative identity disorder (DID)
a condition in which two or more relatively independent personality states appear to exist in one person, including experiences of possession

factitious disorder
a condition in which a person deliberately induces or simulates symptoms of physical or mental illness with no apparent incentive other than attention

factitious disorder imposed on another
a pattern of falsification or production of physical or psychological symptoms in another individual

factitious disorder imposed on self
symptoms of illness are deliberately induced, simulated, or exaggerated, with no apparent external incentive

functional neurological symptom disorder (FNSD)
a condition involving sensory or motor impairment suggestive of a neurological disorder but with no underlying medical cause

iatrogenic disorder
a condition unintentionally produced by a therapist's actions and treatment strategies

illness anxiety disorder
persistent health anxiety and/or concern that one has an undetected physical illness, even when the person has only mild or no physical symptoms

localized amnesia
lack of memory for a specific event or events

malingering
feigning illness for an external purpose

possession
the replacement of a person's sense of personal identity with a supernatural spirit or power

psychogenic
originating from psychological causes

repressed memory
a memory of a traumatic event has been repressed and is, therefore, unavailable for recall

selective amnesia
an inability to remember certain details of an event

somatic symptom and related disorders
a broad grouping of psychological disorders that involve physical symptoms or anxiety over illness, including somatic symptom disorder, illness anxiety disorder, functional neurological symptom disorder, and factitious disorder

somatic symptom disorder (SSD)
a condition involving a pattern of distressing thoughts regarding the seriousness of one's physical symptoms combined with excessive time and concern devoted to worrying about these symptoms

somatic symptom disorder with predominant pain
a condition involving excessive anxiety or persistent concerns over severe or lingering pain

somatic symptoms
physical or bodily symptoms

systematized amnesia
loss of memory for certain categories of information

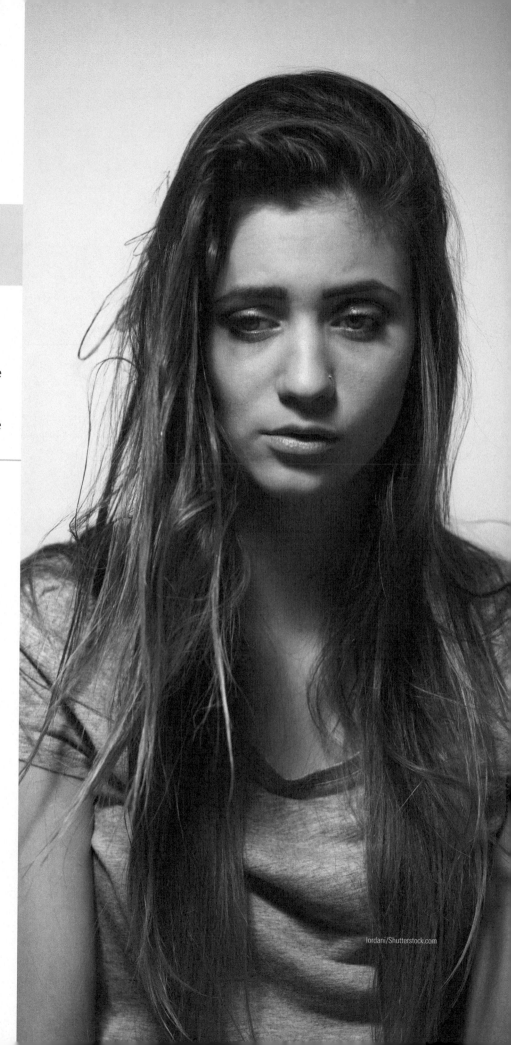

focus
Questions

1 What are symptoms of depression, hypomania, and mania?

2 What are depressive disorders, what causes them, and how are they treated?

3 What are bipolar disorders, what causes them, and how are they treated?

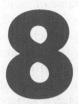

8

Depressive and Bipolar Disorders

Learning Objectives

After studying this chapter, you will be able to . . .

8-1 Describe the symptoms of depression, hypomania, and mania, and important considerations when evaluating mood symptoms.

8-2 Discuss key features of each of the depressive disorders, what causes them, and how they are treated.

8-3 Compare the types of bipolar disorders and explain what causes them and how they are treated.

Chelsea, Raised in a Stable and Loving Family, was an A student and star athlete throughout much of high school. However, in her senior year, she became uncharacteristically irritable, began to miss swimming practice, and fell behind in her school assignments. She seemed uninterested when friends contacted her. When her parents tried to talk to her, Chelsea asked to be left alone and retreated to her bedroom. She spent most of her weekends sleeping. As graduation approached, Chelsea became increasingly withdrawn from family and friends. She felt guilty about how she was treating everyone and finally agreed to meet with a therapist. During her first visit she told the therapist, "I don't know what's wrong with me. Everything had seemed so right, and now everything seems so wrong."

Mood refers to our emotional state or our prevailing frame of mind. Our mood can significantly affect our perceptions of the world, sense of well-being, and interactions with others. Persistent changes in mood, such as the depressive symptoms demonstrated by Chelsea, are concerning, especially when they occur for no apparent reason. You can probably imagine how discouraging it is to want to return to a normal mood, but be unable to do so. As you will learn in this chapter, a variety of factors, including genetic predisposition, early life events, and current stressors, can interact to produce mood changes such as those experienced by Chelsea.

Two groups of mental disorders involve significant mood changes—depressive and bipolar disorders. We include depressive and bipolar disorders in the same chapter because they both entail pervasive, life-altering disturbances in mood. Unfortunately, both depressive and bipolar disorders are associated with an increased risk of suicide, a topic we discuss extensively in Chapter 9.

. . . .

8-1 Symptoms Associated with Depressive and Bipolar Disorders

Most of you experience minor mood changes throughout the day, but are able to stay emotionally balanced and on an even keel. You may also have times where you feel depressed or times when you experience an emotional high—normal reactions to the events going on around you. You may have occasional, brief episodes of more significant mood changes—experiencing overwhelming sadness over the loss of a friendship or feeling extremely energized or even ecstatic when you hear great news. Unlike these temporary, normal emotional reactions, the mood symptoms in depressive and bipolar disorders:

- affect the person's well-being and school, work, or social functioning;
- continue for days, weeks, or months;
- often occur for no apparent reason; and
- involve extreme reactions that cannot be easily explained by what is happening in the person's life.

Depression and mania, opposite ends of a continuum that extends from deep sadness to wild elation, represent the extremes of mood. Whereas depressive disorders involve only one troubling mood (depression), people who live with a bipolar disorder (previously called manic-depression) often cope with two mood extremes—overwhelming depression and periods involving an elevated or abnormally energized mood. Bipolar refers to the fact that the condition involves mood extremes at both emotional "poles." Experiencing these mood extremes on a regular basis can be very distressing and disruptive to everyday life.

Let's begin by looking at the symptoms associated with a depressed or energized mood state (refer to Table 8.1), and how clinicians determine if a person has a depressive or bipolar disorder.

Table 8.1 Symptoms of Depression and Hypomania/Mania

Domain	Depression	Hypomania/Mania
Mood	Sadness, emptiness and worthlessness, apathy, hopelessness	Elevated mood, extreme confidence, grandiosity, irritability, hostility
Cognitive	Pessimism, guilt, difficulty concentrating, negative thinking, suicidal thoughts	Disorientation, racing thoughts, decreased focus and attention, creativity, poor judgment
Behavioral	Social withdrawal, crying, low energy, lowered productivity, agitation, poor hygiene	Overactivity, rapid or incoherent speech, impulsivity, risk-taking behaviors
Physiological	Appetite and weight changes, sleep disturbance, aches and pain, loss of sex drive	High levels of arousal, decreased sleep, increased sex drive

Symptoms of Depression

Depression involves intense sadness or loss of interest in normally enjoyed activities. We can usually tell if someone is depressed because we notice changes in their emotional reactions, or in their thinking, behavior, or physical well-being.

Emotional Symptoms in Depression

> **Case Study**   It's hard to describe the state I was in several months ago. The depression was total—it was as if everything that happened to me passed through this dark filter, and I kept seeing the world through this dark cloud. Nothing was exciting. I felt I was no good, completely worthless, and deserving of nothing. The people who tried to cheer me up just couldn't understand how down I felt. There were many days when I couldn't even make it to class.

The most striking symptom of depression—depressed mood—involves feelings of sadness, emptiness, hopelessness, worthlessness, or low self-esteem. This quote from a college student coming out of a deep depression typifies the hopelessness and emotional numbness that often accompany depression. As this young person so clearly expresses, people experiencing depression have little enthusiasm for things they once enjoyed, including spending time with family and friends. Feeling irritable or anxious and worried is also common.

Cognitive Symptoms in Depression

Certain thoughts and ideas, including pessimistic, self-critical beliefs, are typical among people who are depressed. **Rumination**, continually thinking about upsetting topics or repeatedly reviewing distressing events, often occurs during a depressive episode. Ruminating can intensify feelings of depression, especially when it involves self-criticism, feelings of guilt, or irrational beliefs (Yaroslavsky et al., 2019). Depression can also cause distractibility and interfere with a person's ability to concentrate, remember things, or make decisions (Keefe et al., 2022). These cognitive challenges can lead to feelings of intense frustration, especially when tasks that were previously managed without difficulty suddenly seem overwhelming.

Thoughts of suicide are also common among those who are depressed. This may result from feelings of being a burden to friends and family or a belief that there is little hope for the future or that the emotional pain

Cultural norms can affect how depression is expressed. European Americans tend to display decreased emotional reactivity when depressed (e.g., less smiling), whereas many Asian Americans experience depression through increased internal physiological reactivity (e.g., stomach upset), but display no significant outward change in emotional expression.

Source: Chentsova-Dutton et al., 2010

will never end (Yang et al., 2019). As we discuss in Chapter 9, it is crucial to intervene if someone is feeling suicidal. By encouraging someone who has suicidal thoughts to seek professional assistance, you might help save a life.

Behavioral Symptoms in Depression

Behavioral symptoms such as fatigue, social withdrawal, and reduced motivation are common with depression. Some people who are depressed speak slowly or quietly; they may respond only in short phrases or not respond at all. Some appear agitated and restless, pacing and finding it difficult to sit still. They may cry for no particular reason or in reaction to sadness, frustration, or anger. It may appear that they no longer care about their grooming or personal cleanliness. This occurs because daily activities such as getting out of bed, bathing, dressing, or preparing for work or class may feel overwhelming. Not surprisingly, a person's grades or job performance may slip during a depressive episode.

Physiological Symptoms in Depression

We often focus on the emotional and behavioral changes that occur with depression. However, physiological symptoms are also common during depressive episodes (Lam et al., 2016):

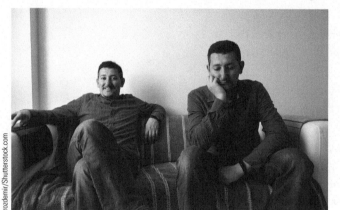

Emotional Changes in Bipolar Disorder

Individuals with bipolar disorder may talk excessively during hypomanic or manic episodes; in contrast, they may withdraw from social interactions when experiencing depression.

- *Appetite and weight changes.* Depression sometimes causes changes in weight due to either increased or decreased eating. While some people have almost no appetite and lose weight, others eat even if they are not hungry (especially sweets and carbohydrates) and find that they are gaining weight.

- *Sleep disturbance.* Many people with depression have difficulty falling asleep or staying asleep. Others sleep much more than usual, but wake up feeling tired and unrefreshed.

- *Unexplained aches and pain.* Headaches, stomachaches, or other body aches commonly occur during depression, especially among those with severe or chronic depression. In some cultural groups, unexplained aches and pains are the main symptoms of depression.

- *Aversion to sexual activity.* Depression often produces dramatically reduced sexual interest and arousal.

Symptoms of Hypomania or Mania

Individuals with bipolar disorder experience mood states characterized by increased energy, emotional changes, and other significant transformations in behavior. This **elevated mood** includes two levels of intensity—hypomania and mania (APA, 2022). The milder form, **hypomania**, is characterized by increased levels of activity or energy combined with a self-important, **expansive mood** or an irritable, agitated mood. Someone with hypomania may appear quite distractible, change topics frequently, have many ideas, talk excessively, or dominate conversations. The person may feel creative and start various projects. Impulsivity and risk taking may also appear during a hypomanic episode. All of these symptoms are uncharacteristic of how the person normally functions.

Mania is a state of even more pronounced mood change involving extremely exaggerated activity levels and emotionality that significantly impair normal functioning. Behaviors demonstrated during mania can range from extreme giddiness, excitement, and **euphoria** (exceptionally elevated mood) to intense irritability, hostility, or agitation. Aside from hypomania being a milder version of mania, another notable difference is that manic episodes cause marked impairment in social or occupational functioning and may involve **psychosis** (loss of contact with reality) and a need for psychiatric hospitalization. When someone is experiencing a manic episode, it is obvious to others that something is amiss; in contrast, hypomania is often more subtle, does not impair normal functioning, and may be evident only to those who know the person well. As with depression, hypomania and mania involve emotional, cognitive, behavioral, and physiological symptoms.

Emotional Symptoms of Hypomania/Mania

People experiencing hypomania may appear to be in unusually high spirits and full of energy and enthusiasm. They also may be uncharacteristically irritable, have a low tolerance for frustration, and overreact with anger or hostility in response to environmental stimuli (e.g., noises, a child crying) or the people around them. People with mania may exhibit **emotional lability** characterized by unstable and rapidly changing emotions and mood. Inappropriate use of humor, poor judgment in expressing feelings or opinions, and **grandiosity** (inflated self-esteem and beliefs of being special, chosen, or superior to others) can result in interpersonal conflicts and aggressive interactions (Serra et al., 2017).

Cognitive Symptoms of Hypomania/Mania

Individuals experiencing hypomania often display energized, goal-oriented behavior at home, school, or work. They may seem excited and talk more than usual, engage in one-sided conversations, and demonstrate little concern about giving others an opportunity to speak. They may have difficulty focusing their attention; demonstrate a flight of ideas or racing thoughts, distractibility, or poor judgment; and fail to recognize the inappropriateness of their behavior (Hukic et al., 2013).

Those experiencing mania are much more likely to appear disoriented and exhibit cognitive difficulties. Their impaired thinking may be apparent from their speech, sometimes referred to as **pressured speech**, which may be rapid, loud, and difficult to understand. Those experiencing mania frequently have extreme difficulty maintaining focus and display a **flight of ideas**; that is, they change topics, become distracted with new thoughts, or make irrelevant or illogical comments.

Behavioral Symptoms of Hypomania/Mania

Individuals experiencing hypomania or mania might appear energetic and productive and display an expansive mood of extreme confidence and self-importance, taking on a variety of complex or creative tasks. In contrast, they might also become easily agitated and react angrily with little provocation; seem uninhibited and act impulsively; or engage in uncharacteristic behaviors such as reckless driving, excessive drinking, illegal drug use, promiscuous conduct, or uncontrolled spending. They may also make impulsive decisions such as changing jobs or developing plans to move to a new location. Similarly, they may have difficulty delaying gratification and insist on following through with their impulsive actions, becoming irritable if family or friends interfere with or encourage them to reconsider their plans. Failure to evaluate the consequences of decisions can lead to unsafe sexual practices or illegal activity. For example, one person described how he felt "on top of the world" as he engaged in "dining and dashing"—ordering an expensive meal and leaving without paying (Carter, 2018). As you might imagine, the behaviors that occur during an energized episode can create significant legal consequences as well as tensions in interpersonal relationships.

During mania, motor movement is often rapid, and speech may be incoherent. Wild excitement, ranting, constant movement, and agitation characterize severe mania. Psychotic symptoms including paranoia, hallucinations, and delusions (false beliefs) may also occur during a manic episode. Individuals experiencing extreme mania may require hospitalization if they become dangerous to themselves or to others.

Physiological Symptoms of Hypomania/Mania

Individuals experiencing hypomania or mania have high levels of physiological arousal that result in intense activity, extreme restlessness, or a need to be constantly "on the go." Increased libido (sex drive) often leads to reckless sexual activity or other impulsive behaviors. A decreased need for sleep is often the first sign of a hypomanic or manic episode; this sleep disturbance often escalates just before an episode and worsens during the episode (Harvey et al., 2015). This arousal results in less sleep, yet the person does not feel tired. During a manic episode, a person may go for days without sleep. The high expenditure of energy and limited sleep characteristic of elevated episodes often result in unplanned weight loss as well as eventual exhaustion.

Evaluating Mood Symptoms

Careful assessment of mood symptoms is essential for accurately diagnosing depressive and bipolar disorders, especially because brief depressive or hypomanic symptoms also occur in people who do not have a mood disorder. Diagnosis is even more complicated because depression occurs in both depressive and bipolar disorders and because the symptoms of these disorders may vary considerably from person to person. Also, irritability occurs in both bipolar and depressive disorders; this symptom overlap further confounds diagnosis, especially when a person's emotional symptoms during hypomania/mania involve quarrelsomeness or agitation. Additionally, people often fail to report hypomanic symptoms to their medical or mental health providers because energetic episodes often do not cause significant problems or impair functioning. For these reasons, when evaluating someone who is depressed, most experienced clinicians are careful to have the client complete a behavioral checklist regarding any hypomanic or manic symptoms.

Diagnosis is further complicated because people experiencing a depressive or hypomanic/manic episode sometimes exhibit symptoms from the opposite pole. For instance, someone who is experiencing mania may cry excessively or talk of suicide; similarly, someone who is depressed may experience extreme restlessness and have racing thoughts. When extreme mood changes such as this occur, the clinician specifies that the mood episode has *mixed features* (Muneer, 2017). Clinicians also ask about the frequency and duration of the mood episodes and about any seasonal changes in mood. They are also interested in whether the symptoms have been mild, moderate, or severe.

Of course, clinicians also consider other factors that can cause mood changes, such as medical conditions or the use or abuse of alcohol, illegal drugs, or prescription medications. Comprehensive assessment prior to diagnosis is important because, as you will see, interventions for depressive and bipolar disorders are quite different. Therapists also monitor symptoms throughout treatment; a diagnosis may change from a depressive disorder to a bipolar disorder if hypomanic or manic symptoms develop. In the next section, we focus on depressive disorders and then conclude the chapter with a discussion of bipolar disorders.

8-2 Depressive Disorders

Depressive disorders, a group of related disorders characterized by depressive symptoms, include major depressive disorder, persistent depressive disorder, and premenstrual dysphoric disorder (Table 8.2).

Diagnosis and Classification of Depressive Disorders

An important consideration when diagnosing a depressive disorder is making sure the person has never experienced an episode of mania or hypomania (refer to Table 8.6 on page 298). Information about such episodes helps the clinician differentiate between a bipolar and a depressive disorder (Shi et al., 2018). When diagnosing depressive disorders, clinicians also consider the severity and chronicity of the depressive symptoms.

Table 8.2 Depressive Disorders

Disorders Chart				
Depressive Disorder	**DSM-5-TR Criteria**	**Prevalence**	**Gender Difference**	**Age of Onset**
Major depressive disorder (MDD)	• Occurrence of at least one major depressive episode (2-week duration) • No history of mania or hypomania	• 14% to 19% • 3 times higher among ages 18 to 29 than over 60	• Twice as high in girls and women	• Any age; average onset in 20s
Persistent depressive disorder (PDD)	• Depressed mood that has lasted for at least 2 years (with no more than 2 months symptom-free)[a]	• 4%, including 3.1% who have chronic depressive symptoms	• Up to 2 times higher in girls and women	• Often childhood or adolescence
Premenstrual dysphoric disorder (PMDD)	• Severe depression, mood swings, anxiety, or irritability occurring before the onset of menses • Improvement of symptoms within a few days of menstruation and minimal or no symptoms following menstruation	• 2% to 5% of women of reproductive age	• Most common in women who have a personal or family history of depression	• Late 20s, although any age after menarche is possible

Source: APA, 2022, 2022; Epperson et al., 2012; Hasin et al., 2018; Kessler et al., 2005

[a] In children and adolescents, mood can be irritable, and diagnosis can occur if symptoms have been present for at least 1 year.

Major Depressive Disorder

> **Case Study** Antonio finally agreed to stop by the university counseling center. His parents were concerned about him, and his roommate also suggested he get some help. Antonio had lost weight and was staying in his room as much as possible, avoiding his friends and often sleeping for hours. Antonio had always been a good student, but was barely passing several of his classes because he was having such difficulty concentrating. Antonio had not told anyone, but he had been feeling incredibly sad and hopeless about his future and worried that he would never find a good job. He had been excited about starting college, but was already counting the days until summer break when he could sleep all day without worrying about missing class.

After seeking help from a therapist at the counseling center, Antonio was diagnosed as having **major depressive disorder (MDD)**. This diagnosis occurs when a person experiences impaired functioning due to a **major depressive episode**, which involves *severe* depressive symptoms that have negatively affected functioning most of the day, nearly every day, for at least 2 full weeks (refer to Table 8.3). According to the DSM-5-TR, a major depressive episode involves a consistent pattern of (a) depressed mood, feelings of sadness, or emptiness and/or (b) loss of interest or pleasure in previously enjoyed activities. The individual must also experience at least four additional changes in functioning involving significant alteration in weight or appetite, atypical sleep patterns, restlessness or sluggishness, low energy, feelings of guilt or worthlessness, difficulty concentrating or making decisions, or preoccupation with death or suicide.

Many people experience **anxious distress** during a depressive episode. For example, Antonio had difficulty functioning not only due to depressive symptoms, but also because of his persistent worry about his future. Individuals who experience anxious distress often feel unusually tense or restless or experience pervasive worries that make it difficult to concentrate. They may also worry that they will lose self-control or that something bad

Table 8.3   DSM-5-TR Criteria for a Major Depressive Disorder

A major depressive disorder involves *a change in functioning that includes at least one of these symptoms most of the day nearly every day over a period of 2 weeks (or longer):*

(a) *depressed mood, feelings of sadness, or emptiness and/or*
(b) *loss of interest or pleasure in previously enjoyed activities.*

The person must *also* experience at least four of these symptoms during the same period:
(a) *significant weight gain or weight loss (without dieting) or increases or decreases in appetite,*
(b) *persistent changes in sleep patterns, involving increased sleep or inability to sleep,*
(c) *observable restlessness or slowing of activity,*
(d) *persistent fatigue or loss of energy,*
(e) *excessive feelings of guilt or worthlessness,*
(f) *persistent difficulty with concentration or decision making, or*
(g) *suicidal behaviors or recurrent thoughts of death or suicide.*

The symptoms cause significant impairment and are not due to the physiological effects of a medical condition, a prescribed medication, or drug or alcohol abuse.

Source: APA, 2022

will happen. It is important for clinicians to inquire about anxious distress because it is associated with longer depressive episodes and a heightened risk of suicide (Sugawara et al., 2019).

Suicide is a significant concern for anyone with MDD. People who feel hopeless may act on suicidal thoughts, especially if they are under the influence of drugs or alcohol (Urban et al., 2020). Up to 45 percent of those with MDD also have a substance-use disorder—a combination that further increases suicide risk (Hasin et al., 2018). Similarly, people who have chronic depressive symptoms or who developed depression in response to grief have increased risk of suicide (APA, 2022).

MDD with a Seasonal Pattern Some people with MDD (and bipolar disorder) report a seasonal pattern to their depressive episodes—they begin to develop depression when daylight decreases as the seasons change. In individuals with this pattern, depressive symptoms typically begin in the fall or winter and remit during the spring or summer (a small number of those affected display the opposite pattern). Seasonal depression typically involves "vegetative depressive symptoms," including low energy, social withdrawal, increased need for sleep, and carbohydrate craving. Winter depressive episodes occur most frequently among younger individuals, in regions with less light in the winter months (northern latitudes), and among those who are sensitive to the influence of environmental light on their circadian rhythm (APA, 2022).

Many clinicians use the term *seasonal affective disorder (SAD)* to refer to this seasonal pattern. It is estimated to affect up to 3 percent of the world's population and is more prevalent in women than men (Majrashi et al., 2020). However, SAD is not an official DSM diagnostic category; the manual instead describes **MDD with a seasonal pattern**, a condition involving at least two seasonal episodes of severe depression ending at a predictable time of year combined with a pattern of depressive episodes that occur seasonally more than nonseasonally. Thus, the many people who experience milder seasonal depressive symptoms would not meet the DSM-5-TR criteria for MDD with a seasonal pattern.

Persistent Depressive Disorder (PDD)

Persistent depressive disorder (PDD) involves chronic depressive symptoms that are present most of the day for more days than not during a 2-year period (with no more than 2 months symptom-free). According to the DSM-5-TR, a diagnosis of PDD requires the ongoing presence of at least two of the following symptoms: feelings of hopelessness; low self-esteem; poor appetite or overeating; low energy or fatigue; difficulty concentrating or making decisions; or sleeping too little or too much. PDD is often associated with negative thinking patterns and a pessimistic outlook on the future. For many, PDD is a lifelong, pervasive disorder with long periods of depression, few periods without symptoms, and poor response to treatment (Schramm et al., 2020).

Premenstrual Dysphoric Disorder

Premenstrual dysphoric disorder (PMDD) is a controversial diagnostic category involving serious symptoms of depression, irritability, and tension that appear the week before menstruation and disappear soon after menstruation begins. Between 3 percent and 8 percent of women meet the criteria for PMDD (Eisenlohr-Moul et al., 2017). A PMDD diagnosis requires the presence of five premenstrual symptoms; at least one of the symptoms must involve significantly depressed mood, mood swings, anger, anxiety, tension, irritability, or increased interpersonal conflict. Other symptoms considered in making a diagnosis include difficulty concentrating; social withdrawal; lack of energy; food cravings or overeating; insomnia or excessive sleepiness;

Did You Know?

Among students completing a U.S. college health survey, 17 percent of college men and 21 percent of college women reported that at some point during the previous 12 months, they had felt "so depressed it was difficult to function."
Source: American College Health Association (ACHA), 2019

feeling overwhelmed; or physical symptoms such as bloating, weight gain, or breast tenderness. These are similar to the physical and emotional symptoms of *premenstrual syndrome*; however, PMDD produces much greater distress and interferes with social, interpersonal, academic, and/or occupational functioning (APA, 2022). Professionals who opposed the addition of this diagnostic category to the DSM expressed concern about designating symptoms of a normal biological function (menstruation) as a psychiatric disorder (Schroll & Lauritsen, 2022).

Depressive Reactions to Grief

Case Study   Mrs. Lee is a 48-year-old married mother of two teenagers who works full-time as a store manager. Over the past 2 months, she has developed symptoms of fatigue, irritability, general aches and pains, loss of appetite, and reduced libido. Mrs. Lee had been her mother's primary caregiver until 4 months ago, when her mother lost her battle with cancer. Her husband is supportive but feels overwhelmed by her depressive symptoms; her children avoid her because of her temper and frequent outbursts of anger. In recent months, Mrs. Lee has stopped attending church and participating in social events. She finally agreed to see her doctor about her symptoms. Although her physical examination was normal, she burst into tears midway through the examination and admitted that she feels that life is hopeless (Lie, 2012).

Loss as a Source of Depression

Mourning the death of a loved one occurs in all cultures and societies, as demonstrated by these women mourning an Iraqi tae kwon do team who were kidnapped and killed. What characteristics or symptoms help distinguish between "normal" grief and major depressive disorder?

Normal grief reactions occur in response to situations such as the death of a loved one or catastrophic events associated with loss such as a natural disaster or sudden serious illness or disability. The DSM-5-TR makes it clear that it is important to distinguish normal grief-related reactions from the severe depression and impaired functioning associated with MDD. Grief often involves feelings of emptiness associated with the loss rather than the more persistent depressed mood or inability to experience pleasure that occurs with MDD. Although normal grief reactions may last for several years, the frequency and intensity of the grief decreases over time. Of course, bereavement can be a significant stressor and result in the development of prolonged grief disorder as we as discussed in Chapter 6.

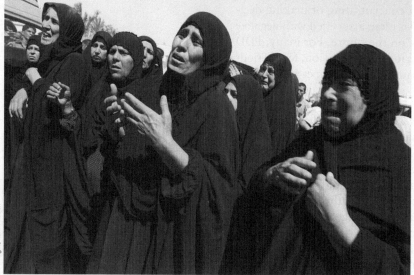

AP Images/Karim Kadim

Prevalence of Depressive Disorders

Depression is one of the most common psychiatric disorders and the second leading cause of disability worldwide, affecting approximately 264 million people each year (World Health Organization [WHO], 2020a). Approximately 21 percent of the U.S. population will experience a major depressive episode at some point in their lives. Women have nearly twice the risk of experiencing major depression compared to men (Hasin et al., 2018). Additionally, approximately 2 percent to 5 percent of women experience symptoms of PMDD during their reproductive years (Epperson et al., 2012). Depressive symptoms are also subject to external stressors. For example, in surveys conducted in 2019, about 8 percent of adults endorsed "having little interest or pleasure in doing things" and "feeling down, depressed or hopeless." In contrast, based on surveys conducted in the summer of 2020 amidst the COVID-19 pandemic and Black Lives Matter demonstrations, the percentage of U.S. respondents who endorsed these same symptoms rose dramatically—with depression affecting almost one third of all adults who responded to the survey (National Center for Health Statistics, 2020).

For many people, depression is a chronic disorder. If depressive symptoms do not completely resolve with treatment, the chances of a relapse or chronic depression are greatly increased. In clinical samples, over three fourths of those with MDD will experience at least one recurrence. Childhood maltreatment, rumination, and residual depressive symptoms after treatment increase the risk of recurrent depressive episodes (Buckman et al., 2018). Approximately 15 percent of those treated for depression fail to demonstrate any significant reduction in symptoms (Berlim & Turecki, 2007); some researchers believe that many of these cases represent undiagnosed bipolar disorder. In one 10-year follow-up of individuals diagnosed with MDD, approximately 19 percent eventually received a bipolar diagnosis; this outcome was most likely for those who had a poor response to antidepressants (Hu et al., 2020). People who are misdiagnosed often experience greater impairment, presumably due to ineffective treatment based on an inaccurate diagnosis.

Etiology of Depressive Disorders

Given the pervasiveness of depressive disorders, a great deal of research has been devoted to searching for answers to why some people develop the distressing symptoms of depression. Consistent with our multipath approach, we will discuss how biological, psychological, social, and sociocultural factors interact in complex ways to cause depressive disorders (Figure 8.1). For instance, we will address the complexity of interactions between genetic susceptibility, timing of stressful life events, and the type of stressors encountered. As you read, keep in mind that environmental factors have more influence on childhood depression, whereas hereditary factors have greater influence in adolescence and adulthood. The transition between middle and late adolescence is considered a time when genetic influences begin to surpass environmental influences (Gobbi et al., 2019).

Biological Dimension

Biological explanations regarding depressive disorders generally focus on neurotransmitters and stress-related hormones, genetic influences, structural or functional brain irregularities, circadian rhythm disruption, or interactions among these factors.

Neurotransmitters and Depressive Disorders Low levels of certain neurotransmitters, including serotonin, norepinephrine, and dopamine, are associated with depression (Schwasinger-Schmidt & Macaluso, 2019). When our biochemical systems are functioning normally, neurotransmitters regulate our emotions and basic physiological processes involving appetite, sleep, energy, and libido; however, biochemical irregularities can produce the physiological symptoms associated with depression. Evidence regarding the importance of neurotransmission in depression comes from a variety of sources. Years ago, it was accidentally discovered that when the drug reserpine was used to treat hypertension, many patients became

Figure 8.1

Multipath Model of Depression

The dimensions interact with one another and combine in different ways to result in depression.

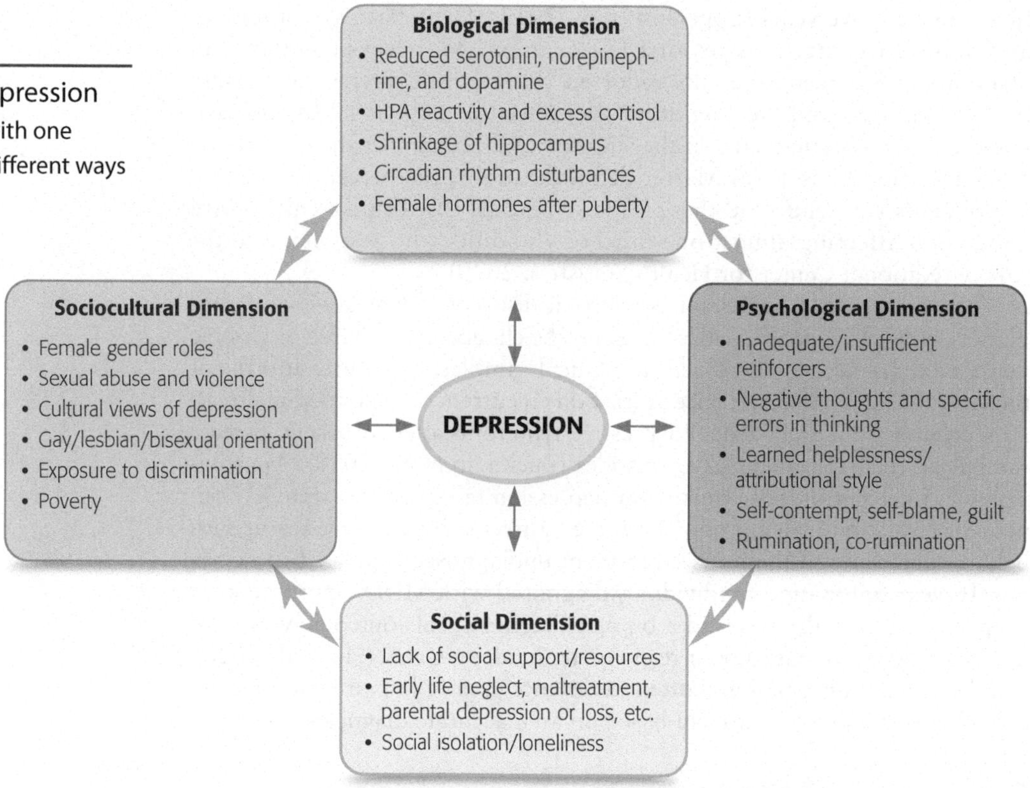

Biological Dimension
- Reduced serotonin, norepineph-rine, and dopamine
- HPA reactivity and excess cortisol
- Shrinkage of hippocampus
- Circadian rhythm disturbances
- Female hormones after puberty

Sociocultural Dimension
- Female gender roles
- Sexual abuse and violence
- Cultural views of depression
- Gay/lesbian/bisexual orientation
- Exposure to discrimination
- Poverty

DEPRESSION

Psychological Dimension
- Inadequate/insufficient reinforcers
- Negative thoughts and specific errors in thinking
- Learned helplessness/attributional style
- Self-contempt, self-blame, guilt
- Rumination, co-rumination

Social Dimension
- Lack of social support/resources
- Early life neglect, maltreatment, parental depression or loss, etc.
- Social isolation/loneliness

depressed (reserpine depletes certain neurotransmitters). Similarly, the drug isoniazid, given to patients with tuberculosis, induced biochemical changes that resulted in mood elevation (Ramachandraih et al., 2011). Findings that antidepressant medications function by increasing the availability of the neurotransmitters norepinephrine and serotonin have also pointed to the role of neurotransmission. Therapies involving electrical stimulation of brain regions that have high concentrations of brain cells that release dopamine have implicated dopamine deficiencies in depression, particularly **treatment-resistant depression** that does not respond to antidepressant medications (Conway et al., 2013).

The Role of Heredity Depression tends to run in families, and the same types of depressive disorders are often found among members of the same family. Genetics are estimated to contribute about half of the variance in susceptibility to depression (Serretti, 2017). Studies comparing the prevalence of depressive disorders among the biological and adoptive families of individuals with depression indicate that the incidence is significantly higher among biological relatives compared to adoptive family members, although the child-rearing environment exerts an equal influence on the development of major depression in children (Kendler et al., 2020). Interestingly, the chances of inheriting depression are greatest for female twins, suggesting gender differences in heritability (Goldberg, 2006). As mentioned previously, genetic influence on depression becomes most evident after puberty. As with many other mental disorders, it appears that many different genes, each with relatively small influence, interact with environmental factors to produce depression.

Cortisol, Stress, and Depression Dysregulation and overactivity of the hypothalamic-pituitary-adrenal (HPA) axis and overproduction of the stress-related hormone cortisol appear to play an important role in

Did You Know?

Chronic depression appears to increase risk of cardiovascular disease. In one study involving over 10,000 individuals who were evaluated every 5 years for over 20 years, those who had the most chronic depressive symptoms were the most likely to develop coronary heart disease.

Source: Brunner et al., 2014

the development of depression in both youth and adults (Juruena et al., 2018). Throughout the world, people with depression have higher levels of cortisol compared to those without depressive symptoms (Shapero et al., 2019). In explaining stress disorders in Chapter 6, we focused on the stress circuitry of the brain and discussed how stressors can increase levels of *cortisol*. Exposure to stress during early development and the resultant increases in cortisol production can increase susceptibility to depression in later life, especially among those who have genetic vulnerability. Many individuals with depression have early life traumas or stressors such as child abuse, neglect, or loss of a parent. In fact, researchers have linked depression to an interaction between childhood adversities and certain genes that increase cortisol release; in other words, environmental stressors appear to trigger these genes, resulting in the release of excess cortisol (Nagy et al., 2018). Thus, genetic predisposition, stress, and the timing of stress can interact to increase cortisol production and produce depressive symptoms.

Research consistently points to the harmful effects of cortisol and other stress-related hormones on biochemical functioning and neuroplasticity in brain regions associated with depression (Detka et al., 2013). But how does cortisol influence depression? The answer is complicated. We know chronic stress and associated high levels of cortisol can damage the hippocampus (i.e., neurons die and fail to regenerate) and interfere with systems involved in our stress response. In fact, excess cortisol may explain why individuals with depression have inhibited neurogenesis (birth of neurons) in the hippocampus (Alves et al., 2017).

An overactive stress response system and excessive cortisol production may also cause depressive symptoms by depleting certain neurotransmitters, particularly serotonin. Additionally, stress can affect the production of enzymes that are necessary for our brains to use serotonin effectively (Jenkins et al., 2016). Of course, these reactions can be circular—depression can result in lifestyle changes (sleep disruption, lack of exercise, alcohol use) that heighten our stress reactivity and further interfere with optimal biochemical functioning.

Functional and Anatomical Brain Changes with Depression   Neuroimaging studies document decreased brain activity and other brain changes in people with depression. For example, brain alterations have been found in the medial prefrontal cortex, anterior cingulate cortex, and hippocampus—areas associated with negative thoughts and memories, rumination, and impairment in executive functioning. These patterns, found in individuals experiencing their first depressive episode as well as in people with chronic depression, can be modified with successful treatment (Zanatta et al., 2019). Ongoing depression is associated with reduced neuroplasticity, including decreased neurogenesis in the hippocampus and in synapses within the cortex (Hayley & Litteljohn, 2013). Researchers have also found that individuals experiencing depression have increased connectivity in the brain regions referred to as the *default mode network*, regions that are associated with a wakeful resting state. Interestingly, antidepressant medications appear to normalize connectivity in this region (Posner et al., 2013).

"Faulty wiring" of emotional circuits may explain why some people experience persistent depression. A meta-analysis of neuroimaging findings concluded that individuals with depression present with different patterns of neural reactivity compared to controls; the pattern of neural activation depends on whether the emotional stimuli are positive or are negative. In some brain regions, for instance, individuals with depression demonstrate heightened activity in response to negative stimuli but reduced activation with positive stimuli (Groenewold et al., 2013). Even those who have the

Did You Know?

Researchers using functional magnetic resonance imaging (fMRI) have found that certain regions of the brain activate when people engage in self-blame. This may explain how guilt and self-blame produce neurological changes associated with depression. Further, focusing on self-kindness and self-compassion can reverse these effects.

Source: Williams et al., 2020

milder depressive symptoms associated with persistent depressive disorder have abnormalities in neurological functioning, including reduced activation in the prefrontal cortex and increased activity in the amygdala (Posner et al., 2013).

In a meta-analysis, the use of cannabis during adolescence was related to a moderately increased risk of developing depression and suicidal behavior later in life. This risk remained even for individuals who curtailed cannabis use. Among this group, neuroanatomic changes were found in areas of the brain containing cannabinoid receptors; the alterations involved decreases in volume in the hippocampus, amygdala, and prefrontal cortex, which may underlie the behavioral and cognitive symptoms of depression (Gobbi et al., 2019).

Circadian Rhythm Disturbances in Depression Our circadian rhythms appear to play a role in physiological disturbances associated with depression, particularly seasonal depression. **Circadian rhythms** are internal biological rhythms, maintained by the hormone melatonin, that influence a number of our bodily processes, including body temperature and sleeping patterns. Depression is associated with disruptions in this system, among individuals both with and without seasonal symptoms (Difrancesco et al., 2019).

Circadian rhythm disturbances affecting sleep can increase risk of depression. For example, insomnia (difficulty falling or staying asleep) increases the risk of developing depression and is related to the severity of depressive symptoms (Asarnow & Manber, 2019). In a study involving twin pairs, excessively short or long sleep duration appeared to activate genes related to depression. Compared to a 27 percent genetic risk of depression for twins with normal sleep patterns, the risk of depressive symptoms increased to 53 percent for those who averaged less than 5 hours and to 49 percent for those who slept more than 10 hours per night (Watson et al., 2014). Disrupted sleep is also linked to the onset of postpartum depression (Okun et al., 2018). Further, it has long been recognized that people with depression have irregularities in rapid eye movement (REM) sleep, the stage of sleep during which dreaming occurs. Reducing the REM sleep of people who demonstrate this pattern can reduce depressive symptoms (Wichniak et al., 2017).

Whether circadian system disturbances, hormonal or neurotransmitter abnormalities, or other brain irregularities exert the greatest influence on depressive disorders cannot be resolved at this time. It certainly appears that complex interactions between biological influences; stressful experiences; and psychological, social, and sociocultural factors influence the development of depression.

Psychological Dimension

A number of psychological theories address the etiology of depression. It is important to note that although these theories may help explain the development of depressive symptoms in some people, they are not necessarily associated with all cases of depression.

Behavioral Explanations Behavioral explanations suggest that depression occurs when people receive insufficient social reinforcement. Losses such as unemployment, divorce, or the death of a friend or family member can reduce available reinforcement (e.g., love, affection, companionship) and produce depression. Consistent with this perspective, behaviorists believe that those affected by depression can reduce their depressive symptoms if they become more physically and socially active, thereby increasing the potential for environmental reinforcement (Bewernick et al., 2017).

Behavioral perspectives regarding depression focus on variables that can increase or decrease a person's chances of receiving positive reinforcement (Lewinsohn et al., 1994). For example, risk of depression is increased when:

- *A person has limited opportunities to engage in activities that are potentially reinforcing.* Opportunities to participate in enjoyable activities may vary depending on a person's age, gender, health, or place of residence.

- *There are few reinforcements available in the person's environment.* Harsh or isolating environments contain fewer possible reinforcers, whereas warm, nurturing environments increase the likelihood of social reinforcement.

- *A person's behavior reduces the likelihood of positive social interactions.* Individuals experiencing depression are less likely to interact in a way that could increase positive reinforcement, such as making eye contact or smiling. They communicate with fewer people, respond less, and are less likely to initiate conversation.

Stressful circumstances can also produce depression by disrupting predictable patterns of social reinforcement and initiating a cycle that further reduces social opportunities and increases vulnerability to depression. For instance, when distressing events result in self-criticism, negative expectancies, and loss of self-confidence, a person may begin to withdraw from social interactions; this social withdrawal may further exacerbate depressive symptoms (Luo et al., 2020).

Paradoxically, positive attributes can also increase the risk of depression. People who are prosocial (e.g., self-sacrificing, willing to promote equality) are more likely to develop symptoms of depression compared to those who are individualist (e.g., self-centered, out for their own personal gain). This depression risk appears to be related to the fact that individuals with prosocial values experience increased stress and activation of the amygdala in situations associated with unfairness and inequality, whereas those with individualist values demonstrate this pattern when other people receive more rewards than they do. The researchers hypothesize that depression occurs more frequently in prosocial individuals because of their empathy and distress over societal inequality (Tanaka et al., 2017).

Cognitive Explanations Depression is a disturbance in thinking rather than a disturbance in mood, according to cognitive explanations of depression. In other words, our internal responses to what is happening around us and the way we interpret our experiences affect our emotions—negative thoughts and errors in thinking result in pessimism, damaging self-views, and feelings of helplessness. According to Aaron Beck's theory of depression, individuals experiencing depression tend to have a negative **self-schema** or way of looking at themselves (Beck, 1976); they have a pessimistic outlook regarding their present experiences and their expectations regarding the future (refer to Table 8.4). Thus, they may draw sweeping conclusions about their ability, performance, or worth from a single experience, or focus on trivial details of an uncomfortable situation. For instance, if no one initiates conversation at a party, someone with a negative self-schema may conclude, "People dislike me." Similarly, if a supervisor makes a minor corrective comment,

Magnification of Events

According to cognitive explanations for depression, people become depressed because of the way they interpret situations. They may overly magnify events that happen to them. In this photo, an adolescent football player sits alone in a locker room after losing a football game.

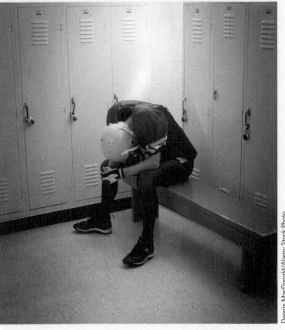

Dennis MacDonald/Alamy Stock Photo

Table 8.4 Beck's Six Types of Faulty Thinking

Arbitrary inference	Drawing conclusions about oneself or the world without sufficient and relevant information. *Example:* A person not hired by a potential employer concludes that they are "totally worthless" and that they will never find a job.
Personalization	Relating external events to one another when there is no objective basis for such a connection. *Example:* Someone who does not receive a response to an e-mail they sent to their supervisor concludes that the supervisor must dislike them.
Overgeneralization	Holding extreme beliefs on the basis of a single incident and applying these inaccurate beliefs to other situations. *Example:* A woman who does not get along with her father believes she will fail in all relationships with men.
Magnification and exaggeration	Overestimating the significance of negative events. *Example:* Someone misses an important social event at work and concludes that all of their coworkers are criticizing them for not attending.
Polarized thinking	An "all-or-nothing," "good or bad," and "either–or" approach to viewing the world. *Example:* Someone feels that they need to be perfect in all they do at work; if they make a mistake, they conclude that they are totally incompetent.
Selective abstraction	Drawing conclusions from very isolated details and events without considering the larger context. *Example:* A student who receives a C on an exam stops attending classes and considers dropping out of school despite having As and Bs in all other courses.

Source: Based on Beck, 1976

the person may focus on the possibility of losing their job, even when the supervisor's overall feedback is highly positive.

These thinking patterns may become so ingrained that they consistently affect a person's emotional reactions. Once this pattern of pessimistic thinking develops, it is easy to succumb to hopelessness and pessimism; in other words, depression can become chronic. Not surprisingly, exaggeration of personal limitations and minimization of accomplishments, achievements, and capabilities is common among those experiencing depression. Such patterns of repetitive negative thinking may increase both the severity of depressive symptoms and their persistence (Spinhoven et al., 2018).

These negative thinking patterns often lead to exaggerated, irrational, or catastrophic thinking involving self-blame and self-criticism. Confirming this line of thought, a meta-analysis involving adolescents found that when negative thinking patterns are reduced through cognitive-behavioral therapies, depression improves (Bell et al., 2023). Individuals with a negative outlook on life not only become stuck in dysfunctional thinking patterns, but also lack the psychological flexibility that would allow them to consider alternative explanations or disengage from negative thoughts (Kashdan & Rottenberg, 2010). They may also experience difficulty using positive events to regulate negative moods. Evidence of a link between cognition and depression is strengthened by studies of memory bias. Researchers testing the theory of cognitive vulnerability to depression found that even when no longer depressed, individuals with a history of depression have more thoughts that are negative and have greater recall of negative information about themselves compared to individuals who have not experienced depression (Romero et al., 2014). People with depression also display the tendency to attribute positive events to external factors and to blame themselves for negative events (Loeffler et al., 2018).

Other cognitive processes also influence depression. For example, individuals with depression often cope with stressful circumstances via rumination rather than active problem solving. Having a ruminative response style increases the likelihood of depressive symptoms among youth and adults, particularly women. As you might imagine, continually

Did You Know?

Individuals who recovered from depression indicated that therapy helped them learn to appraise events in a positive manner, feel "satisfied," cope with adversity, and avoid rumination.

Source: Hoorelbeke et al., 2019

thinking about an upsetting situation keeps the distressing emotions "alive" rather than allowing them to diminish so the person can move on (Hosseinichimeh et al., 2018). **Co-rumination**, the process of constantly talking over problems or negative events with others, also increases the risk for depression. This is most likely to occur among those who have a pattern of seeking constant reassurance from close friends, particularly during periods of high emotional distress (Schwartz-Mette & Smith, 2018). Early negative temperament may influence the tendency to ruminate and thus increase risk of depression. In a group of youth followed from birth through adolescence, negative emotionality at age 1 was associated with self-reported rumination at age 13 and depressive symptoms at ages 13 and 26; the link between rumination and depressive symptoms in this group was particularly strong for girls (Mezulis et al., 2011). Not surprisingly, adolescents and adults who have experienced stressful life events are more likely to develop a pattern of rumination (Michl et al., 2013).

Learned Helplessness and Attributional Style Our **attributional style** (how we explain events that occur in our lives) can have powerful effects on our mood, according to Martin Seligman and his colleagues (Nolen-Hoeksema et al., 1992). Specifically, they suggest that depression is more likely to occur if we display thinking patterns associated with **learned helplessness**—a belief that we have little influence over what happens to us. People who have developed an attributional style of learned helplessness often assume that nothing they do will improve their circumstances, so they give up trying to make any changes—a belief that can result in depressive symptoms.

Individuals with a pessimistic attributional style tend to focus on causes that are *internal*, *stable*, and *global*, according to research on learned helplessness. If something distressing occurs, they might conclude that it is *their* fault, that things will *always* turn out poorly, and that it will affect *all* aspects of their life. Predictably, they are more likely to experience depression. In contrast, those with a positive attributional style focus on explanations that are *external*, *unstable*, and *specific*. If something bad occurs, they may consider it a one-time event resulting from circumstances beyond their control (Loeffler et al., 2018). For instance, suppose that you received a low grade in a math class despite studying extensively. If you had a negative attributional style, you might attribute the low grade to personal factors ("*I* don't do well in math") rather than external factors ("The *teacher* didn't teach very well"). You might also assume the low grade is due to unchangeable factors ("*I'm the type of person* who will never do well in math") rather than a temporary, changeable situation ("My low math grade was due to *my heavy workload this quarter*"). Additionally, you might tend to think globally ("I'm a *lousy student*") rather than specifically ("I'm *struggling with math but am good in other subjects*"). Unfortunately, when someone develops a pattern of making these kinds of negative attributions, they are much more vulnerable to the passivity, apathy, and hopelessness associated with depression.

Factors Associated with Negative Thinking Patterns Cognitive-behavioral theories make an important contribution to understanding how depression might develop. Moreover, patterns of pessimistic thinking often interact with biological and social factors. Further, if we develop a pattern of negative thinking or ruminating, it may have a pervasive influence on the way we look at the world and interact with others.

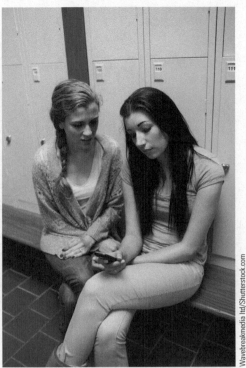

Wavebreakmedia ltd/Shutterstock.com

Talk It Over with a Friend?

People with depression often cope with negative events by ruminating or co-ruminating—constantly talking over their issues with friends. Unfortunately, both coping mechanisms increase the risk for developing depression.

Did You Know?

Among a group of individuals who survived a heart attack, higher scores on a measure of learned helplessness were associated with more depressive symptoms.
Source: Smallheer et al., 2018

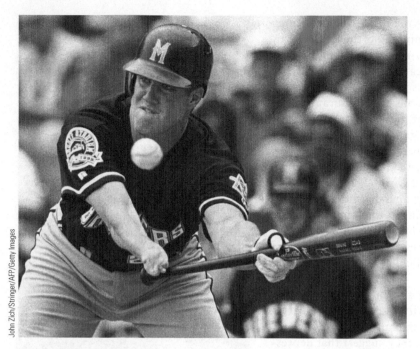
John Zich/Stringer/AFP/Getty Images

Learned Helplessness Leads to Depression

Born without a right hand, former Major League Baseball pitcher Jim Abbott overcame feelings of helplessness and won multiple awards for his determination and courage. According to Martin Seligman, feelings of helplessness can lead to depression. Jim Abbott, however, learned to persevere rather than succumb to helplessness.

As we have mentioned, maltreatment occurring during childhood is associated with increased risk of depression. Early stressful interactions with parents or caregivers may lead to negative thinking patterns. Emotional abuse and neglect in childhood may set the stage for feelings of vulnerability, shame, or inadequacy; beliefs that interpersonal needs will never be met; or expectations that loving someone will lead to rejection (Eberhart, 2011). These cognitive factors can further shape a person's expectations, perspectives, and interpretations of daily situations. Self-contempt, self-criticism, guilt, and shame may also increase vulnerability to depression because emotions such as these can interfere with the development of positive interpersonal relationships.

These maladaptive patterns of thinking are particularly destructive when they influence our self-concept. For example, self-criticism is strongly associated with depression (Zhang, Watson-Singleton, et al., 2019). Similarly, individuals who have experienced a major depressive episode are more likely to have a self-contempt bias in their thinking (a tendency to blame themselves rather than others) compared to individuals without a history of depression (Green et al., 2013). Emotions such as shame and guilt are particularly prominent in individuals with depressive episodes; in one study, individuals with MDD continued to demonstrate neural reactivity in response to thoughts of shame even after their symptoms subsided (Pulcu et al., 2014). Thus, negative thinking patterns can exert lifelong psychological, physiological, and social effects.

Social Dimension

Maltreatment such as parental rejection during early childhood is strongly associated with later depression (Johnco et al., 2021). Adverse childhood experiences (ACEs) appear to modify the expression of genes associated with the HPA axis, increase reactivity to stress, and affect the function and structure of cortical and subcortical areas of the brain (Talarowska, 2020). Further, parental depression appears to exert a strong social influence on intergenerational transmission of depression (Yap et al., 2019). Individuals who fail to develop secure attachments and trusting relationships with caregivers early in life have increased vulnerability to depression when confronted with stressful life events. Among children born by assisted conception, depression in either parent (but especially the mother) increased the likelihood of childhood depression even among children were not biologically related to the depressed parent (Lewis et al., 2011). Parental depression is associated with fewer positive and more negative parent–child interactions; this pattern appears to initiate a cascade of social and psychological risk factors that culminate in depressive symptoms.

Stressful events later in life can also increase the risk of depression. For example, severe acute stress (e.g., serious illness or death of a loved one) that results in inflammatory biological processes and cortisol production has been found to precede the onset of depression in adolescent girls (Slavich et al., 2020). Acute stress is much more likely to cause a first depressive episode than is chronic stress; however, once someone has experienced a serious depression, less severe stressors can subsequently trigger additional depressive episodes.

Chronic social stress often interacts with personal vulnerabilities to produce depression. For instance, individuals who are highly conscientious and who have chronically high levels of work stress coupled with few decision-making opportunities have increased risk of depression (Verboom et al., 2011). Unfortunately, not only does stress increase risk of depression, but depression can also increase social stress. *Stress generation* or engaging in behaviors that lead to stressful events plays an important role in depression. Some individuals increase the risk of depression by generating stressors that are within their control, such as initiating arguments (Mackin et al., 2019).

Why do some people who encounter stressful life events develop depression, whereas others do not? The relationship between stress and depression is complex and interactive. Stress itself may activate a genetic predisposition for depression. As previously discussed, people with a genetic risk have the greatest likelihood of developing depression when they have been exposed to childhood maltreatment. This may explain why some people with genetic predispositions do not develop depression (i.e., significant stressors are absent) and why someone who has encountered the same stressors as a person who becomes depressed does not experience depression (i.e., they do not have the genetic vulnerability).

Social isolation and loneliness seem to contribute to the development of depression. According to the U.S. Surgeon General's Advisory (2023), the U.S. population is undergoing an "an epidemic of loneliness and isolation." About 50 percent of U.S. adults suffer from loneliness with even higher rates reported by young adults. The risk of developing depression is twice as high among adults who report that they often feel lonely versus those who rarely or never feel lonely. Similar findings regarding loneliness and depression are reported for children and adolescents. Conversely, social connection appears to be protective against depression even among those who are at higher risk because of adverse life conditions or stressors.

Distressing social interactions also increase the likelihood of depression. For example, social rejection can lead to depressive symptoms, particularly among those who have genetic vulnerability, prior life stressors, or previous depressive episodes. Vulnerability to the effects of rejection is particularly powerful for people who react to being rebuffed with self-conscious emotions (such as shame or humiliation) or by personalizing the rejection and allowing it to influence their self-concept. Rejection sensitivity also appears to increase alertness for possible disappointing social interactions, which may further exacerbate depression (Kraines et al., 2018).

Sociocultural Dimension

Sociocultural factors found to be associated with depression include race and ethnicity, sexual orientation, and gender. Additionally, people who are struggling financially have high rates of depression. As one individual observed, "we still don't have jobs, we still don't have the things that we need . . . we're a depressed people." Individuals experiencing the lack of security and self-sufficiency associated with poverty often find it difficult, or even impossible, to access the education, employment, or housing that would allow them to envision a more hopeful future and an opportunity to escape the "cycle of poverty." In this manner, discouragement over the systemic stressors associated with chronic poverty can lead to depression (Snell-Rood & Carpenter-Song, 2018).

Can We Immunize People Against Depression?

Just as vaccines can protect people against the flu and other diseases, considerable research now suggests that various interventions can prevent or reduce depressive symptoms. For example, recognizing the strong connection between behaviors associated with depression (withdrawal, listlessness, agitation) and the learned helplessness that develops when aversive situations seem inescapable, positive psychologists have developed programs to "psychologically immunize" children against depression and to combat learned helplessness. People who learn to think optimistically (e.g., recognize how their efforts result in successful outcomes) and cope effectively with disappointments and challenges are much less likely to experience depression (Hoorelbeke et al., 2019).

The Penn Resiliency Program has concentrated on classroom teaching of cognitive-behavioral and social problem-solving skills. Premised on understandings that people's beliefs about events play a critical role in their emotional reactions and behaviors, students are taught to evaluate the accuracy of various thoughts, detect inaccurate thoughts (especially negative beliefs), and consider alternate interpretations of events. Youth also practice coping and problem-solving strategies that can be used in stressful situations (e.g., learning to relax, respond assertively, or negotiate resolutions to conflicts). Overall, the Penn Resiliency Program has had good success in reducing depressive thinking and behaviors, especially among youth with chronic and severe symptoms (Brunwasser & Gillham, 2018). A meta-analysis of resilience-oriented cognitive-behavioral interventions in school settings supported their effectiveness in reducing depressive symptoms in youth (Ma et al., 2020). Components of the programs that make the greatest contribution to a successful outcome are emotional regulation and social skills training (Skeen et al., 2019).

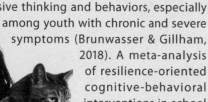

Granger Wootz/Tetra images/Getty Images

Prevention program effects are particularly impressive for high-risk populations, including youth displaying high levels of depressive symptoms (Brière et al., 2014). The outcome is further enhanced when parents are taught depression-prevention strategies (Stice et al., 2009). Programs for adolescent girls target gender-related risk factors such as media messages, negative body image, rumination, and low self-esteem. In one study, the positive effects of this approach were even greater in a mixed gender group (Agam-Bitton et al., 2018).

Other interventions that can help protect against depression include:

- *Mobilizing social support.* Friendships and family support can help youth and adults cope with difficult life circumstances and decrease the incidence of depression (Cheong et al., 2017). Participation in a religious or spiritual community is also associated with decreased risk of depression (Davis & Kiang, 2016), as is trust in neighbors and neighborhood cohesion (McCloskey & Pei, 2019).

- *Increasing positive emotions.* Participating in enjoyable or meaningful activities, reflecting on personal strengths, engaging in positive reappraisal of challenging situations, focusing on gratitude, and performing acts of kindness can significantly increase positive emotions, particularly when multiple strategies are used on an ongoing basis. These practices combined with efforts to boost one's mood by finding pleasure in daily activities ("in-the-moment" pleasure) have the potential to significantly protect against depression (Taylor et al., 2020).

- *Maintaining a healthy lifestyle.* Physical activities such as walking, jogging, weight training, or participating in sports are associated with lower depression risk (Pascoe & Parker, 2019). Exercise, eating a healthy diet (e.g., vegetables, fruit, meat, fish, nuts, legumes, and whole grains), and getting sufficient sleep (7 to 9 hours) are considered the "winning triad" in sustaining mental well-being in people who are at risk for neuropsychiatric disorders such as depression (Briguglio et al., 2020).

In summary, just as a variety of factors contribute to the development of depressive illness, a variety of protective factors can significantly reduce the risk of depression.

Racial and Ethnic Influences on Depression A person's racial or ethnic background may influence a variety of factors associated with depression: descriptions of depressive symptoms, decisions about treatment, client–therapist interactions, and the likelihood of outcomes such as suicide. In some ethnic groups, depression is often expressed in the form of somatic or bodily complaints, rather than as sadness (Giannakopoulou et al., 2021). For instance, many African American and Hispanic women report somatic symptoms when experiencing depression (Lara-Cinisomo et al., 2020).

Do triggers for depression differ among different cultural groups? Greenberger et al. (2000) gained some insight into this question by comparing factors associated with depressed mood among adolescents in China and the United States. In both cultures, certain "culture-general" stressors such as serious illness or family economic distress had similar effects on depressed mood. However, cultural differences emerged for other variables. Depressed mood among Chinese adolescents was frequently associated with poor academic performance or conflicts with parents, perhaps reflecting the Chinese cultural emphasis on family and achievement. In the case of Latinx families in the United States, acculturation conflicts between parents and their adolescent children (e.g., differences in acculturation level and perceptions of obligation to the family) are associated with depressive symptoms (Huq et al., 2016). Similarly, family conflict and intergenerational stress is a risk factor for depression among Chinese American adolescents (Juang et al., 2012). Depression among African American men appears to be associated with stressors such as discrimination, criminal justice involvement, financial insecurity, and less opportunity for upward mobility (Adams et al., 2019).

Perceived discrimination based on race or ethnicity is strongly associated with depression. In a survey conducted in 2019, African Americans had the highest rate of depression of all groups in the United States; these high levels of depression were affected by stressors resulting from racism, including being stopped, questioned, or mistreated by local police, as well as facing predictable, everyday forms of discrimination (Brooks et al., 2020). Given the frequency with which African Americans encounter systemic racism and overt acts of discrimination, it is not surprising that many members of this group experience frequent or persistent depressive episodes; unfortunately, many do not have sufficient trust in the medical establishment to seek treatment (Kim et al., 2015).

Latinx Americans also experience a relatively high prevalence of perceived discrimination and depressive symptoms. Perceived racial discrimination is associated with lower self-esteem and the presence of depressive symptoms among Latinx adolescents (Zeiders et al., 2013). Ethnic-based bullying also increases the likelihood of depression in Latinx children and youth (Lutrick et al., 2020). Not surprisingly, Latinx high school students have high rates (33.7 percent) of experiencing "persistent feeling of sadness and hopelessness" (CDC, 2018a). Among foreign and U.S. born Latinx adults, perceived discrimination and high levels of worry appear to increase depressive symptoms (Zvolensky et al., 2019). However, nurturing community and family relationships are often successful in increasing psychological resilience and lessening the impact of discrimination (Garcini et al., 2020).

Influences of Sexual and Gender Orientation on Depression

Case Study Gabriel, a 24-year-old college upperclassman, began therapy complaining of depressed mood and high anxiety, as well as guilt and disappointment regarding his failure to complete his undergraduate degree on time while his parents continued to pay for his education. . . . Gabriel had experienced anxieties about school when he was an adolescent, in addition to a depressive episode that he attributed to anticipated difficulties in revealing that he was gay to his family. Gabriel insisted that this latter problem had been resolved, in spite of the fact that he had never disclosed his sexual orientation to his father. (Newman, 2010, pp. 25–26)

Societal stressors such as prejudice and discrimination related to identifying as lesbian, gay, bisexual, transgender, or questioning (LGBTQ) can also result in depression. LGBTQ individuals face challenges such as societal, social, family, and personal rejection that may predispose them to the development of higher rates of depression than their non-LGBTQ peers (Johnson et al., 2019). In a national study of college students, 50 percent of transgender or gender nonconforming (TGNC) students had received a diagnosis of depression sometime in their lives (American College Health Association [ACHA], 2022).

As you might expect, lack of family acceptance, bullying, and societal rejection exert a significant effect on the risk of depression in LGBTQ youth (Johnson et al., 2019). TGNC youth often encounter gender-based discrimination and stigmatizing messages associated with their gender identity not only from strangers, but also from family and friends. In one sample of TGNC youth, 33 percent met the criteria for MDD. Those with high levels of internalized transphobia were the most likely to experience depression (Chodzen et al., 2019).

Depression is often associated with a common stressor faced by LGBTQ adolescents and young adults—how and when to disclose their gender identity or sexual orientation to family and friends. As we saw with Gabriel, the decision to *come out* is complex and can create fear of rejection and feelings of social isolation. However, remaining silent about one's sexual orientation or gender identity can result in personal distress and may indirectly affect relationships with friends and family. Unfortunately, negative reactions that sometimes occur during the disclosure process can further increase the risk of depression (Chaney et al., 2011). The prevalence of attempted suicide is much greater for gay, lesbian, or bisexual adolescents compared to their heterosexual peers (21.5 percent vs. 4.2 percent), particularly among youth who report an unsupportive social environment with respect to sexual orientation (Hatzenbuehler, 2011).

Gender and Depressive Disorders Depression is nearly twice as common among women than among men, regardless of region of the world, race and ethnicity, or social class (Salk et al., 2017). In a national study of U.S. college students, 25 percent of the women who responded had received a diagnosis of depression sometime in their lives compared to 12.5 percent of the men (American College Health Association, 2022). Some researchers suggest that the higher prevalence of depression in women is due to sociological variables such as poverty, violence, restrictive gender roles, and discrimination (Salk et al., 2017). Others wonder if women are simply more likely to seek treatment or to discuss their depression with physicians or those conducting surveys regarding emotional well-being.

Some mental health professionals contend that men are as likely as women to experience depression. They suggest that gender disparities in depression rates result from the fact that traditional symptoms of depression (such as sadness and hopelessness) are more likely to be displayed by women, whereas men who are depressed are more likely to display symptoms such as anger, aggression, burying themselves in their work, or substance abuse (Martin et al., 2013). However, evidence suggests that women do, in fact, have higher rates of depression compared to men and

Cultural Differences in Symptoms and Treatment

People from different cultures vary in the ways they express depression. Individuals of Chinese descent often report somatic or bodily complaints instead of psychological symptoms, such as sadness or loss of pleasure. They also are more likely to rely on Chinese medicine and acupuncture to treat their symptoms.

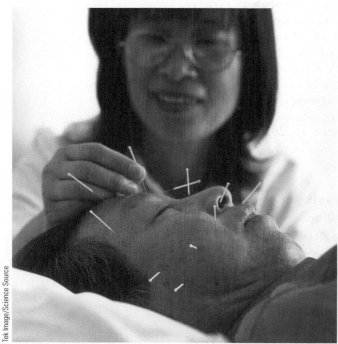

that the differences are real rather than an artifact of self-reports, biases, or externalization of symptoms (Salk et al., 2016). Attempts to explain these differences have focused on physiological, social, and psychological factors (Table 8.5).

Gender differences in depression begin appearing during adolescence and are greatest during the reproductive years. Variations in hormone levels that begin in puberty and continue until menopause appear to influence the development of depression in adolescent girls and women. For instance, many women experience more physiological and stress reactivity just prior to menstruation, suggesting that hormonal factors associated with the menstrual cycle may increase depressive symptoms (Hoyer et al., 2013). Not surprisingly, girls who experience early physical maturity are at particular risk of depression (Hoyt et al., 2020). Additionally, up to 13 percent of women experience depressive mood changes associated with pregnancy (Breese-McCoy, 2011). Menopause is another occasion when women are particularly vulnerable to severe depression, especially when menopause is combined with poor health or negative views regarding aging (Soares, 2019).

Life stressors may interact with physiological factors to influence the development of depression in girls and women. Among a group of children who had undergone early traumatic experiences (such as death, divorce, violence, sexual abuse, or illness), both boys and girls displayed alterations in connectivity in the fear circuitry of the brain (less connectivity between the hippocampus and prefrontal cortex). However, the girls' brains had additional irregularities—reduced connectivity between the amygdala and hippocampus, which may reduce inhibition of fear responses and increase emotional reactivity (Herringa et al., 2013). Although these brain differences most likely represent neuroplastic accommodations designed to allow individuals who experience early life stress to adapt to their environment, these biological changes are linked with both anxiety and depression. Additionally, girls and women have increased risk of encountering certain environmental stressors such as sexual abuse that produce ongoing changes in physiological reactivity; as might be expected, sexual abuse has a strong association with lifetime risk of depression, particularly persistent depression (Garcia-Toro et al., 2013).

Social or psychological factors related to traditional gender roles can also influence the development of depressive disorders. Specifically, social modeling and socialization practices can influence feelings of self-worth.

Table 8.5 Possible Explanations for the Higher Frequency of Depression Among Women

- Women may be more willing to acknowledge and seek help for depression.
- Genetic or hormonal differences may result in higher rates of depression among women.
- Women are subjected to societal factors such as gender role expectations or unequal career opportunities that lead to feelings of helplessness or hopelessness.
- Cognitive styles that increase depression (such as ruminating or co-ruminating) are more common in women.
- Women are more likely to have experienced childhood trauma (sexual abuse, childhood maltreatment) and other stressors associated with depression.

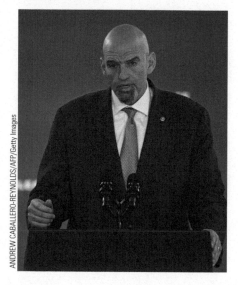

ANDREW CABALLERO-REYNOLDS/AFP/Getty Images

While boys are socialized to strive for autonomy and achievement-oriented goals, girls are encouraged to value social goals and interdependent functioning (e.g., caring about others, not wanting to hurt people's feelings). Therefore, the opinions of others are more likely to influence the self-perceptions of women; this may increase their vulnerability to interpersonal stress, particularly stressors involving close friends or family. Interestingly, some researchers suggest that gender socialization and early social learning also affect gender differences in the regulation and metabolism of stress hormones (Neitzke, 2016). The way women respond to depressed moods also contributes to the severity, chronicity, and frequency of depressive episodes, suggests Nolen-Hoeksema (2012). In her view, women tend to ruminate and amplify their depressive moods, whereas men often find ways to minimize sad feelings through methods such as drinking alcohol. As we have mentioned, rumination is linked to increases in depressive symptoms.

Treatment for Depression

Finding the correct treatment or combination of treatments for depression is very important, because longer depressive episodes are associated with negative long-term outcomes, more frequent depressive episodes, and reduced likelihood of symptom improvement. If depression does not respond to treatment, it is important to inquire about hypomanic/manic symptoms to ensure that the person does not have an undiagnosed bipolar disorder (McIntyre & Calabrese, 2019). We now turn to various treatment strategies used with depressive disorders.

Biomedical Treatments for Depressive Disorders

Biomedical treatments include the use of medication and other interventions that affect various brain systems, such as circadian-related treatments and brain stimulation techniques.

Medication Antidepressant medications increase the availability of certain neurotransmitters. Three classes of antidepressants—the *tricyclics, monoamine oxidase inhibitors* (MAOIs), and *serotonin-norepinephrine reuptake inhibitors* (SNRIs)—block the reabsorption of norepinephrine and serotonin, whereas the *selective serotonin reuptake inhibitors* (SSRIs) block the reuptake of serotonin. *Atypical antidepressants*, a group of unique antidepressant medications, affect other neurotransmitters, including dopamine. Medications within each class are similar in their chemical makeup, but they often differ in their side effects and effectiveness.

Medical providers consider a variety of factors when deciding which antidepressant to prescribe for someone experiencing depression. For example, they take into account the presence of other symptoms (such as anxiety, overeating, or nicotine addiction) that might also be helped by certain antidepressants. They also consider variables such as the person's prior response to antidepressants (or family patterns of response) or desire to avoid certain side effects such as weight gain, sexual side effects, or gastrointestinal problems. The American College of Physicians recommends either cognitive-behavioral therapy or an antidepressant as initial treatment for the acute phase of moderate to severe major depressive disorder. When someone is

Did You Know?

The following rankings were based on prevalence of adults who have ever experienced depression.

Most Depression	Least Depression
1. West Virginia (29%)	1. Hawaii (11.4%)
2. Kentucky (27.6%)	2. California (15.3%)
3. Vermont (26.6%)	3. Maryland (17.2%)
4. Tennessee (26%)	4. South Dakota (17.2%)
5. Arkansas (25.4%)	5. Illinois (17.3%)

Source: Haines (2023)

not responding to initial treatment for depression, a different antidepressant or another type of medication may be added to effect change (Qaseem et al., 2023).

An estimated one third to one half of those who are prescribed antidepressants discontinue their use of the medication due to side effects, often without informing the prescriber. Abrupt discontinuation of antidepressants is associated with withdrawal symptoms such as dizziness, drowsiness, impaired balance, headache, insomnia, confusion, and irritability. Many who discontinue antidepressants find that their depressive symptoms recur, often with greater severity than before taking the medication (Henssler et al., 2019). Researchers who reviewed the literature on this topic found that up to 41 percent of those who discontinued antidepressant medications had a recurrence of depression (Scholten et al., 2020). One of the most concerning side effects involving antidepressants is the possibility of increased risk of suicidality among children, adolescents, and young adults who are prescribed an SSRI (Spielmans et al., 2020).

Despite the popularity of antidepressants, there are many questions about their effectiveness. First, publication bias in research and methodological design flaws involving antidepressant medication is a significant concern. One review of studies evaluating the effectiveness of antidepressants found that although 94 percent of the studies supportive of antidepressants were published and in the public domain, many of the studies that did not support the effectiveness of antidepressants were never published or were written in a manner that gave the false impression of a positive antidepressant outcome (Turner et al., 2008). In a meta-analysis of 522 studies involving antidepressants, one researcher observed, "Publication bias of antidepressant trials is pervasive and distorts the evidence base." The reviewers concluded that due to the pervasiveness of bias, it was difficult to determine if antidepressants do, in fact, have any more benefit than placebo for depression (Munkholm et al., 2019).

Even with this publication bias, the research evidence for antidepressant efficacy is rather weak. In fact, many individuals affected by depression experience little to no improvement with antidepressant medications (MacQueen et al., 2017). Placebos are often as effective as antidepressants in treating mild depression. In fact, a comprehensive study evaluating the effectiveness of antidepressant medication concluded that the benefit of these medications over placebo for treating mild or moderate depression was "minimal" or "nonexistent" (Lewis et al., 2019). In contrast, one large meta-analysis provided support for the effectiveness of antidepressants with premenstrual syndrome and premenstrual dysphoric disorder, although side effects were commonly reported (Marjoribanks et al., 2013). Even when antidepressants are effective, however, they do not cure depression; that is, once medication is stopped, symptoms often return.

Adjunctive treatments (adding something different to the initial treatment) are commonly used to supplement antidepressant use. A trend among prescribers is to add other medications, particularly antipsychotics such as aripiprazole (Abilify) and quetiapine (Seroquel), to boost the effectiveness of antidepressants. Although this adjunctive therapy sometimes produces mild to moderate improvement, caution is urged due to potential side effects of these powerful medications and because the added medication often does not significantly improve a person's quality of life (Spielmans et al., 2013). In fact, one study of adults being treated for depression found that augmenting antidepressants with antipsychotic medication was associated with a 45 percent increased risk of mortality compared to augmenting with a second antidepressant (Gerhard et al., 2020).

The Antidepressant–Suicidality Link: Does the Risk Outweigh the Benefit?

In 2004, the U.S. Food and Drug Administration (FDA) required manufacturers of SSRI antidepressants to provide warnings regarding the possibility of increased risk for suicidal thinking and behavior in children and adolescents taking these medications. In 2007, the FDA expanded the warning to include those ages 18 to 24. The FDA (2007) warned:

> Antidepressants increased the risk compared to placebo of suicidal thinking and behavior in children, adolescents, and young adults in short-term studies of major depressive disorder (MDD) and other psychiatric disorders. . . . All patients being treated with antidepressants for any indication should be monitored appropriately and observed closely for clinical worsening, suicidality, and unusual changes in behavior, especially during the initial few months of a course of drug therapy, or at times of dose changes, either increases or decreases.

Although the data cited by the FDA concluded that suicidal thoughts and behaviors occurred among 4 percent of youth taking antidepressants compared to 2 percent of those taking placebo, some claim that the benefits of using FDA-approved SSRIs in children and adolescents with moderate to severe depression outweigh the risk of suicide and believe the "black box" warning should be removed (Soutullo & Figueroa-Quintana, 2013).

The debate regarding the effect of SSRIs on suicidal thoughts and behavior among those younger than age 25 continues. A comprehensive analysis of data from 12 years of studies on antidepressant use in children and young adults revealed that the suicidal behaviors occurred primarily among youth started on higher-than-average dosages of antidepressants. The authors cautioned clinicians to avoid excessive antidepressant doses and to monitor any young person taking antidepressants for signs of suicidality (Miller et al., 2014). Another group of researchers performed a careful examination of the methodological design of the antidepressant research and concluded that the better-designed studies do, in fact, support an increase in suicidality in youth taking antidepressants and that the black box warning was valid and should remain (Spielmans et al., 2020). Most professionals agree that it is important for treatment providers to remain alert for suicidal ideation in anyone who is depressed, especially during the first months of antidepressant treatment.

For Further Consideration

1. What is your opinion about the FDA warnings regarding antidepressant prescriptions for youth?

2. What factors should be considered when diagnosing and treating children, adolescents, and young adults experiencing depression?

Did You Know?

Almost half (46 percent) of those who responded to an Internet survey regarding depression reported that taking antidepressants had produced a dampening of all emotions, indifference, and feelings of emotional detachment. Among those who experienced this emotional blunting, approximately one third were pleased with this medication side effect.

Source: Goodwin et al., 2017

Omega-3 fatty acid supplements have been found to reduce depressive symptoms and are often used in combination with antidepressant medications (Bozzatello et al., 2019). Further, for many individuals who do not fully respond to antidepressant medication, participating in moderate to intense levels of daily exercise can significantly reduce residual symptoms of depression as well as improve sleep quality and cognitive functioning (Gourgouvelis et al., 2018).

Intravenous administration of the anesthetic ketamine has yielded some promising results for treatment-resistant depression—alleviating the symptoms in some individuals living with severe depression and suicidality in a matter of hours as opposed to the weeks required for antidepressants to become evident. However, intravenous ketamine does not have FDA approval for treating depression, and—due to its addictive properties and side effects such as dissociation, sense of detachment, and "out of the body" experiences—concerns have been raised about this off-label use of a powerful anesthetic. In 2019, the FDA gave fast-track approval for the restricted use of esketamine (a derivative of ketamine delivered via nasal spray) for treatment-resistant depression; this medication, which can be administered only in a hospital or medical office, requires close medical monitoring for several hours after administration. Esketamine has a "black box" warning because side effects such as sedation; difficulty with attention, judgment, and thinking; abuse and misuse; or suicidal thoughts and behaviors are possible (Chen, 2019).

Nontraditional Treatments for Depression Some treatments for depression involve efforts to reset the circadian clock. For example, a night of total sleep deprivation followed by a night of sleep recovery has improved depressive symptoms in some individuals with MDD (Bunney et al., 2015). Additionally, use of specially designed lights is an effective and well-tolerated treatment for those with a seasonal pattern of depression. This therapy involves dawn-light simulation (timer-activated lights that gradually increase in brightness) or daily use of a box, visor, or lighting system that delivers light of a particular intensity for a designated period of time (Nussbaumer-Streit et al., 2019). A well-designed study evaluating treatment for seasonal depression compared light therapy alone to light therapy combined with antidepressants; although both groups made similar improvement (67 percent experienced improvement and approximately half experienced remission of symptoms), light therapy alone produced more rapid improvement and fewer side effects (Lam et al., 2006). Given the comparable effects on seasonal depressive symptoms when comparing light therapy with antidepressants, it appears that light therapy is a viable alternative for people who would prefer to avoid unnecessary medication (Forneris et al., 2019).

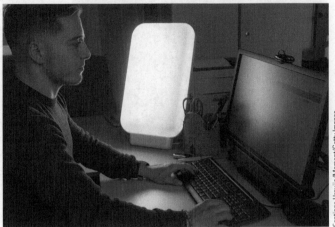

Santiago Urquijo/Moment/Getty Images

The use of probiotics to treat depression has also gained attention following animal and human studies that demonstrate a relationship between the microbiota-gut-brain (MGB) axis, gut microbiota, and MDD. Probiotic use has yielded some promising results in treating depression, but there is a need for further research using well-designed studies (Yong et al., 2020).

Brain Stimulation Therapies Electroconvulsive therapy, vagus nerve stimulation, and deep brain and transcranial magnetic stimulation are sometimes used to treat severe treatment-resistant depression, especially when life-threatening symptoms such as refusal to eat or intense suicidal intent are present. All of these brain stimulation therapies are promising but, unfortunately, their efficacy is based on research with small sample sizes (Makhoul et al., 2021; Munkholm, 2019).

Electroconvulsive therapy (ECT) involves applying moderate electrical voltage to a person's brain in order to produce a very brief seizure; patients undergo anesthesia and are typically treated several times weekly (Bahji et al., 2019). Although ECT has approval from the FDA for use with treatment-resistant depression, the effectiveness of ECT is generally based on low-quality, poorly designed studies, according to a review of meta-analytic studies focused on this procedure. Based on their careful review of the literature, the researchers argued that the use of ECT should be suspended until well-designed studies provide clear support for its benefits, particularly given the frequent occurrence of memory loss as well as the risk of death (Read et al., 2019).

The FDA has also approved vagus nerve stimulation for people with chronic, recurrent depression that has not responded to at least four prior treatment attempts. This technique involves implanting a pacemaker-like device in the chest that then delivers a frequent electronic impulse that

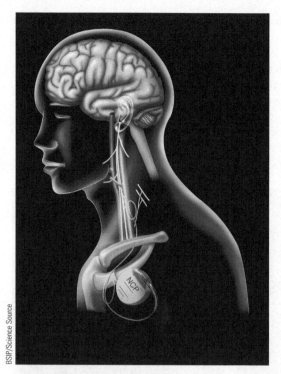

BSIP/Science Source

Treating Depression with Vagus Nerve Stimulation

Vagus nerve stimulation is a newer treatment for severe depression that does not respond to other treatment methods. A neurostimulator, surgically implanted under the skin on the chest, is connected to the left vagus nerve. When activated, the device sends electrical signals along the vagus nerve to the brainstem, which then sends signals to other areas of the brain.

travels from the vagus nerve to the brain. This method of stimulating the vagus nerve has produced improvement in some individuals with treatment-resistant depression (Senova, Rabu, et al., 2019).

Another FDA-approved technique used with treatment-resistant depression is repetitive transcranial magnetic stimulation (rTMS). This noninvasive treatment, which uses magnetic pulses to stimulate specific areas of the brain, has produced moderate improvement in treatment-resistant depression and in maintaining remission of depressive symptoms. The treatment is usually provided 5 days per week over a period of 4 to 6 weeks (Blumberger et al., 2018). Although a meta-analysis concluded that this technique has sufficient research for use with treatment-resistant depression, it is important to note that many patients undergoing a sham procedure also experienced reductions in depression, suggesting the presence of a strong placebo response (Sehatzadeh et al., 2019). Two industry-sponsored research studies comparing rTMS with a sham rTMS procedure found significantly higher positive response rates for rTMS (24 percent and 37 percent) compared to the positive responses from the sham procedure (15 percent and 28 percent); in contrast, a nationally funded study (with no industry ties) found a disappointing positive response rate of 15 percent using rTMS compared to 5 percent with a sham rTMS procedure (McClintock et al., 2018).

Psychological and Behavioral Treatments for Depressive Disorders

Four approaches (behavioral activation, interpersonal therapy, cognitive-behavioral therapy, and mindfulness-based cognitive therapy) have received extensive research support for treating depression. They are considered to be "well-established interventions" (Weersing et al., 2017). As you will see, psychological therapies are continuing to evolve by incorporating techniques from a variety of perspectives. Further, in contrast to the time-limited gains that often occur with antidepressant medication, a variety of psychotherapeutic approaches appear to provide long-lasting relief from depression. That is, effective psychological treatment appears to produce enduring results, whereas medication produces relief from depressive symptoms only during active treatment (Hollon et al., 2019).

Behavioral Activation Therapy Behavioral activation therapy, based on principles of operant conditioning, focuses on helping those who are depressed to increase their participation in enjoyable activities and social interactions—an intervention that subsequently leads to improvements in mood (Dondé et al., 2018). This emphasis is very important because individuals with depression often lack the motivation to participate in social activities. Behavioral activation therapy is based on the idea that depression results from diminished reinforcement. Consistent with this perspective, treatment focuses on increasing exposure to pleasurable events and activities, improving social skills, and facilitating social interactions (Luo et al., 2020). The steps involved in treatment include:

1. identifying and rating different activities in terms of the pleasure or the feelings of self-confidence they might produce;

2. performing some of the selected activities, thereby increasing feelings of pleasure or mastery;

3. identifying day-to-day problems and developing strategies to deal with them; and

4. improving social and assertiveness skills.

Because of the focus on actions that a depressed individual can take rather than talking about problems, this approach is also effective with people from various countries and ethnic backgrounds (Kanter et al., 2012).

Interpersonal Psychotherapy   Interpersonal psychotherapy is an evidence-based treatment focused on current interpersonal problems. Because this approach presumes that depression occurs within an interpersonal context, therapy focuses on relationship issues. Clients learn to evaluate their role in interpersonal conflict and make positive changes in their relationships. By improving communication, identifying role conflicts, and increasing social skills, clients experience more satisfying interactions. Although interpersonal psychotherapy acknowledges the role of early life experiences and trauma, it is oriented primarily toward present, not past, relationships. It has proven to be an efficacious treatment for acute depression; in one study, the symptom reduction was maintained during a 24-month follow-up (Lemmens et al., 2019).

Cognitive-Behavioral Therapy   Cognitive-behavioral therapy (CBT) focuses on altering the negative thought patterns and distorted thinking associated with depression. Cognitive therapists teach clients to identify thoughts that precede upsetting emotions, distance themselves from these thoughts, and examine the accuracy of their beliefs. Clients learn to recognize negative, self-critical thinking and the connection between negative thoughts and negative feelings. They then learn to replace inaccurate beliefs with realistic interpretations. This method of cognitive change has robust research support for the reduction of depressive symptoms (Fitzpatrick et al., 2020). CBT has effectively helped adolescents from diverse backgrounds (Brown et al., 2019), and adapted versions of the therapy are used in non-Western cultures (Khan et al., 2019).

Individuals treated with CBT are less likely to relapse after treatment has stopped compared to individuals taking antidepressants. Adding CBT as an adjunct to medication decreased depressive symptoms in one group of people with treatment-resistant depression—improvement that was maintained at a 12-month follow-up (Nakagawa et al., 2017). Changes in explanatory styles and alterations in negative self-biases may help prevent recurrence of depressive symptoms. Interestingly, a review of brain imaging studies documenting the specific brain changes associated with CBT suggests that many of the neuroplastic modifications associated with CBT involve the anterior cingulate cortex; this finding supports the hypothesis that a significant aspect of CBT is the improved emotional regulation that results from "top down" control of emotions (Franklin et al., 2016).

Abbreviated forms of CBT have also proven effective in reducing depression, including brief training to strengthen cognitive reappraisal so

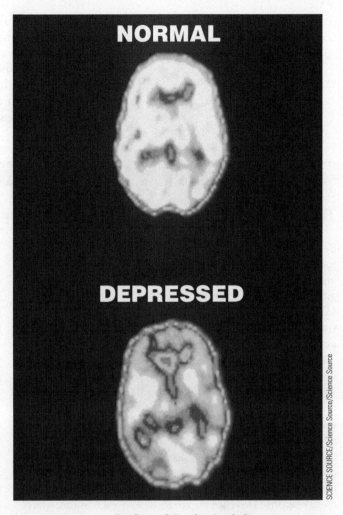

NORMAL

DEPRESSED

Reduced Brain Activity in Depression

These positron emission tomography (PET) scans comparing normal brain activity with the cerebral metabolism of a person with depression demonstrate the same decreased brain activity seen in depressive disorders. Researchers hope that brain scans will soon guide treatment for depressive and bipolar disorders.

that negative thoughts and events are evaluated within a more realistic framework (Shapero et al., 2019). The use of computerized skill-building and cognitive retraining sessions has broadened the reach of CBT skills to a wider audience (Newby et al., 2017). Cognitive bias modification—a guided self-help intervention aimed at minimizing rumination and over-generalization and enhancing specific problem-solving skills—is another low-cost, accessible treatment for depression (Watkins et al., 2012).

Technological Interventions for Depression

Because depression is so prevalent, many researchers have focused on new approaches to early detection and the provision of treatment. One such project involves the use of an artificial intelligence–enabled chatbot for depression screening. The chatbot asked study participants a series of questions (derived from depression inventories) as if it were an actual person conversationally asking the questions. About 79 percent of the participants reported feeling fully satisfied with and engaged with the screening process. The researchers concluded that the use of AI chatbots appears to provide an efficient means of screening for depression in a cost-effective manner (Kaywan et al., 2023). In another study comparing patient preference for online responses generated by an AI chatbot versus an actual physician, the AI answers to patients' questions or comments were preferred by a 4 to 1 ratio. Chatbot responses were rated much higher in empathy and quality of response (Ayers et al., 2023). Results such as these have led to this question: Can AI technology such as this serve as a standalone or as an adjunct screening intervention for individuals experiencing mental health challenges?

Computer-based therapies, which have proven successful in treating anxiety disorders, are now being used in the treatment of depression. Advocates of this approach point to the research supporting the accessibility and effectiveness of these interventions as well as the large number of people with depression who would not otherwise receive any treatment (Wright et al., 2022). A meta-analysis of various studies using computer-based CBT with adults found therapy effects that were equal to face-to-face CBT and superior to attention-only control conditions; symptom improvement continued beyond the treatment period, and satisfaction with treatment was good. Computer-assisted CBT modules have helped prevent depression relapse for up to 2 years after the intervention (Andrews et al., 2010).

Similar positive results occur for children and adolescents participating in computer-based CBT interventions designed to prevent and treat depression. Establishing a format that is interesting for this age group is important, since adherence to traditional Web-based educational formats tends to be low (Achilles et al., 2020). Many of the programs are designed to be engaging, and some programs have been culturally adapted based on suggestions from racially and ethnically diverse youth (Wozney et al., 2017). One interactive computer program designed for adolescents with depression involves participants choosing an avatar to represent themselves in a fantasy world. Participants undertake a series of challenges to restore balance in a world in which GNATs (gloomy, negative, automatic thoughts) rule. Modules in the program focus on finding hope, staying active, dealing with emotions, solving problems, and recognizing and challenging unhelpful thoughts. An avatar guide in the fantasy provides information about the coping strategies needed to move to the next level. Participants who learned strategies to combat negative thoughts and cope with problems though this program made as much progress in reducing depressive symptoms as participants who received face-to-face counseling with a therapist (Merry et al., 2012).

More research is needed to determine the most appropriate use of computer-based interventions and chatbots in screening for and treating depression. One concern expressed about online interventions is that because the programs lack face-to-face contact, there is no clinician to identify signs of severe depression, hypomanic or manic symptoms, or suicidality. Additionally, high dropout rates and failure to complete the full computer intervention are an ongoing concern, particularly with youth or adults who have more severe depressive symptoms (Fleming, Gillham, et al., 2019). Data from behavior change research and input from participants may help researchers develop techniques and modes of delivery that maximize adherence and long-term change (Fleming, Stasiak, et al., 2019).

For Further Consideration

1. What do you consider to be the advantages and disadvantages of AI chatbots and computer-based treatment for assessing mental health needs and treating depression?

2. Do you believe that these limited-contact interventions are a safe alternative for screening for and treating depression, a disorder consistently associated with risk of suicidality?

Mindfulness-Based Cognitive Therapy Mindfulness-based cognitive therapy (MBCT) involves calm awareness of one's present experience, thoughts, and feelings, and promotes an attitude of acceptance rather than judgment, evaluation, or rumination. Mindfulness allows those affected by depression to disrupt the cycle of negative thinking by directing attention to the present moment. Focusing on experiences with curiosity and without judgment prevents the development of maladaptive beliefs and thus reduces depressive thinking (Twohig & Levin, 2017). Additionally, the increases in positive emotions and focus on appreciation of pleasant daily activities appear to have a protective effect against depressive relapse. A randomized clinical trial that assessed supplementing treatment as usual (antidepressant medication and medical monitoring) with the use of a Web-based MBCT app in a group of adults with residual depressive symptoms found that the addition of MBCT resulted in an increased likelihood of remission of depressive symptoms and lower relapse rates compared to those receiving treatment as usual (Segal et al., 2020).

A variant of MBCT is acceptance and commitment therapy (ACT), which incorporates an additional component of encouraging clients to commit to making behavioral changes that are consistent with the individual's needs and values. Clinical studies have found that ACT reduces residual symptoms in chronic depression, is effective in treatment-resistant depression, and lessens the risk of recurrence of depressive symptoms (Østergaard et al., 2020). A promising new approach, Augmented Depression Therapy (AdepT), uses many of the techniques from CBT, behavioral activation therapy, and ACT, but focuses primarily on building a sense of well-being and the ability to experience pleasure, meaning, and connection in life. While many behavioral therapies do a good job of repairing negative mood, they neglect enhancing the clients' positive mood states. In a pilot study, 80 percent of the depressed clients who participated in AdepT no longer met the diagnostic criteria for depression versus 56 percent of the clients treated with "traditional" CBT. These improvements were maintained in an 18-month follow-up (Dunn et al., 2023).

8-3 Bipolar Disorders

Up to this point, we have discussed disorders that involve only depressive symptoms. In this section, we discuss bipolar disorders, a group of disorders that involve episodes of hypomania and mania (refer to Table 8.6) that may alternate with episodes of depression. Although depressive symptoms occur in bipolar disorders, depressive disorders and bipolar disorders are very different conditions. First, bipolar disorders have a very strong genetic component. In fact, there is strong evidence of physiological overlap (i.e., shared biological etiology) between bipolar disorders and schizophrenia (Liebers et al., 2020), a severe mental health disorder involving loss of contact with reality, which we discuss extensively in Chapter 12. Second, people with bipolar disorders respond to medications that have little effect with depressive disorders; in fact, individuals with bipolar disorders often have detrimental experiences if they are prescribed antidepressants prior to a correct diagnosis. Third, the peak age of onset is somewhat earlier for bipolar disorders (teens and early 20s) than for depressive disorders (late 20s). And finally, bipolar disorders occur much less frequently than depressive disorders (refer to Figure 8.2).

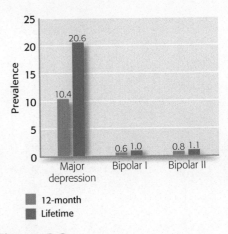

Figure 8.2

12-Month and Lifetime U.S. Prevalence of Major Depressive and Bipolar Disorders

Source: Based on Hasin et al., 2018; Merikangas et al., 2011

Table 8.6 DSM-5-TR Criteria for a Hypomanic or Manic Episode

Hypomanic and manic episodes involve *a distinct period of abnormally and persistently elevated, expansive, or irritable mood and abnormally and persistently increased activity or energy.*

In addition, the person exhibits at least three of the following symptoms (four are required if the mood is irritable rather than elevated or expansive):

1. *Exaggerated self-esteem or feelings of grandiosity and extreme self-importance*
2. *Decreased need for sleep; feeling rested after minimal sleep*
3. *Unusually talkative or seems pressured to keep talking*
4. *Racing thoughts or frequent change of topics or ideas*
5. *Distractibility that may involve attention to unimportant environmental stimuli*
6. *Increased social or work-related goal-directed activity, sexual activity, or physical restlessness*
7. *Impulsive involvement in activities that may have negative consequences (e.g., excessive spending, sexual promiscuity, gambling)*

A hypomanic episode involves continuation of these symptoms for at least 4 consecutive days.

A manic episode involves continuation of these symptoms for at least 1 week (or less if psychiatric hospitalization occurs and shortens the duration of the episode). The manic symptoms are severe enough to require hospitalization or to result in impairment in social or work functioning. Psychotic symptoms may be present.

In both hypomanic and manic episodes, the symptoms are not due to the physiological effects of a medical condition, a prescribed medication, or drug or alcohol abuse.

Source: APA, 2022

Diagnosis and Classification of Bipolar Disorders

Bipolar disorders are diagnosed when careful assessment confirms the presence of hypomanic or manic symptoms. The clinician also inquires about the severity and pattern of any depressive symptoms. Although clinicians are also interested in the frequency of normal mood states, they differentiate between the bipolar diagnostic categories by reviewing the severity of depressive and hypomanic/manic symptoms and the pattern of mood changes. The three types of bipolar disorders are bipolar I, bipolar II, and cyclothymic disorder (refer to Table 8.7).

Bipolar I Disorder

Case Study It took ten years, a suicide attempt, an acute manic episode, and a psychotic break for me to finally get an accurate diagnosis of bipolar disorder. By that time, I was 29, and I had already graduated law school, passed the bar, earned a Master's in Public Health, published my first book and won an award for it. . . . It took roughly a month for me to believe and acknowledge my diagnosis. The antipsychotics worked remarkably fast, and soon, I was confronting the reality of my hallucinations, delusions, and erratic and irrational behavior from the perspective of someone who was neither acutely manic nor psychotic. I couldn't very well deny the diagnosis after looking back at the things I'd done while manic: disrobing in public, yelling obscenities at an infant, trying to give away all my money and belongings—and that's not even the half of it. . . . I'm now able to make a living as a full-time writer. . . . I'm not cured by any stretch. I struggle with this illness every day. . . . Living with bipolar disorder, writing and speaking about it, and gaining strength from others who share in this fight, I've learned never to underestimate the power of compassion, perseverance, resilience and faith. (Moezzi, 2014)

Table 8.7 Bipolar Disorders

DSM-5-TR Disorders Chart				
Disorder	**DSM-5-TR Criteria**	**Lifetime Prevalence**	**Gender Difference**	**Age of Onset**
Bipolar I disorder	• At least one weeklong manic episode • Mixed features or depressive episodes are common, but not required, for diagnosis • Possible psychotic features	• 0.4% to 1.0%	• No major difference, although depressive episodes, rapid cycling, and mixed features are more common in girls and women	• Any age; usually late adolescence or early adulthood, although earlier or later onset is possible
Bipolar II disorder	• At least one major depressive episode • At least one hypomanic episode • No history of mania	• 0.6% to 1.1%	• Mixed results, but appears to occur more frequently in girls and women; rapid cycling and mixed features are more common in girls and women	• Any age; usually early adulthood, but diagnosis often occurs long after onset
Cyclothymic disorder	• Periods involving milder hypomanic symptoms alternating with milder depression for at least 2 years (with no more than 2 months symptom-free)[a] • Symptoms have never met the criteria for a hypomanic, manic, or major depressive episode	• 0.4% to 2.5%	• No difference but women are more likely to seek treatment in clinic settings	• Often adolescence or early adulthood

Source: APA, 2022; Kessler et al., 2005; Merikangas et al., 2007, 2011

[a] In children and adolescents, mood can be irritable and diagnosis can occur if symptoms have been present for at least 1 year.

Melody Moezzi is the author of *Haldol and Hyacinths*, a memoir about her experiences living with bipolar I disorder. **Bipolar I disorder** is diagnosed when someone (with or without a history of severe depression) experiences at least one manic episode (refer to Table 8.6). For a diagnosis of bipolar I disorder, manic symptoms need to significantly affect normal functioning and be present most of the day, nearly every day, for at least 1 week. Manic episodes significantly interfere with common activities and interpersonal interactions. The uncharacteristic behaviors that occur during manic periods often produce feelings of guilt or worthlessness once the episode has ended. Although not everyone with bipolar I experiences depression, it is a common and disabling characteristic of this disorder. Both depressive and manic episodes may involve psychotic symptoms or end in hospitalization. As was the case with Ms. Moezzi, a diagnosis can be a turning point in a person's life—an opportunity to receive help and end the roller coaster of mood swings.

Bipolar II Disorder

Case Study For many years, Phoenix had no idea what was wrong. His depression began in his mid-teens and sometimes lasted for months. In his 20s, he began to have weeks when everything seemed great. He felt energetic, clever, productive, creative, and empowered. He saw himself as athletic, physically strong, and very sexy. He felt unusually social, frequently texting or messaging friends or posting on social media. He was not tired, so he went out dancing and drinking, hooking up with women he met at the local clubs. At work, he had ideas he enthusiastically shared, but he became irritable and impatient when coworkers asked questions or mentioned that his ideas seemed unrealistic. These energized times would sometimes last for weeks. He might then become "grouchy" and easily agitated, crashing into a dark world of depression. It seemed like the depressions were getting longer, and it was getting harder to undo the damage that occurred during his "good times." After years of telling his family to "lay off" and not to worry about him, Phoenix finally agreed that he needed to get some help.

Bipolar II disorder is diagnosed when there has been at least one major depressive episode (refer to Table 8.3) lasting at least 2 weeks and at least one hypomanic episode (refer to Table 8.6) lasting at least 4 consecutive days. The behavior associated with hypomania often surprises, annoys, or creates concern in friends and family. As was the case with Phoenix, those with bipolar II often fail to seek treatment until their mood swings and periods of depression begin to feel overwhelming. Family members are often the first to express concern about the mood swings and uncharacteristic behavior seen during energized episodes.

The primary distinction between bipolar I and bipolar II is the severity of the symptoms during energized episodes (refer to Figure 8.3). A bipolar I diagnosis requires at least one manic episode (including severe impairment that lasts at least 1 week); a bipolar II diagnosis requires at least one major depressive episode and one hypomanic episode, lasting at least 4 days (APA, 2022). Although you may have heard that bipolar II is a "milder" form of bipolar disorder, this is not accurate. The depressive symptoms associated with bipolar II can be as debilitating as the mood extremes that occur in bipolar I. In general, depressive episodes are more prevalent and of greater severity among people living with bipolar II compared to bipolar I (Nierenberg, 2019). Bipolar II is considered an underdiagnosed disorder, in part because many physicians prescribe antidepressants without inquiring about periods of highly energetic, goal-directed activity or other hypomanic symptoms in the individual or among family members (Baldessarini et al., 2020). Assessment instruments that contain self-ratings of hypomanic/manic symptoms and daily mood monitoring can help avoid misdiagnosis.

Cyclothymic Disorder

Cyclothymic disorder involves impairment in functioning resulting from milder hypomanic symptoms that are consistently interspersed with

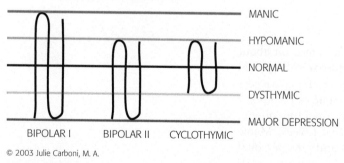

**RANGE OF MOOD SYMPTOMS
IN BIPOLAR DISORDERS**

MANIC

HYPOMANIC

NORMAL

DYSTHYMIC

MAJOR DEPRESSION

BIPOLAR I   BIPOLAR II   CYCLOTHYMIC

© 2003 Julie Carboni, M. A.

Figure 8.3

Mood States Experienced in Bipolar Disorders

Bipolar disorders differ in terms of the range of mood symptoms experienced. The widest range of symptoms occurs with bipolar I, although not everyone with bipolar I experiences depressive episodes.

milder depressed moods for at least 2 years (1 year in children and adolescents). For this diagnosis, the depressive moods must not reach the level of a major depressive episode, and the energized symptoms must not meet the criteria for a hypomanic or manic episode. Additionally, the person must experience mood symptoms at least half of the time and never be symptom-free for more than 2 months. Cyclothymic disorder is similar to persistent depressive disorder because the mood symptoms are chronic; however, with cyclothymic disorder, there are also periods of hypomanic behavior. Some individuals diagnosed with cyclothymic disorder eventually meet the criteria for bipolar II if their mood symptoms become more severe. Cyclothymic disorder is characterized by an early onset (often in the teens) and frequently involves both spontaneous, unpredictable mood swings as well as extreme reactivity to environmental triggers (Perugi et al., 2017).

Features and Conditions Associated with Bipolar Disorder

Bipolar disorder is associated with a variety of features and comorbid conditions. **Mixed features** (i.e., three or more symptoms of hypomania/mania or depression occurring during an episode from the opposite pole) are common with both bipolar I and bipolar II. The presence of mixed features is important to note because the simultaneous occurrence of hypomanic/manic and depressive symptoms increases the risk of impulsive behaviors such as suicidal actions or substance abuse; individuals who demonstrate this pattern of alternating symptoms often require more intensive treatment (Solé et al., 2017). **Rapid cycling**, a pattern where there are four or more mood episodes per year, occurs in some individuals with bipolar disorder; this pattern is especially common among those who develop bipolar symptoms at an early age. Rapid cycling can be triggered by a variety of factors, including sleep deprivation and certain antidepressants (Fountoulakis et al., 2013). Approximately one third of those with bipolar disorder exhibit both mixed features and rapid cycling—a combination that is associated with a more severe and chronic course of the disorder and greater treatment resistance (Köhler et al., 2017).

A variety of conditions are comorbid with bipolar disorders. Both anxiety and substance-use disorders commonly co-occur with bipolar disorder; these conditions often exacerbate mood symptoms, increase functional impairment, and increase the risk of subsequent mood episodes (Prisciandaro et al., 2019). Men with a bipolar disorder have an increased likelihood of having a coexisting substance-use disorder, whereas women with a bipolar diagnosis frequently have eating disorders, particularly binge-eating disorder and bulimia. Those with coexisting conditions tend to develop bipolar disorder earlier and have longer episodes, as well as increased suicidal behavior (McElroy et al., 2011; Suominen et al., 2009).

The suicide risk for people living with bipolar disorders is up to 20 times greater than is found in the general population—a rate exceeding that of most other psychiatric disorders (Baldessarini et al., 2020). Suicide risk is heightened when someone with bipolar disorder takes antidepressant medication without any mood-stabilizing medications; this is most likely to occur when a prescriber is attempting to treat depressive or anxiety symptoms without adequately assessing for episodes of hypomania/mania; when this occurs, the antidepressant may trigger mood changes (e.g., irritation and agitation) and suicidal behaviors (Shim et al., 2017). In addition to increased rates of death from suicide, bipolar disorder is also associated with increased rates of physical illnesses such as hypertension, cardiovascular disease, and diabetes (Yamagata et al., 2017).

Did You Know?

Bipolar disorder is found 10 times more frequently in artists than in the general population. Individuals with bipolar disorder often have enhanced development of certain positive traits—spirituality, empathy, creativity, and resilience. Researchers are considering ways to tap into these strengths to improve treatment outcome.

Source: Greenwood, 2017

Prevalence of Bipolar Disorders

The lifetime prevalence is between 0.4 percent and 1.0 percent for bipolar I and between 0.6 percent and 1.1 percent for bipolar II (refer to Figure 8.2); similarly, cyclothymic disorder has a lifetime prevalence rate between 0.4 percent and 1 percent (APA, 2022; Merikangas et al., 2007). Thus, bipolar disorders are far less prevalent than depressive disorders. It is important to recall, however, that bipolar disorders may be underdiagnosed. It is estimated that about 8.7 percent of women and 7.7 percent of men diagnosed with a depressive disorder will eventually be diagnosed with a bipolar disorder (Musliner & Østergaard, 2018); in many cases, a depressive disorder diagnosis changes to a bipolar diagnosis once hypomanic/manic symptoms come to the attention of the medical or mental health professional who is providing treatment. Although bipolar disorder can begin in childhood, onset more frequently occurs in late adolescence or early adulthood, suggesting that it is particularly important to monitor for signs of depression and hypomania/mania among those in this age range (Vieta et al., 2018).

Research on gender differences in bipolar disorder is mixed. Most researchers agree that there are no marked gender differences in the prevalence of bipolar I (Merikangas et al., 2007) but that depressive and mixed features, bipolar II, and rapid cycling occur more frequently in women (Diflorio & Jones, 2010; Ketter, 2010). Women also have a higher risk that symptoms will recur. As with depressive disorders, reproductive cycle changes, especially childbirth, can precipitate or worsen depressive episodes (Kripke et al., 2015). The transition to menopause is also associated with an increase in the severity of depressive episodes (Perich et al., 2017).

Although bipolar disorders are much less prevalent than depressive disorders, their costs are substantial. Psychosocial functioning and quality of life are adversely affected, especially among those with depressive symptoms (Yatham, Kennedy, et al., 2018). Persisting symptoms and cognitive impairment result in high rates of unemployment (up to 60 percent) among adults with bipolar illness. Relationship problems are common, and the divorce rate is two to three times higher than that in the general population. Furthermore, recurrence of symptoms is common, and relapse rates are high (Wagner-Skacel et al., 2020). In one study, bipolar disorder was associated with 65.5 annual lost workdays per ill worker, compared to 27.2 days for those with major depressive disorder; this is because those with bipolar II disorder often have severe and persistent depressive episodes (Kessler et al., 2006).

Etiology of Bipolar Disorders

What explains the mood roller coaster experienced by those with bipolar disorders? Many of the psychological, social, and sociocultural influences that we have already discussed with respect to the etiology of depressive disorders can also contribute to depressive episodes in bipolar disorder. In this section, we concentrate primarily on factors that contribute to the mood instability and hypomanic/manic symptoms that are unique to bipolar disorders.

Biological Influences

Genetic factors contribute to bipolar disorder—a well-established finding from twin, adoption, and family studies. For example, the chance of developing bipolar I, bipolar II, or cyclothymic disorder when a twin is diagnosed with the condition is quite high—up to 72 percent for identical twins, compared to 14 percent for fraternal twins (Edvardsen et al., 2008). It is important to note that a substantial percentage of individuals with high genetic risk for bipolar disorder (first-degree relatives) remain free of psychopathology during their lifetime. Interestingly, many individuals in this resilient group exhibit brain activation patterns similar to those seen with bipolar illness; however, these abnormalities are accompanied by brain changes indicative of increased neural reserve—a pattern that may reflect adaptive neuroplasticity that succeeds in circumventing the development of bipolar illness (Frangou, 2019).

Bipolar disorders appear to have a complex genetic basis involving interactions among multiple genes, including several genes influenced by the chemical compound lithium. A genome-wide association study found 30 genetic links involving genes related to neural transmission and synaptic connections. In particular, bipolar I appears to have a strong genetic relationship with schizophrenia, whereas bipolar II is strongly related to major depressive disorder (Stahl et al., 2019). Because individuals with bipolar disorders have circadian rhythm abnormalities, it is not surprising that genes that influence our circadian cycle are also linked with vulnerability to bipolar disorder (Takaesu, 2018). Despite the high heritability of bipolar disorders, the exact biological mechanisms by which the various risk genes contribute to the development of these disorders remains unclear. The variability of symptoms among those with bipolar disorders is likely due to varied combinations of risk genes combined with variations in the psychosocial stressors encountered by each individual.

Various neurological abnormalities are associated with bipolar symptoms. For instance, irregularities in the way the brain processes and responds to stimuli associated with reward can influence both manic and depressive symptoms. Consistent with this *dysregulation model of bipolar disorder*, individuals with bipolar disorders may experience hypomanic/manic symptoms after reaching a goal; they also have a tendency to demonstrate anger and irritability in response to obstructed goals. Due to this high sensitivity to reward, mania can develop due to overly ambitious pursuit of goals and the brain dysregulation (i.e., excessive brain activation and increased energy output) that occurs when goals are attained (Nusslock & Alloy, 2017). This same hypersensitivity can cause a shutting down (i.e., deactivation) of motivational systems within the brain in response to perceived failures; this deactivation may produce symptoms of depression, including decreased goal-directed activity, low energy, loss of interest, hopelessness, and sadness (Alloy et al., 2016). Thus, individuals with hypersensitive neurological systems appear to have a vulnerability to bipolar disorder that is triggered by events that activate or deactivate brain systems involved in regulating energy and motivation.

It is likely that multiple biochemical pathways contribute to the symptoms associated with bipolar disorders. In a review of the literature, goal attainment, disrupted circadian cycles, and seasonal increases in light triggered the onset of hypomanic/manic episodes in certain individuals (Proudfoot et al., 2010). Some classes of drugs such as antidepressants (especially SSRIs) and stimulants such as cocaine and methamphetamine can trigger mania, thus implicating certain neurotransmitters (serotonin, norepinephrine, or dopamine) in the etiology of bipolar disorders (Soreff & McInnes, 2014). As with depressive disorders, hormonal influences and disruptions in the stress circuitry of the brain contribute to bipolar symptoms. For example, multiple brain imaging studies have documented elevated glutamate neurotransmission (a neurotransmitter with stimulatory functions) in the brains of individuals with bipolar disorder (Smaragdi et al., 2019).

Did You Know?

In a large population-based study, a diagnosis of cannabis use disorder was associated with an increased risk of developing bipolar disorder and major depressive disorder. The use of cannabis is also associated with an earlier onset of bipolar disorder, a trend toward rapid cycling, and a greater risk of a suicide attempt.

Source: Aas et al., 2014; Jefsen et al., 2023

Evidence from neuroimaging studies also suggests that individuals with bipolar disorders have functional and anatomical brain irregularities, including reduced gray matter, decreased brain activation in regions associated with experiencing and regulating emotions, and increased activation in regions associated with emotional responsiveness (Lu et al., 2019; Zhang et al., 2018). Bipolar I disorder, for example, is associated with atypical brain structure and function in regions of the brain involved with emotional regulation, particularly the limbic system and the amygdala; these abnormalities may explain the onset of mania and the chronic course of the disorder (Caseras et al., 2015).

Psychological Influences

Psychological or individual characteristics can also influence the development and progression of bipolar disorders. Individuals with bipolar disorder tend to cope with stress by disengagement and tend to have limited adaptive coping or problem-solving skills (Fortgang, Hultman, & Cannon, 2016). The personality trait of impulsivity is also strongly associated with bipolar disorder; one study (involving twin pairs in which only one twin has bipolar disorder) found that an impulsive response style was usually present in both twins, not just the twin diagnosed with bipolar illness (Fortgang, Hultman, & Cannon, 2016). Cognitive deficits have also been found in individuals with bipolar disorder and among nonaffected first-degree relatives. These difficulties include the inability to inhibit irrelevant information when trying to achieve a goal; difficulty in holding and manipulating information in the mind; problems in psychological flexibility in response to feedback; and using maladaptive forms of emotional regulation, such as rumination, self-blame, and catastrophizing (Lima et al., 2018). Individuals with bipolar disorders are prone to ruminating about events that occur just prior to or during depressive and hypomanic/manic episodes—a characteristic that may produce or sustain both depressed and energized mood states (Silveira & Kauer-Sant'Anna, 2015).

Social and Sociocultural Influences

Traumatic stressors such as child abuse and bullying during critical periods of brain development may lead to alterations in neurological functioning that increase vulnerability to bipolar disorder (Acosta et al., 2020; Saito et al., 2019). Early life stressors appear to sensitize individuals with genetic vulnerability and lead to the development of mood episodes; this sensitization is associated with emotional reactions to both powerful stressors and relatively minor negative events (Shapero et al., 2017).

A loss of social support or strained social relationships can trigger the onset of either hypomanic/manic or depressive symptoms (Eidelman et al., 2012). In contrast, social support can help people who are undergoing stress to challenge or reframe negative ruminations, thereby reducing the chances of the onset of a mood episode (Owen et al., 2017). Further, social support from family, friends, or a romantic partner increases the likelihood of recovery from bipolar illness (Dunne et al., 2019).

Although the prevalence rate for bipolar disorder is similar across genders, there are differences in the patterns of mood symptoms displayed by men and women. Women are more likely to experience depressive episodes, severe mood symptoms, and sleep difficulties, whereas men are more likely to experience episodes of mania (Williams & McInnis, 2019). Higher rates of mixed mania; suicidal behaviors; and comorbidities such as PTSD, eating disorders, and anxiety disorders are found in women with bipolar disorder, while men with bipolar disorder are more likely to abuse alcohol or other substances (Azorin et al., 2013; Patel et al., 2018).

Commonalities Between Bipolar I Disorder and Schizophrenia

It is now commonly accepted that bipolar I disorder and schizophrenia, both chronic disorders with neurological irregularities and psychotic features, share genetic, neuroanatomical, and cognitive abnormalities. Genome-wide studies have discovered that similar risk alleles contribute to both schizophrenia and bipolar I disorder (Liebers et al., 2020). Additionally, the increased prevalence of either bipolar disorder or schizophrenia among first-degree relatives of individuals with attention-deficit/hyperactivity disorder is attributed to shared genetic factors among the three disorders (Larsson et al., 2013). Neuroimaging comparing the neuroanatomy and neural networks in individuals with schizophrenia and bipolar I disorder reveals similar abnormalities, many of which involve atypically connected or disconnected neural networks associated with the frontal lobe (Ji et al., 2019).

Bipolar disorder and schizophrenia also involve similar cognitive deficits, including confused thought processes and *poor insight* (failure to recognize symptoms of one's own mental illness). In schizophrenia, these difficulties are common throughout the course of the disorder. In bipolar disorder, this lack of insight and failure to recognize the inappropriateness of behavior occurs during hypomanic/manic episodes; insight is usually adequate during depressive episodes (Cassidy, 2010). Neurocognitive deficits that affect psychosocial competence, daily functioning, and work performance are also present in both disorders, although the deficits are usually more severe and more pervasive in schizophrenia and in individuals with bipolar disorder who have experienced a psychotic episode (Menkes et al., 2019).

Treatment for Bipolar Disorders

Treatment for bipolar disorders focuses on the person's primary symptoms. For example, individuals with depressive episodes often benefit from the psychotherapies that are effective with depressive disorders. Because it is currently not possible to "cure" bipolar disorder, therapy attempts to support recovery and eliminate symptoms to the greatest degree possible. As with depressive disorders, lingering or residual symptoms increase the likelihood of relapse and ongoing impairment. Intervention efforts, therefore, target current symptoms, as well as the prevention of future hypomanic/manic and depressive episodes.

Effective treatment incorporates a combination of psychotherapy, mood-stabilizing medications, and psychoeducation geared toward helping those with bipolar disorder (and their family members) understand the importance of taking prescribed medications, using the mood regulation strategies learned in therapy, and normalizing sleep and circadian rhythm patterns (Geddes & Miklowitz, 2013). It is important for those living with bipolar symptoms to remember that although bipolar disorder is a chronic illness, each distressing mood episode is only temporary and that mood fluctuations often become less severe with treatment.

Biomedical Treatments for Bipolar Disorders

Pharmacological treatment for bipolar disorders can be complicated. It is not unusual for individuals with a bipolar disorder to take multiple medications, or to have numerous drug changes before discovering the most effective combination of medications. Choices about medication vary depending on a person's present and past symptoms (e.g., severe mania, severe depression, rapid cycling, mixed or psychotic features). Most agree that medication is an essential component of treatment, not only in managing acute symptoms, but also in preventing relapse.

Mood-stabilizing medications such as lithium are the foundation of treatment for bipolar disorder. Although anticonvulsant and antipsychotic medications with mood-stabilizing properties are also used, lithium is considered the most effective mood-stabilizing medication for those who respond well to its effects, particularly because it also has antisuicidal properties. About one third of people with bipolar disorder respond well to lithium, especially when it is initiated early in the course of the illness (Malhi et al., 2020). Lithium also appears to have neuroprotective effects, reducing the progressive shrinkage of the hippocampus and increasing gray matter density in the hippocampus and amygdala (Won & Kim, 2017). In addition, lithium may be protective against osteoporosis, which is common in individuals with bipolar disorder (Köhler-Forsberg et al., 2022).

Mood stabilizers are usually prescribed on an ongoing basis to prevent recurrence of depressive and/or manic episodes. Antidepressants are occasionally added to deal with depressive symptoms. However, antidepressants are used cautiously with bipolar disorder—although they target depressive symptoms, as noted previously, there is a significant risk the medication will produce or intensify hypomanic/manic symptoms and may induce or increase suicidality (Akinhanmi et al., 2018).

The generally positive results achieved with lithium and some other mood stabilizers may be overshadowed by serious side effects that can occur if blood levels of the medication and other physiological effects are not regularly monitored. Fortunately, blood tests provide the information required to ensure safety and adjust medications or dosages, if necessary. If medications are taken regularly, symptoms of bipolar disorder can often be effectively controlled. When someone abruptly decreases or discontinues a medication, however, mood changes can rapidly recur.

Unfortunately, failure to take medication as prescribed is a major problem associated with lithium and other mood stabilizers. Individuals with bipolar disorder often report discontinuing or adjusting their own medication. This occurs for a variety of reasons, including weight gain; feelings of sedation; difficulty remembering to take medications; a desire to re-create the energetic or excited feelings that occur with hypomania; or a belief that the medication is no longer needed (Levin et al., 2015). Making medication changes against medical advice is most likely to occur when an individual's judgment is impaired by hypomania/mania or by drug or alcohol abuse. Because nonadherence to medication recommendations is common with bipolar illness (estimated to occur in 40 percent to 60 percent of patients), psychoeducation that emphasizes the link between the regular use of medication and long-term improvement is an important aspect of treatment (Sajatovic et al., 2018). A combined psychopharmacological and psychoeducational treatment approach involving a shared decision-making process that includes input from the patient and family members is associated with positive outcomes (Yatham, Kennedy, et al., 2018).

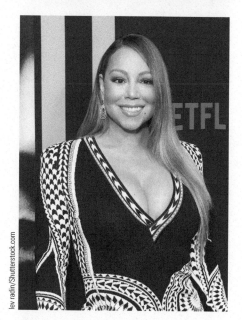

MediaPunch Inc/Alamy Stock Photo

lev radin/Shutterstock.com

Living with Bipolar Disorder

The Grammy-award-winning rapper Ye, formerly known as Kanye West, has made headlines for behaviors associated with bipolar I disorder, symptoms which may have been exacerbated by his challenging work schedule. Mariah Carey, also an extremely successful singer, lives with bipolar II disorder. She has expressed hope that telling the public about her diagnosis will help lift stigma and encourage others struggling with similar symptoms to seek help.

Psychosocial Treatments for Bipolar Disorders

Case Study Learning about bipolar disorder has helped Gabriela manage her symptoms. She takes her mood-stabilizing medications regularly and has an antianxiety medication she uses when anxiety symptoms develop. She tries to go to bed and wake up around the same time each day, and has another medication she takes if she starts waking up alert after only a few hours of sleep, a sign that she might be moving into an energized episode. Gabriela has several friends who have learned about bipolar disorder and who let her know if it seems like her mood is changing. She has also stopped self-medicating with alcohol or marijuana. Instead, she tries to use the mindfulness meditation skills, relaxation, and problem-solving strategies she is learning in therapy. Gabriela realizes that managing her symptoms will be a lifelong challenge, but she is confident that she is learning the strategies she needs to cope when symptoms develop.

Psychological treatments are important adjuncts to medication. As we saw with Gabriela, the self-management and emotional regulation strategies learned in therapy have the potential to significantly enhance recovery and have been found to produce greater efficacy than medication alone (Novick & Swartz, 2019). Educating families about effective communication and problem-solving skills and about the psychological and social factors that contribute to mood instability has the potential to further reduce symptom severity as well as the risk of relapse and hospitalization (Geddes & Miklowitz, 2013).

Individuals with bipolar disorder benefit from learning strategies to help manage their illness. Thus, therapists teach clients to (1) avoid stress and overly ambitious goal setting, (2) practice emotional regulation techniques, (3) identify signs of an impending mood episode, and (4) understand the dangers of substance use and abuse (Miklowitz et al., 2012). Additionally, due to the strong link between sleep deprivation and emotional reactivity, interventions focused on regulating sleep patterns can help prevent the vicious cycle of disrupted sleep leading to mood changes (Eidelman et al., 2010). A smartphone app focused on self-management skills such as taking medications, attending to signs and symptoms, and monitoring sleep and wellness levels, combined with daily check-in with providers, was found to significantly reduce symptoms in adults living with bipolar disorder. Individuals using the app had fewer relapses, less frequent symptoms, and decreased severity of manic and depressive symptoms as compared to individuals in the control group (Goulding et al., 2023). Mindfulness interventions have also proven successful in helping those with bipolar disorder regulate their moods, especially when mindfulness practices are used at the onset of a mood episode (Novick & Swartz, 2019).

One psychoeducational group intervention that has demonstrated success focuses on four main topics: (1) increasing knowledge of bipolar disorder, (2) recognizing mood changes, (3) controlling moods, and (4) changing perspectives about the illness. This intervention helps participants develop self-awareness, feel empowered, have more tolerance for mood swings, increase personal responsibility for managing symptoms, and strengthen their determination to live a "normal and happy life" in spite of the disorder. The group format is beneficial because it allows participants to meet and learn from other people experiencing similar challenges (Davenport et al., 2019).

8-4 Contemporary Trends and Future Directions

Researchers and mental health professionals are directing considerable effort toward preventing depressive and bipolar disorders, with a particular focus on the fact that child maltreatment and other early adverse experiences increase vulnerability to depressive symptoms. Our brains have high neuroplasticity early in life, recording memories of our interactions with the environment so we can effectively adapt to the circumstances we may need to confront. Unfortunately, stressors occurring in early childhood set the stage for brain changes that are associated with depression and mood dysregulation. Researchers are increasingly aware that epigenetic changes that occur during critical periods such as fetal development or early childhood can exert lifelong effects on our physiological reactivity in response to life stressors (Post et al., 2017). Thus, efforts to prevent early childhood stress and trauma are essential if we hope to decrease the prevalence of depressive and bipolar disorders. Some researchers are even hoping to develop medications that increase the brain's neuroplasticity in adulthood, making it possible to undo some of the "faulty wiring" and maladaptive neurological patterns that develop based on damaging early life experiences (Deyama & Duman, 2020).

Accurate diagnosis and effective treatment of depressive and bipolar disorders are also a high priority, especially because the symptoms of these disorders often strike in the prime of a person's life and frequently follow a chronic course. Thus, researchers are searching for the best psychological and medical treatments for those who develop early symptoms of these disorders. For instance, some researchers are attempting to identify psychological factors (e.g., rumination) that increase the risk of a mood disorder so that interventions can occur before these behaviors become habitual (Arditte Hall et al., 2019).

Researchers are also hoping to revolutionize the treatment for bipolar and depressive disorders through **personalized medicine**; once available, this approach would determine a person's vulnerability to developing certain illnesses and identify which therapies would be most effective based on the individual's unique genetic profile or physiological characteristics (Le-Niculescu et al., 2021). Thus, biologically based diagnostic tests rather than subjective symptoms would guide treatment. Personalized medicine will not only improve diagnosis, but will also determine the most efficient treatment with the fewest side effects. Clinicians will be able to choose the most optimal pharmacological and psychotherapeutic treatments at different stages of depressive or bipolar illnesses.

Scientists are making some progress in using genetic testing to determine how an individual might respond to certain medications; however, this work is still in its infancy. It is hoped that at some point in the near future, brain imaging will be able to guide diagnosis and treatment decisions (Haggarty et al., 2020). The use of biological technologies will be particularly helpful in differentiating between recurring major depressive disorder and bipolar II disorder early in the course of the illness so that appropriate treatment can be initiated when symptoms first appear (Han et al., 2019).

Chapter Summary

1 What are the symptoms of depression, hypomania, and mania?

- Depression involves feelings of sadness or emptiness, social withdrawal, loss of interest in activities, pessimism, low energy, and sleep and appetite disturbances.

- Mania produces significant impairment and involves high levels of arousal, elevated or irritable mood, increased activity, poor judgment, grandiosity, and decreased need for sleep. Hypomania refers to milder manic symptoms, which may be accompanied by productive, goal-directed behaviors.

2 What are depressive disorders, what causes them, and how are they treated?

- Depressive disorders are diagnosed only when depressive symptoms occur without a history of hypomania/mania. Depressive disorders include major depressive disorder, persistent depressive disorder, and premenstrual dysphoric disorder.

- Biological factors, including heredity, increase vulnerability to depression. Biochemical irregularities involving neurotransmitters, stress reactivity, and cortisol levels are associated with depression.

- Behavioral explanations for depression focus on reduced reinforcement following losses. Cognitive explanations focus on negative attributions and thinking patterns, irrational beliefs, and rumination.

- Social explanations focus on relationships and interpersonal stressors that increase vulnerability to depression. Early childhood stressors are particularly important.

- Sociocultural explanations have focused on cultural factors, including gender, ethnicity, and sexual orientation.

- Behavioral activation therapy, cognitive-behavioral therapy, and interpersonal psychotherapy have received extensive research support as treatments for depression; mindfulness-based cognitive therapy has also demonstrated promising results. Biomedical treatments include light therapy and electrical stimulation of the brain. Antidepressant medications are frequently used to treat depression; they are most effective with severe depression, but often produce only temporary effects. Psychotherapy is more likely to prevent the return of depressive symptoms.

3 What are bipolar disorders, what causes them, and how are they treated?

- Bipolar disorders involve symptoms of mania or hypomania. Depressive episodes are also common in bipolar disorder.

- Bipolar I involves at least one weeklong manic episode and impaired functioning. Psychotic symptoms are sometimes present. Bipolar II is diagnosed when there is a history of hypomania and at least one major depressive episode. Cyclothymic disorder is a chronic disorder involving milder hypomanic episodes that alternate with depressed mood for at least 2 years.

- Bipolar disorders have a strong genetic basis involving multiple, interacting genes. Biological factors, including neurochemical and neuroanatomical abnormalities and circadian rhythm disturbances, contribute to bipolar disorder. There are many overlaps between bipolar I disorder and schizophrenia.

- The most effective treatment for bipolar disorder is ongoing use of mood-stabilizing medication combined with psychotherapy, psychoeducation, and psychosocial interventions.

Chapter Glossary

anxious distress
symptoms of motor tension, difficulty relaxing, pervasive worries, or feelings that something catastrophic will occur

attributional style
a characteristic way of explaining why a positive or negative event occurred

bipolar I disorder
a diagnosis that involves at least one manic episode that has impaired social or occupational functioning; the person may or may not experience depression or psychotic symptoms

bipolar II disorder
a diagnosis that involves at least one major depressive episode and at least one hypomanic episode

circadian rhythm
an internal clock or daily cycle of internal biological rhythms that influence various bodily processes such as body temperature and sleep–wake cycles

co-rumination
extensively discussing negative feelings or events with peers or others

cyclothymic disorder
a condition involving milder hypomanic symptoms that are consistently interspersed with milder depressed moods for at least 2 years

depression
a mood state characterized by sadness or despair, feelings of worthlessness, and withdrawal from others

elevated mood
a mood state involving exaggerated feelings of confidence, energy, and well-being

emotional lability
unstable and rapidly changing emotions and mood

euphoria
an exceptionally elevated mood; exaggerated feeling of well-being

expansive mood
a mood in which a person may feel extremely confident or self-important and behave impulsively

flight of ideas
rapidly changing or disjointed thoughts

grandiosity
an overvaluation of one's significance or importance

hypomania
a milder form of mania involving increased levels of activity and goal-directed behaviors combined with an elevated, expansive, or irritable mood

learned helplessness
a learned belief that one is helpless and unable to affect outcomes

major depressive disorder (MDD)
a condition diagnosed if someone (without a history of hypomania/mania) experiences a depressive episode involving severe depressive symptoms that have negatively affected functioning most of the day, nearly every day, for at least 2 full weeks

major depressive episode
a period involving severe depressive symptoms that have impaired functioning for at least 2 full weeks

mania
a mental state characterized by very exaggerated activity and emotions, including euphoria, excessive excitement, or irritability that result in impairment in social or occupational functioning

MDD with a seasonal pattern
major depressive episodes that occur seasonally more than non-seasonally; at least two seasonal episodes of severe depression have occurred and ended at a predictable time of year

mixed features
concurrent hypomanic/manic and depressive symptoms

mood
an emotional state or prevailing frame of mind

persistent depressive disorder (PDD)
a condition involving chronic depressive symptoms that are present most of the day for more days than not during a 2-year period with no more than 2 months symptom-free

personalized medicine
the use of a person's genetic profile to guide decisions about prevention and treatment of disease and mental disorders

premenstrual dysphoric disorder (PMDD)
a condition involving distressing and disruptive symptoms of depression, irritability, and tension that occur the week before menstruation

pressured speech
rapid; frenzied; or loud, disjointed communication

psychosis
a condition involving loss of contact with or distorted view of reality

rapid cycling
the occurrence of four or more mood episodes per year

rumination
repeatedly thinking about concerns or details of past events

self-schema
a stable set of beliefs and assumptions about the self that are based on the person's experiences, values, and perceived capabilities

treatment-resistant depression
a depressive episode that has not improved despite an adequate trial of antidepressant medication or other traditional forms of treatment

focus
Questions

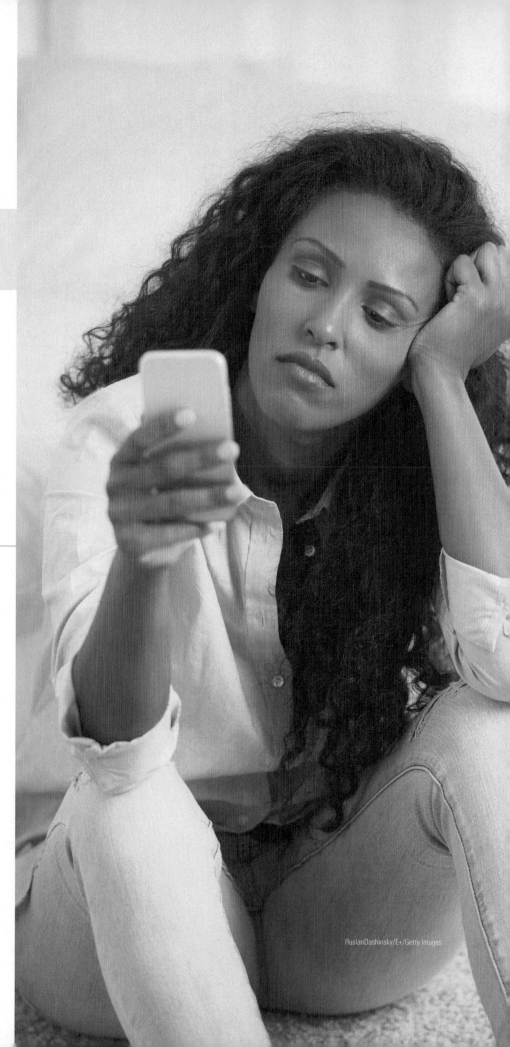

RuslanDashinsky/E+/Getty Images

9

Suicide

Learning Objectives

After studying this chapter, you will be able to . . .

9-1 Summarize what we know about suicide including risk factors associated with suicide among different groups.

9-2 Discuss how suicide affects friends and family.

9-3 Discuss what might cause someone to end their life by suicide.

9-4 Discuss ways in which we can prevent suicide or intervene if someone is experiencing suicidal thoughts.

9-5 Discuss the various moral, ethical, and legal issues surrounding suicide.

9-6 Examine future trends in the field of suicidology.

Late One Evening, Carl Johnson, MD, Left His Downtown Office, got into his Mercedes-Benz S600, and drove toward his expensive suburban home. He was in no hurry, because the house would be empty anyway; his wife had divorced him and moved back East with their children. Although he had been drinking heavily for 2 years before his wife left him, he had always been able to function at work. Now he was unable to stop thinking about his failed marriage. For the past several months, his private practice had declined dramatically. He had once found his work meaningful, but now his patients bored and irritated him. Although he had suffered from depression in the past, this time it was different. The future had never looked so bleak and hopeless. Carl knew he was in serious trouble—he was, after all, a psychiatrist.

Carl parked carelessly, not bothering to press the switch that closed the garage door. Once in the house, he headed directly for his den. There he pulled out a bottle of bourbon and three glasses, filled each glass to the rim, and lined them up along the bar. He drank them down, one after the other, in rapid succession. For a good hour he stood at the window, staring out into the night. Sadly, he made the decision to end his life.

Suicide—the intentional, direct, and conscious taking of one's own life—is as old as human history, so its occurrence is not rare. Suicide is not only a tragic act; it is also difficult to comprehend. Why would someone like Dr. Johnson choose to take his own life? Granted, he was depressed and obviously feeling the loss of his family, but most people under similar circumstances are able to cope and move forward. Why didn't he realize that he had other options? Unfortunately, we will never know the answer. Research on suicide, however, offers clues. First, he had a history of alcohol abuse, a biological factor implicated in suicide. Second, psychological factors such as hopelessness and depression are associated with suicide. Third, social factors clearly influenced Dr. Johnson's mental distress; perhaps the loss of his family made him believe life was no longer meaningful. People who lack or who have ruptured social relationships are more likely to consider suicide. Finally, there are sociocultural aspects to Dr. Johnson's suicide. His gender and occupation are significant factors. Men are more likely to kill themselves compared to women. And occupationally, physicians, particularly psychiatrists, have one of the highest rates of suicide (Anderson, 2018). Clearly, Dr. Johnson was at high risk for suicide on a number of risk dimensions.

Suicide has been extensively researched. We are able to identify suicide risk factors, delineate protective factors, and even develop strategies to successfully intervene with people contemplating suicide. But there is much we don't know. We still have no definitive answer to this question: "Why do people kill themselves?" Although explanations abound for suicide, we can never be entirely certain why people knowingly and deliberately end their own lives. Research suggests that people kill themselves for many different reasons.

Although the DSM does not include suicide as a specific mental disorder, a separate chapter on suicide is provided in this text for several reasons. First, although there is no current diagnostic category for those who contemplate or attempt suicide, some researchers and clinicians believe that suicide and **suicidal ideation**—thoughts about suicide— represent a distinct clinical condition warranting a unique diagnostic label. They point out that incorporating suicide-related thoughts and behaviors as a disorder would allow clinicians to increase their focus on suicide risk assessment (Fehling & Selby, 2021). Such an approach would also permit the use of large health-related databases to identify clinical and biological markers of suicide and to develop intervention strategies (Sisti et al., 2020).

The fact that suicide is the ninth leading cause of death in the United States further reinforces the importance of this topic (Centers for Disease Control and Prevention [CDC], 2023). Unfortunately, throughout history, people have avoided discussing suicide; the shame and stigma involved in taking one's life have produced a "conspiracy of silence." Even mental health professionals find the topic uncomfortable and deeply disturbing. Discussing suicide is of critical importance, however, because death by suicide is an irreversible act. The decision to end one's life by suicide is often an ambivalent one, clouded by many personal and social stressors. Unfortunately, once the action is taken, there is no going back. Many mental health professionals

988 Suicide & Crisis Lifeline

In the United States, the toll-free 988 Suicide & Crisis Lifeline provides 24/7, confidential support to people experiencing suicidal thoughts or other mental health–related distress. The Lifeline supports people who call for themselves as well as anyone who is concerned about a friend or family member who is in crisis.

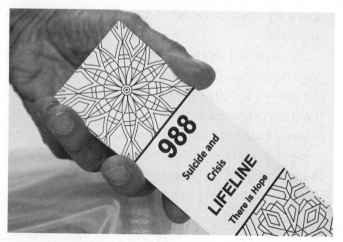

believe that when people who are feeling suicidal are given appropriate support in coping with personal and social crises, their pain lessens and they begin to consider options beyond taking their own life. Most do not want to die; they simply want their pain to end and are unable to appreciate that there are other solutions. Thus, knowledge about factors that influence suicide and strategies to prevent such tragedies is extremely important. Suicide prevention is also crucial because of the devastating psychological effects experienced by the friends and family of those who have ended their lives by suicide.

9-1 Facts About Suicide

People who have died by suicide can no longer share their thoughts, motives, or emotional state. Thus, we must rely on indirect information, such as case records and reports from others, to help us understand what led to their heartbreaking act. Systematically examining information after a person's death in an effort to understand and explain a person's behavior before death is called a **psychological autopsy**. A psychological autopsy is patterned on the medical autopsy, which involves the examination of a body to determine the cause of death. A psychological autopsy attempts to make psychological sense of a suicide by compiling and analyzing background information, including recollections of therapists, interviews with relatives and friends, information obtained from crisis phone calls, social media postings, and messages left in suicide notes (Aquila et al., 2018).

Unfortunately, these sources are not always available or reliable. Often there is no suicide note and no previous contact with a therapist. Additionally, the judgment of friends and family may be clouded by their intense feelings of hurt and shock. Another strategy involves studying those who survive suicide attempts. This method, however, assumes that people who attempt suicide are no different from those who complete the act. Despite these limitations, researchers use all available data to better understand the personal characteristics and demographics linked with suicide, and to develop profiles for at-risk individuals. Table 9.1 summarizes some of the characteristics associated with suicide.

Table 9.1   Common Characteristics of Suicide

1. Belief that things will never change and that suicide is the only solution

2. Desire to escape from psychological pain and distressing thoughts and feelings

3. Triggering events, including intense interpersonal conflict and feelings of depression, hopelessness, guilt, anger, or shame

4. Perceived inability to make progress toward goals or to solve problems; related feelings of failure, worthlessness, and hopelessness

5. Ambivalence about suicide; there is a strong underlying desire to live

6. Suicidal intent communicated directly or indirectly through verbal or behavioral cues

Source: Shneidman, 1998; Van Heeringen & Marusic, 2003

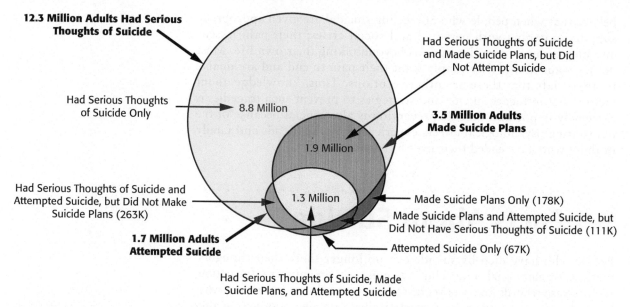

Figure 9.1

U.S. Adults Aged 18 or Older with Serious Thoughts of Suicide, Suicide Plans, or Suicide Attempts in the Past Year, 2021

According to data from the 2021 U.S. National Survey on Drug Use and Health, 12.3 million adults age 18 or older reported having serious thoughts about killing themselves, 3.5 million had made a suicide plan, and 1.7 million had made a nonfatal suicide attempt during the past year.

Source: SAMHSA, 2023

Frequency

Suicidal behavior begins with suicidal ideation, an individual's initial suicidal thoughts. Fleeting suicidal thoughts are not uncommon. For example, in the United States in 2021, an estimated 12.3 million adults seriously thought about suicide, 3.5 million made a plan for suicide, and 1.7 million attempted suicide (CDC, 2023). Although most people who have serious thoughts of suicide never attempt suicide, some people proceed from suicidal ideation to developing a plan; among this group, an even smaller number attempt suicide. Suicide without prior planning is rare (refer to Figure 9.1).

Sadly, every 11 minutes or so, someone in the United States dies by suicide. In 2021, suicide claimed the lives of over 48,000 people in the United States. It is the second leading cause of death for youth ages 10 to 14 and for young adults ages 20 to 34. Suicide rates are increasing across genders, across all racial/ethnic groups, and for all age groups. Men are nearly four times more likely to die by suicide than women (CDC, 2023). Some evidence suggests that coroners are hesitant to label deaths as suicide because of the stigma attached, so the number of actual suicides is believed to be 25 percent to 30 percent higher than that recorded. Many deaths deemed accidental—such as single-auto crashes, drownings, and falls from great heights—may be, in fact, be suicides (Gray et al., 2014).

Methods of Suicide

In 2021, among those who died by suicide in the United States, 55 percent used firearms, 26 percent died from suffocation/hanging, and 12 percent overdosed on poison/drugs (CDC, 2023). Older adolescents most frequently try hanging, jumping, and firearms; girls are more likely to use drug or

Did You Know?

An analysis of suicide attempts and fatalities in San Francisco found that the death rate varied based on the method used: 8 percent for poisoning/drug overdose, 89 percent for hanging/suffocation, 95 percent for firearms, and 98 percent for jumps from the Golden Gate Bridge.

Source: Whitmer & Woods, 2013

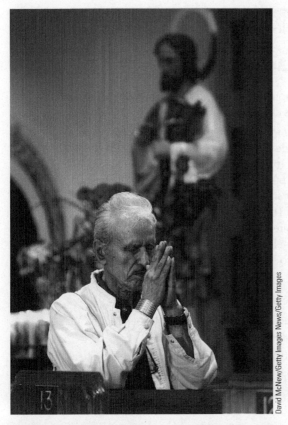
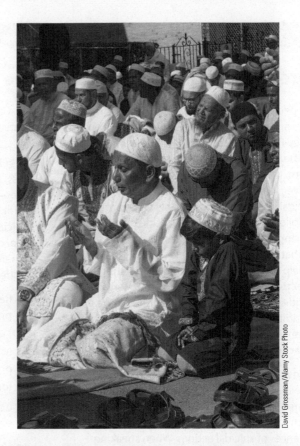

Religion and Suicide

Many religions have strong taboos and sanctions against suicide. In countries in which Catholicism and Islam are strong, for example, the rates of suicide tend to be lower than in countries with fewer religious sanctions against suicide.

alcohol intoxication. Among children younger than age 15, the most common suicide methods involve jumping from buildings or running into traffic. Younger children attempt suicide impulsively and thus use whatever means are most readily available (Hepp et al., 2012). The most common methods of suicide also vary from country to country. For instance, pesticide poisoning is used in 86 percent of all suicides in El Salvador, whereas hanging is common in Japan (69 percent), Kuwait (92 percent), and Poland (91 percent) (Bachmann, 2018).

Occupational Risk Factors

Suicide rates vary across occupations. The jobs with the highest rates of suicide in men include farmworkers, fishermen, lumberjacks, carpenters, miners, electricians, and installers. The lowest rates are reported among librarians and educators. For women, the highest rates of suicide occur for those who were firefighters, police officers, and correctional officers (McIntosh et al., 2016). Among medical professionals, psychiatrists have the highest suicide rate and pediatricians the lowest. It is unknown whether the specialty influences susceptibility or whether people who are prone to suicide are more likely to be attracted to certain specialties. In Canada, the suicide rate for women physicians is higher than that found in their male counterparts (Albuquerque & Tulk, 2019). Researchers speculate that burnout, stress, the availability of drugs, and guilt over medical errors increase the risk of suicide among physicians (Stehman et al., 2019).

Suicide Prevention: Reinforcing Protective Factors

The majority of people who are suicidal are ambivalent about ending their lives and struggle between the wish to live and the wish to die (Oakey-Frost et al., 2023). When helped to understand the origins of their distress and the resources and options available to them, their wish to live can be strengthened. This motivation to live is a key protective mechanism for individuals who are suicidal. One of the most effective ways to prevent someone from following through with a suicide plan is to use a strength-based approach, guided by questions such as: "What are the factors that protect against suicide? How can I use this information to help mobilize coping skills and social support?"

Four protective techniques are especially effective in preventing suicide: (1) reawakening and reinforcing the desire to live, (2) expanding perceptual outlook by reducing suicide myopia, (3) enhancing social connectedness, and (4) increasing the repertoire of coping skills.

1. *Reawakening and reinforcing the desire to live.* Most people possess a natural barrier against suicide. Once we cross that barrier, however, it becomes easier to act against our moral, ethical, or religious upbringing and to ignore the consequences of suicidal actions. When speaking with someone who is contemplating suicide, it helps to reinforce this barrier to prevent it from being crossed; it is especially helpful to focus on concrete actions aimed at connecting the person with friends and loved ones so that purpose and meaning in life can be revived or further developed (Stone et al., 2017).

2. *Expanding perceptual outlook by reducing suicide myopia.* Most people contemplating suicide are overwhelmed by powerful emotions. This often results in confused thinking and a very constricted and narrow perception of problems and options. Conversation can help broaden the person's outlook and prompt consideration of solutions other than suicide. Additionally, our perspective often changes when we engage in interesting or meaningful activities, including volunteer or leisure pursuits, that provide a vision of a more promising future.

3. *Enhancing social connectedness.* Research increasingly reveals that social support; integration with family; and connectedness to schools, peers, and friends are powerful antidotes to suicide (Stone et al., 2017). People who are suicidal often feel lonely, isolated, and disconnected from others, especially those who love them. Many people who consider suicide fail to recognize that friends and family care deeply about them and that there is a purpose to their lives. Therefore, effective interventions often involve reestablishing and strengthening relationships with friends and family. If a client has few social supports, involvement with clubs, support groups (such as NAMI on Campus), volunteer activities, or religious or spiritual pursuits can help fill this void.

4. *Increasing the repertoire of coping skills.* Contemplation of suicide is often associated with difficulty coping with a loss, relationship conflicts, or problematic life events. The more a person is able to regulate emotions and handle difficult situations, the less likely they are to attempt suicide. Therefore, it helps to broaden the person's repertoire of coping strategies and possible steps to take when feeling overwhelmed—actions that can act as a buffer to suicide. Some possible actions might include:

   - Reaching out to supportive friends, family, or professionals

   - Engaging in relaxing, enjoyable, or stress-reducing activities

   - Practicing good self-care, including eating healthy foods, exercising, and getting sufficient sleep

   - Contacting local crisis resources if there is a need for emergency support

Therapists often help clients rehearse what specific actions to take if or when suicidal thoughts emerge. Another possible method of enhancing coping comes from an innovative study using positive psychology techniques: Individuals hospitalized for suicidal thoughts or behaviors participated in exercises involving either (1) gratitude (recalling and writing about recent events for which they were grateful or writing a letter of gratitude to thank someone for a kind act) or (2) personal strengths (taking a survey to identify personal strengths, using one of the strengths for the next 24 hours, and then writing about the experience). Participants exhibited increased optimism and decreased hopelessness, changes that would be predicted to decrease suicidality (Huffman et al., 2014). In summary, it is of critical importance for anyone who has been contemplating or who has attempted suicide to focus on activities that increase optimism and social connection and to realize that there is hope for a positive future once current, overwhelming concerns are resolved.

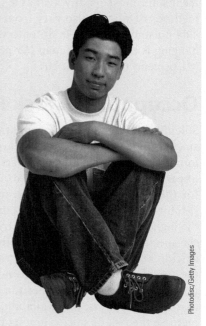

Photodisc/Getty Images

9-2 Effects of Suicide on Friends and Family

Case Study   I probably should have helped a bit more.... I regret not having rung him up or checked up on him. I heard he was doing better, he was picking up again and then they found him hanging. (Bartik et al., 2013, p. 214)

It is estimated that there are from 5 to 80 survivors closely connected to each person who dies by suicide (Cea, 2019). Friends and family of those who have ended their life by suicide often experience a wide range of emotions, including shame, responsibility, and guilt. How do they cope with such feelings? To find out, researchers conducted interviews with people who had lost a friend to suicide, such as the young woman in the case study. These interviews revealed four consistent themes—guilt, attempts to understand and make meaning of the tragedy, development of risky behaviors, and changed relationships with friends. Guilt was common, often involving a desire to have done more or been more available to the friend. The search for meaning often involved attempting to understand why their friend chose suicide, wondering why their friend had not confided in them, and questioning how strong the relationship really was. The woman in the case study, for example, had visited with her friend hours before his suicide and couldn't understand why he hadn't shared his distress with her. Some survivors report engaging in risky behavior, such as substance abuse, after the suicide. For many, friendship patterns changed. Survivors may become afraid to establish close relationships, fearing another loss. Thus, friends of those who have died by suicide may be burdened with unresolved feelings that require mental health intervention.

Family members are also forever changed by a suicide. Parents who lose a child of any age to suicide often feel guilt and responsibility for not being able to protect their loved one. Rates of depression, anxiety, alcohol abuse, and marital difficulties increase, especially during the 2 years following the suicide (Wagner et al., 2021). Recovery from the devastating loss sometimes involves finding a new life purpose. Losing a parent to suicide is also incredibly painful, as is evident in the following case study.

Case Study   I am 27 years old.... I lost my father ... to suicide 26 years ago. He was 53 years old at the time and suffered from depression. I did not know him. I did not know his pain, but I have grown up wondering who he was, what his life was like. I have been haunted with so many questions over the years. Wondering why I wasn't enough for him to live.... As a teenager, this grief, mixed with my own personal struggles, accumulated into a huge messy, confusing ball of emotions. And in my own deepest times of sadness, I convinced myself that I no longer wanted to live. That the pain of life was too great.... I decided I wanted to die. I started swallowing all of the pills.... I remember feeling content in dying. And then, what seems like hours later, but was only minutes later, I felt really, really scared. I started feeling the physical effects of the medication, and it shook me so hard that I went and woke up my mom in the next room and told her what I had done. That I needed her help. That I did not want to die anymore.... I am now a young adult who has known many great joys in life. I have travelled. I have loved.... If my story can help anyone in realizing how serious depression and mental illness is, and how necessary it is to seek help and look for signs, then I am happy to share it. (Diles, 2013)

Depression and Suicide

Paris Jackson, daughter of singer Michael Jackson, was hospitalized after a suicide attempt in January 2014. Like many youth who attempt suicide, she was reportedly overwhelmed by stress and severe depression. Here she attends a party 15 months prior to her suicide attempt.

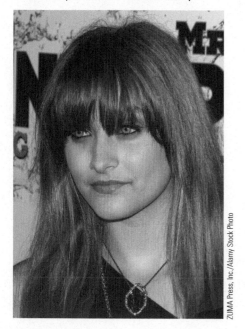

ZUMA Press, Inc./Alamy Stock Photo

As you can imagine from reading this poignant story shared by Katrina Diles, the suicide of a parent can have lifelong effects, even when a child is young at the time of the death. Children who have lost a parent to suicide not only have an increased risk for developing mental health problems, but, like Katrina, they have an increased risk of suicide attempts themselves. Although the suicide risk is greatest if the deceased parent was their mother, children whose fathers died by suicide have an increased likelihood of being hospitalized for depression or anxiety (Kuramoto et al., 2010).

In a study of 26,096 offspring who experienced parental suicide, two different patterns of suicide attempts were found depending on the age of the child when the suicide occurred. For children who lost their parent to suicide during early childhood (up to 12 years of age), the rate of suicide attempts requiring hospitalization steadily increased over decades. In contrast, those who experienced parental suicide during adolescence or early adulthood (13 to 24 years of age) had the highest risk of hospitalization for suicide attempts during the first 2 years after the suicide—a risk that declined over time (Kuramoto et al., 2013). Equally traumatic is the loss of a spouse or life partner due to suicide, as illustrated in the following case.

> **Case Study** My husband of only 8 months took his life in front of me all while I was pregnant with our daughter. Early in our marriage, I noticed he had changed. He had once attempted suicide with his gun in front of me. That time, I'm not exactly sure how I was able to diffuse the situation but we got through it. I didn't know how to take it because I was not educated on signs of suicide or depression. Each time, my husband was extremely intoxicated. I wish I would have known that he was suffering from some type of depression. My husband never asked for help. The day he committed suicide was the saddest day of my life. I keep asking myself why. I wonder why he made me a witness to his suicide. I wonder if he even loved me and the children. I will never know why. I now realize how important it is to get the ones we love the help they need when they show signs. I deeply regret not being aware. (Ester, 2013)

Her husband's decision to end his life has clearly had an everlasting impact on Ester. We can only wonder what the effect has been for her children, including the child born after his death. As these stories demonstrate, those who are left behind after a suicide are forever touched by the traumatic loss of their loved one.

Fortunately, support is available for people affected by suicide, including the hundreds of survivor events sponsored throughout the world by the American Foundation for Suicide Prevention (AFSP). This organization's activities focus on healing through connecting with others; their Web site includes a variety of resources and self-care recommendations (Cea, 2019). Posttraumatic growth has been found with survivors who obtain information about suicide, seek counseling or attend support groups, and engage in self-care while processing their loss (Drapeau et al., 2019).

9-3 Suicide and Specific Populations

In this section, we discuss the occurrence of suicide in various groups: children and adolescents, college students, military personnel, baby boomers, and older adults.

Suicide Among Children and Adolescents

Suicide among young people is an unmentioned tragedy in our society. Sadly, the suicide rate for young people is at its highest since 2000 and appears to be climbing dramatically. In addition, while rates of youth suicide have always been higher for boys than girls, this gap is narrowing. This may be due to the fact that more girls are using hanging/suffocation, a method with greater lethality (Ruch et al., 2019). In one of the first studies focused on suicidality among a community sample of 9- and 10-year-old children, 8 percent reported having thoughts of suicide, nearly 1 percent reported having past or present suicide plans, and 2 percent had made a suicide attempt. The risk for suicidality was higher for youth who had the highest rates of screen time on weekends; in contrast, parental supervision (knowing where children are, what they are doing, and who they are with) appears to be protective against suicidal thoughts (Janiri et al., 2020).

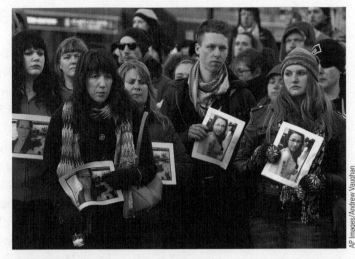

Tragic Consequences of Bullying

Rehtaeh Parsons, of Halifax, Nova Scotia, was taken off life support after attempting to end her life by hanging. Her family says she decided to end her own life following months of bullying, including online distribution of a digital photograph of her taken during an alleged gang rape. Here friends and family are holding pictures of Rehtaeh as they remember her during a community vigil.

Adolescence and young adulthood are often periods of confusing emotions, identity formation, and questioning. It is a difficult and turbulent time for most teenagers, and suicide may seem to be a logical response to the pain and stress of growing up. Many reasons have been proposed for recent increases in suicide among children and teenagers, including escalating substance abuse and social media use (Stone et al., 2018). One analysis of responses to suicidal posts on Twitter revealed that although 62 percent of the initial replies to suicidal posts were supportive, 23 percent were dismissive or, even worse, encouraged the suicide. Although the study did not include data on how the replies affected suicidal behavior, it is certainly possible that unsupportive communication could trigger suicidal actions (O'Dea et al., 2018).

An emerging concern is the significant increase in suicidality among African American children and adolescents. Between the years of 2001 and 2017, the rate of death by suicide increased by 60 percent for African American adolescent boys and by 182 percent for African American adolescent girls. Additionally, in 2017 alone, African American adolescents made over 160,000 suicide attempts severe enough to require medical treatment (Price & Khubchandani, 2019). In another study, young Black children (ages 5 to 12) were found to be twice as likely to die from suicide compared to White children of the same age (Bridge at al., 2018). Advocates within the Black community are stressing the critical importance of identifying the reasons underlying these drastic increases, including understanding barriers to identification and treatment of depression and the role of school experiences such as racial discrimination, low teacher expectations, and inequitable and harsh discipline practices (Lindsey et al., 2017).

The problem of suicidality in youth is complex. The academic environment can function as a major stressor for children and adolescents. Further, conflicts with peers and problems in the family are strongly related to suicidal ideation and depression (Kim, 2020). Homelessness among youth also increases the risk of suicide; this is particularly true for unsheltered youth who cope by using alcohol or drugs, engage in self-blame, or are isolated from others (Gauvin et al., 2019). Other possible explanations for the increase in suicide among children and adolescents include bullying, copycat suicides, and the decreased use of antidepressants with this age group.

The Role of Bullying

Case Study Emilie Olsen had a ready smile, was a straight A student, loved horses, and had a perfect attendance record. At the age of 13, she died by suicide. Her parents said Emilie suffered from relentless bullying regarding her Chinese ethnicity and perceived sexual preference—cruelty that escalated when she was in the fifth and sixth grades. She was jeered by her classmates, called "fake country" for wearing western-style clothes, and told "Chinese people don't wear those clothes." She was also taunted on social media as being "gay." One classmate allegedly followed Emilie into the bathroom, handed her a razor, and told her, "End it." When she was placed in a learning group with the girls who were harassing her, Emilie became more withdrawn, lost interest in her schoolwork, and had a dramatic drop in her grades.

Messages such as "Go kill yourself Emilie" appeared on the school bathroom walls, often making reference to her race and sexual orientation. Emilie wrote to a friend on Facebook, "I['m] causing all this trouble on earth. It hurts when you have to explain yourself to people you don't know or like. You feel them judging you, staring at you, talking about you, and I've made up my mind, I wanna die. . . . I can't please anyone with anything I do. Not even my teachers." Less than 2 weeks later, Emilie died by suicide (Wang, 2016).

Emilie's parents filed a lawsuit against the school district, alleging that the principal and police officers advised them not to talk to the media and not to "stir the pot" with "unfounded rumors." The school district denied the allegations in the suit. An investigative news team found evidence supporting the parents' claim that fellow students repeatedly told Emilie to kill herself, bullied her on social media, scribbled racial and sexual orientation messages on the restroom wall, and physically battered her when at in school (WCPO Staff, 2016).

It is evident from the tragic death of Emilie Olsen that bullying can have serious consequences. Unfortunately, bullying is pervasive, especially during the teen years. Over 20 percent of teens in one study reported being bullied at school, including physical assault; threats; and being the target of teasing, rumors, gossip, or coercion. This statistic is of particular concern because those who are bullied are up to 11 times more likely to consider suicide than those not subjected to bullying. LGBTQ teens are at particularly high risk for both bullying and suicide. Because of the pervasiveness of social media and the inability of the person who is bullied to escape the social environment, cyberbullying seems to be more strongly related to suicide attempts than other forms of bullying (Kuehn et al., 2019). The heartbreak that can result from cyberbullying is evident in the following case study.

Case Study A 14-year-old girl, Andriana Kuch, ended her life a few days after a video showed a group of girls violently attacking her by hitting her on the face with a water bottle and repeatedly punching and kicking her when she fell. This was recorded in the high school hallway with the person taking the video cheering on the attack. Andriana showed her father the video that was circulated online and videos of people taunting and threatening her on TikTok, Instagram, and Snapchat following the attack. Her father contacted the school and local police station to report the incident. No action was taken by either the school or police. He believes she would still be alive if immediate action had been taken. (Rumpf-Whitten, 2023)

It is evident that bullying can lead to tragedy. If people observe bullying, do they intervene? As you might imagine, speaking up against a bully takes courage. Researchers set up an experiment in which two confederates participated in a Facebook discussion with 37 undergraduate women regarding the topic of same-sex marriage; one of the confederates began to bully the other confederate about her comments in the discussion. This resulted in 90.6 percent of the participants attempting to intervene in some way (attacking the bully, changing the subject, offering comfort to the target of bullying, or directly asking that the bullying stop). It is a promising sign that the majority of this group realized that bullying was occurring and tried to intervene (Freis & Gurung, 2013). This supports the view that the most effective way to curtail bullying is to unequivocally state that bullying is occurring and that it needs to stop.

Copycat Suicides

Considerable attention has been directed to suicide contagion or so-called copycat suicides in which youth in a particular school or community attempt suicide in response to the suicide of a peer. Among children and youth 12 to 17 years old, personally knowing someone who died by suicide is associated with an increase in suicidal thoughts and attempts (Swanson & Colman, 2013). Suggestion and imitation seem to play an especially powerful role in the increased risk of suicide among peers following the suicide of a classmate.

Media reports of suicides, especially by celebrities, also seem to spark an increase in suicide, among both youth and adults. In a review of 31 studies, risk of suicide increased by 13 percent after a celebrity died from suicide. When the method of suicide was mentioned, there was a 30 percent increase in suicides using the same method. Even in the case of a noncelebrity suicide, media descriptions of the method of suicide have been associated with an increase in suicides. In contrast, narratives that included alternatives to suicide such as seeking treatment or reaching out for help from a suicide crisis line have been associated with lower suicide rates (Hawley et al. 2023).

This finding illustrates the importance of adhering to media guidelines for the responsible reporting of suicides (Niederkrotenthaler & Till, 2019). Research has indicated that publicizing a suicide may have the effect of glorifying and drawing attention to it. People who are depressed may identify with the pain of someone who ended their life by suicide, increasing their own suicide risk. This pattern appears to be especially true for youngsters who are already thinking about killing themselves; stable, well-adjusted teenagers do not seem to be at risk in these situations. Therefore, best practice guidelines for journalists include not sensationalizing the event, refraining from sharing specific details about the manner of death, and including information on suicide prevention resources (Arkin, 2018).

Decreased Prescribing of Antidepressant Medication

Another explanation for the increase in youth suicides relates to the 2004 U.S. Food and Drug Administration (FDA) warning of an increased suicide risk for children and adolescents taking selective serotonin reuptake inhibitor (SSRI) antidepressants. Although antidepressants can sometimes help youth experiencing depression, the FDA noted an increase in suicidal thoughts and actions among some youth taking SSRIs, and required that a warning to this effect be distributed with all such medication. There is considerable controversy over these actions. Although the effect of SSRIs on the suicide rates in young people is still unresolved (Luft et al., 2018), it remains best practice for medical and mental health professionals to monitor suicidal ideation in anyone who is depressed, especially during the first 4 weeks of medication use. A recent study examining the methodological design of studies focused on antidepressant use with youth came to the conclusion that the better-designed studies confirm an increase in suicidality in youth taking antidepressants and that the black box warning is valid and should remain (Spielmans et al., 2020).

Suicide Among Those Who Serve in the Military

Case Study Leslie McCaddon listened with alarm when she overheard her husband, an Army physician, calling home during a break in his work at a local military hospital, tell their 9-year-old daughter, "Do me a favor . . . Give your mommy a hug and tell her that I love her." A few minutes later, he sent her an e-mail message stating, "This is the hardest e-mail I've ever written . . . Please always tell my children how much I love them, and most importantly, never, ever let them find out how I died . . . I love you." He was later found dead in a room at the hospital where he worked. (Thompson & Gibbs, 2012, p. 24)

Sadly, Leslie McCaddon's husband was battling depression and had reportedly tried to get help multiple times during the week before his death. Many believe the military creates a culture that tends to dismiss and to stigmatize emotional symptoms; this culture may inhibit veterans or those on active duty from seeking help even when dealing with strong emotions such as hostility, anger, hopelessness, or feeling like a burden (Mathes et al., 2020).

Although barriers to seeking and receiving mental health care may contribute to the rates of suicide among members of the military, service members also face other significant influences, including frequent separation from family, deployments, easy access to alcohol and drugs, loss of comrades, and financial or personal problems associated with serving in the military. Mental health issues such as bipolar disorder, opioid use, depression, and PTSD are also significant contributors to military suicide (Veterans Administration [VA], 2019). Additionally, traumatic brain injuries sustained in combat can lead to depression and suicidal thoughts (Bryan & Clemans, 2013).

Suicide risk remains high even after individuals leave the service. U.S. veterans have been found to have a 57.3 percent higher rate of suicide compared to nonveterans (Veterans Administration, 2022). Among 525 military veterans attending college, 46 percent reported having suicidal thoughts at some time during their life, 20 percent had made a suicide plan, 10 percent had frequent thoughts of suicide, 8 percent had made a suicide attempt, and 4 percent indicated that a future suicide attempt was likely or very likely (Rudd et al., 2011). These rates are much higher than those found in the general population. In a comprehensive study analyzing veteran suicides, the Veterans Administration (2016) reported a surge in suicides between 2001 and 2014. While civilian suicides rose 23 percent during this period, veteran suicides increased by 32 percent. Of particular concern was the finding that women who served in the military had 2.4 times the rate of suicide compared to their civilian counterparts. Analysis of suicide rates in subsequent years was equally concerning: The rate of suicide in veterans in 2017 was 1.5 times that of nonveterans (Veterans Administration, 2019). The reasons for the high prevalence of suicidality among military personnel and veterans remain under investigation.

Did You Know?

People who report having nightmares have a fourfold increase in suicide attempts. Experiencing nightmares is more strongly related to suicide risk than are anxiety or depression.

Source: Carr, 2017

Coping with a Suicidal Crisis: A Top Priority

If you or someone you know is experiencing suicidal thoughts, the situation needs to become a top priority. So, what do you? First and foremost, remember that it is important to seek help from someone who has experience dealing with this kind of issue—there is help available day and night. In the United States, you can call or text 988 for the Suicide and Crisis Lifeline, a support network that is available 24/7. You can also use the Lifeline Chat service. A toll-free Spanish-language phone line is available at 1-888-628-9454. These services are free and confidential. You can also contact mental health resources on your campus. Of course, another option is to contact 911 or to go to the local emergency department for immediate assistance. Whether you are the one having the suicidal thoughts or you are concerned that someone else is contemplating suicide, seeking help can make the difference between life and death.

If You Are Having Suicidal Thoughts

What are some things that you can do if you are the one coping with suicidal thoughts? These five steps can help (Jaffe et al., 2013; SAMHSA, 2015):

1. *Promise yourself not to do anything right now.* Even though you are in a lot of emotional pain, make a commitment to yourself that you will wait and put some distance between your suicidal thoughts and any suicidal action. Seeking support can help you keep this commitment. In most situations, suicidal thoughts are associated with mental health problems (such as depression, anxiety, mood swings, or the effects of drugs or alcohol) that can be successfully treated or with temporary problems (such as a relationship breakup, having conflicts with your friends or family, getting bad grades, worries about money) that have solutions. It is likely you will feel much better once these issues are addressed.

2. *Avoid using alcohol or drugs.* It is very important to avoid alcohol or recreational drugs if you are depressed or experiencing suicidal thoughts—they may impair your judgment or make you more likely to act impulsively. Also, they may cause your suicidal thoughts to become even stronger.

3. *Make your environment safe or go to a safe environment.* Try to avoid being alone or thinking about things that make you feel worse. Remove anything you could use to hurt yourself or go somewhere where you know you will be safe.

4. *Remember there is always hope—people who go through hard times find that, with time, their situation improves.* Extreme emotional distress interferes with our ability to consider solutions to problems. No matter how painful your life is right now, if you give yourself time and find support, things will get better—usually *much* better. Reach out for help. Even if you have tried sharing your feelings with someone who

didn't seem to understand, try again. There are people out there who will listen to your concerns with compassion and acceptance, including the people who staff suicide hotlines. They have helped many people like you—they understand.

5. *Don't keep your suicidal feelings to yourself.* Even though it's difficult to discuss your suicidal urges, it is important that you share your thoughts and feelings, including any suicide plans you have made. You can confide in someone you know and trust (a friend, family member, clergy, or therapist, for instance). It also helps to talk with someone experienced in helping people who are having suicidal thoughts. Be honest about what you have been thinking and feeling. Talking can help you put things in perspective—it is very possible that you will discover ways to cope or solutions for some of your worries. Sharing your situation and your thoughts can help you recognize that your distress is temporary and that things will get better. You will find it is a big relief to seek help.

If Someone Else Is Emotionally Distressed or Expressing Suicidal Thoughts

What do you do if someone shares suicidal thoughts with you or if you are with someone who seems very emotionally distressed? By making the person a priority and taking the time to ask, to listen, and to seek help, you may save a life. These steps can help (National Institute of Mental Health [NIMH], 2019a):

1. *Ask—start a conversation so they can share their thoughts and feelings.* If you are concerned about someone, you can start a conversation with openers such as "Are you doing okay? I've been concerned about you" or "You haven't seemed yourself lately. Can we talk about it?" Your goal is to make it clear that you care and want to help. If you are concerned that your friend might be considering suicide, it is important to bring up the topic. You may feel tempted to avoid directly discussing suicide due to fear that if you bring up the subject, you will inadvertently encourage suicidal actions. Nothing could be further from the truth. Someone who is serious about suicide has entertained those thoughts for some time. Our reluctance to discuss suicidal thoughts can have a devastating effect: It prevents a suicidal person from examining the situation more objectively and accessing life-saving help and support. Remember that even if your friend denies suicidal thoughts or plans, that does not necessarily mean there is limited risk; if you feel your friend needs mental health help, continue to encourage them to get that help. If you are unsure what to do after having a conversation, you can contact a suicide hotline, share the specifics of the situation, and seek their advice.

Coping with a Suicidal Crisis: A Top Priority—cont'd

2. *Listen—calmly, empathetically, and without judgment.* Your goal is to allow your friend to talk openly, without fear of being criticized or judged. It is important that you avoid minimizing or discounting what your friend is sharing; avoid arguing or making invalidating comments such as "That's not such a big deal" or "It's not worth killing yourself over that." If your friend is considering suicide, try not to seem frightened, shocked, or overwhelmed by the discussion. Even if the conversation is personally difficult for you, you have an opportunity to help by instilling hope—listening and validating powerful emotions can allow people to move beyond their feelings. You can also help your friend understand that even though the emotional pain may seem unending, the strong feelings they are experiencing can and will get better. Most of the crises we experience in our lives are temporary—suicide is an irreversible solution to a temporary problem.

3. *Seek help.* If you become aware that someone is considering suicide, your goal will be to help connect the person to professional support—as soon as possible. If a suicide attempt seems likely, you can immediately call 911 or call 988 to speak with someone from the Suicide and Crisis Lifeline. Meanwhile, you would stay with the person in a safe environment—somewhere where there is limited access to lethal objects. If your friend has shared any information related to a suicide plan, you would communicate that information to anyone involved in the crisis intervention. This is a situation where getting help is more important than confidentiality; even if you were sworn to secrecy, the main priority is helping your friend stay safe and access needed support. Helping out during a suicidal crisis can be very traumatic. If you are involved in a situation of this nature, consider seeking support from your school's counseling center or local crisis clinic.

For Further Consideration

1. If you were to feel distressed and overwhelmed, who are some people you could confide in? What crisis supports are available at your school or in your city?

2. Why is it so important to check in if you notice that a friend seems withdrawn or is expressing hopelessness? What would you do if you noticed that a classmate or other acquaintance seemed depressed or distressed?

3. For you, what might be the most difficult aspects of helping a friend who shares suicidal thoughts? Would you agree that this is a situation where safety is more important than confidentiality?

Suicide Among College Students

Due to high-profile suicides on several college campuses, national interest in college student suicides has increased (Cramer et al., 2022). When you consider how fortunate college students are to have future opportunities associated with their education, you might wonder why college suicides occur. Was the transition of leaving home, family, and friends; developing new interpersonal relationships; and exposure to a new living arrangement too stressful? Did college work prove too challenging? Were there problems due to drugs and alcohol or a mental health condition? Or did loneliness, isolation, and alienation play a role in their deaths? As with all suicides, we can never be certain.

In a comprehensive study of college student suicide risk, 67,308 students at 108 participating colleges and universities were surveyed about mental health diagnoses, suicidal ideation and attempts, and other demographic factors (Lu, Li, et al., 2019). The study revealed:

- Twenty percent of the students surveyed had thought about suicide and 9 percent had attempted suicide.
- Asian American and multiracial students reported the highest rates of suicidal ideation.

- Transgender students showed elevated rates of suicidal ideation (67 percent), suicide attempts (35 percent), and self-injury (67 percent). Gay/lesbian and bisexual students were two to three times more likely to report suicidal ideation and to attempt suicide than heterosexual students.

- For all students, stress associated with academics, family problems, social relationships, finances, health issues, and personal appearance were strongly related to suicide attempts and to mental health diagnoses.

This study highlights the importance of addressing issues of suicide risk on college campuses. In view of the multiple stressors reported by college students and their relationship to mental health and suicidality, the researchers believe that it is critical to develop programs to inoculate all students against stress during this developmental period; this need is particularly pronounced for highly vulnerable groups such as underrepresented racial or ethnic groups and sexual and gender minorities. Unfortunately, many students who die by suicide do not seek professional help for their distress, despite the ease of access to services through college counseling centers. Students who do share their anguish and thoughts of suicide are most likely to do so with a fellow student (Drum et al., 2009).

Campus prevention and intervention efforts are critically important in identifying students at risk for suicide. Many colleges and universities have developed programs and resources to (1) educate students and staff about warning signs related to suicide; (2) provide counselors, faculty, staff, and students with strategies for intervening if someone appears suicidal; and (3) publicize campus and community resources equipped to deal with a suicidal crisis. Research finds that prevention programs are effective in increasing understanding of suicide and improving help-seeking behaviors (Westefeld, 2018).

Suicide Among Older Adults

Case Study Frank Turkaly took an overdose of tranquilizers. He was a retiree living on disability; had a large amount of debt; had little contact with friends or family; and was coping with depression, diabetes, and high blood pressure. He felt estranged from society—life was different than he had envisioned it in the 1960s and 1970s when the world seemed to have endless possibilities. (Bahrampour, 2013)

In almost all countries, rates of suicide are highest in older adult populations; indeed, suicide rates for elderly men are higher than any other age group (Conejero et al., 2018). In one study comparing rates of suicide among older individuals (age 75 and older) of different ethnic groups, it was found that White men have the highest suicide rate (CDC, 2023).

Aging inevitably results in unwelcome physical changes, including illness and diminishing physical strength. In addition, older adults often encounter a succession of stressful life changes. Bereavement, social isolation, physical ailments, disability and pain, and financial difficulties can increase the risk of suicide in older adults. Older adults who leave suicide notes often express feeling lonely, being socially isolated, or perceiving themselves to be a burden, and they convey frustration over their poor physical or mental health (Cuperfain et al., 2022).

A Matter of Respect

Suicide is less likely to occur among the elderly in cultures that revere and respect people of increasing age. In Asian and African countries and within Indigenous communities, elderhood is equated with greater privilege and status. However, in the United States, growing old is often associated with declining worth and social isolation. What do you think accounts for the high rates of suicide among older adults in the United States?

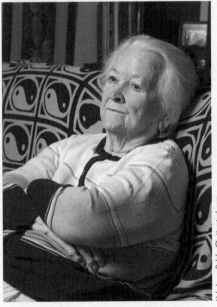

Volodymyr Baleha/Shutterstock.com

Another stressor is the fact that in our youth-oriented society, older adults also face widespread prejudice and discrimination. In fact, internalized ageist stigma has been associated with a reduced will to live (Van Orden & Deming, 2018). This may be especially troubling to those from cultures where elders have traditionally been treated with reverence and respect. Societal mistreatment of older adults may result in depressive symptoms—a depression associated more with "feeling old" than with their actual age or poor physical health (Conejero et al., 2018).

Additionally, elder abuse has increased dramatically. Between 2002 and 2016, assaults of men and women 60 years of age or older rose by 75 percent and 35 percent, respectively. Fifty-eight percent of the perpetrators were family members or acquaintances (Logan et al., 2019). Physical and emotional abuse can result in the elder feeling isolated and devalued. Tragically, elder mistreatment can lead to suicidal behavior (Salvatore et al., 2018).

9-4 A Multipath Perspective of Suicide

A variety of biological, psychological, social, and sociocultural factors can influence a person's decision to end their life by suicide (refer to Figure 9.2). A single risk factor does not cause suicide. Instead, suicide often results from interactions among cumulative or collective influences. Especially when other risk factors are present, a situation, an event, or a series of events can become the final catalyst for suicide.

Biological Dimension

Suicide may have a biological component, according to biochemical and genetic studies. In the mid-1970s, scientists identified a chemical called *5-hydroxyindoleacetic acid* (5-HIAA). This chemical is produced when the body metabolizes serotonin. Low levels of 5-HIAA have been found in people who died from suicide, particularly those who used more violent methods of suicide (Pandey, 2013). This research suggests that reduced availability of serotonin and low serotonin levels are associated with suicide; these abnormalities are also seen in depression. It is also significant that decreased serotonin is linked with increased aggression and impulsivity, characteristics that may increase suicidality (Chadda & Gupta, 2019).

Researchers believe that suicidal tendencies are not simply the result of depression. We already know that some individuals with depression also have low levels of 5-HIAA. What is startling is that low levels of 5-HIAA are found in some people who are suicidal but who have no history of depression, including individuals who have mental disorders other than depression. Researchers believe that low 5-HIAA may indicate a vulnerability to environmental stressors that affect suicidality (Mann et al., 2009). Additionally, researchers compared the levels of neuropeptides (a type of neurotransmitter involved in emotional regulation) in people who died by suicide with levels found in those without suicidal behaviors. Their findings revealed differences in neuropeptide levels between the two groups (Lu, Li, et al., 2019). All of this evidence, of course, is correlational in nature; it does not tell us whether low levels of 5-HIAA or neuropeptide differences cause suicidal behavior—or even whether the two are directly related.

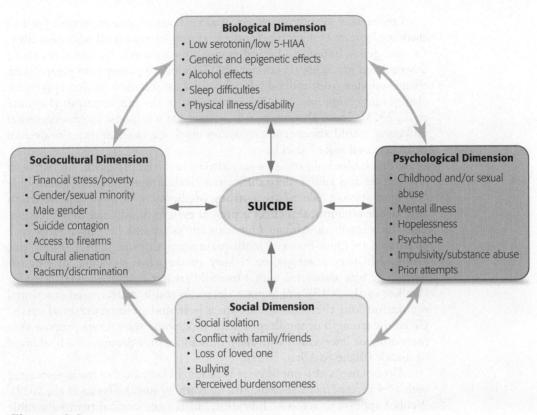

Figure 9.2

Multipath Model of Suicide

A variety of biological, psychological, social, and sociocultural factors may influence a person's decision to end their life by suicide. Cumulative risk factors interact with a situation, an event, or a series of events that become the final catalyst for suicide

Genetics are also implicated in suicidal behavior, but the relationship is complex. Research investigating possible genetic contributions to suicidal behavior suggests that multiple genes are involved, each contributing only small effects, and that suicidal risk is increased when specific genes interact with stressful life events (Antypa et al., 2013). It is likely that these genetic contributions influence both biological processes and certain traits associated with suicide risk. For example, endophenotypes (heritable traits) that are associated with suicide include early-onset major depression, elevated cortisol, serotonin dysfunction, and traits such as aggressive/impulsive tendencies and impaired decision making (Benard et al., 2016).

Some families have higher rates of suicide and suicide attempts (Kenneally et al., 2019). As always, great care must be used in drawing conclusions—increased suicide in the family might be due to factors other than genetics. To separate genetic effects from environmental influences, one group of researchers decided to search for the biological siblings of adoptees who died by suicide (Petersen et al., 2013). The prevalence of suicidal behaviors in this sibling group was significantly higher than a comparison group comprised of siblings of adoptees who died from other causes. This result supports the likelihood of genetic risk factors in suicide. This genetic link to suicide may be expressed in many ways, including traits that increase the potential for suicidality such as stress reactivity or impulsivity. Some researchers believe a gene that regulates interferon production is involved in suicidality, since many people who undergo interferon treatment develop major depressive disorder or suicidal thoughts (Kimbrel et al., 2023).

Did You Know?

People who drink two to four cups of coffee a day have a 50 percent lower rate of suicide, according to a Harvard research study. Caffeine stimulates the central nervous system and boosts neurotransmitters such as dopamine and serotonin; the researchers speculate that this may produce a mild antidepressant effect and thus lower suicide rates.

Source: Lucas et al., 2013

Epigenetic research (the study of alterations in gene expression) is also shedding light on biological processes that may be associated with suicidality. Certain genes known to be influenced by epigenetic factors seem to be dysregulated in suicide (Lutz et al., 2017). Similarly, analysis of postmortem tissue samples from individuals who died by suicide revealed epigenetic changes involving unique DNA alterations in the hippocampus (Labonté et al., 2013). These alterations, which represent a response to environmental influences, could affect gene expression involving characteristics associated with increased risk of suicide.

Other biological processes may also be involved in suicide. Among both adolescents and adults, sleep difficulties (including nightmares and trouble falling or staying asleep) are a strong predictor of both suicidal ideation and suicide attempts; this effect is present even in the absence of depression. One study involving African American adults admitted for psychiatric care confirmed this link between inadequate sleep and suicidality; among this group, a history of struggling to stay awake while working, driving, or socializing was associated with a fourfold greater risk for suicidal behavior (Walker et al., 2019). Inadequate sleep can result in decreased emotional regulation and thereby exacerbate a personal or interpersonal crisis. Given the strength of the sleep–suicide link, some researchers propose that preventing or intervening with sleep difficulties may decrease the likelihood of suicide (Blake & Allen, 2019).

Alcohol use is also implicated in suicide. In fact, alcohol use is associated with a 94 percent increase in the risk of death by suicide (Isaacs et al., 2022). Alcohol appears to act as a "lubricant," increasing suicidality in vulnerable individuals. Alcohol reduces the inhibitory control of our prefrontal cortex; raises our pain threshold; and affects brain regions, such as the limbic system, that are responsible for our emotions and mood. Thus, when emotionality is increased and the prefrontal cortex is less able to inhibit these strong emotions, the risk of suicide rises. In addition, alcohol raises dopamine levels and decreases serotonin levels, a pattern associated with poor impulse control and aggression. This combination of factors can increase the risk of suicide. However, we know that much more than biological factors is involved in suicide.

Psychological Dimension

Case Study Two teenage boys sexually assaulted a 15-year-old girl who passed out after drinking alcohol; they wrote on intimate parts of her body and then circulated a cell phone picture of her. In a Facebook message, she wrote, "I have a reputation for a night I don't even remember and the whole school knows." She later died by suicide. (Associated Press, 2015)

This teen who was sexually assaulted was faced with a multitude of psychological stressors, including shame and humiliation. Psychological pain associated with maltreatment in childhood, particularly sexual abuse and emotional abuse, is a consistent risk factor for suicide in adolescents and adults (Miller et al., 2013). In fact, men and women who experienced physical abuse in childhood are about five times more likely to have suicidal ideation compared to those not subjected to such abuse (Fuller-Thompson, 2012). College women who are survivors of sexual assault have a three-fold greater risk of suicidality than women who have never been assaulted (Dworkin et al., 2020). *Rumination* is linked with increased suicide risk, ideation, and attempts, particularly when the repetitive focus on a topic

Did You Know?

While undergoing fMRI scans, suicidal and nonsuicidal young adults were presented with words that were either positive, neutral, or associated with death and suicide. Using data derived from analyzing differences in cerebral blood flow patterns between the two groups, there was a 91 percent success rate in a follow-up investigation using fMRI scans to differentiate between suicidal and nonsuicidal subjects.

Source: Just et al., 2017

Investigating the Decision to Proceed with a Suicidal Act

How does someone with suicidal ideation make the decision to end their life? For obvious reasons, it is challenging to answer this question in an ethical manner. Since we are unable to assess the thinking of individuals who die by suicide, Franklin et al. (2019) wanted to determine if an analogue approach might provide some insight into understanding suicidal decision-making. Using virtual reality to better understand how someone with suicidal ideation makes the choice to take an action that would result in death, they designed a study in which undergraduate students had the opportunity to virtually participate in two suicide scenes: (1) walking into a building, going into an elevator, riding up several hundred feet, seeing a long plank as they exit the elevator, walking onto the plank, stepping off, and plummeting to the ground; and (2) going into an apartment with a gun in hand, facing a wall, pointing the gun at one's face and pulling the trigger with a resultant flash and loud bang that end the scene. The participants also had the choice of not performing the suicidal act by virtually pressing the elevator button to return to the ground floor in the first scene or by shooting at a blue barrel instead of their face in the second scene. Of the participants, 9.5 percent chose to complete one of the suicide scenarios, and 1.12 percent chose to participate in both scenarios.

All participants were questioned about their reasoning for participating in or avoiding the suicidal act. The researchers believe that research such as this will provide important clues about characteristics of people who follow through with suicidal acts, particularly if future research includes people with suicidal ideation. Although this may be a technological advance in the study of suicide, the study calls into question whether virtual reality investigations might function as a "dry run" for suicidal individuals, perhaps increasing the "acquired capacity" to perform a suicidal act.

For Further Consideration

1. What role can virtual reality play in the study of suicide?

2. What do you think you would have learned about yourself if you had participated in this study?

3. What concerns do you have about the impact on the participants in such a study?

4. Should future research include suicidal individuals in such a study? Why or why not?

takes the form of brooding (Holdaway et al., 2018). Other psychological factors contributing to suicide include shame, discouragement, distress over academic or social pressures, and other life stressors that seem overwhelming (Lu, Li, et al., 2019).

Further, many people who die by suicide have a history of mental illness; the risk is particularly high with depression, bipolar disorder, schizophrenia, eating disorders, some anxiety disorders, some personality disorders, and substance abuse (APA, 2022). For those who do not have a mental disorder, personal problems that precipitate social withdrawal can raise suicide risk (Bachmann, 2018).

Depression and Hopelessness

Suicidal thoughts sometimes develop when someone is experiencing the overwhelming hopelessness, fatigue, and loss of pleasure associated with depression. These intense feelings can lead to suicidal acts, especially when they are combined with a willingness to withstand pain (Rogers & Joiner, 2019). Shneidman (1998) described these feelings as a **"psychache,"** an intolerable pain created from an absence of joy. It is an acute state that encompasses shame, guilt, humiliation, loneliness, and fear. Psychache has, in fact, been strongly linked with suicidal ideation, even more so than depression or hopelessness (Lambert et al., 2020).

We know that having a depressive disorder is associated with suicidal thoughts and behaviors, but what about milder symptoms of depression? In a sample of 12,395 adolescents from 11 countries, 29 percent had symptoms of mild depression and another 10.5 percent had symptoms severe enough to meet the criteria for a depressive disorder; those with mild depression had

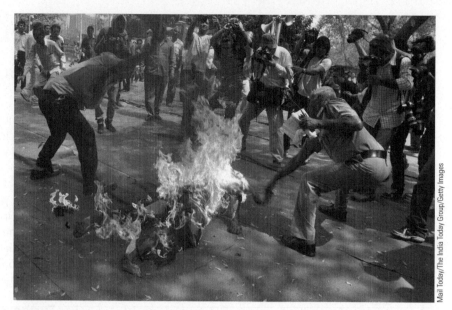

Politically Motivated Suicide

In some cultures, self-immolation is conducted as a form of protest against the government. In this photo, a Tibetan man is engulfed in flames after setting himself on fire to protest China's control over Tibet.

three times more suicidal thoughts compared to adolescents without depressive symptoms, whereas those with more severe depression had nine times more suicidal thoughts (Balazs et al., 2013). Thus, even milder depression may increase suicide risk. Although depression is associated with suicidal thoughts and behavior, the relationship is complex. For example, in some cases, the limited energy seen in severe depression makes suicide less likely. The danger period often comes when the depression begins to lift. Energy and motivation increase, enhancing the likelihood of follow-through with suicide plans.

Drug and Alcohol Use

Substance use involving alcohol, cocaine, cannabis, opioids, amphetamines, or sedatives increases the risk of suicide for men and, even more so, for women (Bohnert et al., 2017). The use of opioids and opioid-use disorder seem to have a particularly strong relationship to suicide. In one analysis, more than 40 percent of suicides and overdose deaths involved opioids (Bohnert & Ilgen, 2019). Cannabis use during adolescence is associated with depression and suicidal ideation in young adulthood; these findings are concerning because of the increasing use of cannabis among adolescents (Gobbi et al., 2019).

One of the most consistently reported correlates of suicidal behavior is alcohol consumption. In one study, 71 percent of men and 43 percent of women who had a drinking problem had attempted suicide (Dambrauskiene et al., 2019). Further, as many as 70 percent of people who attempt suicide drink alcohol before the act, and autopsies of individuals who died by suicide suggest that many were legally intoxicated. Not only does alcohol have biological effects such as decreasing judgment, it also has psychological effects such as lowering inhibitions related to the fear of death, thus making it easier to carry out suicide plans (Conner & Bagge, 2019). Heavy alcohol consumption, such as binge drinking, also seems to deepen feelings of remorse during dry periods, resulting in an increased risk even when the person is sober.

Several classic studies, however, suggest another explanation for the effects of alcohol: The strength of the relationship between alcohol and suicide may result from "alcohol-induced myopia," a constriction of cognitive and perceptual processes (Bayless & Harvey, 2017). Alcohol use may increase personal distress by focusing a person's thoughts on negative aspects of their personal situation. Alcohol does seem to constrict cognitive and perceptual processes. Although drinking may relieve depression and anxiety by distracting the person from problems, it is equally likely to intensify distress by narrowing the person's focus and increasing attention to personal challenges (Sevincer & Oettingen, 2014). Thus, a psychological link between alcohol and suicide may be due to the myopic qualities of alcohol exaggerating a previously existing depressed state.

Social Dimension

Case Study Ten-year-old Tammy Jimenez was the youngest of three girls—a loner who had attempted suicide at least twice in the previous 2 years. Tammy's parents always seemed to be arguing and threatening divorce. Her father often lashed out at the children when he was intoxicated. One evening in late February, Tammy was struck and killed by a truck when she darted out into the highway that passed by her home. The incident was declared an accident. However, her older sister reported that Tammy had deliberately killed herself. On the evening of her death, an argument with her father had upset and angered her. Her sister said that seconds before Tammy ran out onto the highway, she cried out that no one wanted her around and that she wanted to die.

As in Tammy's tragic death, many suicides are interpersonal in nature and occur following relationship conflicts. Social factors that separate people or make them less connected to families, friends, religious institutions, or communities can also increase susceptibility to suicide. For example, unhappiness over a broken relationship, marital discord, disputes with parents, and recent bereavements all increase suicide risk (Stewart et al., 2019). Family instability, stress, and a chaotic family atmosphere are factors in suicide attempts by younger children, as we saw in the death of Tammy. Children who consider suicide are more likely to have experienced physical or sexual abuse, emotional neglect, unpredictable traumatic events, and/or the loss of a significant parenting figure (Sousa et al., 2017; Wan et al., 2019). Other adverse childhood experiences such as neglect, experiencing or witnessing violence, or having a family member attempt or die by suicide are also associated with an increased risk of suicide ideation and planning among adolescents. Among one group of high school students who had experienced sexual violence, nearly one third made a suicide attempt (Anderson et al., 2022).

It is not surprising that suicide prevention efforts often focus on increasing social support and connectedness as well as on decreasing social isolation. Lizbeth, a Latina immigrant whose language barrier made it difficult to establish friendships, linked her suicide attempt directly to her experience of thwarted belongingness, explaining, "Nobody supports me. I have no one to talk to. So, I just want to die so I don't have to be with all of this" (Gulbas et al., 2019).

The case of Lizbeth demonstrates one of the social factors associated with suicide in Thomas Joiner's interpersonal-psychological theory of suicide (Horton et al., 2016; Joiner et al., 2009). In an attempt to integrate

Myth Suicides occur more frequently during the holiday season because of depression, loneliness, and a feeling of disconnection from significant others.

Reality Despite media reports that there are more suicides over the holiday season, the suicide rate in the United States is lowest during the month of December, with suicide rates peaking in the spring and fall. There is an increase in suicidal behavior on New Year's Day, whereas fewer suicidal acts occur on Independence Day, Thanksgiving, and Christmas. Some researchers are concerned that the perpetuation of the holiday suicide myth may result in an actual increase in suicides due to a "contagion" effect.

Source: Beauchamp et al., 2014

the many influences associated with suicide, Joiner proposed that two social factors are strongly associated with suicide attempts: (a) perceived burdensomeness—feelings of being a burden to family, friends, or society; and (b) thwarted belongingness—feelings of alienation and a lack of meaningful connections to others. How important are interpersonal relationship issues in suicides? Investigators studied 100 suicide attempters to determine if some type of negative life event occurred within 48 hours of the attempt. As predicted by Joiner's theory, many reported recent interpersonal issues with a partner or other relationship conflicts (Bagge et al., 2013). Another study also found that the perception of being a burden was an antecedent for suicidality among military service members (Crowell-Williamson et al., 2019).

A unique third condition must exist before a suicide attempt occurs, according to Joiner's theory: the acquired capacity for suicide. People must experience a reduction in fear of taking their own life that is sufficient to overcome self-preservation reflexes. Unfortunately, repeated exposure to traumatic life events (physical or emotional abuse, rape, bullying, exposure to wartime atrocities, etc.) may result in habituation to painful life circumstances and may lower the fear of inflicting self-injury; this is the acquired capacity for suicide. Studies have found that people who attempt suicide do indeed report higher levels of fearlessness and pain insensitivity, as well as greater frequency of painful life events (Smith et al., 2010). In one study, individuals with a history of attempted suicide tolerated holding their breath and holding their hand under ice cold water longer than a matched psychiatric sample without a history of suicide attempts. These results support the view that the "numbing" of physical sensations may represent an acquired capacity (DeVille et al., 2020). For adolescents, acquired capacity increases with continued exposure to negative experiences, a focus on suicidal thoughts and plans, and self-injurious acts (Holland et al., 2017).

Marital Status

A stable marriage or relationship makes suicide less likely (Kyung-Sook et al., 2018). Additionally, for women, having children decreases suicide risk (Denney, 2010). Not surprisingly, people who are divorced, separated, or widowed have higher suicide rates than those who are married (Navaneelan, 2013). In fact, the death of a spouse is associated with a 50 percent higher risk of suicide for men, and divorced men have a 39 percent higher risk of suicide compared to married men (Denney et al., 2009).

Sociocultural Dimension

French sociologist Émile Durkheim (1897/1951) studied suicides in different countries, across different periods, and proposed one of the first sociocultural explanations of suicide. Suicide, as theorized by Durkheim, results from an inability to integrate oneself with society. In Durkheim's view, failing to maintain close ties with the community deprives a person of the support systems that are necessary for adaptive functioning. Without such support, the person becomes isolated and alienated from other people. Some **suicidologists** believe that our modern, mobile, and technological society, which deemphasizes the importance of extended families and a sense of community, is partially responsible for increased suicide rates.

Suicide Bombings

In the aftermath of a suicide bombing in Baghdad, two men try desperately to move a car to clear the way for help. These events have become an all too common sight in Iraq.

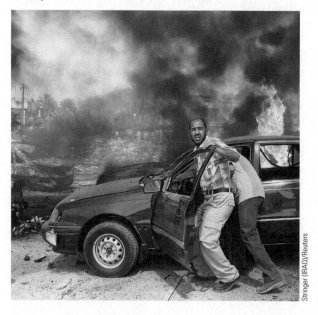

Stringer (IRAQ)/Reuters

Ethnic and Cultural Variables

Suicidal ideation and rates of suicide vary among ethnic groups in the United States. The rates of suicide are highest among American Indian/Alaska Native people, followed by non-Hispanic Whites; they are lowest among Blacks, Asian Americans, and Latinx Americans (AFSP, 2020). Between 2018 and 2021, suicide rates significantly increased among American Indian/Alaska Natives (an increase of 26 percent) and among Blacks (an increase of 19.2 percent), and they declined by 3.9 percent among Whites (Stone et al., 2023).

Suicide rates for men of color are from three to four times higher than for their female counterparts. Native American/Alaska Native and European American boys and men have the highest rates of suicide; rates are much lower among African American, Hispanic American, and Asian American/Pacific Islander boys and men (AFSP, 2020). Although women in all groups have lower rates of suicide compared to men, the pattern of ethnic distribution among women is quite similar to that seen with men (refer to Figure 9.3).

Everyday experiences with discrimination, such as those frequently encountered by people of color, not only link directly to increased risk of suicidal ideation but also appear to exert an indirect influence by increasing the risk of anxiety and depression (Kwon & Han, 2019). Thus, it is not surprising that for all ethnic groups, those who report the highest levels of discrimination have the greatest likelihood of experiencing suicidal thoughts, plans, or attempts (Oh et al., 2019). Cumulative experiences of racial or ethnic discrimination appear to have a particularly strong effect on young adult Latinas, particularly those with a history of traumatic stress and depression (Polanco-Roman et al., 2019).

Social change and social disorganization, which reduces integration with one's community, may predispose members of a particular group to suicide. A regrettable example of this is the disorganization imposed on Native Americans by U.S. society: Families were deprived of their lands, torn apart, and forced to live on reservations, while their children were sent to boarding schools only to become trapped on the margins of two different cultural traditions. Many Native Americans became alienated and isolated from their communities and from larger society (Sue et al., 2022).

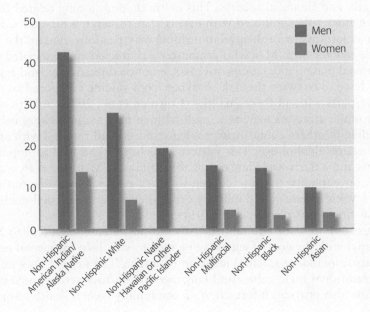

Figure 9.3

Age-Adjusted Rates of Suicide by Gender/Race/Ethnicity: United States, 2021

There are significant between-group differences in suicide rates within the United States—between men and women and between different ethnic and racial groups.

Source: CDC, 2023

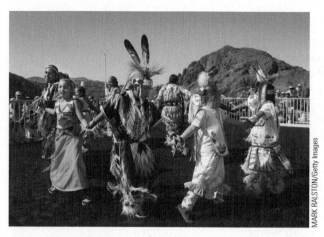

Native American and Proud of It

Efforts to combat high suicide rates among Native American youth have focused on efforts to increase ethnic pride and validation of cultural wisdom and traditions. Many tribes are attempting to build resilience by connecting children and adolescents with their cultural heritage. Here Native American children perform a traditional dance.

MARK RALSTON/Getty Images

Risk factors for suicide among Asian/Pacific Islanders include alcohol and substance use, historical trauma, mental health issues such as depression, loss of cultural identity and community, and internalized stigma (Allen et al., 2018; O'Keefe & Reger, 2017). During the COVID pandemic, anti-Asian incidents increased by nearly 150 percent, ranging from online harassment to physical assaults. This resulted in increases in depression and suicidal ideation (Zhou et al., 2021).

In contrast, aspects of the African American culture such as close family relationships, strong community connections, and religious and personal values that discourage suicide may decrease suicide risk. Similarly, the strong social connections and religiosity seen in Latinx communities may account for the lower incidence of suicide. Conversely, the perception that suicide would bring shame to the family might account for the relatively low suicide rates among Asian Americans (Sue et al., 2022).

Gender and Sexual Orientation

Worldwide, men are about twice as likely as women to die by suicide, although women and girls have higher rates of suicidal thoughts and suicide attempts (Bachmann, 2018). In the United States, men are about four times more likely to die by suicide than women (CDC, 2023). Recent findings indicate that the U.S. gender gap in death by suicide is narrowing, however, particularly within the 10- to 19-year-old age group. Even though boys continue to choose methods with greater lethality such as firearms and hanging/suffocation while drug overdose/poisoning remains the most common method used by girls, death by hanging/suffocation has increased among girls (Ruch et al., 2019).

Although the use of lethal methods partially explains the high rate of suicide among boys and men, the issue is more complex. Suicide among men is particularly perplexing because many men who die by suicide have no history of mental illness and no previous suicide attempts (Kaplan et al., 2012). One possible explanation is that most men are socialized to believe they must meet perceived societal expectations such as self-sufficiency, strength, and financial success. This cultural conditioning related to the male gender role combined with events that threaten a masculine ideal (such as job loss or broken relationships) may partially explain the high suicide rate for men. Men who demonstrate characteristics associated with traditional masculinity (competitiveness, emotional restriction, and aggression) have over twice the risk of dying from suicide compared to their counterparts without these qualities (Coleman et al., 2020). Additionally, when under stress or experiencing loss, men may avoid seeking help or confiding in others about their problems and instead respond with anger, violence, or alcohol use. This pattern of behavior can lead to impulsive actions and a narrowed view of possible solutions. Men may also acquire a greater capacity for suicide due to work-related exposure to death (e.g., law enforcement and military careers) and access to lethal methods, such as firearms (Coleman et al., 2011).

A group in Colorado launched a multimedia campaign (called Man Therapy) with the goal of encouraging men to seek help for mental health concerns, including suicidal ideation or intent. The project uses humor and traditional male values and language to confront serious issues; the Web site also provides information on community mental health resources

(Spencer-Thomas, 2018). In a similar attempt to engage masculine concepts, the U.S. Department of Veterans Affairs initiated a campaign with the slogan "It takes the strength and courage of a warrior to ask for help."

Suicide risk is also significantly elevated within the LGBTQ community. For example, as compared to their cisgender and heterosexual peers, LGBTQ youth have higher rates of suicide attempts. In a 2021 survey of U.S. high school students, 26.3 percent of the gay and lesbian students surveyed reported that they had attempted suicide, a rate five times higher than that reported by heterosexual students (5.2 percent) (CDC, 2023). A large population-based study on sexual minority and transgender students in Canada found that transgender youth experienced high rates of bullying and cyberbullying and were 7.6 times more likely to attempt suicide compared to their cisgender peers. Among other significant findings, cisgender girls attracted to girls had 3.3 times the risk of suicide, adolescents attracted to multiple genders had 2.8 times the risk of suicide attempts, and youth questioning their sexual orientation had twice the risk of attempted suicide (Kingsbury et al., 2022).

The sense of alienation and isolation experienced by many LGBTQ youth and adults may explain their increased suicide risk (di Giacomo et al., 2018). There is additional concern that laws that prohibit school personnel from discussing sexual orientation or gender nonconformity or that deny the provision of gender-affirming medical treatments may result in increased distress among and more prejudice, discrimination, and bullying directed toward members of the LGBTQ community.

Social support from adults, peers, and other allies can decrease the risk of suicidality among LGBTQ youth. The strongest protective supports involve acceptance from parents and family members followed by peer acceptance. For transgender and nonbinary youth, peer acceptance is especially impactful. Further, having even one supportive adult can significantly reduce the odds of a suicide attempt (Price & Green, 2023).

Socioeconomic Stressors

Environmental and economic issues can have a significant impact on suicide rates. Mental health issues often arise during natural disasters. In Puerto Rico, for example, the rate of suicide increased by 29 percent after the destruction caused by Hurricane Maria. After telephone service was reestablished, over 5,000 of the people who made calls to the local mental health helpline expressed suicidal thoughts (Acevedo, 2018). Suicide rates and alcohol-involved suicides also increase during economic recessions, particularly among those experiencing poverty and unemployment (Kerr et al., 2017) and those who declare bankruptcy (Kidger, 2011). Consistent with these data, unemployed adults are over twice as likely to have serious thoughts of suicide, and over four times more likely to make suicide plans or attempt suicide compared to fully employed adults. Also, individuals who qualify for Medicaid (subsidized medical assistance for those with low income) have higher suicide rates compared to those who can afford health insurance (Substance Abuse and Mental Health Services Administration [SAMHSA], 2012). These economic conditions may increase anxiety, depression, and alcohol consumption, leading to suicidal behavior.

Religious Affiliation

Religious affiliation appears to influence certain aspects of suicidal behavior. In a review of 87 studies examining religion and suicide, religious affiliation and attendance appears to protect against suicide attempts and suicide but not against suicidal ideation (Lawrence et al., 2016). Although it may be that religiosity is protective because some religions view suicide to be sinful or immoral, it is also possible that connection with a spiritual community provides the supportive elements of a larger social network. The children of parents with strong religious beliefs have been found to have an 80 percent lower risk of suicide ideation or attempts than children whose parents feel religion is unimportant. Interestingly, this association exists independent of the children's own religious beliefs (Svob et al., 2018).

9-5 Preventing Suicide

Suicide is irreversible, of course, so prevention is critical. Early detection and successful intervention rely on understanding risk and protective factors associated with suicide (refer to Table 9.2). Suicide prevention can occur at several levels. Someone in crisis can self-refer for help, or referrals can originate from concerned family, friends, or coworkers. One promising intervention is gatekeeper training; with this model, designated people within a system (such as schools or the military) learn about risk factors associated with suicide and methods for screening people at high risk (CDC, 2022). If screening results are suggestive of suicide risk, comprehensive assessment and intervention occur. Screening and risk assessment within communities of color are most effective when nontraditional risk factors such as societal rejection, community violence, or racism are incorporated into the screening or assessment process (Molock et al., 2023).

Working with a potentially suicidal individual is a three-step process that involves (1) knowing which factors increase the likelihood of suicide; (2) determining whether there is high, moderate, or low probability that the person will act on the suicide wish; and (3) implementing appropriate actions (Isaac et al., 2009). Figure 9.4 summarizes the process of assessing risk and intervening based on different levels of risk. People trained in working with individuals who are suicidal often begin by looking for clues to suicidal intent.

Table 9.2 Risk and Protective Factors in Suicide Assessment and Intervention

Risk Factors	Protective Factors
• Previous suicide intent or attempt; self-injurious behavior or talk about suicide, dying, or self-harm	• Good emotional regulation, problem-solving, and conflict-resolution skills
• Substance abuse, chronic pain or physical illness, insomnia, and certain mental disorders	• Willingness to talk about problems
• Hopelessness, shame, humiliation, despair, anxiety/panic, self-loathing; impulsive or aggressive tendencies	• Cultural and religious beliefs that discourage suicide
• Recent loss or significant traumatic event, including a failed relationship, bereavement, or unemployment	• Open to seeking treatment for mental, physical, or substance-use disorders
• Relational conflicts, loneliness, and social isolation	• Family and community support
• Seeking out or easy access to lethal methods, especially guns	• Connection to or responsibility for children or beloved pets
• Family turmoil; history of physical or sexual abuse	• Restricted access to lethal means of suicide
• Family members, peers, or favored celebrities who have died from suicide	

Source: CDC, 2019b

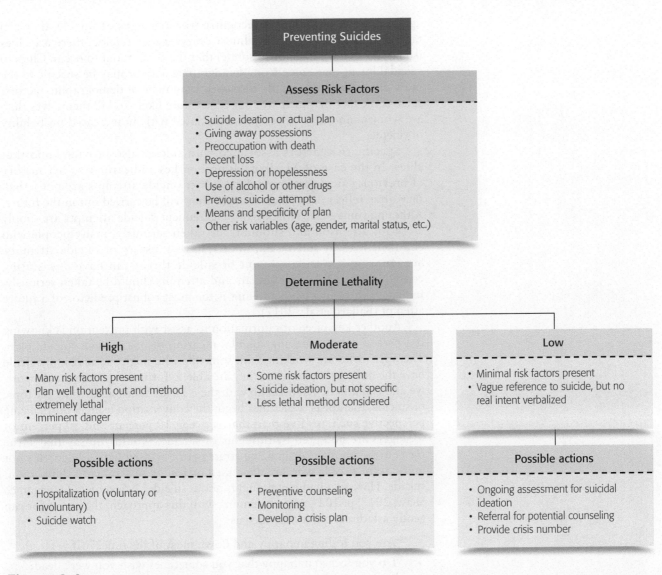

Figure 9.4

The Process of Preventing Suicide

Suicide prevention involves the careful assessment of risk factors to determine lethality—the probability that a person will choose to end their life. Working with an individual who is potentially suicidal is a three-step process that involves (1) knowing what risk factors are associated with suicide; (2) determining whether there is high, moderate, or low probability that the person will act on suicidal thoughts; and (3) implementing appropriate actions.

Clues to Suicidal Intent

Case Study   At the height of her acting career, Marilyn Monroe took a large number of barbiturates, and then called people to tell them she was in trouble. She had made similar suicide attempts in the past and had always been rescued. This time help came too late. Had she truly wanted to die? Could something have been done to prevent her death? (Fernández-Cabana et al., 2013)

Preventing suicide depends on recognizing signs of potential suicide. Therapists, friends, family, or those trained in gatekeeper programs (such as the programs used on many college campuses) are the first line of defense against suicide—when they recognize warning signs of suicide, they can take actions to intervene. In almost every case of suicide, there are clues (some subtle and some not so subtle) that the act is about to occur. Clues to suicidal intent may come from demographic data or may be specific to the individual. We have already discussed a number of demographic factors, such as the fact that men are four times more likely to kill themselves than are women, and that older age is associated with an increased probability of suicide.

Specific risk factors associated with suicide also provide important clues. In the case of Marilyn Monroe, a key indicator was her history of previous suicide attempts. Even when suicide attempts are not lethal, they often reflect deep suicidal intent that will be carried out in the future. Although some believe the myth that frequent suicide attempts are simply a cry for attention and shouldn't be taken seriously, many people who end their lives by suicide do, in fact, have a history of suicide attempts. So, ignoring a suicide attempt or suicide threat can have devastating consequences. All suicide threats and attempts should be taken seriously. In fact, a previous suicide attempt is the most robust predictor of a future attempt (Ballard et al., 2017).

Another key piece of information to assist with prevention is knowing if a person is experiencing suicidal ideation or has made a suicide plan. Therapists who are working with someone who might be at risk of suicide have the most influence when they are able to form and maintain a supportive and empathetic relationship with their client. When addressing the topic of suicide, therapists sometimes begin the conversation using a normalizing perspective such as "I've read that between 10 percent and 50 percent of teenagers are bothered by thoughts of suicide. Would you say that's true for you?" A similar normalizing strategy can be used with adults: "It's not unusual for people who are depressed or feeling miserable to think about suicide. Have you had any thoughts about suicide?" (Sommers-Flanagan & Shaw, 2017, p. 102). After beginning with this approach, the counselor can gently ask direct questions, such as:

"Are you feeling unhappy and down most of the time?" (If yes . . .)

"Do you feel so unhappy that you sometimes wish you were dead?" (If yes . . .)

"Have you ever thought about taking your own life?" (If yes . . .)

"What methods have you thought about using to kill yourself?" (If the client specifies a method . . .)

"When do you plan to do this?"

This openness will not adversely affect those who are suicidal. Instead, direct and straightforward discussion may help diminish distress and allow someone contemplating suicide to consider problems and situations from a broader perspective—especially if an empathetic and normalizing stance had been taken in the beginning. Many people considering suicide are relieved to be able to discuss a taboo topic openly and honestly, and to have someone help them look at their situation more objectively. Additionally, the amount of detail involved in a suicide plan is a clue to the potential seriousness of the situation. A person who provides specific details, such as method, time, or place, is much more at risk than someone who has no detailed plan.

Suicide potential further increases if the person has direct access to the means of suicide, such as a loaded pistol. Also, suicide is often preceded by a precipitating event. Triggers such as the breakup of an important relationship, perceiving oneself to be a burden, difficulties at school or at work, public humiliation, loss of a loved one, family discord, chronic pain, or terminal illness may contribute to a person's decision to end their life.

Many people contemplating suicide verbally communicate their intent. Some people make very direct statements: "I wish I were dead" or "If this happens again, I'll kill myself." Others make indirect statements: "I've had it," "Everyone would be better off without me," "I'm so tired of feeling depressed," or "I've been thinking a lot about death lately." Sometimes these communications occur in person, but it is equally likely for messages to be sent via e-mail, text, or social media posts, sometimes shortly before the suicidal act.

Although some clues are very direct, many indications are much more subtle. Indirect behavioral clues include withdrawal, restlessness or changes in sleep patterns, reckless behavior, increased drinking or drug use, giving away possessions, or a prolonged or unexpected farewell. Concern is greatest when behavior deviates from what is normal for the person. Some clinicians divide warning signs into two categories: (a) early signs, such as depression, expressions of guilt or remorse, tension or anxiety, insomnia, or loss of appetite, and (b) critical signs, such as sudden changes in behavior (uncharacteristic risk taking or calmness after a period of anxiety or depression), unusual or unexpected contact with family or friends, saying goodbye, giving away belongings, putting affairs in order, direct or indirect threats, and actual attempts (Smith et al., 2013). Recognizing clues to intent is a critical first step—the next step is seeking immediate help if you believe someone is at risk of dying by suicide.

Suicide Hotlines

National agencies and local communities that sponsor suicide prevention centers and suicide hotlines recognize that a suicidal crisis requiring immediate preventive assistance can occur at any time, day or night. These resources are available to those considering suicide and to people concerned about a friend, family member, or coworker. Suicide hotlines typically operate 24 hours a day, 7 days a week. Because most contacts are by phone, crisis lines publicize their numbers throughout the community. One well-known hotline in the United States is the 988 Suicide and Crisis Lifeline, a national network that provides 24/7 free and confidential phone and text support for children, teens, and adults experiencing emotional distress. This project also includes a specialized pilot program providing text and chat services for lesbian, gay, bisexual, transgender, queer, questioning, and other sexual and gender minority youth and young adults.

Volunteers, paraprofessionals, and mental health professionals who staff suicide prevention centers are trained in a variety of crisis intervention techniques, including:

1. *Maintaining contact and establishing a relationship.* Establishing a good relationship with a suicidal caller by demonstrating interest and concern and keeping the caller on the line increases the chances that the caller will realize there are solutions other than suicide.

2. *Obtaining necessary information.* The worker elicits demographic data and the caller's name and address. This information is very valuable in case there is an urgent need to locate the caller.

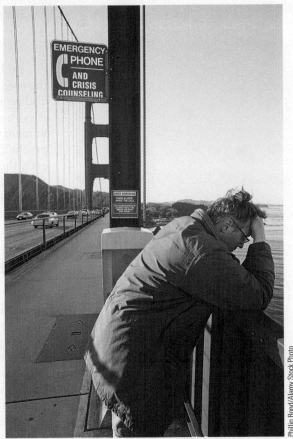

Phillip Bond/Alamy Stock Photo

Intervening Before It Is Too Late

Suicide prevention centers and the 988 Suicide & Crisis Lifeline operate 24 hours a day, 7 days a week, with well-trained crisis workers available to provide immediate support.

3. *Evaluating suicidal potential.* The staff person taking the call must quickly determine the seriousness of the caller's self-destructive intent. Most centers use **lethality** rating scales to help workers determine suicide potential. These usually contain questions about age, gender, onset of symptoms, situational plight, prior suicidal behavior, and access to lethal methods.

4. *Clarifying the nature of the caller's distress.* Crisis workers help callers (1) clarify the exact nature of their concerns, (2) recognize that they may be under so much duress that they are not thinking clearly, and (3) realize that there are other solutions besides suicide. Because feelings of hopelessness often interfere with logical thinking, a key goal is to help callers recognize that there are options they might not have considered. When callers seem disoriented or confused, workers ask very specific questions to help bring them back to reality.

5. *Assessing strengths and resources.* In developing a crisis plan, workers often mobilize a caller's strengths or available resources. In their agitation and distress, callers may forget coping strategies that have helped them previously. The worker explores potential social resources, including family, friends, and coworkers, as well as professional resources such as doctors, clergy, and therapists.

6. *Recommending and initiating an action plan.* Besides being supportive, crisis workers are highly directive in developing a course of action. Whether the recommendation entails immediately seeing the person, calling the person's family, or referring the person for a crisis counseling appointment the next day, the worker presents a systematic plan of action.

Both the approach and the order of these steps will vary depending on the needs of the individual caller and the potential lethality of the situation. Today, hundreds of suicide hotlines function in the United States. There is evidence that suicide prevention efforts such as these can help meet the immediate needs of callers—reducing suicidal thoughts and decreasing psychological pain and feelings of hopelessness (Tyson et al., 2016). However, the key to enhancing the success of suicide prevention efforts is the availability of mental health services during and immediately after a crisis. Many centers provide crisis treatment. Centers that lack such resources develop cooperative service arrangements with community mental health agencies equipped to provide crisis services.

Suicide Crisis Intervention

Suicide crisis intervention can be highly successful for (1) those who independently seek professional help for suicidal ideation; (2) clients who bring suicidal thoughts or intentions to the attention of their therapist; and (3) people encouraged to seek professional help by concerned family, friends, teachers, or coworkers. In addition to preventing suicide, the goal is to resolve feelings of hopelessness and concerns about immediate life crises. Crisis workers focus on the person's emotional pain and operate under the assumption that anyone considering suicide is ambivalent about the act; they exert great effort to preserve the drive to live (Vatne & Naden, 2016). They may point out that the person's willingness to share their despair and thoughts of suicide reflects a desire for help and a desire to live.

Similarly, the person intervening may explain that suicidal thoughts often represent the depth of a person's feelings rather than a true intent to take action, particularly considering the finality of death. They may also reassure the suicidal person that although it may seem that the pain will go on forever, there are resources to help them cope and resolve whatever feels so overwhelming. Although discussions often begin by validating the person's emotional anguish, the conversation moves on to practical matters such as ideas for decreasing stress and managing immediate problems. Unlike traditional psychotherapy, in which sessions are spaced out and treatment is provided on a more leisurely long-term basis, crisis intervention personnel recognize the immediacy of the person's need for hope and support.

An approach sometimes used in interventions with someone expressing suicidal intent is a "no-harm" agreement, sometimes referred to as a "no-suicide contract" or "suicide-prevention contract." Typically, this is a written agreement developed between the suicidal person and a therapist or the person involved in crisis intervention. Generally, the agreement involves a commitment that the suicidal person will not engage in self-harm for a designated period of time; a plan is also developed in the event that suicidal impulses continue. Although agreements such as these are frequently used, there is a lack of research supporting their effectiveness. In fact, the use of a no-harm agreement may lead to liability issues for the therapist if the person proceeds with suicide. Instead, therapists often develop a broad safety plan that may include actions such as journaling and calling a friend or a crisis helpline (Caldwell, 2019).

In some cases, the safest plan for those with strong suicidal urges is temporary hospitalization. In a hospital environment, there is close monitoring and the opportunity to receive assistance from a psychiatric team until the immediate crisis has passed. The hospital team also helps determine what supports are needed once patients leave the hospital. After returning to a more stable emotional state and with the immediate risk of suicide behind them, patients can begin more traditional outpatient treatment. Relatives and friends are often enlisted to help monitor their loved one's safety and well-being following hospitalization and are given guidance on how to provide support between therapy sessions and whom to notify if problems arise outside of the hospital.

Psychotherapy for Suicidal Individuals

Treatment for those who have attempted suicide or who have suicidal ideation often involves both medication (which will vary depending on the underlying mental disorder) and psychotherapy. Psychotherapy techniques proven to reduce suicide risk include cognitive-behavioral therapy (CBT) and dialectical behavior therapy (DBT). The CBT program focuses on vulnerabilities associated with suicide such as feelings of hopelessness; social isolation; poor impulse control; poor problem solving; and difficulty refuting thoughts, images, and beliefs associated with suicide. One cognitive-behavioral program, developed to treat suicidality in veterans, addresses two factors related to suicidal risk—"thwarted belongingness" and "perceived burden." Cognitive-behavioral techniques are used to question thoughts such as "No one wants me around," and more realistic thoughts are identified and substituted. The veterans are then presented with ambiguous scenarios that they practice resolving in a positive manner. This program has demonstrated success in reducing suicidality (Short et al., 2019).

Dialectical behavior therapy (DBT) is also effective with severely suicidal individuals. DBT focuses on helping clients accept their current lives and the emotional anguish they feel. An important goal for suicidal clients is learning to regulate and tolerate their emotions rather than allowing emotions to overwhelm them and result in a suicidal act. A meta-analysis of 18 DBT studies confirmed that DBT significantly reduces self-directed violence (DeCou et al., 2019).

Cognitive-behavioral therapy for suicide prevention, an innovative program for suicidal adolescents, combines features of both CBT and DBT (Asarnow et al., 2017). Risk factors and stressors, including emotional, cognitive, behavioral, and interpersonal processes that occurred just before and after the suicide attempt or suicidal crisis, are discussed. Other difficulties such as an inability to regulate emotions, poor problem-solving skills, or negative thoughts and beliefs are also identified. The treatment program includes:

1. *Chain analysis*—During this phase, the client describes all the events, stressors, thoughts, interpersonal conflicts, and other factors, such as drug use, that led to the suicide attempt. This information allows the mental health professional to devise a specific treatment plan based on the client's unique circumstances. The adolescent's family members also participate in a similar chain analysis.

2. *Safety planning*—Clients work with the therapist to develop a prioritized list of internal and external coping strategies and social supports that can be relied on during a suicidal crisis.

3. *Psychoeducation*—The client and family learn about suicide prevention, safety issues, and strategies for regulating emotions. Parents are taught how to actively listen and validate feelings, problem-solve, and participate in self-care.

4. *Building hope and addressing reasons for living*—The therapist helps the client focus on reasons for staying alive such as friends and family, plans for the future, or things the client would like to do or accomplish. Coping strategies make more sense when there is hope for the future.

5. *Learning and using adaptive strategies from CBT and DBT to deal with specific problems*—The client is given homework that involves making use of strategies learned in therapy.

This program is not only effective in reducing suicide attempts and self-harm, but also has the additional benefit of strengthening the bond between the adolescents and their parents.

Recovery After a Suicide Attempt

Case Study   On the morning of December 25, 2000, Terry Wise tried to kill herself. She awoke two days later in the intensive care unit. The death of Terry's husband from Lou Gehrig's disease was a trigger for her suicide attempt.... Terry was overwhelmed by an intense emotional pain that had been building for years ... suicide felt like a way to end the pain. (SAMHSA, 2015, p. 1)

Case Study   Jordan was only 16 when he was diagnosed with depression. Jordan said that he hated himself. As an African American, he felt that he didn't fit in with the mostly White students in his school, and he felt like a failure if he didn't get the grades he and his parents wanted him to achieve ... after his suicide attempt, he ended up in a coma. (SAMHSA, 2015, p. 5)

Both Terry and Jordan survived their suicide attempts and are now speakers who travel the country helping others who are struggling with suicide. As with many suicide survivors, they found the strength to recover despite the increased stressors following their survival. The aftermath of a suicide attempt often includes continuation of the emotional pain that led to the suicidal act, sometimes exacerbated by reactions from family and friends; complicated emotions, including relief, anger, embarrassment, shame, or guilt; and feeling alone and isolated. Therefore, it is of critical importance for anyone who has attempted suicide to focus on activities that increase optimism and social connection and to realize that there is

Going Deeper

Do People Have a Right to Die?

Under what conditions, if any, should people have the right to take their own lives? Is suicide acceptable if someone has a terminal illness, degenerating physical condition, poor quality of life, or "unbearable psychological anguish"? We will present examples of such situations for you to consider.

Physician-Assisted Suicide

Physician-assisted suicide for terminal conditions (referred to as death with dignity) is permitted by legislation in Oregon, Washington, Vermont, California, Colorado, the District of Columbia, Hawaii, Maine, Montana, New Mexico, and New Jersey. There are strict rules associated with these laws. For example, in Oregon and Washington, it is permitted only if:

- two physicians confirm that the person has a terminal condition and less than 6 months to live;
- two verbal requests and one written request are made in the presence of witnesses; and
- the individual is of sound mind (a mental health evaluation may be required).

People who have requested physician-assisted suicide in Oregon based their decision on concerns about a deteriorating quality of life, loss of ability to engage in activities that make life enjoyable, loss of autonomy, and loss of dignity (Oregon Public Health Division, 2013).

Suicide Because of "Unbearable Psychological Anguish"

At the age of 29, Aurelia Brouwers drank a substance given to her by a physician and lay down to die. She did not have a terminal illness but had unbearable psychological pain. Aurelia had been diagnosed with numerous psychiatric disorders and had made about 20 serious suicide attempts. She claimed that she never once experienced happiness during her life.

Voluntary euthanasia is against the law in most countries but is permitted in the Netherlands for suffering that is "unbearable with no likelihood of change" and where there is "no reasonable alternative." Aurelia's psychiatrist and doctor would not endorse her request to end her life, since it did not involve a terminal illness; therefore, she applied to the End-of-Life Clinic in The Hague, a city in the Netherlands—a facility that was willing to consider rejected applications. The review process often takes years, and only about 10 percent of psychiatric applications are approved. The vast majority of approved cases involve terminal illnesses. However, in 2017, there were 83 people who were euthanized because of extreme psychological suffering. Aurelia's death provoked a huge outcry in the Netherlands and around the world regarding euthanasia for "unbearable psychiatric suffering," with many opponents questioning if it was a "a reasonable alternative" for a nonterminal psychiatric condition. Canada is now entering into the fray. Beginning in March, 2024, medical assistance for dying (physician-assisted suicide) will be permitted for individuals with a "grievous and irremediable" mental illness who request and qualify for this intervention (Yasgur, 2023).

For Further Consideration

1. Under what circumstances do individuals have the right to elect to die? Are declining physical or mental conditions a sufficient reason for assisted suicide?

2. Instead of the term *assisted suicide*, some are using the term *voluntary assisted dying*. Does this change in terminology affect your views on the topic?

3. How would you define "unbearable psychological anguish"? Do you believe it is possible to accurately conclude that a person's emotional distress will never improve?

4. Should someone like Aurelia who reported suffering from unremitting psychological pain be forced to take medications or undergo other treatments?

hope for a positive future. During this very vulnerable period, steps that may assist a survivor move toward recovery and develop resilience include (SAMHSA, 2015; Sokol et al., 2022):

- *Choosing life*: Making the emotional decision to live by embracing hope and recognizing that adversity is temporary
- *Optimizing identity*: Understanding one's life history and affirming oneself as a valued individual with strengths, weaknesses, and the potential for growth
- *Rediscovering meaning*: Embracing the meaning and purpose of life through spirituality, religion, or a sense of a higher purpose
- *Cultivating and reestablishing connections*: Family, friends, and support groups can help reduce feelings of loneliness; the American Association of Suicidality Web site contains information that helps families and friends as well as survivors move forward
- *Making a plan to stay safe*: Thoughts of suicide might remain after a suicide attempt, especially when the survivor encounters challenges. It helps when survivors develop a specific plan that they can refer to when there is a need to consider realistic options for dealing with problems, including a list of coping strategies and resources to assist in the event of another suicidal crisis
- *Nurturing empowerment*: Developing a broader set of emotional regulation and problem-solving skills for dealing with common challenges such as with a loss, relationship conflicts, or problematic life events; broadening the person's repertoire of coping strategies and identifying steps to take when feeling overwhelmed can increase resilience and act as a buffer to suicide
- *Moving toward a hopeful future*: Reconnecting with reasons for living can help build hope; some survivors create a "hope box" to serve as a physical reminder of the things in life that bring joy—a way to lift their spirits when they feel overwhelmed or depressed; positive emotions are also generated by making a list of reasons to feel grateful or identifying personal strengths and using one each day

9-6 Moral, Ethical, and Legal Issues Surrounding Suicide

Case Study In September 2003, after the release of his book *I Ask the Right to Die*, 21-year-old Vincent Humbert's mother administered an overdose of sedatives into his intravenous line, causing his death (Smith, 2003). Humbert, a French citizen, had serious physical injuries resulting from a traffic accident. He regained consciousness after 9 months in a coma, and was able to hear, think, and reason; however, his only means of communication was with his thumb. With that one thumb, he pointed to letters of the alphabet and wrote a special appeal to then French president Jacques Chirac asking for the right to die. His case, and the arrest of his mother for assisting with his death, set off an international debate about the morality and legality of euthanasia.

Ironically, medical science has added fuel to the right-to-die movement. Along with medical technology that extends life comes the reality that we are increasingly lengthening the process of dying. This prolongation has caused many people, especially those who are elderly or terminally ill, to fear being kept alive by artificial means, with no thought to their desires or dignity. Humane and sensitive physicians who believe that the resulting quality of life does not merit heroic measures, but whose training impels them to sustain life, are caught in the middle of this conflict. In many states, they may face a civil or criminal lawsuit if they agree to allow a patient to die, particularly if the person has no **advance directive** regarding the use of resuscitation or machinery to prolong life.

This brings us to a significant question: Do people have the right to choose suicide? The act of suicide seems to violate what many of us believe regarding the sanctity of life. Many segments of the population consider suicide immoral. Within the United States, many states have laws against suicide. Of course, such laws are difficult to enforce, because the deceased are not around to prosecute. Many are beginning to question the legitimacy of such sanctions, however, and are openly advocating a person's right to suicide. In November 1998, Oregon voters passed the first physician-assisted suicide act granting physicians the legal right to help end the lives of terminally ill patients who wish to die by suicide. This legislation and similar laws in other states have intensified the debate over whether it is morally, ethically, and legally permissible to allow relatives, friends, or physicians to provide support, means, and actions to carry out a suicide.

Proponents of the right to suicide believe that it can be a rational act and that medical professionals should be allowed to help such patients without fear of legal or professional repercussions. Others argue, however, that suicide is not rational, that many who choose suicide are mentally ill, and that determining "rationality" is fraught with hazards. Some voice the fear that if suicide is legalized, patients will be coerced by relatives intent on collecting inheritances or who believe the patient has become a burden. Other critics of assisted suicide fear that in response to medical cost control, medical professionals might encourage people who are terminally ill to choose assisted suicide, and that those who are poor and disadvantaged would receive the most encouragement.

Major problems also exist in defining the subjective term *quality of life* as the criterion for deciding between life and death. At what point do we consider quality of life sufficiently poor to justify terminating it? Should society allow people who have been severely injured or disfigured to end their own lives? What about people who are intellectually disabled or seriously mentally ill? Could it be argued that their quality of life is equally poor? Moreover, who decides whether a person is terminally ill? There are recorded cases of "incurable" patients who recovered spontaneously or who responded to newly discovered treatments.

Such questions deal with ethics and human values, and they have no easy answers. Yet mental health practitioners cannot avoid these issues. Like their medical counterparts, mental health professionals are trained to intervene to prevent suicide. Strong social, religious, and legal sanctions support this position. Many therapists work with clients who have strong suicidal intent—clients who are not terminally ill but, for a variety of reasons, view suicide as the answer to their emotional distress. In most

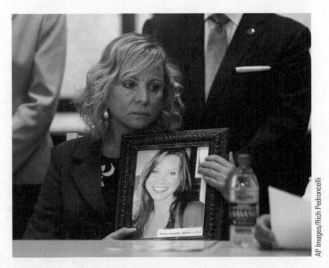

AP Images/Rich Pedroncelli

Suicide and Terminal Illness

Brittany Maynard, diagnosed with an untreatable form of brain cancer, became an advocate for "death with dignity" after learning that her home state did not allow physician-assisted suicide for terminal conditions. Brittany moved to Oregon, where she ended her life on November 1, 2014. In this photo, Brittany's mother holds a photo of her daughter.

situations, their deaths would bring immense pain and suffering to their loved ones. Moreover, as we have discussed, most people who attempt suicide are ambivalent about the act, or find that their suicidal urges pass when their life circumstances improve. Clearly, suicide brings up a number of important social and legal issues and challenges the personal value systems of those considering suicide, their family members, medical and mental health professionals, and those who devise and enforce our laws.

9-7 Contemporary Trends and Future Directions

Suicide is a global concern—over 700,000 people take their own life each year (World Health Organization [WHO], 2021). Each death brings incredible pain for the families and friends left behind. Given the tragic nature of suicide, researchers across the globe are devoting considerable energy to understanding this perplexing phenomenon. Many research endeavors focus on the multiple risk factors that underlie the propensity to consider and engage in suicidal behaviors. Other efforts involve searching for ways to most effectively detect and intervene with individuals contemplating suicide.

Researchers continue to investigate the best methods for predicting who is at risk for suicide. A reliance on self-report or therapist judgment can be flawed because many individuals do not report suicidal ideations or intentions. An innovative approach to understanding and predicting suicidal behavior involves the use of algorithms and artificial intelligence to analyze enormous data sets. In one study, anonymous information from the electronic medical records of veterans who died by suicide were compared with data from (1) veterans who used mental health services but did not die by suicide and (2) veterans who did not use mental health services or die by suicide. Differences between the groups were identified, and a predictive algorithm was developed that was able to differentiate between the groups with 65 percent accuracy (Poulin et al., 2014). Similarly, the electronic health records and clinical notes for over 1,725,000 individuals were analyzed, including data from 20,246 patients who had suicidal behavior. Computer-based comparisons between the groups led to the development of an algorithm that successfully identified nearly half of all suicides and suicidal behavior 3 to 4 years in advance of the event (Barak-Corren, 2017). A cross-cultural study similarly reported the successful use of a machine prediction model in identifying suicide risk in a group of 59,984 Korean adolescents. The predictions were based on 26 variables, including sociodemographic characteristics, health-related lifestyle factors, and specific psychological stressors. The machine-learning program had an accuracy rate of nearly 80 percent in distinguishing between suicidal and nonsuicidal students (Jung, Park, et al., 2019).

Machine-learning programs—capable of sorting through countless pieces of data, identifying significant variables, and developing predictive algorithms—appear to have the capacity to add to our understanding of factors underlying suicide. However, some researchers express concern about the low sensitivity and low predictive power of suicide prediction models, arguing that the information they provide has not yet been effectively linked to effective individualized suicide intervention (Kessler et al., 2020).

Another group of researchers employed sophisticated linguistic-based prediction models to analyze social media posts—comparing data from users who attempted suicide with matched controls who did not. With the goal of detecting social precursors to suicidal behavior, the research team, relying on data from 18- to 24-year-old women who agreed to have their Facebook posts reviewed, succeeded in identifying key words and phrases associated with later suicidality (Coppersmith et al., 2018). Successful identification of characteristics associated with risk paves the way for early intervention. Of course, further research is needed to determine if the findings apply to other groups of Facebook users. Further, this group of researchers made no attempt to identify language associated with imminent suicide risk.

Taking a very different approach, Facebook worked with suicide experts to develop an automated suicide prevention algorithm focused on real-time analysis of all Facebook posts—an intervention precipitated by a cluster of live-streamed suicides on their platform. Once a user's post is flagged due to words or phrases suggestive of suicide, Facebook's content moderators analyze the individual's social media history. If the team detects the potential for "imminent harm," they either send resource information to the person or notify local emergency responders—who then intervene. The issue that emerges from efforts such as this is the relative importance of personal privacy versus the opportunity to prevent suicide. Further, there is no systematic research to evaluate the validity and reliability of Facebook's approach to using digital data to intervene because the algorithm lacks real-world data such as medical records to confirm the link between risk analysis and the ultimate outcome—actual suicidal behavior. Additionally, it does not address the many impulsive suicides that occur without warning (Goggin, 2019). There is some optimism that the use of technology and innovative programs will reduce suicide, but privacy issues will remain at the forefront of these efforts.

Chapter Summary

1 What do we know about suicide?

- Suicide is the intentional, direct, and conscious taking of one's own life. The topic is often avoided, even among those directly affected by a suicide.

- A variety of demographic and specific risk factors are associated with suicide.

- Although women make more suicide attempts, men are more likely to kill themselves.

2 How does suicide affect friends and family?

- Suicide can affect surviving friends and family for years—feelings of guilt and responsibility are common.

3 How is suicide unique in different age groups?

- In recent years, childhood and adolescent suicides have increased at an alarming rate.

- Suicide among college students is also a serious concern.

- Suicide rates are high among the baby boomer generation and other older adults.

4 What might cause someone to end their life by suicide?

- Genetic risk and biochemical abnormalities involving serotonin and neuropeptides are associated with suicide; alcohol use also exerts biological effects that increase suicide risk.

- Psychological factors include mental disturbance, depression, hopelessness, psychache, and suicide myopia resulting from excessive alcohol consumption.

- Lack of positive social relationships, feelings of loneliness and disconnection, interpersonal conflicts, and loss of a significant other can increase the chances of suicide.

- Ethnicity, economic downturns, male gender, and LGBTQ identity and other demographic variables are all associated with increased risk of suicide.

5 How can we prevent suicide?

- The best way to prevent suicide is to recognize risk factors and intervene before suicide occurs.

- Crisis intervention strategies can help individuals who are contemplating suicide become more hopeful and consider other options. Intensive short-term therapy is used to stabilize the immediate crisis.

- Suicide prevention centers and the 988 Suicide and Crisis Lifeline operate 24 hours a day to provide intervention services to people contemplating suicide.

- After a suicidal crisis has been resolved, ongoing therapy can help teach coping skills and treat underlying mental disorders. Cognitive-behavioral therapy (CBT) and dialectical behavior therapy (DBT) can help reduce suicidal ideation and suicide attempts.

- Suicide survivors benefit from a focus on activities that increase optimism and social connection.

6 Are there situations in which suicide should be an option?

- A few states allow physician-assisted suicide for carefully screened people who are terminally ill and wish to end their suffering.

7 What are future directions in the field of suicidology?

- Researchers worldwide are attempting to stem the tide of suicide by focusing on risk factors associated with suicide and effective methods of intervention.

- There is hope that the use of technology and innovative programs that analyze medical records and social media posts will eventually succeed in reducing the number of suicides.

Chapter Glossary

advance directive
written health care instructions specifying the treatments a person is willing to have or not have if unable to make decisions because of mental or physical incapacity

lethality
the capability of causing death

psychache
a term created to describe the unbearable psychological hurt, pain, and anguish associated with suicide

psychological autopsy
the systematic examination of existing information after a person's death for the purpose of understanding and explaining the person's behavior before death

suicidal ideation
thoughts about suicide

suicide
the intentional, direct, and conscious taking of one's own life

suicidologist
a professional who studies the manifestation, dynamics, and prevention of suicide

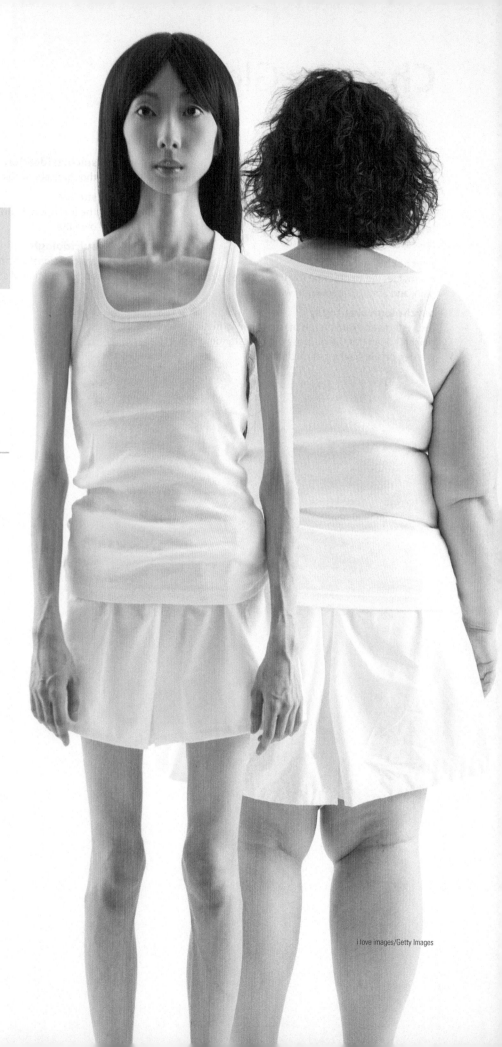

focus Questions

1 What kinds of eating disorders exist?

2 What are some causes of eating disorders?

3 What are some treatment options for eating disorders?

4 What causes obesity, and how is it treated?

i love images/Getty Images

10

Eating Disorders

Learning Objectives

After studying this chapter, you will be able to . . .

10-1 Summarize key features of the various eating disorders.

10-2 Discuss each of the multipath explanations for eating disorders.

10-3 Describe some treatment options for specific eating disorders.

10-4 Discuss some causes of and treatment options for obesity.

I Looked in the Bathroom Mirror and a Skull Stared Back. At 5 ft 7 in. and 40 lb, Rachael Farrokh was deemed a "hospital liability"—her anorexia had progressed too far for them to treat. She found only one facility that specialized in refeeding individuals with extremely low body weight. Because of the cost for treatment, she appealed for help on online, saying, "I'm not someone who ever asks for help but I need your help . . . Otherwise I don't have a shot and I'm ready to get better" (Dovey, 2015).

I Purge About Four Times a Day. . . . I have to be skinny, I want to be skinny. . . . I feel guilty and stupid if I don't purge everything out of my stomach. . . . I'm really scared. I don't want to die.

My Friends and I Put on Weight During Our First Semester of College. . . . We ate dinner as a group, trying to stick to salad and grilled chicken, until one of us said, "Screw it," and we shared a heaping bowl of our favorite makeshift dessert: marshmallow fluff and butter melted in the dining hall microwave then mixed with sugary cereal and chocolate chips.

A cross the globe, **disordered eating** behaviors such as extreme dieting, binge eating, self-induced vomiting, excessive exercising, and use of laxatives is becoming increasingly prevalent. In a review of 32 studies of eating disorders among youth in 16 different countries, more than 30 percent of girls and 17 percent of boys reported disordered eating. Among U.S. adolescents, 57 percent of girls and 31 percent of boys had engaged in unhealthy weight control measures (Simone et al., 2022). Twelve-month prevalence estimates of disordered eating in U.S. college students are around 54 percent for college women and 19 percent for college men (Harrer et al., 2020). Over 90 percent of college women have attempted to control their weight through dieting, and 25 percent have used purging as a weight control method (Anorexia Nervosa and Associated Disorders, 2014). Weight and body shape concerns are now common not only among young White women and girls (the group most affected by eating disorders) but also among older women, men and boys, and people of color.

In this chapter, we will discuss disordered eating patterns such as those presented at the beginning of this chapter, and you will learn about the characteristics, causes, and treatment of eating disorders. We also include a discussion of obesity, another food-related condition with serious physical and psychological consequences.

10-1 Eating Disorders

Preoccupation with weight and body dimensions or reliance on food as a coping mechanism can become extreme and lead to eating disorders such as anorexia nervosa, bulimia nervosa, or binge-eating disorder (Table 10.1). These conditions are associated with significant stress. For example, suicide attempts are up to six times higher among individuals with an eating disorder (Udo et al., 2019). We begin our discussion of eating disorders with a focus on a life-threatening condition: anorexia nervosa.

Anorexia Nervosa

Case Study   Portia DeGeneres, known for her starring roles in the television shows *Scandal*, *Arrested Development*, and *Better Off Ted*, weighed 82 pounds, at 5 ft 7 in. tall, when coping with an eating disorder in her mid-20s. In her quest to become a model, she became consumed with binge eating, purging, exercising, dieting, and using laxatives. In her autobiography, *Unbearable Lightness: A Story of Loss and Gain*, DeGeneres recounts eating only 300 calories per day, taking up to 20 laxatives a day, and exercising for hours. She received a "wake-up call" when her brother broke down and said he was afraid she was going to die. When she collapsed on a movie set, her doctors said her organs were close to failing. These events prompted her to seek help and make changes in her life. With the development of self-confidence and self-acceptance, and coming out as a lesbian, DeGeneres now maintains a normal weight (de Rossi, 2010).

One of the most obvious symptoms of **anorexia nervosa** is extreme thinness. Individuals with this disorder starve themselves, relentlessly pursue thinness, and detest weight gain. Their body image is distorted

Table 10.1 Eating Disorders

Disorder	DSM-5-TR Criteria	Prevalence and Gender Difference	Age of Onset
Disorders Chart			
Anorexia nervosa types: • Restricting • Binge-eating/purging	• Restricted caloric intake resulting in body weight significantly below the minimum normal weight for one's age and height • Intense fear of gaining weight or becoming fat, which does not diminish even with weight loss • Body image distortion (not recognizing one's thinness) or self-evaluation unduly influenced by weight	• Lifetime prevalence 0.6% to 0.8% • Much higher rates in women • About 90% in clinical samples are girls or women	• Usually after puberty or in early adulthood
• Bulimia nervosa	• Recurrent episodes of binge eating and compensatory behaviors (one or more times per week for 3 or more months) • Loss of control over eating behavior when bingeing • Use of vomiting, exercise, laxatives, or fasting to control weight • Self-evaluation unduly influenced by weight or body shape	• Up to 2.6% • Much higher rates in girls or women	• Late adolescence or early adulthood
• Binge-eating disorder (BED)	• Recurrent episodes of binge eating (one or more binges a week for 3 or more months) • Loss of control when bingeing • Eating until uncomfortably full or when not hungry • No regular use of inappropriate compensatory activities to control weight • Marked distress (guilt, embarrassment, depression) over bingeing	• Lifetime prevalence 0.85% to 2.8%; • About 20% to 40% in weight control clinics have this disorder • 2 to 3 times more prevalent in women than in men	• Late adolescence or early 20s

Source: Data from APA, 2022; Benjamin et al., 2019; Galmiche et al., 2019

(i.e., they see themselves as overweight), and they deny the seriousness of the physical effects of their low body weight.

Anorexia nervosa has been recognized for centuries. It occurs primarily in adolescent girls and young women, although up to 10 percent of those with this condition are boys or men (APA, 2022). A characteristic of anorexia nervosa is that most people with the disorder, even when clearly emaciated, continue to insist they are overweight. Some may acknowledge that they are thin but maintain that some parts of their bodies are too fat. This cognitive distortion regarding their body, shape, and weight results in behaviors such as excessive mirror and weight checking. When other people begin to express concerns about their emaciated appearance, they may wear large clothes to hide their shape and avoid social events and people who comment on their weight loss (Sproch & Anderson, 2018).

Subtypes of Anorexia Nervosa

Although the popular view of an individual with anorexia nervosa is a person who eats very little, there are actually two subtypes of the disorder: the restricting type and the binge-eating/purging type. Those with the *restricting type* pursue weight loss through severe dieting and/or exercising. Individuals with the *binge-eating/purging type* frequently binge eat and then use self-induced vomiting, laxatives, or

Portia DeGeneres's eating disorder had its roots in attempts to meet an idealized standard of beauty as well as turmoil over her sexual orientation.

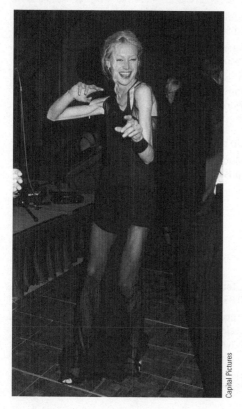

Capital Pictures

diuretics to avoid weight gain. Although both groups vigorously pursue thinness, they differ in some aspects. Those with the restricting type of anorexia nervosa are more introverted and tend to deny psychological distress or feelings of hunger. Those with the binge-eating/purging type are more extroverted and impulsive; report more anxiety, depression, and guilt; often have a strong appetite; and tend to be older (Sansone & Sansone, 2011).

Physical Complications and Associated Characteristics

Anorexia nervosa is associated with serious medical complications. Portia DeGeneres experienced osteoporosis (weakening of the bones) and cirrhosis of the liver and was near death as a result of her condition. Rachael Farrokh, the 40-pound woman discussed at the beginning of the chapter, suffered a heart attack, liver failure, and breathing difficulties. As these cases demonstrate, self-starvation produces a variety of physical problems including irregular heart rate, low blood pressure and the severe heart damage that occurs when the body is forced to use muscles as a source of energy. Other physical changes include extreme fatigue, dry skin, brittle hair, low body temperature, and kidney disease. Those who **purge** often develop enlarged salivary glands, resulting in a "chipmunk look" to the face (National Institute of Mental Health [NIMH], 2014). Many of these conditions can be reversed with proper nutrition and medical care (Mehler et al., 2023). Another medical finding associated with anorexia nervosa are brain changes involving a reduction of cortical thickness two to four times greater than that found in other mental illnesses (Walton et al., 2022).

The mortality rate among those with anorexia is up to six times higher than that of the general population due to suicide, substance abuse, and the effects of starvation (Cliffe et al., 2020). About 20 percent have concurrent nonsuicidal self-injury behavior (Davico et al., 2019). Depression, anxiety, impulse control problems, obsessive-compulsive symptoms, and loss of sexual interest also occur concurrently with anorexia nervosa (Kountza et al., 2018). Many individuals with anorexia nervosa tend to suppress their emotions and to ruminate, behaviors that may maintain disordered eating patterns (Prefit et al., 2019).

Course and Outcome

The course of anorexia nervosa is highly variable and can range from full recovery after one episode to a fluctuating pattern of weight gain and relapse to a chronic and deteriorating course ending in death. Approximately 50 percent of those with this diagnosis experience relapse, and 20 percent have a protracted illness (Kaye & Bulik, 2021). Rachael Farrokh (from the case presented earlier) survived and has nearly reached her previous weight of 125 pounds. She is still frail and fragile but is recovering. However, others with anorexia may not be as fortunate. In one sample, 6 percent of individuals with anorexia nervosa died within 15 years of their diagnosis (Demmler et al., 2020). Onset in adolescence is associated with more positive outcomes, although there is a high risk for the development of other psychiatric disorders (Jagielska & Kacperska, 2017). In a 30-year follow-up of 47 youth with adolescent onset anorexia nervosa in Sweden, 64 percent made a full recovery from anorexia, although the average duration for the disorder was 10 years (Dobrescu et al., 2020). Little is known about the long-term outlook for men with anorexia; the few results are conflicting or inconclusive (Strobel et al., 2018).

Anorexia's Web

- Drink ice-cold water ("Your body has to burn calories to keep your temperature up") and hot water with bouillon cubes ("only 5 calories a cube, and they taste wonderful").

- "Starvation is fulfilling. . . . The greatest enjoyment of food is actually found when never a morsel passes the lips."

- "I will be thin, at all costs. It is the most important thing—nothing else matters."

Tips to reduce caloric intake, testimonials regarding the satisfaction of not eating, ways to conceal thinness from friends and family members, and rules to remain thin are part of pro-ana (anorexia) and pro-mia (bulimia) Web sites (Boniel-Nissim & Latzer, 2016). Some of the screen names used in online discussion groups include "thinspiration," "puking pals," "disappearing acts," and "anorexiangel." Participants on the Anorexic Nation Web sites talk about how it is important to have friends who are like them and argue that anorexia is a lifestyle choice, not an illness. In one study, 43 percent of those who visited the Web sites indicated that they received emotional support: "I kind of lost all of my friends at school and in my neighborhood but I still have my pro-ana and pro-mia friends" (Csipke & Horne, 2007, p. 202).

Such Web sites are visited by thousands of people each day, including many adolescents experimenting with disordered eating. Exposure to these Web sites is associated with increases in body dissatisfaction, dieting, and negative emotional states (Rodgers et al., 2016). Medical experts are deeply concerned that the sites are increasing the incidence of eating disorders, especially among susceptible individuals.

For Further Consideration

1. How much danger do you feel these Web sites pose to people with and without eating disorders?

2. What types of messages from these Web sites might resonate with young girls?

3. What kinds of restrictions, if any, should be placed on pro-ana and pro-mia Web sites?

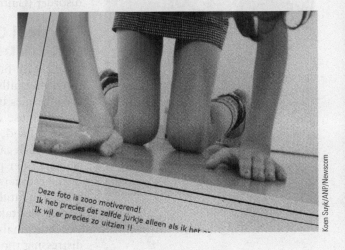

Deze foto is zooo motiverend!
Ik heb precies dat zelfde jurkje alleen als ik het ~~
Ik wil er precies zo uitzien !!

Koen Suyk/ANP/Newscom

Bulimia Nervosa

Case Study A 35-year-old Latina immigrant had nightly binge-eating episodes, where she mechanically looked for foods in her kitchen and ate until she felt "stuffed." During the binges, she felt "out of control," had limited awareness, and consumed over 3,000 calories of food. Purging occurred at least once a week. She engaged in excessive exercising to compensate for her weight gain and became distressed if she didn't exercise. She also reported daily mood swings, along with feelings of depression, worthlessness, and guilt, which resulted in frequent crying spells (Lui, 2017).

Bulimia nervosa is an eating disorder characterized by (a) recurrent episodes of **binge eating** (consumption of large quantities of food) that occur at least once a week for 3 months or more and (b) a loss of control over eating during the binge episode. Individuals with bulimia nervosa attempt to avoid weight gain by vomiting; using laxatives, diuretics, or enemas; restricting food intake; or engaging in excessive exercise or physical activity. A final diagnostic criterion is that the individual's self-evaluation is strongly influenced by their weight or body shape (APA, 2022).

People with bulimia realize that their eating patterns are not normal, and are distressed by that knowledge. Eating episodes sometimes continue

Popular singer Kesha, who has battled body image issues since middle school, has participated in intensive inpatient treatment for an eating disorder. Her eating disorder reportedly developed in response to criticism about her weight from individuals managing her career.

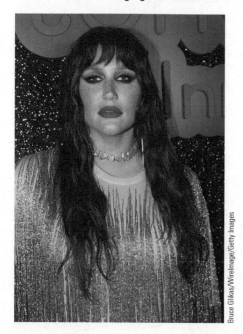

Bruce Glikas/WireImage/Getty Images

until they develop abdominal pain or induce vomiting. They often feel disgusted or ashamed of their eating and hide it from others. Some individuals eat nothing during the day but lose control and binge eat in the late afternoon or evening. For those who vomit or use laxatives to compensate for overeating, the temporary relief from physical discomfort or fear of weight gain is overshadowed by feelings of shame and despair. Binge-eating episodes may be followed by a commitment to fasting, severely restricting eating, or engaging in excessive exercising or other physical activity (Lui, 2017). Most people who have bulimia nervosa maintain a normal weight but have frequent weight fluctuations (Costandache et al., 2023).

Bulimia nervosa is much more prevalent than anorexia nervosa. Up to 2.6 percent of women have bulimia at some point in their lifetime, and an additional 10 percent of women report some bulimic symptoms but do not meet all the criteria for the diagnosis. The incidence of bulimia appears to be increasing, particularly in urban areas. Although fewer men and boys exhibit bulimia, they comprise up to 10 percent of those affected by the disorder (Galmiche et al., 2019).

Physical Complications and Associated Characteristics

People with bulimia use a variety of measures—fasting, self-induced vomiting, diet pills, laxatives, and exercise—to control the weight gain that accompanies binge eating. Side effects from self-induced vomiting or from excessive use of laxatives include erosion of tooth enamel from vomited stomach acid; dehydration; swollen salivary glands; and lowered potassium, which can weaken the heart and cause heart irregularities and cardiac arrest. Other possible gastrointestinal disturbances include inflammation of the esophagus, stomach, and rectal area (Gravina et al., 2018). Cases involving fatal stomach ruptures have been reported when sodium bicarbonate was taken to relieve indigestion and bloating (Han et al., 2022).

Individuals with bulimia nervosa often use eating as a way of coping with distressing thoughts or external stressors. As one woman stated, "Purging was the biggest part of my day. . . . It was my release from the stress and monotony of my life" (Erdely, 2004, p. 117). There is a close relationship between emotional states and disturbed eating. For example, among individuals with bulimia, negative moods such as sadness, hostility, and fear often occur before bingeing and purging episodes, and temporarily decrease after these activities (Berg et al., 2013). Thus, bulimic behaviors may represent maladaptive attempts at emotional regulation. Psychiatric comorbidities are common and include anxiety disorders, depression, borderline personality, self-harm, and substance abuse (Costandache et al., 2023).

According to the Office of Women's Health (2022), girls and women with bulimia may also demonstrate behavior changes such as:

- Retreating to the bathroom right after eating (to throw up)
- Exercising a lot, even in bad weather or when hurt or tired
- Acting moody, sad, or hopeless
- Not wanting to go out with friends or engage in activities that were previously enjoyed

Many individuals with bulimia are impulsive, engage in risky behaviors, and abuse drugs (Pearson et al., 2016). Suicidal thoughts are common in individuals with bulimia nervosa, and those with this disorder are seven times more likely to commit suicide as compared to the general population (Smith et al., 2018).

Course and Outcome

Bulimia nervosa has a somewhat later onset than anorexia nervosa, often beginning in late adolescence or early adult life. Outcome studies have revealed a mixed course, although the prognosis is more positive than for anorexia nervosa. In a 22-year follow-up of one group of individuals diagnosed with bulimia, 68 percent of the participants no longer demonstrated bulimic symptoms (Eddy et al., 2017). Individuals with greater emotional stability and positive social support have better outcomes, whereas psychosocial stress and low social status increase the likelihood of continued difficulties (Steinhausen & Weber, 2009).

Binge-Eating Disorder

Case Study Ms. A., a 38-year-old African American woman, was single, lived alone, and was employed as a personnel manager. She weighed 292 pounds. Her chief reason for coming to the clinic was that she felt her eating was out of control, and as a result, she had gained approximately 80 pounds over the previous year. A typical binge episode consisted of the ingestion of two pieces of chicken, one small bowl of salad, two servings of mashed potatoes, one hamburger, one large serving of french fries, one large chocolate shake, one large bag of potato chips, and 15 to 20 small cookies—all within a 2-hour period. She was embarrassed by how much she was eating, and felt disgusted with herself and very guilty after eating. (Goldfein et al., 2000, p. 1052)

Binge-eating disorder (BED) is similar to bulimia nervosa in that it involves binge eating, an accompanying feeling of loss of control, and marked distress over eating during the episodes. (Refer to Table 10.2 for questions used to assess for various eating disorders.) To be diagnosed with BED, an individual must have a history of binge-eating episodes at least once a week for a period of 3 months. Additionally, those with BED exhibit at least three of the following with binge-eating episodes: eating more rapidly than normal; uncomfortable feeling of fullness; eating large amounts of food even when not hungry; eating alone due to embarrassment about the quantity eaten; or feeling depressed or guilty after binge eating. Unlike bulimia nervosa, those with BED do not use compensatory behaviors such as vomiting, excessive exercising, or fasting (APA, 2022).

Approximately 4 percent of adults have been diagnosed with BED at some point in their lives, with women and girls having a 1.5 times greater likelihood of receiving this diagnosis compared to men and boys (Galmiche et al., 2019). Adolescents show the highest past-year prevalence—up to 3.6 percent in girls, 1.5 percent in gender-diverse youth, and 1.2 percent in boys (Giel et al., 2022).

BED is the most common eating disorder across racial and ethnic groups in the United States, especially among Black women, who are twice as likely as White women to have BED (5 percent vs 2.5 percent, respectively). Over 30 percent of Black women with obesity have BED (Goode et al., 2022). The onset of BED is similar to that of bulimia nervosa in that it typically begins in late adolescence or early adulthood. Overeating in childhood increases the risk of binge-eating episodes during adolescence and the eventual development of BED (Herle et al., 2020).

Body Revolution 2013

Aware of societal pressures on weight, Lady Gaga, who struggled with bulimia and anorexia in her teens, launched a project called Body Revolution 2013 to help her fans accept their bodies rather than focus on perceived shortcomings. Lady Gaga has since gained weight and reports feeling happier than ever with her body.

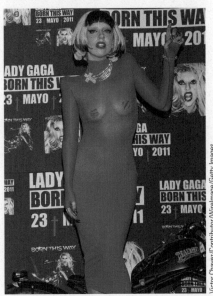

Victor Chavez/Contributor/WireImage/Getty Images

Table 10.2 Do You Have an Eating Disorder?

Questions for Possible Anorexia Nervosa
1. Are you considered to be underweight by others? (Screening question. If yes, continue to next questions.)
2. Are you intensely fearful of gaining weight or becoming fat even though you are underweight?
3. Do you feel that your body or a part of your body is too fat?
4. Do you diet, exercise, or make yourself vomit or take laxatives to lose weight even though you are underweight?

Questions for Possible Bulimia Nervosa
1. Do you have binges in which you eat a lot of food? (Screening question. If yes, continue to next questions.)
2. When you engage in binge eating, do you feel a lack of control over eating?
3. Do you make yourself vomit, take laxatives, or exercise excessively because of overeating?
4. Are you very dissatisfied with your body shape or weight?

Questions for Possible Binge-Eating Disorder
1. Do you have episodes of binge eating in which you eat a lot of food?
2. When you have a binge-eating episode, do you feel a lack of control over eating?

3. When you have a binge-eating episode, do three or more of the following apply?
  a. You eat more rapidly than usual.
  b. You eat until uncomfortably full.
  c. You eat large amounts even when not hungry.
  d. You eat alone because of embarrassment from overeating.
  e. You feel disgusted, depressed, or guilty about binge eating.

4. Do you feel great distress regarding your binge eating?

Note: These questions are derived from the diagnostic criteria for eating disorders (APA, 2022).

Physical Complications and Associated Characteristics

In contrast to those with bulimia nervosa, individuals with BED are often overweight. Thus, complications from BED include medical conditions associated with obesity, such as type 2 diabetes, high blood pressure, and high cholesterol levels. Many individuals who participate in weight control programs have BED.

Those who expect that eating will help relieve emotional distress are more likely to engage in binge eating (De Young et al., 2014). For this reason, binge-eating episodes are often preceded by distressing emotions such as guilt, depression, or disgust; although overeating may temporarily provide a distraction from these feelings, they quickly reappear (or even intensify) after a binge-eating episode (Schaefer et al., 2020). Individuals with BED who become obese tend to have significant difficulty not only regulating negative emotions but also controlling impulsive behavior. Further, they have difficulty self-monitoring their eating behavior, which allows binges to occur (Aloi et al., 2020).

Course and Outcome

There is limited information on the natural course of BED, although remission rates appear to be higher than with anorexia nervosa or bulimia nervosa. In one study, most individuals with BED made a full recovery over

Does Emotional Eating Really Provide Comfort?

- When you are feeling depressed or unhappy, do you start to snack?
- Do you eat more when you are under stress?
- When working on a boring task, do you look for something to eat?
- When you are feeling irritated or angry, does food make you feel better?
- Do you eat more when you have nothing else to do?

You are probably familiar with the concept of emotional eating—mindlessly consuming unhealthy foods in response to stressful circumstances or negative moods. You may also be aware that some people have a decreased appetite when they are feeling stressed. Rather than looking for comfort foods, they have little interest in eating and may even forget meals. So why do some of us turn to emotional eating? Can eating foods high in sugar, fat, and salt actually improve your mood?

Although consuming junk food may provide temporary comfort—transient feelings of gratification and distraction, or a brief improvement in mood—emotional snacking is often followed by embarrassment regarding the loss of self-control or by guilt over unhealthy eating (Volkow et al., 2013). Further, when a pattern of emotional eating develops, changes in brain reward pathways may begin to modify normal hunger signals as well as feelings of fullness and result in disordered eating patterns (van Strien, 2018). In fact, a consistent pattern of emotional eating can lead to a binge-eating disorder (Turton et al., 2017).

What causes some people to develop the habit of turning to food when experiencing emotional discomfort? Some researchers argue that emotional eating stems from an interaction between individual genetic vulnerabilities, ineffective coping strategies, and the rewarding nature of certain foods (van Strien, 2018). Studies of gender differences in emotional eating suggest that college women are more likely to turn to comfort food when they are stressed, whereas college men turned to food when they are anxious or bored. Further,

women are much more likely to experience guilt following emotional eating (Bennett et al., 2013).

Understanding emotional eating is important not only because of its relationship with eating disorders but also because of the health effects resulting from excessive caloric intake. As the health care system focuses more on prevention and early intervention, there is interest in targeting emotional eating because it is a modifiable risk factor. Not surprisingly, interventions that result in decreases in emotional eating are associated with weight reduction in individuals trying to lose weight (Braden et al., 2016).

How can people effectively self-soothe and seek comfort in ways that don't involve food? In contrast with physiological hunger, emotional eating often comes on rapidly and intensely in response to a stressful event or uncomfortable feelings. When this happens, it helps if you take a moment to identify the emotional need you are experiencing—in other words, what are you really hungry for? If you want to break a pattern of emotional eating, you might try strategies such as recognizing specific triggers associated with your emotional eating, recognizing true hunger signals and eating mindfully (eating slowly and paying attention to what you are eating) while reminding yourself that food is nourishment.

The more you are able to use effective emotional regulation and problem-solving techniques when you are feeling anxious, tense, stressed, or bored, the less likely you are to turn to food for comfort. Options such as exercising, meditating, spending time with friends, or distracting yourself with a pleasant activity can not only assist you to regulate emotions but also help in maintaining a healthy weight.

For Further Consideration

1. Would emotional eating become less common if we taught emotional regulation strategies to children and adolescents?

2. What strategies have you found to be effective for preventing emotional eating?

---

a 5-year period, even without treatment, with only 18 percent continuing to demonstrate an eating disorder of clinical severity. However, their weight remained high, including 39 percent who were obese (Fairburn et al., 2000). Adolescents with BED appear to have the most promising prognosis, with few meeting the criteria for the disorder over time (Giel et al., 2022).

Other Specified Feeding or Eating Disorders

The category **other specified feeding or eating disorders** includes seriously disordered eating patterns that do not fully meet the criteria for anorexia nervosa, bulimia nervosa, or binge-eating disorder. This is the most commonly diagnosed eating disorder, accounting for up to 40 percent of eating disorder diagnoses (Galmiche et al., 2019). Examples of people who fit in this category include the following:

- Individuals of normal weight who meet the other criteria for anorexia nervosa
- Individuals who meet the criteria for bulimia nervosa or binge-eating disorder, except that binge eating occurs less than once a week or has been present for less than 3 months
- Individuals with *night-eating syndrome*, a distressing pattern of binge eating late at night or after awakening from sleep
- Individuals who do not binge but frequently purge (self-induced vomiting; misuse of laxatives, diuretics, or enemas) as a means to control weight

Other specified feeding or eating disorders is a problematic diagnostic category because it includes a variety of symptoms and nonspecific symptom severity. Although individuals with this diagnosis may feel that their condition is not particularly serious, many experience significant health complications. Over one third have comorbid psychiatric disorders (Mustelin et al., 2016). Additionally, up to one third of those who receive this diagnosis will eventually meet the diagnostic criteria for bulimia nervosa or binge-eating disorder (Stice et al., 2013). As with other eating disorders, this category is associated with an increased risk of mortality and higher risk of suicide (Crow et al., 2009).

10-2 Etiology of Eating Disorders

The search for the causal factors associated with eating disorders is complicated because biological, psychological, social, and sociocultural factors interact to produce vulnerability to these disorders. We examine each of these influences to determine how they might explain the development of the severe dieting, binge-eating, and purging behaviors found in eating disorders. Understanding etiology involves looking for conditions that both precede the development of disordered eating and maintain the disorder. Keeping this in mind, we use the multipath model (Figure 10.1) to consider the risk factors associated with eating disorders.

Psychological Dimension

Numerous psychological risk factors increase an individual's chances of developing an eating disorder. For instance, certain eating patterns displayed by children during the first 10 years of their lives increase the risk of experiencing an eating disorder in adolescence: Children who overeat may develop a binge-eating disorder, whereas picky undereaters are more likely to present with anorexia nervosa (Herle et al., 2020). Additionally, obese children are more likely to cope with feelings of stress or boredom by engaging in emotional eating or eating when bored (Thaker et al., 2020). Further, the preoccupation with weight and shape that often arises in early adolescence appears to be a core aspect of disordered eating and is strongly linked to severe dieting, binge eating, or maintaining an unhealthy weight

Is Orthorexia a New Eating Disorder?

Veganism gave me a feeling of physical wellness and complete control . . . my dedication to the plant-based diet had evolved into obsession. I had started an Instagram account . . . chronicling my vegan adventures, and posted photos of bright, colorful salads and mason jars filled to the brim with blended, green concoctions. . . . I was an absolute wreck to be around. I couldn't sleep because I was so full of anxiety about what I was going to eat the next day and what foods I had to avoid. My hair was thinning, my skin was a mess (and orange from too much beta-carotene), and my face was gaunter than gaunt. I looked and felt like a shadow of my former self. . . . Once I started to let go of that addiction to emptiness and purity, I started to live again. (Younger, 2015)

Social media and other online sources tout many types of diets and food (paleo, keto, detoxing, apple cider vinegar, etc.) as having health benefits. Organic foods are promoted for "clean eating," and fats, carbohydrates, and processed foods are rejected (Birch, 2019). Under what conditions does "healthy" eating become an eating disorder? While the DSM has not listed "orthorexia nervosa" as a disorder, other sources have listed possible criteria for its diagnosis (Thomas, 2019):

- Obsession over foods that are "healthy and pure"
- Intrusive, recurrent thoughts regarding food
- Spending an inordinate amount of time planning, obtaining, and preparing "healthy" foods
- Hypersensitivity to "unpure" foods
- "Clean eating" has become central to one's life

It is estimated that almost 7 percent of U.S. adults have the characteristics associated with "orthorexia nervosa." Despite the focus on healthy food intake, many professionals are concerned that this rigid eating style and extreme obsession with food quality and purity can have negative health and psychological consequences (Zickgraf & Barrada, 2022).

For Further Consideration

1. How would you distinguish healthy eating from orthorexia?
2. Should orthorexia be included as a diagnosis in the next DSM?
3. What has created the orthorexia phenomenon in U.S. society?

(Askew et al., 2020). Up to 84 percent of adolescents experience body dissatisfaction (Baker et al., 2019). For both men and women, characteristics such as passivity, low self-esteem, dependence, and lack of assertiveness are associated with dysfunctional eating patterns (Arcelus et al., 2013). Other characteristics linked with eating disorders include perfectionism, impulsivity, depression, lack of self-confidence, and use of control over eating as a method of dealing with stress (Soidla & Akkermann, 2020).

Maladaptive perfectionism is a risk factor that appears to interact with body dissatisfaction to influence the development of anorexia nervosa and other eating disorders. Maladaptive perfectionism involves two characteristics: (a) inflexible high standards and (b) negative self-evaluation following mistakes. As you might imagine, imposing perfectionist standards on one's own weight, shape, or food intake could result in disordered eating. Not surprisingly, perfectionistic traits in early childhood are associated with the eventual development of anorexia nervosa (Dahlenburg et al., 2019).

Not only do individuals with eating disorders appear to have interpersonal anxiety and perfectionistic tendencies, they also possess "self-uncertainty," which involves a low self-concept and limited sense of self (von Lojewski & Abraham, 2014). Restrictive food intake in anorexia nervosa may represent an effort to demonstrate self-control or to improve self-esteem and body image. One woman stated, "I started to become aware that the anorexia wasn't a choice—it was a reaction. As a teenage girl, the only thing I could control was my body because I had no power" (Wetzler et al., 2020).

Figure 10.1

Multipath Model of Eating Disorders

The dimensions interact with one another and combine in different ways to result in an eating disorder.

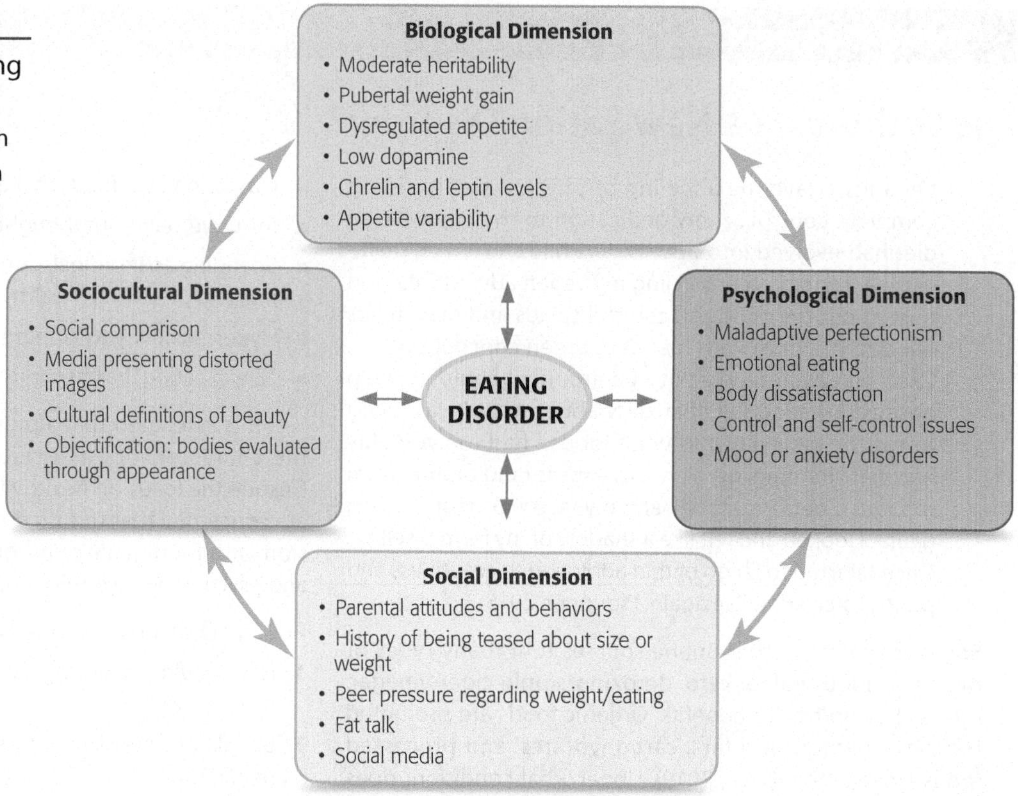

Biological Dimension
- Moderate heritability
- Pubertal weight gain
- Dysregulated appetite
- Low dopamine
- Ghrelin and leptin levels
- Appetite variability

Sociocultural Dimension
- Social comparison
- Media presenting distorted images
- Cultural definitions of beauty
- Objectification: bodies evaluated through appearance

EATING DISORDER

Psychological Dimension
- Maladaptive perfectionism
- Emotional eating
- Body dissatisfaction
- Control and self-control issues
- Mood or anxiety disorders

Social Dimension
- Parental attitudes and behaviors
- History of being teased about size or weight
- Peer pressure regarding weight/eating
- Fat talk
- Social media

Continuum Video Project

Sara: Bulimia Nervosa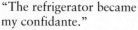

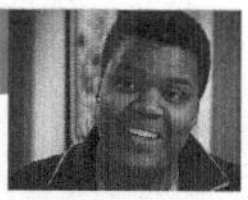

"The refrigerator became my confidante."

Access the Continuum Video Project at www.cengagebrain.com

Perceived or actual inadequacies in interpersonal skills are also associated with eating disorders, particularly when combined with maladaptive perfectionism (Ferrier-Auerbach & Martens, 2009). Many individuals with BED have internalized societal weight biases and stigma associated with weight—a factor that contributes to their emotional distress and binge eating (Gmeiner & Warschburger, 2022). Interestingly, in one sample of women with binge-eating disorder, their level of body dissatisfaction significantly increased following exposure to a stressful situation involving social evaluation (a mock job interview), whereas women in the control group (overweight women without a history of binge eating) did not demonstrate a similar sense of personal inadequacy (Naumann et al., 2018).

Mood disorders such as depression often accompany eating disorders. Rates of depression are also higher in relatives of individuals with eating disorders than in control populations, suggesting that, in some cases, disordered eating may be a symptom of depression (Sloan et al., 2017). At this point, we still do not know the precise relationship between depression and eating disorders. Depression may be the result, not the cause, of disordered eating. It is apparent, however, that individuals with eating disorders often use food as a means of handling stress, unhappiness, or anxiety. This maladaptive reaction then maintains dysfunctional eating, particularly when food is perceived as a source of comfort and a way to counteract depression and other negative feelings. As you might predict, individuals who believe eating will relieve negative emotions are more likely to binge (McCuen-Wurst et al., 2018).

Social Dimension

Can certain relationship patterns increase the likelihood of developing an eating disorder? Some individuals coping with eating disorders report that their parents or family members frequently criticized them or had negative reactions to their eating patterns (Rienecke & Richmond, 2017). In this manner, negative family relationships may produce a self-critical style that causes depression and body dissatisfaction. Further, teasing and criticism about weight or body shape by family members may increase body discomfort and exacerbate eating problems.

Family members can also unintentionally produce pressure to be thin through frequent discussions of weight and a focus on diet or exercise. For instance, mothers who diet are indirectly transmitting the message of the importance of slimness and a thin-ideal to their daughters (Keel et al., 2013). This relationship was seen in a study in which mothers and their preadolescent daughters were asked to view thin-ideal advertisements in magazines together; one group of mothers was instructed to make negative comments regarding their own weight or shape, whereas the control group of mothers made no such comments. The daughters' level of body esteem, body satisfaction, and eating attitudes were assessed before and after the experimental manipulation. During the follow-up assessment, the daughters of mothers who made negative comments about their own appearance scored lower on body satisfaction and expressed more problematic eating attitudes compared to girls whose mothers had not made negative comments (Handford et al., 2018). There is little doubt that parents play an important role in communicating appearance-based standards to their children; high expectations and negative attitudes or teasing about a child's weight have a strong relationship to eating disorders in both girls and boys (Barakat et al., 2023).

Kate Winslet Photoshopped?

Actress Kate Winslet, pictured on the right, has frequently been the target of image manipulation. *Harper's Bazaar* has been accused of grafting Winslet's head onto another woman's body for the cover shot on the left. Why do magazines go to such lengths in their portrayal of thinness?

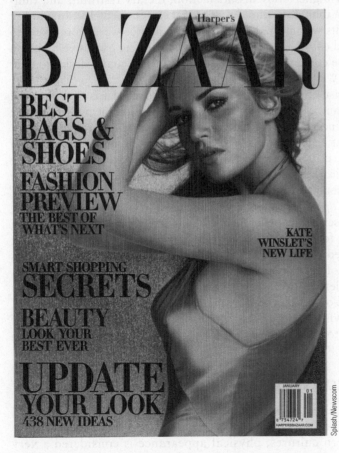

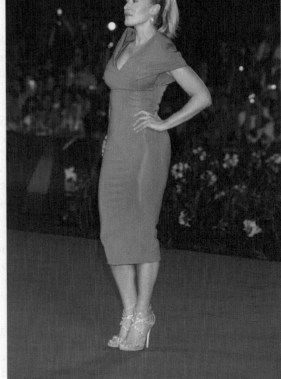

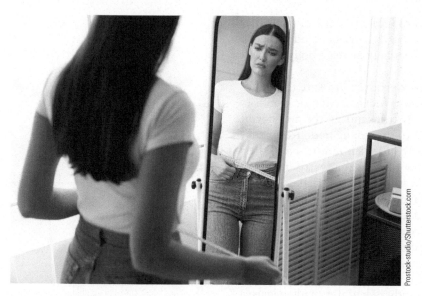

Body Consciousness

Women and girls are socialized to be conscious of their bodies. Although most of the attention has been directed to concerns over appearance among young White girls, rates of disordered eating and body dissatisfaction are also high among Latina and American Indian girls.

Did You Know?

When calorie labels were placed on the right side of the menu, U.S. college students made food choices without considering the calories. However, when the labels were on the left side, participants made food choices that reduced their caloric intake by 24 percent. When this experiment was conducted with Hebrew-speaking Israelis (who read the menu from right to left), the opposite effect occurred.

Source: Dalles et al., 2019

Peers can also produce pressure to lose weight, particularly when exposure to the ideal of thinness occurs during a critical period of development such as adolescence or early adulthood. In one longitudinal study, girls who reported that their friends were very focused on dieting at the beginning of the study were most likely to engage in extreme dieting and unhealthy weight control behaviors 5 years later (Eisenberg & Neumark-Sztainer, 2010). Similarly, women whose college friends and roommates focused on dieting were more likely to exhibit disordered eating during adulthood even though their friendships, life roles, and the living environment had changed (Keel et al., 2013). Among college-age women, "fat talk" is common. It involves the discussion of being overweight with friends who usually deny this observation. Although women who engage in "fat talk" believe it makes them feel better about their bodies, this pattern of conversation can increase body dissatisfaction and lower self-esteem (Rudigera & Winstead, 2013). Similarly, among a group of men who self-identified as athletes, eating disorder symptoms were most common among the men who reported engaging in appearance-focused conversations involving "fat talk" (Ahlich et al., 2019).

Social media has also been implicated in disordered eating. For instance, 13-year-old girls who regularly shared self-images on social media had significantly higher body dissatisfaction, dietary restraint, and thin-body idealization than girls who did not (McLean et al., 2015). In another study, participants who posted digitally edited photos were more likely to have anxiety and eating disorder symptoms, including excessive focus on weight and shape concerns, restrictive caloric intake, and a desire to constantly exercise (Wick & Keel, 2020).

We are increasingly recognizing that appearance standards are influenced by social media and a desire to look attractive to an online audience. One 22-year-old influencer received a record number of views and responses for a TikTok video that began with a clip of her flat stomach and protruding hip bones. She received many responses from people comparing their body size with hers. Subliminal messages such as this regarding the purported importance of slimness can prompt body checking and disordered eating (Adigun, 2022).

A new term, *appearance-related social media consciousness*, or ASMC, was coined to describe the phenomenon of obsessively selecting and editing selfies, checking for appearance flaws or imperfections, and monitoring likes on uploaded personal photos and selfies. These ASMC behaviors increase the risk of developing or continuing disordered eating. Individuals who report high levels of ASMC have high levels of body surveillance, body comparison, self-objectification, and depression (Choukas-Bradley et al., 2019). Women who report greater interest in and digital manipulation of their online photos also have an increased tendency toward engaging in bulimic behavior (Cohen et al., 2018).

Sociocultural Dimension

A great deal of research has focused on the influence of sociocultural norms and values in the etiology of eating disorders. In the United States and most Western cultures, physical appearance is considered a very important attribute, and women and girls are socialized to be conscious of their body shape and weight. At an early age, girls are sexualized and objectified through movies, television, music videos, song lyrics, magazines, and advertising (refer to Figure 10.2). Following this socialization process, body dissatisfaction arises when someone's weight or body shape differs considerably from the imagined ideal that has become ingrained in our psyche via television, movies, advertisements, or social media (Aparicio-Martinez et al., 2019). Thus, teenage girls often strive to be very thin; although an extremely slender body type is far from the norm (refer to Table 10.3 for data on the average weights of adults in the United States), it is consistent with body images portrayed in the media. Men are also subject to body image pressures. For example, men who highly value personal attractiveness and appearance report decreased body satisfaction when exposed to TV commercials featuring muscular men (Hargreaves & Tiggemann, 2009).

What kind of predisposition or characteristic leads some people to interpret images of thinness in the media as evidence of their own inadequacy? Are people who develop eating disorders chronically self-conscious to begin with, or do they develop eating disorders because their social environment makes them chronically self-conscious? How does exposure to portrayals of thinness in the mass media influence the values and norms of young people? The development of disordered eating and preoccupation with body image appears to involve multiple, intersecting processes incorporating these factors (Stice et al., 2017).

A process of *social comparison* occurs in which women and girls begin to evaluate themselves according to external standards (refer to Figure 10.3). Because these standards are unattainable for most women, body dissatisfaction occurs. Studies on the topic suggest that one third of the women in the United States are dissatisfied with their body shape and weight (Fallon et al., 2014). When women compare their body shape or weight to other women, those with high body dissatisfaction report increased feelings of guilt and depression and a process of social withdrawal. To relieve these distressing feelings, they begin to consider "solutions" such as dieting, purging, and extreme exercise. Thus, social comparison appears to be a strong risk factor for eating disorders, especially among women who are dissatisfied with their bodies (Stice et al., 2017).

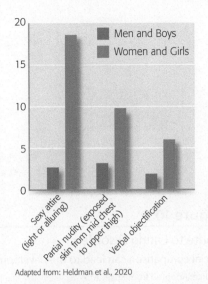

Adapted from: Heldman et al., 2020

Figure 10.2

Objectification of Women and Girls

In family films (those with a G, PG, or PG-13 rating), women and girls often are "scantily clad" and very attractive, and they have an unrealistic body shape. Does this contribute to the objectification of girls and women?

Table 10.3 Average Weight for U.S. Women and Men in 2000 and 2018*

	2000	2018
Women	163.8	170.8
Men	189.4	199.8
By Ethnicity and Gender		
European American women	161.9	170.9
African American women	185.9	188.5
Mexican American women	157.5	172.0
Asian American women	*	135.0
European American men	192.3	203.4
African American men	188.7	200.4
Mexican American men	177.9	196.0
Asian American men	*	168.1

Source: Fryar et al., 2018, 2021
*Data not available for Asian Americans in 2000

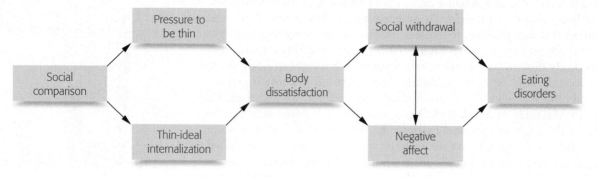

Figure 10.3

Route to Eating Disorders

Social comparison can lead to the development of eating disorders.

Source: Adapted from Stice, 2017

As noted in the beginning of the chapter, mass media portrayals of lean, muscular male bodies are increasing. Further, we are seeing a gradual shift away from traditional measures of masculinity, such as wealth and power, to physical appearance. Given this trend, body image dissatisfaction is also increasing among men. Between 10 percent and 30 percent of men report body dissatisfaction, and many adolescent boys are dissatisfied with their muscularity (Quittkat et al., 2019). This trend has also resulted in adolescent boys focusing on muscle-enhancing behaviors such as the use of protein powders, steroids, and muscle-building exercise (Field et al., 2014).

Compared to heterosexual men, gay men tend to place greater emphasis on physical attractiveness. This focus on physical attributes leads to concern over body size, muscularity, body fat distribution, and a greater prevalence of disturbed eating patterns. Exposure to media images of lean, muscular men is associated with the use of steroids to gain muscles and the use of purging to become lean, practices that occur more frequently among gay youth and

Ideal Male Bodies?

Most men and boys would prefer to be heavier and more muscular. Will the increased media focus on physically powerful men increase body image distortion and dissatisfaction among men?

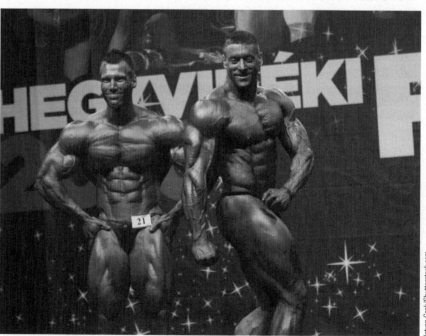

Istvan Csak/Shutterstock.com

gay men compared to their heterosexual counterparts (Calzo et al., 2017). Further, gay men who use social media are more focused on muscularity and the possible use of steroids compared to gay men who do not engage with social media; additionally, the social media users have more body dissatisfaction and eating disorder symptoms (Griffiths et al., 2018).

Previous studies have reported that lesbians are less preoccupied with physical appearance, have a better body image, have lower levels of body dissatisfaction, and embrace a larger ideal body size compared to heterosexual women (Alvy, 2013; Boehmer et al., 2007). A meta-analysis focused on eating disorders among sexual minority women concluded that although lesbians continued to have less preoccupation with thinness and less body dissatisfaction compared to heterosexual women, they had higher rates of binge eating and purging (Meneguzzo et al., 2018).

Underrepresented Ethnic Groups and Eating Disorders

Do cultural values and standards affect body dissatisfaction and eating disorders? Within the United States, there are definite ethnic differences in body dissatisfaction and susceptibility to eating disorders. In general, acculturation to mainstream U.S. values appears to increase the risk of developing an eating disorder, particularly among those who have internalized societal values concerning attractiveness (Schaefer et al., 2018). For instance, one study documented that Asian American women, many of whom have been influenced by Western standards of beauty, are affected not only by weight and body shape concerns but also by social comparisons based on height, facial features, and skin tone (Yu et al., 2019). In another study, European American and Asian American college women reported greater frequency of body checking and thin-ideal internalization than their African American and Latina peers (White & Warren, 2013). Although some Latinas have levels of body dissatisfaction equal to that of their White counterparts, Latina girls with a strong ethnic identity are less apt to experience body dissatisfaction when exposed to images of thin White women (Schooler & Daniels, 2014).

African American girls and women display much less body dissatisfaction than other comparison groups. Although they tend to be heavier than their White counterparts, they are more satisfied with their body size,

Did You Know?

In one study, individuals who used digital technology to record their food intake and exercise had significantly higher scores for eating disorder symptoms and compulsive exercising than nonusers; this was particularly true for those who were focused on their weight and shape rather than health and fitness.

Source: Plateau et al., 2018

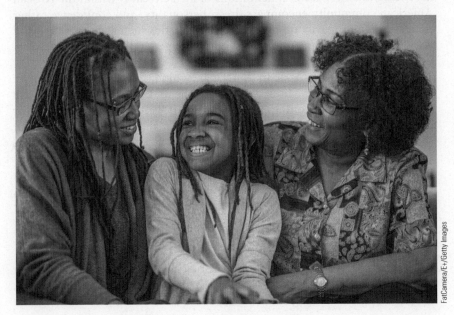

FatCamera/E+/Getty Images

Beauty Standards

African American women have a greater acceptance of heavier body sizes than European American women do. In addition, they adopt a broader definition of beauty that includes attitude, personality, and style. Thus, African American girls have less social pressure and more realistic body expectations.

Table 10.4 Differences in Body Image and Weight Concerns Among African American and European American Women and Girls

	African Americans	European Americans
Influence of media	Less affected by media images of thin women	Compared body with those portrayed by media
Body image	Perceived selves to be thinner than they actually were	Perceived selves to be heavier than they actually were
Attitude toward dieting	Believed that it is better to be a little overweight than underweight	Believed in the importance of dieting to produce a slender body; feared being overweight
Definition of beauty	Good grooming, style, and overall attractiveness; beauty is having the right attitude and personality	Slim; 5 ft 7 in.; 100 to 110 lb; a perfect body can lead to success and the good life
Being overweight	Of those who were overweight, 40% considered their figures attractive or very attractive	Those who believed they did not have a weight problem were underweight
Age and beauty	Believed they would get more beautiful with age	Believed that beauty is fleeting and decreases with age

Source: Boyington et al., 2008; Desmond et al., 1989; Fiery et al., 2016; Hughs, 2023; Quick & Byrd-Bredbenner, 2014; Schaefer et al., 2018

weight, and appearance and are less interested in being thin (Quick & Byrd-Bredbenner, 2014). In a study evaluating the ethnic identity and self-esteem of African American, European American, and Latina adolescent girls, high ethnic identity and high self-esteem appeared to protect against disordered eating among the African American girls (Rhea & Thatcher, 2013). Nearly two thirds of overweight or obese African American women in one study reported high self-esteem compared to 41 percent of average-sized or thin European American women (*Washington Post*, 2012). Table 10.4 compares some differences in body image and weight concerns between African American and European American women.

Why are African American women and girls somewhat insulated from unrealistic standards of thinness? It is possible that several cultural factors exert a protective influence. First, because many do not identify with European American women and girls, media messages of thinness may have less influence. Second, definitions of attractiveness within the African American community encompass dress, personality, and confidence rather than focusing primarily on physical characteristics such as body shape and weight. Third, African American women are generally less influenced by gender-restrictive messages (Schaefer et al., 2018).

However, not all African American women and girls are immune to thin-ideal messages. In a study of sixth- and seventh-grade African American girls (of whom approximately half were either overweight or obese), 60 percent expressed body dissatisfaction and a desire to lose weight (Buckingham-Howes et al., 2018). With respect to disordered eating, African American girls do diet, binge, and purge, but with less frequency than other groups (Howard et al., 2017). And although African American women are less likely to experience anorexia nervosa or bulimia nervosa, they are as likely as other groups of women to have binge-eating disorder (Franko et al., 2012).

Cross-Cultural Studies on Eating Disorders

Although far fewer reports of eating disorders are found in Latin American and Asian countries compared to European countries, Israel, and Australia, the incidence is increasing (Kolar et al., 2016). Of concern is the finding that body dissatisfaction and disordered eating increase among women and girls from other countries when they are exposed to Western values (Shekriladze et al., 2019). For instance, although fuller figures have traditionally been equated with beauty in South Africa, when Black teenage girls in this region were exposed to Western standards of thinness, there was a dramatic increase in eating disorders (Simmons, 2002). Asian countries have also reported increases in body shape concerns and disordered eating attitudes following exposure to Western media and online sources (Guo et al., 2022).

Cultural values and norms affect views on body shape and size. Our perspectives on what is considered a normal weight are influenced by our cultural beliefs and practices. Historically, eating disorders in Chinese populations have been rare because plumpness in women and girls has been considered desirable and attractive. However, in Hong Kong, individuals with eating disorders are now demonstrating a fat-phobic pattern similar to that seen in Western countries (Pike & Dunne, 2015).

Becker (2004) studied the impact of television on adolescent girls living in a rural community in western Fiji. Traditional Fijian cultural norms support robust appetites and body sizes. Food and feasts are socially important, and plump bodies are considered aesthetically pleasing. After 3 years of exposure to Western television programs, the Fijian girls expressed admiration for Western standards: "The actresses and all those girls, especially those European girls, I admire them and want to be like them. I want their body. I want their size" (p. 546). The girls also paid attention to TV commercials advertising exercise equipment, which portrayed the ease with which weight could be lost. "When they show exercising on TV . . . I feel I should . . . lose my weight" (p. 542). The media exposure dramatically increased body dissatisfaction and purging among Fijian girls (Becker et al., 2002). Media exposure to Western standards of beauty has also altered peer norms and has contributed to an increase in eating disorders in other Fijian communities (Gerbasi et al., 2014).

Biological Dimension

At this point, we have considered the psychological, social, and sociocultural dimensions associated with eating disorders. Although people are exposed to many of these influences, why do only a small percentage go on to develop anorexia nervosa, bulimia nervosa, or binge-eating disorders? Considering biological factors and possible gene × environment interactions helps us answer this question. For instance, if someone has a genetic predisposition toward severe dieting, exposure to certain environmental factors (e.g., family pressures or societal emphasis on being thin) may increase the risk of developing an eating disorder. Conversely, those without the predisposition might find severe dieting to be extremely aversive, which would decrease the risk of restrictive eating. In this section, we consider possible genetic influences on eating disorders.

Disordered eating appears to run in families. Female relatives of those with anorexia nervosa are 11 times more likely to develop the disorder than those without a family relationship. Increased family risk is also found for bulimia nervosa and binge-eating disorder. Estimates for heritability based on twin studies are about: 50 percent to 60 percent for anorexia nervosa; 60 percent for bulimia nervosa; and 40 percent to 60 percent for binge-eating disorder; the remaining variance would be explained by various environmental influences (Bulik et al., 2019; Himmerich et al., 2019).

The largest genetic study of anorexia nervosa (involving 17,000 individuals with the illness and 55,000 matched controls) identified eight areas in the human genome associated with metabolism and weight. Based on these genetic findings, it is hypothesized that individuals with this genotype avoid eating and develop anorexia nervosa because malfunctioning metabolic processes override hunger signals. Even after successful weight restoration, it is difficult for those with anorexia to maintain a healthy weight. As one researcher observed, "Recovery from anorexia nervosa is fighting an uphill battle against their biology" (Watson et al., 2019).

Genetic influences such as these may be triggered by physical changes, such as those occurring during puberty. In a sample of twins, the heritability of anorexia appeared to be low among preadolescent teens but was substantial after puberty. This suggests that either the process of puberty itself or social processes associated with puberty (e.g., increasing awareness of sexuality and body shape) may influence the expression of genes for disordered eating through gene × environment interactions (O'Connor et al., 2020).

Genetics may also influence the availability of neurotransmitters associated with eating behaviors. Research has focused on dopamine, which is considered the primary neurotransmitter involved in the reinforcing effects of food (Volkow et al., 2017). Low levels of dopamine can increase hunger, whereas greater dopamine availability can decrease appetite. Differences in dopamine levels may explain why those with bulimia nervosa are more attentive to food stimuli and why individuals with anorexia nervosa demonstrate less appetitive response to food images (Brooks et al., 2011). Additionally, having genes associated with lower dopamine availability may interact with adverse childhood rearing experiences to result in emotional eating patterns (van Strien et al., 2010).

Although dopamine seems like a promising lead in explaining eating disorders, other neurotransmitters such as serotonin (which can help signal satiety and thus regulate appetite) also appear to be involved (Donovan & Tecott, 2013). Ghrelin, a gastrointestinal hormone capable of stimulating hunger, regulating taste sensation, and increasing interest in food, is also a focus of research. When the appetitive circuitry is operating normally, ghrelin levels rise before meals and decrease after eating. Ghrelin works in conjunction with leptin, a hormone that signals satiety and suppresses appetite. Abnormalities in these hormones have been found in those with eating disorders. Manipulating ghrelin levels as a method of promoting weight gain in those with anorexia nervosa or decreasing interest in food for those with who eat excessively is being explored as a mechanism for treating obesity and eating disorders (Müller & Tschöp, 2013). More research is needed to determine the precise relationship between genetic factors, neurotransmitters, and environmental influences.

Altered functioning of the *appetitive neural circuitry* (brain structures and processes that mediate appetite) also appears to influence disordered eating patterns. Magnetic resonance imaging (MRI) scans were used to study neural regions associated with response to pleasant-tasting foods. Women who had recovered from anorexia nervosa or bulimia nervosa were compared with women without these disorders in their response to the sweet taste of sucrose. As compared to the control group, the women who had recovered from anorexia nervosa exhibited a significantly diminished response to sucrose, whereas those who had recovered from bulimia nervosa demonstrated a highly elevated response to the sweet flavor. Thus, the restricted eating in anorexia nervosa and overeating in bulimia nervosa may be due to alterations in appetitive neural circuitry that affect the reward aspects of taste (Oberndorfer et al., 2013).

Women who have recovered from anorexia nervosa also display several differences in brain circuitry compared to healthy women. The women who had experienced anorexia nervosa had reduced activity in the part of the brain that motivates reward-seeking, even when it was time to eat. They also exhibited increased activation of the cognitive control circuitry (an area associated with appetite control) when it was time for a meal. People with anorexia nervosa may not experience hunger, even when starving, due to this insufficient activation of the reward circuitry and the increased activation of the cognitive "self-control" circuitry that reduces their desire to eat (Wierenga et al., 2015).

10-3 Treatment of Eating Disorders

Although there are some similarities in treatment strategies used for anorexia nervosa, bulimia nervosa, and binge-eating disorder, treatment of each of these disorders involves unique approaches and priorities. With all eating disorders, remission is most likely to occur when there is a reduction in symptoms early in the treatment process (Pellizzer et al., 2019).

Treatment of Anorexia Nervosa

Case Study A young woman who began treatment for anorexia nervosa weighing 81 pounds reported:

I did gain 25 pounds, the target weight of my therapist and nutritionist. But every day was really difficult. I would go and cry. A big part of anorexia is fear. Fear of fat, fear of eating. But [my therapist] taught me about societal pressures to be ultra-thin that come from the media, TV, advertising. . . . She talked me through what I was thinking and how I had completely dissociated my mind from my body. . . . I'm slowly reintroducing foods one thing at a time. I'd like to think I am completely better, but I'm not. I'm still extremely self-conscious about my appearance. But I now know I have a problem and my family and I are finding ways to cope with it. (Bryant, 2001, p. B4)

As you have seen, eating disorders, especially anorexia nervosa, can be life threatening. Weight gain is vital for a successful outcome. Unfortunately, as is evident from this case study, it can be extremely difficult to change eating patterns. Because anorexia nervosa is a complex disorder, there is a need for teamwork among physicians, nutritionists, psychiatrists, and therapists. Treatment is provided in either an outpatient or a hospital setting, depending on the weight and health of the individual.

Because patients who are treated for anorexia nervosa are starving, the initial goal is to restore weight and address the medical complications associated with starvation. The physical condition of the person is carefully monitored because sudden and severe physiological reactions can occur during refeeding. During the weight restoration period, new foods are introduced to supplement food choices that are not sufficiently high in calories (Herpertz-Dahlmann, 2021). Because these foods may be considered "forbidden," phobic-like reactions can occur. One woman described her response to eating spaghetti in the following manner: "My chest is tight, my stomach just feels very full . . . I feel like I want to cry. I'm trying to control my breathing or else I'll start hyperventilating" (Battiste & Effron, 2012). As you can see, the thought of ingesting a high-calorie food can be very distressing and require a great deal of psychological support. Those with anorexia nervosa are often terrified of gaining weight and need the opportunity to discuss these reactions in therapy.

Psychological interventions provide emotional support and help the client (a) understand and cooperate with nutritional and physical rehabilitation, (b) identify and question the dysfunctional attitudes related to the eating disorder, (c) improve interpersonal and social functioning, and (d) address other psychological disorders or conflicts that reinforce disordered eating behavior. Focusing on improving quality of life and mood disorder symptoms is particularly important in treating severe cases of anorexia nervosa (Hay, 2020).

Family therapy is an important and effective component in the treatment of anorexia nervosa (Couturier et al., 2020). The importance of family therapy was demonstrated in the case of an 18-year-old woman who remained emaciated despite inpatient treatment, dietary training, and cognitive-behavioral therapy. Her family was enlisted to assist with her recovery by participating in family therapy. The therapist focused on (a) helping the family understand that anorexia nervosa is a serious disease, (b) exploring healthier methods for family communication, (c) having the parents assist in the refeeding process by planning meals, and (d) reducing parental criticism regarding eating patterns. The parents were encouraged to help their daughter develop skills, attitudes, and activities appropriate to her developmental stage. With the addition of family therapy, the woman was able to gain more than 22 pounds (Sim et al., 2004).

Treatment of Bulimia Nervosa

During the initial assessment of individuals with bulimia nervosa, physical conditions that result from purging are identified and treated; these may include dental erosion, muscle weakness, cardiac arrhythmias, dehydration, electrolyte imbalance, or gastrointestinal problems involving the stomach or esophagus. As with anorexia nervosa, treatment often involves an interdisciplinary team that includes a physician and a therapist. Normalizing patterns of food intake and eliminating the binge–purge cycle is a primary goal of treatment (Office on Women's Health, 2022).

Cognitive-behavioral approaches can help individuals with bulimia develop a sense of self-control and reduce binge–purge symptoms. Cognitive-behavioral treatment involves encouraging the consumption of three balanced meals a day, reducing rigid food rules and body image concerns, identifying triggers for binge eating, and developing strategies for coping with emotional distress (Couturier et al., 2020). Adding exposure and response prevention procedures to therapy (i.e., exposure to cues associated with binge eating and prevention of purging following a binge-eating episode) appears to improve long-term outcomes for individuals with bulimia (McIntosh et al., 2010). Antidepressant medications such as selective serotonin reuptake inhibitors (SSRIs) are sometimes helpful in treating bulimia (Bello & Yeomans, 2018).

Treatment of Binge-Eating Disorder

Case Study   Mrs. A. had very rigid rules concerning eating that, when violated, would result in her "going the whole nine yards." Two types of triggers were identified for her binges—emotional distress (anger, anxiety, sadness, or frustration) and work stress (long hours, deadlines). Interventions were applied to help her deal with her stressors and develop more flexible rules regarding eating. First, she learned about obesity, proper nutrition, and physical exercise. Her body weight was recorded weekly, and a healthy pattern of three meals and two snacks a day was implemented. She used a food diary to record the type and amount of food consumed and her psychological state preceding eating. Second, her therapist used cognitive strategies to help change her disordered beliefs about eating. Mrs. A. made a list of "forbidden" foods and ranked them in order of "dangerousness." Gradually these foods were introduced into normal eating routines, beginning with those perceived as being least dangerous.

The prejudices of society about body size were discussed, and realistic expectations about change were addressed. Mrs. A. was asked to observe attractive individuals with a larger body size so that she could consider positive qualities rather than focusing solely on the body. After performing this "homework," she discovered that overweight women can look attractive and began to buy more fashionable clothes for herself. She was astonished at the positive reactions and comments from friends and coworkers and attributed the attention to her confidence and improved body image (Goldfein et al., 2000).

Treatments for binge-eating disorder are similar to those for bulimia nervosa, although binge-eating disorder presents fewer physical complications because of the lack of purging. Individuals with binge-eating disorder do differ in some ways from those with bulimia nervosa. Most are overweight and have to deal with societal prejudices regarding their weight. Due to the health consequences of excess weight, many therapy programs also focus on healthy approaches to weight loss. As we saw in the case study, treatment involves nutritional education as well as having the client identify triggers for overeating and then practicing strategies to reduce eating binges.

Antidepressant medications are sometimes effective in reducing or stopping binge eating; however, psychological interventions tend to produce the best long-term results. At this time, medication is seen as an add-on to cognitive-behavioral therapy rather than a primary treatment (Brownley et al., 2016). Although cognitive-behavioral therapy (CBT) can produce significant reductions in binge eating, it has less effect on weight reduction (Hilbert et al., 2012). CBT has also begun to incorporate strategies for addressing interpersonal difficulties and regulating negative emotions that can trigger binge eating and purging, a focus similar to the emotional regulation and distress tolerance skills taught in dialectical behavior therapy (Giel et al., 2022).

Preventing Eating Disorders

Prevention programs are attempting to reduce the incidence of eating disorders and disordered eating patterns. Programs geared toward women and girls target protective factors such as social support and strong social bonds as well as characteristics such as self-determination, autonomy, and social competence. Girls who have a sense of personal power and who recognize their positive personal qualities are less likely to exhibit disordered eating or become obsessed with their weight or body shape (Wacker & Dolbin-MacNab, 2020). Programs designed to reduce body dissatisfaction help women and girls to accept not only their weight and body shape but also their overall appearance. Interventions such as the Body Project Program that attempt to achieve this goal emphasize:

- increasing awareness of societal messages of what it means to be a woman and the role the media plays in creating unrealistic views of an ideal body;

- exploring ways to resist pressures to conform to unrealistic standards;

- developing a more positive body image by eliminating "fat talk" and teasing about body size;

- incorporating moderate eating and exercising into a healthy lifestyle;

- increasing comfort in openly expressing feelings to peers and family members;

- developing healthy ways of coping with stress and pressure; and

- increasing assertiveness skills.

These topics are addressed through group discussions and the use of videos, magazines, and examples from mass media (Chapman et al., 2010).

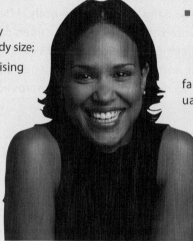
Kevin Peterson/Photodisc/Getty Images

There has been less focus on preventing eating disorders in men and boys. Programs are attempting to fill this gap by focusing on:

- expanding the definition of masculinity to include pro-social characteristics such as caring, nurturance, and cooperation;

- examining beliefs regarding what it means to be a man (e.g., needing to be brave and strong, remaining unemotional, taking charge) and understanding how these beliefs affect men's feelings about their bodies;

- learning to challenge the muscular body ideal;

- identifying and developing a positive sense of self that include qualities other than appearance;

  - developing a broader range of emotions and feelings and learning to express them in a healthy manner; and

    - developing skills to effectively deal with stressors (Bauer et al., 2019; Friedman, 2007).

It is hoped that bolstering protective factors such as social support, critical evaluation of unrealistic societal messages, and coping and communications skills will help stem the tide of eating disorders. Further, ongoing efforts to transform U.S. societal norms and eradicate systemic racism should help reduce racial disparities in access to health care and quality food as well as prevent the chronic stress associated with everyday discrimination.

10-4 Obesity

Case Study Eileen Isotalo wore large dark clothes to hide the shape of her body. She was able to lose weight but would gain it back. She was unable to curb her appetite, describing it as a "drive to eat" and a "craving for food." Even when she successfully lost weight with medication, she felt ashamed because of not being able to accomplish the loss through will power (Kolata, 2023).

Obesity is defined as having a **body mass index (BMI)** greater than 30. Our BMI, an estimate of our body fat, is calculated based on our height and weight. The DSM does not yet recognize obesity as a specific disorder, despite its devastating medical and psychological consequences. Some researchers believe that forms of obesity that are characterized by an excessive drive for food, such as that experienced by Eileen Isotalo in the case study, should be recognized as a "food or fat addiction" (Florio et al., 2022). We include obesity in this chapter because it is often accompanied by depression and anxiety, low self-esteem, poor body image, and unhealthy eating patterns. Obesity is also related to a greater risk of developing neurocognitive disorders such as vascular dementia and Alzheimer's disease (Flores-Cordero et al., 2022).

The worldwide prevalence of obesity nearly tripled between 1975 and 2023, with obesity now representing a phenomenon that affects more than 650 million individuals (World Health Organization [WHO], 2023). According to BMI standards, 42 percent of U.S. adults are obese, with 9.2 percent being severely obese. Asian Americans adults have the lowest obesity rate (16.1 percent) compared with White (41.4 percent), Latinx (45.6 percent), and Black (49.9 percent) adults. Obesity rates among Native American and Alaska Native adults are also a significant concern (CDC, 2022). Figure 10.4 indicates self-reported obesity among U.S. adults in various states in 2022 (CDC, 2023).

Severe obesity has significantly increased among children ages 2 to 5 years; additionally, there is an upward trend toward obesity occurring among youth between ages 6 and 19, especially African American and Hispanic American youth (Skinner et al., 2018). Among U.S. youth, obesity prevalence is higher in Black (24.8 percent) and Hispanic (26.2 percent) youth as compared to White (16.6 percent) and Asian (9 percent) youth (CDC, 2022).

There is growing recognition that obesity is not the result of being lazy or lacking self-control. Rather than blaming individuals who are obese for their excess weight, it is more accurate to consider obesity as a disease with specific symptoms, abnormal physiological processes, and associated health risks (Rubino et al., 2020). Being overweight or obese increases the risk of high cholesterol and triglyceride levels, type 2 diabetes, cancer, coronary heart disease, stroke, gallbladder disease, arthritis, sleep apnea, and respiratory problems (Warren et al., 2019). Among adolescents, it is also associated with reduced cognitive performance and acceleration of brain

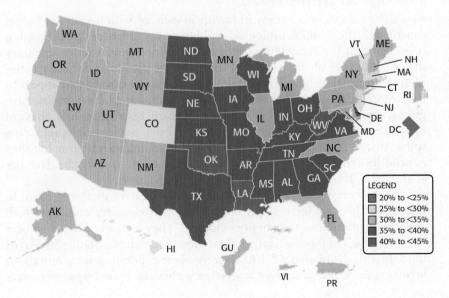

Figure 10.4

Prevalence of Self-Reported Obesity Among U. S. Adults by State and Territory, 2022

Source: CDC, 2023

changes associated with aging (Chan et al., 2013). In addition, children and adolescents who are overweight or obese have an increased risk of developing an eating disorder (Stabouli et al., 2021).

Childhood obesity has a significant health impact, especially for girls. Girls who are obese are nine times more likely to develop high blood pressure compared to their peers who are not obese, whereas boys have a threefold increase in risk (Ortiz, 2011). Being overweight or obese in childhood is associated with an increased risk of coronary heart disease in adulthood. Paradoxically, in a review of 97 studies involving nearly 3 million adults age 65 and older, being overweight was not associated with an increase in mortality; in fact, overweight individuals died at a slightly lower rate than those of normal weight, and older adults with mild obesity died no more frequently than their normal-weight peers (Flegal et al., 2013). In a study of Swedish adults, the BMI with the lowest mortality rate was in the middle of the overweight classification. It is not clear why overweight adults have a healthier outcome than those of "normal" weight (Afzal et al., 2016).

Etiology of Obesity

Obesity stems from many causes, including genetic and biological factors; our sedentary lifestyle combined with easy access to attractive, high-calorie foods; and some of the same disturbed eating patterns seen in eating disorders. Thus, obesity is a product of biological, psychological, social, and sociocultural influences, as presented in Figure 10.5. How these dimensions interact is still a matter of debate. For instance, one theory, termed the thrifty genotype hypothesis, points to the role of both genetics and the environment in accounting for the rapid rise in obesity (Hollstein et al., 2019). According to this perspective, certain genes helped our ancestors survive famines by storing body fat. These same genes, however, may be dysfunctional in an environment in which high-fat foods are now plentiful. Researchers suggest that individuals with "thrifty genes" display lower-than-average energy expenditure both when fasting and when overeating compared to those without this genetic characteristic (Reinhardt et al., 2016). Although "thrifty genes" and access to foods can account for some cases of obesity, other factors must be involved because rates of obesity also vary according to variables such as income level, gender, and ethnicity.

Biological Dimension

Researchers focus on a variety of factors associated with obesity, including genetic influences and neurological and hormonal functioning. Although it is evident that the availability of high-calorie foods and a more sedentary lifestyle influence obesity, some individuals have particular difficulty maintaining a normal weight. For example, African American women appear to have more difficulty losing weight when participating in weight-loss programs, even when they follow prescribed calorie restrictions and physical activity recommendations. It is hypothesized that some people, including some African American women, have a lower resting metabolism and thus expend less energy than other people attempting to lose weight (DeLany et al., 2013; Toledo et al., 2018).

Obesity may involve more than just the excessive intake of food. In fact, researchers are increasingly implicating neurocircuitry associated with appetite regulation in the obesity epidemic. They consider obesity to be a "neurobiological disease" rather than merely a matter of faulty intake of food. In a study involving 2,100 severely obese children, genetic mutations involving the KSR2 gene were associated with an increased sense of hunger

Myth Body mass index standards represent unvarying thresholds that remain constant from year to year.

Reality In 1998, the BMI cutoff scores were lowered for all weight classes. This resulted in a sudden increase in the prevalence of individuals considered overweight or obese. For example, the BMI cutoff for the category of overweight was lowered from 27 to 25. This resulted in millions of Americans being added to the overweight category—an overnight increase of 42 percent.

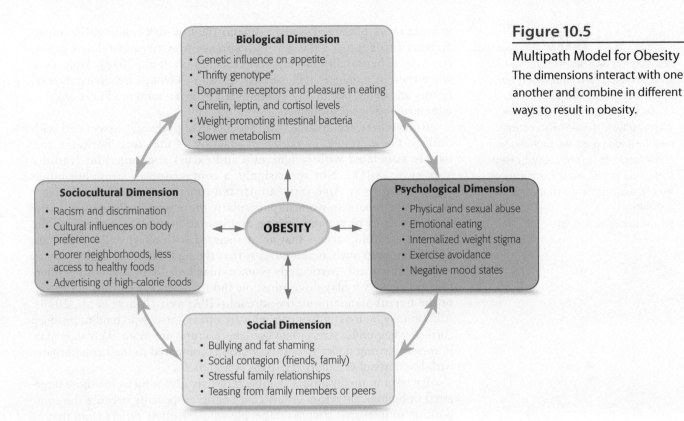

Figure 10.5

Multipath Model for Obesity
The dimensions interact with one another and combine in different ways to result in obesity.

Biological Dimension
- Genetic influence on appetite
- "Thrifty genotype"
- Dopamine receptors and pleasure in eating
- Ghrelin, leptin, and cortisol levels
- Weight-promoting intestinal bacteria
- Slower metabolism

Sociocultural Dimension
- Racism and discrimination
- Cultural influences on body preference
- Poorer neighborhoods, less access to healthy foods
- Advertising of high-calorie foods

OBESITY

Psychological Dimension
- Physical and sexual abuse
- Emotional eating
- Internalized weight stigma
- Exercise avoidance
- Negative mood states

Social Dimension
- Bullying and fat shaming
- Social contagion (friends, family)
- Stressful family relationships
- Teasing from family members or peers

and a slower metabolism (Pearce et al., 2013). Further, genetic variants have been identified that appear to be associated with increases in body fat storage (Krishnan et al., 2018).

In another genetic study, individuals with a high-risk variant of the FTO gene—an allele associated with increased food intake—had a 70 percent greater chance of becoming obese compared to individuals with a low-risk version of the gene. Individuals with the high-risk allele found pictures of high-fat foods more appealing than those with the low-risk gene; additionally, the hormone ghrelin (responsible for stimulating hunger) was slow to decline after eating and then rose more rapidly in those with the high-risk variant (Karra et al., 2013). The appetite-regulating hormone, leptin, is also implicated in obesity. For example, a group of children who weighed more than 200 pounds by age 10 were found to have a chromosomal abnormality that affected nine of the genes that influence leptin production (Bochukova et al., 2010).

Even if you inherit a high-risk genetic profile for obesity, the environment plays a large role in determining the degree of its expression. Most Samoans have a genetic variation strongly related to obesity that is extremely rare in other populations. However, the degree of genetic expression is dependent on environmental factors. In 2003, 68 percent of the men and 84 percent of the women in Samoa were overweight or obese. Seven years later, the prevalence rates for obesity had increased to 80 percent and 91 percent, respectively, likely resulting from greater access to high-calorie foods and an increasingly sedentary lifestyle. One of the researchers pointed out that "Samoans weren't obese 200 years ago" (Minster et al., 2016).

Similarly, the degree of expression of a genetic predisposition to obesity differed among twins raised in either a high- or low-obesogenic environment (determined by the availability of healthy or unhealthy foods, physical activity opportunities, and parental rules around television watching and use of other media). Whereas the heritability of high BMI was 86 percent

BMI may not be a dependable measure for biological health. Nearly 50 percent of overweight, 29 percent of obese, and 16 percent of severely obese individuals were metabolically healthy (blood pressure, triglyceride, cholesterol, etc.) in one study. Interestingly, over 30 percent of the normal weight subjects were metabolically unhealthy.

Source: Tomiyama et al., 2016

in a high-risk obesogenic environment, the low-risk home environment appeared to suppress the genetic expression of obesity-related genes, resulting in heritability of 36 percent (Schrempft et al., 2018). Thus, even when there is a genetic risk, obesity is also influenced by environmental factors and could potentially be prevented by behavioral modifications that minimize obesogenic influences.

Researchers are investigating biochemical pathways associated with obesity. For example, increased production of the stress hormone cortisol is associated with weight gain and excess abdominal fat (van der Valk et al., 2018). Not surprisingly, a comparison of stress hormones between European American and African American women revealed that the African American women (particularly those who had experienced the highest rates of recent and lifelong discrimination) had higher levels of the stress-related biomarkers that are associated with obesity (Cedillo et al., 2020). Findings such as this suggest that the high rates of obesity seen in African Americans, particularly women, may be a by-product of the interplay between everyday discrimination and the resultant chronic activation of the hypothalamic-pituitary-adrenal (HPA) axis (Lehrer et al., 2020). Additionally, among individuals who are obese, those who tend to produce cortisol when under stress (high cortisol reactors) are more likely to engage in comfort eating under stressful conditions compared to their counterparts with less cortisol reactivity (Herhaus et al., 2020).

Bacteria in the intestines (gut bacteria) are also a focus for those interested in biological factors influencing obesity, especially because the composition of intestinal bacteria in people who are obese differs from that of those who are slim. Researchers are learning that bacteria affect our metabolism and the conversion of the food we consume into fat. Because our diet can affect the type of bacteria we have in our intestines, dietary changes incorporating healthier food selections can influence the makeup of gut bacteria, increasing the microorganisms that promote leanness instead of obesity (Rastelli et al., 2018).

Researchers have used mice to demonstrate that intestinal bacteria can cause obesity. In an intriguing study, researchers obtained gut bacteria from human twins, selecting twin pairs in which one twin was thin and the other obese. They then transferred the bacteria into mice. Amazingly, several weeks later, the mice with bacteria from the obese twins began to gain weight and demonstrated metabolic changes associated with obesity; mice who received bacteria from slender twins stayed thin (Ridaura et al., 2013). Research will now attempt to identify exactly which microorganisms in the intestines produce this effect, and if bacterial manipulation can help treat obesity. Overall, evidence is accumulating that there are significant genetic and biological influences that result in a predisposition toward developing obesity. Such information helps explain why losing weight is so difficult for some people.

Psychological Dimension

Physical and sexual abuse during childhood increases the risk for obesity. In a study involving 57,321 nurses, over 8 percent reported severe physical abuse in childhood and 5.3 percent reported severe sexual abuse. Those who experienced childhood abuse had a greater risk of being overweight and engaging in out-of-control eating. It is possible that such a background increases the tendency to use eating as a means of coping with stressful emotions (Mason et al., 2013). Adverse childhood experiences (ACEs) have also been associated with obesity in childhood; the association is particularly strong for girls who have been experienced sexual abuse and for children who have been subjected to multiple ACEs (Schroeder et al., 2021).

Children and adults who are obese often report feeling stressed, anxious, or depressed. These responses are likely associated with the "fat shaming" and weight stigma that exist in society and the related harassment and prejudice that occur in school and work environments (Robinson et al., 2020). Discrimination related to obesity increases depression and decreases life satisfaction in adults who struggle with weight control, and it is also associated with avoidance of physical activity, low self-esteem, and substance abuse (Jackson et al., 2015). The stigma with obesity can become internalized. Further, the stigma associated with obesity may prevent some individuals from seeking medical assistance or discussing weight concerns with physicians or other health care providers (Stanford et al., 2018). Education that reframes obesity as a chronic, but treatable, medical condition involving heredity, biological homeostatic conditions, and other nonbehavioral factors (rather than a lack of willpower) may help reduce the internalized stigma of children and adults who find it extremely challenging to lose weight (English & Vallis, 2023).

Social Dimension

Social stressors during childhood such as bullying and "fat shaming" can increase the risk of weight issues (Lynch et al., 2018). Children bullied during elementary or secondary school are more likely to be overweight at age 18 compared to their nonbullied classmates. The risk is especially high for children bullied throughout their school years, with the risk of obesity nearly twice that experienced by their nonbullied peers (Baldwin et al., 2016). Additionally, stressful social interactions are common among youth already struggling with weight issues, since classmates often ostracize children and adolescents who are overweight. Given the relationship of obesity to weight-related stigma, a vicious cycle often develops that maintains obesity. First, environmental stressors produce physiological stress reactions that lead to obesity. Obesity then leads to weight-related stigma that produces more stress, thereby reinforcing the cycle (Tomiyama, 2019).

Fear of victimization, bullying, or ridicule may lead overweight youth to avoid social or physical activities that could assist with weight reduction. Almost two thirds of adolescents attending a weight-loss camp reported weight-based victimization, with the majority of perpetrators being friends and peers. More than half of the adolescents reported that bullying from peers involved social media or texting. The adolescents also reported that physical education and other teachers, sport coaches, and family members engaged in teasing and bullying regarding weight (Puhl et al., 2013). Thus, it is not surprising that those who face weight discrimination are more likely to become or remain obese than individuals who do not face such discrimination (Stanford et al., 2018).

Stress within the family has also been associated with excess weight during childhood, adolescence, and even adulthood. Longitudinal follow-up found that teens who had a "poor relationship" with their mothers during their early years were twice as likely to become obese during adolescence compared to those who reported having a positive relationship with their mothers (Anderson et al., 2012). Teasing by family members about weight issues is also associated with obesity (Pearlman et al., 2019). Family eating patterns and attitudes may also influence food intake in children. For instance, in families where parents provide an authoritative (warm, responsive, and fair) mealtime atmosphere, adolescents are less likely to become overweight or obese (Ardakani et al., 2023).

Can social contagion spread obesity to friends, families, or communities? Christakis and Fowler (2007) followed the social networks of 12,067 adults over a period of 32 years to determine social factors associated with

Plus Size Models—A Passing Fad?

Fashion model Whitney Thompson, an ambassador for the National Eating Disorders Association, is worried that the use of full-figured models is only a temporary phenomenon. Is she right?

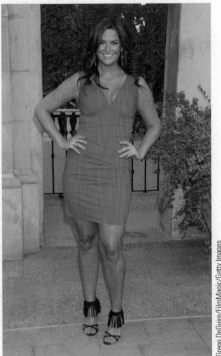

Gregg DeGuire/FilmMagic/Getty Images

obesity. They wanted to determine if a person's friends, siblings, partners, or neighbors had an impact on weight gain. Some of the findings were quite surprising. If someone a person considers a friend becomes obese, the person's chances of becoming obese increase by 57 percent. If both individuals consider each other friends, the chances increase by 171 percent. The chances of an individual becoming obese also increase by 40 percent when an adult sibling became obese or by 37 percent when a spouse became obese. These findings suggest that people influence others in their social network regarding the acceptability of weight gain (Datar et al., 2023). The same effect was found in military families who moved to military bases that differed in obesity rates. There was greater weight gain in both parents and their children among families who moved to a base with higher obesity rates compared to those who moved to installations with low rates of obesity. This association between higher levels of community obesity and weight gain was most pronounced for the families who stayed longest in their military community (Datar & Nicosia, 2018).

Significant increases in pediatric obesity during the COVID pandemic have been attributed to factors such as social isolation, disrupted routines, and decreased opportunity to exercise. The weight gain was especially pronounced among youth from low-income families, suggesting that preexisting social inequalities associated with obesity were exacerbated during the pandemic (Betts et al., 2023).

Sociocultural Dimension

Attitudes regarding food and acceptable weight are often developed in the home and community. In some ethnic groups, there is less pressure to remain thin, and being moderately overweight is not a big concern. Overall, rates of obesity tend to be highest among underrepresented racial or ethnic groups (CDC, 2020). As noted earlier, among African Americans, there is greater acceptance of fuller figures, which may partially account for the fact that African American women have the highest rates of obesity of any group. Although most overweight African American women would prefer to weigh less, they tend to underestimate their body size and do not express high levels of body dissatisfaction until they are nearly obese (Baruth et al., 2015).

Rates of obesity also tend to be higher among individuals with fewer financial resources. This may occur because people living in poorer neighborhoods often have limited access to parks, playgrounds, and sports (Frederick et al., 2014). Similarly, the availability of high-calorie, lower-cost foods may contribute to obesity in communities where there are fewer options to purchase healthy, fresh food. However, the most significant factor affecting obesity in marginalized populations may be discrimination—both everyday discrimination and the long-term effects of traumatic discriminatory events.

The overeating that leads to obesity may represent a method of coping with these pervasive social stressors. Thus, discussions of obesity need to consider the chronic impact of inadequate social, economic, and health care systems, as well as social disadvantage related to race, ethnicity, and poverty (Kumanyika, 2019). For example, among African American youth, increased BMI is associated with experiences of racial discrimination, especially for African American girls (Nelson et al., 2018). Further, a study found that the BMI of African American adolescents was inversely associated with their parents' exposure to stressors related to community safety—the children of parents who perceived more safety-related environmental stressors had a higher BMI (Allport et al., 2019). This points to one of the means by which discrimination is linked to weight gain—the constant need for vigilance (i.e., being on the watch for danger or difficulties) that occurs in oppressed communities. For instance, a study of Black women in Chicago revealed a strong association between a woman's waist circumference and use of vigilance as a means of coping with racism (Hicken et al., 2018). As you might imagine, this vigilance not only involves wariness of potential discrimination toward oneself but also includes chronic worry about racism directed toward friends and family members, a concern that intersects with the very real issue of personal and community safety.

Treatment for Obesity

Treatments for obesity have included dieting, lifestyle changes, medications, and surgery. In general, dieting alone may produce short-term weight loss but tends to be ineffective in the long term; some individuals gain back more weight than was lost. When dieters significantly reduce their caloric intake, their overall metabolic rate is lowered and hormones that increase appetite are released. Even a year after dieting, the hormonally based appetite stimulation effect may still be present. Most adults would be better off not dieting, because weight fluctuations create considerable stress on the body. The "yo-yo" effect in dieting (cycles of weight gain and loss) is associated with increased risk of cardiovascular disease and stroke, as well as decreased immune system function. Weight reduction is most successful when there are lifestyle changes that include the consumption of low-energy-density foods—foods containing water, fiber, and proteins such as fruits, vegetables, and legumes. These foods are more effective in helping people maintain or lose weight because they have fewer calories and stimulate more energy expenditure than high-energy-density foods such as processed products that are high in fat or sugar (Benton & Young, 2017). Given the link between certain intestinal bacteria and obesity, the use of probiotics is also increasingly used to treat obesity (Cai et al., 2023).

Comprehensive lifestyle intervention programs appear to be the most promising form of treatment for obesity. Collaborative care programs that include behavioral and problem-solving strategies combined with antidepressants, if necessary, have produced reductions in both BMI and depression (Ma et al., 2019). Participants who took part in a structured 6-month lifestyle intervention program (healthy diet, physical activity, behavioral therapy, and at least 14 individual or group counseling sessions) lost up to 18 pounds and improved their cardiovascular health and quality of life. Follow-up participation in a weight-loss maintenance program allowed the participants to avoid regaining weight by encouraging the continuation of physical activity and healthy food choices (Wadden et al., 2020).

Lifestyle interventions have also been successful with children. A meta-analysis of 64 studies that included dietary changes, physical activity, and behavioral interventions found that many of the children who engaged in these programs not only lost weight but also improved their self-esteem and body image (Gow et al., 2020). Not surprisingly, researchers have found that lifestyle changes can attenuate the genetic predisposition for weight gain (Wang et al., 2018). Given the higher prevalence of obesity among populations of color, there is increasing interest in developing comprehensive

Childhood Obesity

In response to increasing rates of obesity in China, overweight children are enrolled in summer camps designed to encourage weight loss. The boys pictured here are participating in their camp's daily exercise program.

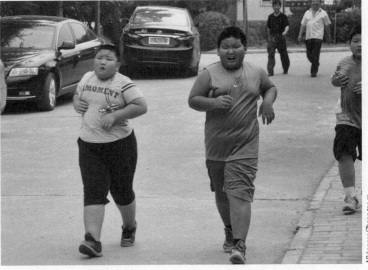

AP Images/Zhang tao zz

treatment programs geared to socially marginalized communities that are dealing with inadequate food systems and a variety of social stressors that include racism, income disparities, and limited access to health care (Byrd et al., 2018).

Surgical methods such as gastric banding (placing an adjustable inflatable band around the upper stomach) or gastric bypass (creating a small pouch from the upper stomach and attaching it to the intestine) are used in the treatment of severe obesity. These methods facilitate weight loss by severely limiting the amount of food that can be consumed and appear to promote changes in intestinal bacteria that are conducive to weight loss (Martinou et al., 2022). Although gastric bypass seems to be more effective for weight loss, there are many possible complications. Long-term follow-up studies indicate that bariatric surgical procedures provide substantial and durable weight loss, but there is often a need for follow-up surgeries (O'Brien et al., 2019). Endoscopic sleeve gastroplasty, a newer, minimally invasive procedure that involves inserting a suturing device down the throat and placing sutures into the stomach, is considered a safe and effective procedure. With all of these interventions, the individual is expected to make lifestyle changes involving diet and exercise to ensure long-term success (de Miranda Neto et al., 2020). Dietary counseling is also recommended to ensure adequate intake of essential nutrients when adjusting to a lifelong modified diet (Shah et al., 2013).

Medications are becoming an increasingly popular alternative for individuals who are obese or who are significantly overweight. For example, medications containing semaglutide (e.g., Wegovy, Ozempic, Rybelsus), administered via weekly injections, are being prescribed for the management of obesity. They are also used when someone who is significantly overweight has other weight-related conditions such as high blood pressure, high cholesterol, or type 2 diabetes. These medications target areas of the brain that regulate appetite and food intake. They create a sensation of fullness and slow digestion of food. Side effects involve a variety of gastrointestinal symptoms. One group of patients taking one of these medications (Wegovy) lost about 15 percent of their body weight over a 68-week period (Kosiborod et al., 2023). For most individuals, the weight stays off only when using the medication. For example, in one study of adults who had been receiving semaglutide injections, participants regained about two-thirds of their lost weight after discontinuing the medication (Wilding et al., 2022).

The American Academy of Pediatrics (AAP) has provided guidelines for the treatment of obesity in children and adolescents (Hampl et al., 2023):

- For children 2 to 5 years of age and older, comprehensive intervention including motivational interviewing, parent–child involvement, cognitive behavioral therapy, physical activity treatment, and face-to-face interaction with the child and parents is recommended.

- For children 8 to 11 years of age and older, medication may be offered as an adjunct to behavioral and lifestyle treatment.

- For youth 13 years and older with severe obesity, evaluation for bariatric surgery can be considered.

These guidelines have been controversial and do not have broad acceptance. Given the limited availability of comprehensive obesity treatment programs, critics express concern that health care providers may find it easier to provide medication or offer surgery as interventions.

Concern is also expressed over the use of medication for young children and surgery for youth as young as 13 years of age, particularly given the lack of long-term studies evaluating these interventions with children. In addition, consideration must be given to the long-term medical needs, lifestyle changes, and nutritional requirements associated with bariatric surgery (Volpe & Kean, 2023). Further, the emphasis on medical interventions may increase weight stigma and disproportionately affect youth and adults who cannot afford these treatments.

Other problems exist with the AAP guidelines. The determination of obesity is based solely on BMI scores, which the American Medical Association considers a problematic measure for determining "healthy" weight or obesity. BMI is based primarily on people of European descent and does not adequately predict disease risk for other ethnic and racial groups. In addition, BMI by itself is an incomplete measure of health risk and does not take into account other important risk factors such as body composition, belly fat, and waist circumference (Berg, 2023).

10-5 Contemporary Trends and Future Directions

It is clear that media depictions of thin women have a negative impact on the body satisfaction of women and girls and are a major contributor to eating disorders. Similarly, images of idealized masculine bodies are affecting the body image of boys and men. To counter the impact of unrealistic images, physicians and mental health advocates in many countries are demanding that advertisers include more images of people of varying sizes and weights. Research is finding that exposure to more normative body images can produce a shift toward more realistic body preference (Ogden et al., 2020). Promoting a wider range of body types in mass media and advertising may promote healthier lifestyles and greatly reduce the body dissatisfaction that is so rampant in society today.

Researchers are also developing online resources to counteract Web sites that encourage disordered eating. For instance, one such resource offers an online support group for children, adolescents, and young adults who are struggling with eating and weight issues. This anonymous social network is easily accessible and provides medical information and advice about nutrition, coping with weight concerns, and healthy ways to manage eating. Members can share success stories, team up with a weight-loss buddy, or post in chat rooms and on message boards. The goal of Web sites such as these is to help children, adolescents, and young adults receive positive social support in their attempts to lose weight and to combat the isolation and discrimination that overweight individuals face. Such supportive programs can help people struggling with obesity or disordered eating who may be too embarrassed to talk to health care providers or others about weight issues.

Innovative research is also examining the use of technology to guide lifestyle changes. For example, a game-like smartphone app focused on activity tracking has been effective in significantly increasing engagement in physical activities. Participants received points and social rewards from family members or friends for attaining goals. Making participation more game-like, self-competitive, and social increased the participants' motivation to continue the physical activities (Patel et al., 2019). A chatbot designed to simulate human conversation based on a cognitive-behavioral eating disorders treatment program was successful in reducing women's concerns over weight and body shape as compared to a wait-list control group. This reduction remained evident at a 6-month follow-up, suggesting that this may be an effective and low-cost intervention to prevent and intervene with eating disorders (Fitzsimmons-Craft et al., 2022). Similarly, a guided chatbot mini-intervention consisting of one session that focused on having a healthy body resulted in improved body image and was rated by participants as enjoyable and easy to use (Nemesure et al., 2023). These interventions have the potential to prevent or reduce the probability of developing an eating disorder.

The COVID-19 pandemic spotlighted and generated conversations about health disparities and the disproportionate and serious impact of illness on African Americans, Native Americans, and Latinx Americans. Given the high prevalence of obesity and related health conditions within these communities, it has become increasingly evident that research and intervention directed toward the complex and systemic societal factors contributing to these health disparities is long overdue. This topic will be an essential component of future efforts to decrease rates of disordered eating and obesity within marginalized populations.

Chapter Summary

1 What kinds of eating disorders exist?

- Individuals with anorexia nervosa exhibit severe body image distortion. They are afraid of getting fat, and they engage in self-starvation. There are two subtypes of anorexia nervosa: the restricting type and the binge-eating/purging type.

- Individuals with bulimia nervosa engage in recurrent binge eating; feel a loss of control over eating; and use vomiting, exercise, or laxatives to attempt to control weight.

- Individuals with binge-eating disorder also engage in recurrent binge eating and feel a loss of control over eating; however, they do not regularly use purging or exercise to counteract the effects of overeating and are often overweight.

- Individuals who display atypical patterns of severely disordered eating that do not fully meet the criteria for anorexia nervosa, bulimia nervosa, or binge-eating disorder are given the diagnosis of other specified feeding or eating disorders.

2 What are some causes of eating disorders?

- Genetic influences, neurotransmitter dysfunction, abnormal neural circuitry, and intestinal bacteria are implicated in eating disorders.

- It is believed that societal emphasis on thinness plays a key role in the prevalence of eating disorders.

- Parental attitudes regarding the importance of thinness and peer attitudes about body size and weight can contribute to disordered eating.

- Countries that are influenced by Western standards have seen an increasing incidence of eating disorders.

3 What are some treatment options for eating disorders?

- Many of the therapies for eating disorders attempt to teach clients to identify the impact of societal messages regarding thinness and encourage them to develop healthier goals and values.

- For individuals with anorexia nervosa, medical as well as psychological treatment is necessary, because the body is in starvation mode. The goal is to help clients gain weight, normalize their eating patterns, understand and alter their thoughts related to body image, and develop healthier methods of dealing with stress.

- With both bulimia nervosa and binge-eating disorder, therapy involves normalizing eating patterns, developing a more positive body image, and learning to deal with stress in a healthier fashion.

- With bulimia nervosa, medical assistance may be required because of the physiological changes associated with purging.

- Because many people with binge-eating disorder are overweight or obese, weight reduction strategies are often included in treatment.

4 What causes obesity, and how is it treated?

- The causes of obesity vary from individual to individual and involve combinations of biological predispositions and psychological, social, and sociocultural influences.

- In general, lifestyle changes that include reduced intake of high-calorie foods combined with exercise have proven to be the most effective treatment for obesity. Some individuals with extreme obesity have benefited from gastric surgery.

Chapter Glossary

anorexia nervosa
an eating disorder characterized by low body weight, an intense fear of becoming obese, and body image distortion

binge eating
rapid consumption of large quantities of food

binge-eating disorder (BED)
an eating disorder that involves the consumption of large amounts of food over a short period of time with accompanying feelings of loss of control and distress over the excess eating

body mass index (BMI)
an estimate of body fat calculated on the basis of a person's height and weight

bulimia nervosa
an eating disorder in which episodes involving rapid consumption of large quantities of food and a loss of control over eating are followed by purging, excessive exercise, or fasting in an attempt to compensate for binges

disordered eating
physically or psychologically unhealthy eating behavior such as chronic overeating or dieting

obesity
a condition involving a body mass index (BMI) greater than 30

other specified feeding or eating disorders
a seriously disturbed eating pattern that does not fully meet criteria for another eating disorder diagnosis

purge
to rid the body of unwanted calories by means such as self-induced vomiting or misuse of laxatives, diuretics, or other medications

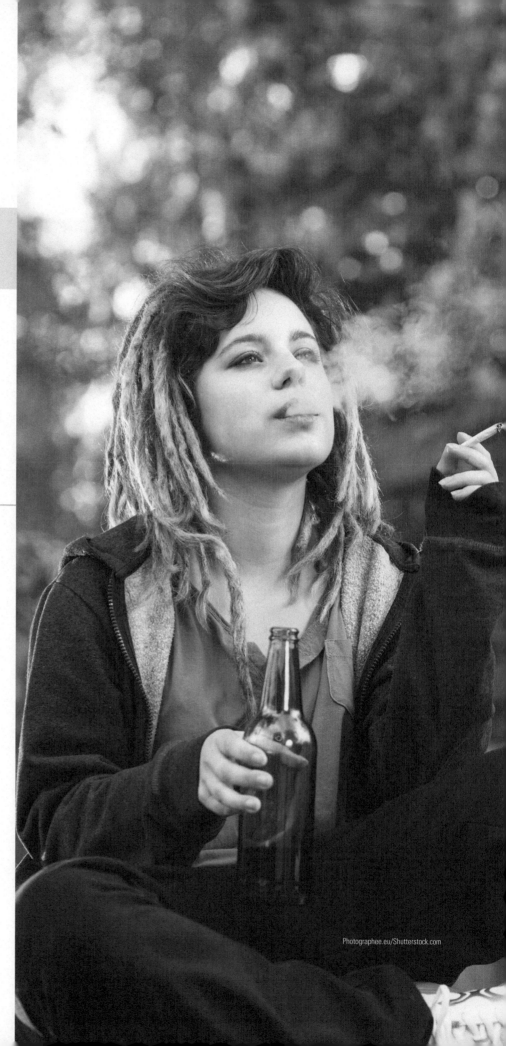

focus Questions

1 What are substance-use disorders?
2 What substances are associated with addiction?
3 Why do people develop substance-use disorders?
4 What kinds of interventions and treatments for substance-use disorders are most effective?
5 Can behaviors such as gambling be addictive?

11

Substance-Related and Other Addictive Disorders

Learning Objectives

After studying this chapter, you will be able to . . .

11-1 Describe how the DSM-5-TR defines a substance-use disorder.

11-2 Identify substances that are associated with addiction and describe some of the specific properties and concerns associated with each of these substances.

11-3 Discuss reasons why people develop substance-use disorders.

11-4 Describe the types of interventions and treatments that are most effective for treating substance-use disorders.

11-5 Describe characteristics of gambling disorder and debate whether behavioral addictions should be included in the DSM.

Jay, Age 20, Was Arrested for Initiating a Fight and was brought to the emergency department due to his extreme agitation and violent behavior. When medical staff attempted to evaluate his condition, he yelled and made threats if anyone approached him. Periods of calm alternated with extreme emotionality and aggressive outbursts. At times, Jay sobbed uncontrollably and talked about suicide. When Jay eventually calmed down, he shared that he had smoked some "really great pot" earlier that day. He was eventually transferred to the inpatient psychiatric unit, where the staff was able to obtain a urine sample. Jay tested positive for both cannabis and PCP. Apparently, someone had laced the marijuana he had smoked with PCP (Schmetze & McGrath, 2014).

Throughout history, people have used a variety of chemical substances to alter their mood, level of consciousness, and/or behavior. People in the United States, for example, purchase vast quantities of alcohol, tobacco, prescription medications, and illegal drugs. These substances can lead to addiction or acute psychiatric symptoms such as those experienced by Jay. Each year, the Substance Abuse and Mental Health Services Administration (SAMHSA) obtains information regarding the use of various substances from interviews with approximately 67,500 adolescents and adults throughout the United States. Based on data obtained in 2021, the researchers estimated that 164.8 million adolescents and adults—60.2 percent of people in the United States age 12 or older—had used at least one substance (i.e., tobacco, alcohol, or illicit drugs) in the previous month (Figure 11.1). The data also suggest that in 2021, there were 61.2 million adolescents and adults—21.9 percent of the population—who used federally defined illicit drugs such as cannabis, cocaine, or illegally obtained prescription medications (Figure 11.2). Addiction specialists are particularly concerned that young adults (ages 18 to 25) are reporting high rates of marijuana use, as well as heavy drinking and nonmedical use of prescription drugs (SAMHSA, 2022). Although the use of illicit drugs among youth declined during the COVID pandemic, there has been a dramatic postpandemic rise in drug use and overdose deaths among U.S. teens ages 14 to 18; as with

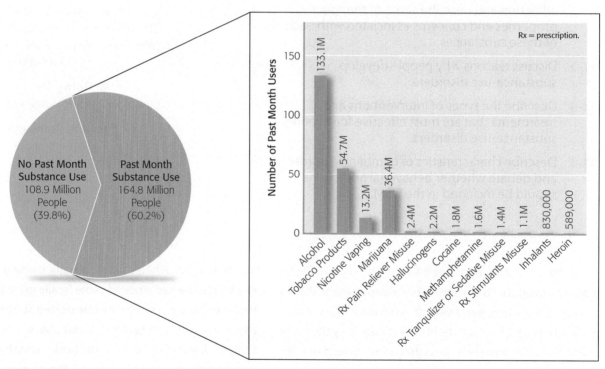

Note: The estimated numbers of current users of different substances are not mutually exclusive because people could have more than one type of substance in the past month.

Figure 11.1

Past Month Substance Use Among People Age 12 or Older in 2021

Data from a nationwide survey in the United States reveal that approximately 60.2 percent of people age 12 or older had used a substance in the previous month. Of the estimated 164.8 million people with past-month substance use, approximately 133.1 million people drank alcohol, 54.7 million used a tobacco product, and 36.4 million people used marijuana.

Source: SAMHSA, 2022

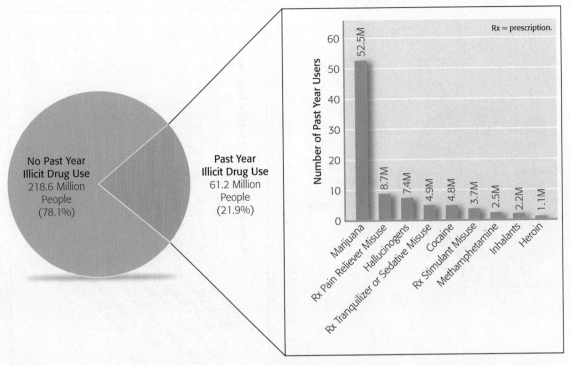

Note: The estimated numbers of past year users of different illicit drugs are not mutually exclusive because people could have used more than one type of illicit drug in the past year.

Figure 11.2

Past-Year Illicit Drug Use Among People Age 12 or Older in 2021

Many users of illicit drugs use more than one substance. Although federal law still deems marijuana an illicit, controlled substance, legalization in numerous states has led to a significant rise in marijuana use. In contrast, there has been a downward trend in heroin use and a significant decrease in the misuse of pain medications, including opioids.

Source: SAMHSA, 2022

the increase in overdose deaths among adults, many of these deaths are attributed to fentanyl use or unintentional fentanyl ingestion from fentanyl-laced pills purchased on the black market (Miech et al., 2023).

As these statistics suggest, **substance abuse**, the excessive or harmful use of drugs or alcohol, is pervasive in our society. In 2021, an estimated 46.3 million adolescents and adults (16.5 percent of the U.S. population age 12 and up) met the criteria for a **substance-use disorder** at some time during the year. As you will find in Figure 11.3, alcohol is the most commonly abused substance, followed by misused prescription medications and marijuana (SAMHSA, 2022).

You may wonder which substances are considered the most dangerous. A comprehensive analysis (conducted prior to the introduction of fentanyl) concluded that heroin, crack cocaine, and methamphetamine present the greatest danger for the user, but that alcohol is the most dangerous drug when both personal and societal consequences are considered (Nutt et al., 2010). As you proceed through this chapter, consider the individual and societal effects of the substances discussed, as well as the vast number of people affected directly and indirectly by substance abuse.

We first examine the various substances involved in substance-use disorders. We next use the multipath perspective to understand possible causes of drug and alcohol addiction. We then review addiction treatment and conclude with a focus on other addictions, including gambling disorder.

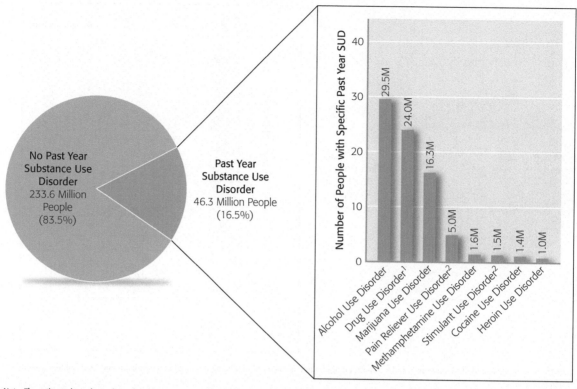

Note: The estimated numbers of people with substance use disorders are not mutually exclusive because people could have use disorders for more than one substance.

[1] Includes data from all past year users of marijuana, cocaine, heroin, hallucinogens, inhalants, methamphetamine, and prescription psychotherapeutic drugs (i.e., pain relievers, tranquilizers, stimulants, or sedatives).

[2] Includes data from all past year users of the specific prescription drug.

Figure 11.3

People Age 12 or Older with a Past-Year Substance-Use Disorder in 2021

In 2021, approximately 46.3 million people age 12 or older had a substance-use disorder, including 29.5 million who had an alcohol-use disorder and 24 million who abused other substances, including marijuana, prescription medications, methamphetamine, cocaine, and heroin.

Source: SAMHSA, 2022

11-1 Substance-Related Disorders

Substance-related disorders arise when **psychoactive substances**—substances that alter moods, thought processes, or other psychological states—are used excessively. Heavy substance use causes changes in the brain that result in the behaviors that characterize addiction (Hammoud & Jimenez-Shahed, 2019). **Addiction** involves compulsive drug-seeking behavior and a loss of control over drug use. Once addiction develops, it is difficult to stop using the substance, not only because of the pleasurable feelings associated with use but also because of the **withdrawal** symptoms—negative psychological and physiological effects such as shaking, irritability, or emotional distress—that occur when use is discontinued.

What causes these withdrawal symptoms? Withdrawal occurs when chronic exposure to a substance results in **physiological dependence**—our bodies adapt, and we need the substance to feel normal. In other words, withdrawal symptoms develop if we have become accustomed to regular use of a substance and then we suddenly stop. Different substances produce different withdrawal symptoms. Evidence of either withdrawal symptoms or **tolerance**, which involves a progressive decrease in the effectiveness of the substance, indicates that physiological dependence has developed.

The DSM-5-TR incorporates all of these concepts into the criteria for diagnosing a substance-use disorder. The DSM-5-TR differentiates substance-use disorders based on the substance used, such as alcohol-use disorder, cannabis-use disorder, or hallucinogen-use disorder. A substance-use disorder is considered mild when two to three of the designated symptoms are present and moderate if there are four to five symptoms. The presence of six or more symptoms indicates a severe substance-use disorder (refer to Table 11.1).

The DSM-5-TR also outlines the specific effects of intoxication and withdrawal associated with different substances. **Intoxication** refers to the distinct and recognizable pattern of problematic behavioral or psychological changes associated with the use or abuse of a substance. For example, some of the DSM-5-TR criteria for alcohol intoxication (slurred speech, unsteady gait, inappropriate sexual or aggressive behavior, etc.) differ from descriptors of cannabis intoxication (increased appetite, euphoria, sensation of slowed time, social withdrawal, etc.). Similarly, the withdrawal symptoms differ: Alcohol withdrawal produces agitation, sweating, insomnia, hand tremor, and hallucinations, whereas cannabis withdrawal can result in irritability, anger, or aggression; decreased appetite; or depressed mood. As you might imagine, many emergency department visits are the result of intoxication or withdrawal from various substances.

Table 11.1 DSM-5-TR Criteria for a Substance-Use Disorder

According to the DSM-5-TR, a substance-use disorder may be an appropriate diagnosis when *at least two* of the following characteristics occur within a 12-month period and cause significant impairment or distress:

- the quantity of the substance used or the amount of time spent using is often greater than intended;
- efforts to control use of the substance are unsuccessful due to a persistent desire for the substance;
- considerable time is spent using the substance, recovering from its effects, or attempting to obtain the substance;
- a strong desire, craving, or urge to use the substance is present;
- substance use interferes with major role obligations at work, school, or home;
- use of the substance continues despite harmful social or interpersonal effects caused or made worse by substance use;
- participation in social, work, or leisure activities is given up or reduced due to substance use;
- substance use occurs in situations where substance use may be physically hazardous;
- continued substance use occurs despite knowledge that the substance is causing physical or psychological problems or making these problems worse;
- tolerance for the substance develops, including a need for increasing quantities of the substance to achieve intoxication or desired effects or a noticeable decrease in effects when using the same amount of the substance;
- after heavy or sustained use of a substance, reduction in or abstinence from the substance results in withdrawal symptoms or precipitates resumption of use of the substance or similar substances to relieve or avoid withdrawal symptoms.

Adapted from APA, 2022

Substance use may cause depression, anxiety, sleep difficulties, or psychotic disorders in individuals who have never previously experienced such symptoms, as occurred with Jay in the introductory vignette. For example, users of marijuana may develop a cannabis-induced psychotic disorder, cannabis-induced sleep disorder, or cannabis-induced anxiety disorder. These substance/medication-induced disorders develop within 1 month of using the substance and involve a constellation of symptoms that are unique to each substance.

In summary, based on their chemical makeup, different substances produce different psychological and physical effects along with different symptoms of intoxication and withdrawal, as well as increased susceptibility to certain mental disorders. We now move on to discuss the various substances that can lead to the development of a substance-use disorder.

11-2 Substances Associated with Abuse

Substances that are abused include prescription medications used to treat anxiety, insomnia, or pain; legal substances such as alcohol, caffeine, tobacco, and household chemicals; and illegal substances such as cocaine and heroin. Most of the substances discussed in this chapter can create significant physical, social, and psychological problems. Table 11.2 lists abused substances and their effects, as well as their addictive potential.

Table 11.2 Commonly Abused Substances

Substance	Short-Term Effects[a]	Addictive Potential
Central Nervous System Depressants		
Alcohol	Relaxation, impaired judgment	High
Opioids	Pain relief, sedation, drowsiness	High
Sedatives, hypnotics, anxiolytics	Sedation, drowsiness, reduced anxiety, impaired judgment	Moderate to high
Central Nervous System Stimulants		
Caffeine	Energy, enhanced attention	Moderate
Amphetamines	Energy, euphoria, enhanced attention	High
Cocaine	Energy, euphoria	High
Hallucinogens		
LSD, psilocybin, mescaline, salvia	Altered perceptions, sensory distortions	Low
Dissociative Anesthetics		
Phencyclidine (PCP)	Confusion, sensory distortions, feelings of detachment	Moderate
Ketamine, methoxetamine (MXE)	Confusion, sensory distortions, feelings of detachment	Moderate
Dextromethorphan (DXM)	Confusion, sensory distortions, feelings of detachment	Moderate
Substances with Multiple Effects		
Nicotine	Energy, relaxation	High
Cannabis	Relaxation, euphoria, sensory distortions	Moderate
Inhalants	Disorientation	Variable
Ecstasy (MDMA)	Energy, sensory distortions, feelings of connection	Moderate
Gamma hydroxybutyrate (GHB)	Relaxation, euphoria, enhanced strength	High

[a]Specific effects depend on the quantity used, the extent of previous use, and other substances concurrently ingested, as well as on the experiences, expectancies, and personality of the person using the substance.

Depressants

Depressants cause the central nervous system to slow down. Individuals taking depressants may feel relaxed and sociable due to lowered interpersonal inhibitions. Let's begin by examining the most widely used depressant—alcohol.

Alcohol

Case Study   Jim, a married father of two teenage sons, recently lost his job, in large part due to his heavy drinking. Jim began drinking in high school, hoping it would help him feel less anxious in social situations; at first, he disliked the taste of alcohol but forced himself to continue drinking. Over the next several years, Jim acquired the ability to consume large amounts of alcohol and was proud of his drinking capacity. He remained anxious about social gatherings, but after a few drinks he became the "life of the party." His heavy drinking continued throughout college.

Soon after Jim married and began his career, he began drinking throughout the week, claiming drinking was the only way he could relax. He attributed his increased drinking to pressures at work and a desire to feel comfortable in social situations. Despite frequent arguments with his wife regarding his alcohol use, the loss of his job because he was drinking at work, and a physician's warning that alcohol was causing liver damage, Jim could not control his alcohol consumption.

Jim's problem drinking is typical of many people who develop an alcohol-use disorder. Although he initially found the taste of alcohol unpleasant, he continued drinking. Heavy drinking served a purpose: He believed it helped him fit in socially and reduced his anxiety in work and social situations. His preoccupation with alcohol and deterioration in social and occupational functioning are also characteristic of problem drinkers. Jim continued to drink despite obvious negative consequences, including arguments with family members, the loss of his job, and health problems. Like many with an alcohol-use disorder, Jim claimed that he did not have a serious problem with drinking. Do you think things would have turned out differently if Jim had sought professional help for his anxiety rather than trying to self-medicate with alcohol?

We begin our discussion of alcohol by clarifying terminology. One drink is defined as 12 ounces of beer, 5 ounces of wine, or 1.5 ounces of hard liquor. **Moderate drinking** refers to lower-risk patterns of drinking, generally no more than one drink for women or two drinks for men. **Heavy drinking** involves the consumption of more than two drinks per day or 14 drinks per week for men and more than one drink per day or 7 drinks per week for women. **Binge drinking** is episodic drinking involving five or more drinks on a single occasion for men and four or more drinks for women. It should be noted that researchers have consistently found that drinkers often underestimate the quantity of alcohol that they are consuming, especially once they have started drinking (Kirouac et al., 2019).

A 2022 SAMHSA survey of individuals age 12 and older suggests that although 52 percent of this group consumed at least one alcoholic drink in the previous month, the vast majority of adolescents and adults (about 80 percent) do not drink excessively—they either abstain or drink in moderation. However, 45 percent of those who do consume alcohol engage

Did You Know?

Among adults who engage in binge drinking, 25 percent report doing so weekly, and 25 percent consumed at least eight drinks during a binge drinking episode.
Source: Bohm et al., 2021

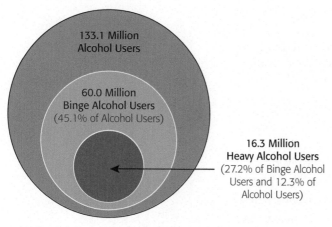

Note: Binge Alcohol Use is defined as drinking five or more drinks (for men) or four or more drinks (for women) on the same occasion on at least 1 day in the past 30 days. Heavy Alcohol Use is defined as binge drinking on the same occasion on 5 or more days in the past 30 days; all heavy alcohol users are also binge alcohol users.

Figure 11.4

Current, Binge, and Heavy Alcohol Use Among People Age 12 or Older in 2021

In 2021, among the estimated 133 million U.S. Americans age 12 or older who consumed alcohol in the previous month, about 45 percent engaged in binge drinking, and 27 percent of the binge drinkers reported that their heavy alcohol use included at least five binge-drinking episodes during the month.

Source: SAMHSA, 2022

in binge drinking, including 12.3 percent who engage in "heavy alcohol use," which is defined by SAMHSA as binge drinking 5 or more days per month (refer to Figure 11.4). In other words, about one in five U.S. Americans age 12 and older engage in binge drinking (SAMHSA, 2022).

Men and boys are more likely to consume alcohol and participate in binge and heavy drinking compared to women and girls. However, problematic drinking among young women is increasing. Ethnic group data reveal that Asian Americans have the lowest levels of excessive drinking (SAMHSA, 2022). In the past, Black students have consistently demonstrated the lowest rates of drug and alcohol use compared to White and Latinx students. However, data from 2022 reveal a significant reversal, with Black teens reporting higher use of alcohol and many other drugs compared to other racial groups (Miech et al., 2023).

Let's focus on statistics for the college-age population. Binge drinking and heavy drinking are especially problematic among young adults (ages 18 to 25), with 29.2 percent of those in this age group engaging in binge drinking, including 7.1 percent who binge drink at least 5 days per month (SAMHSA, 2022). College students also engage in other unsafe drinking practices such as skipping meals to compensate for high-caloric binge drinking or to deliberately get drunk faster, a practice that not only hastens intoxication but also increases the risk of dehydration, blackouts, seizures, and cardiac arrest (Piazza-Gardner & Barry, 2013).

How does alcohol affect the body? Once swallowed, alcohol is quickly absorbed into the bloodstream and begins to depress central nervous system functioning. When the blood alcohol level, or alcohol content in the bloodstream, is about 0.1 percent—for many, the equivalent of drinking 3 ounces of whiskey or three glasses of beer—muscular coordination and judgment are impaired. Higher levels of blood alcohol, 0.3 percent in some individuals, can result in a loss of consciousness or even death (refer to Figure 11.5). Alcohol lowers inhibitions, impairs judgment, and can increase aggression and impulsivity. These psychological effects may partially explain why alcohol is frequently associated with suicidal behavior (Conner & Bagge, 2019).

Some people become physiologically dependent on alcohol. That is, if they stop drinking, alcohol withdrawal symptoms (e.g., headache, fatigue, sweating, body tremors, and mood changes) develop. The toxicity and central nervous system damage associated with chronic alcohol abuse can lead to extreme withdrawal symptoms, including a life-threatening condition called **delirium tremens**, which begins with profound anxiety, agitation, and confusion followed by seizures, disorientation, hallucinations, or extreme lethargy (Long et al., 2017).

Our bodies produce "cleanup" enzymes, including aldehyde dehydrogenase (ALDH), to counteract toxins that build up as our bodies metabolize alcohol. Production of ALDH is affected by gender (men, especially younger men, produce more than women) and genetic makeup (some people, especially people with Asian or African ancestry, produce less ALDH). Recently ingested food, beverages, and medications also affect how we metabolize alcohol. For instance, carbonated beverages and aspirin accelerate alcohol absorption and reduce the efficiency of the ALDH cleanup, whereas food slows absorption, giving the enzymes more time to work. Intoxication occurs more rapidly in those who have a low body weight or consume alcohol rapidly. Large amounts of alcohol consumed quickly can result in impaired breathing, coma, and death; this condition, known as **alcohol poisoning**, can be exacerbated by the vomiting and dehydration that occur as the body attempts to rid itself of excess alcohol (National Institute on Alcohol and Alcoholism, 2023).

Now, let's talk about people who have an alcohol-use disorder (refer to Table 11.1 and recall that impaired functioning and two of the symptoms may reflect an alcohol-use disorder). The lifetime prevalence of alcohol-use disorder in the U.S. adult population is 18 percent. Although men are twice as likely to develop this disorder, **alcoholism** in women progresses more rapidly (Agabio et al., 2017).

There are multiple physiological consequences associated with excessive alcohol use. Tolerance to alcohol develops rapidly, so drinkers who want to feel the effects of alcohol often increase their intake. Unfortunately, tolerance does not decrease the toxicity of alcohol, so heavy drinkers progressively expose their brains and bodies to greater physiological risk. Neurological effects include impaired motor skills, reduced reasoning and judgment, memory deficits, distractibility, and reduced motivation. Additionally, alcohol affects the liver and the entire cardiovascular system; for this reason, excessive alcohol use increases the risk of heart attack, heart arrhythmias, and congestive heart failure (Whitman et al., 2017). People with alcoholism who continue to drink also demonstrate declines in neurological functioning. Although sustained **abstinence** can lead to cognitive improvement, those who were heavy drinkers often demonstrate ongoing intellectual impairment (Hammoud & Jimenez-Shahed, 2019).

In stark contrast to the stereotype of someone who is homeless and living on the streets due to alcohol addiction, many people with an alcohol-use disorder are able to function without obvious disruption to their life—many of these individuals with so-called *high-functioning alcoholism* work, raise families, and maintain social relationships. Although aware of the negative physical and social consequences of their drinking, and distressed over their inability to control their alcohol intake, they often deny they have a problem with alcohol or hide their drinking. It is common for individuals with alcohol-use disorder to alternate between periods of excessive drinking and sobriety, often in an attempt to prove to themselves or their families that they can abstain (Witkiewitz et al., 2019).

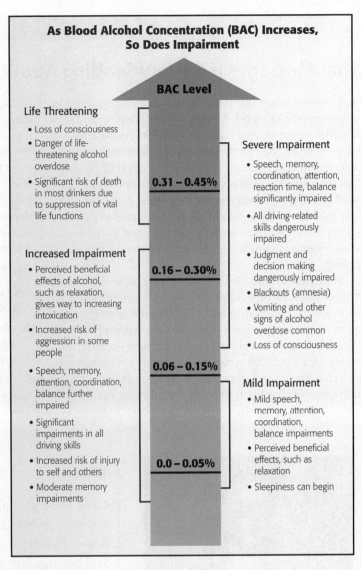

As Blood Alcohol Concentration (BAC) Increases, So Does Impairment

BAC Level

Life Threatening
- Loss of consciousness
- Danger of life-threatening alcohol overdose
- Significant risk of death in most drinkers due to suppression of vital life functions

0.31 – 0.45%

Increased Impairment
- Perceived beneficial effects of alcohol, such as relaxation, gives way to increasing intoxication
- Increased risk of aggression in some people
- Speech, memory, attention, coordination, balance further impaired
- Significant impairments in all driving skills
- Increased risk of injury to self and others
- Moderate memory impairments

0.16 – 0.30%

0.06 – 0.15%

Severe Impairment
- Speech, memory, coordination, attention, reaction time, balance significantly impaired
- All driving-related skills dangerously impaired
- Judgment and decision making dangerously impaired
- Blackouts (amnesia)
- Vomiting and other signs of alcohol overdose common
- Loss of consciousness

Mild Impairment
- Mild speech, memory, attention, coordination, balance impairments
- Perceived beneficial effects, such as relaxation
- Sleepiness can begin

0.0 – 0.05%

Figure 11.5

Alcohol Effects on Blood Alcohol Concentration
Excessive drinking can result in a variety of consequences, including motor incoordination, impaired judgment, and even death.

Source: National Institute on Alcohol and Alcoholism, 2023

Did You Know?

In the United States, approximately one alcohol-related car fatality occurs every 50 minutes. In 2016, of the drivers responsible for a fatal crash, 62 percent had blood alcohol levels above the legal limit.

Source: National Highway Traffic Safety Administration, 2017

What Messages Is Society Sending About Alcohol Use?

What messages are we sending regarding alcohol use in contemporary society? Alcohol advertising and media glamorization of alcohol is pervasive. The myth persists that "everyone drinks," despite the fact that the majority of American adults consume alcohol only occasionally or not at all. Although efforts to prevent alcohol abuse stress the personal and societal risk of underage drinking and excessive alcohol consumption, these messages receive only minimal attention. Should we be making more effort to balance marketing and social media messages with information regarding the potential dangers of alcohol?

Professionals focused on addiction prevention assert that we need to find innovative ways to nullify societal messages that normalize and even glamorize alcohol use and to heighten awareness of risk factors, especially among those who are most vulnerable to addiction—adolescents and young adults. This is particularly important because we know that alcohol and other substances exert powerful effects on the developing brain through the mid-20s. Further, the college years are a very high-risk period for beginning the addiction process because students who participate in underage alcohol use often drink heavily (SAMHSA, 2022). Given the data on heavy drinking among college students, there is a need for new strategies for educating students about alcohol and the addiction process. Although alcohol-abuse prevention campaigns are attempting to reduce the frequency of drinking, it will be difficult to reduce the prevalence of alcohol abuse as long as our society at large tolerates binge drinking and underage alcohol consumption.

For Further Consideration

1. In what ways does the college environment influence decisions to participate in heavy or underage drinking?

2. What issues associated with alcohol use and abuse have the most relevance for college students, and how can these be incorporated into prevention messages?

3. What kinds of prevention efforts do you think would be the most effective on your college campus?

Opioids

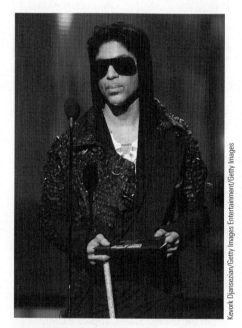

Kevork Djansezian/Getty Images Entertainment/Getty Images

The Sudden Loss of a Music Legend

Fans across the world were dismayed at the news of the overdose death of legendary singer Prince, who is pictured here performing at the 55th Annual Grammy Awards Ceremony several years before his demise.

Case Study   Prince, the legendary singer and performer, was living with hip pain associated with a lifetime of energetic and physically demanding stage performances. In April 2016, several months before his 58th birthday, Prince was found unresponsive on the floor of an elevator at Paisley Park, his estate in Minnesota. The coroner ruled that he died from fentanyl toxicity after toxicology reports revealed high amounts of fentanyl in his system. Prince had reportedly developed an opioid addiction following hip surgery in 2010 (Browne, 2018).

Opioids (sometimes called narcotics) are typically prescribed for the management of pain. Heroin and opium, both derived from the opium plant, are the best-known illicit opioids. All opioids (including the medications morphine, codeine, oxycodone, and fentanyl) are highly addictive and require careful medical management. Prescriptions for opioids rose dramatically beginning in the late 1990s when pharmaceutical industry representatives failed to acknowledge their high potential for addiction and convinced prescribers that opioids were a safe option for the management of pain. A pattern of liberal prescribing, combined with the highly addictive nature of these medications, resulted in their widespread misuse and the resultant deaths and addiction that have come to be known as the opioid epidemic. Of additional concern is the fact that over half of all opioid prescriptions are written for individuals who have a concurrent mood or anxiety disorder, a group that is particularly vulnerable to self-medicating (Davis et al., 2017).

Prescription opioids are considered a **gateway drug**—a substance that leads to the use of more dangerous drugs. Many people who abuse opioids begin their habit with prescribed medication, eventually buying prescription drugs illegally or trying less expensive and even more lethal opioids—heroin or fentanyl (Palamar & Shearston, 2018). This may have been what occurred with Prince and his eventual use of a powerful opioid, fentanyl, for pain management. Those who misuse prescription opioids often rationalize their use because the substances are prescription medications. Given the increase in opioid-use disorders since physicians were first allowed to prescribe opioids for pain management in patients without cancer, many physicians now question whether the benefits of prescribing opioids outweigh the addictive risks.

Opioids produce both euphoria and drowsiness. Tolerance builds quickly, resulting in dependency and a need for increased doses to achieve desired effects. Opioid withdrawal symptoms (including restlessness, muscle pain, insomnia, and cold flashes) are often severe. Lethargy, fatigue, anxiety, and disturbed sleep may persist for months, and drug craving can persist for years. Unfortunately, deaths from accidental opioid overdose are common and often involve concurrent use of alcohol and/or other drugs.

Some U.S. states are disproportionately affected by the opioid crisis and drug overdose deaths (Figure 11.6). Prior to the COVID pandemic, prescription opioid misuse was declining. Even so, in 2018, an average of 41 people died each day in the United States from overdoses involving prescription opioids. Despite the increasing community use of the emergency opioid antidote naloxone (administered by an injection or nasal spray to rapidly reverse an opioid overdose), opioids are still involved in over two thirds of all drug overdose fatalities (Wilson et al., 2020).

Although strengthened regulations and guidelines have reduced opioid prescribing, the misuse of illegally obtained prescription opioids and illicitly manufactured opioids (especially fentanyl pills and heroin laced with fentanyl) has become an increasing concern. Fentanyl, the highly lethal painkiller that killed Prince, is 50 to 100 times more powerful than morphine and highly addictive. Unfortunately, these dangerous synthetic opioids have become increasingly popular on the black market and are purchased by users looking for a substance that produces a fast-acting, euphoric high. In many cases, people found with fentanyl in their system had no idea that their street drugs had been laced with this addictive substance. Even a small dose of fentanyl can result in almost immediate death; the decline in prescription opioid–related fatalities seen prior to the COVID pandemic has been replaced by a postpandemic surge in deaths due to synthetic opioids such as fentanyl (Baumgartner & Radley, 2023). Even more alarming is the emergence of nitazenes (nicknamed Frankenstein opioids), a powerful class of novel synthetic opioids which are 1000 times more potent than morphine. In emergency room visits, those who overdosed on this drug class were more likely to have cardiac arrest, require intubation, or die.

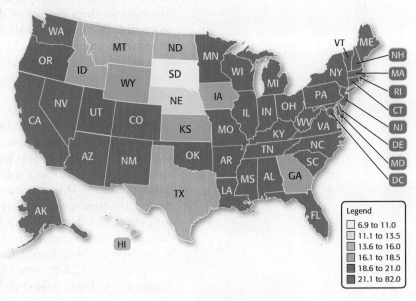

Legend
- 6.9 to 11.0
- 11.1 to 13.5
- 13.6 to 16.0
- 16.1 to 18.5
- 18.6 to 21.0
- 21.1 to 82.0

Figure 11.6

Rates of Drug Overdose Deaths by State per 100,000 Population in 2020

This map illustrates how the rate of drug overdose deaths per 100,000 population varies significantly between the states, a reflection of regional differences in opioid misuse. Of the 91,799 drug overdose deaths that occurred in the United States in 2020, over 70 percent involved an opioid.

Source: CDC, 2023

Two or more doses of naloxone are often needed to reverse a nitazene overdose (Amaducci et al., 2023).

Sedatives, Hypnotics, and Anxiolytics

Sedatives, including hypnotics (sleeping pills) and anxiolytics (antianxiety medications), have calming effects and are prescribed to reduce muscle tension, insomnia, agitation, and anxiety. **Hypnotics** induce sleep and combat insomnia. **Anxiolytics** are used to treat anxiety; they are sometimes referred to as minor tranquilizers, so named to distinguish them from the major tranquilizing medications used with psychotic disorders. The drug classes of *barbiturates*, such as Seconal and phenobarbital, and *benzodiazepines*, such as Valium, Ativan, and Xanax, provide rapid anxiety-reducing effects when used in moderate doses; higher doses are prescribed to produce hypnotic, or sleep-inducing, effects.

Sedative, hypnotic, or anxiolytic substance-use disorder can develop if someone takes high prescription doses, or deliberately misuses or illegally obtains these medications. Individuals who have difficulty dealing with stress or who experience anxiety or insomnia are particularly prone to overusing and becoming dependent on sedatives. Additionally, some use sedatives recreationally or to counteract cocaine withdrawal symptoms (Sola et al., 2010). Sedatives are quite dangerous when misused. Even in low doses, they cause drowsiness, impaired judgment, and diminished motor skills. As with opioids, systems are in place to monitor their legal use in an attempt to reduce the risk of drug dependence; however, misuse is difficult to control due to their availability via illegal drug markets. Excessive use of sedatives can lead to accidental overdose and death. Combining alcohol with sedatives can be especially dangerous because alcohol compounds their depressant effects, slowing breathing and increasing the risk of coma or death.

There is high potential for tolerance and physiological dependence with all sedatives; when they are discontinued, sedative withdrawal can produce insomnia, nervousness, headache, and drowsiness. Due to concerns regarding addictive potential and lethality with overdose, many medical practitioners avoid prescribing sedatives to treat anxiety, and instead prescribe antidepressants. This stance is supported by data from a 35,000-participant national survey revealing that individuals prescribed sedatives for anxiety are twice as likely to develop a sedative-use disorder (Fenton et al., 2010). Young adults are the most likely group to misuse sedatives; in one comprehensive survey, among those who took prescription sedatives in the previous year, 42.8 percent of those ages 18 to 25 reported that they had engaged in sedative misuse (Schepis et al., 2018).

Stimulants

Stimulants, substances that speed up central nervous system activity, are used for a variety of reasons: to produce feelings of euphoria and well-being, improve mental and physical performance, reduce appetite, and prevent sleep. Unwanted physiological effects include heart arrhythmias, dizziness, tremors, and sweating. Psychological side effects can include anxiety, restlessness, agitation, hostility, and paranoia. Binge use of illicit stimulants is common, with sequential high doses leading to exhaustion and acute psychotic symptoms. Tolerance to the stimulant effects develops rapidly, leading to increased use. Stimulant withdrawal can produce depression, anxiety, and extreme fatigue. Our discussion begins with a commonly used mild stimulant, caffeine.

Caffeine

Case Study   I use energy drinks to stay awake while I study at night. I am noticing that I need more and more energy drinks to stay awake and keep alert. It's getting to the point where I need over four or five cans to get through a night, when normally it would take me only one can.

Caffeine is a stimulant found in coffee, chocolate, tea, and soft drinks. It is the most widely consumed psychoactive substance in the world, prized by almost every culture for increasing attentiveness. As seen in the case example, we often develop tolerance to caffeine and need more to produce the desired effect. Caffeine intoxication can produce symptoms such as restlessness, nervousness, insomnia, and cardiac arrhythmia. Caffeine withdrawal symptoms include headache, fatigue, irritability, and difficulty with concentration. The DSM-5-TR contains a proposed diagnostic category of caffeine-use disorder for those who display impairment due to caffeine addiction (APA, 2022).

About 90 percent of adults in North America use caffeine every day. Caffeine is usually consumed in moderate doses (a cup of tea has 40 to 60 mg, coffee has 70 to 175 mg, and cola has 30 to 50 mg), but caffeine intake has increased due to the widespread marketing and consumption of energy drinks. Energy beverages, now a multibillion-dollar industry, typically have 70 to 240 mg of caffeine in addition to sweeteners and energy-boosting additives (National Institutes of Health [NIH], 2018). Frequent consumption of energy drinks can produce caffeine intoxication and caffeine withdrawal symptoms or even more serious health consequences if combined with alcohol or illicit drugs (De Sanctis et al., 2017). The habitual use of energy drinks among adolescents is a particular concern because many habitual users tend to minimize the potential danger of using other substances. Further, high schoolers who frequently consume energy drinks are significantly more likely to initiate marijuana use compared to peers who consume energy drinks infrequently or not at all (Leal & Jackson, 2019).

Amphetamines

Amphetamines, also known as "uppers," significantly speed up central nervous system activity. Some amphetamines, such as Ritalin, Adderall, and Dexedrine, which are prescribed to treat attention and sleep disorders, are increasingly used illicitly, particularly by young adults; an estimated 1.3 percent of the adolescent and adult population have misused these medications (SAMHSA, 2022). Amphetamines have high addictive potential, particularly when taken intravenously or nasally ("snorting"), or in high doses. Although amphetamines can induce feelings of euphoria and confidence, negative effects such as agitation, psychosis, and assaultive or suicidal behaviors also occur. Abstinence produces psychological and physical discomfort, which often leads to cravings and a return to drug use (May et al., 2020).

Methamphetamine ("meth"), a particularly dangerous amphetamine that is eaten, snorted,

Methamphetamine Effects

This pair of mug shots is part of the Faces of Meth project started when justice officials noticed the significant physical decline among methamphetamine users who were arrested more than once. As demonstrated here, many of the second (later) mug shots clearly demonstrate the gauntness and facial lesions associated with ongoing methamphetamine use.

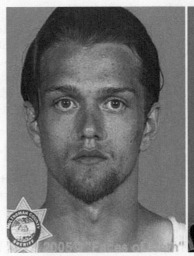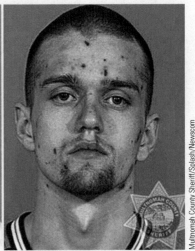

Multnomah County Sheriff/Splash/Newscom

injected, or heated and smoked in rock "crystal" form, is used by 0.9 percent of the U.S. adolescent and adult population (SAMHSA, 2022). Popular due to its low cost and rapid euphoric effects, methamphetamine has serious health consequences, including permanent damage to the heart, lungs, and immune system. In addition to the profound dental and aging effects of methamphetamine, significant psychological changes also occur, including psychosis, depression, suicide, and violent behavior. As with the other stimulants, methamphetamine has high potential for abuse and addiction (Papageorgiou et al., 2019).

Cocaine

Case Study A 49-year-old woman previously diagnosed with congestive heart failure was admitted to the hospital with a severe cough and labored breathing. She reported that she had never smoked cigarettes; consumed alcohol; or used drugs other than cocaine, which she had been smoking for 30 years. Due to her severe emphysema and continued cocaine use, she was not a candidate for heart transplantation. She died from respiratory failure and cardiac arrest (Vahid & Marik, 2007).

Cocaine, a stimulant extracted from the coca plant, induces feelings of energy and euphoria. Crack is a potent form of cocaine produced by heating cocaine with other substances ("freebasing"); it is sold in small, solid pieces ("rocks") and is typically smoked. Crack produces immediate but short-lived effects. Cocaine has a high potential for addiction, sometimes after only a short period of use. In 2021, there were an estimated 4.8 million people who used cocaine in the United States (1.7 percent of the population), with about 1.4 million demonstrating a cocaine-use disorder (SAMHSA, 2022).

Due to cocaine's intense effects, cocaine withdrawal causes lethargy and depression; those who are experiencing withdrawal often take multiple doses in rapid succession trying to re-create the high. The constant desire for cocaine coupled with the high monetary cost and need for increased doses to achieve a high can cause those who are addicted to resort to crime to feed their habit. Because cocaine stimulates the sympathetic nervous system, side effects that include irregular heartbeat, heart attack, stroke, and death may occur. Individuals who use cocaine sometimes experience acute psychiatric symptoms such as delusions, paranoia, and hallucinations; more chronic difficulties such as anxiety, depression, sexual dysfunction, and sleep disturbance also occur. Similar to the woman in the case example, regular users of cocaine often have a shortened life span (Sanvisens et al., 2021).

Hallucinogens

Hallucinogens are substances that can produce vivid sensory experiences, including hallucinations. Traditional hallucinogens are derived from natural sources: lysergic acid diethylamide (LSD) from a grain fungus, psilocybin from mushrooms, mescaline from the peyote cactus, and salvia from an herb in

Cocaine Addiction from Mother to Child

Women who use drugs during pregnancy sometimes give birth to babies who are underweight, addicted to drugs, and at risk for serious developmental problems. Pictured here is a newborn baby being monitored as they go through cocaine withdrawal symptoms.

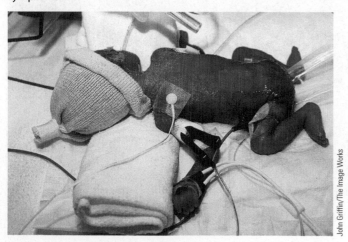

John Griffin/The Image Works

Stimulants and Performance Enhancement: A New Source of Addiction?

The nonmedical use of prescription medications is on the rise, including illicit use of stimulant medications by high school and college students as well as young professionals who want to enhance their functioning and outperform the competition. This concern is supported by the fact that 18- to 25-year-olds have the highest rate of emergency department visits resulting from nonmedical use of prescription stimulants. As is true with marijuana and alcohol use, many college students overestimate the true prevalence of illicit stimulant use, an inaccurate perception that increases the likelihood of misuse (Fossos-Wong et al., 2022). Heightening the concern about stimulant diversion and misuse on college campuses is the finding that many of these same students also report other substance use. These concerns have prompted some researchers to explore the utility of on-campus health campaigns highlighting the health and legal risks associated with the diversion and misuse of prescription stimulants (Su et al., 2020).

In contrast to the minority of college students who engage in stimulant misuse, a majority of university students indicate that they have no intention of using stimulants to avoid sleep or enhance performance; this decision involves both health risks and ethical considerations (Sattler et al., 2013). Some physicians are also speaking out against stimulant use, pointing out their addictive potential and possible effects on the developing brain.

For Further Consideration

1. What do you think are the biggest concerns arising from the illicit use of prescription medications to enhance performance?

2. Do you believe an educational campaign regarding stimulant misuse is needed at your school?

the mint family. Natural hallucinogens have been used in cultural ceremonies and religious rites for thousands of years. Some synthetic drugs (such as PCP, ketamine, and Ecstasy) have hallucinogenic effects combined with other properties (e.g., stimulant or tranquilizing effects) and are discussed later in the chapter. Some hallucinogens appear to be effective in reducing symptoms in disorders such as major depressive disorder, although researchers are carefully monitoring potential side effects from the use of these substances (Goodwin et al., 2022). Approximately 7.4 million people, about 2.6 percent of the U.S. adolescent and adult population, used hallucinogens in 2022 (SAMHSA, 2022). A small percentage of those who use hallucinogens develop *hallucinogen persisting perception disorder*, in which they experience distressing recurrence of hallucinations or other sensations weeks or even years after drug intake (Ford et al., 2022).

The effects and emotional reactions from hallucinogen use can vary significantly, even for the same person. The altered state that hallucinogens produce is sometimes pleasant but can be an extremely traumatic experience. "Good trips" are associated with sharpened visual and auditory perception, heightened sensation, and perceptions of profound insight. "Bad trips" can produce severe depression, disorientation, delusions, and sensory distortions that result in fear and panic. Hallucinogens are not addictive and therefore do not cause compulsive drug-seeking behavior. However, tolerance does develop, so users frequently need larger quantities to re-create the initial effects of the drug (Olsen, 2022). Large doses are not typically fatal, although there are reports of people who have unwittingly ended their lives while under the influence of hallucinogens.

Dissociative Anesthetics

Phencyclidine (known as PCP) and ketamine (sometimes referred to as Special K), both highly dangerous and potentially addictive substances, are classified as **dissociative anesthetics**; developed for use as anesthetics

Did You Know?

Oregon became the first state to decriminalize possession of small amounts of hallucinogenic drugs and hard drugs such as cocaine, heroin, and methamphetamine. Instead of being considered a criminal act, offenders will be fined $100, a penalty that will be waived if they agree to undergo substance abuse assessment
Source: Loew & Barreda, 2020

in veterinary medicine, they produce a dreamlike detachment in humans. PCP and ketamine are very similar chemically, and they have the potential to produce a *phencyclidine-use disorder*. They have dissociative, stimulant, depressant, amnesic, and hallucinogenic properties. PCP and ketamine are among the most dangerous of the so-called *club drugs*, a term that comes from the popular use of certain drugs at dance clubs. These drugs cause disconnection, perceptual distortion, euphoria, and confusion, as well as delusions, hostility, and violent psychotic behavior, as seen in the case of Jay discussed at the beginning of the chapter. Additionally, frequent users demonstrate cognitive and memory deficits as well as depressive, dissociative, and delusional symptoms; delusions can persist even after cessation of use (Bertron et al., 2018).

Dextromethorphan (DXM), an active ingredient in many over-the-counter cold medications and cough suppressants, is another frequently misused dissociative anesthetic. Despite industry efforts to control misuse of these products, "robotripping" still occurs as adolescents and young adults use cough and cold medicines to get high (Stanciu et al., 2016). Effects of DXM abuse can include disorientation, confusion, agitation, paranoia, and psychosis. The large quantities consumed by those who misuse DXM can result in **hyperthermia** (elevated body temperature), high blood pressure, and heart arrhythmia; as with PCP and ketamine, health consequences are intensified when DXM is combined with alcohol or other drugs. A practice of concern to medical personnel and drug enforcement officials is the ingestion of "lean" or "sizzurp," which is a dangerous mixture comprised of a potent cough syrup, carbonated soda, and hard candy (Palamar, 2019).

Substances with Mixed Chemical Properties

A number of abused substances have varied effects on the brain and central nervous system. We begin by briefly discussing nicotine, an addictive drug with both depressant and stimulant features. We then discuss cannabis; inhalants; and designer drugs, including Ecstasy, as well as the unique dangers involved when substances are combined.

Nicotine

Nicotine, a drug most commonly associated with cigarette smoking, is highly addictive and can result in a tobacco-use disorder. For most people, nicotine acts as both a stimulant and a sedative. Almost 54.7 million adults and adolescents (22 percent of the population) use tobacco products, primarily cigarettes. Many current tobacco users find it extremely difficult to quit due to the strength of their nicotine addiction (SAMHSA, 2022).

Nicotine releases both adrenaline and dopamine, which deliver a burst of energy and feelings of pleasure, respectively. A smoker's first cigarette of the day produces the greatest stimulant effect; as the day progresses, euphoric effects decrease (Benowitz, 2010). As tolerance develops, more nicotine is needed to experience energy, pleasure, and relaxation. Those who attempt to stop smoking often go through tobacco withdrawal symptoms, which include difficulty concentrating, restlessness, anxiety, depressed mood, and irritability. Globally, more than 8 million people die each year due to tobacco use. It is considered the single most preventable cause of premature death (World Health Organization [WHO], 2023).

Smoking's Effects on the Lungs

A New York City exhibit of real, whole human body specimens provides an actual view of the healthy lungs and heart of a nonsmoker versus the blackened lungs and heart of a smoker. The human body specimens are preserved through a revolutionary technique called polymer preservation. All bodies are from people who died of natural causes.

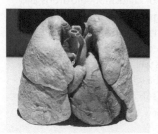 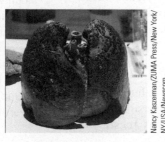

Nancy Kaszerman/ZUMA Press/New York/ NY/USA/Newscom

Vaping, first introduced to the U.S. market almost two decades ago, has gained popularity among nonsmokers and those trying to quit smoking. Vaping involves inhaling the aerosols produced by a heated liquid contained in battery-powered devices such as e-cigarettes, "mods," e-hookahs, Juuls, and e-pens. The liquid is often infused with flavors, and sometimes with nicotine or cannabis oil. Proponents of e-cigarettes argue that they provide smokers with an alternative, less-harmful source of nicotine, whereas others express concern because vaping has introduced many nonsmokers to the addictive effects of nicotine. The rate of experimentation and use of vaping devices has been increasing rapidly, particularly among adolescents; in a Monitoring the Future survey, about 27 percent of 12th graders reported vaping in the previous month (Miech et al., 2023).

In the spring of 2019, vaping became the topic of much discussion when medical professionals began reporting cases of severe lung injury and death among users of vaping devices, concluding that e-cigarette or vaping use-associated lung injury (EVALI) was likely the result of one or more additives used in vaping products. Health advocates, concerned about EVALI and other vaping-related health issues, are calling for effective testing and regulation of vaping products (Banks et al., 2023).

Cannabis

Cannabis is the botanical name for a plant that contains a chemical (delta-9-tetrahydrocannabinol, referred to as THC) that can produce stimulant, depressant, and hallucinogenic effects. Marijuana, a well-known THC product, is derived from the leaves and flowering top of the cannabis plant, whereas hashish, which contains particularly high levels of THC, comes from the pressed resin of the plant. Growing conditions influence THC content, as do the plant's chemical and medicinal properties. Cannabis produces feelings of euphoria, tranquility, and passivity combined with mild perceptual and sensory distortions but can also increase anxiety and depression. Some individuals develop chronic psychotic symptoms or schizophrenia triggered by cannabis, especially when use occurs at a young age (West & Sharif, 2023). Use of cannabis is also associated with depressive disorders. However, there may be a bidirectional relationship in that cannabis users may be more likely to develop depression and depression may lead to the use of cannabis (Langlois et al., 2021).

Marijuana is the most commonly used illicit drug worldwide (United Nations Office on Drugs and Crime, 2020). In the United States, an estimated 52.5 million adults and adolescents use marijuana, with approximately 2.6 million initiating marijuana use in 2022 (refer to Figure 11.7). Marijuana consumption is especially widespread among adolescents and young adults, in part due to the significant increase in daily marijuana use among those ages 18 to 25, particularly women (SAMHSA, 2022). The annual Monitoring the Future survey of high school students in 2022 revealed that 19.5 percent of 10th graders and 30.7 percent of 12th graders used marijuana in the previous year (Miech et al., 2023).

These statistics are of particular concern because many addiction specialists view cannabis as a gateway drug associated with later use of other illicit substances; this is especially true for those who use marijuana to cope with serious life stressors (McCutcheon & Watts, 2018). Additionally, marijuana has addictive potential and is the drug most frequently associated with a substance-use disorder diagnosis. Further, frequent marijuana use often occurs concurrently with heavy alcohol use and opioid misuse in adolescents and young adults. Approximately 10 percent

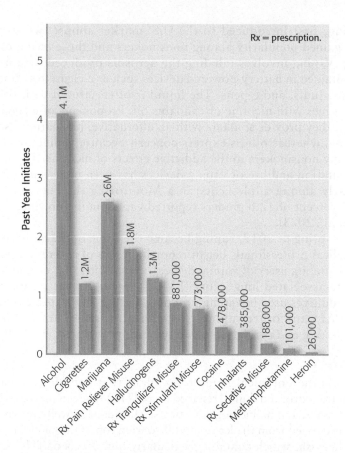

Rx = prescription.

Past Year Initiates

Alcohol 4.1M
Cigarettes 1.2M
Marijuana 2.6M
Rx Pain Reliever Misuse 1.8M
Hallucinogens 1.3M
Rx Tranquilizer Misuse 881,000
Rx Stimulant Misuse 773,000
Cocaine 478,000
Inhalants 385,000
Rx Sedative Misuse 188,000
Methamphetamine 101,000
Heroin 26,000

Note: Estimates for prescription pain relievers, prescription tranquilizers, prescription stimulants, and prescription sedatives are for the initiation of misuse.

Figure 11.7

First-Time Substance Use in 2021

Among the adolescents and adults who first used a substance during 2021, alcohol and marijuana were the substances most frequently involved in first-time use.

Source: SAMHSA, 2022

of those who use marijuana become dependent on the drug, and more than 16.3 million adolescents and adults demonstrated a cannabis-use disorder in 2021 (SAMHSA, 2022). A unique characteristic of marijuana dependence is a pervasive lack of concern regarding the consequences of drug use. Cannabis withdrawal symptoms include irritability, anxiety, insomnia, restlessness, and depression, as well as distressing physical symptoms such as stomach pain, tremors, sweating, fever, and headache. Withdrawal symptoms cause many users to return to cannabis use or to resort to using other drugs (Zehra et al., 2018).

Long-term use of cannabis is associated with impaired judgment, memory, and concentration. Diminished cognitive functioning involving attention, memory, and learning can persist for years, especially for those who begin use during adolescence. These cognitive effects may be more pronounced and persistent in adolescents because their brains are undergoing a critical period of development, thus increasing their vulnerability to the effects of the drug (Testai et al., 2022).

Did You Know?

Marijuana use doubles the risk of having a fatal car accident; if the driver consumes alcohol, this risk is further increased.

Source: Brady & Li, 2014

A Closer Look at Legalizing Pot

Although possession of cannabis remains illegal under federal law, discussions about legalizing marijuana are occurring across the United States. Despite the fact that the Food and Drug Administration does not consider cannabis a safe or effective medical treatment, 33 states now allow the production and distribution of marijuana for certain medical conditions. Furthermore, many municipalities have decriminalized the possession of marijuana for personal use, and voters in multiple states have gone further—legalizing the commercialization, production, and sale of cannabis and allowing adults age 21 and older to possess small quantities of marijuana for personal use.

Proponents of legalization contend that marijuana is safe and poses fewer serious health consequences than legal substances such as alcohol or tobacco. Additionally, they emphasize the benefits associated with the taxation and regulation of marijuana sales. They also hope that legalization will allow law enforcement officials to focus on other priorities. Professionals in the addiction field are attempting to counter the assertion that cannabis use poses limited physical or psychological risk. Instead, they emphasize that marijuana is a potent, addictive substance that can have long-term negative effects on brain functioning. They also express concern that the increased availability of marijuana combined with the potency of today's cannabis will lead to a variety of health and personal problems, including addiction (D'Souza et al., 2020).

Many researchers are concerned that the legalization of marijuana will normalize the use of marijuana and increase usage rates; this group strongly advocates for public education regarding the health consequences associated with cannabis. Although data from the University of Michigan's Monitoring the Future survey reveal that marijuana use has not increased among adolescents, the researchers did express concern about the significant decrease in the number of high school students who believe that marijuana poses health risks, with only 28 percent of 12th graders in 2021 indicating that regular marijuana use is potentially harmful (Miech et al., 2023). Mental health professionals are also concerned that increased cannabis use will lead to increases in psychotic disorders, especially for those who initiate marijuana use during adolescence (Gonçalves-Pinho et al., 2020).

There is little doubt that the debate will continue as marijuana use becomes more prevalent. Further, states that have legalized marijuana are now contending with issues such as oversight of the marijuana industry and penalties for legal violations involving public or underage use, as well as traffic safety infringements.

For Further Consideration

1. If chemicals in cannabis are found to be safe and effective for certain medical conditions, should they be distributed in herbal form by marijuana dispensaries or prepared in a standardized manner and dispensed in pill or liquid form by pharmacies?

2. What methods of research can we use to assess the effects of laws allowing the recreational or medical use of marijuana? What outcome variables should researchers monitor?

Inhalants

Case Study   "The spray makes me talk slow. Besides the headache I get when I'm not doing it, it makes me slower. The high is good but it makes me slow. When it's wearing off, it makes me like I am stupid. I have to talk slow because the words don't come out. . . .

"Sometimes I get suicidal. I don't know why. I just do. I just don't give a damn. I just get out in the street in front of cars. Sometimes I remember that I'm doing it and sometimes I don't know it. When I do know it, I don't give a damn. I just want to stop my life because the headaches I get when I stop the spray paint just make me crazy." (Ramos, 1998, p. 14)

Inhalant abusers become intoxicated from chemical vapors found in a variety of common household products, including solvents (paint removers, gasoline, lighter fluid), office supplies (marker pens, correction fluids), aerosol sprays (spray paints, hair spray), and compressed air products (computer and electronics duster sprays). Inhalation of these substances (known as "huffing") is accomplished through sniffing fumes from containers, bags, or balloons; directly inhaling aerosol sprays; or using inhalant-soaked rags.

Inhalant use affected about 2.2 million adolescents and adults in 2021 and was most common among those ages 12 to 17 (SAMHSA, 2022). The use of inhalants by children and adolescents was once considered a silent epidemic; however, the rate of use appears to be declining (Miech et al., 2023). Experimental use of inhalants in younger adolescents typically occurs before experimentation with tobacco or alcohol. Fortunately, experimentation with inhalants does not appear to be a gateway to more serious drug use, although those who chronically abuse inhalants often initiate marijuana and cocaine use (Ding et al., 2009).

The immediate effects of inhalants vary depending on the chemicals involved; typical effects include impaired coordination and judgment, euphoria, dizziness, and slurred speech. The intoxicating effects of inhalants are brief, resulting in repeated huffing to extend intoxication. Hypoxia (oxygen deprivation) results in persistent cognitive deficits such as the severe memory impairment and slow information processing seen in the case study. Any episode of inhalant use, even in first-time users, can result in stroke, acute respiratory distress, or sudden heart failure (referred to as "sudden sniffing death"). Fatal outcomes are most common with gasoline, benzine, compressed air products, aerosol sprays, butane, propane, and nitrous oxide (Radparvar, 2023).

Inhalant use produces a number of emotional and interpersonal difficulties, including paranoid thinking and suicidal ideation. In one sample of inhalant abusers, 67 percent had contemplated suicide and 20 percent had attempted suicide (Howard, Perron, Sacco, et al., 2010). Additionally, chronic inhalant abuse is associated with high levels of anxiety and depression, as well as antisocial behavior and interpersonal violence (Howard, Perron, Vaughn, et al., 2010).

Designer Drugs

The term *designer drugs* refers to substances manufactured as recreational drugs using a variety of chemicals; these synthetic drugs are created to mimic the effects of hallucinogenic or stimulant drugs while evading legal restrictions. Many of these drugs are available in the form of pills, powders, or liquids and are sold on the street or over the Internet under a variety of product names (Luethi & Liechti, 2020).

Designer drugs include substances such as the following:

- Ecstasy (methylenedioxymethamphetamine, or MDMA)
- Synthetic marijuana, made from a combination of herbs and chemicals
- MDPV marketed as "bath salts" or "plant food"
- DOM, known as STP or Serenity, Tranquility, and Peace
- Bromo-Dragonfly or B-fly, with persistent hallucinogenic effects
- Methoxetamine or MXE, with effects similar to PCP and ketamine

One of the major concerns with these substances is that they can affect multiple systems of the body. For example, "bath salts" are a relatively inexpensive, human-made substance that mimics the chemical properties of the khat plant. The cardiac and neurological effects of these illicit products have been responsible for tens of thousands of emergency department visits throughout the United States (Palamar et al., 2019). Concern about the dangers of synthetic marijuana and bath salts has led to federal efforts to ban the importation and sale of the chemicals used in their manufacture. Unfortunately, efforts at regulation often result in the manufacture of new substances using novel combinations of unregulated chemicals.

Ecstasy Ecstasy (methylenedioxymethamphetamine, or MDMA), which has both stimulant and hallucinogenic properties, is a designer drug that has gained popularity as a party drug. Short-term effects of Ecstasy, including euphoria, mild sensory and cognitive distortion, and feelings of intimacy and well-being, are often followed by intense depression. Users frequently experience hyperthermia or the need to suck on lollipops or pacifiers to counteract involuntary jaw spasms and teeth clenching. Following a period of increasing use, Ecstasy use among high school students has been decreasing, with only 1.9 percent of high school seniors reporting using the drug in the previous year (Miech et al., 2023).

Promising research into MDMA-assisted psychotherapy using prescribed doses of MDMA for the treatment of mental disorders such as depression and PTSD has led to the possibility that the FDA may approve the use of MDMA as an adjunct to psychotherapy sessions (Reardon, 2023). Although Ecstasy has the potential for addiction and memory loss when taken in high quantities (3 mg/kg or more), the low doses that are usually used in clinical studies do not appear to produce these adverse effects (Pantoni et al., 2022).

Unfortunately, street drugs identified as ecstasy often have other substances that may result in severe toxicity even with first time use (Figurasin & Maguire, 2022). A review of 82 cases in which Ecstasy was a cause of death revealed the following: Ecstasy was the sole cause of death in 23 percent of the cases, combined drug toxicity caused 59 percent of the deaths, and significant cardiovascular changes contributed to the remaining deaths. Surprisingly, despite the youth of the those who died, *atherosclerosis* (hardening of the arteries, a condition typically associated with aging) was found in 58 percent of decedents. This effect, typically seen in cocaine and methamphetamine users, may relate to the stimulant properties of Ecstasy (Kaye et al., 2009).

Club Drugs Many of the designer drugs, including Ecstasy and substances such as PCP, ketamine, and Rohypnol, are considered club drugs because they are often used in a club or party context. Club drugs are used to induce energy and excitement, reduce inhibitions, and create feelings of well-being and connection with others. Although positive effects may last for hours, they are typically followed by a crash—lethargy, low motivation, and fatigue. Unfortunately, energy exertion in a warm environment intensifies harmful effects of drug use, particularly hyperthermia and dehydration. Extreme depression and anxiety or acute physical symptoms (associated with dehydration or changes in blood pressure and heart rhythm) can occur. These effects are most probable when club drugs are combined or taken with alcohol.

Cocaine is also used within the club drug culture. In one large sample of individuals using drugs in a club context, 90 percent reported cocaine use; in fact, 59 percent demonstrated cocaine dependence (Parsons et al., 2009). Another common club drug with high addictive potential is gamma hydroxybutyrate (GHB), a substance used primarily by men because of its purported strength-enhancing properties. Because GHB (sometimes referred to as liquid ecstasy) is a central nervous system depressant with strong sedative effects, it is particularly dangerous when combined with alcohol. For those who become physiologically dependent on GHB, withdrawal symptoms can be life threatening (Kamal et al., 2016).

Opening Up About Addiction

Justin Bieber now acknowledges heavy marijuana use beginning in his early teens followed by increasing episodes of drinking alcohol and using a wide variety of drugs. Bieber reports he finally decided to get sober because he felt like he was dying during a very dark period in his early 20s.

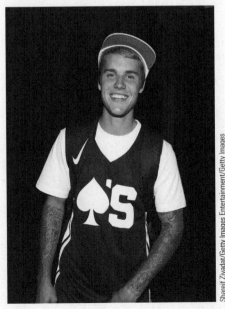

Combining Multiple Substances

Case Study   Kelly M., age 17, was hospitalized after her mother found her unconscious from an overdose of tranquilizers; her blood alcohol level was 0.15. The overdose was apparently accidental. Kelly was regularly using tranquilizers to help her relax and relieve her stress. Arguments with her mother would precipitate heavy use of the drugs. Eventually she found that she needed more of the pills to relax and began stealing money to buy them from classmates. She sometimes used alcohol as a substitute for or in combination with the tranquilizers. Her mother reported that she had no knowledge of her daughter's drug misuse or alcohol use, although she had noticed that Kelly was increasingly isolated and sleepy. Hospital personnel informed Kelly of the dangers of sedatives, especially when combined with alcohol, and recommended that she begin substance abuse treatment.

Dangerous interactions can occur when substances are combined. Chemicals taken simultaneously may exhibit a **synergistic effect**; interactions between the substances intensify effects or create unique side effects. For instance, when tranquilizers are combined with alcohol, both substances depress the central nervous system, and the synergistic effect can result in respiratory distress or even death. Furthermore, some substances (such as alcohol) may reduce judgment, resulting in excessive (or lethal) use of other drugs. Equally dangerous is the use of one drug to counteract the effects of another substance, such as taking stimulants and later taking a sleeping pill to counteract insomnia from the stimulant.

Of particular concern is multiple drug use involving Ecstasy. One group of rave attendees taking Ecstasy tested positive for an average of four other drugs; those who illicitly manufacture drugs such as Ecstasy often adulterate them with other substances, a factor that may have affected the findings (Black et al., 2009). Increased intoxication also occurs when combining alcohol and energy drinks. Research suggests that students who combine alcohol and caffeine have more heavy-drinking episodes, drunkenness, and alcohol-related consequences such as sexual assault, physical injury, and driving while intoxicated (Kponee et al., 2014).

11-3 Etiology of Substance-Use Disorders

Why do people abuse substances, despite knowing that alcohol and drug abuse can have devastating consequences? What leads people down the path to drug or alcohol addiction? In general, the progression from initial substance use to substance abuse follows a typical sequence. First, an individual decides to experiment with alcohol or drugs—perhaps to satisfy curiosity, enhance self-confidence, rebel against authorities, imitate others, or conform to social pressure. Second, the substance begins to serve an important purpose (such as to reduce anxiety, produce feelings of pleasure, or enhance social relationships) and so consumption continues. Third, brain chemistry becomes altered from substance use. In many cases,

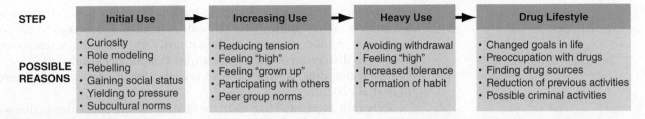

STEP	Initial Use		Increasing Use		Heavy Use		Drug Lifestyle
POSSIBLE REASONS	• Curiosity • Role modeling • Rebelling • Gaining social status • Yielding to pressure • Subcultural norms		• Reducing tension • Feeling "high" • Feeling "grown up" • Participating with others • Peer group norms		• Avoiding withdrawal • Feeling "high" • Increased tolerance • Formation of habit		• Changed goals in life • Preoccupation with drugs • Finding drug sources • Reduction of previous activities • Possible criminal activities

Figure 11.8

Typical Progression Toward Drug Abuse or Dependence

The progression from initial substance use to substance abuse typically begins with curiosity about a drug's effects and casual experimentation.

physiological dependency develops, resulting in craving for the substance and withdrawal symptoms if use is discontinued; it also becomes difficult to experience pleasure without the substance. Fourth, lifestyle changes occur due to chronic substance use. These changes may include loss of interest in previous activities and social relationships as well as preoccupation with opportunities to use the substance (Figure 11.8). Consistent with the multipath model, all four phases—biological, psychological, social, and sociocultural influences—are involved (Figure 11.9).

Psychological Dimension

Coping with psychological stress and emotional symptoms appears to be a major motive for substance use. Of the 44.1 million adults with a substance-use disorder in 2021, almost half had a concurrent psychiatric disorder (SAMHSA, 2022). Individuals with psychiatric symptoms often

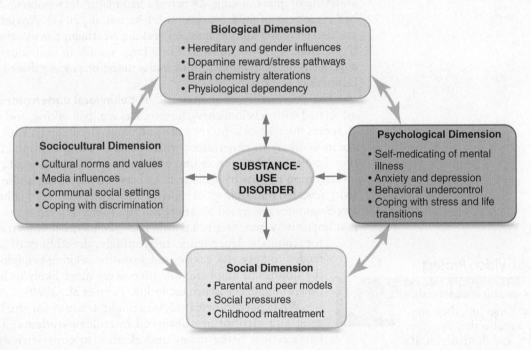

Figure 11.9

Multipath Model of Substance-Use Disorders

The dimensions interact with one another and combine in different ways to result in a substance-use disorder.

use drugs and alcohol in an attempt to regulate emotions such as depression and anxiety. When adolescents or adults use alcohol or drugs to reduce unpleasant physical or emotional sensations, they often obtain temporary relief from distressing feelings. Each time this happens, substance use is reinforced and, thus, is more likely to become a habitual method of coping (May et al., 2020).

Research suggests that four categories of life stressors influence substance use and the development of substance-use disorders: (a) general life stress (e.g., relationship or work difficulties), (b) stress resulting from trauma or catastrophic events, (c) childhood stressors or maltreatment, and (d) the stress of everyday discrimination based on being a member of a racially/ethnically underrepresented group or a gender/sexual minority (Stepp et al., 2021). For example, individuals with posttraumatic stress disorder often report using drugs or alcohol to cope with their ongoing emotional and physical reactivity (Dworkin et al., 2018). In one study of people undergoing drug treatment, those with the most severe posttraumatic stress disorder symptoms—especially hyperarousal and reexperiencing the trauma—reported the greatest dependence on marijuana, supporting the self-medication hypothesis (Villagonzalo et al., 2011). Similarly, a large number of problem drinkers report using alcohol to cope with mood symptoms; those with this pattern have an increased likelihood of developing an alcohol-use disorder (Turner et al., 2018).

Internalizing disorders such as depression and anxiety often precede substance use and abuse (Palmisano & Pandey, 2017). For instance, in a longitudinal study involving low-income adults seen at a public health clinic, symptoms of stress, depression, and anxiety preceded and predicted binge drinking, illegal drug use, and smoking (Walsh et al., 2013). Anxiety and depressive symptoms that begin in early childhood and persist into adulthood appear to increase the risk of alcohol abuse, particularly when accompanied by social withdrawal (Hussong et al., 2011). Among individuals trying to quit smoking, 24 percent had major depression and 17 percent had symptoms of mild depression (Hebert et al., 2011). Anxiety diagnoses are also common among smokers seeking treatment for nicotine addiction (Piper et al., 2010). Almost half of a large sample of individuals who were dependent on methamphetamine had a mood or anxiety disorder (Glasner-Edwards et al., 2010).

The personality characteristic of **behavioral undercontrol**, which is associated with rebelliousness, novelty seeking, risk taking, and impulsivity, increases the risk of substance use and abuse. Individuals with these traits are more likely to experiment with substances and continue use because they find the effects rewarding and exciting (Waddell et al., 2022). An investigation of possible genetic links between substance abuse and impulsivity revealed that siblings of individuals with addiction to either heroin or amphetamines possessed a variety of impulsivity-related traits, suggesting that impulsivity may be a behavioral *endophenotype* that increases the risk for stimulant dependence. Interestingly, the siblings of heroin users tended to have risk-taking and sensation-seeking behaviors, whereas the siblings of amphetamine users were more likely to have a more general impulsive approach to life (Long et al., 2020).

What psychological factors might account for the increases in drug and alcohol use observed in college students? Undergraduates report using drugs and alcohol to cope with anxiety and depression; academic, social, and financial pressures; as well as social changes such as being away from home for the first time, living in a new environment, and having increased responsibility (Sloane et al., 2010). College students high in impulsivity and behavioral undercontrol, particularly those in fraternities or sororities, are especially vulnerable to alcohol dependence (Grekin & Sher, 2006). Similarly, college students with high levels of sensation seeking are more likely to exhibit alcohol or cannabis dependence (Kaynak et al., 2013). Impulsivity has a particularly strong association with alcohol abuse among college students who are also risk takers and poor planners (Banks & Zapolski, 2017). Although some college students decrease their alcohol use after drinking has resulted in distressing consequences, negative events associated with drinking—such as sexual assault, embarrassment over behavior while intoxicated, and poor academic performance—can also lead to increased drinking or to drug use (Dams-O'Conner et al., 2006).

Social Dimension

The influence of social factors on substance abuse varies across the life span, exerting different effects at different ages. Experiencing stressful events in childhood, including neglect and emotional, physical, and sexual abuse, is strongly associated with heavy drinking, especially for those with multiple victimization experiences. This relationship appears particularly strong for African Americans (Lee & Chen, 2017). One variable linking child abuse with risk for substance-use disorders is the increasing use of alcohol and marijuana during adolescence among individuals exposed to childhood maltreatment (Yoon et al., 2020). Childhood trauma may increase the likelihood of impulsive behaviors in response to distress, such as turning to substances as a means of coping. Not surprisingly, in one study, adolescents with parents who have an alcohol-use disorder reported drinking heavily and drinking alone, with the goal of becoming intoxicated in order to forget their problems (Chalder et al., 2006).

As you might expect, adolescence and early adulthood are particularly vulnerable periods with respect to social influences on substance use, even for those without other life stressors. Patterns of alcohol or drug abuse often begin in early adolescence. Among one group of adolescents who were dependent on alcohol or other drugs by late adolescence, the mean age of onset of drinking or illicit drug use was 14 (Swendsen et al., 2012). Various social factors affect decisions to initiate drinking or drug use, including pressure from peers, a wish to fit in socially, attempts to rebel and challenge authority, a desire to assert independence or escape from societal or parental pressures for achievement, or interest in having fun or taking risks (Gallegos et al., 2020). Adolescent boys often report that drugs help them "relax socially" and "have more fun at parties." Associating with friends who get drunk increases high-risk drinking. Best friends and older siblings can exert a particularly strong influence with respect to substance use (Schuler et al., 2019).

Family attitudes and behaviors toward drinking and drugs (including the use of prescription medication) affect adolescents' likelihood of experimenting with substances. As you might imagine, when parents use drugs or alcohol liberally, so do their children. Additionally, adolescents who receive less parental monitoring have increased substance use, as do those whose parents feel unable to enforce rules or influence decisions related to substance use and those whose parents believe cultural myths such as "All adolescents experiment" or "It's okay to have teens drink at home" (Cope et al., 2017).

College presents its own unique set of environmental influences, particularly for younger students. Many of you are probably aware that the first year of college is an especially vulnerable transitional period for students who have recently graduated from high school. Students are free from parental supervision, have easy access to alcohol, and are often surrounded by classmates who engage in heavy drinking. Unofficial social events that promote partying and peers who minimize the consequences of drinking further contribute to college drinking (Krieger et al., 2018). Social media also increases the acceptability and frequency of alcohol use in college. Exposure to online postings about alcohol can lead students to misjudge the prevalence of college drinking and increase their likelihood of experimenting with alcohol or illicit drugs (Groth et al., 2017). In general, college students and other young adults significantly overestimate the extent of alcohol and marijuana use by their peers, thus inflating the social acceptability of substance use. Not surprisingly, those who overestimate peer use of alcohol and marijuana have an increased likelihood of using these substances (Bertholet et al., 2013).

Sociocultural Dimension

Although substance use varies according to sociocultural factors such as gender, age, socioeconomic status, ethnicity, religion, and nationality, the use and abuse of alcohol and other substances pervades all social classes. Certain substances—alcohol; nicotine; and, to some extent, marijuana and prescription drugs—are an accepted part of U.S. culture, as we have seen from prevalence data. Additionally, the data suggest that drug and alcohol use have become a normative part of adolescent culture (Miech et al., 2023). Declines in the number of teens who view substance use as harmful and increases in peer approval for getting high are associated with increased use of substances in social situations and party environments. Further, adolescents whose peer group lacks school commitment and connectedness are particularly prone to engaging in substance use with their peers (Latimer & Zur, 2010).

Communal social settings, such as those associated with fraternities and sororities, can also influence the use of alcohol. In one study, binge drinking rates (during the prior 2 weeks) were compared between nonfraternity college students and fraternity and sorority members, further comparing those who lived either at or outside the fraternity/sorority house. Among men living at the fraternity, 82 percent had engaged in binge drinking, compared with 64 percent of fraternity members living elsewhere and 51 percent of their nonfraternity peers. Among women living at a sorority, 50 percent had engaged in binge drinking, compared with 44 percent of the sorority members living elsewhere and 23 percent of their nonsorority peers. The social norms for drinking within a fraternity or sorority setting appear to influence drinking patterns (McCabe et al., 2018).

It is common to encounter marketing messages for alcohol and prescription drugs, as well as depictions of these products in songs, movies, television, and social media. Social acceptance of drug or alcohol use is increasing, whereas warnings from parents, schools, and antidrug advertising are decreasing. The effects of media images involving substance use can be very powerful. For instance, exposure to movies depicting alcohol use is associated with earlier onset of drinking in adolescents (Jackson et al., 2018). Similarly, factors such as perceived prevalence of smoking and exposure to smokers in movies are associated with increased prevalence of initiating smoking (Leonardi-Bee et al., 2016). Some researchers believe that the effect is strong enough to require presenting antitobacco messages before any movie with tobacco images. Similarly, there is concern that public debate regarding the legalization of marijuana appears to be normalizing its social acceptability, with resultant increases in use (Johnston et al., 2020).

Did You Know?

People in the United States spent almost $421 billion on prescription medications in 2021.

Source: Parasrampuria & Murphy, 2022

Use and abuse of alcohol and illicit drugs vary both within and between ethnic groups, as discussed earlier. Cultural values affect not only the substances used and amount consumed but also the cultural tolerance of substance abuse. African American 12th graders were most likely to have used alcohol (57 percent) compared to European Americans (32 percent) and Latinx Americans (41 percent). There has been a reversal of trends from previous years when African American teens were least likely to drink alcohol (Miech et al., 2023).

Factors affecting the variability in substance use between ethnic groups include increased availability of alcohol in urban areas in which many members of ethnically underrepresented groups reside; social and economic disadvantage, including limited job opportunities and inadequate health care; community safety concerns; and stress associated with racial discrimination and acculturation (Chartier & Caetano, 2010). Substance abuse within Native American communities has been linked with the historical trauma of colonization, loss of cultural heritage and ancestral lands, and ongoing systemic racism and oppression (Skewes & Blume, 2019). The experience of unfair treatment and racial discrimination is associated with increased risk of substance-use disorders among Asian Americans, African Americans, and Latinx Americans, especially among those who develop a pattern of using substances as a coping mechanism (Vu et al., 2019). Among Latinx adults, discrimination appears to increase the risk of alcohol abuse for women and drug abuse for men and is also linked to heavier smoking and difficulty with smoking cessation (Kendzor et al., 2014; Otiniano-Verissimo et al., 2014). Discrimination may also account for the finding that among all immigrant groups in the United States, more time in the United States is associated with increased prevalence of alcohol use and abuse (Szaflarski et al., 2019).

Although psychological, social, and sociocultural influences have a pronounced effect on both the initiation and the continuation of substance use, this question remains: Why are some individuals able to use drugs or alcohol in moderation, whereas others succumb to heavy use and addiction? Biological explanations provide considerable insight into this issue, as we explain in the following section.

Biological Dimension

Biological factors affect the development of substance-use disorders in various ways. First, substance use alters brain functioning. Some drugs (such as cannabis) produce changes by mimicking the actions of various neurotransmitters. Other drugs (such as stimulants) flood the brain with dopamine and alter the dopamine reward circuit, the neurological pathway associated with pleasure. Feelings of euphoria or contentment ensue. The "high" resulting from excessive dopamine reinforces continued drug use. Eventually, substance use crowds out other pleasures and turns into an all-consuming, compulsive desire.

Effects of Cocaine Use

These positron emission tomography scan images compare the cerebral metabolic activity of a control subject (top row) with those of a person who formerly abused cocaine at 10 days after discontinuing the substance (middle row) and after 100 days of abstinence (bottom row). Red and yellow areas reveal efficient brain activity, whereas blue regions indicate minimal brain activity. After 100 days of abstinence, brain activity is improved but remains far from normal.

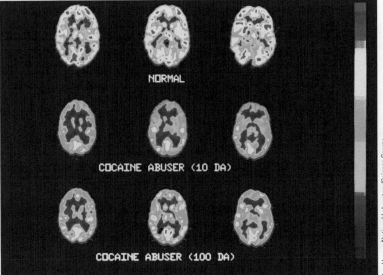

Brookhaven National Laboratory/Science Source

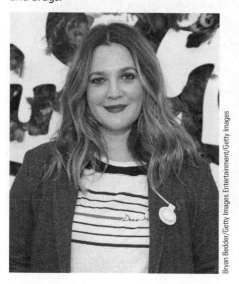
When exposed to excessive dopamine, brain cells adapt to the overstimulation by decreasing the number of dopamine receptors. The brain goes into this self-protective mode in order to maintain equilibrium. As the brain becomes less sensitive to the effects of dopamine and drug tolerance develops, the brain requires more of the substance to re-create the original "high." This decreased sensitivity to dopamine means that drugs and alcohol (as well as other normally enjoyable activities) become increasingly ineffective at producing feelings of pleasure (Everitt & Robbins, 2016).

Furthermore, substance-induced changes in the prefrontal cortex result in impaired judgment and decision making. These changes also reduce self-control, making it difficult for individuals with a substance-use disorder to resist cravings. Thus, compulsive drug-seeking behavior ensues without consideration of negative consequences. Adolescence through early adulthood is a critical period for nuanced development of the prefrontal cortex; when drug or alcohol use affects this process, disruptions in reasoning, goal setting, and impulse control can lead to a lifelong pattern of neurological dysregulation and substance abuse (Guerri & Pascual, 2019).

Genetic factors also play an important role in the development of substance abuse. There is strong evidence based on twin studies and analyses of family patterns of addiction that substance abuse runs in families. However, because family members usually share both genetic and environmental influences, researchers face the challenge of somehow separating the contributions of these two sets of factors. Kendler and Prescott (2006), using data from more than 4,500 pairs of identical and fraternal twins to isolate genetic and environmental factors involved in substance abuse, concluded the following:

- Genetic factors accounted for 56 percent of the risk of alcohol dependence and 55 percent of the risk of nicotine dependence.
- Genetic factors accounted for 75 percent of the risk of misusing other drugs, with cannabis dependence having the strongest genetic risk.

Although collective findings support the importance of heredity in the etiology of substance use, the manner by which specific genes or gene combinations influence addiction is complex. For example, genetics influence personality traits such as impulsivity, risk taking, and novelty seeking that increase the likelihood that someone will experiment with drugs or alcohol, as well as protective characteristics such as self-control.

We also know that genes affect individual responses to specific drugs and the risk of drug dependence. For instance, one person may be susceptible to alcoholism, whereas another has a genetic risk of marijuana dependence. And some gene combinations produce the risk of addiction to multiple substances. Additionally, genetic variations can influence the degree of pleasure (or aversion) experienced during initial use of specific substances, as well as the negative and positive effects of ongoing use. For example, in a comprehensive longitudinal study, teens who experimented with smoking and who had high genetic risk for smoking were 43 percent more likely to enjoy smoking and to progress to heavy smoking compared to those without these high-risk genes (Belsky et al., 2013). Genetics can also influence the degree to which someone is affected by a substance: Individuals who have the short allele of the serotonin transporter 5-HTTLPR genotype (which we have discussed in relation to depression and anxiety) tend to have a diminished response to alcohol, which results in heavier drinking behavior and an increased likelihood of developing a substance-use disorder (Cope et al., 2017).

Genes can also decrease the risk of substance abuse. For example, some people have genetic variations associated with decreased production of the alcohol cleanup enzyme ALDH; when individuals with this variant consume alcohol, toxins from metabolized alcohol accumulate and cause unpleasant physical reactions. This naturally occurring effect makes alcohol consumption aversive and thus reduces the risk of alcoholism. The protective effects of ALDH variations are quite strong in some individuals and occur primarily in individuals with African or Asian ancestry (Edenberg & McClintick, 2018).

Sex differences in the physiological effects of substances are also important in understanding addiction. Women who use drugs or alcohol experience a more rapid progression to addiction compared to men, are more reactive to drug-related cues, and are more susceptible to relapse. Investigation into the neurobiological basis of these sex differences has implicated the effects of estrogen, which can influence dopamine levels and susceptibility to the reinforcing effects of addictive substances. Other physiological differences may explain the more rapid development of alcoholism that occurs in women: Women tend to weigh less, produce fewer enzymes to metabolize alcohol, possess less total body fluid to dilute alcohol in the blood, and are more likely to limit food intake—factors that can increase toxicity and physiological changes associated with alcohol dependence. Further, sex differences in physiological reactions to stress (combined with differential exposure to traumatic life events) may help explain the more severe course of alcoholism in women (Milic et al., 2018).

In summary, gender and genetic predispositions, as well as physiological changes from heavy or chronic substance exposure, influence susceptibility to addiction. However, many factors beyond physiological effects contribute to the development and maintenance of substance abuse. The psychological, social, and sociocultural explanations previously discussed provide substantial insight into forces involved in decisions to initiate substance use, factors that can also influence continued use and response to treatment.

11-4 Treatment for Substance-Use Disorders

Many of us have friends, family members, or acquaintances recovering from addiction to drugs or to alcohol. In fact, tens of millions of adolescents and adults in the United States are now in recovery, living free from the addictive behaviors that previously controlled their lives. Many different methods lead to recovery and sustain recovery (Kelly et al., 2017). There is a huge disparity, however, between the millions of people in the United States who have a current substance-use disorder and the relatively small percentage who are receiving some form of intervention. Unfortunately, many who recognize that they have a serious substance-abuse problem are unable to seek help, often because cost and access are significant barriers.

Treatment and supportive interventions take place in a variety of settings, including self-help groups, mental health clinics, and inpatient and outpatient recovery programs. Self-help group meetings are the most common means of substance-abuse intervention in the United States, with many individuals participating in groups such as Alcoholics Anonymous (AA) and Narcotics Anonymous. Rather than specialized treatment, self-help groups provide a

Curbing the Tide of Substance Abuse

Substance-use disorders are unique among mental disorders because they are completely preventable—refraining from substance use *guarantees* that a substance-use disorder will not occur. In fact, some individuals with family members who have substance-use disorders decide to never tempt fate—to never use substances—thus halting familial patterns of addiction. Unfortunately, because substance abuse is a complex issue affected by a variety of processes operating over time, the solution is often not so simple.

We know that each day in the United States, many youth experiment with illicit drugs for the first time. Thus, a key to developing resilience is providing young people with the tools to refrain from such experimentation. Programs developed to prevent substance use and abuse often target critical periods of change—especially transitions during adolescence and early adulthood. Because youth develop within the broader context of family, school, community, and cultural groups, programs supporting healthy development typically aim at enhancing protective factors in a variety of areas (Banks et al., 2019; Kuntsche & Kuntsche, 2016), including the following:

- *Family*—Encouraging parents to build strong family relationships, articulate expected behavior (including abstinence from substance use), monitor activities and friendships, communicate positive cultural values, and interact with schools and other institutions

- *Individual assets*—Helping youth develop a positive identity; acquire constructive values; and build social competencies, including healthy strategies for coping with stress or adversity

- *Schools*—Providing students with effective learning opportunities regarding abused substances and how substance-use disorders develop and skills for resisting peer pressure

- *Community connections*—Developing community activities that help youth strengthen interpersonal connections and develop a sense of purpose

Communities, schools, and families play a crucial role in any effort to reduce the prevalence of substance abuse. For youth facing systemic societal oppression, the strengthening of ethnic pride and connection with spiritual practices can significantly enhance resilience (Banks et al., 2019). Preventing early experimentation with substances can have far-reaching consequences, not only in terms of decreasing the likelihood of substance abuse but also in terms of preventing detrimental effects on the academic and social competence of youth.

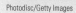
Photodisc/Getty Images

supportive approach to addiction, emphasizing fellowship and spiritual awareness to support abstinence. Self-help groups are often included as a component of ongoing treatment or as a mechanism to support sustained recovery once abstinence has been achieved.

Treatment is most effective when it incorporates best practices based on high-quality addiction research. Additionally, the inclusion of integrated care that addresses underlying emotional difficulties enhances treatment outcome (Fadus et al., 2019). Goals of treatment include achieving sustained abstinence; maintaining a drug-free lifestyle; and functioning productively in family, work, and other environments. This requires changing habits, minimizing thoughts of drugs or alcohol and substance-related social activities, and learning to cope with daily activities and stressors without substance use. Additionally, because drugs so often disrupt multiple aspects of an individual's life, there is a need to rebuild relationships with family, friends, and colleagues.

Most alcohol and drug treatment programs have two phases. In the first phase, called **detoxification**, the user ceases or reduces use of the substance. If the person is physiologically dependent on the substance, medical supervision may be necessary to help manage withdrawal symptoms. In the second phase, intervention focuses on preventing **relapse**, a return to use of the substance. Support is very important at this stage because relapse is common among those attempting to recover from alcohol or drug addiction.

Understanding and Preventing Relapse

Relapse prevention considers the physiological and psychological withdrawal symptoms a person might be experiencing, as well as neurological changes that occurred due to substance use; these physiological changes can influence motivation, impulsivity, learning, or memory. **Neuroplasticity**, the ability of the brain to change its structure and function in response to experience, is an important concept in addiction treatment. Just as the brain of someone who has an addiction became conditioned to needing a substance, treatment and abstinence can help recondition the brain, create new neural pathways, and undo changes caused by addiction. Sustained abstinence is necessary for permanent neurological changes to occur and is thus essential for maximizing treatment results.

Relapse prevention is a critical component of effective treatment because many individuals with substance-use disorders discontinue treatment when craving occurs. A single lapse in abstinence often leads to complete relapse. Many therapists view relapse not as a treatment failure but as an indicator that treatment needs to be intensified. People in treatment sometimes take medications to help prevent withdrawal symptoms, craving, and relapse. Medications prescribed vary depending on the substance abused. It is important to remember that although medication can assist with cravings and withdrawal, medication alone—given the complexities of addiction—is not sufficient to prevent relapse.

Contingency management procedures in which participants receive either voucher or cash incentives for verified abstinence, adherence to treatment goals, or compliance with a prescribed medication plan can significantly reduce relapse. Contingency programs also increase treatment participation and maximize behaviors that are incompatible with substance use, such as exercising, attending school, or learning new job skills. Verifying abstinence via toxicology screening is an important component of these interventions. One contingency management technique allows participants to accrue points on a credit card by attending various components of treatment and then use the card to purchase desired activities such as driving lessons, gym membership, or cinema tickets (Moss et al., 2020).

An approach that is effective in setting the stage for successful treatment and preventing relapse is **motivational enhancement therapy** (DiClemente et al., 2017). This method addresses a common barrier to effective treatment—ambivalence about giving up substance use. Unless this ambivalence is resolved, change is slow and short-lived. Motivational interviewing helps clients consider both the advantages and disadvantages of continued substance use; once there is a commitment to change, relapse risk is reduced and therapy moves forward with an emphasis on life modifications that increase the likelihood of abstinence (D'Amico et al., 2018).

As we have covered in our exploration of the etiology of substance abuse, the development of addiction is a complicated process that is made even more complex by the addictive characteristics of different substances. What all substances have in common are the long-lasting, difficult-to-reverse physiological and psychological changes that occur with chronic use. Some people are very susceptible to environmental triggers associated with drugs or alcohol, so treatment strategies that help people avoid or cope

Did You Know?

Life changes needed for long-term recovery include:

- eliminating cues associated with substance use;
- learning to manage drug craving;
- developing skills to cope with stress, depression, or anxiety;
- learning effective interpersonal skills;
- rebuilding family relationships;
- cultivating friendships with those who are not using substances;
- developing new hobbies and activities;
- addressing financial issues; and
- enhancing job skills.

with such triggers can reduce drug-seeking behavior and relapse (Robinson et al., 2014). Thus, effective treatment targets the variety of psychological, social, and sociocultural factors associated with continued substance use. In the following sections, we discuss research-validated treatment for the most commonly abused substances: alcohol, opioids, stimulants (including cocaine), cannabis, and nicotine.

Treatment for Alcohol-Use Disorder

Alcoholics Anonymous (AA) is a no-cost, peer-led intervention for alcoholism. The AA fellowship regards alcoholism as a disease and advocates total abstinence. Thus, it is not surprising that there is a strong association between regular attendance at AA meetings and decreased alcohol use. In a comprehensive review of studies comparing the effects of AA with mental health treatment, AA participation was more strongly associated with positive long-term outcomes compared to professional treatment without AA support. AA members not only obtain ideas for sustaining abstinence but also build strong social connections (Kelly et al., 2020). The Recovery Community Center model, a newer peer-operated approach to addiction treatment, involves the creation of a centralized location that houses AA meetings, sober social activities, and community agencies.

Consistent with the position of AA, alcoholism specialists who believe alcoholism is a disease argue that chronic alcohol use changes brain functioning in fundamental and long-lasting ways and that people who are recovering from alcoholism must completely abstain from drinking because any consumption will set off the disease process (Wollschlaeger, 2007). On the other hand, proponents of **controlled drinking** assume that, under the right conditions, people with alcoholism can learn to limit their drinking to appropriate levels. In a meta-analysis of studies comparing abstinence and controlled, low-risk use of alcohol, no outcome differences were found between the two treatment approaches on variables such as the severity of drinking and the probability of relapse. The controlled drinking approach appears to be most successful when people follow recommended low-risk limits rather than self-defined reductions (Henssler et al., 2021).

Medications are frequently used to treat alcohol abuse. Antabuse (disulfiram), a medication that produces an aversion to alcohol by creating highly unpleasant symptoms if alcohol is consumed, has been used for decades. Although it can be effective in those who take it as prescribed, many people avoid taking Antabuse once they have experienced the adverse effects caused by drinking (Skinner et al., 2014). The medication acamprosate (which also produces unpleasant symptoms when combined with alcohol) is also used to assist with abstinence, especially among those who have undergone detoxification. Additionally, naltrexone, a medication used to reduce desire for and pleasure in using alcohol, is sometimes effective in reducing heavy drinking, especially for individuals who stopped drinking before starting the medication. Nalmefene, a more recently approved medication, is a harm-control measure that is prescribed with the goal of reducing heavy drinking in individuals who have not achieved abstinence. In general, these medications have only low to medium effectiveness (Palpacuer et al., 2018).

Given the modest effects associated with pharmaceutical intervention, Mann and Hermann (2010) proposed an individualized approach to assessing the effectiveness of medications—assessing medication effects with subgroups of people with alcoholism based on biologically defined endophenotypes. They give the example of naltrexone being more effective with carriers of a specific gene variant and in those individuals with the strongest MRI evidence of brain reactivity in response to pictures of alcohol. Similarly, Ooteman et al. (2009) found that genetic characteristics of individuals undergoing alcohol treatment were associated with differential response to both acamprosate and naltrexone.

Overall, psychological and pharmacological approaches to alcohol treatment demonstrate only modest effects (Akbar et al., 2018; Klimas et al., 2018). Interventions supported by research offer the greatest promise. For instance, a comprehensive analysis of interventions to decrease college drinking revealed that individual, face-to-face conversations using motivational interviewing and providing information correcting misperceptions of social norms regarding drinking yielded the greatest reduction in alcohol-related problems (Carey et al., 2007). The use of these methods combined with challenging positive expectancies regarding alcohol use also successfully reduced heavy drinking in another group of students (Wood et al., 2007). More research regarding treatments for alcoholism, as well as more access to alcohol treatment, is needed. This is particularly important because a decision to enter treatment appears to be a crucial change point for those with alcohol dependence.

Treatment for Opioid-Use Disorder

Case Study After several months of denying the seriousness of his heroin habit, Gary B. finally enrolled in a residential treatment program that featured methadone maintenance, peer support, cognitive-behavioral therapy, and job retraining. Although Gary initially responded well to the program, he soon began to feel depressed. The staff reassured him that experiencing depression during opioid withdrawal is common. Gary began taking an antidepressant medication and started working with a psychologist for individual therapy. Psychotherapy helped Gary identify unhealthy relationships in his life and examine the parallels between his dependence on these relationships and his dependence on drugs. He also began to understand how he often turned to drugs to escape his problems. The therapy then focused on practicing coping skills and exploring healthy alternatives to drug use. Gary worked hard during his therapy and made considerable progress.

Gary was satisfied with the changes he was making in his life until the day he realized that he was eagerly looking forward to his daily methadone dose. Although Gary had friends who had become addicted to methadone, it was a shock when it happened to him. He decided almost immediately to terminate his methadone maintenance program. The withdrawal process was physically and mentally painful, and Gary often doubted his ability to function without methadone. However, by joining a support group composed of others who were discontinuing opioid use, he was eventually able to complete methadone withdrawal. Gary had never imagined that the most difficult part of his heroin treatment would be giving up methadone.

Physicians working with individuals who misuse prescription opioids often attempt to minimize withdrawal symptoms by gradually tapering the dose while simultaneously suggesting alternative methods of pain management (Davis et al., 2020). Due to the strong symptoms that can occur with opioid withdrawal, physicians sometimes decide to prescribe synthetic opioids such as methadone to reduce cravings without producing euphoria.

Overcoming Addiction

Former Boston Celtic Chris Herren struggled with substance abuse for much of his basketball career. He has been drug-free and alcohol-free since August 1, 2008; attends daily meetings to support his sobriety; and speaks to the public about the dangers of addiction. In this photo, Herren pumps his fist in the air following a Celtics victory over the Atlanta Hawks.

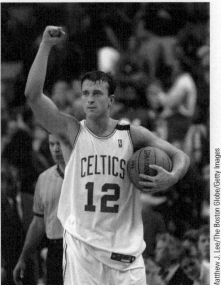

Matthew J. Lee/The Boston Globe/Getty Images

As was evident in the case study, methadone may seem like a simple solution to the problem of prescription opioid abuse or heroin addiction; however, it has an important drawback—tolerance develops, resulting in an addictive need for methadone. Although methadone is still used for treatment of opioid-use disorders, alternative medications are now available. For example, buprenorphine is a less-addictive synthetic opioid that can ease opioid withdrawal and prevent cravings and relapse. Buprenorphine is most effective when the dose is reduced slowly and additional support is provided (Cisewski et al., 2019).

Opioid addiction is often associated with psychological drug dependence and feelings of being overwhelmed and unable to cope with daily activities. Thus, it is not surprising that being married and having a close relationship with one's spouse predicted better treatment outcome for heroin users (Heinz et al., 2009). Contingency management with incentives for abstinence and individual and family counseling also improve treatment outcomes.

Treatment for Stimulant-Use Disorder

There are currently no effective pharmacological interventions for stimulant abuse. One approach that has found some success with individuals receiving treatment for stimulant dependence is the use of incentives for stimulant-free toxicology reports (Carroll et al., 2016). One group of researchers found that teaching people who use cocaine strategies for coping with temptations and high-risk situations was beneficial not only in lowering cocaine use but also in lowering the amount of cocaine used during a relapse (Rohsenow et al., 2000). Efforts are ongoing to find effective treatments for stimulant abuse, particularly because misuse of stimulants is so hard on the brain and entire vascular system (Bachi et al., 2017).

Treatment for Cannabis-Use Disorder

Cannabis-use disorder is difficult to treat because individuals who are dependent on marijuana not only resist engaging in treatment but also have trouble initiating and maintaining abstinence. In view of the cognitive and motivational deficits associated with marijuana use, some researchers advocate using short, frequent therapy sessions and focusing on increased self-efficacy (Munsey, 2010). Individuals who are attempting to stop cannabis use are most successful when they understand the potential negative outcomes associated with continued cannabis use and believe they have the strength to resist using cannabis even when experiencing distressing emotions (Gullo et al., 2017). In general, most psychosocial interventions for cannabis dependence fail to achieve abstinence. In one review of treatment studies, intensive intervention involving a combination of cognitive-behavioral therapy, motivational enhancement therapy, and abstinence-based incentives increased the likelihood of a successful outcome (Gates et al., 2016). Periodic maintenance check-ins following treatment can be helpful in sustaining abstinence (Walker et al., 2015).

Increases in treatment admissions and the recognition of a cannabis withdrawal syndrome have led to the use of various medications to assist in minimizing the nausea, stomach pain, and insomnia associated with withdrawal. Researchers are also searching for medications to reduce cravings, with a particular focus on the brain systems uniquely affected by THC, particularly the cannabinoid system (Brezing & Levin, 2018).

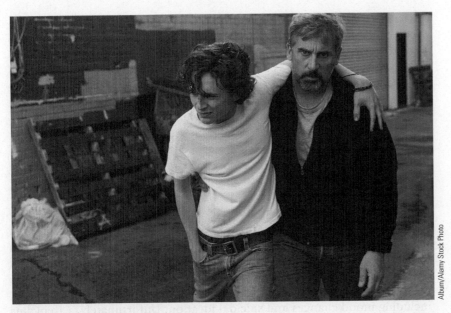

Album/Alamy Stock Photo

A Harrowing Path to Recovery

The movie *Beautiful Boy* is based on the memoir of journalist David Sheff, who watched his son Nic's downward spiral into substance abuse, including a severe addiction to methamphetamine. The movie also depicts the father's emotional struggle as he attempted to help his son overcome his addiction.

Treatment for Tobacco-Use Disorder

Smoking is associated with increased mortality, even among people who smoke only a few cigarettes each day (Inoue-Choi et al., 2017). Unfortunately, due to the highly addictive nature of nicotine, even when smoking cessation occurs, relapse to smoking remains high. In fact, although a vast majority of smokers (70 percent) would like to quit smoking, only a small minority (3 percent) succeed at sustained cessation (Jordan & Xi, 2018). Relapse rates and withdrawal-related discomfort are higher in people who also have depression, anxiety, or other substance-use disorders; thus, it is important to address underlying emotional issues.

Various psychological strategies have been used to assist in reducing the urge to smoke by teaching alternative methods for coping with distressing emotions. This is important because some smokers have difficulty tolerating negative moods and thus return to smoking when they feel depressed or anxious (Lerman & Audrain-McGovern, 2010). One successful four-session intervention (SMART—Smoking Treatment and Anxiety Management Program) recognizes that anxiety sensitivity (fear of aversive anxiety symptoms) can be a barrier to smoking cessation and directly teaches methods of coping with everyday anxiety and the negative feelings associated with tobacco withdrawal (Zvolensk et al., 2018). Intervention to address anxiety issues is particularly important in smokers with anxiety disorders because they have greater nicotine dependence and are less responsive to standard pharmacological interventions (Piper et al., 2010).

Some cessation approaches focus on gradually reducing the quantity of cigarettes smoked or the use of medications that assist with smoking reductions. For example, electronic cigarettes are sometimes used to help smokers ease tobacco withdrawal symptoms as they quit smoking; however, the evidence suggests that the use of e-cigarettes does not lead to cessation of nicotine intake (Patil et al., 2020). Three pharmaceutical products used for smoking cessation—nicotine replacement, bupropion, and varenicline—have variable success. The newest medication, varenicline (marketed as Chantix), aids smoking cessation by reducing cue-activated cravings and withdrawal symptoms, as well as decreasing smoking satisfaction by blocking the reward network in the brain. Nicotine replacement therapy (NRT) involves delivering increasingly smaller doses of nicotine using a patch, inhaler, nasal spray, gum, or sublingual tablet. The goal of NRT is to reduce the urge to smoke and avoid relapse by preventing withdrawal symptoms.

Bupropion (marketed under the name Zyban as an antismoking agent and Wellbutrin as an antidepressant) is frequently mentioned in the smoking cessation literature. Bupropion reduces activation of brain regions associated with craving, even in the presence of smoking-related cues. As with many antidepressant medications, caution is urged in the use of bupropion and varenicline due to concerns about side effects, including mood changes and suicidal ideation. Unfortunately, varenicline demonstrates only modest long-term effectiveness (18 percent to 30 percent sustained smoking cessation), and NRT and bupropion have even less success (Jordan & Xi, 2018).

Women have a more difficult time with smoking cessation compared to men; one variable that appears to influence success is the phase of the menstrual cycle at the time of smoking cessation (Weinberger et al., 2015). Other factors that appear to make it more difficult for women to stop smoking include stress and negative mood, enjoyment of the routine of smoking, sensitivity to smoking cues, and fear of weight gain (Perkins, 2009). A study investigating methods to help women who were concerned about weight gain achieve cessation found success when bupropion was used in combination with cognitive-behavioral therapy focused on the issue of weight control (Levine et al., 2010).

11-5 Gambling Disorder and Other Addictions

Gambling disorder, involving a compulsive desire to engage in gambling activities despite negative consequences, is the first non-substance-related addiction included in the DSM. In contrast to people who occasionally gamble without negative consequences, people with a gambling disorder experience distress or impairment in social or professional functioning due to their gambling. A gambling disorder may be diagnosed when someone exhibits at least four of the following characteristics over a 12-month period:

- Needs to bet larger quantities of money to achieve the desired excitement
- Feels irritable or restless following attempts to reduce or stop gambling
- Is unsuccessful when attempting to control, reduce, or stop gambling

- Experiences frequent preoccupation with gambling, including previous or future gambling activities
- Turns to gambling when feeling upset or distressed
- Returns for more gambling, trying to break even after losing money
- Deceives others to conceal the extent of involvement with gambling
- Has risked or lost jobs, relationships, or important opportunities because of gambling
- Turns to others for money due to financial desperation resulting from gambling

Gambling disorder may be mild (four to five of the symptoms), moderately severe (six to seven symptoms), or severe (eight to nine symptoms). A person can have persistent or chronic symptoms or distinct episodes of pathological gambling. Some people with gambling disorder tend to be impulsive and overconfident, whereas others gamble when feeling depressed or lonely. Gambling disorder is relatively uncommon, with a lifetime prevalence of less than 1 percent (APA, 2022).

Some people develop a gambling disorder gradually, whereas others rapidly progress to pathological gambling. Some individuals with gambling disorder prefer games of strategy (such as poker or sports betting), whereas others choose nonstrategic games (such as slot machines), with the latter group experiencing more aversion to loss and less-effective decision making when gambling. Although gambling disorder has been associated with impulsivity, understanding underlying emotional issues may be as important as addressing poor impulse control in managing problem gambling (Lorains et al., 2014). Given the fact that much of the research on gambling has focused on men, there is a call for research into the unique factors that influence the development of patterns of gambling and gambling addiction in women (McCarthy et al., 2019).

Group approaches to therapy, including facilitated 12-step groups and cognitive-behavioral therapy (focusing on changing dysfunctional cognitions and reactivity to triggers associated with gambling), have produced decreases in gambling behavior (Marceaux & Melville, 2011). Improving financial management skills is also an important component of treatment. Similar to trends in treatment for substance-use disorders, researchers are attempting to use neuroimaging and monitoring of brain changes associated with addiction-related cues to determine which treatments are most effective for gambling addiction. For instance, fMRI imaging may provide insight into which treatments increase impulse control and the ability to cope with distressing emotions, as well as decrease reactivity to cues associated with gambling (Moccia et al., 2017).

Internet Gaming Disorder

The DSM-5-TR includes Internet gaming disorder—a condition involving excessive and prolonged engagement in computerized or Internet games either alone or with other players—as a proposed diagnostic category. Although gambling and associated financial difficulties are not involved, the criteria are very similar to those for gambling disorder, including the fact that gaming interferes with social relationships and day-to-day responsibilities (APA, 2022). Internet gaming disorder is a significant concern in Asian countries and is most common among adolescent boys. Cognitive-behavioral treatment approaches include both a focus on behavioral change and treatment of underlying emotions such as anxiety and depression (Stevens et al., 2019).

There is much debate about whether Internet gaming and other excessive behaviors (such as compulsive sex, eating, buying, or Internet use) constitute an addiction. Because some compulsive behaviors share behavioral and neurological similarities with substance addiction (disrupting biological processes associated with sensitivity to reward and reducing impulse control), some researchers propose that they should, in fact, be considered addictions (Hasanović et al., 2021). Some argue that classification of these behaviors as addictions would provide reliable definitions for research, destigmatize people distressed by these behaviors, and facilitate the development of preventive and treatment strategies (Fineberg et al., 2022). Time will tell if the mental health profession heads in the direction of broadening the definition of addiction. Certainly, inclusion of gambling disorder and a proposal for Internet gaming disorder in the DSM-5-TR are a step in that direction.

11-6 Contemporary Trends and Future Directions

Research into addiction remains a high priority given the significant personal and societal toll that results from substance-use and gambling disorders. Researchers continue to focus on the individual and environmental circumstances that increase risk for experimentation with alcohol and illegal substances, including the ways in which media and social media directly and indirectly promote the use of substances, particularly alcohol. Because so many people with substance-use disorders begin experimenting during early adolescence, professionals in the addiction field continue their efforts to educate youth regarding the potential dangers of substance use, particularly the effects of substance use early in life when the brain is still developing. Researchers are prioritizing interventions that (a) allow parents to more accurately estimate their children's use of alcohol or other substances and (b) enhance communication between parents and their children regarding the potential consequences of substance use.

The collection of annual survey data highlights national trends in substance use and helps guide prevention and intervention efforts. These data also provide insight into any consequences of significant policy changes, such as the decriminalization and legalization of marijuana. Researchers who follow these trends caution that it is particularly important to monitor newly introduced substances or products (such as vaping) because their popularity can grow quickly during the "honeymoon period" when the supposed benefits of a substance are rapidly communicated via informal networks, long before information about potential dangers emerges (Johnston et al., 2020).

It is apparent that there is a considerable gap between those needing and those receiving treatment. Thus, developing affordable, accessible, and culturally relevant treatment opportunities is crucial if we hope to decrease the number of individuals and families affected by addiction. The importance of broadening and deepening prevention and intervention efforts in communities and subcultures with a high prevalence of drug or alcohol abuse has become increasingly evident. This will require addressing systemic factors associated with substance abuse, including poverty, racism, and all forms of discrimination. Participants in racial and social justice movements have articulated the transformational societal changes that will be needed if we wish to decrease the burden of oppression faced by marginalized communities. Addressing substance abuse in this manner will require open dialogue with all stakeholders within local communities and support systems. This will also necessitate a commitment from residential and community-based recovery programs to incorporate an antiracist framework into the provision of services (Matsuzaka & Knapp, 2019).

A move in this direction is reflected in the development of an academic–community partnership involving Native American tribal members and researchers from a local university. Their common goal is to develop culturally relevant substance abuse interventions. The program development began with the input of tribal members, who described their local tribal customs and shared their knowledge about substance use and recovery on the reservation. Their observations and wisdom served as the foundation for a sustainable, community-driven intervention program. This culturally sensitive program emphasizes a holistic approach to recovery based upon values that are important to the tribe, including spiritual and interpersonal harmony (Skewes et al., 2019).

Researchers are also continuing to use current technology such as neuroimaging techniques to help assess the effectiveness of addiction treatments (Moccia et al., 2017). A promising development is the National Drug Abuse Treatment Clinical Trials Network, which facilitates the sharing of research regarding psychological, pharmacological, and integrated treatments. Professionals and researchers in the field of addiction hope that easy access to electronic health records will accelerate research on effective interventions within various communities and diverse populations (Wu, Payne, et al., 2019).

Chapter Summary

1 What are substance-use disorders?

- People often use chemical substances that alter their mood, level of consciousness, or behavior.
- The use of such substances is considered a disorder when there is a maladaptive pattern of recurrent use over a 12-month period and the person is unable to reduce or cease intake of the substance despite social, occupational, psychological, medical, or safety problems.

2 What substances are associated with addiction?

- Substances are classified on the basis of their effects. Substances that are abused include depressants, stimulants, hallucinogens, dissociative anesthetics, and substances with multiple properties.
- Widely used depressants include alcohol, opioids (such as heroin, fentanyl, and prescription pain relievers such as oxycodone), and prescription medications that produce sedation and relief from anxiety.
- Stimulants energize the central nervous system, often inducing elation, grandiosity, hyperactivity, agitation, and appetite suppression. Amphetamines, cocaine, and caffeine are all stimulants.
- Hallucinogens produce altered states of consciousness, perceptual distortions, and sometimes hallucinations. Included in this category are LSD, psilocybin, and mescaline.
- Dissociative anesthetics produce a dreamlike detachment. Phencyclidine (PCP), ketamine, and dextromethorphan (DXM) are included in this category.
- Substances with multiple chemical properties include nicotine, cannabis, inhalants, and Ecstasy.

3 Why do people develop substance-use disorders?

- No single factor accounts for the development of a substance-use disorder. Biological, psychological, social, and sociocultural factors are all important.
- In terms of biological factors, heredity can significantly affect the risk of developing a substance-use disorder. Additionally, chronic drug or alcohol use alters brain chemistry, crowds out other pleasures, impairs decision making, and produces a compulsive desire for the substance.

- Psychological approaches to understanding substance-use disorders have emphasized personality characteristics such as behavioral undercontrol and self-medicating with substances to cope with stressful emotions and life transitions.
- Social factors are important in the initiation of substance use. Teenagers and adults use drugs because of parental models, social pressures from peers, and a desire for increased feelings of comfort and confidence in social relationships.
- Sociocultural factors affecting alcohol and drug use include media influences, cultural and subcultural norms, and societal stressors such as discrimination.

4 What kinds of interventions and treatments for substance-use disorders are most effective?

- The complex nature of addiction underscores the importance of a research-based, multifaceted treatment approach that is tailored to the individual's specific substance-use disorder and any concurrent social, emotional, or medical problems.
- Treatment for substance-use disorders has had mixed success. Intervening earlier in the addiction process increases success.
- Even after physiological withdrawal from a substance, individuals who abuse substances often relapse. Relapse prevention is enhanced through the use of motivational enhancement techniques to increase readiness for change, combined with pharmacological products to minimize withdrawal symptoms and with incentives for abstinence. Relapse indicates that longer-lasting or more intensive treatment is needed.

5 Can behaviors such as gambling be addictive?

- The definition of addiction has expanded to include behavioral addictions.
- The DSM-5-TR includes gambling disorder, a compulsive desire to engage in gambling activities despite negative consequences, as a diagnostic category.
- Internet gaming disorder, which involves excessive engagement in computerized or Internet games, is a proposed diagnostic category.

Chapter Glossary

abstinence
restraint from the use of alcohol, drugs, or other addictive substances

addiction
compulsive drug-seeking behavior and a loss of control over drug use

alcohol poisoning
potentially life-threatening, toxic effects resulting from rapidly consuming alcohol or ingesting a large quantity of alcohol

alcoholism
a condition in which the individual is dependent on alcohol and has difficulty controlling drinking

anxiolytics
a class of medications that reduce anxiety

behavioral undercontrol
a personality trait associated with rebelliousness, novelty seeking, risk taking, and impulsivity

binge drinking
episodic intake of five or more alcoholic beverages for men or four or more drinks for women

controlled drinking
consuming no more than a predetermined amount of alcohol

delirium tremens
life-threatening withdrawal symptoms that can result from chronic alcohol use

depressant
a substance that causes a slowing of responses and generalized depression of the central nervous system

detoxification
the phase of alcohol or drug treatment during which the body is purged of intoxicating substances

dissociative anesthetic
a substance that produces a dreamlike detachment

gateway drug
a substance that leads to the use of additional substances that are even more lethal

hallucinogen
a substance that induces perceptual distortions and heightens sensory awareness

heavy drinking
chronic alcohol intake of more than two drinks per day for men and more than one drink per day for women

hyperthermia
significantly elevated body temperature

hypnotics
a class of medications that induce sleep

intoxication
a condition involving problem behaviors or psychological changes that occur with excessive substance use

moderate drinking
a lower-risk pattern of alcohol intake (no more than one or two drinks per day)

motivational enhancement therapy
a therapeutic approach that addresses ambivalence and helps clients consider the advantages and disadvantages of changing their behavior

neuroplasticity
the ability of the brain to change its structure and function in response to experience

opioid
a painkilling agent that depresses the central nervous system, such as heroin and prescription pain relievers

physiological dependence
a state of adaptation that occurs after chronic exposure to a substance; can result in craving and withdrawal symptoms

psychoactive substance
a substance that alters mood, thought processes, and/or other psychological states

relapse
a return to drug or alcohol use after a period of abstinence

sedatives
a class of drugs that have a calming or sedating effect

stimulant
a substance that energizes the central nervous system

substance abuse
a pattern of excessive or harmful use of any substance for mood-altering purposes

substance-use disorder
a condition in which cognitive, behavioral, and physiological symptoms contribute to the continued use of alcohol or drugs despite significant substance-related problems

synergistic effect
the result of chemicals (or substances) interacting to multiply one another's effects

tolerance
decreases in the effects of a substance that occur after chronic use

withdrawal
the adverse physical and psychological symptoms that occur after reducing or ceasing intake of a substance

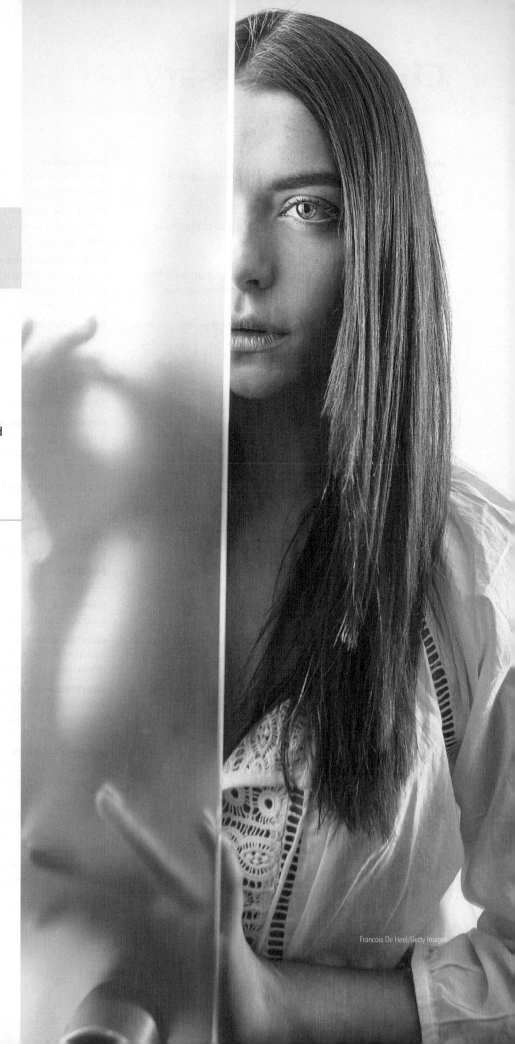

focus
Questions

1. What are the symptoms associated with schizophrenia spectrum disorders?

2. Is there much chance of recovery from schizophrenia?

3. What causes schizophrenia?

4. What treatments are currently available for schizophrenia, and are they effective?

5. How do other psychotic disorders differ from schizophrenia?

Francois De Heel/Getty Images

12

Schizophrenia Spectrum Disorders

Learning Objectives

After studying this chapter, you will be able to . . .

12-1 Describe the symptoms of schizophrenia spectrum disorders.

12-2 Debate the potential for recovery from schizophrenia.

12-3 Discuss the factors associated with the development of schizophrenia.

12-4 Describe the treatments currently available for schizophrenia and discuss their effectiveness.

12-5 Differentiate between schizophrenia and the other psychotic disorders.

At the Age of 8, Elyn Saks began to experience the hallucinations and fears of being attacked that have accompanied her throughout her life. She understood the importance of not talking openly about what ran through her mind. In fact, she was able to hide her delusional thoughts and hallucinations and maintain top grades throughout college. In graduate school, she experienced full-blown psychotic episodes (e.g., believing that someone had infiltrated her research and dancing on the roof of the law library) that resulted in her hospitalization and subsequent diagnosis of schizophrenia. Many of her symptoms persisted even after she began treatment. During one period, she believed her therapist had been replaced by an evil person with an identical appearance. In her book *The Center Cannot Hold: My Journey Through Madness*, Saks (2007) recounts her experiences with mental illness, describing schizophrenia as a "slow fog" that becomes thicker over time.

Saks's struggle with schizophrenia, as well as her experience with forced treatment, resulted in an intense interest in mental health and the law. Her doctors had painted a bleak picture of her future. They believed that she would not complete her degree or be able to hold a job or get married. However, Saks did marry and complete graduate school. She is a professor of law, psychology, and psychiatry at the University of Southern California and the founder and director of the Saks Institute for Mental Health Law, Policy and Ethics, a research institute dedicated to interdisciplinary collaboration involving scholars and policymakers who are focused on issues of mental health and mental illness.

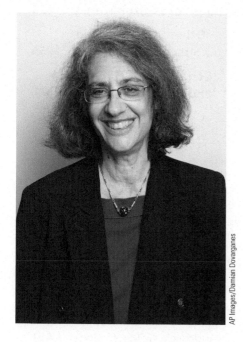

AP Images/Damian Dovarganes

ike Elyn Saks, individuals with **schizophrenia** and some of the related disorders on the **schizophrenia spectrum** experience specific symptoms, including:

- an impaired sense of reality known as **psychosis;**
- hallucinations (seeing or hearing things that are not actually present) and delusions (false beliefs);
- impaired cognitive processes (including confused speech);
- unusual or disorganized motor behavior; and
- uncommon behaviors that affect social interactions.

Although schizophrenia itself is considered a serious mental illness, the schizophrenia spectrum disorders vary in severity, duration of symptoms, causes, and outcome. One of the major challenges with schizophrenia and related disorders is **anosognosia**, an inability of those living with the condition to recognize their own mental confusion. This impaired awareness of illness is often why individuals living with schizophrenia fail to comprehend the importance of seeking treatment or complying with medical recommendations.

These disorders, particularly schizophrenia, receive a great deal of attention because they profoundly affect the individual, as well as family members and friends. People who have undergone a psychotic episode often mention that the experience is very confusing and damaging to their self-confidence. Initial psychotic episodes can be particularly scary because the person has no explanation for what is occurring. Psychosis is highly distressing because the hallucinations seem real and the delusions seem logical. The period after a psychotic breakdown is often full of chaos and confusion, especially if the individual is separated from family and friends due to hospitalization.

A diagnosis of schizophrenia in a member of the family affects all members of the unit. Common family experiences after an initial diagnosis include feelings of despair, worry that they might have somehow contributed to the illness, feelings of being unable to talk about their experiences with friends and family due to the stigma of mental illness, and economic strain. In the following first-person account, Eric Sundstrom presents a personal perspective on the distressing changes he witnessed in his older sister after she developed schizophrenia.

Case Study My family spent 3 years in Holland when my sister was in middle school. I think she was truly happy then, forming friendships and teaching me about the things she loved. It seems incredible she was once an ordinary girl, full of vibrant personality. I still remember how she taught me to read, using a now-ancient copy of *The Cat in the Hat*. When our family returned to America, all of her friends signed the clogs for her to remember them by. The clogs and a few memories are my only window into who she was then and who she should be now. (Sundstrom, 2004, p. 191)

Eric recalls how his sister developed delusions and unpredictable behavior during her sophomore year in high school. Auditory hallucinations insulted her and commanded her to break things. One day, his sister's hallucinations intensified and, following the commands, she began to destroy items throughout the house. After Eric and his brother cleaned up the broken glass and silently began eating their dinner, they realized that their sister had thoughtfully baked quiche for them—one side filled with vegetables for his brother and the other side plain, the way he liked it. Eric felt a profound sense of loss for the person that existed before the illness struck. As you can imagine, when psychotic symptoms develop, the experience can be confusing, frightening, and heart wrenching for everyone involved.

In this chapter, we begin with an in-depth discussion of symptoms associated with schizophrenia and other disorders on the schizophrenia spectrum. We then discuss the diagnosis, etiology, and treatment of schizophrenia and conclude with an overview of other disorders on the schizophrenia spectrum.

12-1 Symptoms of Schizophrenia Spectrum Disorders

The symptoms associated with schizophrenia spectrum disorders fall into four categories: *positive symptoms*, *cognitive symptoms*, *psychomotor abnormalities*, and *negative symptoms* (Cayouette et al., 2023).

Positive Symptoms

Case Study   Over a month before he committed a mass shooting at the Washington Navy Yard, Aaron Alexis called police to report that three people—two men and one woman—were following him. He explained that he was unable to sleep because these people talked to him through the walls, ceiling, and floors of his hotel room. He also reported that they were using a microwave to send vibrations into his body. (Winter, 2013)

Positive symptoms associated with schizophrenia spectrum disorders involve delusions, hallucinations, disordered thinking, incoherent communication, and peculiar behavior. The term *positive symptoms* refers to the "added" sensations and behaviors associated with schizophrenia. These experiences can range in severity and duration. In the case above, Alexis experienced two positive symptoms: auditory hallucinations (hearing voices) and a delusion that three people were following him, keeping him awake, and sending vibrations into his body.

Delusions

Many individuals with psychotic disorders experience delusions. **Delusions** are false beliefs that are firmly and consistently held despite disconfirming evidence or logic. Individuals experiencing delusions are not able to distinguish between their private thoughts and external reality. Lack of insight is particularly common among individuals experiencing delusions; in other words, they do not recognize that their thoughts or beliefs are extremely illogical. In the following case study, therapists attempted to rationally discuss a graduate student's delusion that rats were inside his head, consuming a section of his brain.

Although some individuals with delusions, like Erin, attempt to maintain some sense of logic, most are either unaware or only moderately aware that their delusions or other symptoms are illogical or reflective of mental illness (Figure 12.1).

A variety of delusional themes occur in schizophrenia spectrum disorders, including:

- *Delusions of grandeur*: Individuals may believe they are someone famous or powerful (from the present or the past).
- *Delusions of control*: Individuals may believe that other people, animals, or objects are trying to influence or control them.
- *Delusions of thought broadcasting*: Individuals may believe that others can hear or can control their thoughts.
- *Delusions of persecution*: Individuals may believe that others are plotting against, mistreating, or even trying to kill them.
- *Delusions of reference*: Individuals may believe they are the center of attention or that all happenings revolve around them.
- *Delusions of thought withdrawal*: Individuals may believe that someone or something is removing thoughts from their mind.

A common delusion involves **paranoid ideation**, or suspiciousness about the actions or motives of others as presented in the following case.

Figure 12.1

Lack of Awareness of Psychotic Symptoms in Individuals with Schizophrenia

Most individuals with schizophrenia are unaware or only somewhat aware that they have signs or symptoms of mental illness. The symptoms they are most unaware of include asociality, delusions, and restricted affect.

Source: Amador, X. (2006). Percentage of patients with schizophrenia who were unaware of these signs and symptoms of their illness. http://mentalillnesspolicy.org/medical/lack-of-insight-schizophrenia.pdf. Used by permission of Dr. Xavier Amador.

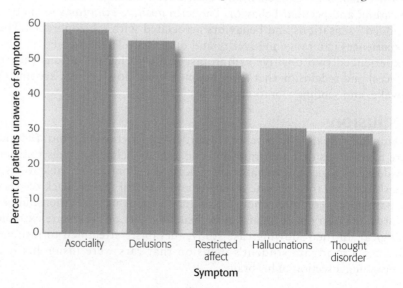

Case Study   I was convinced that a foreign agency was sending people out to get rid of me. I was so convinced because I kept receiving messages from them via a device planted inside my brain.... I decided to strike first: to kill myself so they wouldn't have a chance to carry out their plans and kill me. (Kean, 2011, p. 4)

Those with paranoid thinking often experience **persecutory delusions,** or beliefs that others are plotting against them, talking about them, or out to harm them in some way. The man in the case study was so concerned about the conspiracy against him that he decided to take his own life to prevent their plot from succeeding. Fortunately, he received help before his delusional thinking resulted in suicide. Those with paranoid ideation often have high levels of anxiety and worry, as well as angry reactions to perceived persecution (Diaconescu et al., 2019). They are suspicious, and their delusional thinking causes them to misinterpret the behavior and motives of others. A busy clerk who fails to offer help is part of a plot to mistreat them. A telephone call that was a wrong number is an act of harassment or an attempt to monitor their comings and goings. As you can imagine, such interpretations can further reinforce paranoid thinking.

Delusions can produce strong emotional reactions such as fear, depression, or anger. Those with persecutory delusions may respond to perceived threats by leaving "dangerous" situations, avoiding areas where they might be attacked, or becoming more vigilant. Paradoxically, these "safety" behaviors may prevent them from encountering **disconfirmatory evidence** (information that contradicts the delusional belief), thus reinforcing the idea that the lack of catastrophe was due to their cautionary behaviors. In one sample of individuals with delusions, between 80 percent and 90 percent had engaged in safety-seeking behavior in the previous month (Gaynor et al., 2013).

Delusions may involve a single theme or multiple topics, as was the case for one woman who believed that celebrities were talking to her through

Painting by Someone With Schizophrenia

The inner turmoil and private fantasies of people with schizophrenia are often revealed in their artwork. This painting was created by an individual with schizophrenia. What do you think the painting symbolizes?

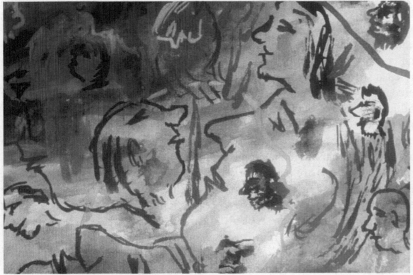

BSIP/Universal Images Group/Getty Images

the television, that her deceased husband was still alive and cheating on her, and that her internal organs were getting infected (Mahgoub & Hossain, 2006). Delusions may include plausible themes, such as being followed or spied on, as well as bizarre beliefs, such as plots to remove internal organs or perform mind control. The strength of delusional beliefs and their effects on the person's life can vary significantly. Delusions have less impact when the individual is able to consider alternative explanations for the delusion or acknowledge that others may question the accuracy of the belief.

Capgras delusion, named after the person who first reported it, is a rare type of delusion involving a belief in the existence of identical doubles who replace significant others. The mother of one woman with Capgras delusion explained how her daughter would phone her and ask questions such as what she had worn as a Halloween costume at the age of 12 or who had attended a specific birthday party: "She was testing me because she didn't think I was her mother. . . . No matter what question I answered, she was just sobbing" (Stark, 2004). The daughter believed that an impostor in a bodysuit had kidnapped her mother and was then pretending to be her mother. Elyn Saks, described at the beginning of this chapter, had Capgras delusion when she believed that an evil double had replaced her therapist. In her case, the delusion was a symptom of her chronic schizophrenia. However, Capgras delusion is also found with brief forms of psychosis that develop suddenly after an emotionally distressing event and often involves a person with whom the individual has close emotional ties (Salvatore et al., 2014).

Hallucinations

Case Study An individual describes their experience with auditory hallucinations while hospitalized with schizophrenia:

"You're alone," an insidious voice told me. "You're going to get what's coming to you." . . . No one moved or looked startled. It was just me hearing the voice. . . . I had seen others screaming back at their voices. . . . I did not want to look mad, like them. . . . Never admit you hear voices. . . . Never question your diagnosis or disagree with your psychiatrist . . . or you will never be discharged. (Gray, 2008, p. 1006)

A **hallucination** is a perception of a nonexistent or absent stimuli; it may involve a single sensory modality or a combination of modalities, including hearing (*auditory hallucination*), seeing (*visual hallucination*), smelling (*olfactory hallucination*), touching (*tactile hallucination*), or tasting (*gustatory hallucination*). Auditory hallucinations are most common; the voices can be malicious or benevolent or involve both qualities. As you can surmise from the case study, some individuals with hallucinations recognize that their perceptions are not real and try their best to "look normal" even when the hallucinations are occurring. Although individuals with psychosis sometimes jump to a conclusion or make quick decisions based on the perceived "truthfulness" of a hallucination, they also report that it is easier to ignore hallucinations that are inconsistent with their beliefs (Dudley et al., 2016).

Hallucinations are particularly distressing when they involve dominant, insulting voices. These hallucinations can be quite unsettling; those who hear destructive voices often try to cope by ignoring them or by keeping busy with other activities. Not all auditory hallucinations are upsetting, however. One individual reported hearing encouraging voices: "I thought I could hear the voice of God, and it was God who told me to refer myself for mental health help" (Jepson, 2013, p. 483).

Should We Challenge Delusions and Hallucinations?

The doctor asked a patient who insisted that he was dead: "Look. Dead men don't bleed, right?" When the man agreed, the doctor pricked the man's finger, and showed him the blood. The patient said, "What do you know, dead men do bleed after all." (Walkup, 1995, p. 323)

Clinicians are often unsure about whether to challenge psychotic symptoms. Some contend that delusions and hallucinations serve an adaptive function and that any attempt to change them would be useless or even dangerous. The example of the man who believed he was dead demonstrates the apparent futility of using logic with delusions. However, many clinicians have found that some clients respond well to challenges to their hallucinations and delusions (Ross et al., 2011).

Coltheart et al. (2007) used a "gentle and tactful offering of evidence" to successfully treat a man who believed his wife was not his wife but was, instead, his business partner. The man was asked to entertain the possibility that the woman was actually his wife. The therapist pointed out that the woman was wearing a wedding ring identical to the one he had bought for his wife. The man said that the woman probably bought the ring from the same shop. He was then shown that the initials engraved in the ring were those of his wife. Within 1 week, he accepted the fact that the woman was his wife. This approach of gently presenting contradictory information and having clients consider alternative explanations appears to be a successful approach to weakening delusions.

For Further Consideration

1. Should we challenge psychotic symptoms? If so, what is the best way of doing so?

2. In what ways might hallucinations or delusions serve an adaptive function?

Auditory hallucinations seem very real to the individual experiencing them and sometimes involve relationship-like qualities (Perona-Garcelán et al., 2020). In one study of individuals hospitalized with acute psychosis, 61 percent of respondents reported that the voice they heard had a distinct gender; 46 percent believed that the voice was that of a friend, family member, or acquaintance; and 80 percent reported having back-and-forth conversations with the voice. Most believed the voices were independent entities. Some even conducted "research" to test the reality of the voices. One woman said she initially thought that the voice might be her own but rejected it when the voice called her "Mommy," something she would not call herself. Another woman explained, "They are not imaginary. They see what I do. They tell me that I'm baking a cake. They must be there. How else would they know what I'm doing?" (Garrett & Silva, 2003, p. 447).

The strength of hallucinations and delusions can vary significantly among individuals experiencing psychosis. Some believe in them 100 percent, whereas others are less certain. Further, some individuals are able to combat delusions and hallucinations by testing out the reality of their thinking. For example, when faced with delusions or hallucinations, one person learned to ask himself, "What's the evidence for that?" (Saks, 2013).

People with symptoms such as hallucinations or delusions often do not understand that their symptoms are the result of mental illness. This anosognosia or lack of insight is most common among those with severe symptoms and those who had difficulties functioning before the onset of their mental illness. Those who lack insight have a greater likelihood of experiencing poor compliance with treatment recommendations and lower levels of community functioning. Anosognosia may not be present in all areas of functioning. For example, some individuals might be unaware that their thinking is delusional, yet might recognize that the voices they are hearing are hallucinations (Konstantakopoulos, 2019). Although better insight increases compliance with treatment and results in a better prognosis for improvement, awareness of having a serious mental illness can lead to depression, feelings of hopelessness, self-stigma, and an increased risk of

Did You Know?

In an effort to increase empathy for people experiencing psychosis, pharmacy students were asked to perform a series of mental tasks while listening to an audio tape simulating auditory hallucinations. The participants reported feeling stressed and anxious; they also had difficulty with memory and concentration. All of the students agreed that the demonstration increased their empathy for people living with mental illness.
Source: Skoy et al., 2016

suicide. Therapists can assist clients who have gained insight into their illness by focusing on the potential for recovery when treatment recommendations are followed (Lysaker et al., 2018).

Cognitive Symptoms

Disordered thinking, communication, and speech are common cognitive characteristics of schizophrenia. The cognitive symptoms are generally present even before the onset of the first psychotic episode. They also tend to persist even with treatment and are found (to a lesser degree) among nonpsychotic relatives of individuals with schizophrenia (Silberstein & Harvey, 2019).

When disordered thinking occurs, individuals with psychosis have trouble inhibiting verbalizations that are loosely connected to previous words or thoughts. Thus, there is no hierarchical structure or organization to their thinking (Manschreck et al., 2012). Individuals experiencing these symptoms may change topics, speak in an unintelligible manner, or reply tangentially to questions. This **loosening of associations**, also referred to as *cognitive slippage*, involves a continual shifting from topic to topic without any apparent logical or meaningful connection between thoughts. Disorganized communication often includes the incoherent speech or idiosyncratic responses demonstrated in the following case study.

Case Study   INTERVIEWER: "You just must be an emotional person, that's all." PATIENT: "Well, not very much I mean, what if I were dead? It's a funeral age. Well, I . . . um. Now I had my toenails operated on. They got infected and I wasn't able to do it. But they wouldn't let me at my tools." (Thomas, 1995, p. 289)

The beginning phrase in the person's first sentence appears appropriate to the interviewer's comment. However, the reference to death later in the sentence is not. Loosening of associations is also apparent in the references to a funeral age, toenails, and tools, since none of these thoughts are related to the interviewer's conversational focus.

Individuals with schizophrenia also demonstrate *overinclusiveness* in their thinking. For instance, when asked to sort cards with pictures of animals, fruit, clothing, and body parts into piles of things that go together, one man placed an ear, apple, pineapple, pear, strawberry, lips, orange, and banana together in a category he named "something to eat." When asked the reason for including the ear and lips in the "something to eat" category, he explained that an ear allows you to hear a person asking for fruit, and lips allow you to ask for and eat fruit (Doughty et al., 2009). In another study, individuals with schizophrenia wore a head-mounted virtual reality display that gave them the sense of going through a neighborhood, a shopping center, and a market. Fifty incoherencies such as a mooing dog, an upside-down house, and a red cloud were presented during the journey. Almost 90 percent of those with schizophrenia failed to detect these inconsistencies. Even when the inconsistencies were identified, about two thirds of the participants had difficulty explaining them (Sorkin et al., 2008). Another cognitive characteristic is that people with schizophrenia may respond to words or phrases in a very concrete manner. For example, a saying such as "a rolling stone gathers no moss" might be interpreted as meaning no more than "moss cannot grow on a rock that is rolling."

Individuals with schizophrenia often demonstrate moderately severe to severe impairment in executive functioning—deficits in the ability to sustain attention, to absorb and interpret information, to make decisions, and to carry out tasks. Difficulties with social-cognitive skills; social perspective taking; and understanding one's own and other's thoughts, motivations, and emotions are also common. These neurocognitive deficits play a significant role in the difficulties that individuals with schizophrenia experience in the areas of work and schooling (Seidman et al., 2016).

Psychomotor Abnormalities

Case Study A man was brought into the emergency department standing stiff as a statue with one arm hand held up. He was verbally unresponsive and stayed that way for several days. After successful treatment, the man had said he had heard a voice from the sky that told him he could stop flooding in the city by holding up his hand. (Ruiz, 2021)

The symptoms of schizophrenia that involve motor functions, such as those in this case study, can be extremely distressing to family members. This man was experiencing an episode of **catatonia**, a condition involving extremes in activity level, peculiar body movements or postures, strange gestures and grimaces, or a combination of these (refer to Figure 12.2 for symptoms associated with catatonia).

People experiencing *withdrawn catatonia* are extremely unresponsive, despite appearing to be awake and aware of all that is going on around them. They may exhibit prolonged periods of stupor and mutism. Some may adopt and maintain strange postures and refuse to move or change position. They may stand for hours at a time, perhaps with one arm stretched out to the side. They also may lie on the floor or sit awkwardly on a chair, staring, aware of what is occurring but not responding or moving. If someone attempts to change the

An Episode of Withdrawn Catatonia

The woman in the wheelchair is experiencing a form of catatonia that involves unresponsiveness and the adoption of a rigid body posture. Positions such as this are sometimes held for hours, days, weeks, or even months at a time.

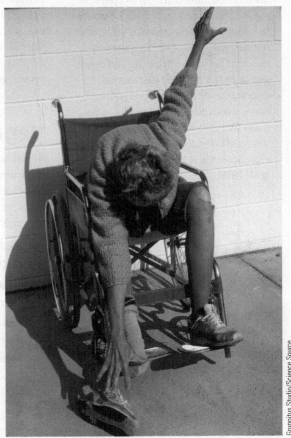

Grunnitus Studio/Science Source

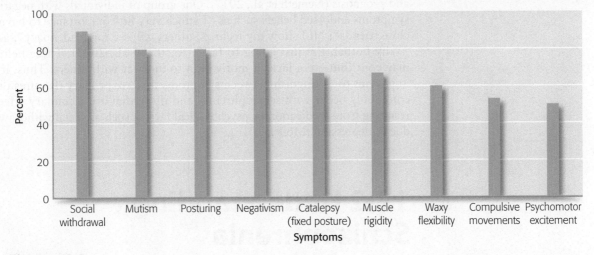

Figure 12.2

Prevalence of Symptoms in 30 Young Patients with Catatonia

Catatonic symptoms can vary significantly.

Source: Cornic et al., 2007

person's position, they may persistently resist. Others exhibit a waxy flexibility, allowing their bodies to be arranged in almost any position and then remaining in that position for long periods. The extreme withdrawal associated with a catatonic episode can be life-threatening when it results in inadequate food or liquid intake.

In contrast with the stupor associated with withdrawn catatonia, people displaying *excited catatonia* have disorganized behavior and may be agitated, hyperactive, and/or lack inhibitions. In this less common version of catatonia, they may talk and shout constantly, moving or running until they drop from exhaustion. They may appear to be acting "silly" and display loud, inappropriate laughter. They sleep little and are continually on the go. Their behavior can become dangerous and involve violent actions (Walther et al., 2019).

Negative Symptoms

Negative symptoms of schizophrenia involve deficits in typical human functioning such as decreased ability to initiate actions or speech, express emotions, or feel pleasure (Cella et al., 2017). The term *negative* is used because certain behaviors or experiences are diminished or lost from a person's life once schizophrenia develops. Negative symptoms include:

- **avolition**: profound apathy, including an inability to initiate or persist in goal-directed behavior;
- **alogia**: a lack of meaningful speech;
- **asociality:** minimal interest in social relationships;
- **anhedonia**: reduced ability to experience pleasure from positive events; and
- **diminished emotional expression**: reduced display of emotion involving facial expressions, voice intonation, or gestures in situations in which emotional reactions are expected.

Negative symptoms are common in individuals with schizophrenia spectrum disorders. In fact, over half of those diagnosed with schizophrenia display negative symptoms (Sicras-Mainar et al., 2014). Negative symptoms are more common in men and are associated with poor social functioning and prognosis (Németh et al., 2017). One group of individuals with negative symptoms endorsed beliefs such as "I attach very little importance to having close friends"; "If I show my feelings, others will see my inadequacy"; and "Why bother, I'm just going to fail" (Rector et al., 2005). These beliefs may contribute to a lack of motivation to interact with others. Thus, it is important to distinguish between symptoms that are primary (features that commonly occur with schizophrenia) and those that are secondary effects resulting from medication or psychological factors such as social withdrawal due to depression (Möller, 2016).

12-2 Understanding Schizophrenia

According to the DSM-5-TR, a diagnosis of schizophrenia requires the presence of two of the following: delusions, hallucinations, disorganized speech, gross motor disturbances, or negative symptoms. At least one of the two indicators must be delusions, hallucinations, or disorganized speech (refer to Table 12.3, on page 466). Additionally, there is deterioration from a previous level of functioning in areas such as work, interpersonal relationships, or self-care. The symptoms must be present most of the time for at least 1 month, and the disturbance must persist for at least 6 months, unless the symptoms subside due to successful treatment (APA, 2022). Because the lifetime prevalence rate of schizophrenia in the United States is about 1 percent, this disorder affects millions of people (Alnaes et al., 2019).

Although sudden onset of psychotic behaviors can occur in previously well-functioning people, in most cases of schizophrenia, there is evidence of impairment in **premorbid** functioning; that is, individuals often demonstrate some abnormalities before the onset of major symptoms (Sheffield et al., 2018). Similarly, most people with schizophrenia recover from an illness episode gradually rather than suddenly. The typical course of schizophrenia consists of three phases: prodromal, active, and residual.

The **prodromal phase** includes the onset and buildup of schizophrenic symptoms. Social withdrawal and isolation, peculiar behaviors, inappropriate affect, poor communication patterns, and neglect of personal grooming may become evident during this phase. Friends and relatives often notice these differences and consider the changes in behavior as odd or peculiar. Psychosocial stressors or excessive demands on the individual in the prodromal phase may result in the onset of prominent psychotic symptoms, or the *active phase* of schizophrenia. In this phase, the person presents with full-blown symptoms of schizophrenia, including severe disturbances in thinking, significant deterioration in social relationships, and restricted or markedly inappropriate emotional expression. Eventually, the person may enter the *residual phase*, in which the symptoms are no longer prominent. In the residual phase, the psychotic behavior and symptom severity decline. Frequently, the individual once again demonstrates the milder impairment exhibited in the prodromal phase. Although long-term studies have found that many people with schizophrenia can lead productive lives, only about 20 percent show complete recovery (Onitsuka et al., 2022). (Figure 12.3 presents different courses schizophrenia may take.)

Long-Term Outcome Studies

What are the chances of recovering from or experiencing significant symptom improvement after an episode of schizophrenia? In a 5-year follow-up of older Dutch individuals hospitalized for schizophrenia symptoms, nearly 50 percent were in remission; only 4 percent had deteriorated (Lange et al., 2019). Similarly, in a 3-year follow-up study of Chinese patients in Hong Kong, 45 percent had a sustained remission of psychotic symptoms (Chang et al., 2013). In a longer term 20-year study, periods of 1 or more years of recovery were found for 13 percent of patients who displayed negative symptoms and for 63 percent of those who never displayed negative symptoms (Strauss et al., 2010). Researchers have celebrated findings of even better outcomes for individuals who participated in comprehensive programs focused on early identification and treatment for first-episode psychosis (Correll et al., 2018).

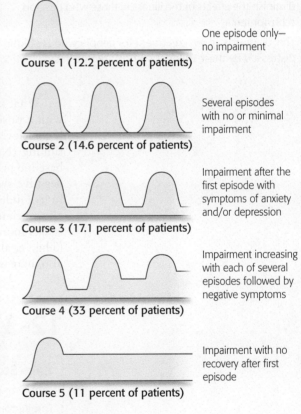

Course 1 (12.2 percent of patients)
One episode only—no impairment

Course 2 (14.6 percent of patients)
Several episodes with no or minimal impairment

Course 3 (17.1 percent of patients)
Impairment after the first episode with symptoms of anxiety and/or depression

Course 4 (33 percent of patients)
Impairment increasing with each of several episodes followed by negative symptoms

Course 5 (11 percent of patients)
Impairment with no recovery after first episode

Figure 12.3

Varying Outcomes with Schizophrenia

This figure indicates five trajectories and outcomes experienced by individuals with schizophrenia during a 15-year follow-up study.

Source: Wiersma et al., 1998

Attenuated Psychosis Syndrome: A Beneficial or Harmful Diagnosis?

A proposed diagnostic category, attenuated psychosis syndrome, has generated considerable discussion and debate. **Attenuated psychosis syndrome** involves symptoms such as distressing or disabling delusions, hallucinations, or disorganized speech that have emerged or become progressively worse over the previous year and that occur at least once per week; these symptoms are less severe and more transient than those experienced by individuals with schizophrenia. Despite these symptoms, the individual is able to stay in touch with reality (APA, 2022). Whether these "milder" signs of psychosis should warrant a psychiatric diagnosis is at the heart of extensive debate. Those in favor of this diagnostic category make several arguments (Pani & Keefe, 2019):

1. Symptoms of attenuated psychosis syndrome occurring in childhood and adolescence increase the risk for schizophrenia and other psychiatric impairment in adulthood.

2. Rapid deterioration often occurs during the early years of psychosis, so early intervention and treatment might diminish the effects of the illness in those who develop schizophrenia.

3. This diagnosis allows treatment for people who are highly distressed by these milder psychotic symptoms.

Opponents of including the attenuated psychosis syndrome diagnosis in the DSM argue that many individuals with this diagnosis will not develop a psychotic disorder ("false positives") and that premature diagnosis could result in unnecessary stigma and unwarranted use of antipsychotic medications (Zachar et al., 2020). They also point out that psychotic-type experiences are present not only in those with schizophrenia spectrum disorders but also in the general population (Hodgekins et al., 2018; Maijer et al., 2018). For example, reports of psychotic symptoms such as beliefs of persecution, thought interference, and auditory hallucinations are common among adolescents but, in most cases, are only transitory (Legge et al., 2019). Because of the controversy, the DSM-5 workgroup decided to include attenuated psychosis syndrome as a "condition that requires further research" rather than a specific diagnostic category.

For Further Consideration

1. What is your opinion about including attenuated psychosis syndrome as a specific diagnosis?

2. What position do you believe pharmaceutical companies will take regarding inclusion of the attenuated psychosis syndrome diagnosis when it is time to revise the DSM?

What factors influence recovery from schizophrenia? Factors associated with a positive outcome include gender (women have a better outcome), higher levels of education, and having a higher premorbid level of functioning (Novick et al., 2016). In a 10-year follow-up study examining baseline predictors associated with recovery, researchers found that fewer negative symptoms, a prior history of good work performance and ability to live independently, and lower levels of depression and aggression were all associated with improved outcome (Shrivastava et al., 2010). Recovery is also more likely for those who are married or have a network of friends (Sibitz et al., 2011). Lower levels of self-stigmatization and negative beliefs also increase the chances of recovery (Kao et al., 2017).

12-3 Etiology of Schizophrenia

Case Study   A 13-year-old boy who was having behavioral and academic problems in school was taking part in a series of family therapy sessions. Family communication was negative in tone, with a great deal of blaming. Near the end of one session, the boy suddenly broke down and cried out, "I don't want to be like her." He was referring to his mother, who had been receiving treatment for schizophrenia. Her unpredictable behavior frightened him, and he was concerned that his friends would find out about her condition. But his greatest fear was that he would inherit the disorder. Sobbing, he turned to the therapist and asked, "Am I going to be crazy, too?"

If you were the therapist in the case study, how would you respond? At the end of this section on the etiology of schizophrenia, you should be able to reach your own conclusion about what to tell the boy. Schizophrenia and other psychotic conditions are best understood using a multipath model that integrates heredity (genetic influences on brain structure and neurocognitive functioning), psychological characteristics, cognitive processes, and social adversities such as social or economic disadvantage. To develop an accurate etiological framework, all of these dimensions must be considered, as presented in Figure 12.4.

Although we discuss the biological, psychological, social, and sociocultural dimensions separately, keep in mind that each dimension interacts with the others. For instance, emotional or sexual abuse, cannabis use, and trauma are all hypothesized to affect brain functioning in those susceptible to schizophrenia. In one sample, each of these factors independently increased the risk of persistent psychotic symptoms. Moreover, the risk was particularly elevated for individuals who were exposed to all three influences (Stilo & Murray, 2019).

The interactive model of schizophrenia (refer to Figure 12.5) demonstrates how an underlying biological vulnerability combined with other risk characteristics (e.g., male sex, young age) can result in the development of prodromal symptoms of schizophrenia. As time progresses, psychotic features may appear or intensify if additional environmental risk factors (e.g., cannabis use, trauma, abuse, bullying) occur. If the environmental exposures are chronic or severe, the risk of developing schizophrenia further increases. With these complexities in mind, we now begin the discussion of specific risk factors associated with schizophrenia.

Obstacles to Recovery

The film *The Soloist* is based on the true story of Nathaniel Ayers (pictured on the left), a homeless musician living with schizophrenia. When *Los Angeles Times* columnist Steve Lopez attempted to help Ayers after writing an acclaimed series of articles about the talented musician, he ran into many of the obstacles facing people who are homeless and mentally ill.

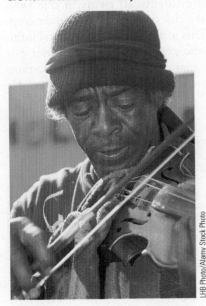

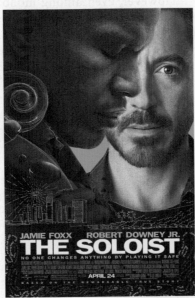

Figure 12.4

Multipath Model of Schizophrenia
The dimensions interact with one another and combine in different ways to result in schizophrenia.

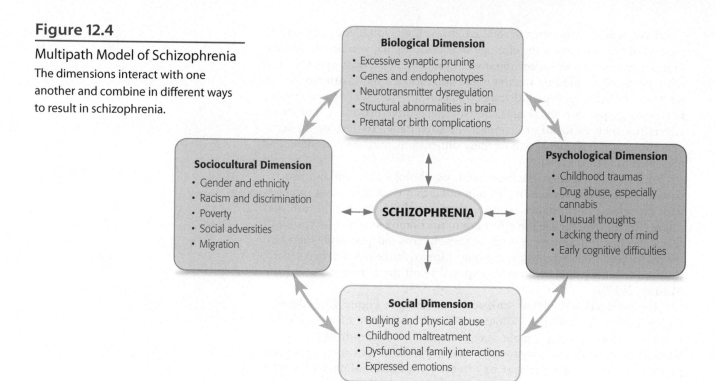

Biological Dimension
- Excessive synaptic pruning
- Genes and endophenotypes
- Neurotransmitter dysregulation
- Structural abnormalities in brain
- Prenatal or birth complications

Sociocultural Dimension
- Gender and ethnicity
- Racism and discrimination
- Poverty
- Social adversities
- Migration

SCHIZOPHRENIA

Psychological Dimension
- Childhood traumas
- Drug abuse, especially cannabis
- Unusual thoughts
- Lacking theory of mind
- Early cognitive difficulties

Social Dimension
- Bullying and physical abuse
- Childhood maltreatment
- Dysfunctional family interactions
- Expressed emotions

Biological Dimension

Genetics and heredity play an important role in the development of schizophrenia. Interactions between genes and the environment during gestation and early life set the stage for the development and functioning of neural structures. In terms of genetic influences, researchers have found that closer blood relatives of individuals diagnosed with schizophrenia run a greater risk of developing the disorder (Figure 12.6). Thus, the boy described in the case study earlier who is concerned about developing schizophrenia like his mother has a 16 percent chance of being diagnosed with schizophrenia, whereas his mother's nieces or nephews have only a 4 percent chance. (The risk for the general population is 1 percent.)

However, even among monozygotic (identical) twins, if one twin receives the diagnosis of schizophrenia, the risk of the second twin developing the disorder is less than 50 percent. This is because environmental influences also play a significant role in genetic expression of the disorder. For example, low birth weight and other pregnancy and delivery complications are associated with an increased risk for schizophrenia. Yet most people

Figure 12.5

Interactive Variables and the Onset of Clinical Psychosis

This model demonstrates how psychological and social factors may interact with genetic vulnerability to result in psychosis.

Source: Dominguez et al., 2010

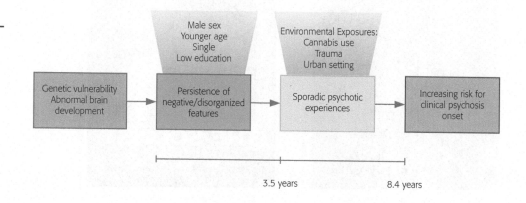

Male sex
Younger age
Single
Low education

Environmental Exposures:
Cannabis use
Trauma
Urban setting

Genetic vulnerability
Abnormal brain development

Persistence of negative/disorganized features

Sporadic psychotic experiences

Increasing risk for clinical psychosis onset

3.5 years   8.4 years

who are exposed to these types of early life complications never develop the disorder. Instead, it is primarily among those with genetic susceptibility that complications occurring prenatally or during birth present a risk (Forsyth et al., 2013).

Genetic Linkage Studies

Whereas past research focused on identifying the specific gene or genes that cause schizophrenia, the disorder is now understood to result from interactions among a large number of different genes; single genes appear to make only minor contributions toward the illness. Researchers are now identifying different genetic regions suspected to be associated with psychosis. For example, various alleles of the C4 gene can exist on one section of chromosome 6; several of these C4 alleles are now believed to have a strong association with schizophrenia. During typical brain development, when these alleles of the C4 gene are turned on during late adolescence, the "pruning" of excessive synapses or brain connections formed during childhood begins. It is hypothesized that some of the symptoms in schizophrenia result from an abnormal and overactive pruning process. In mice genetically engineered to have C4 allele abnormalities, the pruning process was indeed overactive, eliminating important brain connections. Interestingly, the neurological pruning process normally occurs during late adolescence or early adulthood, the time period during which initial symptoms of psychosis are most likely to appear (Sekar et al., 2016). Supporting these findings, PET scans have demonstrated that individuals with schizophrenia have weakened synaptic activity in areas of the cortex that are related to specific symptoms; it is hypothesized that these abnormalities could be the result of excessive pruning (Onwordi et al., 2020).

Polygenetic risk scores focusing on which combination of genes might help explain genetic risk are increasingly used in the study of schizophrenia. This is accomplished by comparing the genome variants of individuals with and without the disorder. One study relied on demographic, clinical, and genetic data for 540 individuals with schizophrenia and 844 control subjects from the National Institute of Mental Health data pool (Dickinson et al., 2020). Analyzing IQ scores before and after illness, the researchers identified three cognitive trajectory subgroups (refer to Figure 12.7):

1. *Cognitively stable adolescent development* (37 percent). This subgroup had no difficulties in early academic and cognitive functioning, a mild course of illness, and the best employment record compared to the other subgroups.

2. *Adolescent disruption of previous cognitive development* (44 percent). This subgroup had the most severe symptoms and significant decline in cognitive functioning after diagnosis, low levels of employment, and a genetic profile indicating significant risk of developing schizophrenia.

3. *Preadolescent cognitive impairment* (19 percent). This subgroup had continuous cognitive impairment, including childhood learning problems. They completed less schooling and had low rates of employment.

Endophenotypes

Another strategy in genetic research in schizophrenia involves a focus on the specific characteristics or traits demonstrated by those diagnosed with the disorder. This approach involves the identification and study of

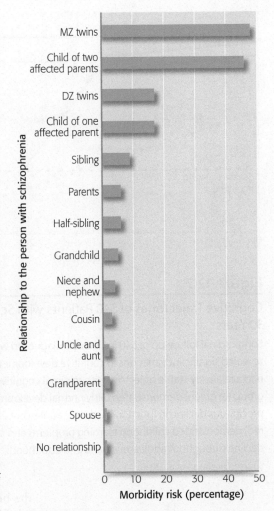

Figure 12.6

Risk of Schizophrenia Among Blood Relatives of Individuals Diagnosed with Schizophrenia

This figure reflects the estimate of the lifetime risk of developing schizophrenia—a risk that is strongly correlated with the degree of genetic influence.

Source: Data from Gottesman, 1978, 1991

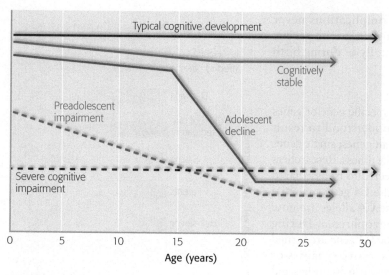

Figure 12.7

Cognitive Trajectories of 540 Patients with Schizophrenia Over 30 Years

Longitudinal follow-up of 540 individuals diagnosed with schizophrenia revealed significant variations in cognitive development; one group (in blue) had a relatively stable trajectory with minimal cognitive decline, another group (in green) demonstrated fairly normal development followed by a precipitous decline in functioning during adolescence, and a third group (in red) demonstrated childhood learning problems and continuous cognitive decline throughout adolescence and into adulthood.

Source: Dickinson et al., 2020

endophenotypes—measurable, heritable traits. Endophenotypes are hypothesized to underlie heritable illnesses (such as schizophrenia) and thus exist in the individual before the disorder, while symptoms are present, and following remission. Researchers have identified several possible endophenotypes associated with schizophrenia—characteristics found with higher frequency, although in milder forms, among "non-ill" relatives of individuals with schizophrenia. These traits include irregularities in working memory, executive function, sustained attention, and verbal memory (Blokland et al., 2018).

Neurostructures

How do genes produce a vulnerability to schizophrenia? Clues to the ways in which a person's genome might increase susceptibility have involved the identification of structural and neurochemical differences between individuals with and without schizophrenia. For instance, in individuals with schizophrenia, fMRI scans have found that areas of the limbic system associated with emotions are overactive in response to neutral stimuli. This may lead to hypervigilance, delusional thoughts, and a tendency to respond to situations as "threatening" (Dugré et al., 2019). Additionally, dysfunctions in the striatum (the part of the brain where corrective feedback occurs) may explain the difficulties modifying illogical thoughts or delusions associated with schizophrenia (Karcher et al., 2019).

Individuals with schizophrenia have gray matter loss in the cortex, amygdala, hippocampus, thalamus, and other areas of the brain (Haijma et al., 2013), as well as enlargement of the ventricles in the brain (Chung et al., 2017). Not surprisingly, individuals with schizophrenia who have the greatest loss of gray matter also demonstrate the most significant cognitive deficits (Van Rheenen et al., 2018). White matter abnormalities affecting the connectivity between different areas of the brain are also evident and may explain the widespread cognitive and perceptual disruption associated with schizophrenia (Klauser et al., 2017).

A striking loss of brain cells in the cortex over a period of 6 years among young people with schizophrenia was reported in a longitudinal study comparing brain changes in youth with and without schizophrenia. The loss was so rapid that it was likened to a "forest fire" (Thompson et al., 2001). Part of this loss may be due to excessive synaptic pruning, an acceleration of the process that typically occurs in later adolescence and early adulthood. Fortunately, this rate of gray matter loss appears to slow down in later years (Cropley et al., 2017). Healthy siblings of adolescents with child-onset schizophrenia demonstrated similar cortical loss that also normalized in later adulthood (Ordóñez, Luscher, & Gogtay, 2016).

How might decreased cortex volume and enlarged ventricles explain symptoms of schizophrenia? These structural characteristics may result in atypical or weak connectivity between the various brain regions, leading to reductions in integrative functioning within the brain and impaired cognitive processing (Salgado-Pineda et al., 2007). Thus, ineffective communication between different brain regions may lead to the **cognitive symptoms** (e.g., disorganized speech and impairment in memory, decision making, and problem solving), negative symptoms (e.g., lack of drive or initiative), and positive symptoms (e.g., delusions and hallucinations) that are found in schizophrenia. Although some of the abnormalities found in the brains of individuals with schizophrenia may result from the use of antipsychotic medication rather than the disorder itself, scientists have found structural abnormalities in individuals with schizophrenia who never took antipsychotic medication (Davidson, 2018).

Biochemical Influences

Abnormalities in certain neurotransmitters (chemicals that allow brain cells to communicate with one another), including dopamine, serotonin, GABA, and glutamate, have also been linked to schizophrenia. Their alteration can lead to abnormal functioning of neurocircuitry throughout the brain, thereby producing cognitive, behavioral, and social dysfunction (Yang & Tsai, 2017). Researchers are particularly interested in the neurotransmitter dopamine. According to the **dopamine hypothesis**, schizophrenia develops due to excessive dopamine-related activity in certain areas of the brain (Kokkinou et al., 2020). Support for the dopamine hypothesis has come from research with three types of drugs: phenothiazines, L-dopa, and amphetamines.

- *Phenothiazines* are conventional antipsychotic drugs that decrease the severity of disordered thinking, decrease social withdrawal, alleviate hallucinations, and improve the mood of individuals with schizophrenia. Phenothiazines reduce dopamine activity in the brain by blocking dopamine receptor sites.

- *L-dopa* is used to treat symptoms of Parkinson's disease, such as muscle and limb rigidity and tremors. L-dopa increases levels of dopamine; schizophrenic-like side effects often occur in individuals with Parkinson's disease who take this medication. (In contrast, the phenothiazines, which reduce dopamine activity, can produce side effects that resemble Parkinson's disease.)

- *Amphetamines* are stimulants that increase the availability of dopamine and norepinephrine (another neurotransmitter) in the brain. When individuals not diagnosed with schizophrenia use amphetamines, they sometimes present with symptoms very much like those of acute paranoid schizophrenia. Also, even small doses of amphetamine can increase the severity of symptoms in individuals diagnosed with schizophrenia.

Thus, one group of drugs that blocks dopamine reception has the effect of reducing the severity of schizophrenic symptoms, whereas two drugs that increase dopamine availability either produce or worsen these symptoms. Such evidence suggests that excess dopamine may be responsible for schizophrenic symptoms.

The evidence is not clear-cut, however. Phenothiazines are not effective in treating many cases of schizophrenia, and newer antipsychotics such as clozapine and risperidone work mainly by blocking serotonin receptors rather than dopamine receptors. In addition, individuals with schizophrenia often have decreased glutamate levels, and abuse of drugs such as ketamine, which binds to glutamate, can also produce psychotic symptoms (Yang & Tsai, 2017). This suggests that researchers may be looking for an oversimplified explanation by focusing on dopamine alone without considering the interactive biochemical functioning that occurs throughout the brain.

Because schizophrenia involves multiple neurochemicals and brain regions, it is unlikely that one "magic bullet" medication will successfully treat all forms of schizophrenia.

The use of cocaine, amphetamines, alcohol, and especially cannabis can produce a temporary, substance-induced psychotic episode as well as increase the risk of developing schizophrenia. In one study, the percentage of individuals who developed schizophrenia after experiencing substance-induced psychosis was highest for cannabis (35 percent) followed by hallucinogens (26 percent), amphetamines (22 percent), opioids (12 percent), alcohol (10 percent), and sedatives (9 percent) (Murrie et al., 2020). Cannabis has a strong association with the onset of psychotic symptoms in vulnerable individuals and may worsen symptoms in those with psychotic disorders (West & Sharif, 2023). During the past two decades, the number of cases of schizophrenia associated with cannabis-use disorder has increased 3 or 4 fold, probably due the greater use of and higher potency of cannabis (Hjorthøj et al., 2021).

The effects of cannabis occur in a dose-dependent manner—the higher the intake of cannabis, the greater the likelihood of psychotic symptoms. Heavy, chronic, and early use of cannabis has been consistently associated with psychosis-related symptoms and reduced attention, memory, and cognitive flexibility (D'Souza et al., 2020). Use of high-potency forms of cannabis also increases the risk of psychosis (Di Forti et al., 2019). Among cannabis users who develop schizophrenia, the onset of psychosis is nearly 3 years earlier in comparison to nonusers (Large et al., 2011). In one study of individuals (mostly young men) who experienced an episode of psychosis, 46 percent were cannabis users. During a 5-year follow-up period, the group who used cannabis had "substantially worse clinical outcomes," including more frequent and compulsory hospitalizations, more days hospitalized, and more treatment failure and relapse (Patel et al., 2016).

Cannabis use is associated with structural changes in the brain similar to those found in schizophrenia, including reductions in grey matter (Lawrie, 2018) and altered connectivity throughout the brain (Sami et al., 2020). Researchers have proposed that cannabis interacts with a schizophrenia risk gene (ZNF804A) to trigger psychosis (Soler et al., 2019). Of particular concern is the finding that cannabis alters the neurotransmission pathways associated with psychosis and interferes with the overall neurodevelopment of the adolescent brain (Vaucher et al., 2018).

Although the prevalence of schizophrenia is roughly equal between men and women, the age of onset is about 4 to 6 years earlier in men. The gender ratio shifts by the mid-40s and 50s, when the percentage of women receiving a schizophrenia diagnosis begins to exceed that of men; this trend is especially pronounced among individuals diagnosed in their mid-60s and later (Ordóñez, Loeb, et al., 2016). Researchers have hypothesized that the later age of onset found in women is because the protective effects of estrogen diminish after menopause (Sommer et al., 2023).

A variety of studies support the view that estrogen appears to protect against psychotic symptoms. In a study of premenopausal women with schizophrenia, significant improvements in psychotic symptoms were observed during the luteal phase of their menstrual cycle (the period after ovulation), when estrogen levels are highest (Bergemann et al., 2008). Use of an estrogen patch as an adjunct to antipsychotic medication in women of child-bearing age results in a greater reduction of symptoms compared to antipsychotic medication alone, especially among women approaching menopause (Weiser et al., 2019). Further, women with schizophrenia who have estrogen replacement therapy for menopausal symptoms also report improved cognitive functioning (Bergemann et al., 2008).

Because the **concordance rate**—the likelihood that both members of a twin pair demonstrate the same characteristic—is less than 50 percent when one identical twin has schizophrenia, other factors that are not shared between the twins must also play a role. Conditions influencing prenatal or postnatal neurodevelopment that have been associated with schizophrenia include pregnancy and birth complications, prenatal infections such as influenza and measles, and head trauma (Stilo & Murray, 2019). Although a variety of biological influences appear to increase susceptibility to schizophrenia, specific psychological, social, and sociocultural variables can also influence development of the disorder. We now examine these influences.

Psychological Dimension

Individuals who develop schizophrenia often have cognitive attributes, dysfunctional beliefs, and interpersonal functioning that may predispose them to the development of psychotic symptoms. For example, characteristics such as deficits in empathy (understanding the feelings of others) or a tendency to focus only on one's own thoughts and feelings may compromise social interactions (Silberstein & Harvey, 2019). These attributes may also affect nonverbal communication. For instance, individuals with schizophrenia tend to gesture less when speaking and nod less frequently when listening compared to individuals without the disorder. Such a communication pattern may interfere with the development of interpersonal rapport and emotional connection (Lavelle et al., 2013). Among healthy adolescents, poorer interpersonal functioning during adolescence predicted perceptual abnormalities and delusional thinking later in life (Collip et al., 2013).

These communication problems and the lack of insight that frequently occurs with schizophrenia may result, in part, from deficits in the **theory of mind**—the ability to recognize that others have emotions, beliefs, and desires that may be different from one's own. Thus, individuals with schizophrenia may operate based on their own perspectives, without understanding that others have their own point of view (Charernboon, 2020). As you might imagine, this could create major difficulties in communication and interpersonal interactions.

Early cognitive deficits are also associated with schizophrenia. Numerous studies have documented an association between early developmental delay and schizophrenia (Stilo & Murray, 2019). One large prospective population study found that infants who later developed schizophrenia were slower to smile, lift their heads, sit, crawl, and walk compared to infants who did not develop schizophrenia (Sørensen et al., 2010). Similarly, early behavioral disturbances and cognitive and language deficits were evident in a substantial minority of preteen youth who were later diagnosed with schizophrenia (Seidman & Mirsky, 2017). Further, low cognitive ability test scores in childhood and adolescence predicted the presence of psychotic-like experiences and clinically significant psychotic symptoms in middle age; the low scores may represent early evidence of abnormalities in neural development (Barnett et al., 2012). Additionally, in a group of young men, a decline in verbal ability between ages 13 and 18 was associated with an increased risk of developing a psychotic disorder (MacCabe et al., 2013). These cognitive decrements may be an indication of brain abnormalities that result in less "cognitive reserve" and reduced opportunity for the brain to bounce back from the neurological changes associated with schizophrenia (Barnett et al., 2012).

Certain personal cognitive processes involving misattributions or negative attitudes can lead to or maintain psychotic symptoms such as delusions. For instance, negative symptoms such as limited motivation

Continuum Video Project

Andre: Schizophrenia

"I believe that other people are pathological liars, and I'm not. So why should I even have to listen to them?"

Access the Continuum Video Project in MindTap.

Table 12.1 Negative Expectancy Appraisals Associated with Negative Symptoms

Negative Symptom	Low Self-Efficacy (Success)	Low Satisfaction (Pleasure)	Low Expectation for Acceptance	Low Available Resources
Restricted affect	If I show my feelings, others will see my inadequacy.	I don't feel the way I used to.	My face appears stiff and contorted to others.	I don't have the ability to express my feelings.
Alogia	I'm not going to find the right words to express myself.	I take so long to get my point across that it's boring.	I'm going to sound weird, stupid, or strange.	It takes too much effort to talk.
Avolition	Why bother—I'm just going to fail.	It's more trouble than it's worth.	It's best not to get involved.	It takes too much effort to try.

Source: Rector et al., 2005, p. 254

and **restricted affect** may be associated with individuals' beliefs that they are worthless and that their condition is hopeless (Beck et al., 2013). The combination of having low expectations for pleasure or success combined with low motivation may maintain negative symptoms. In fact, some researchers, hypothesizing that faulty interpretation of events may be the primary cause of the distress and disability associated with schizophrenia, have found that individuals diagnosed with schizophrenia have a tendency to interpret emotionally ambiguous stimuli as negative and to attend to information that supports these distressing beliefs (Yiend et al., 2019). In other words, pessimistic interpretations may produce and maintain negative symptoms. Table 12.1 presents patterns of thinking that may be associated with negative symptoms. Along with negative attentional bias, maladaptive emotional regulation strategies such as worry, rumination, and suppression of emotions may maintain and exacerbate positive symptoms (Liu et al., 2020).

Social Dimension

The role of social relationships in the development of schizophrenia has been extensively studied. In fact, not long ago, dysfunctional family patterns, rather than biology, were considered the primary cause of schizophrenia. Unfortunately, blaming families for schizophrenia still occurs today. One parent whose son was hospitalized for psychosis heard a nurse say, "Well, no wonder he's ill—look at the state of his mother." The staff member apparently failed to understand that the mother's state of mind was the result of weeks of stress attempting to help her adult son cope with his psychotic symptoms prior to his hospitalization (Wainwright et al., 2014, p. 8). It is quite probable, however, that among individuals with a biological predisposition, the social environment can increase the risk of schizophrenia. We will consider social factors that are associated with increased vulnerability to schizophrenia.

Certain social events such as maltreatment during childhood or other significant social stressors may alter neurodevelopment in a manner that increases susceptibility to schizophrenia and to the appearance of psychotic symptoms. Childhood adversities have been found to be related to structural changes in the brain such as a smaller volume of the hippocampus and amygdala (Barker, Bois, Johnstone, et al., 2016) and alterations in the cortex (Barker, Bois, Neilson, et al., 2016). There is also an additive interaction of genetic liability with adversities such as sexual abuse, emotional abuse, emotional neglect, and childhood bullying. In a longitudinal study focused on 2,232 twins, those who experienced maltreatment by an adult or bullying by peers had a higher risk of psychotic symptoms at age 12 (refer to Figure 12.8); the risk was magnified among those exposed to both bullying and maltreatment (Guloksuz et al., 2019). Being bullied by a sibling during childhood has also been linked to an increased risk of developing a psychotic disorder (Dantchev et al., 2018).

In one sample of 12-year-old children followed from age 7, the risk of psychotic symptoms doubled for those who were bullied between ages 8 and 10; the association was stronger with more severe or chronic forms of bullying (Schreier et al., 2009). Another study found a similar dose-dependent relationship between the severity of bullying and the risk for psychotic experiences in school-age adolescents—the more severe the bullying, the greater the risk of schizophrenia. The study reported another finding that has important implications for prevention programs—the psychotic symptoms in affected youth often decreased or subsided if the bullying stopped (Kelleher et al., 2013).

Relationships with caregivers within the home can also influence the development of schizophrenia. Individuals with psychosis were three times more likely to report severe physical abuse from mothers before 12 years of age than were individuals without psychosis (Fisher et al., 2010). In contrast, among adolescents with symptoms that appeared to put them "at imminent risk" for the onset of psychosis, positive remarks and warmth expressed by caregivers were associated with decreases in negative and disorganized symptoms and improvement in social functioning (O'Brien et al., 2006). Children at higher biological risk for schizophrenia may be more sensitive to the effects of both adverse and healthy child-rearing patterns.

Expressed emotion (EE), a negative communication pattern found among some relatives of individuals with schizophrenia, has been associated with higher relapse rates in individuals diagnosed with schizophrenia (Cechnicki et al., 2013; Hinojosa-Marqués et al., 2019). EE is determined by a variety of factors, including critical comments made by relatives; statements of dislike or resentment directed toward the individual with schizophrenia by family members; and statements reflecting emotional overinvolvement, overconcern, or overprotectiveness with respect to the family member with schizophrenia. Although high EE has been associated with an increased risk of relapse, the studies are correlational in nature and are therefore subject to different interpretations.

- A high EE environment is stressful and may lead directly to relapse in the family member who has schizophrenia.

- An individual who is more severely ill has a greater chance of relapse and may cause more negative or high EE communication patterns in relatives.

- The effects of EE and illness are bidirectional: Odd behaviors or symptoms of schizophrenia may increase the likelihood that family members criticize, overprotect, or react to the symptoms with frustration, which in turn produces increases in psychotic symptoms.

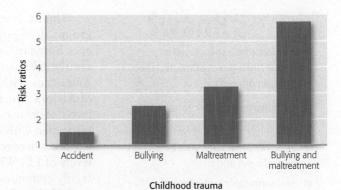

Figure 12.8

Risk of Psychotic Symptoms at Age 11 Associated with Cumulative Childhood Trauma

Youth exposed to both bullying and childhood maltreatment demonstrate a significantly increased risk of developing psychotic symptoms.

Source: Arseneault et al., 2011

Individuals who experienced a psychotic breakdown attributed their emotional collapse to:

- drug use (especially cannabis),
- recent trauma (e.g., sexual assault),
- personal sensitivity (e.g., bottling up feelings), and
- problems during childhood (e.g., child abuse).

Source: Dudley et al., 2009

The EE construct appears to have less meaning for different cultural groups. It is possible that this occurs because cultural factors may influence how family members view and react to the symptoms. For instance, family criticism scores were not associated with relapse for Mexican Americans with schizophrenia (Rosenfarb et al., 2006). Among a sample of African Americans and European Americans with schizophrenia, high levels of critical and intrusive behavior by family members (high EE) were associated with *better* outcomes for African American clients over a 2-year period, whereas European American clients had better outcomes with low levels of EE. Within some African American families, seemingly negative family communication may, in fact, reflect caring and concern (Rosenfarb et al., 2006). Lopez and associates (2004) concluded that different cultural groups interpret family communication processes—such as emotional over-protection or overinvolvement—differently. In fact, therapists who focus on reducing critical and intrusive communication patterns in culturally diverse families may inadvertently increase family stress. Family therapists have moved away from the expressed emotions perspective and instead are collaborating with family members in finding ways to support their loved one after a schizophrenia diagnosis (McFarlane, 2016).

Sociocultural Dimension

There are significant ethnic differences in the rates of schizophrenia. For example, follow-up of a large birth cohort in the United States revealed that African Americans were two to three times more likely to receive a diagnosis of schizophrenia compared to European Americans (Bresnahan et al., 2007). Another study found that Hispanic and African Americans are more likely to receive a diagnosis of schizophrenia than non-Hispanic White Americans. Further, African Americans are most likely to display positive symptoms and disorganized thoughts even when undergoing treatment (Hamilton et al., 2018).

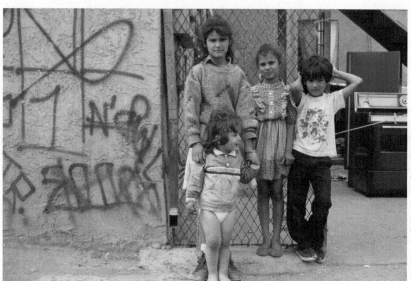

Visions of America/Universal Images Group/Getty Images

Socioeconomic Status and Schizophrenia

Schizophrenia is much more prevalent in poorer neighborhoods. Some believe that the increased stress from living in poverty may be the cause; others believe that individuals with schizophrenia move into poorer neighborhoods because of their decreased ability to function in society.

Why is there a consistently higher rate of schizophrenia within the African American community? Although some wonder if these findings reflect clinician bias rather than actual differences in rates of the disorder, African Americans are more likely to be diagnosed with schizophrenia even when assessment data and clinical interviews are reanalyzed by clinicians unaware of the ethnicity of clients (Sabbag et al., 2015). However, it is quite possible that previous discriminatory experiences lead to cultural mistrust and a "healthy paranoia" that is picked up during clinical assessments. In other words, discriminatory experiences may cause African Americans to react in a manner that represents a normative response to ongoing discrimination, yet their responses may appear delusional to clinicians who do not understand these sociocultural realities (Gara et al., 2012). In an effort to explain the development of psychosis in Latinx and African American individuals, Anglin and colleagues (2021) have proposed an integrative model that includes sociocultural, environmental, and individual level stressors that contribute to a psychosis endophenotype (refer to Figure 12.9).

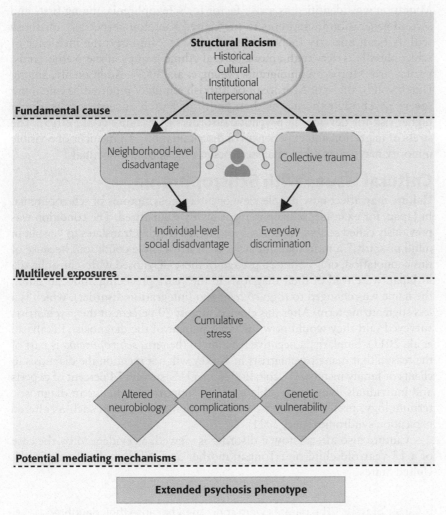

Figure 12.9

Hypothesized Model Linking Systemic Racism and Psychosis in the United States

This hypothesized model linking systemic racism and the development of psychosis can also apply to other marginalized groups that face discrimination and oppression.

Source: Anglin et al., 2021

A number of other social factors have been identified as risk factors for schizophrenia, such as being unemployed, of lower socioeconomic status and educational level, and living in impoverished urban areas (Kirkbride et al., 2017). These forms of social adversity, especially when combined with other risk factors, appear to produce an increased risk of developing schizophrenia compared to those not exposed to these adversities (Morgan et al., 2019). Interestingly, living among members of one's own ethnic group reduces the risk of experiencing psychotic symptoms. Residing in a neighborhood or community with others of the same ethnic background may serve as a buffer to social adversity and reduce the risk of developing psychotic symptoms (Das-Munshi et al., 2012).

Immigration experiences also appear to increase susceptibility to schizophrenia. In general, immigrants and their descendants are more than twice as likely to have psychotic symptoms compared to nonimmigrants, with refugees having the greatest likelihood of developing schizophrenia (Hollander et al., 2016). Immigrant groups, particularly those of African descent, have the highest rates of schizophrenia in Western Europe (Oduola et al., 2019). Migration was identified as a risk factor for schizophrenia among first- and second-generation immigrants to the United Kingdom, especially for those with African ancestry (Schofield et al., 2011). Similarly, the incidence of schizophrenia is very high among several ethnic groups in the Netherlands, particularly Moroccan immigrants (Veling et al., 2007). Additionally, among Dutch youth, those of Moroccan or Turkish ethnicity reported having more severe psychotic experiences than youth of Dutch ancestry, indicating a higher risk for developing psychotic disorders (Adriaanse et al., 2015). The stress of migration and experiences of discrimination as a member of a visible minority may act as additional stressors in predisposed individuals.

Cultural Issues With Schizophrenia

Culture may affect how people view or interpret symptoms of schizophrenia. In Japan, for example, schizophrenia is highly stigmatized. The condition was previously called *seishin-bunretsu-byou*, which roughly translates to "a split in mind or spirit," a term that implies it is an irreversible condition. Because of this connotation, only about 20 percent of those diagnosed with schizophrenia in Japan were told of their diagnosis in the years preceding 2000. In 2002, the name was changed to *togo-shitcho-sho* (integration disorder), which is a less stigmatizing term. After this change, almost 70 percent of the psychiatrists surveyed said they would now inform a patient of the diagnosis (Takahashi et al., 2011). Similarly, a negative reaction to the term *schizophrenia* is part of the reason that many psychiatrists in Turkey will not mention the diagnosis to clients or family members (Ucok, 2007). In a U.S. survey, 74 percent of experts and individuals living with schizophrenia supported a change in diagnostic terminology, preferring the use of a less-stigmatizing term such as altered perception syndrome (Ruiz, 2021).

Culture also affects how a disorder is viewed, as evidenced by the case of a 13-year-old child of a Tongan mother and White father living in the United States.

Case Study The parents were concerned because their daughter began to isolate herself and appeared to have visual hallucinations, was observed talking to herself, and reported hearing voices of a woman who sounded like her mother and a man who sounded like her dead grandfather. Although she demonstrated some improvement after taking antipsychotic medication, the girl still reported that people were talking about her and ghosts were disturbing her.

The mother decided that her daughter suffered from "fakama-haki," a culture-bound syndrome in which deceased relatives can inflict illness or possess the living when customs have been neglected; she arranged a trip to Tonga so her daughter could properly mourn at her grandfather's gravesite. Additionally, for 5 days, a traditional healer ("witch doctor") treated the girl with herbal potions that induced vomiting. When the girl was reevaluated after she returned to the United States, there were no symptoms of psychosis. Follow-up contact revealed that the girl was continuing to do well. (Takeuchi, 2000)

This case is interesting because pharmaceutical intervention was only minimally successful, whereas traditional healing seemed to be effective. Although it is also possible that the disorder was time-limited, there is no doubt that taking into account cultural beliefs might enhance the understanding and treatment of psychotic symptoms.

As noted throughout this book, the study of cross-cultural perspectives on psychopathology is important because belief systems influence views of etiology and treatment. In India, for instance, the belief in supernatural causation of schizophrenia is widespread, with nearly two thirds of one group of patients believing that their illness was a result of "black magic" or "punishment from God." Although most sought traditional medical treatment for their condition, they also sought assistance from religious institutions or Indigenous healers (Jacob & Kuruvilla, 2018).

In a cross-cultural study of individuals with schizophrenia from four ethnic groups (Anglos in the United Kingdom, African Caribbeans, Bangladeshis, and West Africans), distinct differences in explanatory models were found for the disorder (Table 12.2) (McCabe & Priebe, 2004). The different explanations endorsed by the participants included biological (e.g., physical illness or substance abuse), social (e.g., interpersonal problems, stress, negative childhood events, personality), supernatural (e.g., evil forces, black magic), and various nonspecific explanations. Anglos from the United Kingdom were the most likely to attribute the condition to biological causes and least likely to believe in supernatural forces; in contrast, a substantial number of individuals from the other cultural groups supported supernatural causes. Differing views on etiology also influenced their receptiveness to taking medication for their symptoms. Those who cited biological causes felt that medication was the correct treatment, whereas those who supported a supernatural explanation preferred alternative forms of treatment, such as spiritual intervention. Thus, views of etiology can affect our understanding of schizophrenia, including its severity, prognosis, and appropriate treatment.

Table 12.2 Explanatory Models of Illness in Schizophrenia Among Four Ethnic Groups

	Biological Explanation	Social Explanation	Supernatural Explanation	Nonspecific Explanation
African Caribbean	6.7%	60.0%	20.0%	23.3%
Bangladeshi	0.0%	42.3%	26.9%	30.8%
West African	10.7%	31.0%	28.6%	21.4%
Anglo (in the United Kingdom)	34.5%	31.0%	0.0%	34.5%

Source: McCabe & Priebe, 2004

Instilling Hope After a Schizophrenia Diagnosis

Case Study Susan suffered 7 months of continuous psychosis and had to drop out of her PhD program. As she recovered, she desperately wanted to be a professor but no longer had the energy to do research and write. Instead, she decided to write a nonfiction book on pirates. When it became clear that she could not complete a book, she wrote articles for historical and pirate reenactment magazines. She began to find joy in her life again. However, the extensive research required for her articles felt overwhelming and she began to think of herself as a failure. She searched for another outlet and started to write poetry—a task she could complete at her own pace. Repurposing her previous research on pirates, Susan decided to write poems on that topic for children. After two years of hard work, she completed the book, *Pirates and Spooks Beware*. Her second book for adults came out in 2020. As Susan reflected, "I found my little place in the universe at last. My own garden to tend and bring to blossom. . . . Mental illness doesn't have to be the one definition of who we are. It may be a disability we have to cope with, but it also may bring opportunities we never expected to make life bright and enjoyable." (Weiner, 2019)

Schizophrenia is no longer viewed as a chronic disorder with an inevitably poor prognosis. About 25 percent of those diagnosed with schizophrenia will experience complete recovery, with many others demonstrating different degrees of recovery (Hancock et al., 2018). Studies indicate that comprehensive, early intervention can lead to significant functional and social recovery. Over half will achieve remission of symptoms, nearly one quarter will regain social functioning, and nearly 20 percent will achieve both (Onitsuka et al., 2022). Even among the most chronically ill, a sizable minority have feelings of optimism and happiness (Edmonds et al., 2018). This newer perspective, referred to as the *recovery model*, mobilizes optimism and collaborative support for recovery. It also envisions substantial return of function for many individuals with schizophrenia. The model views schizophrenia as a chronic medical condition, such as diabetes or heart disease, which may interfere with optimal functioning but does not define the individual. The recovery model is based on the following assumptions (Bellack, 2006; Hancock et al., 2018):

■ Recovery is an ongoing positive journey even when there are ups and downs.

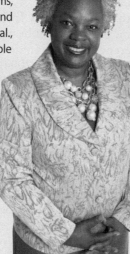

Hogan Imaging/Shutterstock.com

■ Healing involves separating one's identity from the illness and developing the ability to take an active role in one's recovery.

  ■ Empowerment of the individual helps correct the sense of powerlessness and dependence that results from traditional mental health care.

    ■ When complete recovery is not possible, it is still important to establish or strengthen social connections.

      ■ It is crucial to seek and find hope, optimism, self-determination, self-respect, and happiness during the process.

Recovery may include—but does not require—a complete remission of symptoms. Recovery is a process that involves overcoming the label of a "mental health patient" through personal growth, self-direction, identifying and building on strengths, assumption of responsibility for self-care, and establishment of a personally fulfilling and meaningful life. It is learning to productively engage in important life roles, such as partner, friend, spouse, worker, and parent.

12-4 Treatment of Schizophrenia

Through the years, schizophrenia has been treated by a variety of means, including performing a **prefrontal lobotomy**—an outdated surgical procedure in which the frontal lobes were disconnected from the remainder of the brain. The research and clinical perspective on people with schizophrenia has since shifted from a focus on illness and deficit to one of recovery and promotion of health, competencies, independence, and self-determination. Thus, schizophrenia is now treated from a much more holistic perspective, including medications, cognitive-behavioral therapies, and cognitive enhancement therapy.

Antipsychotic Medications

Case Study Peter, a 29-year-old man, was diagnosed with chronic paranoid schizophrenia.... When on medication, he heard voices talking about him and felt that his phone was bugged. When off medication, he had constant hallucinations and his behavior became unpredictable.... He was on 10 milligrams of haloperidol (Haldol) three times a day.... Peter complained that he had been quite restless, and did not want to take the medication. Over the next 6 months, Peter's psychiatrist gradually reduced Peter's medication to 4 milligrams per day.... At this dose, Peter continued to have bothersome symptoms, but they remained moderate.... He was no longer restless. (Liberman et al., 1994, p. 94)

The case study demonstrates that **antipsychotic medication** can be effective in reducing the intensity of hallucination, delusions, and other symptoms associated with schizophrenia. Many consider the 1955 introduction of *Thorazine*, the first antipsychotic drug, to be the beginning of a new era in treating schizophrenia. For the first time, a medication was available that sufficiently relaxed even those most severely affected by schizophrenia and helped organize their thoughts to the point that straitjackets were no longer needed for physical restraint. The **first-generation antipsychotics** (also called *conventional* or *typical antipsychotics*) are still viewed as effective treatments for schizophrenia, although their use has been largely supplanted by the newer **atypical antipsychotics**, medications with somewhat different chemical properties compared to the earlier drugs. Although medications have improved the lives of many with schizophrenia, they do not cure the disorder. Unfortunately, up to one third of those with schizophrenia do not benefit at all from antipsychotic medication. This treatment-resistant population has been found to have higher polygenetic risk scores than treatment-responsive patients and, thus, may constitute an illness subgroup requiring alternative interventions (Zhang, Robinson, et al., 2019).

Conventional antipsychotic medications (such as chlorpromazine [Thorazine] or haloperidol [Haldol]) have dopaminergic receptor–blocking capabilities (i.e., they reduce dopamine levels), a factor that led to the dopamine hypothesis of schizophrenia. The newer atypical antipsychotics (such as risperidone [Risperdal], olanzapine [Zyprexa], quetiapine [Seroquel], and aripiprazole [Abilify]) act on both dopamine and serotonin receptors. These newer medications are purportedly less likely to produce serious side effects such as the rigidity, muscle spasms, tremors, and restlessness that occur with the older antipsychotics. Complaints from those taking these medications include weight gain (62 percent) as well as feelings of restlessness (61 percent) and excessive sedation (59 percent) (Achtyes et al., 2018). One of the dangerous side effects of these newer antipsychotic medications is an enhanced risk of cardiovascular conditions, such as heart arrhythmia or elevated blood pressure. Further, atypical antipsychotic medications

Did You Know?

Cannabidiol (CBD), a nonintoxicating extract from cannabis, appears to normalize brain activity in regions of the brain associated with psychotic symptoms. Its action is opposite of the psychosis-inducing properties of cannabis that contains THC. Researchers hope cannabidiol extracts will eventually be approved as an alternative to current antipsychotic medications.
Source: O'Neill et al., 2020

Did You Know?

In one study, 28 percent of the participants had positive attitudes about their psychotic symptoms, including "hearing voices." Some participants reported discontinuing their antipsychotic medications so their symptoms would return.
Source: Moritz et al., 2013

appear to increase the risk of **metabolic syndrome**, a condition associated with obesity, diabetes, high cholesterol, and cardiovascular events such as heart attacks and strokes (Jaberi et al., 2020).

There is also concern that antipsychotic medications may have mixed effects on cognitive functioning and motivation. Some individuals taking antipsychotics report that their thinking is slowed down; that their emotions are not as intense; and that the medications weaken their hallucinations and delusions, allowing them to think more clearly. Others are concerned that the antipsychotics negatively affect their motivation and ability to function; they report feeling numb, overwhelmingly sleepy, and unable to act normally (Thompson et al., 2020).

Individuals taking antipsychotics, particularly first-generation antipsychotics, sometimes experience other distressing effects, including **extrapyramidal symptoms**, which include *parkinsonism* (muscle tremors, shakiness, and immobility), *dystonia* (involuntary muscle contractions involving the limbs and tongue), *akathisia* (motor restlessness), and *neuroleptic malignant syndrome* (fever, muscle rigidity, and physiological dysregulation, which can be fatal if untreated). Other symptoms may involve the loss of facial expression, shuffling gait, tremors of the hand, rigidity of the body, and poor balance. Although many symptoms are reversible once medication is stopped, some symptoms (e.g., involuntary movements) can be permanent (Casey, 2006). In one study involving 4,621 people taking antipsychotics, 12.6 percent had hospitalizations, emergency department visits, and increased health care costs resulting from extrapyramidal symptoms (Abouzaid et al., 2014).

Tardive dyskinesia is another side effect associated with antipsychotics. This chronic condition involves involuntary and rhythmic movements of the tongue; chewing, lip smacking, and other facial movements; and jerking movements of the limbs. The risk of developing this disorder is greatest for those who take antipsychotic medications over an extended period. Valbenazine, approved in 2017 by the FDA as a treatment for tardive dyskinesia, can diminish some of the distressing symptoms caused by this condition (Arya et al., 2019).

Close monitoring of undesirable reactions is important because side effects may affect a person's willingness to continue treatment (Stroup & Gray, 2018). In fact, from one half to three quarters of patients discontinue use of antipsychotics for a variety of reasons (Moritz et al., 2013):

- Too many side effects (80 percent)
- Belief that they do not need antipsychotics (58 percent)
- Mistrust of the physician or therapist (31 percent)
- Rejection of medication in general (28 percent)
- Friends or relatives advised them not to take the medication (20 percent)

Due to all of the concerns about the side effects of antipsychotics, questions have arisen about whether it is possible for individuals with schizophrenia to function successfully after reducing or discontinuing their antipsychotic medication. The current treatment guidelines recommend that medication be continued for 1 year after the remission of symptoms in the case of first-episode psychosis. Many patients, however, wish to stop medications once the symptoms have been resolved. Although there is a tendency for relapse in the first 6 to 10 months among individuals with schizophrenia who discontinue their medication, some individuals who discontinue after 3 years of stability have favorable outcomes (Alvarez-Jimenez et al., 2016). Thus, it appears that continuous medication may not be needed for some individuals with schizophrenia. Unfortunately, at this time we have no way to determine which individuals can achieve long-term stability or remission after discontinuing antipsychotic medication.

Dose reduction may be another option. In one group of individuals with schizophrenia, reducing the dosage of antipsychotic medication by half resulted in a significant improvement in cognitive functioning, including verbal memory and processing speed (Takeuchi et al., 2012). In a 7-year follow-up study, dose-reduction patients were twice as likely to recover compared to patients receiving ongoing maintenance medication (Wunderink et al., 2013). More gradual dose-reduction appears to further reduce psychotic relapses (Bogers et al., 2023). A 4-year randomized control study is currently underway involving a group of young adults who had an early episode of psychosis, comparing those who receive continuous medication with those who have their dosages tapered, reduced, and (when possible) eventually discontinued. In the latter group, if signs of relapse develop, medication levels will be adjusted. This study should provide a more definitive answer regarding the outcome with medication maintenance versus discontinuation (Begemann et al., 2020).

Although medications can reduce many symptoms of schizophrenia, one fact is clear. Individuals with schizophrenia who are discharged from protective hospital environments are often confronted with real-world stress once they return to the community. Experiencing chronic stress or external stressors can result in the return of psychotic symptoms and rehospitalization (Bhattacharyya et al., 2023); medication alone is often not enough to help those with schizophrenia function in their natural environments. For this reason, other therapeutic interventions are included as part of a comprehensive treatment program.

Going Deeper

The Marketing of Atypical Antipsychotic Medications

Television advertising has suggested that the addition of a specific medication may be helpful for individuals with symptoms of depression who have not yet benefited from an antidepressant. The fact that the medication being advertised is an atypical antipsychotic is not mentioned. Advertising also does not mention that combining some of the newer atypical antipsychotics with antidepressants has been found to increase mortality risk (Gerhard et al., 2020).

Atypical antipsychotics such as quetiapine (Seroquel), aripiprazole (Abilify), olanzapine (Zyprexa), and risperidone (Risperdal) are profitable drugs that are heavily promoted by pharmaceutical companies. They are among the top-selling class of medications in the United States. This is partly the result of prescribing antipsychotics "off-label"; that is, the drug is used for a condition, for an age group, or at a dosage that is not FDA approved (Vijay et al., 2018). For example, antipsychotics are prescribed for a range of mental disorders, including attentional, conduct, depressive, and anxiety disorders, although they have never been evaluated or approved for use with these conditions (Zito et al., 2013).

Multiple studies have found that off-label use of antipsychotics results in more adverse drug reactions compared to the medications approved to treat specific conditions. According to the FDA Adverse Reporting System, there have been 5,398 complaints involving hospitalizations and life-threatening complications associated with Abilify, including suicidal ideation. Further, Abilify has also been associated with compulsive behaviors, including gambling, shopping, and hypersexuality (Cornell, 2017). The increased use of atypical antipsychotic medications is also of concern due to their association with troublesome side effects such as weight gain, hyperlipidemia, and increased risk for type 2 diabetes (Sultan et al., 2019). Findings such as these have led many to question whether the benefits of off-label use of antipsychotics are worth the risk.

For Further Consideration

1. Should regulations be in place to protect consumers from the increasing off-label use of antipsychotic medications?

2. Should physicians and psychiatrists be required to inform patients when antipsychotics have not been approved for the treatment of their specific condition?

Psychosocial Therapy

> **Case Study** Philip's psychotic symptoms were significantly reduced with medication. However, he was unable to obtain employment because of cognitive and behavioral peculiarities. He did not seem to understand social conventions such as appropriate conversational topics or attire. His therapist suggested that his clothing (sweatshirt, exercise pants, headband, and worn sneakers) might be inappropriate for job interviews. He coached Philip to observe attire worn by individuals in different businesses. He also gave Philip opportunities to practice engaging in informal conversation and answering job interview questions. When interviewing for a landscape job, Philip wore a work shirt, blue jeans, and construction boots and was hired by the landscaping contractor. (Heinssen & Cuthbert, 2001)

Psychotherapeutic work with individuals with schizophrenia often focuses on the direct teaching of adaptive conversational, behavioral, and social skills. Heinssen and Cuthbert (2001) found that eccentricities in the appearance, attire, and communication patterns of individuals with schizophrenia, as well as a lack of discretion in discussing their illness, can impede employment or the establishment of social networks. Social communication may also be problematic because of difficulties with emotional perception and understanding the beliefs and attitudes of others. Thus, it is beneficial when communication skills are taught directly and practiced in role-play situations, as occurred with Philip in the case study.

A number of programs have been developed to deal with the interpersonal deficiencies found in individuals with schizophrenia, including social cognition and interaction training (SCIT), a 20-week group intervention focused on improving emotional recognition, social interaction skills, and quality of life. SCIT participants engage with an online program focused on communication skills and then practice these skills in a group setting, an approach that has resulted in significantly improved social skills (Gordon et al., 2018). A similar program, Work-Focused Cognitive Behavioral Therapy, which was developed for severely ill patients, provides 12 group sessions focused on obtaining and maintaining work in a competitive environment. The program covers topics such as increasing positive attitudes toward work, bolstering coping and problem-solving skills, and improving social interactions skills. A 6-month follow-up of one group found that 73 percent of the participants were able to obtain steady work (Kukla et al., 2019).

Another program, metacognitive training (MCT), aims to ameliorate the neurocognitive deficits found in individuals with schizophrenia such as the tendency to jump to a false conclusion. The MCT modules focus on identifying possible cognitive bias and increasing flexibility with thinking processes. This training material is culturally sensitive and available at no cost. A meta-analysis showed that MCT can reduce hallucinations and delusions and improve negative symptoms and self-esteem. Follow-up studies have shown sustained effectiveness for at least one year (Penney et al., 2022). Other therapies such as cognitive-behavioral therapy often incorporate elements of metacognitive training (Martiadis et al., 2023).

Cognitive-Behavioral Therapy

Major advances have been made in the use of cognitive and behavioral strategies in treating the symptoms of schizophrenia; this is particularly important for those who do not respond to medication. Therapists teach coping skills that allow clients to manage their positive and negative symptoms, as well as the cognitive challenges associated with schizophrenia. An 18-month follow-up of 216 individuals with persisting psychotic symptoms found that those receiving cognitive-behavioral therapy demonstrated 183 days of normal functioning, compared to 106 days of normal functioning for those who received the typical intervention of medication and periodic contact with a psychiatric nurse (van der Gaag et al., 2011).

Can cognitive-behavioral therapy prevent or delay psychotic episodes in individuals with ultrahigh-risk symptoms? Fifty-eight high-risk individuals were randomly assigned to either CBT or treatment as usual (TAU). The CBT included modules over 30 individual weekly sessions that covered: psychoeducation and goal setting; assessment and engagement; normalization of psychotic-like experiences; cognitive restructuring for automatic, maladaptive thoughts; skills for emotion management; interventions on worry, anxiety, depression, and social skills; and relapse prevention strategies. In contrast, the TAU group received 30 weeks of individual sessions that included empathetic supportive listening, paraphrasing, and validation of the experiences of the participants. When the participants were contacted 14 months after the intervention, 10.3 percent of the participants in the CBT group had developed a psychotic episode versus 27.5 percent in the TAU group. Further, CBT was nearly twice as effective as supportive therapy in reducing depression and anxiety in the participants (Pozza & Dèttore, 2020).

The following case study provides an example of symptoms of schizophrenia that might be effectively addressed with cognitive-behavioral treatment strategies.

> **Case Study** A young African American woman with auditory hallucinations, paranoid delusions, delusions of reference, a history of childhood verbal and physical abuse, and adult sexual assault felt extremely hopeless about her prospects for developing social ties. She believed that her "persecutors" had informed others of her socially undesirable activities. . . . She often loudly screamed at the voices she was hearing. . . . When she did leave her home, she often covered her head with a black kerchief and wore dark sunglasses, partly in an effort to disguise herself from her persecutors. (Cather, 2005, p. 260)

Cognitive-behavioral treatment to address concerns such as those experienced by this young woman involves some of the following steps:

- *Psychoeducation and engagement*: The therapist explains the therapy and works to foster a safe and collaborative method of looking at causes of distress, drawing out the client's understanding of stressors and ways of coping.

- *Assessment and normalization*: Clients are encouraged to discuss their fears and anxieties; the therapist shares information about how symptoms are formed and maintained. In the preceding case study, the therapist helped the woman make sense of her persecutory delusions. The therapist explained that those who have experienced abuse often internalize beliefs that they are responsible for the abuse, and that her view that she was "bad" led her to expect negative reactions from others and the subsequent need to disguise herself.

- *Cognitive restructuring and identification of negative beliefs*: The therapist explains to the client the link between personal beliefs and emotional distress, and the ways that beliefs such as "Nobody will like me if I tell them about my voices" can be disputed and changed

Did You Know?

When individuals with anhedonia (difficulty experiencing positive emotions) are taught to "savor" past, present, and future events, their mood improves and they become less apathetic.

Source: Favrod et al., 2015

Paintings and sculptures by William Scott, who has been diagnosed with schizophrenia and an autism spectrum disorder, are sold around the world at cutting-edge art galleries. Scott is pictured here with a self-portrait.

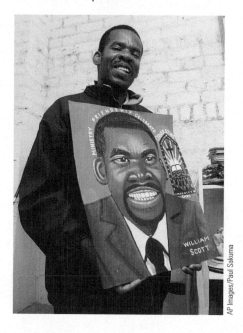

to "I can't demand that everyone like me. Some people will and some won't." This reinterpretation often leads to decreases in feelings of depression.

- *Normalization:* The therapist works with the client to normalize and decatastrophize the psychotic experiences. Information that many people can have unusual experiences may reduce a client's sense of isolation.

- *Collaborative analysis of symptoms:* Once a strong therapeutic alliance has been established, the therapist begins critical discussions of the client's symptoms, such as "If voices come from your head, why can't others hear them?" Evidence for and against the maladaptive beliefs is discussed, combined with information about how beliefs are maintained when someone comes to inaccurate conclusions about events or experiences.

- *Development of alternative explanations:* The therapist helps the client develop alternatives to previous maladaptive assumptions, using the client's ideas whenever possible.

Instead of trying to eliminate or combat hallucinations, therapists teach clients to accept them in a nonjudgmental manner. In mindfulness training, clients learn to let go of angry or fearful responses to psychotic symptoms; instead, they are taught to let the psychotic symptoms come into consciousness without reacting (e.g., just noticing and accepting the voices or thoughts rather than believing them or acting on them). This process enhances feelings of self-control and significantly reduces negative emotions (Aust & Bradshaw, 2017). This approach was used with men who had heard malevolent and powerful voices for more than 30 years. Their attempts to stop the voices or to distract themselves were ineffective. After undergoing mindfulness training, the men were less distressed with the voices and more confident in their ability to live with them (Taylor et al., 2009). Similarly, malevolent and persecuting voices became less disturbing when individuals with schizophrenia learned to access positive emotions such as warmth and contentment during psychotic episodes (Mayhew & Gilbert, 2008).

Treatment programs that work specifically on the neurocognitive deficits found in individuals with schizophrenia are also producing positive results. *Integrated psychological therapy (IPT)* is a computer-based program that specifically targets deficits such as basic impairments in neurocognition (e.g., attention, verbal memory, cognitive flexibility, concept formation), deficits in social cognition (e.g., social-emotional perception, emotional expression), impaired interpersonal communication (e.g., verbal fluency and executive functioning), and difficulties solving day-to-day problems. These deficits occur in most cases of schizophrenia and impede functional recovery. The neurocognitive and social focus of these integrated programs not only results in improvements in overall functioning but also appears to help prevent the return of serious illness, particularly when the intervention incorporates exercises focusing on personal experiences and everyday life situations and encourages participants to practice the skills learned in multiple environments. One group of individuals who received IPT had a relapse rate of 24 percent compared to the 54 percent who relapsed after receiving typical treatment (Mueller et al., 2020). Further, in a meta-analysis of 36 treatment studies, patients undergoing IPT experienced greater reductions in negative symptoms and more improvement in neurocognition, social cognition, and psychosocial functioning compared to treatment as usual (Roder et al., 2011).

Interventions Focusing on Family Communication and Education

More than half of those recovering from a psychotic episode return to live with their families, and new psychological interventions address this fact. Family intervention programs have not only reduced relapse rates but have also lowered the cost of care. They also improve the quality of life of family caregivers (Verma et al., 2019). Most family programs include the following components:

- educating family members about schizophrenia;
- demonstrating concern and empathy for all family members;
- avoiding blaming the family or pathologizing their coping efforts;
- identifying the strengths and competencies of the client and family members;
- teaching skills for solving problems and managing stress within the family;
- providing family members with strategies for coping with the symptoms of mental illness and its repercussions on the family; and
- strengthening the communication skills of all family members (Grácio et al., 2018).

Family intervention programs with these components have successfully reduced relapse rates by up to 50 percent (McFarlane, 2016). An innovative, interactive web-based program incorporates online education, advice, and suggestions for problematic issues by means of a network of connections between families as well as experts in the field. An ongoing randomized outcome study of this method is currently focused on variables such as improvements in family communication and the well-being of all family members (Sin et al., 2020).

Overall, the best outcome occurs when individuals with schizophrenia have access to treatment that includes closely monitored use of medication, cognitive-behavioral therapy, neurocognitive training, family therapy, and direct support within the individual's school or work environment.

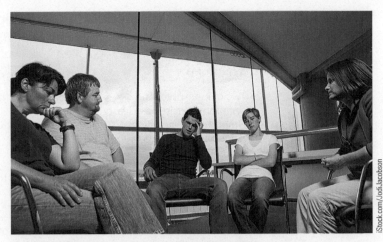

Family Communication and Education

Therapy that includes the family members of individuals with schizophrenia reduces relapse rates and is more effective than drug treatment alone.

12-5 Other Schizophrenia Spectrum Disorders

Additional disorders on the schizophrenia spectrum include delusional disorder, brief psychotic disorder, schizophreniform disorder, and schizoaffective disorder (refer to Table 12.3). These spectrum disorders include some or all of the symptoms we discussed at the beginning of this chapter, but differ from schizophrenia in a variety of ways, including the

Table 12.3 Schizophrenia Spectrum and Other Psychotic Disorders

Disorders Chart				
Disorder	**Symptoms**	**Prevalence**	**Gender Differences**	**Age of Onset**
Schizophrenia	Two or more psychotic symptoms persisting at least 6 months and including delusions, hallucinations, or disorganized speech	• About 1% of the population	About equal	• 18 to 24 for men • 24 to 35 for women
Delusional disorder	One or more delusions for at least 1 month	• About 0.03% to 0.2%	About equal	• More prevalent in older adults
Brief psychotic disorder	One or more psychotic symptoms lasting less than 1 month and including delusions, hallucinations, or disorganized speech	• From 2% to 7% of new cases of psychosis • Higher in developing countries	Somewhat more common in women, especially postpartum	• Most common in 30s
Schizophreniform disorder	Two or more of psychotic symptoms, of which at least one must be delusions, hallucinations, or disorganized speech for at least 1 month but less than 6 months	• Much lower rate than schizophrenia. • Higher in developing countries	About equal	• 18 to 24 for men • 24 to 35 for women
Schizoaffective disorder	Episode of mania or major depression concurrent with delusions, hallucinations, or disorganized speech; psychotic symptoms persist after the mood episode ends	• About 0.32%	More women	• Usually early adulthood

Source: APA, 2022; Bhalla, 2013; Brannon & Bienenfeld, 2012; Memon, 2013

specific symptoms involved, the duration of symptoms, and/or the presence of additional symptoms. With all of the schizophrenia spectrum disorders, clinicians must first rule out the possibility that the symptoms are the result of medication side effects, medical conditions, substance use or abuse, or other mental disorders.

Delusional Disorder

Case Study Janet was working as an intern and studying for her master's degree when she became convinced that the people living in the apartment above her were making noises because they disapproved of her intense sexual desires. Janet reacted angrily, shouting at her neighbors and knocking on the ceiling. She believed that her colleagues and Facebook friends also disapproved of her for the same reasons. (Salvatore et al., 2012)

Delusional disorder is characterized by persistent delusions that are not accompanied by other unusual or odd behaviors—other than those related to the delusional theme. According to the DSM-5-TR, the delusions must persist for at least 1 month (APA, 2022). Because Janet experienced persisting delusions but had no other evidence of psychosis, she received a diagnosis of delusional disorder. Delusional disorder is distinct from the other psychotic disorders due to the absence of additional disturbances in thoughts or perceptions, beyond occasional hallucinations that may be associated with the delusion (e.g., sensations of insects crawling on the skin within the context of a delusion that one's home is infested with insects).

Delusional disorder is rarely diagnosed (the prevalence is 0.03 percent to 0.2 percent); however, it is believed that many with the disorder do not perceive they have a problem and therefore do not seek assistance. People with delusional disorder generally behave normally when they are not discussing or reacting to their delusional ideas. Common themes involved in delusional disorders include the following (Chopra & Bienenfeld, 2011):

- *Erotomania*: The belief that someone is in love with the individual; this delusion typically has a romantic rather than sexual focus
- *Grandiosity*: The conviction that one has great, unrecognized talent, special abilities, or a relationship with an important person or deity
- *Jealousy*: The conviction that one's spouse or partner is being unfaithful
- *Persecution*: The belief that one is being conspired or plotted against
- *Somatic concerns*: The conviction that one has body odor, is malformed, or is infested by insects or parasites.

In a rare form of delusional disorder (shared psychotic delusion), a person who has a close relationship with an individual with delusional or psychotic beliefs comes to accept those beliefs, as demonstrated in the following case.

Case Study A 28-year-old woman and her mother both shared the delusion that the daughter had been given poisoned food and was hypnotized by a man so that he could rape her. They appeared at an emergency department together, with the mother requesting that the daughter be "dehypnotized." (Mahgoub & Hossain, 2006)

Shared delusions (sometimes referred to as *folie à deux*) are more prevalent among those who are socially isolated. In the preceding case, the daughter never married, lived with and was submissive to her mother, and had no close relationships with others. The pattern generally involves a family member or partner acquiring the delusional belief from the dominant individual. Individuals who take on someone else's false beliefs are often younger, are highly suggestible, are more passive, and possess lower self-esteem (Al Saif & Al Khalili, 2020). In many cases, an individual who shares another person's delusional views loses faith in those beliefs when the two individuals are separated.

A decreased ability to obtain feedback correcting a false belief, combined with preexisting personality traits of suspiciousness, may increase a person's susceptibility to developing a delusional disorder. For example, hearing impairment in early adolescence is associated with an increased risk of developing delusions (van der Werf et al., 2011). There is a significant genetic relationship between delusional disorder and schizophrenia; a small proportion of those with the disorder eventually develop schizophrenia (APA, 2022). Delusional disorder is difficult to treat. Antipsychotic medications and cognitive-behavioral therapy have been tried in some cases, but there is scant evidence regarding their effectiveness (Skelton et al., 2015).

Brief Psychotic Disorder

Case Study Eve was a 20-year-old student studying forensic medicine when she first experienced a chaotic world of delusions. She believed that her body was decaying, deteriorating, and rotting away. She feared seeing her reflection in mirrors, worried that it would show that her skin was falling apart and would reveal a rotted monster. She pasted paper over windows and smashed the mirror in the bathroom. She splashed perfume over everything to hide the stench of her rotting body. She stayed in constant motion because she believed that remaining still would cause her body to deteriorate more quickly. At some point all she could do was scream.

During an interview after she was hospitalized, Eve was asked if she was aware that something was wrong. She replied that the disturbances produced by the delusions were so strong that she could not logically evaluate the experience. Eve received a diagnosis of brief psychotic disorder, and the psychiatrist prescribed an antipsychotic medication, an antidepressant, and a sleeping aid. Within 2.5 weeks, her symptoms had subsided and she moved back in with her family. (Purse, 2013)

A DSM-5-TR diagnosis of **brief psychotic disorder** requires the presence of one or more psychotic symptoms, including at least one symptom involving delusions, hallucinations, or disorganized speech, that continue for at least 1 day but last less than 1 month. The symptoms sometimes occur during pregnancy or within 4 weeks of childbirth (APA, 2022). Because of the abrupt and distressing nature of the disorder, prevention of self-harm through hospitalization and use of antipsychotic drugs is sometimes necessary (Memon, 2013). If there is rapid symptom remission after administration of antipsychotic medication, differential diagnosis becomes more difficult.

A significant stressor often precedes the onset of symptoms, although in some cases a precipitating event is not apparent. Eve experienced a number of stressors before her psychotic episode. She had just lost her best friend to an accident, was struggling with academic demands, was juggling two jobs, had moved into a new apartment, was dealing with the divorce of her parents, and was coping with a recent break-up.

Brief psychotic disorder accounts for up to 7 percent of individuals who seek help for first-time psychotic symptoms. In contrast to schizophrenia and other psychotic disorders, there is often a full return to normal functioning after the episode, although relapses are common. If the psychotic symptoms persist, another diagnosis from the schizophrenia spectrum may be appropriate (APA, 2022).

Schizophreniform Disorder

According to the DSM-5-TR, a diagnosis of **schizophreniform disorder** requires the presence of two or more of the following symptoms: delusions, hallucinations, disorganized speech, gross motor disturbances, or negative symptoms. At least one of these symptoms must involve delusions, hallucinations, or disorganized speech. This condition lasts between 1 and 6 months (APA, 2022).

Schizophreniform disorder occurs equally in men and women and shares some of the anatomical and neural deficits found in schizophrenia (Bhalla & Ahmed, 2011). Like schizophrenia, the onset peaks at around

Morgellons Disease: Delusional Parasitosis or Physical Disease?

More than 20 years ago, "Mary Leitao plucked a fiber that looked like a dandelion fluff from a sore under her two-year-old son's lips. . . . Sometimes the fibers were white, and sometimes they were black, red, or blue." Leitao was frustrated by the inability of physicians to diagnose her son's skin condition. In fact, many of the professionals she consulted indicated that they could find no evidence of disease or infection. Frustrated by the medical establishment, Leitao put a description of the condition on a Web site in 2001, calling it Morgellons disease after a 17th-century French medical study involving children with similar symptoms (Middelveen et al., 2018).

The Web site has since compiled 11,000 worldwide reports of the condition among adults and children. Sufferers report granules and fiber-like threads emerging from the skin at the site of itching; sensations of crawling, stinging, or biting; and rashes and skin lesions that do not heal. Some describe the fibers as "inorganic but alive" and report that the fibers pull back from a lit match (Browne, 2011). Symptoms such as vision difficulties, joint pain, fatigue, mental confusion, and short-term memory difficulties have been reported in connection with Morgellons disease (CDC, 2011). Singer and songwriter Joni Mitchell explained, "I have this weird, incurable disease that seems like it's from outer space. Fibers in a variety of colors protrude out of my skin like mushrooms after a rainstorm: They cannot be forensically identified as animal, vegetable or mineral" (Nelson, 2017).

What could cause this disorder? Many dermatologists, physicians, and psychiatrists believe that Morgellons disease results from self-inflicted injury or is a somatic type of delusional disorder such as *delusional parasitosis*, a condition in which individuals (often those with psychosis or a substance-use disorder) maintain a delusional belief that they are afflicted with living organisms or other pathogens (Hylwa & Ronkainen, 2018).

Some physicians, however, believe there is an underlying physical disorder associated with spirochetal infection, citing those with Morgellons symptoms who test positive for Lyme disease or whose symptoms are alleviated with antibacterial or antiparasitic medications. Other individuals with Morgellons symptoms present with evidence of immune system deficiency and markers of chronic inflammation (Middelveen et al., 2018).

Because of the controversy and the increasing number of complaints, the CDC initiated an investigation into the characteristics and epidemiologic data related to Morgellons, including psychological testing, environmental analysis, examination of skin biopsies, and laboratory study of fibers or threads obtained from numerous people (CDC, 2011). Researchers concluded that no medical condition or infection could explain the reported symptoms and that the skin lesions were probably produced by scratching. Fibers found at the site of skin inflammation were cotton or nylon, not organisms. Psychological tests revealed that individuals studied were more likely to be depressed and more attentive to physical symptoms than the general population, but that they were not delusional (Pearson et al., 2012). Many researchers believe that Morgellons disease is a psychogenic condition that spread as a result of passionate discussion of its symptoms on social media and the Internet (Nunziato et al., 2021).

For Further Consideration

1. Are Internet Web sites or social media posts on diseases such as Morgellons creating disorders among vulnerable individuals, or do they provide comfort for those with an actual disease?

2. Do you believe that individuals reporting symptoms of Morgellons are suffering from a somatic delusion?

---

18 to 24 years of age in men and 24 to 35 years of age in women. Good prognostic signs for schizophreniform disorder include an abrupt onset of symptoms, good premorbid functioning, and the absence of negative symptoms. As with schizophrenia, there is a significant risk of suicide, especially when the disorder is accompanied by depression (Bhalla, 2013). One third of individuals with this diagnosis recover within the 6-month time frame, and the other two thirds eventually receive a diagnosis of schizophrenia or schizoaffective disorder (APA, 2022).

Brief psychotic disorder and schizophreniform disorder share many commonalities with schizophrenia (refer to Table 12.4) and are often considered **provisional diagnoses**. For example, an initial diagnosis of brief psychotic disorder may change to schizophreniform disorder if symptoms last longer than 1 month and to schizophrenia if they last longer than 6 months and impair social or occupational functioning.

Table 12.4 Comparison of Brief Psychotic Disorder, Schizophreniform Disorder, and Schizophrenia

	Brief Psychotic Disorder	Schizophreniform Disorder	Schizophrenia
Duration	Less than 1 month	Less than 6 months	6 months or more
Psychosocial stressor	Likely present	Usually present	May or may not be present
Onset of symptoms	Abrupt onset of psychotic symptoms	Often abrupt psychotic symptoms	Gradual onset of psychotic symptoms
Outcome	Return to premorbid functioning	Possible return to premorbid functioning	Occasional return to premorbid functioning
Risk factors	More common in women	Some increased risk of schizophrenia among family members	Higher prevalence of schizophrenia among family members

Source: APA, 2022; Bhalla & Ahmed, 2011; Memon, 2013

Schizoaffective Disorder

Case Study By her last year of college, Beth Baxter, M.D., an honors student and class president, knew there was something wrong with her brain; during the previous 4 years, she had routinely slept only 4 hours a night. . . . She fought suicidal urges and had made several half-hearted suicide attempts. In her second year of medical school, she became convinced that the songs being played on the radio were carrying messages to her. Her grades began to slip for the first time, so she took a break and visited her grandparents' cattle ranch in Texas. While there, she went missing. She had left for an imagined meeting with friends, following "messages" she heard on the radio. Found wandering a day later, she was picked up by police on the side of a highway. While hospitalized, she was diagnosed with bipolar disorder. She managed to return and graduate from medical school, hiring a tutor to talk through all of her class notes. After her residency, Dr. Baxter became increasingly depressed and suicidal; she tried to slash her neck and was hospitalized for a year. Due to the extent of her psychotic symptoms, her diagnosis was changed to schizoaffective disorder. She gradually began to recover, encouraged by a hospital psychiatrist who gave her hope for a full recovery. The psychiatrist was correct in her optimism. Dr. Baxter is now a psychiatrist herself, with a successful private practice. She understands the importance of taking her medications regularly to control her symptoms. (Solovitch, 2014)

Schizoaffective disorder is diagnosed when someone demonstrates psychotic symptoms that meet the diagnostic criteria for schizophrenia combined with symptoms of a major depressive or manic episode that continue for the majority of the time the schizophrenic symptoms are present. Additionally, according to the DSM-5-TR, the psychotic features must continue for at least 2 weeks after symptoms of the manic or depressive episode have subsided. Thus, schizoaffective disorder has features of both schizophrenia and a depressive or bipolar disorder (Rink et al., 2016). If the individual has experienced manic episodes, the clinician specifies that the client has the bipolar subtype of schizoaffective disorder rather than the depressive subtype. Diagnosis is difficult because many people with depressive or bipolar disorders experience hallucinations or delusions during a manic or depressive episode. However, individuals with mood disorders do not have psychotic symptoms in the absence of a major mood episode. Schizoaffective disorder continues to be a controversial diagnosis, particularly because few research studies exist that shed light on its etiology, course, or treatment. While some experts view it as an independent disorder, others believe it is best understood as a form of schizophrenia or a type of mood disorder (Miller & Black, 2019).

Schizoaffective disorder is relatively rare, occurring in only 0.32 percent of the population, and is more prevalent in women (Brannon & Bienenfeld, 2016). Younger individuals with this disorder tend to have the bipolar subtype, whereas older adults are more likely to have the depressive subtype. As with schizophrenia, the age of onset is later for women than men. In a twin study, schizoaffective disorder and schizophrenia demonstrated substantial familial overlap (Cardno & Owen, 2014). Similar biochemical and brain structure abnormalities have been found in individuals with schizoaffective disorder and schizophrenia (Radonic et al., 2011). The prognosis with schizoaffective disorder, including degree of social disability, is better than that associated with schizophrenia but somewhat worse than the prognosis for bipolar or depressive disorders (Brannon & Bienenfeld, 2016). Treatment includes antipsychotic medication combined with mood stabilizers and individual and group psychotherapies.

12-6 Contemporary Trends and Future Directions

Two trends are evident in the field of schizophrenia: (1) the move from pessimistic views regarding outcome for the disorder to the recovery model and (2) the early identification and treatment of individuals at high risk for developing schizophrenia. Dr. Elyn Saks, who has faced a lifelong struggle with schizophrenia, is part of the first trend. As she notes:

> Although I fought my diagnosis for years, I came to accept that I have schizophrenia and will be in treatment for the rest of my life. . . . What I refused to accept was my prognosis. . . . There are others with schizophrenia and active symptoms such as delusions and hallucinations who have significant academic and professional achievement. (Saks, 2013)

Because of her success, Dr. Saks has had to contend with disbelief at her diagnosis and claims from others that she could not possibly have schizophrenia. In response, she asks doubters to "please tell that to the delusions crowding my mind." She and some of her colleagues are studying individuals living with schizophrenia who are leading productive lives. This group includes graduate students, managers, technicians, and professionals. More than 75 percent of the group has been hospitalized from two to five times because of their illness. In spite of this, with medication and therapy, these individuals are examples of the principles of the recovery model—it is not necessary to be completely free of symptoms in order to live and work in accordance with one's potential (Saks, 2013).

Researchers are also emphasizing the importance of early identification and integrated treatment for first-episode psychosis. Early identification is important. Longer duration without treatment is related to greater impairment of cognitive functioning and lower quality of life (Rebhi et al., 2019). Despite the effectiveness of early intervention, one study reported that in the year after an initial psychotic episode, 61 percent of those with a schizophrenia spectrum disorder had not received any antipsychotic medication and 41 percent had not received any individual therapy. Mortality rates for the group (excluding those who died because of physical illness) was 18 times higher than a matched age cohort from the general population (Schoenbaum et al., 2017).

One integrated early intervention program that demonstrated encouraging results linked adolescents and young adults diagnosed with schizophrenia to vocational and educational services and provided individual and family therapy shortly after diagnosis. Compared to those receiving treatment as usual, individuals in the integrated intervention group were much more likely to be employed, live in mainstream housing, and demonstrate improved emotional well-being (Tsiachristas et al., 2016). Similarly, positive results were achieved by the National Institute of Mental Health (NIMH) Recovery After an Initial Schizophrenia Episode (RAISE) program that includes personalized medication management, family psychoeducation, resilience-focused individual therapy, and support for education and employment. As compared to those receiving traditional community care, the RAISE participants experienced greater improvement in quality of life, interpersonal relationships, sense of purpose, and emotional engagement. Further, they were more likely to be working or going to school (Kane et al., 2016). In a 5-year follow-up, participants in the RAISE program continued to have more improvement compared to those who received treatment as usual (Robinson et al., 2022). Early intervention programs that include integrated services are increasing optimism for the outcome of people with psychosis. Effectiveness may be further increased by including cognitive-behavioral therapy or cognitive enhancement therapies within the integrated models.

Chapter Summary

1 What are the symptoms associated with schizophrenia spectrum disorders?

- Positive symptoms involve "added" sensations and behaviors such as unusual thoughts or perceptions, such as delusions, hallucinations, disordered thinking, and bizarre behavior.
- Cognitive symptoms include disorganized speech and problems with attention, memory, and developing plans of action.
- Abnormal psychomotor behaviors such as catatonia may occur in those with schizophrenia.
- Negative symptoms include certain behaviors or experiences are that are diminished or lost from a person's life such as decreased ability to initiate actions (avolition) or speech (alogia), express emotions, or feel pleasure.

2 Is there much chance of recovery from schizophrenia?

- The prognosis for schizophrenia is variable and is associated with premorbid levels of functioning. Many individuals with schizophrenia experience minimal lasting impairment and recover enough to lead productive lives.

3 What causes schizophrenia?

- Multiple factors are associated with the development of schizophrenia. Biological risk factors include genetics and abnormalities in neurotransmitters or brain structures. Early negative childhood experiences, use of substances such as cannabis and amphetamines, and sociocultural stressors may interact with genetic predisposition to produce schizophrenia.

4 What treatments are currently available for schizophrenia, and are they effective?

- Schizophrenia involves both biological and psychological factors; treatment that combines medication with psychotherapy appears to hold the most promise.
- Drug therapy usually involves conventional antipsychotics or the newer atypical antipsychotics.
- The accompanying psychosocial therapy consists of either supportive counseling or behavioral therapy, with an emphasis on cognitive and social skills training and facilitation of positive communication between those with schizophrenia and their family members. Cognitive enhancement therapies focus on improving the cognitive deficits found in people with schizophrenia.

5 How do other psychotic disorders differ from schizophrenia?

- Delusional disorder is characterized by persistent delusions and the absence of other unusual or odd behaviors.
- Brief psychotic disorder is usually associated with a stressor and is characterized by psychotic symptoms that last less than 1 month.
- Schizophreniform disorder is characterized by psychotic symptoms that are usually associated with a stressor and that last from 1 to 6 months.
- Schizoaffective disorder involves symptoms of schizophrenia combined with episodes of major depression or mania.

Chapter Glossary

alogia
lack of meaningful speech

anhedonia
inability to experience pleasure from previously enjoyed activities

anosognosia
a lack of awareness of or insight into one's own mental dysfunction

antipsychotic medication
medicine developed to counteract symptoms of psychosis

asociality
minimal interest in social relationships

attenuated psychosis syndrome
a condition being researched that involves distressing or disabling early signs of delusions, hallucinations, or disorganized speech that emerged or became progressively worse over the previous year; reality testing remains fairly intact

atypical antipsychotics
newer antipsychotic medications that are less likely to produce the side effects associated with first-generation antipsychotics

avolition
lack of motivation; an inability to take action or become goal oriented

brief psychotic disorder
a condition characterized by psychotic episodes with a duration of at least 1 day but less than 1 month

catatonia
a condition characterized by marked disturbance in motor activity ranging from extreme excitement to motoric immobility

cognitive symptoms
symptoms of schizophrenia associated with problems with attention, memory, and developing a plan of action

concordance rate
the likelihood that both members of a twin pair experience the same characteristic

delusion
a false belief that is firmly and consistently held

delusional disorder
persistent delusions without other unusual or odd behaviors; tactile and olfactory hallucinations related to the delusional theme may be present

diminished emotional expression
reduced display of observable verbal and nonverbal behaviors that communicate internal emotions

disconfirmatory evidence
information that contradicts a delusional belief

dopamine hypothesis
the suggestion that schizophrenia may result from excess dopamine activity at certain synaptic sites

endophenotypes
measurable characteristics (neurochemical, endocrinological, neuroanatomical, cognitive, or neuropsychological) that can give clues regarding the specific genes involved in a disorder

expressed emotion (EE)
a negative communication pattern found among some relatives of individuals with schizophrenia

extrapyramidal symptoms
side effects such as restlessness, involuntary movements, and muscular tension produced by antipsychotic medications

first-generation antipsychotics
a group of medications originally developed to combat psychotic symptoms by reducing dopamine levels in the brain; also called *conventional* or *typical antipsychotics*

hallucination
a sensory experience (such as an image, sound, smell, or taste) that seems real but that does not exist outside of the mind

loosening of associations
continual shifting from topic to topic without any apparent logical or meaningful connection between thoughts

metabolic syndrome
a medical condition associated with obesity, diabetes, high cholesterol, and hypertension

negative symptoms
symptoms of schizophrenia associated with an inability or decreased ability to initiate actions or speech, express emotions, or feel pleasure

paranoid ideation
suspiciousness about the actions or motives of others

persecutory delusions
beliefs of being targeted by others

positive symptoms
symptoms of schizophrenia that involve unusual thoughts or perceptions, such as delusions, hallucinations, disordered thinking, or atypical behavior

prefrontal lobotomy
a surgical procedure in which the frontal lobes are disconnected from the remainder of the brain

premorbid
before the onset of major symptoms

prodromal phase
early signs of illness have developed but are not sufficiently apparent for diagnosis

provisional diagnosis
an initial diagnosis based on currently available information

psychosis
a condition involving loss of contact with or distorted view of reality

restricted affect
severely diminished or limited emotional responsiveness

schizoaffective disorder
a condition involving the existence of symptoms of schizophrenia and either major depressive or manic symptoms

schizophrenia
a disorder characterized by severely impaired cognitive processes, disordered thinking and behaviors, and social withdrawal

schizophrenia spectrum
a group of disorders that range in severity and that have similar clinical features, including some degree of reality distortion

schizophreniform disorder
psychotic episodes with a duration of at least 1 month but less than 6 months

theory of mind
the ability to recognize that others have emotions, beliefs, and desires that may be different from one's own

focus
Questions

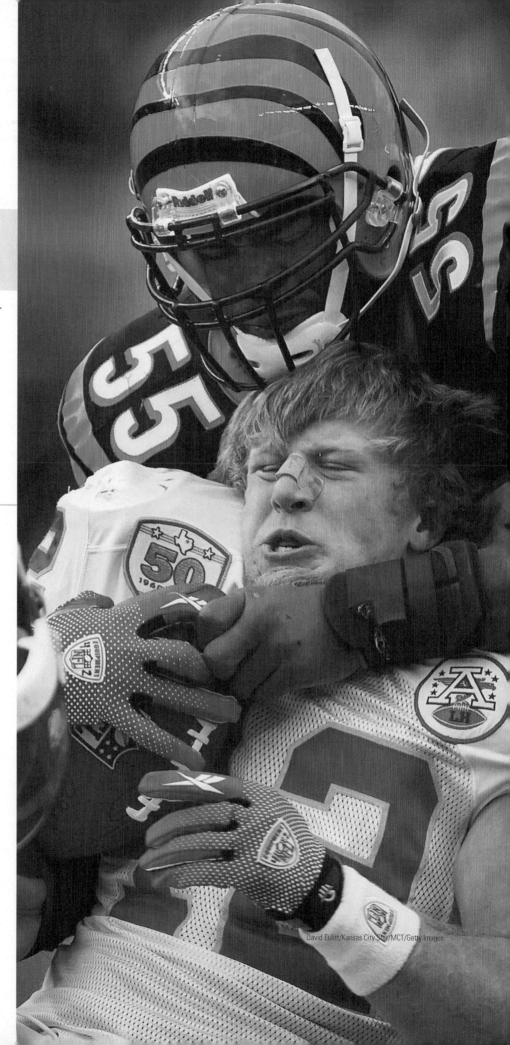

David Eulitt/Kansas City Star/MCT/Getty Images

13

Neurocognitive and Sleep–Wake Disorders

Learning Objectives

After studying this chapter, you will be able to . . .

13-1 Explain how we can determine whether someone has a neurocognitive disorder and discuss the three different types of neurocognitive disorders.

13-2 Summarize the key features of the various neurodegenerative and event-based neurocognitive disorders.

13-3 Describe some current treatments for neurocognitive disorders.

13-4 Compare and contrast the various sleep–wake disorders and discuss some of the treatments for these conditions.

Mr. C., Age 42, Was in a Coma for 2 Weeks After Falling from a Ladder. Before his fall, he was respectful, reliable, and easygoing. After the fall, socially inappropriate and impulsive behaviors, such as getting into arguments and groping women, occurred frequently and interfered with all aspects of his life. Brain scans and neuropsychological testing documented residual brain injury, including damage to the frontal lobe of his brain, an area associated with decision making and impulse control. Although additional rehabilitation resulted in significant improvement in his cognitive skills, lasting effects from the injury prevented complete recovery (Rao et al., 2007).

M r. C.'s life changed significantly after he fell and hit his head. Like many others who have experienced serious head trauma, Mr. C. qualifies for a diagnosis of **neurocognitive disorder** due to traumatic brain injury. Neurocognitive disorders result from transient (temporary) or permanent brain dysfunction triggered by changes in brain structure or biochemical processes within the brain. These structural and chemical changes result in impaired thinking, memory, or perception. Changes in behavior and emotional stability, as seen in the case of Mr. C., are also common among individuals diagnosed with a neurocognitive disorder. In fact, many individuals who sustain severe injury to the front regions of the brain display impulsive behavior, including saying or doing things without thinking. As you can imagine, these changes in functioning can be very frustrating for everyone involved.

In this chapter, we discuss the assessment of neurocognitive functioning and then focus on how the DSM-5-TR classifies neurocognitive disorders, as well as some of the causes for these disorders and methods of prevention, treatment, and rehabilitation. We also discuss sleep–wake disorders, many of which have a neurological basis.

13-1 Types of Neurocognitive Disorders

Although the DSM-5-TR defines only three major categories of neurocognitive disorders (major neurocognitive disorder, mild neurocognitive disorder, and delirium), the classification system recognizes that the symptoms of these disorders result from many disease processes or medical conditions. Therefore, medical assessment and determining specific etiology are important components of the diagnostic process. Thus, before we present the specific neurocognitive disorders outlined in the DSM-5-TR, we discuss an important first step—assessing and documenting a person's adaptive, day-to-day mental functioning.

The Assessment of Brain Damage and Neurocognitive Functioning

Medical professionals and medical procedures play a key role in assessing and diagnosing neurocognitive disorders. Physicians sometimes evaluate patients for brain damage during hospitalization following a traumatic event. Additionally, physicians may initiate assessment when an individual or family member is concerned about declining memory or other changes in mental functioning.

Clinicians begin by gathering background information, paying particular attention to mental changes involving memory, thinking, or self-help skills. They carefully evaluate overall thinking skills, personality characteristics, and adaptive coping, as well as behaviors and emotional reactivity. They rule out sensory conditions (such as impaired hearing or vision) or emotional factors (such as depression) as the primary cause of the cognitive decline. Assessment frequently involves screening of mental status, including memory and attentional skills and orientation to time and place. Additionally, psychologists may perform more extensive neuropsychological testing to pinpoint areas of cognitive difficulty or to evaluate emotional functioning. The goal is to see how a person's cognitive skills and adaptive behaviors compare with others of the same gender, age range, and educational level.

Medical professionals attempt to identify and treat any physical conditions that may be causing the symptoms. In some cases, something as simple as a urinary tract infection can impair cognitive functioning. Similarly, blood tests can detect medical conditions such as impaired thyroid or liver functioning or low levels of vitamin B_{12}. Structural and functional neurological testing procedures discussed in Chapter 3, such as electroencephalograph (EEG), computed tomography (CT), magnetic resonance imaging (MRI), and positron emission tomography (PET), are sometimes used to assess current brain functioning, as well as to monitor progression of **brain pathology**. Physicians decide which tests to use based on the person's specific symptoms, as well as the risks and benefits of the procedures.

After reviewing all of the data from medical and psychological tests, the professionals involved have a much better understanding of probable causes of the impairment. Neuropsychological testing and standardized cognitive screening also provide objective information about the severity of cognitive difficulties. Comprehensive baseline assessments allow clinicians to monitor changes in functioning. Although neuropsychological and neurological tests can assist with diagnosis, they provide limited information regarding prognosis or the predicted course of the disorder. Even when there is no cure, early diagnosis may provide an opportunity for interventions that delay the progression of a condition or allow the individual to make decisions about future care needs before symptoms worsen.

We will now review the three major categories of neurocognitive disorders described in the DSM-5-TR: (a) major neurocognitive disorder, (b) mild neurocognitive disorder, and (c) delirium (refer to Table 13.1).

Major Neurocognitive Disorder

Case Study   After retiring from a successful and demanding career as a company executive, Mr. P. filled his leisure time reading poetry, going to the theater, swimming, diving, and hiking. However, when Mr. P. was in his late 70s, his wife and daughters noticed that he seemed to lose interest in these activities. He also became forgetful, easily confused, and began to require assistance with daily tasks. He was easily agitated and complained that he felt trapped and lost. He lamented, "I feel like I am losing myself. What is happening to me?" (Sarafidou, 2018)

Table 13.1   Neurocognitive Disorders

Disorder	DSM-5-TR Criteria
Major neurocognitive disorder	Significant decline in performance in one or more cognitive areas; the deficits are severe enough to interfere with independence
Mild neurocognitive disorder[a]	Modest decline in performance in one or more cognitive areas; some compensatory strategies may be required to maintain independence
Delirium[b]	Sudden changes in cognition, including diminished awareness and impaired attention and focus

[a] Mild and major neurocognitive disorder are sometimes earlier and later stages of the same physiological condition.

[b] Delirium can occur with major and mild neurocognitive disorders but can also occur independent of these conditions.

Source: Based on information from APA, 2022

Individuals diagnosed with **major neurocognitive disorder** exhibit *significant* decline in both of the following:

- one or more areas of cognitive functioning, involving attention and focus, decision making and judgment, language, learning and memory, visual perception, or social understanding (Table 13.2); and
- the ability to independently meet the demands of daily living (this can involve more complex skills such as managing bills or medications).

The evidence from cognitive screening, neuropsychological testing, and interviews with the individual and others knowledgeable about the person's functioning must confirm that the person is demonstrating a significant skill deficit that represents a decline from prior levels of functioning. When known, clinicians specify the underlying medical circumstances causing the disorder. In the case of Mr. P., screening tests and input from his family members revealed a concerning deterioration in many areas of functioning. Although diagnosis of major neurocognitive disorder requires a significant deficit in only one cognitive area, deficits in multiple areas are common.

Dementia is the decline in mental functioning and self-help skills that results from the death of brain cells associated with a major neurocognitive disorder. People with dementia may forget past events or the names of significant others. They may also display difficulties with problem solving and impulse control. Agitation due to confusion or frustration is also common (World Health Organization, 2023a). Dementia typically has a gradual onset followed by continuing cognitive decline.

Age is the most studied and the strongest risk factor for dementia. The longer a person lives, the greater the chance of developing dementia. Although there is not a significant difference between women and men in the proportion who are diagnosed with dementia at any given age, due to their longer life expectancy, women in the United States have a greater lifetime risk of dementia (37 percent) compared to men (24 percent). Consistent with concerns about overall health disparities between racial/ethnic and socioeconomic groups within the United States, people who are White or who are well-educated tend to develop dementia much later in life, whereas people of color or who are less educated have both an earlier age of onset and a higher lifetime risk of exhibiting declines in neurocognitive functioning (Hale et al., 2020). As we discussed in Chapter 7, when people live with social conditions (such as poverty or racial discrimination) that result in ongoing stress, the result may be compromised health and cumulative physiological dysregulation that eventually result in cognitive impairment or dementia (Forrester et al., 2019).

Table 13.2 Areas of Possible Neurocognitive Dysfunction

Cognitive Domain	Skills Affected
Complex attention	Focus, planning, working memory
Executive ability	Decision making, mental flexibility
Learning and memory	Long-term and recent memory; ability to learn new tasks
Language	Understanding and use of language
Visual-perceptual ability	Construction, visual perception
Social cognition	Recognition of emotions, understanding of social situations, behavioral self-control

Source: APA, 2022

Mild Neurocognitive Disorder

Individuals diagnosed with **mild neurocognitive disorder** demonstrate a *modest* decline in at least one major cognitive area (refer to Table 13.2). The degree of cognitive impairment is more subtle than that seen in major neurocognitive disorder. Individuals with a mild neurocognitive disorder are often able to participate in their normal activities, although they may require extra time or effort to complete complex tasks. Although accommodations to maintain independence may be required (e.g., hiring someone to manage finances), overall independent functioning is not compromised.

Mild neurocognitive disorder is considered an intermediate stage between normal aging and major neurocognitive disorder or dementia. One of the challenges in diagnosing mild neurocognitive disorder is ensuring that the symptoms are, in fact, a disorder and not the effects of physical or emotional difficulties associated with aging. The primary difference is that the cognitive slowing and occasional memory lapses associated with normal aging have a minimal effect on daily functioning compared to the declines associated with mild or major neurocognitive disorder (refer to comparisons in Table 13.3).

The principal distinction between major and mild neurocognitive disorder is the severity of the decline in cognitive and independent functioning. In fact, mild and major neurocognitive disorders are sometimes earlier and later stages of the same disease process. For example, someone in the early stages of a progressive disorder such as Alzheimer disease may initially remain independent and display only moderate changes in cognitive functioning. As the disease progresses, however, the symptoms will increase in severity and begin to affect independent functioning. Unfortunately, the mild cognitive impairment associated with early dementia often goes undiagnosed; when this occurs, those affected do not have the benefit of receiving practical information about the condition or the opportunity to plan for future care before experiencing more severe cognitive difficulties.

Table 13.3   Normal Aging or Neurocognitive Disorder?

Normal Aging	Neurocognitive Disorder
Is independent in most activities, but may need occasional assistance with electronic devices, etc.	Has difficulty or requires assistance with normal, day-to-day activities
Occasionally misplaces things and locates them after searching	Places items in unusual locations; may not recall objects are missing or may accuse others of stealing
Occasionally forgets a name, word, or appointment	Frequently forgets words or recently learned information; uses incorrect words; repeats the same questions or comments
Is slower to complete mental or physical activities	Has difficulty performing familiar tasks
Acknowledges occasional forgetfulness	Is unaware or unconcerned about memory difficulties
Experiences occasional distractibility	Exercises poor judgment; fails to remember important dates or details
Continues interacting socially; occasionally feels tired	Exhibits decreasing social skills, declining social interest, and passivity; difficulty following or contributing to conversations
Occasionally gets lost	Experiences increasing disorientation and confusion; becomes lost or unaware of present location
Undergoes normal changes in mood	Has personality changes or drastic mood shifts; may seem apathetic, anxious, confused, or depressed

In some situations, a diagnosis is upgraded from major to mild neurocognitive disorder; this might occur when someone experiences partial recovery from a stroke or traumatic brain injury or was experiencing a temporary, treatable medical or psychological condition that caused transient cognitive decline. Treatment of these nondegenerative conditions may result in a return to normal functioning (Mehta & Herath, 2019). Unfortunately, individuals with either major or mild neurocognitive disorder (and people without any previous cognitive impairment) can experience an abrupt decline in functioning if they experience an episode of delirium, the third type of neurocognitive disorder.

Delirium

Case Study Police brought an 18-year-old high school senior to the emergency department after he was picked up wandering in traffic. He was angry, agitated, and aggressive. In a rambling, disjointed manner he explained that he had been using "speed." In the emergency room he had difficulty focusing his attention, frequently needed questions repeated, and was disoriented as to time and place. (Spitzer et al., 1994, p. 162)

Delirium is an acute state of confusion characterized by disorientation and impaired attentional skills. This disturbance in a person's mental abilities results from physiological factors such as medication reactions, alcohol or drug intoxication or withdrawal, or exposure to toxins (APA, 2022). Delirium can emerge in the context of a major or mild neurocognitive disorder, but it often appears independently as seen in the case of the teenager using drugs. Delirium differs from mild and major neurocognitive disorder based on its core characteristics (disturbance in awareness and difficulty focusing, maintaining, or shifting attention), as well as its abrupt onset and fluctuating course. Delirium typically develops over a period of several hours or days. Symptoms can be mild or quite severe, and can be brief or last for several months. People experiencing delirium often have significant cognitive difficulties, including confusion regarding where they are or the time of day. Wandering attention; disorganized thinking; and rambling, irrelevant, or incoherent speech may be present. Psychotic symptoms such as delusions or hallucinations may also occur. Symptoms of delirium fluctuate and can range from agitation and combativeness to drowsy, unresponsive behavior.

Because delirium is caused by relatively sudden neurological dysfunction, treatment involves identifying the underlying cause. Possible causes include high fever; severe dehydration or malnutrition; acute infection; sensitivity to a medication or combination of medications; alcohol, drug, or inhalant intoxication; physiological withdrawal from alcohol, sedatives, or sleeping medications; or brain changes associated with a neurocognitive disorder. Delirium also develops in some sleep–wake disorders, a topic we discuss later in the chapter. Additionally, when people are ill or elderly, they are more likely to develop delirium with medical illness, severe stress, or surgical procedures. Given the multiple stressors experienced during hospitalization (illness, sleep deprivation, recovery from surgery and anesthetics),

Hospital Delirium

Delirium is frequently experienced by individuals who are hospitalized, especially those who are seriously ill and receiving intensive care. Here a daughter comforts her father in the critical care unit in Denver, Colorado.

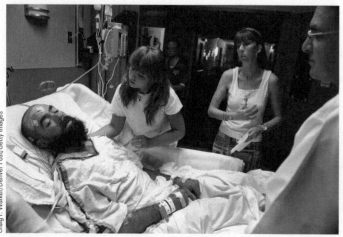

Craig F. Walker/Denver Post/Getty Images

episodes of hospital-associated delirium are common, especially among older adults. Delirium associated with hospitalization is presented in the following case study.

Case Study Justin Kaplan, an alert 84-year-old Pulitzer Prize–winning historian hospitalized after contracting pneumonia, describes an episode of delirium in which he fought with aliens: "Thousands of tiny little creatures, some on horseback, waving arms, carrying weapons like some grand Renaissance battle." In an attempt to "attack the aliens," Kaplan fell out of bed, injuring himself. He later threatened to kill his wife and kicked a nurse who was trying to restrain him. Once his medical condition improved, the delirium subsided. (Belluck, 2010)

As you can see from the case of Mr. Kaplan, the severe symptoms of hospital delirium can distress loved ones, especially because there is usually no prior history of such behavior. Hospital delirium is more common in older individuals and can result in longer hospital stays, lower rates of survival, and persistent cognitive impairment (Krämer et al., 2022). Fortunately, many hospitals attempt to detect and intervene with delirium in its earliest stages to prevent these consequences.

13-2 Etiology of Neurocognitive Disorders

Neurocognitive disorders result from a variety of medical conditions. Therefore, rather than an etiological discussion using our multipath model, we focus on some of the *sources* of neurocognitive disorders. We do this because, in most cases, neurocognitive disorders involve an identified or suspected medical condition or disease process. As you will see, some neurocognitive disorders involve neurodegenerative conditions in which symptoms become worse over time (Table 13.4), whereas others involve specific events such as stroke or head injury (Table 13.5). **Neurodegeneration** refers

Table 13.4 Neurodegenerative Disorders

Etiology	Characteristics
Alzheimer disease	Declining cognitive functioning, including early, prominent memory impairment
Dementia with Lewy bodies	Visual hallucinations, fluctuating cognitive impairment, dysfunction in motor skills
Parkinson disease	Tremor, muscle rigidity, slow movement, and possible cognitive decline
Huntington disease	Involuntary movement, cognitive decline, and emotional instability
Frontotemporal lobar degeneration	Brain degeneration in frontal or temporal lobes that includes variants that affect language, behavior, or motor skills
AIDS dementia complex	Cognitive decline due to HIV or AIDS

Table 13.5 Event Causes of Neurocognitive Disorders

Etiology	Characteristics
Ischemic stroke	Blockage of blood flow in the brain
Hemorrhagic stroke	Bleeding within the brain
Traumatic brain injury	Head wound or trauma
Substance abuse	Results from oxygen deprivation or other factors associated with intoxication, withdrawal, or chronic substance use

to progressive brain damage due to neurochemical abnormalities and the death of brain cells. In contrast with the recovery that is possible in cases of stroke, traumatic brain injury, or substance abuse, individuals with neurodegenerative disorders exhibit a pattern of decline in function rather than improvement. Neurodegenerative disorders vary greatly in terms of age of onset, skills affected, and course of the disorder. It is not unusual for people with a neurodegenerative disorder to have brain abnormalities associated with more than one condition.

As we discuss the various medical conditions associated with neurocognitive disorders, it is important to remember that even with the same underlying brain condition, a variety of factors can influence outcome. For example, people with similar brain trauma may recover quite differently, depending on their personalities, their coping skills, and the availability of resources such as rehabilitation and family support. Additionally, the disruptions in brain function seen in neurocognitive disorders can lead to a variety of behavioral and emotional changes; factors such as apathy, depression, anxiety, or difficulty with impulse control can significantly affect recovery. Furthermore, insensitivity or impatience directed toward

Focus on Resilience

Can We Prevent Brain Damage?

Given the serious consequences of neurocognitive disorders, you may wonder: "Is there anything that can be done to reduce the chances of experiencing a stroke, suffering a head injury, or developing a degenerative disorder?" The answer is yes, especially when prevention efforts begin at an early age. For instance, the use of car seats and seat belts can help prevent head injury, as can the use of safe practices and properly fitting protective headgear during sports (Trefan et al., 2016). Similarly, allowing the brain to rest and recover after a blow to the head or a concussion can reduce the likelihood of long-term brain damage (American Academy of Neurology, 2020).

Lifestyle changes focused on maintaining a healthy cardiovascular system such as exercising regularly and eating a well-balanced diet also

Kevin Peterson/Photodisc/Getty Images

reduce the risk of both stroke and dementia (Gardener et al., 2016). A healthy lifestyle protects against dementia not only by reducing risk factors but also by promoting neurogenesis, the formation of new brain cells (Hueston et al., 2017). Prevention efforts focus on modifiable risk factors (e.g., avoiding smoking and excessive consumption of salt, sugar, saturated fats, and alcohol), because these unhealthy behaviors account for the majority of the risk of stroke and much of the risk of dementia (Kivipelto et al., 2018). Regular participation in cognitively stimulating activities across the life span (especially during early and middle adulthood) is also associated with fewer pathological brain changes (less beta-amyloid) later in life (Landau et al., 2012). Prevention efforts can make a significant difference in maintaining brain health.

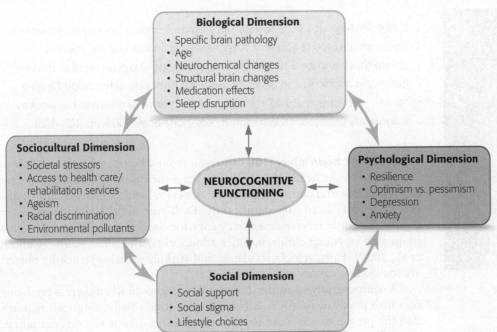

Figure 13.1

Multipath Model of
Neurocognitive Disorders
The dimensions interact with
specific brain pathology to
produce the symptoms and
pattern of recovery seen
in various neurocognitive
disorders.

Biological Dimension
- Specific brain pathology
- Age
- Neurochemical changes
- Structural brain changes
- Medication effects
- Sleep disruption

Sociocultural Dimension
- Societal stressors
- Access to health care/ rehabilitation services
- Ageism
- Racial discrimination
- Environmental pollutants

NEUROCOGNITIVE FUNCTIONING

Psychological Dimension
- Resilience
- Optimism vs. pessimism
- Depression
- Anxiety

Social Dimension
- Social support
- Social stigma
- Lifestyle choices

people with neurocognitive disorders can add to their stress and negatively affect their functioning. Indeed, stress can exacerbate symptoms that stem from the brain pathology itself. From the perspective of our multipath model, the specific brain pathology is the primary biological factor for each condition; however, psychological, social, and sociocultural factors can interact with the neurological condition to affect outcome, as presented in Figure 13.1. We now begin our discussion of medical conditions that can result in a neurocognitive disorder.

Neurocognitive Disorder due to Traumatic Brain Injury

Case Study   United States Representative Gabrielle Giffords, age 40, was shot in the head at point-blank range on January 8, 2011. The bullet entered into and exited from the left side of her brain. Following surgery, Representative Giffords remained in a **medically induced coma**, a state of deep sedation that allows time for the brain to heal. Part of her skull was removed to accommodate the anticipated swelling of her brain and to prevent further damage. Giffords's purposeful movements and responsiveness to simple commands were early, encouraging signs. Although extensive therapy helped Giffords regain many language and motor skills, she officially resigned her congressional seat, recognizing that she needed to continue to participate in specialized cognitive and physical rehabilitation in order to maximize her recovery.

Case Study   At age 53, H. N. sustained multiple injuries, including mild bleeding in the brain, when he was hit by a car. Although his initial delirium subsided, other behavioral changes, including pervasive apathy punctuated by angry outbursts, persisted for months. Subsequent MRI scans revealed damage in the orbitofrontal cortex, an area of the brain involved in emotion and decision making. (adapted from Namiki et al., 2008, p. 475)

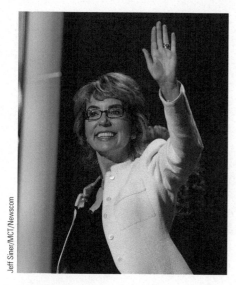

Recovery from Traumatic Brain Injury

Gabrielle Giffords, a former U.S. Congress member, sustained a brain injury from a gunshot in 2011. Here Giffords waves to the delegates at the 2012 Democratic National Convention, where she captivated the audience by reciting the Pledge of Allegiance in a halting but strong voice while holding her right hand over her heart with the help of her stronger left hand.

Case Study P. J. M., a 38-year-old woman, remained in a coma for several weeks after a bicycle accident. After regaining consciousness, she had severe short- and long-term memory deficits (including no recall of the year before her accident) and difficulty using the right side of her body. Despite some improvement, P. J. M. remains unable to drive or return to her work as a university professor. (adapted from Rathbone et al., 2009, pp. 407–408)

Traumatic brain injury (TBI) can result from a bump, jolt, blow, or physical wound to the head. As you can see from the cases presented, the degree of impairment and course of recovery associated with a neurocognitive disorder due to TBI can vary significantly. Each year in the United States, over 2 million people receive emergency care for head injury; TBI occurs most frequently in young children, older adolescents, and older adults (Capizzi et al., 2020). Falls, vehicle accidents, and striking or being struck by objects are the leading causes of TBI (Figure 13.2).

A neurocognitive disorder due to TBI is diagnosed when there is persisting cognitive impairment due to a brain injury; additionally, diagnosis requires that the person experienced loss of consciousness, amnesia, disorientation, or confusion following the event or received neurological testing that documented brain dysfunction (APA, 2022). The effects of TBI can be temporary or permanent and can result in mild to severe cognitive impairment. You have probably heard stories about people who have made a remarkable recovery following TBI. For example, the much-publicized progress of Gabrielle Giffords after her injury demonstrates the capacity for brain recovery. In her case, immediate intervention, an excellent rehabilitation program, personal resilience, and social support all played a key role in her progress. Similar conditions facilitated the recovery of news anchor Bob Woodruff, who sustained a life-threatening brain injury resulting from a roadside bomb explosion while he was covering the war in Iraq. After surgery, he spent 36 days in a medically induced coma. He underwent extensive rehabilitation and was able to return to work as a television news reporter. In both cases, prompt medical attention and surgery played an important role in survival and recovery.

Figure 13.2

Leading Causes of Traumatic Brain Injury
* These data do not include injuries that occurred during military deployment.
Source: Taylor et al., 2017

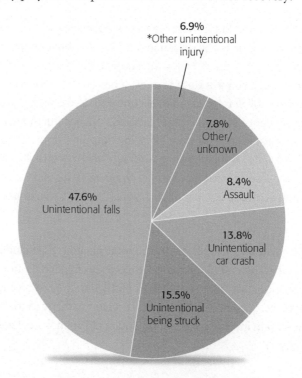

Just How Safe Are Contact Sports?

How important is it for those involved in sports to know about concussion? Injuries resulting from team sports are increasingly sparking public concern. The suicides of Pennsylvania college football player Owen Thomas, age 21, and NFL linebacker Junior Seau, age 43, garnered attention when their autopsies revealed evidence of the degenerative brain condition chronic traumatic encephalopathy (CTE), likely resulting from repeated head injuries incurred while playing football. An autopsy on former Cincinnati Bengals player Chris Henry, age 26, who died after falling out of a truck, also revealed CTE. Amazingly, none of these athletes were ever diagnosed with a concussion during their years in football. How could such significant brain damage occur at such a young age, particularly with no history of concussion?

A groundbreaking study involving a high school football team shed some light on the issue (Talavage et al., 2014). Researchers compared cognitive testing and brain imaging of the players (obtained before, during, and after the football season) with data regarding the frequency and intensity of head impact during the football season (obtained by equipping the players' helmets with special impact-monitoring sensors). As expected, players who had experienced a concussion during the season experienced MRI changes and related cognitive declines. However, so did half of the other players; data from the impact-monitoring sensors revealed that the players who experienced brain changes but no recorded concussions had sustained multiple impacts during the season. For example, one affected player had experienced 1,600 significant head blows during the season. A similarly designed study involving college varsity football and ice hockey players wearing instrumented helmets revealed that those with more measured instances of physical contact and head impact

displayed deterioration in performance on tests involving verbal learning and reaction time. The researchers concluded that repetitive head impact throughout a single sports season has the potential to impair learning in college athletes (McAllister et al., 2012). Interestingly, concussions and repetitive head impacts in collegiate football are disproportionally higher during preseason compared to the regular season (McCrea et al., 2021).

Professional medical organizations have created guidelines for school-age athletes suspected of having a concussion. Recommendations include immediate removal from play and restriction of physical activity for at least 7 to 10 days. Return to play should occur only after all acute symptoms subside and a health professional knowledgeable about head injury agrees that it is safe to resume athletic activities (American Academy of Neurology, 2020). If followed, these guidelines could significantly increase safety for athletes. Careful monitoring of athletes with possible neurological damage (e.g., headache, confusion, poor balance, speech, vision, or hearing difficulties) is certainly a step in the right direction. However, it is equally important to minimize the frequency of impact injuries because repetitive head impact increases the likelihood of long-term neurological consequences (Stemper et al., 2019).

For Further Consideration

1. Are there adequate protections in place for athletes who experience a blow to the head but display no symptoms of a concussion?

2. Are the potential dangers of head injuries in sports such as basketball, soccer, baseball, hockey, or cycling receiving sufficient attention?

A far different outcome resulted from what initially appeared to be a minor head injury sustained by actress Natasha Richardson. Her first symptom, a headache, did not appear until almost an hour after she hit the back of her head during a ski lesson; however, unrecognized neurological injury (i.e., bleeding between the skull and brain) resulted in her rapid and unexpected death. Sometimes referred to as the "talk and die" syndrome, such an injury can have severe, even fatal, consequences. All of these stories highlight the importance of immediate medical intervention when a head injury occurs.

As seen in the case studies, the severity, duration, and symptoms of TBI can vary significantly depending on the extent and location of the brain damage, as well as the person's age. Symptoms can include headaches, disorientation, confusion, memory loss, deficits in attention, poor concentration, fatigue, and irritability, as well as emotional and behavioral changes. Generally, the greater the damage to brain tissue or cells, the more impaired the functioning.

Chronic Traumatic Encephalopathy and Suicide

An autopsy of Junior Seau, a former NFL linebacker who committed suicide in May, 2012, revealed that he suffered from chronic traumatic encephalopathy, a condition resulting from recurrent head trauma that can lead to depression and cognitive difficulties. Autopsies on other NFL players who committed suicide have revealed similar brain pathology.

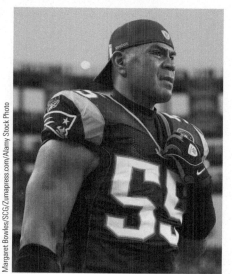

Margaret Bowles/SCG/Zumapress.com/Alamy Stock Photo

Acute head injuries include concussions, contusions, and cerebral lacerations. **Concussion**, the most common form of traumatic brain injury, refers to trauma-induced changes in brain functioning, typically caused by a blow to the head. The injury affects the functioning of neurons and causes disorientation or loss of consciousness. Symptoms of concussion can include headache, dizziness, nausea, impaired coordination, and sensitivity to light. Following a concussion, physicians recommend resting, minimizing stimulation or mental challenge, and refraining from any activity that can produce subsequent head injury (American Academy of Neurology, 2020). Symptoms of a concussion are usually temporary, lasting no longer than a few weeks; however, in some cases they persist for much longer. Amnesia for events prior to a concussion appears to be a strong predictor of severity of impairment following a concussion (Jackson & Starling, 2019). It is estimated that U.S. children and adults incur almost 4 million concussions per year while involved in competitive sports or recreational activities; however, as many as half of these concussions go unreported and untreated (Baldwin et al., 2018).

A **cerebral contusion** (bruising of the brain) results when the brain strikes the skull with sufficient force to cause bruising. Unlike the disruption in cellular functioning seen in a concussion, contusions involve actual tissue damage in the areas bruised. Symptoms are similar to those seen with a concussion. Contusions and concussions commonly occur together. When someone receives a blow to the head, brain injury often occurs both at the site of impact and on the opposite side of the brain (i.e., the initial blow causes the brain to move and hit the other side of the skull). Neuroimaging can detect brain damage and monitor swelling. Unfortunately, brain imaging cannot always detect the more subtle changes caused by damage to neurons (a concussion), mild bruising of brain tissue (a contusion), or mild bleeding within the brain.

A **cerebral laceration** is an open head injury in which brain tissue is torn, pierced, or ruptured, usually from a skull fracture or an object that has penetrated the skull. As with a contusion, damage is localized and immediate medical care focuses on reducing bleeding and preventing swelling. As with other brain injuries, symptoms of cerebral lacerations can be quite serious, depending on the location of the injury, the extent of damage to the brain tissue, the amount of hemorrhaging or swelling within the brain, and the medical care received.

Severe brain trauma can have long-term effects, and, as you saw in the introductory case studies, recovery does not always ensure a return to prior levels of functioning. Along with the physical or cognitive difficulties produced by the injury, sleep difficulties and emotional symptoms commonly associated with TBI (e.g., depression, anxiety, irritability, or apathy) can also affect recuperation (Misch & Raukar, 2020). In some cases, the brain trauma sets off a cascade of events within the brain that cause progressive mental deterioration.

Chronic Traumatic Encephalopathy

Case Study   A highly decorated military officer was known for his competence, reliability, and emotional stability. During his career, he participated in multiple training exercises and in combat situations that involved exposure to bombs and improvised explosive devices (IEDs) detonating in close proximity. He had frequent headaches and began to have difficulty with memory and mental focus. Eventually, his speech became jumbled, and he moved slowly and became uncharacteristically angry. He died by suicide. Although an MRI scan performed 1 month before his death showed nothing abnormal, his autopsy revealed a unique pattern of abnormalities seen in other veterans exposed to blast injuries. (Shively et al., 2016)

Chronic traumatic encephalopathy (CTE) is a degenerative condition associated with traumatic brain injury. CTE occurs when abnormal deposits of a normally occurring brain substance, tau protein, begin to clump together, causing both gray and white matter to slowly and progressively atrophy. Not only does the pathology associated with the head trauma persist, but the damage also spreads within the brain, causing progressive, long-term debilitating effects. This condition occurs in individuals who have experienced brain injury resulting from incidents involving impact to the head or from explosive blast–related injuries associated with military combat. The risk of developing CTE is increased among those who experience multiple episodes of brain injury—such as athletes participating in contact sports or military personnel exposed to combat (McKee et al., 2023; Vanltallie, 2019).

The various stages of CTE (refer to Figure 13.3) include the following cognitive and psychological symptoms (Fesharaki-Zadeh, 2019):

Stage I: Headache and loss of attention and concentration

Stage II: Depression, explosive outbursts, and short-term memory loss

Stage III: Cognitive impairment, including difficulties with planning and impulse control

Stage IV: Dementia, word-finding difficulty, and aggression

Similar to the neurodegenerative disorders we discuss later in the chapter, the neurological damage associated with CTE progresses slowly over decades, eventually resulting in dementia. When someone with a history of head trauma (particularly cumulative head trauma) demonstrates this constellation of cognitive and emotional symptoms, CTE may be suspected, but a CTE diagnosis can be confirmed only by an autopsy of the brain. A puzzling new development—the postmortem discovery of brain pathology associated with CTE in individuals with no history of neurotrauma—has baffled researchers and will require further research (Iverson et al., 2019).

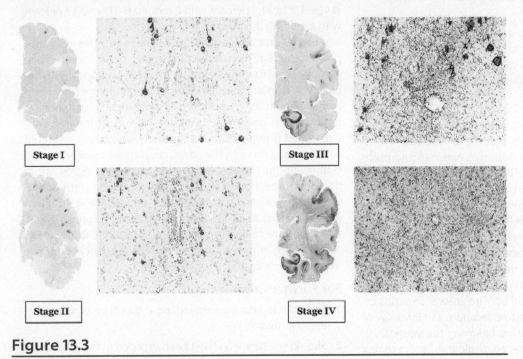

Stage I

Stage II

Stage III

Stage IV

Figure 13.3

Stages of Chronic Traumatic Encephalopathy

Postmortem analysis of tissue from brain donations from former athletes and military personnel has increased our understanding of the four stages of chronic traumatic encephalopathy.

Source: Fesharaki-Zadeh, 2019

Traumatic Brain Injury Among Combat Veterans

Many members of the armed forces involved in conflicts in the Middle East have experienced serious brain injuries. John Barnes, pictured here, incurred a traumatic brain injury in Iraq when mortar shrapnel entered his brain. Due to extensive damage involving his frontal lobe, Barnes continues to exhibit impulsive behavior and lack of inhibition.

Vascular Neurocognitive Disorders

Vascular neurocognitive disorders can result from a one-time **cardiovascular** event such as a stroke or from unnoticed, ongoing disruptions to blood flow within the brain. Vascular neurocognitive disorders often begin with **atherosclerosis**, thickening of the arteries resulting from a buildup of plaque. This **plaque** (composed of fat, cholesterol, and other substances) accumulates over time, thickens, and narrows artery walls; the result is reduced blood flow

---

Going Deeper

Head Injury: What Do Soldiers Need to Know?

- A 28-year-old soldier with six separate blast-related concussions reports that he has daily headaches and difficulty performing simple mental tasks.

- After a bomb explosion hurled an army enlistee against a wall, he continued working despite being dazed and suffering shrapnel wounds. Confusion, headaches, and problems with balance persisted for months; he later developed seizures.

- The driver of a vehicle hit by a roadside bomb did not appear to be seriously injured. However, in the months following the explosion, his speech was slurred and he had difficulty reading and completing simple tasks (Miller & Zwerdling, 2010).

A confidential survey conducted by the Rand Corporation (2010) revealed that almost 20 percent of veterans returning from Iraq and Afghanistan reported experiencing probable traumatic brain injury (TBI) during combat—injuries caused by blasts from hidden land mines and improvised explosive devices. These explosions cause complex brain damage, including (a) scattered brain injury resulting from shock waves that bruise the brain and damage nerve pathways, (b) penetrating injury from fragments of shrapnel or flying debris, and (c) injury from being thrown by the blast (Champion et al., 2009). Just what are the long-term risks from head injuries sustained in combat? The answer depends on many factors, including the source, location, and intensity of the injury, as well as interventions following the injury. Civilians treated for TBI are encouraged to allow the brain to rest to facilitate full recovery. However, in combat situations, mild head injuries are often not recognized, documented, and treated; soldiers frequently return immediately to combat (Murray et al., 2005). Even when good care is available, we need to recognize that some veterans will experience ongoing and often progressive psychological and cognitive difficulties long after they leave the military. The likelihood that a veteran will develop long-term disability depends on the severity of the brain injury, ranging from 65.6 percent of those with a severe TBI to 31.4 percent with a moderate TBI and 12 percent with a mild TBI (Agimi et al., 2021).

Long-term consequences of these injuries may also place soldiers at risk for the progressive brain degeneration associated with chronic traumatic encephalopathy (Elder et al., 2019). In a longitudinal study comparing the 5-year outcome for military veterans who experienced an apparently mild concussion following blast exposure compared with a matched group of combat veterans who never exhibited concussive symptoms, the nonconcussed group exhibited no significant impairment. In contrast, the blast-injured group demonstrated significant disability involving both cognitive and psychiatric symptoms and reduced life satisfaction (Mac Donald et al., 2019). Both scientists and veterans' affairs advocates are calling for enhanced treatment strategies to alleviate the long-term and costly consequences of these wartime injuries.

For Further Consideration

1. Should standard recommendations for TBI for civilians also apply to soldiers?

2. Should veterans who have been exposed to blast injuries receive long-term monitoring for emotional or cognitive symptoms associated with CTE?

to the brain and other organs. Predominant cognitive symptoms of vascular neurocognitive disorder involve difficulties with complex attention, information processing, planning, and problem solving. Changes in motivation, personality, or mood are also common.

Stroke

> **Case Study** Kate McCarron's stroke symptoms started on a Friday, with a little tingle in her leg. On Saturday, McCarron, age 46, felt uncharacteristically tired. Sunday, she seemed a bit under the weather. Monday, her left side felt numb. Tuesday morning, she couldn't move her left side. She was rushed to the hospital. A small blood vessel leading to a deep part of her brain was closing, choking off a region of her brain that controlled motion. (Dworkin, 2009)

A **stroke** occurs when there is an obstruction in blood flow to or within the brain; the sudden halt of blood flow results in death of neurons and loss of brain function. Each year more than 795,000 people in the United States have a stroke. Of those who survive a stroke, over half become seriously disabled. Although immediate medical attention and careful management of neurological complications from stroke (e.g., bleeding or swelling within the brain) can improve outcome, stroke remains a leading cause of death in the United States; stroke risk and mortality from stroke are particularly high for African American and Pacific Islander adults (CDC, 2023e).

There are two major types of strokes: *hemorrhagic strokes* and *ischemic strokes*. A **hemorrhagic stroke**, unrelated to plaque buildup, occurs when a blood vessel bursts and bleeds into the brain. An **ischemic stroke** is caused by a clot or severe narrowing of the arteries; approximately 87 percent of strokes are ischemic (CDC, 2023). A **transient ischemic attack (TIA)** is a "mini-stroke" or "warning stroke" resulting from temporary blockage of blood vessels in the brain; symptoms often last for only a few minutes. Seeking medical attention for transient stroke symptoms is important because these episodes often precede an ischemic stroke (American Stroke Association, 2023). When people seek emergency medical care for stroke symptoms, medications can dissolve the clot and prevent serious brain damage. In both ischemic and hemorrhagic strokes, brain damage occurs when brain cells die due to lack of blood, oxygen, and nutrients (Figure 13.4).

Strokes can occur at any age; in fact, the risk of someone under age 50 having an ischemic stroke has been steadily increasing. This increase appears to be due to significant increases in traditional risk factors among this group, including hypertension, obesity, diabetes, high cholesterol, and smoking (George et al., 2017). Cigarette smoking is a major contributor in about one in four strokes; however, when young adults experience a stroke, the contribution of smoking approaches 50 percent. An analysis of worldwide data revealed that men and women who smoke have a 60 percent to 80 percent increase in stroke risk; not surprisingly, countries that have seen a decrease in the rates of smoking have also seen decreases in the risk of having a deadly hemorrhagic stroke (Nicholson et al., 2019). Use of oral contraceptives (i.e., "the pill") can increase stroke risk, particularly when there are other risk factors such as smoking or hypertension (Carlton et al., 2018). Worldwide data regarding stroke risk point to additional modifiable factors that contribute to stroke, including an unhealthy diet, a sedentary lifestyle, and heavy drinking (Donkor, 2018). Certain biomarkers in the blood (e.g., proteins and enzymes associated with inflammation in the arteries) are now used to identify individuals at risk for ischemic stroke (Hu, Liu, et al., 2019).

Did You Know?

Postmortem analysis of the donated brains of over 100 National Football League players revealed that 99 percent had pathology findings consistent with chronic traumatic encephalopathy, with the majority displaying severe damage.
Source: Mez et al., 2017

Figure 13.4

Types of Stroke
Ischemic strokes resulting from a blocked artery account for approximately 87 percent of all strokes.

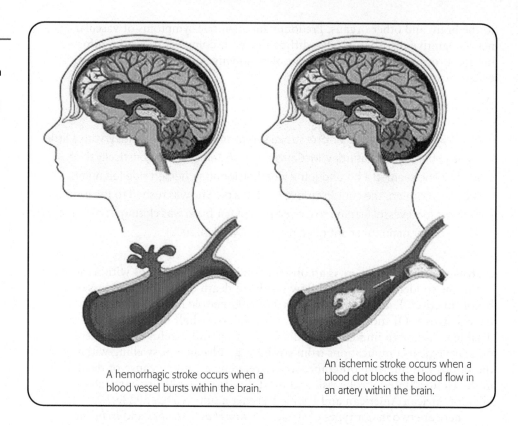

A hemorrhagic stroke occurs when a blood vessel bursts within the brain.

An ischemic stroke occurs when a blood clot blocks the blood flow in an artery within the brain.

Stroke is not only a leading cause of death but also a significant cause of disability. Prompt medical intervention decreases the chances of death and vastly improves prognosis; this underscores the importance of recognizing signs of a stroke (Table 13.6). Because many people do not recognize stroke symptoms (e.g., slurred speech, blurry vision, vertigo, or numbness on one side of the body), or hesitate to treat these symptoms as an emergency, public health campaigns continue to stress the importance of immediate intervention. Additionally, many are unaware that women may display unique stroke symptoms, including fainting, sudden nausea, overall weakness, or shortness of breath (American Stroke Association, 2023).

Stroke survivors who do not receive immediate intervention often require long-term care because residual physical and psychological symptoms impair independent functioning. Strokes damaging the left side of the brain typically affect speech and language proficiency, as well as

Table 13.6 Stroke Symptoms: Know When to Act

Recognizing stroke symptoms and seeking immediate medical attention can significantly improve outcomes for both ischemic and hemorrhagic strokes.

- Numbness or weakness, including drooping of facial features or weakness on one side of the body

- Confusion or difficulty understanding questions or conversation

- Slurred or incoherent speech

- Vision difficulty in one or both eyes

- Sudden dizziness, loss of balance, or difficulty with coordination

- Severe headache with no known cause

physical movement on the right half of the body. Strokes occurring within the right hemisphere can increase impulsivity and impair judgment, short-term memory, and motor movement on the left side of the body. Visual problems (blurry or double vision) may also occur in those with a right-hemisphere stroke. Cognitive, behavioral, and emotional changes that occur following stroke depend not only on the extent of brain damage but also on the individual's personality, emotional resilience, and coping skills. Some stroke survivors experience frustration and depression, whereas others actively and optimistically participate in therapeutic rehabilitation activities. Unfortunately, the onset of depression after stroke is not uncommon, especially when the stroke is serious or there is a prior history of depression. Further, depression following an ischemic stroke is associated with an increased likelihood of a subsequent stroke (Wu, Zhou, et al., 2019).

Vascular Dementia

Vascular dementia results from a series of small asymptomatic (symptomless) strokes or other conditions that interfere with optimal blood flow to the brain. When small bleeds in the brain (microbleeds) or a decrease in blood flow from small clots or narrowed arteries occur, the resulting brain damage often leads to neurodegeneration and a resultant deterioration in intellectual and physical abilities. Increasing confusion and disorientation are often the first signs of this condition. The severity of symptoms depends on the extent of the damage and the brain regions involved. Vascular dementia is the second most common type of dementia, estimated to account for 5 percent to 10 percent of cases of dementia. This condition often coexists with Alzheimer disease because lifestyle risk factors such as hypertension, diabetes, and smoking increase the risk of both disorders (Alzheimer's Association, 2023).

Neurocognitive Disorder due to Substance Abuse

Use or abuse of drugs or alcohol can result in delirium or more chronic brain dysfunction. Delirium is associated with extreme intoxication, drug or alcohol withdrawal, use of multiple substances, or inhalant use (due to oxygen deprivation or the toxicity of substances inhaled). Symptoms consistent with mild neurocognitive disorder are common in individuals with a history of heavy substance use and those who continue using after age 50 (APA, 2022). Although the symptoms frequently continue during initial abstinence, they often improve if the person remains sober. For example, many of the deficits associated with alcohol-induced neurocognitive disorder require a full year of abstinence before they fully subside; however, older individuals and chronic substance users are less likely to recover full brain function (Schulte et al., 2014).

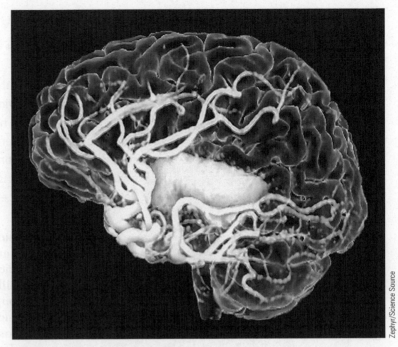

Zephyr/Science Source

Results of a Stroke on the Brain

The brain damage associated with a stroke is caused by blockages that cause an interruption in the brain's blood supply or by the leakage of blood through blood vessel walls. Here, a three-dimensional magnetic resonance angiogram scan reveals a human brain after a hemorrhagic stroke. Major arteries are in white. The central region in yellow is an area in which bleeding occurred.

Neurocognitive Disorder due to Alzheimer Disease

Case Study Elizabeth R., a 46-year-old woman diagnosed with Alzheimer disease, is trying to cope with her increasing memory difficulties. She writes notes to herself and rehearses conversations, anticipating what might be said. After reading only a few sentences, she forgets what she has read. She sometimes forgets where the bathroom is located in her own house and is depressed by the realization that she is becoming a burden to her family. (Clark et al., 1984, p. 60)

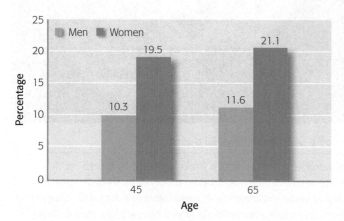

Figure 13.5

Estimated Lifetime Risk for Alzheimer Dementia, by Gender at Age 45 and Age 65

The longer life expectancy of women is associated with a greater risk of developing Alzheimer disease.

Source: Alzheimer's Association, 2023

Alzheimer disease (AD), the most prevalent neurodegenerative disorder, affected more than 6 million U.S. Americans in 2020. It is estimated that by 2050 over 13 million adults in the United States will have AD. Although AD can strike adults in midlife, risk of the disease significantly increases with age; over three fourths of those diagnosed with AD in the United States are age 75 or older. Given their greater longevity, women account for approximately two thirds of all cases of the disorder in the United States (Alzheimer's Research Association, 2023) (refer to Figure 13.5).

AD usually begins gradually and involves a pattern of progressive cognitive decline. Although clinicians sometimes make a diagnosis of mild or major neurocognitive disorder due to AD by incorporating biological data such as genetic testing into the diagnostic process, they often rely on subjective reports regarding observed declines in cognitive and self-help skills. The main feature of AD is memory impairment; however, clinicians avoid diagnosing AD based solely on memory difficulties. Without clear physiological indicators (e.g., evidence of genetic mutations or biomarkers associated with AD), it is not yet possible to predict which patients with mild memory impairment will develop AD (Weller & Budson, 2018). Individuals seeking treatment for impaired memory develop AD at a rate of 12 percent to 15 percent per year; however, individuals with memory impairment in the general population (i.e., not just those who seek treatment) are less likely to develop AD, and, in cases involving a transient medical condition, the symptoms disappear (APA, 2022).

Characteristics of Alzheimer Disease

Memory and learning impairments associated with AD develop quite gradually, followed by a progressive decline in other areas of cognitive functioning. Unfortunately, the physiological processes that produce AD begin years before the onset of cognitive difficulties. As early symptoms—memory dysfunction, irritability, and cognitive impairment—gradually worsen, other symptoms such as social withdrawal, depression, apathy, delusions, impulsive behaviors, and neglect of personal hygiene often appear. Some individuals with AD become loving and childlike, whereas others become increasingly agitated and combative. At present, no curative or disease-reversing interventions exist for AD.

As we saw in the case of Elizabeth, deterioration of memory is one of the most disturbing symptoms for those who have AD and for their family members. Initially, those affected may forget appointments, phone numbers, and addresses, but as AD progresses, they lose track of the time of day, have trouble remembering recent and past events, and forget who they are. But even when memory is gone, emotions remain. In fact, researchers have found that although those with AD may forget details of an emotional event (such as the plot of a sad movie), the emotions of the experience continue (Feinstein et al., 2010). Overlearned skills such as guitar playing or singing often remain during the later stages of Alzheimer disease even as memories fade and behavioral changes occur. In describing her experiences watching her husband's cognitive decline, the wife of singer Tony Bennett stated, "There's a lot about him that I miss . . . But when he sings, he's still the old Tony" (Nolfi, 2021).

Other Factors Affecting Memory Loss

A common concern of older adults is whether occasional memory lapses are signs of AD. Memory loss occurs for a variety of reasons. In some cases, it is an early symptom of AD. However, occasional lapses of memory are common in healthy adults. As we age, neurons are gradually lost, our brains become smaller, and we process information more slowly. Thus, occasional difficulty with memory or learning new material is normal. Many older adults experience only minimal decline in cognitive function; this is because as we age, we continue to generate new brain cells and the brain reorganizes itself in a way that maximizes cognitive efficiency (Sampedro-Piquero et al., 2018).

Memory loss and confusion can also result from temporary conditions such as severe stress, infection, or reactions to prescription drugs. Medications sometimes interact with one another or with certain foods to produce side effects, including memory impairment. In addition, various physical conditions and nutritional deficiencies can produce memory loss and symptoms resembling dementia. This type of memory loss usually disappears once the medical condition is diagnosed and treated.

Alzheimer Disease and the Brain

Individuals with AD exhibit a variety of changes in the brain that begin years before symptoms develop. Brain autopsies of people with AD reveal two irregularities—neurofibrillary tangles and beta-amyloid plaques. These abnormalities affect metabolic processes and the health of neurons in the

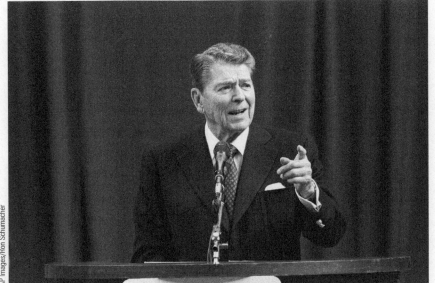

AP Images/Ron Schumacher

Did You Know?

Difficulty identifying smells such as lemon, banana, and cinnamon may be an early sign of Alzheimer disease.

Source: Jung et al., 2019

Did Alzheimer Disease Affect His Presidency?

Former President Ronald Reagan was diagnosed with Alzheimer disease at age 83. Many believe he began to exhibit symptoms of the disease, such as memory difficulties, while still in office. Five years prior to the diagnosis, Reagan was treated for a traumatic head injury that occurred when he was thrown from a horse. Some have speculated that this head injury accelerated the progression of his Alzheimer disease.

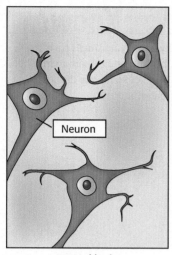

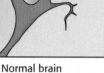

Normal brain

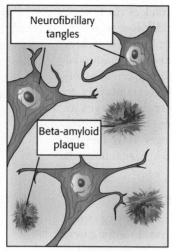

Alzheimer's brain

Figure 13.6

Brain Changes Associated with Alzheimer Disease

Autopsies of the brains of individuals with Alzheimer disease reveal beta-amyloid plaques in the spaces between neurons and neurofibrillary tangles inside nerve cells. These brain changes begin years before symptoms of the disease appear.

hippocampus and in areas of the cortex associated with memory and cognition. **Neurofibrillary tangles**, found inside nerve cells, are composed of twisted fibers of *tau*, a protein that has important functions in healthy cells; in those with AD, biochemical alterations in tau protein result in a clumping of the protein within the cell. As the abnormal accumulation of tau protein continues to result in neurofibrillary tangles, dysfunctional cellular communication produces mild cognitive symptoms, followed by progressive cognitive decline and impairment in daily functioning.

Additionally, **beta-amyloid plaques** develop when beta-amyloid proteins aggregate in the spaces between neurons (refer to Figure 13.6). Once the beta-amyloid deposits appear and begin to multiply, neurodegeneration accelerates. Neurofibrillary tangles and beta-amyloid plaques are associated with decreased neurogenesis (reduced production of new brain cells), as well as inflammation, loss of cellular connections, and other changes that eventually result in the death of neurons and shrinking of the brain (Saha & Sen, 2019). We are learning more about this process due to advances in single-photon emission computed tomography (SPECT) and positron emission tomography (PET) imaging that allow the detection and monitoring of beta-amyloid plaques, tau protein accumulation, and neuroinflammation in the living brain (Valotassiou et al., 2018). Not long ago, it was impossible to diagnose AD before autopsy, even when a person had multiple indicators suggestive of AD (e.g., memory loss or brain scans demonstrating brain shrinkage). However, there is increased hope for early diagnosis given some significant advances in the ability to monitor tau and beta-amyloid proteins in blood plasma and in cerebrospinal fluid (the liquid that surrounds the brain and spinal cord) as well as to detect beta-amyloid plaques via PET and SPECT imaging (Stevenson-Hoare et al., 2023).

Etiology of Alzheimer Disease

A number of factors increase the risk of AD, including both hereditary and environmental influences. We are learning more about risk genes associated with AD, particularly the APOE-e4 gene, which is carried by about 20 percent to 30 percent of the U.S. population. Our bodies produce a chemical, apolipoprotein E (ApoE), that helps clear beta-amyloid by-products from the brain. The gene associated with this process (the APOE gene) has three variants (alleles). One of these variants, the e4 allele of the APOE gene, is associated with decreased production of ApoE, which increases the risk for the beta-amyloid accumulations associated with AD. Although the APOE-e4 allele increases the likelihood of developing AD, people with this genotype do not necessarily develop AD; however, risk is further increased when the APOE-e4 allele is inherited from both parents (Alzheimer's Association, 2023).

Researchers have also identified genetic mutations that directly cause *autosomal-dominant Alzheimer disease*; these uncommon, deterministic genes are responsible for the multigenerational inheritance of early-onset AD in some families. Individuals affected by these mutations usually develop AD in midlife, sometimes as early as the mid-30s. People who inherit these mutations appear to produce large quantities of a stickier version of the beta-amyloid protein that exits more slowly from the brain. Carriers of the rare autosomal-dominant genes associated with early-onset AD have visible AD biomarkers in their cerebrospinal fluid, reinforcing other findings that demonstrate that the pathologies associated with AD begin decades before the onset of overt symptoms (Schindler et al., 2019). As you might imagine, following the progression of biomarkers in asymptomatic individuals is of great interest to researchers.

Lifestyle variables that increase the likelihood of stroke and cardiovascular disease also increase risk of AD. Researchers interested in determining how dietary intake affects beta-amyloid have found that a diet high in saturated fat results in increases in circulating beta-amyloid and reductions of ApoE, the chemical that helps clear the brain of beta-amyloid by-products, resulting in a 39 percent increase in the risk for AD (Ruan et al., 2018). In a 10-year study, adults (age 60 or older) with normal cognition underwent ApoE genotyping and were surveyed regarding their health habits and lifestyle (nutritional choices, regular exercising, active social life, cognitive activities, etc.). In the follow-up assessment, a healthy lifestyle was associated with a lower probability of progression to mild cognitive impairment or dementia, even among the 20 percent of the participants who had the ApoE genotype (Jia et al., 2023).

There is also a link between sleep and the amount of beta-amyloid in the brain. Insomnia is related to reports of memory decline in middle-aged and older adults and often precedes mild cognitive impairment and dementia (Zhao et al., 2022). In one study, even one night of sleep deprivation was associated with higher beta-amyloid accumulation in healthy adults (Shokri-Kojori et al., 2018). Similarly, older adult volunteers who reported poor sleep quality or quantity had more beta-amyloid deposits in the brain compared to those reporting adequate sleep (Spira et al., 2013). Additionally, in a group of asymptomatic individuals involved in an ongoing study, those with evidence of beta-amyloid abnormalities had the poorest documented sleep quality (Ju et al., 2013). These findings are consistent with data suggesting that beta-amyloid and other proteins are cleared from the brain during sleep. Researchers are attempting to determine if the buildup of beta-amyloid plaque disrupts sleep or if loss of sleep contributes to the development of beta-amyloid plaque (Lloret et al., 2020). There is growing evidence that individuals who eventually develop AD demonstrate changes in sleep patterns (disrupted sleep and increased wakefulness) years before the onset of cognitive symptoms and that the sleep disturbance first results from the buildup of tau protein, which leads to a cascade of neurological changes, including the buildup of beta-amyloid plaque (Holth et al., 2017).

Continuum Video Project

Myriam: Alzheimer Disease

"I'm going to forget their names. I'm going to forget who they are. Alzheimer's is eating away at my brain."

Access the Continuum Video Project in MindTap.

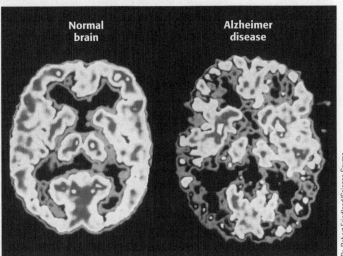

Normal brain

Alzheimer disease

Dr. Robert Friedland/Science Source

Alzheimer Disease

As can be seen in these PET scans comparing brain activity between someone with Alzheimer disease and a healthy control, Alzheimer disease causes degeneration and death of nerve cells and significantly reduces metabolic activity in the brain. The associated brain dysfunction results in symptoms such as memory loss, disorientation, and personality change.

Neurocognitive Disorder due to Dementia with Lewy Bodies

Case Study Before taking his own life, acclaimed actor and comedian Robin Williams was tormented by unexplained psychological symptoms, including extreme paranoia and emotional distress. He was diagnosed with Parkinson disease 3 months prior to his death. An autopsy performed after his death revealed that Lewy bodies had destroyed neurons throughout his brain and brainstem, thus explaining the acute memory difficulties, confusion, and out-of-character fear and anxiety he had experienced during the last year of his life. (Williams, 2016)

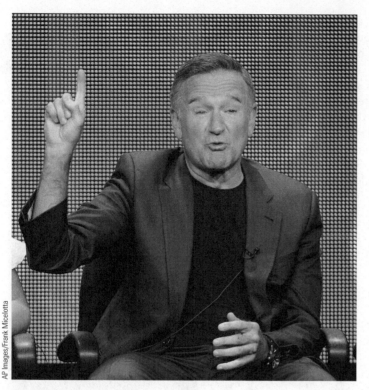

Dementia with Lewy bodies (DLB), the second most common form of degenerative dementia, affects approximately 1.4 million adults in the United States. DLB results in significant cognitive decline combined with psychiatric symptoms and the development of unusual movements similar to those seen in Parkinson disease, a disorder we discuss later in the chapter. Characteristics of DLB include:

- impaired thinking and significant fluctuations in attention and alertness (e.g., staring spells and periods of extreme drowsiness);

- recurrent, detailed visual hallucinations and other psychiatric symptoms, including depression, apathy, anxiety, agitation, delusions, and paranoia;

- impaired mobility that occurs after the onset of cognitive decline (e.g., frequent falls, a shuffling gait, muscular rigidity, and slowed movement); and

- difficulties with regulation of blood pressure, digestion, and sleep, including physically acting out dreams during sleep.

A Tragic Loss

Fans throughout the world responded to the news of Robin Williams's suicide with shock and sadness. An autopsy revealed the presence of Lewy bodies, which likely caused the changes in his psychological functioning. Known for his philanthropy and zany comedic style, Williams appears here in July 2013, about a year before he died.

Like Robin Williams, individuals with DLB have brain cell irregularities, called Lewy bodies, which result from the buildup of abnormal proteins in the nuclei of neurons. These unique cell structures (named after Frederick Lewy, who first discovered them) are also present in Parkinson disease. When Lewy bodies develop in the cortex, they deplete the neurotransmitter acetylcholine (associated with neuroplasticity, memory, and attention), resulting in the perceptual, cognitive, and behavioral symptoms seen in DLB and in later stages of Parkinson disease. Lewy bodies in the brainstem cause the depletion of dopamine and result in the unique motor dysfunction associated with both Parkinson disease and DLB (refer to Figure 13.7).

The incidence of DLB increases with age and occurs more frequently in men. Although DLB may account for up to one third of all dementias, postmortem studies have revealed that only about 30 percent of people with DLB are accurately diagnosed while they are alive. This occurs because

Figure 13.7

Dopamine Levels in a Normal Neuron and a Lewy Body–Affected Neuron

Parkinson disease and dementia with Lewy bodies both involve damage to neurons that produce dopamine and resultant impairment in movement and balance.

Source: Editorial Team. (February 23, 2017).

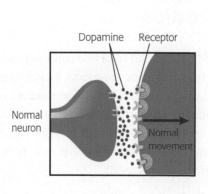

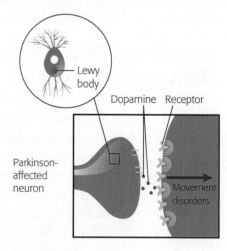

many physicians are unfamiliar with the disorder, there is overlap of symptoms with other neurodegenerative disorders, and DLB can be confirmed only by autopsy. Differential diagnosis is complicated by the fact that some people with DLB have a mixed dementia, involving both Lewy bodies and the amyloid plaques and tau protein tangles seen in AD. Accurate diagnosis is important because certain medications can worsen DLB symptoms (Lewy Body Dementia Association, 2023).

Neurocognitive Disorder due to Frontotemporal Lobar Degeneration

Frontotemporal lobar degeneration (FTLD), the fourth leading cause of dementia, is characterized by progressive declines in language, behavior, and/or motor skills; these deficits result from degeneration and atrophy in the frontal and temporal lobes of the brain. FTLD has several variants that involve behavioral, language, or movement symptoms. Symptoms associated with the three variants include (a) significant changes in behavior, personality, and social skills (e.g., impulsive or uninhibited actions, apathy, loss of empathy, repetitive behavior patterns); (b) progressive difficulty with fluent speech or understanding of language; and (c) muscular rigidity, clumsiness, or other motoric abnormalities. Difficulty in planning or organizing activities and a lack of recognition of declining abilities occurs with all three variants.

The average age of onset for FTLD is between 45 and 64 years, making it the leading cause of early-onset dementia. Those who first present with behavioral and personality changes sometimes receive a psychiatric diagnosis before it becomes clear that they have a neurodegenerative disorder; diagnosis often occurs after neuroimaging reveals the patterns of atrophy in the frontal or temporal lobes that are characteristic of FTLD. Genetic mutations appear to contribute to FTLD, with up to 40 percent of individuals with FTLD reporting a family history of neurodegenerative illness (Association for Frontotemporal Degeneration, 2023).

Neurocognitive Disorder due to Parkinson Disease

Parkinson disease (PD) involves four primary symptoms: (a) tremor of the hands, arms, legs, jaw, and/or face; (b) rigidity and stiffness of the limbs and trunk; (c) slowness in initiating movement; and (d) impaired balance and awkward gait (Parkinson's Foundation, 2023). Frequent nightmares or distressing dreams are reported by individuals with PD and may be prodromal symptoms of the disorder (Otaiku, 2022). As the disease progresses, the increasing severity of the tremors and incoordination can interfere with daily activities. The symptoms of PD result from the buildup of Lewy body proteins, which damage and destroy dopamine-producing neurons in the brainstem and midbrain (affecting motor movement) and cause depletion of the neurotransmitter acetylcholine in the cortex (affecting cognitive skills). As the disease progresses, personality changes may occur and psychiatric symptoms may arise, including hallucinations, delusions, depression, and/or anxiety. Mild cognitive impairment may also develop, which presents in the same manner as dementia with Lewy bodies. The primary difference between dementia associated with PD and that seen in DLB is the timing of the motor symptoms. Parkinson disease dementia is the diagnosis when motor difficulties develop at least 1 year prior to any notable cognitive decline (Lewy Body Dementia Association, 2023).

Bruce Willis's Battle with Dementia

Actor Bruce Willis, who has made over $5 billion for movies such as *Die Hard* and the *Sixth Sense*, stepped away from acting because of communication difficulties. In 2023, the 67-year-old actor received a diagnosis of frontotemporal lobar degeneration, a progressive disorder that is currently without a cure.

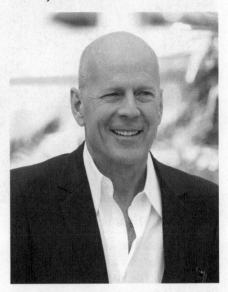

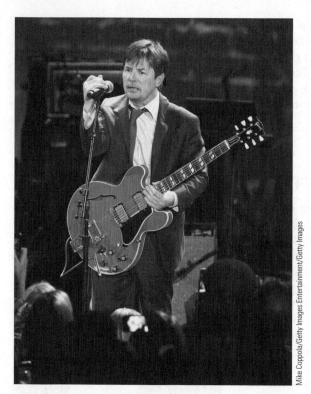

Parkinson Disease

Actor Michael J. Fox, who has Parkinson disease, performs at a benefit for the Michael J. Fox Foundation for Parkinson's Research in New York City.

PD is the most common neurodegenerative movement disorder, affecting almost 1 million individuals in the United States and about 10 million worldwide. The severity and progression of symptoms varies significantly from person to person. The prevalence of PD increases with age; only a small percentage (4 percent) of individuals are diagnosed with PD before age 50. Men are 1.5 times more likely to develop PD compared to women, but the reasons for this discrepancy are unclear (Parkinson's Foundation, 2023).

Because genetic mutations account for only a small percentage of PD cases, researchers are trying to better understand what causes the pattern of brain cell death seen in the disease. Studies have revealed that occupational exposure to herbicides and pesticides or certain toxins (including those contained in solvents and household cleaners) appears to increase the likelihood of developing PD (Ball et al., 2019). PD occurs more frequently in the northern Midwest and the Northeast and in urban settings; this geographic distribution has raised questions about whether environmental toxins common to these areas are associated with the development of the disorder (Marras et al., 2018). Research is beginning to support the hypothesis that the biochemical processes associated with PD (and other neurodegenerative disorders) may, in fact, arise in the gut (i.e., within the enteric nervous system) and that altered microbiota contribute to both neuroinflammation and neurodegeneration (Doroszkiewicz et al., 2021).

Neurocognitive Disorder due to Huntington Disease

Case Study A 35-year-old man was seen at a neurological clinic because of jerky involuntary movements. They would begin in the right arm, followed by movements in the left arm, then spread to the lower limbs, and finally the neck and head. The movements only occurred during wakefulness and disappeared during sleep. His walking had a dancelike characteristic. Behavioral changes also occurred with outbursts of anger, aggression, insomnia, and depression. During the disturbances in mood, his movement symptoms increased. (Singh, 2022)

Huntington disease (HD) is a rare, genetically transmitted degenerative disorder characterized by involuntary movement, progressive dementia, and emotional instability as seen in the man in the case study. Age of onset is variable; although onset ranges from childhood to late in life, HD generally begins during midlife (APA, 2022). Initial symptoms often involve neurocognitive decline and changes in personality and emotional stability. The progressive cognitive deficits associated with HD typically begin with difficulties in executive functioning involving complex attention, planning, and problem solving. Additionally, many individuals with HD become uncharacteristically apathetic, moody, and quarrelsome. As the disorder progresses, physical symptoms such as facial grimaces, difficulty speaking, and abrupt, repetitive movements often develop. Eventually, the severity of motor and cognitive impairment results in total dependency and the need for full-time care. There is no effective treatment for HD; death typically occurs within 20 years of the onset of symptoms (McColgan & Tabrizi, 2018).

Because HD is transmitted from parent to child through a dominant genetic mutation, the offspring of someone with HD have about a 50/50 chance of carrying the gene and developing the disorder. Predictive genetic testing is available for family members who want to know if they have inherited the gene that produces HD.

Neurocognitive Disorder due to HIV Infection

Many people know about the serious complications associated with HIV infection and AIDS (acquired immune deficiency syndrome), including susceptibility to diseases, physical deterioration, and death. Relatively few people realize that cognitive impairment is sometimes the first sign of an untreated HIV infection that has crossed the blood–brain barrier and is producing inflammation throughout the brain and central nervous system. In serious cases, when the HIV infection becomes increasingly active within the brain and produces significant brain dysfunction, a diagnosis of HIV-associated neurocognitive disorder is made. Symptoms can vary but often include slower mental processing, difficulty with complex mental tasks, and difficulty concentrating or learning new information (APA, 2022).

Although the antiretroviral therapies used to treat HIV infection and AIDS can prevent or delay the onset of the severe cognitive dysfunction associated with HIV-associated neurocognitive disorder, HIV-related neurochemical imbalances and other brain changes still occur in many of those taking antiretroviral medications. Executive functioning and working memory are often compromised and can affect daily living skills.

Going Deeper

Genetic Testing: Helpful or Harmful?

DNA testing is now available to provide information regarding risk for a variety of neurocognitive disorders. Genotyping (gathering information about specific genes by examining an individual's DNA) brings up a number of interconnected issues. When genotyping is performed on individuals who have a family member with a *genetically determined* condition such as Huntington disease (HD) or early-onset Alzheimer disease (AD), the outcome of the test reveals life-changing information—they know *with certainty* if they will develop the disorder afflicting their parent or other family members. In cases where genetic tests indicate only *possible* risk (e.g., the APOE-e4 genotype associated with later-onset AD), clinicians often discourage genetic testing due to concerns that knowledge of possible risk can be more harmful than helpful. For instance, someone who learns that they have the APOE-e4 genotype knows there is approximately a 25 percent chance of developing AD—not the 100 percent risk revealed through genotype analysis involving HD or early-onset AD (Marshe et al., 2019).

Those who encourage genetic testing for individuals who may carry *deterministic genes* (e.g., when family members have HD or early-onset AD) emphasize benefits such as being able to plan for the future, including decisions about whether or not to have children. However, others discourage such testing because of the social and economic stigma associated with these conditions and the lack of specific treatments or interventions if gene mutations are detected (*The Lancet Neurology*, 2010). Those who support genetic testing when there is *possible* risk of AD (e.g., families who have the APOE-e4 genotype) believe that learning about an increased risk of AD may motivate lifestyle changes that ultimately reduce the risk of developing the disease. Additionally, individuals with the APOE-e4 genotype may be able to participate in research studies aimed at preventing or slowing the progression of AD. Once such interventions exist, some of the debate may subside.

For Further Consideration

1. If your parent had Huntington disease or early-onset Alzheimer disease, would you want to know if you would eventually develop the disorder?

2. If one of your family members had later-onset Alzheimer disease, would you want to know if you carried the APOE-e4 genotype and had a 25 percent risk of developing the disorder?

The declines in cognitive functioning are further exacerbated when cardiovascular disease is also present (Sacktor, 2018). Researchers hope that the prevalence of HIV-related neurocognitive disorder will decrease once antiretroviral medications are able to efficiently penetrate the brain and central nervous system (Kopstein & Mohlman, 2020).

13-3 Treatment Considerations with Neurocognitive Disorders

Because neurocognitive disorders have many different causes and are associated with different symptoms and dysfunctions, treatment approaches vary widely. First, any underlying medical conditions are addressed. Beyond that, the major interventions for neurocognitive disorders include rehabilitation services, biological interventions, cognitive and behavioral treatment, lifestyle changes, and environmental support.

Rehabilitation Services

The key to recovery for those affected by stroke or TBI is participation in comprehensive, sustained rehabilitation services. Physical, occupational, speech, and language therapy help individuals relearn skills or compensate for lost abilities. Rehabilitative interventions are often guided by the individual's physical and cognitive strengths, as well as deficits. A person's commitment to and participation in therapy plays an important role in recovery. Depression, pessimism, and anxiety can stall progress. Fortunately, those participating in rehabilitation often feel encouraged when the brain begins to reorganize and skills return. Neuroimaging techniques are

Effective Rehabilitation

This army veteran is undergoing treatment at the Warrior Recovery Center for a traumatic brain injury he sustained while deployed in Afghanistan. The program uses multiple therapies, including computer applications that focus on improving attention and processing speed.

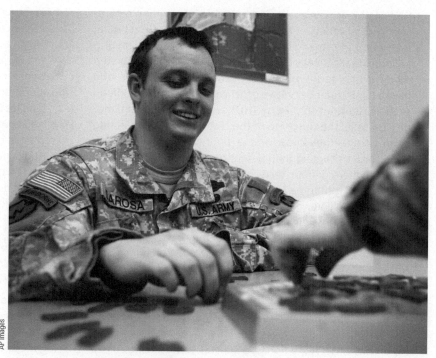

AP Images

increasingly used to document brain changes achieved through rehabilitation; in fact, neuroimaging can help determine which physical and occupational therapies best enhance brain recovery.

Biological Treatment

Medications can help prevent, control, or reduce the symptoms of some neurocognitive disorders. Treating vitamin deficiencies can also improve or reduce symptoms in some conditions. For instance, higher blood levels of an amino acid, homocysteine, are associated with increased risk of AD. Fortunately, certain vitamins, such as vitamin B_{12}, can decrease homocysteine levels (Smith et al., 2018). MRI scans of individuals with mild cognitive impairment taking high doses of B vitamins over a 2-year period revealed that brain atrophy was slowed by about 30 percent; atrophy was reduced the most (up to 53 percent) in those with the highest initial levels of homocysteine (Smith et al., 2010).

Medications, including levodopa, a drug that increases dopamine availability, can provide relief from both cognitive and physical symptoms of PD; however, this class of medication can also produce hallucinations and other psychotic symptoms (Reich & Savitt, 2019). For this reason, physicians often delay pharmacological treatment for PD until it is certain that the benefits clearly outweigh the risks. Deep brain stimulation is sometimes successful in improving physical symptoms of PD, including tremors and impaired mobility. However, the treatment also seems to increase impulsivity (Lo Buono et al., 2021). Gene therapy (using a virus to introduce a working version of a gene into a targeted neuron) is also being tested with PD patients with the goal of sufficiently modifying brain cells so that they once again produce and transmit dopamine (Barker & Björklund, 2023).

Two medications have received FDA approval for the treatment of people in the early stages of AD when there is confirmation of beta-amyloid plaques in the brain. Both medications, which are administered via intravenous infusion, aim to slow the progression of the disease by reducing the production of beta-amyloid (Alzheimer's Association, 2023). Unfortunately, these medications do not restore or reverse cognitive loss. Thus, efforts continue to focus on preventing the development of dementia by avoiding the development of beta-amyloid and tau protein irregularities in those at high risk for AD. Other proposed treatments for AD are still in the early stages, including deep brain stimulation to improve neural circuit function (Tatulian, 2022).

Cognitive and Behavioral Treatment

Cognitive deficits and emotional changes caused by neurocognitive disorders (e.g., emotional reactivity and diminished ability to concentrate) can hinder recovery and interfere with well-being. For example, depression, common among those with vascular neurocognitive conditions, can decrease follow-through with treatment recommendations and increase risk of subsequent strokes (Sibolt et al., 2013).

Psychotherapy can enhance coping and participation in rehabilitation efforts. For instance, a cognitive-behavioral treatment identifying life stressors and teaching the participants self-care, stress management, and relaxation techniques has helped decrease depression and anxiety in individuals with PD (Egan et al., 2015). Cognitive and behavioral therapy techniques can also reduce the frequency or severity of problem behaviors associated with neurocognitive disorders, such as aggression or socially inappropriate conduct. Strategies may include teaching the individual social skills,

Did You Know?

Among dementia-free older adults, the regular use of the internet (up to two hours daily) was associated with just half the risk of developing dementia vs non-users. However, dementia risk also seemed to increase for those who were on the internet for over two hours a day.

Source: Cho et al., 2023

adjusting complex tasks, or simplifying the environment to avoid confusion and frustration. Additionally, preliminary research has demonstrated slower cognitive decline and positive neurological changes in individuals with mild neurocognitive impairment who participated in a meditation and mindfulness-based stress reduction program (Russell-Williams et al., 2018).

Lifestyle Changes

Lifestyle changes can help prevent or reduce the progression of some neurocognitive disorders. Among one group of adults with early-stage AD, those with good cardiovascular fitness had less brain atrophy than those who did not exercise regularly (Cass, 2017). Intervention for vascular neurocognitive disorders often targets smoking cessation; weight reduction; and blood sugar, cholesterol, or blood pressure control. Making changes in these modifiable risk factors can also slow cognitive decline with AD (Tariq & Barber, 2018). One longitudinal study focused on a cohort of older adults with normal cognitive function who were assessed for dementia risk based on their genetic profiles. Not surprisingly, participants who had either a genetic risk or an unhealthy lifestyle were more likely to develop dementia compared to those without these risks. However, when those with a high genetic risk had a favorable lifestyle (no smoking or excessive alcohol consumption, regular exercise, healthy diet), the risk of developing dementia was decreased compared to those with an equally high genetic risk but an unfavorable lifestyle (Lourida et al., 2019). In a study involving people diagnosed with either mild cognitive impairment or AD, participants who took part in a physical activity program for a period of 6 months showed no cognitive deterioration; in contrast, patients in the control group showed a significant decline. When the physical activity was discontinued, the slowing of cognitive deterioration remained evident in the mild cognitive impairment group but not for those with AD. The latter group may need a more consistent exercise program to maintain the benefit (Fonte et al., 2019).

Increased social interaction and mental stimulation involving enjoyable, social activities and hobbies that provide an opportunity to concentrate and use memory skills can slow cognitive decline in individuals with dementia, with those participating in the greatest number of activities receiving the most benefits (Krell-Roesch et al., 2019). However, the use of specific cognitive training programs does not have strong research support, nor does the training appear to generalize to daily living activities among individuals exhibiting cognitive decline (Lövdén et al., 2013).

Environmental Support

Although rehabilitation can be very effective with acute conditions such as TBI or stroke, neurodegenerative disorders involving dementia or impaired motor skills are irreversible and best managed by providing a supportive environment. There are many ways to help those with declining abilities to feel happier and to live comfortably and with dignity. Further, modifying the environment can increase safety and comfort while decreasing confusion and agitation. For instance, exposure to bright lighting throughout the day can improve sleep and decrease anxiety and

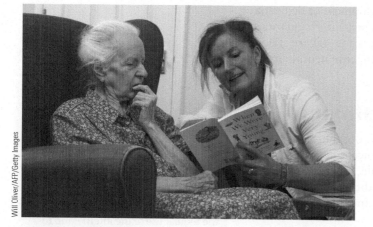

Will Oliver/AFP/Getty Images

Connecting with Positive Memories

Although dementia cannot be cured, individuals with the condition benefit from social contact and activities associated with positive memories. Here a volunteer reads poetry to a woman with dementia.

depression in individuals with dementia (Onega et al., 2018). Techniques such as writing answers to repeatedly asked questions or labeling family photos can decrease frustration resulting from memory difficulties. Family visits enhance the lives of those with dementia because emotional memories (e.g., happiness at seeing a loved one) persist even when the visit itself is no longer recalled (Feinstein et al., 2010).

Family and friends who provide care may themselves need support. They may feel overwhelmed, helpless, frustrated, anxious, or even angry at having to take care of someone with a neurocognitive impairment. Caring for someone with dementia or another degenerative condition can be very stressful, especially because of the need for constant supervision and extensive assistance with personal care. Sometimes, agonizing decisions must be made about whether the affected individual can remain at home versus living in a skilled nursing or assisted-living facility.

13-4 Sleep–Wake Disorders

Sleep is an important topic because sleep difficulties increase the risk of high blood pressure, obesity, diabetes, stroke, and heart disease as well as psychiatric disorders (Liu et al., 2016). In contrast, good-quality sleep is associated with mental and physical resilience. Although most adults require 7 to 9 hours of sleep per night to function optimally (refer to Table 13.7), obtaining restful and adequate sleep is difficult for many adults, particularly people living with mental illness. Based on self-reports of sleep duration, about one third of adults—an estimated 83.6 million people—sleep less than 7 hours per night (Liu et al., 2016).

What is a normal sleep pattern? Normal sleep has two phases: *Non–rapid eye movement (NREM) sleep* is a deep sleep state in which the muscles are relaxed and breathing and heart rate are slowed; during this stage, our bodies perform important functions such as building bone and muscle, repairing tissues, and strengthening the immune system. The second phase is *rapid eye movement (REM) sleep*, in which breathing, heart rate, and brain activity increase. REM sleep, which is associated with dreaming, occupies about 10 percent to 25 percent of sleep and usually alternates with NREM sleep every 90 minutes (Bollu, 2019).

Many of us experience occasional interruptions in normal sleep patterns, daytime sleepiness, or periodic difficulty falling or staying asleep, particularly after a traumatic experience or when dealing with stressful circumstances. Not surprisingly, many college students report having some sleep disturbance (Milojevich & Lukowski, 2016). However, in most cases, these difficulties are temporary and do not interfere with daytime functioning.

Table 13.7   How Much Sleep Do You Really Need?

Age	Sleep Needs
Preschoolers (3 to 5 years)	10 to 13 hours
Elementary children (5 to 10 years)	9 to 12 hours
Adolescents (10 to 17 years)	8 to 10 hours
Adults	7 to 9 hours

Source: National Sleep Foundation, 2023

Did You Know?

Sleep patterns vary by geographic region. Adults in the Great Plains states are more likely to get adequate sleep, whereas the southeastern United States and Appalachian Mountain regions have the lowest rates of healthy sleep patterns.
Source: Liu et al., 2016

Table 13.8 Sleep–Wake Disorders

Disorder	Characteristics
Dyssomnias	
Insomnia disorder	Difficulty falling asleep or remaining asleep
Hypersomnolence disorder	Difficulty waking up after sleeping, excessive daytime sleepiness, or waking up unrefreshed after prolonged nighttime sleep
Narcolepsy	Sudden sleep or overwhelming need for sleep in the daytime despite sleeping adequately during the night
Obstructive sleep apnea	Breathing-related sleep disorder involving partial or complete upper-airway obstruction
Circadian rhythm sleep disorder	Disrupted biological sleep–wake cycle
Parasomnias	
Non–rapid eye movement (NREM) sleep arousal disorders	Episodes of incomplete arousal during NREM sleep, including night terrors and sleepwalking
Nightmare disorder	Frightening dreams with themes of danger that produce awakening
REM sleep behavior disorder	Motor behaviors and vocalizations occur during REM sleep

When excessive sleepiness, ongoing problems initiating or maintaining sleep, or other sleep abnormalities result in daytime distress and impairment, the individual may meet the criteria for one of the sleep disorders. There are two major categories of sleep disorders: dyssomnias and parasomnias (refer to Table 13.8). We will discuss some of the disorders from each of these categories.

Dyssomnias

Dyssomnias involve difficulties in falling asleep or maintaining sleep, as well as excessive sleepiness during the day. They include insomnia disorder, hypersomnolence disorder, narcolepsy, obstructive sleep apnea (a breathing-related sleep disorder), and circadian-rhythm sleep–wake disorder.

Insomnia Disorder

Case Study It happens two or three times a week. I get in bed, turn off the light and wait to fall asleep . . . and wait . . . and wait. It might be two or three hours before I drop off. And even then, I might wake up a couple of hours later to go through the whole thing again. (Lemonick, 2004, p. 100)

Insomnia disorder, the most prevalent of all sleep disorders, involves a distressing and disruptive pattern of difficulty falling asleep or remaining asleep. Various factors cause insomnia, including stress, worry, or anxiety. In fact, insomnia is now considered by many researchers to be a disorder of chronic and systemic hyperarousal associated with racing brain waves, rapid heart rate, elevated body temperature, and hormonal dysfunction (Pillai et al., 2016). Insomnia is also the most common sleep disorder among children and adolescents (Dewald-Kaufmann et al., 2019). Older adults and women also have high rates of insomnia (APA, 2022).

Excessive daytime sleepiness is a common result of chronic insomnia and may impair cognitive functioning and alertness, driver safety, performance at work, and enjoyment of family or recreational activities. The economic costs of chronic insomnia, such as poor work performance and increased likelihood of accidents or need for health care, are estimated to exceed $100 billion per year (Wickwire et al., 2016). Many individuals with insomnia have comorbid physical or mental health conditions. For example, people receiving treatment for cancer often have significant difficulty with sleep, a factor that can inhibit recovery by suppressing the immune system or impeding the restorative processes that occur during sleep (Walker & Borniger, 2019).

Hypersomnolence Disorder

Case Study A 27-year-old carpenter sought help because he always felt tired. He was sometimes able to resist falling asleep in important situations but had several car accidents related to sleepiness. He sometimes slept for several hours during the day but did not feel refreshed after sleeping. His excessive daytime sleepiness began during adolescence, when he often fell asleep after returning from school and slept until morning. (Bassetti & Aldrich, 1997)

Hypersomnolence (excessive sleepiness) disorder is characterized by a pattern of difficulty waking up after sleeping, excessive daytime sleepiness, or prolonged nighttime sleep with a tendency to wake up unrefreshed. Those with this disorder sleep at least 7 hours but, as seen in the case vignette, may lapse into sleep or feel compelled to nap during the day; however, naps do not provide relief from sleepiness. Many individuals with hypersomnolence disorder experience **sleep inertia**, which involves significant grogginess and impaired alertness on awakening (Hilditch & McHill, 2019). How common is hypersomnolence disorder? Among 16,000 U.S. adults interviewed about sleep symptoms, 27.8 percent reported experiencing periodic excessive sleepiness; 1.5 percent of the group reported symptoms consistent with hypersomnolence disorder (Ohayon, Dauvilliers, & Reynolds, 2012).

Narcolepsy

Case Study A 14-year-old adolescent falls asleep 30 times or more per day, often in class, and has gone missing when operating on "dreamlike autopilot." She takes medication to reduce the excessive daytime sleepiness and the episodes of muscle weakness associated with her narcolepsy. (Francis, 2014)

Narcolepsy, a very rare sleep disorder, results in an irresistible or overwhelming need for sleep in the daytime even when adequate sleep occurs during the night. Drowsiness or sudden sleep can occur without warning. Individuals with narcolepsy often go immediately into REM sleep, whereas a normal sleep cycle begins with 90 minutes of NREM sleep. Surprisingly, in one sample, narcolepsy went undiagnosed for up to 16 years for men and 28 years for women (Won et al., 2014). Narcolepsy results from a loss of neurons in the hypothalamus; the missing neurons normally produce orexin, a neuropeptide that regulates arousal and wakefulness. Research has further explored the possibility that this neuronal damage is the result of an autoimmune process (Mahoney et al., 2019).

Did You Know?

High social media use is linked with poor sleep quality and poor mental health; however, more research is needed about the directionality of the relationship between these variables.

Source: Alonzo et al., 2021

Many individuals with narcolepsy experience *cataplexy*, a sudden loss of muscle function, varying from slight muscular weakness to complete physical collapse that can last for seconds or minutes; the person remains completely conscious during these episodes. Cataplexy is often triggered by laughter or by emotional states such as anger or fear. Those with narcolepsy also experience other disruptive sleep–wake symptoms, including disturbed sleep, sleep paralysis, and hallucinations (Bassetti et al., 2019).

Obstructive Sleep Apnea

Case Study Forty-year-old Mike Palomar suffers from constant sleepiness and struggles to complete daily activities. He can fall asleep at any moment, is unable control his weight, and feels sluggish. His wife complains of his loud snoring and is alarmed when he appears to stop breathing during sleep. During a sleep assessment it was found that he had 78 breathing pauses each hour. (Simons, 2014)

Mike Palomar was surprised when he received the diagnosis of **obstructive sleep apnea (OSA)**, a common breathing-related sleep disorder. When asleep, those with this condition experience a collapse of the soft tissue in the rear of the throat, resulting in partial or complete upper-airway obstruction. The obstruction repeatedly interferes with breathing during sleep. After detecting low levels of oxygen, the brain sends a signal to resume breathing, which results in snoring or gasping for breath. Having extra tissue around the airway due to excessive weight increases vulnerability to OSA (Patel, 2019).

Symptoms of OSA include disruptive snoring, breathing pauses, snorting or gasping, and excessive daytime sleepiness. OSA can cause high blood pressure, cardiovascular disease, and weight gain and is associated with increased risk of stroke (Lau et al., 2019). Sleep apnea is also associated with shortened telomere length, suggesting that the condition may accelerate cellular aging (Carroll et al., 2019).

OSA is a relatively common disorder that remains undiagnosed in about 90 percent of women and 80 percent of men with the condition (Downey et al., 2013). In the general population the prevalence of OSA is estimated to range from 3 percent to 7 percent in men and 2 percent to 5 percent in women and is most prevalent among older adults (Lurie, 2011).

Circadian Rhythm Sleep Disorder

Circadian rhythm sleep disorder is a pattern of recurrent sleep disturbance caused by a disrupted biological sleep–wake cycle or a mismatch between environmental demands and a person's internal clock. Circadian rhythm sleep disorder can result in insomnia or excessive sleepiness. **Circadian rhythms** are internal biological rhythms that influence a number of our bodily processes, including sleeping patterns. Our circadian rhythms are influenced by light, which also affects production of the sleep-inducing hormone, melatonin. Many of us have experienced jet lag, a temporary disruption in circadian rhythm that results from travel between time zones. Shift work can also dysregulate a person's circadian rhythm if the work schedule is in opposition to sleep-regulating cues associated with sunlight. Over 36 percent of night-shift workers and 26 percent of rotating workers experience disruptions in the normal circadian rhythm pattern (Sack et al., 2007). Although there is little information on the prevalence of circadian rhythm sleep disorder, it does occur with more frequency in older adults, especially individuals affected by a neurocognitive disorder (Kim & Duffy, 2018).

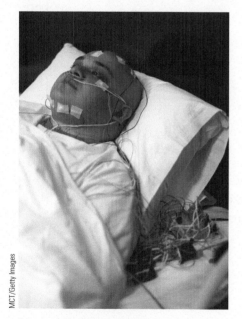

MCT/Getty Images

Studying Biological Functioning During Sleep

Emmanuel Michael, age 29, prepares for a sleep disorder test at a University of Chicago clinic. Sleep evaluations usually involve an overnight stay at a sleep disorders clinic so that technicians can monitor biological changes that occur during sleep.

Parasomnias

Parasomnias involve unusual behaviors or events occurring during sleep or the sleep–wake transition; in other words, the physiological systems associated with sleep do not function normally. The parasomnias include non–rapid eye movement (NREM) sleep arousal disorders, nightmare disorder, and rapid eye movement (REM) sleep behavior disorder (APA, 2022).

Non–Rapid Eye Movement (NREM) Sleep Arousal Disorders

Non–rapid eye movement (NREM) sleep arousal disorders involve simultaneous wakefulness and NREM sleep; these episodes of incomplete arousal, which involve talking or motor activity with eyes open but minimal conscious awareness, occur early in the night and usually last no more than 10 minutes. In general, there is little or no memory of the episode the next day. Many individuals exhibit both subtypes of this disorder: sleep terrors and sleepwalking.

Sleep Terrors   **Sleep terrors** are abrupt episodes of intense fear that occur during deep sleep. Those who experience sleep terrors often cry out in panic but are not fully aroused. They display physiological symptoms such as sweating, rapid breathing, or increased heart rate and are confused, incoherent, and difficult to calm. They often become more agitated if awakened. Sleep terrors occur during NREM sleep, whereas nightmares typically occur during the dreaming that happens during REM sleep. People usually recall details of a nightmare but are unlikely to recall a sleep terror episode. Sleep terrors occur in up to 6 percent of children and are most common in youth between 4 and 12 years of age (Leung et al., 2020).

Sleepwalking   Sleepwalking typically involves sitting up or walking during sleep; someone who is sleepwalking usually has a blank stare, does not respond if spoken to, and is not easily awakened. Sleepwalking occurs in a state of reduced alertness and involves behaviors requiring little complexity. During sleepwalking episodes, some individuals eat or engage in sexual activity (without conscious awareness) or unusual behavior such as urinating in inappropriate places. Sleepwalking may also develop as a side effect of certain medications, particularly medications used for insomnia and narcolepsy (Stallman et al., 2018).

Repeated sleepwalking episodes causing distress and impairment affect up to 5 percent of the adult population. Sleepwalking behavior peaks in childhood, with between 10 percent and 30 percent of children experiencing at least one episode of sleepwalking. This disorder tends to disappear during early adolescence but may continue into adulthood (APA, 2022).

Nightmare Disorder

Nightmare disorder involves dreams with themes of danger that are frightening enough to produce awakening. These story-like episodes occur almost exclusively during REM sleep. Nightmares often involve threats to our survival or sense of security. The fear and anxiety associated with the nightmare cause the person to become alert; hyperarousal and distress from the dream often make it difficult for the person to resume sleep.

Nightmares are most common during adolescence and young adulthood and are more prevalent in women; approximately 4 percent of adults experience distressing nightmares. Individuals with psychiatric disorders, particularly those with PTSD, have a greater likelihood of experiencing nightmare disorder (Morgenthaler et al., 2018).

REM Sleep Behavior Disorder

REM sleep behavior disorder involves vocalizations and motor behavior (often of a violent nature) during REM sleep. The movement or speaking is often associated with the content of a person's dreams. Sometimes, people with this disorder scream and hit or otherwise injure their sleeping partner. Once awakened, the person is alert and oriented (APA, 2022). REM sleep behavior disorder often precedes the onset of degenerative neurological disorders such as Alzheimer and Parkinson disease, as well as dementia with Lewy bodies (Zhang et al., 2020).

Etiology of Sleep–Wake Disorders

Problems in sleep can result from neurological vulnerabilities; psychological factors such as stress, anxiety, and depression; environmental factors such as noise, light, or other stimuli; or from various health or behavioral habits, including substance use or abuse. Clinicians assessing someone for a sleep disorder inquire about the age of onset, predisposing characteristics (being a light sleeper, family history of sleep problems, current stressors, illnesses, or medications), lifestyle, and daily activity patterns. They also seek input from the bed partner about any observations of snoring, breathing pattern changes, or movement or verbalizations during sleep.

Dyssomnias tend to be associated with lifestyle and psychological factors, including the following:

- Intrusive, uncontrollable thoughts associated with stress, worry, anxiety, or depression and preoccupation with sleep and distress over sleep difficulties. For example, in one sample of sleep-disordered adolescents, catastrophizing thoughts regarding interpersonal relationships and school performance played a key role in delayed sleep onset (Hiller et al., 2014).

- Lifestyle factors, such as irregular schedules resulting from shift work, retirement, napping, early bedtimes, or long periods spent in bed.

- Activities that interfere with sleep, such as exercising or consuming heavy meals, caffeine, or alcohol in the evening.

- Medical conditions such as congestive heart failure or stroke.

- Drug or alcohol abuse and psychiatric conditions, particularly depression, PTSD, and anxiety disorders (Lubit et al., 2013).

Many people with sleep disorders, particularly parasomnias, have family members with sleep difficulties (APA, 2022). Based on twin studies, the heritability of insomnia is estimated to be 59 percent in women and 38 percent in men (Lind et al., 2015). A genetic predisposition to physiological arousal, coupled with preoccupation with getting enough sleep and distress when unable to sleep, can create a vicious cycle that results in insomnia and the disruption of normal sleep patterns (Harvey et al., 2015). Epigenetic processes affecting biological rhythms and physiological processes associated with sleep are also implicated in the etiology of sleep–wake disorders (Qureshi & Mehler, 2014). There is less known about etiology with the parasomnias; fortunately, parasomnias often remit spontaneously.

Treatment of Sleep–Wake Disorders

Treatment for insomnia involves techniques that help people psychologically and physically prepare for a good night's sleep (Liu et al., 2016). Successful strategies include the following:

- Maintaining a regular sleep–wake schedule
- Exercising regularly but not too late in the day
- Avoiding excessive caffeine or long naps during the day, as well as heavy meals, alcohol, or nicotine within 2 hours of sleep
- Creating a relaxed attitude or frame of mind when going to bed and practicing relaxation procedures and mindfulness techniques to calm the body and the mind
- Minimizing worry about sleep and avoiding clock-watching if unable to sleep
- Eliminating distractions and competing behaviors from the bedroom, thus creating a sleep-conducive environment and strengthening the association between the bedroom and sleep; going to sleep only when sleepy; avoiding use of the bed for anything except sleep (and sex); and leaving the bedroom if unable to sleep, returning only when sleepy

Cognitive-behavioral therapy (CBT) is effective for the treatment of insomnia; additionally, CBT results in the increased ability to cope with stress and reduces symptoms associated with comorbid psychiatric disorders such as anxiety or depression (Friedrich et al., 2018). For mild sleep apnea, recommendations include avoiding alcohol or medications that make it harder for the throat to remain open during sleep; losing weight (if overweight); and sleeping on the side rather than the back, as this position is more likely to keep the throat open. People with moderate to severe sleep apnea often use a continuous positive airway pressure mask—a device that forces air through the nasal passages to prevent the throat from collapsing during sleep (Calik, 2016). A meta-analysis of interventions for obstructive sleep apnea revealed that exercises such as aerobics and resistance training can reduce the severity of symptoms, reduce daytime sleepiness, and improve cardiopulmonary fitness. Exercise may promote upper airway muscle activation and reduce pharyngeal collapse during sleeping (Peng et al., 2022).

Medications are often used to treat sleep disorders. Medications that maintain alertness treat the symptoms of excessive sleepiness seen in narcolepsy, sleep apnea, and sleepiness due to shift work (Savarese & Di Perri, 2020). Sodium oxybate can help control the cataplexy or sudden muscle weakness associated with narcolepsy and is now approved for use with both adults and children (Kushida et al., 2022). The sedating properties of clonazepam (a benzodiazepine) and the sleep-inducing effects of the hormone melatonin are sometimes successful in reducing the aggressive movement that occurs in REM sleep behavior disorder; melatonin produces fewer adverse effects compared to clonazepam (St. Louis & Boeve, 2017).

A variety of sleep-inducing medications such as zolpidem (Ambien), zaleplon (Sonata), and eszopiclone (Lunesta)

Treatment for Obstructive Sleep Apnea

Continuous positive airway pressure (CPAP) therapy is often used to treat obstructive sleep apnea. Here a man sleeps as the machine keeps his airways open by providing steady air pressure.

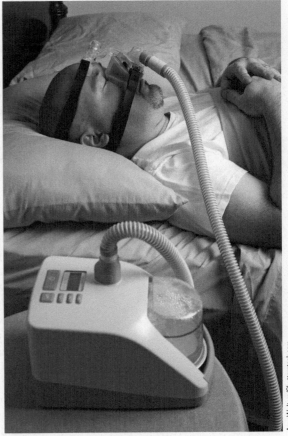

Amy Walters/Shutterstock.com

are used to treat insomnia. However, sedative effects may persist after the person awakens and result in motor incoordination, cognitive confusion, and traffic accidents. Antidepressant medications are also used to treat underlying symptoms of anxiety or depression that interfere with sleep. Antianxiety medications (benzodiazepines) are prescribed with caution due to the increased likelihood of drug dependence (Sateia et al., 2017).

13-5 Contemporary Trends and Future Directions

There is extensive research occurring related to neurocognitive and, to a lesser extent, sleep–wake disorders. The increasing economic and psychological burden associated with these conditions has invigorated the search for methods of prevention and treatment. Simultaneously, medical professionals continue to emphasize lifestyle changes we can make to reduce our vulnerability to neurocognitive and sleep–wake disorders. Of course, there are also ongoing efforts to learn more about how environmental factors, such as toxins or head injuries, trigger neurodegenerative disorders.

Researchers are addressing these disorders from a variety of perspectives, sharing and building on studies from across the globe. Because symptoms of the degenerative neurocognitive disorders do not appear until significant cell death and brain damage have already occurred, researchers continue to focus on identification of early biomarkers associated with neurodegeneration, particular specific pathologies (such as those associated with tau protein), which are implicated in the development and acceleration of a broad range of damaging physiological processes (VandeVrede et al., 2020). Some innovators are researching the use of passive immunotherapy in which specific antibodies are used to enhance the power of the body's immune response to clear destructive tau and beta-amyloid proteins from the brain (Vander Zanden & Chi, 2020). Some teams are contributing to the discussion by addressing the role of epigenetic dysregulation in neurodegenerative disorders, hoping that insight gained from research on one disorder will advance our understanding of related disorders (Hwang et al., 2017).

Additionally, there is a continued shift from research focused on treatment to research addressing early identification and intervention with neurodegenerative disorders; this includes therapies to prevent the onset of biological processes associated with neurodegenerative conditions or to stop degenerative processes once they begin. For example, researchers have begun to use specialized positron emission tomography (PET) imaging to detect and monitor beta-amyloid and tau protein abnormalities in the living brain. Advances such as these will allow clinicians to detect brain abnormalities in high-risk individuals even before symptoms develop, and to assess the effectiveness of prevention or intervention efforts (Stern et al., 2019). Biomarkers are also being identified for Parkinson disease, with the goal of implementing interventions as early as possible (American Parkinson Disease Association, 2023). Given our increased recognition that exposure to fine particulate matter from air pollution, especially from wildfires and agricultural activity, is associated with an increased likelihood of developing dementia, interventions to reduce pollution exposure may lead to decreases in the life-long risk of developing a neurodegenerative disorder (Zhang et al., 2023).

Researchers are focusing considerable energy on the effects of our modern lifestyle (e.g., insufficient sleep, poor diet, and limited physical activity) on brain function and neurodegenerative disorders. Microorganisms that are found in our intestines have a significant effect on physical and mental functioning; for this reason, scientists are also continuing to explore the link between the gut microbiome and neurodegenerative disorders (Askarova et al., 2020). Further, researchers interested in the use of dietary interventions to prevent Alzheimer disease are concentrating on the ways in which specific diets (e.g., Mediterranean or ketogenic diet) reduce or delay cognitive impairment (Vinciguerra et al., 2020).

As we learn more about how genes are expressed, it is hoped that advances in gene therapy (inserting genes into a person's existing cells in order to silence or to inhibit overexpression of the gene) will revolutionize treatment and prevention efforts. Researchers are identifying which genes to target, with the goal of halting neurodegenerative disease processes or even delaying or preventing the development of neurocognitive disorders (Sudhakar & Richardson, 2019). In addition to these biological advances, researchers are also investigating behavioral indicators (e.g., apathy, depression, and sleep disturbance) that may signal the early onset of neurodegeneration and neurocognitive decline (Clement et al., 2020).

Researchers have increasingly emphasized the bidirectional relationship between sleep impairment and both psychiatric and neurocognitive disorders with the hope that treatment or prevention of sleep disorders can avert the development of disabling conditions (Wang & Holtzman, 2020). This is particularly important given the increasing evidence that sleep disorders increase the risk of, or even directly contribute to, some psychiatric disorders, including anxiety and depressive, bipolar, and trauma-related disorders as well as conditions associated with aging such as Alzheimer disease (Anderson & Bradley, 2013). Further, sleep difficulties (particularly nightmares and insomnia) are associated with an increased likelihood of both suicidal ideation and suicide attempts even when a person does not appear to be experiencing depression. Given this association, suicide researchers are also examining ways to intervene with sleep difficulties (Blake & Allen, 2020). Finding effective treatments is also a priority due to the economic costs of inadequate sleep (Hafner et al., 2017).

Recognizing that the hours that college students spend socializing, working on assignments, and studying for tests can result in sleep deprivation and failure to function optimally, some colleges and universities are raising awareness about the importance of improving sleep habits and prioritizing adequate sleep. Some schools have implemented successful programs that combine cognitive-behavioral therapy with relaxation techniques, mindfulness, and hypnotherapy (Friedrich & Schlarb, 2018). In general, mindfulness and meditation continue to be a focus of research because they are low-cost methods with broad benefits, including improved sleep, improved cognition, and increased feelings of well-being (Russell-Williams et al., 2018).

Chapter Summary

1 How can we determine whether someone has a neurocognitive disorder?

- The effects of brain damage vary greatly. The most common symptoms include confusion; attentional deficits; and impairments in consciousness, memory, and judgment.

- Brain damage is assessed using interviews, psychological tests, neurological tests, and other observational or biological measures.

2 What are the different types of neurocognitive disorders?

- There are three main types of neurocognitive disorders: major neurocognitive disorder, mild neurocognitive disorder, and delirium.

- Major neurocognitive disorder involves significant declines in independent-care skills and cognitive functioning.

- In mild neurocognitive disorder, cognitive declines are subtle and independent functioning is not compromised.

- Delirium is an acute condition characterized by diminished awareness, disorientation, and impaired attentional skills.

3 What are the causes of neurocognitive disorders?

- Various events or conditions can cause neurocognitive disorders, including head injuries, substance abuse, and lack of blood flow to the brain.

- The incidence of memory problems and cognitive disorders increases with age. However, many older adults do not experience any significant cognitive decline.

- Neurocognitive disorders caused by neurodegenerative processes include conditions involving dementia (e.g., Alzheimer disease, vascular cognitive impairment, dementia with Lewy bodies, frontotemporal lobar degeneration) and disorders such as Parkinson disease and Huntington disease that cause significant motor dysfunction.

4 What treatments are available for neurocognitive disorders?

- Treatment strategies include physical rehabilitation and cognitive and behavioral therapy. Medications sometimes help control symptoms or slow the progression of some neurocognitive disorders.

5 What do we know about disorders that affect our sleep?

- When excessive sleepiness, ongoing problems initiating or maintaining sleep, or other sleep abnormalities result in daytime distress and impairment, the individual may meet the criteria for one of the sleep disorders.

- Dyssomnias involve difficulties falling asleep or maintaining sleep and excessive daytime sleepiness. They include insomnia disorder, hypersomnolence disorder, narcolepsy, obstructive sleep apnea, and circadian-rhythm sleep–wake disorder.

- Parasomnias involve unusual behaviors or events during sleep or the sleep–wake transition. They include non–rapid eye movement (NREM) sleep arousal disorders, nightmare disorder, and rapid eye movement (REM) sleep behavior disorder.

- Much more is known about the etiology and treatment of the dyssomnias; treatment often focuses on making lifestyle changes, managing stress and worry, and developing a home environment conducive to sleep.

Chapter Glossary

Alzheimer disease
dementia involving memory loss and other declines in cognitive and adaptive functioning

atherosclerosis
clogging of the arteries resulting from a buildup of plaque

beta-amyloid plaques
clumps of beta-amyloid proteins found in the spaces between neurons

brain pathology
a dysfunction or disease of the brain

cardiovascular
pertaining to the heart and blood vessels

cerebral contusion
bruising of the brain, often resulting from a blow that causes the brain to forcefully strike the skull

cerebral laceration
an open head injury in which brain tissue is torn, pierced, or ruptured

chronic traumatic encephalopathy (CTE)
a progressive, degenerative condition involving brain damage resulting from multiple episodes of head trauma

circadian rhythm
internal biological rhythms that influence bodily processes such as the sleep–wake cycle

circadian rhythm sleep disorder
sleep disturbance due to a disrupted sleep–wake cycle

concussion
trauma-induced changes in brain functioning, typically caused by a blow to the head

delirium
an acute state of confusion involving diminished awareness, disorientation, and impaired attentional skills

dementia
condition with symptoms involving deterioration in cognition and independent functioning

dementia with Lewy bodies (DLB)
dementia involving visual hallucinations, cognitive fluctuations, and atypical movements

dyssomnias
disorders involving abnormalities in the quality, amount, or timing of sleep

frontotemporal lobar degeneration (FTLD)
dementia involving degeneration in the frontal and temporal lobes of the brain causing declines in language, behavior, or motor skills

hemorrhagic stroke
a stroke involving leakage of blood into the brain

Huntington disease
a genetic disease characterized by involuntary twitching movements and eventual dementia

hypersomnolence (excessive sleepiness) disorder
a condition involving difficulty waking up after sleeping and excessive daytime sleepiness or prolonged unrefreshing sleep

insomnia disorder
chronic difficulty falling asleep or remaining asleep

ischemic stroke
a stroke due to reduced blood supply caused by a clot or severe narrowing of the arteries supplying blood to the brain

major neurocognitive disorder
a condition involving significant decline in independent living skills and in one or more areas of cognitive functioning

medically induced coma
a deliberately induced state of deep sedation that allows the brain to rest and heal

mild neurocognitive disorder
a condition involving a modest decline in at least one major cognitive area

neurocognitive disorder
a disorder that occurs when brain dysfunction affects thinking processes, memory, consciousness, or perception

neurodegeneration
declining brain functioning due to progressive loss of brain structure, neurochemical abnormalities, or the death of neurons

neurofibrillary tangles
twisted fibers of tau protein found inside nerve cells

nightmare disorder
a condition involving frightening dreams that produce awakening

obstructive sleep apnea (OSA)
a breathing-related sleep disorder involving partial or complete upper-airway obstruction

parasomnias
sleep abnormalities occurring during sleep or in the sleep–wake transition

Parkinson disease
a progressive disorder characterized by poorly controlled motor movements that are sometimes accompanied by cognitive decline and psychiatric symptoms

plaque
sticky material (composed of fat, cholesterol, and other substances) that builds up on the walls of veins or arteries

REM sleep behavior disorder
a condition involving dream-related vocalizations and motor behavior that occur during REM sleep

sleep inertia
significant grogginess and impaired alertness after sleeping or napping

sleep terrors
episodes of intense fear that occur during deep sleep

stroke
a sudden halting of blood flow to a portion of the brain, leading to brain damage

transient ischemic attack (TIA)
a "mini-stroke" resulting from temporary blockage of arteries

traumatic brain injury (TBI)
a physical wound or internal injury to the brain

vascular dementia
progressive mental deterioration associated with impaired blood flow to the brain

vascular neurocognitive disorder
a condition involving cognitive impairment due to reduced blood flow to the brain

focus
Questions

1 What are normal sexual behaviors?

2 What do we know about normal sexual responses and sexual dysfunction?

3 What causes gender dysphoria, and how is it treated?

4 What are paraphilic disorders, what causes them, and how are they treated?

5 What factors are associated with rape?

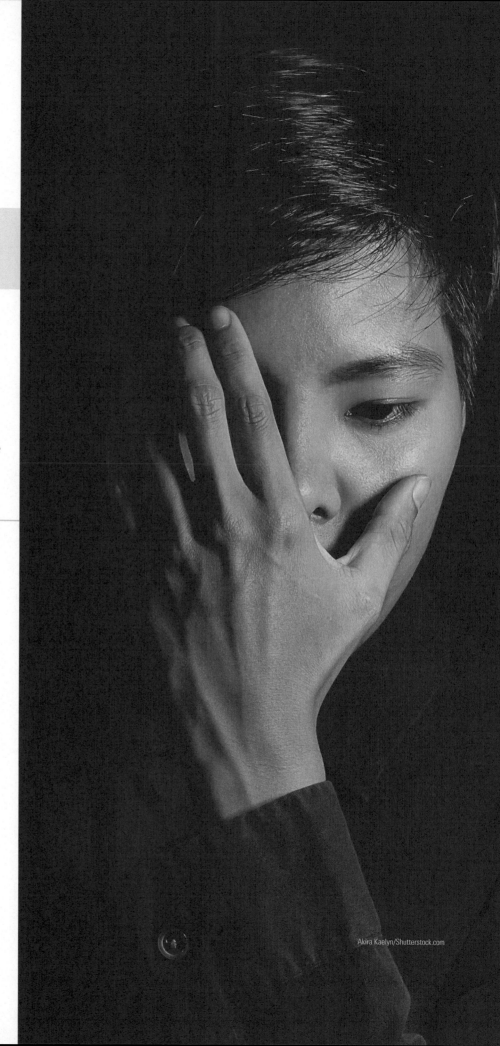

Akira Kaelyn/Shutterstock.com

14

Sexual Dysfunctions, Gender Dysphoria, and Paraphilic Disorders

Learning Objectives

After studying this chapter, you will be able to . . .

14-1 Discuss what is known about normal sexual responses and sexual dysfunction.

14-2 Outline the various sexual dysfunctions, including treatment and factors associated with their development.

14-3 Describe normal variations in gender expression and explain the causes of and treatments for gender dysphoria.

14-4 Describe the paraphilic disorders, what causes them, and how they are treated.

14-5 Discuss the characteristics of individuals who perpetrate rape and the effect of rape on sexual assault survivors.

Christina and Jeremiah Decided to Seek Therapy after only 8 months of marriage. Both were extremely dissatisfied with their sex life. Jeremiah complained that Christina never initiated sex, found excuses to avoid sexual contact, and appeared to fake orgasms during intercourse. Christina complained that Jeremiah's lovemaking was often brief, perfunctory, and without affection. During the therapy sessions, it became clear that Christina had never had a strong interest in sex and seldom became aroused during intercourse. Although Jeremiah had never had a problem maintaining an erection, sex with Christina had become progressively distressing, as he often had difficulty getting hard enough for penetration. Before initiating sex, Jeremiah began to drink heavily to give him "courage" to approach Christina and to alleviate his guilt at "forcing her to have sex." These encounters were often humiliating, as he felt that Christina only agreed to have sex out of pity.

The case of Christina and Jeremiah demonstrates the psychological and physiological complexities associated with one of the three groups of disorders discussed in this chapter: *sexual dysfunctions*, which involve problems in the normal sexual response cycle. The other disorders we discuss are *gender dysphoria* (distress resulting from an incongruence between a person's gender identity and assigned gender) and *paraphilic disorders* (problematic sexual interests, urges, and behaviors). We begin with a discussion about what constitutes "normal" sexual behavior and conclude the chapter with a discussion of rape, a deviant behavior that has a significant effect on society.

14-1 What Is "Normal" Sexual Behavior?

Many people have difficulty dealing with the topic of sexual behavior in an open and direct manner. However, such discussion is important because sex is an integral part of our lives, and because many myths and taboos surround the topic. Much of our understanding of human sexual physiology, practices, and customs comes from the classic studies of researchers such as Alfred Kinsey and his colleagues (Kinsey et al., 1953) and William Masters and Virginia Johnson (1966, 1970), who brought the topic of sexuality to the forefront during the 20th century. Further studies such as the *Janus Report on Sexual Behavior* (Janus & Janus, 1993); the National Survey of Sexual Health and Behavior (2023); and the work of contemporary sex researchers has added to our knowledge of sexual functioning.

Despite the quantity of research on the topic, distinguishing between harmless variations in sexual preferences and behavior of concern is often challenging. Definitions of normal sexual behavior vary widely and are influenced by both moral and legal judgments. For example, more than one fifth of U.S. states still have laws against oral or anal sex, with statutes that describe these practices using wording such as "lewd and lascivious," "unnatural and perverted," and "a crime against nature" (Rude, 2022). However, most people in contemporary society would not classify these sexual practices as deviant. For example, in one survey, over 75 percent of the adult respondents reported engaging in oral sex (Habel et al., 2018). Surveys such as this provide important information about typical sexual practices and have helped clarify what constitutes normal sexual behavior.

Understanding what is "normal" is important when diagnosing sexual problems and behaviors. However, making this differentiation is not an easy task. As you might imagine, it is difficult to define what constitutes "normal" sexual interest, behavior, fantasies, or frequency of sexual activity. To take one example, people report tremendous variation in frequency of sexual outlet or release, according to research by Kinsey and colleagues (1948). One man reported that he had ejaculated only once in 30 years, and another claimed to have averaged 30 orgasms per week for 30 years. Such wide variations make it difficult to determine when to categorize someone as having atypical sexual behavior. Also, using number of orgasms (via intercourse or masturbation) to determine whether or not someone's sexual behavior is "normal" may introduce gender bias into the definition of "normal" sexual desire, since men masturbate and experience more frequent orgasms compared to women. Further, some people may have a high sex drive but not engage in sexual activities, whereas others

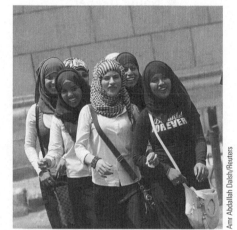

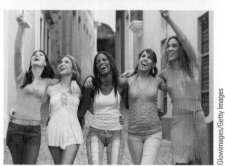

Cultural Influences and Sexuality

Sexuality is influenced by how it is viewed in different cultures. Some societies have very rigid social, cultural, and religious taboos associated with exposure of the human body, whereas other societies are more open. Note the dress and behavioral differences between the young women shown here.

Is Hypersexual Behavior a Sexual Disorder?

We have all seen media reports of celebrities and political figures who have engaged in repetitive, socially unacceptable sexual activities despite the potential for life-changing personal or professional consequences. They appear to have little self-control over their sexual behaviors and continue seeking sex even when harmful consequences occur (Walton et al., 2015). Given the impairment and distress that can result from excessive sexuality, the working group revising the DSM considered the inclusion of "hypersexual disorder." Although there was a decision not to incorporate this diagnosis in the DSM-5, most clinicians and researchers agree that some people do have an obsession with sex that resembles an addiction and interferes with optimal functioning.

These individuals have recurrent sexual fantasies and urges and often report that they compulsively engage in sexual activity in response to depression, anxiety, boredom, irritability, or stressful life events. Additionally, they have considerable difficulty reducing or controlling sexual urges, activities, and fantasies, even when the behaviors cause physical or emotional harm to themselves or others (Todd, 2018). In one survey of U.S. adults, 10.3 percent of men and 7 percent of women endorsed clinically relevant levels of distress and/or impairment associated with difficulty controlling sexual feelings, urges, and behavior (Dickenson et al., 2018). A German national survey revealed that 4.9 percent of men and 3 percent of women reported "intense and recurring sexual impulses or sexual urges" that were difficult to control and resulted in sexual behavior (Briken et al., 2022).

Although "hypersexual disorder" was not included as a diagnostic category in the DSM, a diagnosis of "compulsive sexual behavior disorder" is included in the ICD-11 and involves criteria that include:

(a) irresistible, persistent, and repetitive sexual impulses or urges;

(b) the sexual activity has become central to the person's life;

(c) an inability to reduce these activities even though they result in adverse consequences; and

(d) these behaviors are present for 6 months or more.

It is likely that discussions about hypersexual behavior will continue when it is once again time to revise the DSM. In the meantime, therapists will continue to work with clients who exhibit this behavioral pattern.

For Further Consideration

1. What do you believe are the pros and cons of having "compulsive sexual behavior" recognized as a psychiatric disorder?

2. Why do you believe some professionals consider hypersexuality a real disorder while others contend it is simply an excuse for bad behavior?

3. Should promiscuity or compulsive use of masturbation or online pornography be considered hypersexual behavior?

---

may have little sexual interest but engage in frequent sexual behaviors for the sake of their partners.

There is disagreement as to whether low-frequency sexual behavior should be considered "abnormal." Approximately 0.4 percent to 3.3 percent of individuals are *asexual*; that is, they show a lack of sexual attraction or interest in being sexual with others. However, about three quarters of this group report having romantic attraction, and many are in relationships (Antonsen et al., 2020). The asexual identity appears to be relatively stable (Su & Zheng, 2023). An online support community, Asexuality Visibility and Education Network, seeks to reduce public stigma about asexuality and affirm that lack of sexual interest is a normal variant of human sexual behavior. Some individuals (including some who identify as asexual) consider themselves to be aromantic due to their lack of romantic attraction or interest in commitment to a life partner (Carvalho & Rodrigues, 2022).

Since it is not easy to delineate "normal" sexual behavior, it is not surprising that definitions of sexual disorders are also inexact. In fact, over the past century, psychiatrists in the United States and Europe have pathologized and de-pathologized a variety of sexual preferences, desires, and behaviors. Revised definitions of what constitutes pathological behaviors or normative sexual practices often occur during the periodic updating of psychiatric classification systems such as the DSM.

If legal, moral, and statistical models are unable to adequately differentiate between normal and abnormal sexual behavior, can we simply state that sexual behavior is deviant if it is a threat to society, causes distress to participants, or impairs social or occupational functioning? Using this definition, there would be no objection to defining child sexual abuse, which includes elements of distress and victimization, as deviant behavior. But what about sexual arousal to an inanimate object (fetishism)? This behavior is not a threat to society and frequently does not cause distress to the people involved. Many would argue that there is no need for society or psychiatric classification systems to consider these behaviors as indicative of a mental disorder. There is even greater controversy as to whether gender dysphoria should be considered a psychiatric disorder, especially because much of the suffering associated with this condition stems from discrimination and negative societal reactions. In short, the ambiguities and controversies surrounding all classification systems are particularly relevant with respect to the three groups of disorders discussed in this chapter.

The Sexual Response Cycle

Understanding and treating sexual dysfunctions requires consideration of the normal sexual response cycle, which traditionally consists of four stages: appetitive (interest and desire), arousal, orgasm, and resolution (Figure 14.1). Empirical findings suggest that it is difficult to distinguish between the desire of the appetitive and arousal stages, because they seem to overlap. Desire and interest, for example, may precede or follow arousal. Although we use a four-stage description, it is best to view the appetitive and arousal stages as intertwined and interactive.

1. The *appetitive phase* is characterized by a person's interest in sexual activity. The person begins to have thoughts or fantasies about sex, feels attracted to another person, or daydreams about sex.

2. The *arousal phase* involves heightened and intensified arousal resulting from specific and direct sexual stimulation. In a male, blood flow increases in the penis, resulting in an erection. In a

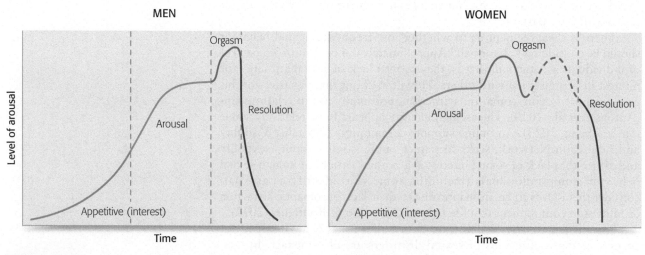

Figure 14.1

Human Sexual Response Cycle

The studies of Masters and Johnson reveal similar normal sexual response cycles for men and women. Note that women may experience more than one orgasm. Sexual disorders may occur at any of the phases but seldom at the resolution phase.

female, the breasts swell, nipples become erect, blood engorges the genital region, and the clitoris expands.

3. The *orgasm phase* is characterized by involuntary muscular contractions throughout the body and the eventual release of sexual tension. In males, muscles at the base of the penis contract, propelling semen through the penis. In females, the outer third of the vagina contracts rhythmically.

4. The *resolution phase* is characterized by relaxation of the body after orgasm. Males enter a refractory period during which they are unresponsive to sexual stimulation. However, females are capable of multiple orgasms with continued stimulation.

Problems may occur in any of the phases of the sexual response cycle, although they are rare in the resolution phase.

14-2 Sexual Dysfunctions

A **sexual dysfunction** is a recurrent and persistent disruption of any part of the normal sexual response cycle involving sexual interest, arousal, or response. The DSM-5-TR requires that the symptoms associated with a sexual dysfunction be present for at least 6 months and be accompanied by significant distress. People who have no interest in sexual activity or who are unconcerned about an inability to experience an orgasm, for instance, would not receive a sexual dysfunction diagnosis. Also, if the sexual problem is mainly due to severe interpersonal relationship problems or another mental condition such as an anxiety disorder, a sexual dysfunction diagnosis would not be made.

Approximately 40 percent to 45 percent of adult women and 20 percent to 30 percent of adult men have experienced at least one sexual dysfunction. The most frequent sexual dysfunctions for women involve desire or arousal; for men, it is premature (early) ejaculation and erectile dysfunction. Women are also more likely to experience multiple sexual dysfunctions than men are (McCabe et al., 2016). In a study of young adults in France, 48 percent of women and 23 percent of men reported at least one sexual dysfunction. Pain during intercourse, lack of sexual desire, difficulty reaching orgasm, and lack of pleasure during intercourse were the most common complaints among women respondents. For men, the primary problem involved premature ejaculation (Moreau et al., 2016). The 12-month prevalence of sexual problems in adults is summarized in Table 14.1.

Table 14.1 Past Year Prevalence of Sexual Disorders in Men and Women in Germany

Condition	Women (%)	Men (%)
Lack of interest in sex	27.1	14.7
Inability to reach orgasm	23.1	12.4
Early ejaculation	N/A	11.7
Pain during sex	10.9	N/A
Sexual arousal problem	23.4	N/A
Delayed ejaculation	N/A	9.7
Erectile difficulties	N/A	13.6

Source: Briken et al., 2020

Sexual dysfunctions can be *lifelong* (evident during initial sexual experiences), *acquired* (developed after successful sexual experiences), *generalized* (occurring in nearly all situations), or *situational* (occurring with certain partners, situations, or types of stimulation). According to the DSM-5-TR, "If severe relationship distress, partner violence, or significant stressors better explain the sexual difficulties, then a sexual dysfunction diagnosis is not made" (p. 478). As indicated in Table 14.2, the DSM-5-TR includes dysfunctions associated with sexual interest and arousal, orgasm, and pain during sex. For gender diverse individuals, the diagnosis of sexual dysfunction is not dependent on the individual's specific sex or gender. Instead, diagnoses such as erectile dysfunction, ejaculatory issues, and genito-pelvic pain disorder are based on current anatomy (APA, 2022).

Sexual Interest/Arousal Disorders

Sexual interest/arousal disorders involve problems with sexual excitement, including difficulties with feelings of sexual pleasure or the physiological changes associated with the appetitive and arousal phases. They include:

- **male hypoactive sexual desire disorder**, which is characterized by little or no interest in sexual activities, either actual or fantasized, and
- **female sexual interest/arousal disorder**, which is characterized by little or no interest in sexual activities, either actual or fantasized, and/or a lack of or diminished arousal to sexual cues during nearly all sexual activities.

A diagnosis is made only if the individual feels clinically distressed by their lack of sexual interest or desire. Some clinicians estimate that

Table 14.2   Sexual Dysfunctions

DSM-5-TR Disorders Chart			
Dysfunction[a]	**DSM-5-TR Definition**	**Prevalence**	**Associated Features**
Male hypoactive sexual desire	Recurrent lack of sexual interest	Up to 15% of men have transient episodes; less than 6% have chronic symptoms	Increasing prevalence with age
Erectile dysfunction	Inability to attain or maintain erection sufficient for sexual activity	13% to 75% dependent on age	Low self-esteem or lack of confidence; fear of failure
Premature ejaculation	Ejaculation prior to or within 1 minute after vaginal penetration	Up to 30% indicate concern	Fear of not satisfying partner; but only 1% to 3% meet the criteria
Delayed ejaculation	Persistent delay or absence of ejaculation nearly all the time during partnered sex activity	1% to 5% of men	Partner may feel less attractive; feelings of frustration
Female sexual interest/arousal disorder	Little or no sexual interest or arousal for sexual activity	30% with symptoms, but many do not experience distress	Problems with arousal, pain, orgasm; relationship problems
Female orgasmic disorder	Persistent delay or inability to attain an orgasm in nearly all sexual encounters	8% to 72% from surveys; nearly 10% never achieve an orgasm in their lifetime	Only mildly related to women's sexual satisfaction
Genito-pelvic pain/penetration disorder	Difficulty with vaginal penetration, fear of pain, tightening of pelvic muscles	10% to 28% of women report painful intercourse	Fear of penetration; avoidance of sexual activities

[a]All dysfunctions require that the individuals experience "clinically significant distress."

Source: APA, 2022; Carvalheira et al., 2014; Pazmany et al., 2013

40 percent to 50 percent of all sexual difficulties involve deficits in interest; this is one of the most common complaints of couples seeking sex therapy (Hogue et al., 2019). The condition is more than twice as common in women as in men (Vowels et al., 2021). Low sexual interest may be the consequence of pain during intercourse or another sexual dysfunction such as erectile disorder or premature ejaculation (Meissner et al., 2019). As previously mentioned, according to the DSM-5-TR, a diagnosis of sexual dysfunction is not appropriate when factors such as severe relationship problems, other mental disorders, or significant stressors play a key role in the sexual difficulties.

This distinction is important because sexual interest or arousal difficulties are often associated with depression or anxiety, relationship issues with the current partner, or stressful life events. In a sample of men between the ages of 18 and 75, a distressing lack of sexual interest was reported by 14.5 percent of the participants, with stress involving work or professional activities being a common explanation for reduced interest in sex (Carvalheira et al., 2014). In one group of women, 31 percent reported experiencing a lack of sexual interest; in many cases, their disinterest resulted from negative attitudes regarding sex or distressing early sexual experiences (McCabe & Goldhammer, 2013). Relationship issues are also an important consideration. Low social interest has been found in women who perceive inequities with their partners in activities such as the performance of household chores (Harris et al., 2022).

Although people with sexual interest/arousal disorders are often capable of experiencing orgasm, they have little interest in, or derive minimal pleasure from, sexual activity. In the following case, relationship problems contributed to the couple's sexual difficulties.

Case Study After 5 years of marriage, Rhonda and Michael decided to seek sex therapy because of their unsatisfactory sex life. Although they had enjoyed sex for the first year of their marriage, sexual intercourse had progressively declined: For the past 3 years, they have had little or no sexual contact. Rhonda described Michael as "unloving, cold, angry, controlling, and demanding" and explained to the therapist that she does not love or feel sexually interested in Michael. Michael described Rhonda as "punitive, angry, and a vengeful person" and believes she is punishing him for a brief affair he had with a coworker early in their marriage. Correspondingly, he feels angry, resentful, and cheated of a "normal sex life."

In this case, should Rhonda receive a female sexual interest/arousal disorder diagnosis because of her low sexual desire and limited sexual interest in Michael? Most clinicians would question the legitimacy of such a diagnosis because her lack of desire appears to result from severe relationship difficulties. These interpersonal problems, rather than Rhonda's lack of sexual interest, would be the most appropriate focus of treatment.

Erectile Disorder

Case Study A 20-year-old college student was experiencing acquired erectile dysfunction. His first episode of erectile difficulty occurred when he attempted sexual intercourse after drinking heavily. Although he knew that his sexual performance was affected by alcohol, he began to have doubts about his sexual ability. During a subsequent sexual encounter, his anxiety and worry increased. When he failed in this next coital encounter, even though he had not been drinking, his anxiety level rose even more. When his erectile difficulties continued, he decided to seek therapy.

In men, inhibited sexual excitement takes the form of an **erectile disorder**, defined as a frequent inability to attain or maintain an erection sufficient for sexual intercourse or other sexual activity. As was the case of the student seeking therapy, a man with erectile dysfunction may feel fully aroused yet be unable to engage in intercourse. The prevalence of this disorder increases with age, with over half of men ages 40 to 70 reporting some degree of erectile dysfunction (Anderson et al., 2022). Although complaints regarding erectile dysfunction are common among older men, the incidence is increasing in younger individuals, with up to 30 percent of young men in one study reporting erectile difficulties (Nguyen et al., 2017).

In the past, people often attributed erectile dysfunction to psychological causes ("It's all in the head"). However, studies indicate that a large percentage of erectile dysfunction is due to limited blood flow caused by

Can Internet Porn Cause Sexual Dysfunction?

At the age of 23, Gabe "freaked out" when he was unable to respond sexually to his "extremely attractive" girlfriend. He worried that his frequent watching of Internet pornography had caused a condition call PIED (porn-induced erectile dysfunction). Even taking Viagra and Cialis did not improve his sexual performance. Gabe began viewing pornography in early adolescence. "I would get out of middle school and come home as fast as I could, and watch porn—look up whatever I could for about three or four hours before my parents got home from work . . . I was watching every type of porn that you could think of" (James & O'Shea, 2014).

Does watching Internet porn lead to sexual problems? There is some evidence that erectile dysfunction is increasing among adolescent boys and young men such as Gabe. In one study, 45.3 percent of male adolescents had experienced erectile dysfunction (O'Sullivan et al., 2016). Similarly, 21.5 percent of a group of young men reported experiencing some degree of erectile difficulties (Jacobs et al., 2021). Could the availability and consumption of Internet porn be responsible for the increased frequency of erectile dysfunction? And if so, do the effects depend on conditions such as age of exposure, frequency of exposure, or type of pornographic material? These questions are not easily answered, as contradictory findings exist.

In a comprehensive review of research on the relationship between Internet porn and sexual dysfunctions, Park et al. (2016) reported the following findings from different studies:

- Half of one group of subjects recruited from bars and bathhouses where video porn was omnipresent reported they could only respond sexually to novel or extreme pornographic material.

- Over half of another group of men who were compulsive Internet porn users reported erectile dysfunction; they also reported diminished attraction to women but not to sexually explicit videos.

- Internet porn users appear to require more novel and "kinky" content to become sexually aroused. Once their sexual arousal became conditioned to the ongoing sexual novelty within the videos, it becomes more difficult for live sexual partners to meet this requirement.

- Men who begin to require pornography for sexual arousal (such as Gabe in the case study) are able to recover sexual functioning with a partner after abstaining from porn for a lengthy period of time.

Park and colleagues believe that the limitless novelty and variety of Internet porn results in a "supernormal stimulus," beyond that which our brains were evolved to pursue. The sexual conditioning to this ever-changing and extraordinarily exciting stimulus does not easily transfer to real-life sexual situations. Because of this, arousal does not occur or diminishes rapidly with a sexual partner. Park also believes that there may be a critical sexual developmental phase early in life (adolescence) where the exposure to porn has its greatest influence. Other reviewers (Dwulit & Rzymski, 2019; Rowland et al., 2023) find little evidence that viewing porn is related to sexual dysfunctions but some evidence that it may lead to less sexual satisfaction.

For Further Consideration

1. Do you believe there is a relationship between Internet porn and sexual dysfunctions? If so, what do you think are possible remedies?

2. Should adolescents receive education regarding the possible effects of excessive pornography exposure?

vascular insufficiency. A meta-analysis of 25 studies involving 154,794 men found that men with erectile dysfunction were more likely to develop coronary vascular disease (43 percent), coronary heart disease (59 percent), or stroke (34 percent); they also experienced greater mortality (Zhao, Hong, et al., 2019). These studies indicate that erectile dysfunction is often more than just psychological and may indicate a significant health condition.

Determining whether erectile dysfunction is primarily biological or psychological is often difficult. One procedure used to make this distinction involves recording *nocturnal penile tumescence*—the frequent, spontaneous erections that occur in healthy men during sleep. If a man has a physiological problem, he is unlikely to have these spontaneous erections during sleep. If sleep studies confirm normal erectile activity during sleep, there is reason to conclude that the erectile problems are psychological, not physiological, in nature (Lin et al., 2018). In many cases, however, both physical and psychological factors influence erectile difficulties.

Orgasmic Disorders

Orgasmic disorders affect both men and women. Those with this condition experience difficulty achieving or an inability to achieve a satisfactory orgasm after entering the excitement phase and receiving adequate sexual stimulation. *Female orgasmic disorder* is quite different from organismic difficulties experienced by men. In men, the symptoms of orgasmic dysfunction are subsumed under the diagnostic categories of *delayed ejaculation* and *premature (early) ejaculation*.

Female Orgasmic Disorder

A woman with **female orgasmic disorder** experiences persistent delay or inability to achieve an orgasm or a "markedly reduced intensity of orgasmic sensations" on nearly all occasions of sexual activity; for a diagnosis, these symptoms must have lasted for a minimum of 6 months. Female orgasmic disorder is a frequently reported sexual problem for women. In fact, approximately 10 percent of all women have never achieved an orgasm (APA, 2022).

Most women require clitoral stimulation to achieve an orgasm; this may be one of the reasons that only a small percentage of women report consistently experiencing orgasm during sexual intercourse. The diagnosis of female orgasmic disorder is given only if the woman has difficulty achieving an orgasm through clitoral stimulation. In one study suggesting a physiologic cause, a group of women with female orgasmic disorder were found to be less sensitive to vibratory clitoral stimulations compared to women with other sexual dysfunctions (Gruenwald et al., 2020).

Delayed Ejaculation

Delayed ejaculation is the persistent delay or absence of ejaculation after the excitement phase has been reached and sexual activity has been adequate in focus, intensity, and duration. This diagnosis is typically given only when a man experiences a delay or inability to ejaculate during partnered sexual activity, even with full arousal (Abdel-Hamid & Ali, 2018). For a disorder to be diagnosed, delayed ejaculation must have occurred 75 percent to 100 percent of the time for at least

Did You Know?

Two urologists viewed almost 200 YouTube videos discussing treatments for premature ejaculation. After rating the information provided by each video as either reliable or unreliable, only 30 percent were deemed reliable in terms of the information presented.
Source: Gul & Diri, 2019

6 months. Due to a lack of consensus in the research, the diagnostic criteria do not address what constitutes a "delay" (APA, 2022). As noted, men who have this dysfunction are usually able to ejaculate when masturbating.

Premature (Early) Ejaculation

In contrast to delayed ejaculation, **premature (early) ejaculation** involves a distressing and recurrent pattern of having an orgasm with minimal sexual stimulation before, during, or shortly after vaginal penetration; the diagnostic criterion specifies that ejaculation must occur within approximately 1 minute of penetration or attempted penetration. It is estimated that 1 percent to 3 percent of men meet the criteria for a premature ejaculation diagnosis (APA, 2022). However, there are differing opinions about the definition—some believe it should depend on the individual's subjective response of "being too early" or that the time reference should be revised to longer than 1 minute. Depending on the definition, the lifetime prevalence of premature (early) ejaculation can reach as high as 75 percent (El-Hamd et al., 2019). Men who experience premature ejaculation report lower satisfaction with intercourse, poor self-confidence, and personal distress (Siroosbakht et al., 2019).

Genito-Pelvic Pain/Penetration Disorder

According to the DSM-5-TR, **genito-pelvic pain/penetration disorder** may be diagnosed when a woman experiences distress and difficulty associated with vaginal penetration during intercourse, pain in the genital or pelvic region during intercourse (**dyspareunia**), fear of pain or vaginal penetration, or tension in the pelvic muscles (APA, 2022). The pain and distress associated with genito-pelvic pain/penetration disorder is not caused exclusively by lack of lubrication or by the rare condition, **vaginismus**, which results when involuntary spasms of the outer third of the vaginal wall prevent or interfere with sexual intercourse.

Painful intercourse is relatively common in women under age 40 and is estimated to affect between 15 percent and 21 percent of women in this age group; the prevalence increases in postmenopausal women (Gross & Brubaker, 2022). As compared to a control group of pain-free women, a sample of women with dyspareunia reported significantly higher levels of distress over their body image and genitals (Pazmany et al., 2013). As you might expect, many women with genito-pelvic pain/penetration disorder also experience reduced sexual arousal.

Etiology of Sexual Dysfunctions

Sexual dysfunctions clearly demonstrate the complex interaction of various etiological factors. Let's return to the case of Jeremiah and Christina from the opening of this chapter to understand how various etiological factors can contribute to sexual dysfunction. (You may wish to reread the case in order to follow this multipath analysis.)

Sexual Flirtation Common Among Teens

Direct expressions of sexual interest are discouraged in many cultures. Flirting, however, allows for indirect, playful, and romantic sexual overtures toward others. It may occur through verbal communication (tone of voice, pace, and intonation) or body language (eye contact, open stances, hair flicking, or brief touching).

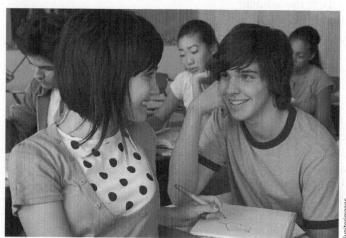

Jupiterimages

Case Study Analysis   Christina and Jerimiah sought sex therapy because Christina did not seem to desire or enjoy sex. Additionally, Jeremiah was experiencing erectile difficulties for the first time in his life. The therapist concluded that these problems were not primarily the result of severe relationship distress. Christina was diagnosed as having a sexual interest/arousal disorder and Jeremiah an erectile disorder. The possibility that Christina could also be experiencing an orgasmic disorder was entertained but eliminated as therapy progressed. It appeared that she was quite capable of being aroused and orgasmic under the right conditions.

Their sexual difficulties involved a variety of interacting factors. Christina's limited interest in sex increasingly strained their sexual relationship and caused Jeremiah, who felt anger, guilt, and humiliation, to experience difficulty maintaining an erection. After a while, Jerimiah began to drink before initiating sex, which decreased his inhibition; although drinking gave him the courage to initiate sex with a reluctant partner, alcohol is a central nervous system depressant, a factor that made it more difficult for him to achieve an erection.

When Jeremiah was able to become erect, he quickly entered Christina for fear of losing the erection, and in turn appeared "brief" and "perfunctory" in lovemaking. This resulted in Christina feeling hurt and rejected. Additionally, the brevity of the sexual encounter did not allow Christina to become sexually aroused; this resulted in insufficient lubrication, painful intercourse, and an inability to achieve an orgasm. Christina then began to fake orgasms in order to please Jeremiah, who was further humiliated because he realized she was pretending. He not only blamed himself for the failure but also felt humiliated. As a man, Jeremiah was also affected by cultural scripts—social and cultural beliefs that guide attitudes and behaviors—that associate masculinity with sexual potency. Thus, he began to equate his inability to satisfy Christina with "not being a real man." Given all of these influences, they both found their sexual encounters increasingly unpleasant, a factor that added stress to their relationship and further decreased Christina's interest in sex.

As you can see, Jeremiah and Christina's sexual disorders are intertwined and cannot be viewed in isolation. Although the problems began with Christina's low sexual interest, they escalated as Jeremiah began experiencing difficulties achieving and maintaining an erection. Consistent with our case example, research suggests that difficulties with sexual interest, desire, and performance are due to interactions among biological, psychological, social, and sociocultural factors as reflected in our multipath model (Figure 14.2).

Biological Dimension

Environmental and relationship variables may influence sexual dysfunction to a greater degree than biological factors do (Burri, 2013). However, sexual hormones can play a significant role in sexual responsiveness. For example, in men with medical conditions that diminish the production of sex hormones, lower levels of testosterone can affect sexual desire and erectile dysfunction (Rastrelli et al., 2018). Also, prescription use of the ovarian hormone, estradiol, or the male hormone, testosterone, is associated with increased sexual desire in peri- and post-menopausal women (Goldstein et al., 2017). The relationship between hormones and sexual behavior, however, is complex. In one study of healthy men and women, higher

Figure 14.2

Multipath Model of Sexual Dysfunctions

The dimensions interact with one another and combine in different ways to result in a specific sexual dysfunction.

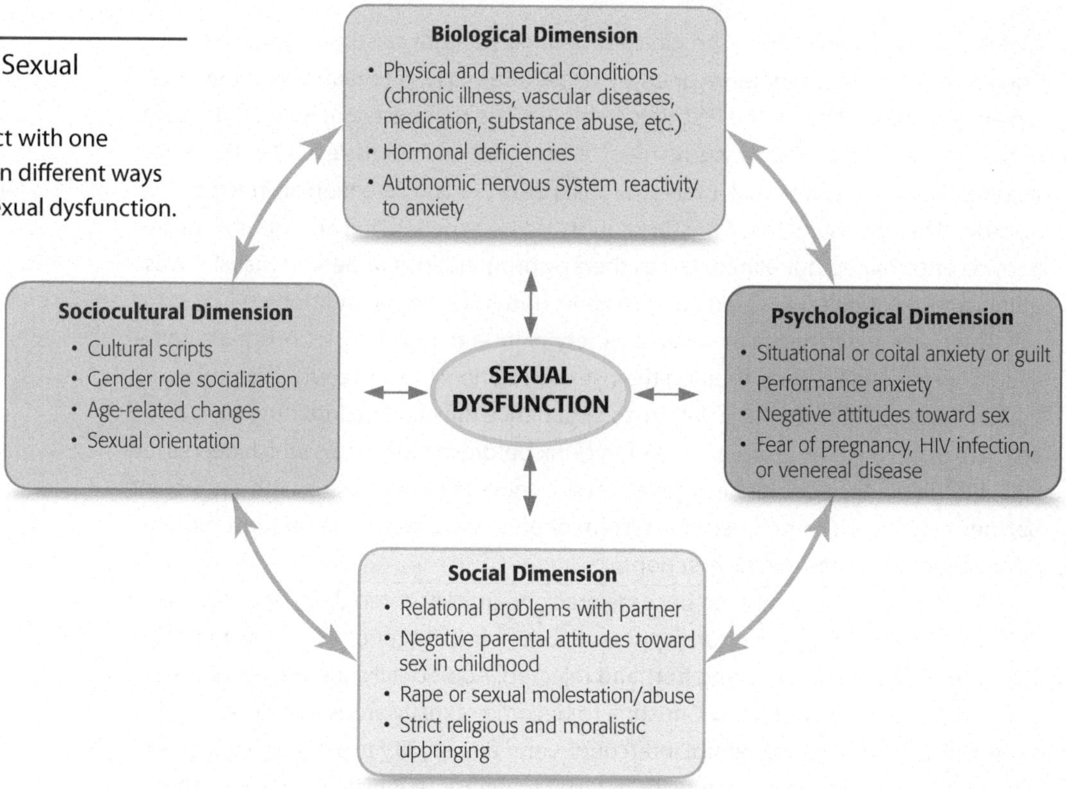

Biological Dimension
- Physical and medical conditions (chronic illness, vascular diseases, medication, substance abuse, etc.)
- Hormonal deficiencies
- Autonomic nervous system reactivity to anxiety

Sociocultural Dimension
- Cultural scripts
- Gender role socialization
- Age-related changes
- Sexual orientation

SEXUAL DYSFUNCTION

Psychological Dimension
- Situational or coital anxiety or guilt
- Performance anxiety
- Negative attitudes toward sex
- Fear of pregnancy, HIV infection, or venereal disease

Social Dimension
- Relational problems with partner
- Negative parental attitudes toward sex in childhood
- Rape or sexual molestation/abuse
- Strict religious and moralistic upbringing

testosterone levels in women were associated with increased sexual desire as evidenced by masturbatory behavior, but not activity with a partner. In contrast, no significant correlation was found between testosterone level and sexual desire in men (van Anders, 2012).

Sexual dysfunction in both men and women is affected by modifiable health or lifestyle conditions such as obesity, smoking, or the use of alcohol or recreational drugs. For instance, obesity is associated with erectile dysfunction in men and reduced sexual desire in women, possibly due to associated conditions such as vascular disease, which can decrease blood flow to the genitals. Additionally, smoking appears to have a negative effect on sex hormones, and alcohol is a central nervous system depressant, which can affect sexual responsiveness (Mollaioli et al., 2020). Antidepressant medications, especially the SSRIs, are also associated with sexual dysfunctions, as are certain medical conditions and other prescribed medications (Rothmore, 2020). However, not everyone who takes antidepressant medication, consumes alcohol, or is ill has a sexual dysfunction. In some people these factors may combine with a predisposing personal history or with current stressors to produce problems in sexual function. A complete physical workup—including a medical history, physical exam, and laboratory evaluation—is a necessary first step in assessment. For instance, genito-pelvic pain/penetration disorder is often caused by gynecological conditions such as endometriosis (Rossi et al., 2022).

Psychological Dimension

Sexual dysfunctions may result from psychological factors alone or from a combination of psychological and biological factors. Psychological causes for sexual dysfunctions include predisposing or historical factors, as well as current problems and concerns. Stressful situations and the presence of anxiety, depression, and trauma-related disorders tend to inhibit sexual responding and functioning in both women and men (Grotto et al., 2016).

Did You Know?

A survey of X-rated film actresses revealed that they were more likely to be bisexual, enjoy sex, have more sexual partners, use more drugs, and have higher self-esteem than a matched sample of women. They were also less likely to have experienced childhood abuse.

Source: Griffith et al., 2013

For example, veterans of the wars in Iraq and Afghanistan who were subsequently diagnosed with posttraumatic stress disorder (PTSD) were over three times more likely to have a sexual dysfunction compared to veterans without the disorder (Breyer et al., 2014). Guilt, anger, or resentment toward a partner can also interfere with sexual performance (Westheimer & Lopater, 2005). As was the case for Jeremiah and Christina, having a partner with a sexual dysfunction further increases the risk of sexual difficulties in the other partner (Jiann et al., 2013).

Apprehension about sexual performance plays a key role in erectile disorder (Jiang et al., 2020). Men with erectile dysfunction often report anxiety over sexual overtures, including a fear of failing sexually or being judged as sexually inferior, as well as anxiety over the size of their genitals. Performance anxiety and taking on a "spectator role" can exacerbate erectile dysfunction. For instance, if a man experiences a problem achieving or maintaining an erection, he may then begin to worry that it will happen again. Instead of enjoying the next sexual encounter and becoming aroused, he monitors or observes his own reactions ("Am I getting an erection?") and becomes a spectator who is anxious and detached from the situation. This can result in sexual failure and increased anxiety during future sexual encounters.

Situational anxiety or emotional factors resulting from sexual abuse or other traumatic childhood sexual experiences often interfere with sexual functioning in women. Other factors associated with sexual dysfunction in women include having a sexually inexperienced or dysfunctional partner; fear of being an undesirable sexual partner; worry that they will never be able to attain orgasm; concern about pregnancy or sexually transmitted disease; an inability to accept the partner, either emotionally or physically; and misinformation or ignorance about sexuality or sexual techniques (Jiann et al., 2013).

Negative thoughts such as "my partner doesn't really care about me" and dysfunctional beliefs such as "sexual desire is sinful" also play a role in female sexual dysfunction. Such thoughts and beliefs are associated with sexual interest/arousal and orgasmic difficulties, as well as painful intercourse (Carvalho et al., 2013). Women who are self-consciousness about their attractiveness or who focus excessively on their bodies may experience more difficulty with sexual arousal. Women are also more likely than men to have higher levels of body dissatisfaction and a greater concern over physical appearance (Carvalheira et al., 2016). They are also more likely to blame themselves rather than their partner for sexual difficulties (Stephenson & Meston, 2016).

Social Dimension

Social upbringing and current relationships both influence sexual functioning. The attitudes parents display toward sex and their expression of affection toward each other can affect their children's attitudes. A strict religious upbringing is associated with sexual dysfunction in both men and women (Carvalho et al., 2013). Traumatic sexual experiences involving rape or sexual abuse during childhood or adolescence are also factors to consider. Women who have been raped or molested as children may find it difficult to trust and establish intimacy and may exhibit sexual dysfunction (Buster, 2013). Sexual dysfunction in one partner decreases sexual satisfaction and increases the chances of sexual dysfunction in the other partner (Balon, 2017).

Relationship issues are often at the forefront of sexual disorders. Marital satisfaction, for example, is associated with greater levels of sexual arousal and sexual frequency between partners, whereas relationship

Did You Know?

In a study of online sexual activity experiences of college students in Canada, Germany, Sweden, and the United States:

- 89 percent reported accessing sexual information (e.g., safer sex, infections, sexual dysfunctions);

- 77 percent reported accessing sexual entertainment (e.g., erotic stories, pornographic pictures and videos);

- 48 percent reported browsing for sexual products; and

- 31 percent had engaged in cybersex.

Source: Döring et al., 2017

dissatisfaction can lead to sexual interest and arousal disorders. Specifically, sexual satisfaction is increased when relationships are caring, warm, and affectionate and when couples communicate openly about sex and sexual activities (McCool-Myers et al., 2018). Men and women may define sexual satisfaction differently. For many women, closeness to a partner is more important than the frequency of orgasms or the intensity of sexual arousal.

Sociocultural Dimension

A variety of sociocultural factors can influence sexual attitudes, behavior, and functioning. Although the human sexual response cycle is similar for women and men, gender differences are clearly present: Women have different sexual fantasies than men, are more attuned to relationships in the sexual encounter, and take longer than men to become aroused (Safarinejad, 2006). Likewise, gender may interact with other factors that affect sexual interest or arousal. Sex researchers and clinicians who do not take into account these gender differences may unfairly portray women as having a sexual dysfunction.

Cultural expectations can also play a role in sexual dysfunction. Through the process of gender role socialization, we learn cultural scripts about sex—social and cultural beliefs and expectancies regarding sexual behavior (Masters et al., 2013). In U.S. society, men are taught to be sexually assertive, whereas women are socialized to avoid initiating sex directly. Cultural scripts for men in the United States may include "sexual potency in men is a sign of masculinity," "the bigger the sex organ, the better," and "strong and virile men do not show feelings." For women, scripts include "nice women don't initiate sex," "women should be restrained and proper in lovemaking," "men are only after one thing," and "it is the woman's responsibility to take care of contraception." Because these scripts often guide our sexual attitudes and behaviors, they can exert a major influence on sexual functioning.

Cultural scripts also exist in other nations. For instance, people in Asian countries consistently report the lowest frequency of sexual intercourse. Guilt regarding sex may be a contributing factor. In a study of European Canadian and Chinese Canadian women, the former group reported less sexual guilt and greater sexual desire. Further, Chinese Canadian women who showed greater acculturation to Western standards reported less guilt and greater sexual desire than their less acculturated counterparts. Cultural differences in sex guilt may be a means by which ethnicity affects reported sexual desire (Woo et al., 2012).

Sexual orientation is also a sociocultural influence that may affect sexual responsiveness and sexual dysfunction in gay men and lesbians. For example, problems among heterosexuals often involve issues with sexual intercourse, whereas sexual concerns among lesbians and gay men may focus on other issues (e.g., aversion toward oral sex or anal eroticism) or power dynamics in a same-sex relationship (McDonagh et al., 2016). Gay men with sexual dysfunction may be influenced by conservative or judgmental societal beliefs and stressors associated with being a member of a sexual minority (Grabski et al., 2019). Similarly, lesbian women may be affected by a belief that their sexual desire is a sin (Peixoto & Nobre, 2014). Lesbians and gay men must also deal with societal or internalized homophobia, which may inhibit openly expressing affection toward sexual partners. Finally, gay men continue to face the association between sexual activity and HIV infection. These broader contextual issues may create diminished sexual interest or desire, sexual aversion, or negative feelings toward sexual activity.

Did You Know?

Data from U.S. surveys indicate:

- The percentage of adults who report having engaged in sex with someone of the same gender has doubled from the early 1990s to 2014 (changing from 3.6 percent to 8.7 percent for women and from 4.5 percent to 8.2 percent for men).

- Increases in same-sex activity were largest among White Americans, with little change among Black Americans.

Source: Twenge et al., 2016

Treatment of Sexual Dysfunctions

Many approaches are used to treat sexual dysfunctions, including biological interventions and psychological treatment approaches.

Biological Interventions

Discovering underlying biological issues is an important first step in treating sexual dysfunction. Biological interventions may include hormone replacement, special medications, or mechanical means to improve sexual functioning. For instance, men with physiologically based erectile dysfunction are sometimes treated with penile implants. The penile implant is an inflatable device that, once expanded, produces an erection sufficient for intercourse and ejaculation (refer to Table 14.3). Penile implants appear to be well tolerated with a high degree of patient satisfaction, although many men eventually experience physical complications (Chierigo et al., 2019).

Medications are also used to treat erectile disorder. One form of medical treatment for erectile dysfunction involves injecting medication (Alprostadil) into the penis or inserting a suppository with the medication into the opening at the tip of the penis (Krzastek et al., 2019). Within a very short time, blood flow to the area is increased and the man gets an erection, which may last from 1 to 4 hours. These methods do have some side effects, including prolonged erections and bruising of the penis.

Oral medications such as Viagra, Levitra, and Cialis are frequently used to treat erectile disorder (El-Wakeel et al., 2020). Unlike injectables, Viagra and its competitors do not produce an erection in the absence of sexual stimuli. If a man becomes aroused, the drugs enable the body to follow through the sexual response cycle to completion. The medications do not improve sexual functioning in normally functioning men, nor do they lead to a stiffer erection. However, it is possible that these drugs may act as a placebo in men without erectile dysfunction and thereby improve sexual arousal and performance by stimulating their expectations and fantasies; this psychological boost may then lead to subjective feelings of enhanced pleasure. Viagra has, in fact, been found to increase the level of confidence of men engaging in sexual activity (Seftel et al., 2014).

Although biological treatments are increasingly important in treating sexual dysfunctions, these treatments deemphasize the role of psychological and social factors. Because relationship, sociocultural, and psychological factors are often involved, treatment needs to include more than medications or other biological means to boost sexual interest or desire. In one study, group therapy plus Viagra was more effective than Viagra alone for treating erectile dysfunction (Read & Mati, 2013).

Finding medications to treat female disorders such as low sexual desire has been controversial and not particularly successful. Addyi (flibanserin), developed to activate brain regions associated with sexual desire, was blocked twice by the U.S. Food and Drug Administration (FDA) due to concern about the drug's limited effectiveness and negative side effects such as dizziness, fatigue, and nausea (Pollack, 2015). Addyi has since received FDA approval. Research suggests that Addyi appears to improve sexual desire, arousal, and orgasm in about 50 percent of premenstrual and 40 percent of postmenstrual women; this compares to improvement in 34 percent of premenstrual and 29 percent of postmenstrual women who were given a placebo (Pettigrew & Novick, 2021). Addyi comes with a "black box" warning suggesting that women discontinue drinking alcohol at least 2 hours before taking their daily dose of the medication. A second drug, Vyleesi, was approved as an additional option for women with low

Table 14.3 Treating Erectile Disorder: Medical Interventions

Treatment	Primary Agent	Effects	Drawbacks
Oral medication	Viagra, Levitra, or Cialis	Taken as a pill; enhances blood flow to the penis and allows many users to achieve normal erections; the drugs are taken before sex, and stimulation is needed for an erection	Medication side effects, including head or stomach pain or nasal congestion
Surgery	Vascular surgery	Corrects venous leak from a groin injury by repairing arteries to boost blood supply in the penis; restores the ability to have a normal erection	Minimal problems when used appropriately with diagnosed condition
Suppository	Muse (alprostadil)	Tiny pellet is inserted into the penis by means of an applicator 5 to 10 minutes before sex; erections can last an hour	Penile aching, minor urethral bleeding or spotting, dizziness, and leg-vein swelling
Injection therapy	Vasodilating drugs, including Caverject or Edex (alprostadil)	Drug is injected directly into the base of the penis 10 minutes to 2 hours before sex, depending on the drug; the drug helps relax smooth-muscle tissues and creates an erection in up to 90% of patients; erection lasts about an hour	Pain, bleeding, and scar tissue formation; erections may not readily subside
Devices	Vacuum pump	Creates negative air pressure around the penis to induce the flow of blood, which is then trapped by an elastic band encircling the shaft; pump is used just before sex; erection lasts until band is removed	Some difficulty in ejaculation; penis can become cool and appear constricted in color; apparatus can be clumsy to use
	Penile implants	Considered a last resort; a penile prosthesis is implanted in the penis, enabling men to literally "pump themselves up" by pulling blood into it	Swelling or infection; destruction of spongy tissue inside the penis

sexual desire. It is injected under the skin of the abdomen or thigh at least 45 minutes before sexual activity. As with Addyi, side effects can occur; approximately 40 percent of women in the clinical trial reported nausea. Effectiveness studies demonstrated that a successful outcome occurred in 25 percent of the women taking the medication versus 17 percent in the placebo control group (FDA, 2019).

Psychological Treatment Approaches

Psychological interventions have been effective in treating sexual dysfunction, especially for female sexual interest/arousal disorders and female orgasmic disorder. General psychological treatment approaches for improving a couple's sexual relationship include the following components (Frühauf et al., 2013; Goldstein et al., 2017):

- *Education*: The therapist helps the client replace sexual myths and misconceptions with accurate information about sexual anatomy and functioning.

- *Anxiety reduction*: The therapist teaches strategies to minimize anxiety. The therapist explains that constantly observing and evaluating one's performance can interfere with sexual functioning.

- *Maladaptive thoughts and beliefs*: The therapist helps the client identify and change negative thoughts and beliefs that interfere with sexual enjoyment.

- *Structured behavioral exercises*: The therapist gives a series of graded tasks that gradually increase the amount of sexual interaction between the partners. Each partner takes turns touching and being touched over different parts of the body except for the genital regions. Later the partners fondle the body and genital regions without making demands for sexual arousal or orgasm. Successful sexual intercourse and orgasm are the final stage of the structured exercises.

- *Communication training*: The therapist teaches the partners appropriate ways of communicating their sexual wishes to each other and strategies for effectively resolving relationship conflicts.

In addition to these general psychological treatments, sex therapists can also focus on specific aspects of sexual dysfunction. Some specific nonmedical treatments for other dysfunctions include:

- *Female orgasmic dysfunction*: Behavioral exercises, cognitive mindfulness-based skills (e.g., focusing on the present experience, noticing negative thoughts but not dwelling on them), and communication training have been successful in treating sexual arousal disorders in women (Brotto et al., 2016). Masturbation appears to be the most effective way for women with orgasmic dysfunction to achieve an orgasm. The procedure involves education about sexual anatomy, visual and tactile self-exploration, use of sexual fantasies and images, and masturbation, both individually and with a partner. High success rates are reported with this procedure, especially for women who have never experienced an orgasm. However, this approach does not necessarily lead to a woman's ability to achieve orgasm during sexual intercourse (Salmani et al., 2015).

- *Premature ejaculation*: In one technique, the partner stimulates the penis until the man feels the sensation of impending ejaculation. At this point, the partner momentarily stops the stimulation and then continues it again. This pattern is repeated until the man can tolerate increasingly greater periods of stimulation before ejaculation (Martin et al., 2017). This stop–start process has also been effective when practiced using a vibrator without a partner (Ventus et al., 2019).

- *Vaginismus*: Treatment involves deconditioning the involuntary spasms or closure of the vaginal muscle by having the woman relax and then inserting successively larger dilators. In a meta-analysis of studies on vaginismus, a successful outcome (penetrative intercourse) occurred in about 80 percent of the women treated (Maseroli et al., 2018).

Further, mindfulness-based therapies that focus on nonjudgmental, present-moment awareness have been successful in improving sexual arousal and desire in women by reducing anxiety and negative cognitive schemas related to sex (Jaderek & Lew-Starowicz, 2019). Similarly, mindfulness strategies have helped men with situational erectile dysfunction (Bossio et al., 2018).

14-3 Gender Dysphoria

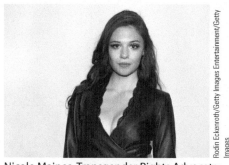

Nicole Maines, Transgender Rights Advocate

Case Study   Nicole Maines, an actress and transgender rights activist, showed interest in Barbie dolls and other "girl" toys in early childhood. Before the age of 3, Maines told her father, "Daddy, I hate my penis." At age 6, Maines insisted on wearing a pink princess dress to a party. Just before entering fifth grade, Maines changed her name to Nicole. During high school, Nicole started taking female hormones, began dating, and experienced her first kiss. (Pols, 2015)

Our gender identity—the gender we identify with emotionally and intellectually—typically emerges at a young age and is an integral part of who we are. Any discussion of psychopathology related to gender identity needs to begin with an understanding of gender diversity, particularly because greater cultural openness in the United States and other countries is allowing increasing numbers of people to comfortably embrace nontraditional **gender expression**. Although most people have a **cisgender** identity, in which their gender identification and expression conform with traditional gender categories and their sex assigned at birth, many people self-identify as gender nonconforming. This latter group includes individuals with a **nonbinary** gender identity who do not identify as a man or a woman, but rather with a fluid spectrum of gender expression; this group sometimes self-identifies as genderqueer.

Over 1 million U.S. adults recognize that their innate emotional and psychological identity as male or female (or nonbinary) is inconsistent with their sex assigned at birth and thus identify as **transgender** (Meerwijk & Sevelius, 2017). Although previous estimates suggested that between 0.17 percent and 1.3 percent of the U.S. population would be considered to have a transgender identity (Connolly et al., 2016), U.S. high school students are identifying themselves as transgender at an increasing rate, with an estimated 1.8 percent prevalence of expressed transgenderism among this group; in addition, another 1.6 percent describe themselves as questioning their gender (Scheim et al., 2022). Current survey methods may underestimate the prevalence of those whose expressed gender does not align with their sex assigned at birth, since many gender diverse youth do not identify with the word *transgender* (Meerwijk & Sevelius, 2017).

Gender incongruence is experienced differently at different ages, and individuals are more likely to express a transgender identity once they become more familiar with the concept of incongruous gender identity. Transgender individuals often begin to experience gender-role conflicts early in childhood. As was true for Nicole, children assigned male at birth may demonstrate disgust with their penis and be interested in toys and activities considered "feminine." They may prefer playing with girls and avoid the aggressive activities commonly enjoyed by boys. Children assigned female at birth may insist that they have a penis or will grow one and may exhibit an avid interest in rough-and-tumble play. Nonconformity with stereotypical gender role behavior should not, however, be confused with the pervasive gender conflicts experienced by those with a transgender identity (Parekh, 2016). The *strength*, *pervasiveness*, and *persistence* of gender-incongruent feelings and behaviors are key features of transgenderism.

Individuals with a consistent transgender identity who decide to make a social transition to their internalized gender often begin with a name change accompanied by changes in the way they dress or behave. Thus, transgender girls or women move away from their assigned male identity, and transgender boys or men begin to renounce their assigned female identity. Many transgender individuals, like Nicole Maines, express anguish prior to making a gender transition but adjust well once their outwardly expressed gender aligns with their internal identity. Some eventually decide to pursue gender-affirming medical interventions, which involve changing their physical characteristics through medical procedures such as gender-affirming hormone therapy or surgeries that change their existing external genitalia to those of the other sex. In one study of transgender youth, most participants were aware of gender conflicts early in life and had taken steps toward social transitioning by changing their names and other outward expressions of gender (Kuper et al., 2019).

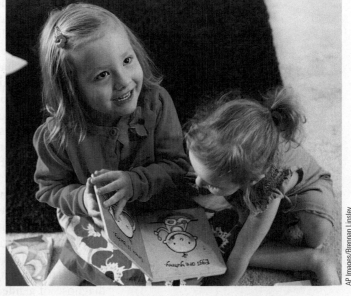

Life as a Transgender Girl

Coy Mathis, left, plays with her sister at their home in Colorado. Coy has self-identified as a girl since early childhood.

Understanding Gender Dysphoria

Transgender individuals sometimes meet the criteria for **gender dysphoria**—a condition characterized by ongoing distress and impairment in functioning that results from the marked incongruence (mismatch) between a person's experienced or expressed gender and the **assigned gender** at birth. In other words, individuals who experience gender dysphoria have serious emotional distress associated with their transgender experience (refer to Table 14.4).

Individuals with gender dysphoria often display a strong dislike of their sexual anatomy, a desire for sexual characteristics of their experienced gender, and rejection of objects or activities associated with their assigned gender. In rare cases, the experienced gender is nonbinary (APA, 2022).

Table 14.4 DSM-5-TR Criteria for Gender Dysphoria

Gender dysphoria is manifested by at least two of the following for a period lasting at least 6 months:

(a) a marked difference between experienced or expressed gender and one's own sex characteristics
(b) a strong desire to be rid of one's primary and/or secondary sex characteristics
(c) a strong desire to have the sex characteristics of the other gender
(d) a strong desire to be a different gender
(e) a strong desire to be treated as a different gender
(f) a strong conviction that one has the typical feelings and reactions of a different gender

The condition is associated with clinically significant distress or impairment in social, occupational, or other important areas of functioning.
Based on APA (2022).

Diagnoses of gender dysphoria are relatively rare, however, because many transgender individuals do not experience significant distress or impairment in functioning or do not seek treatment. The prevalence of gender dysphoria ranges from 0.1 percent to 0.6 percent for both individuals assigned male at birth and individuals assigned female at birth (APA, 2022).

Adults who develop gender dysphoria are responding to intense, lifelong feelings of gender incongruence. They may have long-standing preoccupation with the idea of eliminating their biologically based sexual characteristics and acquiring those of their experienced gender. As physiological maturation progresses during puberty, dislike for and desire to be rid of their sexual anatomy may strengthen, thus increasing their distress. As their personal identity develops during adolescence, their emotions and reactions may increasingly resemble those of their experienced gender, a factor that further increases gender incongruence. During adolescence and early adulthood, they may find it increasingly important to be treated and accepted as a member of their experienced gender. It is often under these circumstances that the distress associated with gender incongruence leads them to seek treatment. In some cases, a diagnosis of gender dysphoria is required before an insurance company will approve reimbursement for gender-affirming treatment.

Individuals with a transgender identity are often aware of the mismatch between their assigned gender and experienced gender years before sexual interests develop during puberty. Gender identity and **sexual orientation** are not the same thing—the sexual orientation of someone with a transgender identity can be heterosexual, gay, lesbian, bisexual, or asexual. For example, when television personality and Olympic gold medal winner Caitlyn Jenner first publicly spoke about her decision to transition to a woman, she pointed out the difference between gender identity and sexual orientation. "Sexuality is who you're attracted to, who turns you on—gender identity is who you are, what is in your soul" (Donnelly, 2015).

Etiology of Gender Dysphoria

In all likelihood, a number of variables interact to produce gender dysphoria. Although having a gender identity different from that associated with one's birth-assigned sex is a normal biological variation, societal intolerance of this diversity can result in a variety of distressing experiences. As family members and society become more aware and accepting of gender variations, we can hope that both social and physical transition will become easier, thus diminishing distress over gender incongruence.

Biological Influences on Transgender Development

Biological research suggests that genetics may be involved in the development of a transgender identity, including a gene associated with estrogen reception in female to male transgenderism (Cortés-Cortés et al., 2017). Researchers have also linked several genes responsible for sex hormone signaling with feminized characteristics in transgender women (Foreman et al., 2019). Neurohormonal factors also appear to be associated with transgenderism. In animal studies, for instance, the presence or absence of testosterone early in life appears to influence the organization of brain centers that govern gender-related behavioral patterns. In humans assigned female at birth, early exposure to testosterone has resulted in a more masculine behavior pattern. Thus, it does appear that gender orientation can be influenced by a lack or an excess of sex hormones. Interestingly, a study involving physiological indicators of prenatal testosterone exposure found that

Continuum Video Project

Dean: **Gender Dysphoria**

"The more I tried to be a girl, it just wasn't right."

Access the Continuum Video Project in MindTap.

transgender girls with an early-onset transgender identity appeared to have had less exposure to testosterone compared to a group of cisgender boys who served as matched controls; in fact, the physiological patterns of these transgender girls were similar to cisgender girls (Burke, Menks, Cohen-Kettenis et al., 2014).

The transgender experience may be more than a hormone imbalance. In one study, sex hormone levels were found to be consistent with the gender assigned at birth in transgender youth; this raises doubt that biology alone determines masculine and feminine behaviors (Olson et al., 2015). Although research data on hormonal levels are contradictory, physiological influences on sex differentiation within the brain are believed to be the primary explanation for transgenderism (Kreukels & Guillamon, 2016).

Researchers are also looking into any specific neurological characteristics associated with a transgender identity. Neuroimaging using functional magnetic resonance imaging (fMRI) to compare transgender individuals who had not yet undergone treatment with matched controls revealed differences in brain connectivity between the groups; however, the neurological differences observed in participants with a transgender identify did not provide insight into the etiology of transgenderism. Instead, the findings suggested that transgender individuals may dissociate (detach) bodily emotion from body image, possibly as a way of coping with their lifelong gender incongruence (Lin et al., 2014). Previous studies have also revealed brain alterations in transgender adults—unique patterns that are associated with psychosocial distress and social exclusion (Ku et al., 2013).

Psychological and Social Factors Influencing Gender Dysphoria

Psychological and social explanations for gender dysphoria must also be viewed with caution. Early researchers based their work on case studies and hypothesized that childhood experiences influence the development of a transgender identity and gender dysphoria. Factors proposed to contribute to a transgender identity in children assigned male at birth include parental encouragement of feminine behavior, discouragement of the development of autonomy, excessive attention and overprotection by the mother, the absence of male role models, a relatively powerless or absent father figure, a lack of exposure to male playmates, and encouragement to cross-dress (Zucker & Cohen-Ketteris, 2008). Of course, psychosocial stressors such as stigma, lack of societal acceptance, or difficulty obtaining adequate health care are much more plausible explanations for the distress and impairment associated with gender dysphoria. Sexual assault also disproportionately affects transgender people. In one sample of transgender adults, 77 percent of the respondents reported sexual victimization experiences occurring after puberty, and 21 percent had been raped (Kolp et al., 2020).

Transgender individuals often face discrimination and negative reactions from family members and the community. Transgender individuals in one study reported significant social stressors, including:

- traumatic experiences within the family such as bullying and coercion against transitioning, including the withdrawal of financial support;
- interpersonal negativity in the community, including being called names or being referred to as "it"; and
- fear of physical harassment or assault when using public restrooms (Burnes et al., 2016).

Rejection of an individual's gender identity can be psychologically damaging. Being subjected to negative responses during the process of

Midlife Gender Transition

Caitlyn Jenner, who won an Olympic gold medal in the 1976 decathlon, publicly disclosed her gender transition during a television interview in 2015. Jenner, who is pictured here attending a fashion event in Los Angeles, made the transition with support from her family and friends.

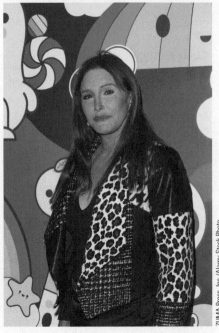

ZUMA Press, Inc./Alamy Stock Photo

becoming aware of and navigating gender identity issues can seriously affect the individual and their relationships with friends and family, resulting in an overwhelming sense of isolation. Transgender youth have been found to have a two- to threefold increase in risk of depression, anxiety disorder, suicidal ideation, suicide attempt, and self-harm compared to cisgender matched controls (Reisner et al., 2015). Similarly, in a nationwide survey of high school students, transgender participants reported significantly more depression, suicidality, and interpersonal victimization compared to their cisgender peers (refer to Figure 14.3) (Trevor Project, 2019). Some transgender individuals are pressured by family or religious organizations to engage in conversion therapy, an intervention aimed at changing a person's gender identity to align with their sex assigned at birth. Participation in this "therapy" is associated with severe psychological distress and increased risk of suicide attempts (Turban et al., 2020).

Mental health professionals are concerned that the amplified politicalization of gender incongruity and the increasingly hostile social environment that transgender individuals are facing will have a negative impact on the psychological well-being of the transgender population in the United States. As of June 2023, numerous U.S. states had passed more than 30 bills that target gender-affirming treatment, prohibit participation in school sports, restrict bathroom use, ban the discussion of gender identity in school, and mandate that teachers "out" trans students to their parents or guardians (Sprayregen, 2023).

Acceptance from family, peers, and the community is vital and can prevent gender dysphoria. Not surprisingly, socially transitioned transgender children who are supported in their identity show no difference in anxiety or depression compared to their cisgender peers (Olson et al., 2016). Transgender individuals with strong social connections have more resilience to psychosocial stressors, whereas those who have internalized transphobia

Figure 14.3

Past Year Prevalence of Depression, Suicidality, and Victimization Among Transgender High School Students

Transgender youth reported significantly increased rates of depression, suicidality, and victimization compared to their cisgender peers. Approximately one third of the transgender youth reported attempting suicide or being a target of sexual violence in the previous year, and more than half reported a two-week period of depression.

Source: *The Trevor Project Research Brief: Data on Transgender Youth. February 2019.*

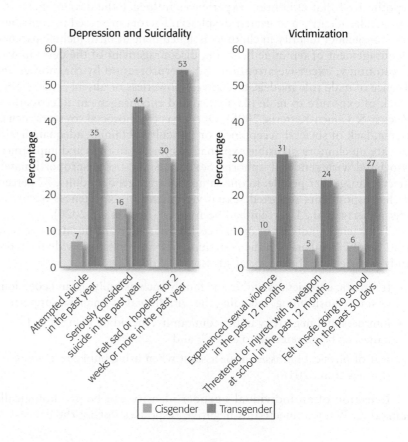

often develop anxiety and depression (Kolp et al., 2020). The support provided by online communities has the potential to increase resilience and enhance healthy development among transgender adolescents and adults (Selkie et al., 2020).

Treatment of Gender Dysphoria

Case Study Transgender teen Leelah Alcorn stepped in front of a semitrailer, leaving behind a suicide note mentioning that her family never accepted her transition. Her mother continued to refer to Leelah by her birth name, Josh, stating that God doesn't make mistakes and that Leelah would never be a girl. In her suicide note, Leelah wrote, "Either I live the rest of my life as a lonely man who wishes he were a woman or I live my life as a lonelier woman who hates herself. There's no winning. There's no way out. The only way I will rest in peace is if one day transgender people aren't treated the way I was, they're treated like humans, with valid feelings and human rights. Gender needs to be taught about in schools, the earlier the better. My death needs to mean something. My death needs to be counted in the number of transgender people who commit suicide this year. I want someone to look at that number . . . and fix it. Fix society. Please." (Mikkelson, 2014)

As in the case of Leelah, the decision to come out sometimes leads to rejection. The subsequent social isolation and emotional turmoil can have a profound impact on the person's emotional well-being. For this reason, both individual and family therapy are important when treating youth with gender dysphoria. Fortunately, many health organizations are developing or strengthening training for professionals regarding the importance of providing gender-affirmative care to transgender youth (Oransky et al., 2019).

There are conflicting opinions regarding how parents should approach a young child who consistently expresses gender dissatisfaction or who persistently displays gender nonconforming behavior. The range of possible responses include:

- allowing the gender development to occur without pressure or expectation regarding the outcome,
- openly affirming the child's expressed gender identity, or
- encouraging the child to align with the sex identified at birth.

In the treatment of older children with gender dysphoria, there is greater consensus—the goal is to accept and support the child's experienced gender identity as well as help them learn to deal with stressors associated with their decision to socially transition (American Psychological Association, 2015). Many experts believe that for children of any age who are "consistent, persistent, and insistent" in expressing a cross-gender identity, family and school systems can help facilitate a positive transitional experience (Snow, 2015). Further, allowing transgender children to live a life congruent with their experienced gender (e.g., accepting a name change and addressing the child by the preferred name or supporting gender-congruent clothing and hairstyles) does not appear to have any negative effects on the child's mental health (Durwood et al., 2017). In one study of youth who made a social gender transition, 7.3 percent detransitioned at least once during the five-year period included in the study. In the final analysis, 97 percent of the youth continued to identify as transgender or nonbinary (Olson et al., 2022).

A variety of medical options are available to assist with gender transitioning. Many transgender people rely on gender-affirming hormone therapy (taking hormones associated with their experienced gender) beginning in adolescence. Pubertal-suppressing hormone therapy has been found to decrease suicidality and improve the mental health of transgender youth (Turban et al., 2020). In a randomized clinical trial involving transgender and gender diverse adults seeking masculinization, testosterone therapy resulted in a reduction in gender dysphoria, depression, and suicidality (Nolan et al., 2023). Although this type of medical intervention is associated with improved emotional well-being, there appears to be an increased risk of alcohol abuse in transgender men, perhaps due to the incongruence between a transgender man's biologically based physiology and societal norms regarding alcohol consumption in men (Tomita et al., 2019).

About one third of transgender adults make the decision to undergo gender-affirming surgery (Kailas et al., 2017). The surgery for those who were assigned female at birth involves removal of the breasts, and, in some cases, individuals choose to have surgery to construct a penis. For those who were assigned male at birth, the genital surgeries involve altering the penis and scrotum and constructing female genitalia.

The vast majority of those who undergo gender affirming surgery appear to be satisfied with the outcome; only about 0.6 percent of transgender women and 0.3 percent of transgender men report regretting their decision (Wiepjes et al., 2018). In a nationwide survey of 27,715 transgender and gender diverse adults, 12.8 percent had undergone one or more types of gender-affirming surgery. Those who had the surgery were less likely to suffer from severe psychological distress, binge on alcohol, experience suicidal ideation, or attempt suicide compared to those who did not undergo surgery (Almazan & Keuroghlian, 2021).

Some professionals and members of the public have expressed concern about the increasing number of young people who are identifying as transgender and receiving puberty-blocking or cross-sex hormones as the first line of treatment, particularly when youth sometimes change their mind about making a gender transition. An additional concern is that without comprehensive and competent assessment by well-trained professionals, youth with other mental health conditions might be misdiagnosed as having gender dysphoria (Rojas Saffie & Eyzaguirre Bauerle, 2023).

Recognizing these concerns, many clinics and professionals use the *WPATH Standards of Care for the Health of Transgender and Gender Diverse People* when making treatment decisions involving transgender and gender diverse youth and adults (Coleman et al., 2022). These evidence-based guidelines involve:

- A thorough assessment by a mental health gender specialist who is knowledgeable about gender dysphoria and trained to make differential psychiatric diagnoses. The therapist is required to "identify and exclude other possible causes of apparent gender incongruence prior to the initiation of gender-affirming treatments."

- For prepubertal youth, psychological support is provided to further understand the reasons for gender confusion or conflict; no medical interventions are recommended.

- At the initial signs of puberty, some youth may be eligible for puberty blockers which would pause puberty, allowing time for further exploration of the adolescent's gender identity.

- Individuals who are assessed and treated after going through puberty may be eligible for feminizing or masculinizing hormone treatment; the dosage is increased very gradually to allow the individual to assess the effects and to stop treatment, if desired.
- Adults may elect gender-affirming surgical procedures only after they complete at least 1 year of hormone treatment, are satisfied with the results, and are certain of their desire for surgery.

During each of these steps, ongoing evaluations occur to make certain that the individual wants to continue. These guidelines are especially important in determining who qualifies for more invasive treatment, thus reducing the need for de-transitioning.

14-4 Paraphilic Disorders

A **paraphilia** is a condition in which a person's sexual arousal and gratification depends on fantasies or behavior involving socially unacceptable objects, situations, or individuals. According to the DSM-5-TR, paraphilias involve sexual interest in non-normative targets or "distorted components of human courtship behavior." The intense and persistent sexual interest associated with a paraphilia can involve unusual erotic behaviors (such as spanking or whipping) or socially unacceptable erotic targets (such as children, animals, or inanimate objects). A **paraphilic disorder** is diagnosed only when the paraphilia harms, or risks harming, others (and is acted on) or causes the individual to experience distress or impairment in social or other areas of functioning. Thus, the DSM-5-TR makes a clear distinction between paraphilias and paraphilic disorders. Such a distinction prevents labeling behavior as pathological just because it is not common behavior. Therefore, a paraphilic disorder is *not* diagnosed if a paraphilia:

1. involves only urges or fantasies, but has not been acted on;
2. has not harmed others or created the potential to harm others;
3. does not impair the person's social, occupational, or other areas of functioning; or
4. does not create anxiety, shame, guilt, loneliness, or sexual frustration or in other ways distress the person.

When the fantasies, urges, or behaviors associated with a paraphilia do not cause personal distress or do not have the potential to harm others, psychiatric diagnosis and intervention are not warranted. Additionally, for a paraphilic disorder diagnosis, the dysfunctional paraphilic behaviors must have persisted for at least 6 months.

In some cases, diagnosis occurs because the person is severely distressed by or has experienced impairment in social or occupational functioning due to the paraphilia. In other situations, paraphilic disorder is diagnosed when there is evidence or disclosure confirming that the person has acted on paraphilic urges that caused harm, or created risk of harm, to others. This often involves reports from witnesses because many individuals arrested for paraphilic behavior deny engaging in the behavior or otherwise proclaim their innocence. In many cases, paraphilias that harm or interfere with the well-being of others result in arrest.

In all cases, paraphilic disorders are associated with recurrent urges, behaviors, or fantasies involving any of the following three categories (refer to Table 14.5):

1. nonhuman objects, as in fetishistic and transvestic disorders;
2. nonconsenting others, as in exhibitionistic, voyeuristic, frotteuristic (rubbing against others for sexual arousal), and pedophilic disorders; or
3. real or simulated suffering or humiliation, as in sexual sadism and sexual masochism disorders.

It is not unusual for people with paraphilic disorders to have multiple paraphilias (Baur et al., 2016). Some men who have committed incest, for example, have also molested nonrelatives, exposed themselves, raped adult women, and engaged in voyeurism. In most cultures, paraphilias seem to be much more prevalent in men than in women (Fisher & Marwaha, 2020). This finding has led some to speculate that biological factors may account for the unequal distribution.

Table 14.5 Paraphilic Disorders

DSM-5-TR Disorders Chart			
Paraphilia Category	**DSM Definition[a]**	**Prevalence[b]**	**Associated Features**
Nonhuman objects	**Fetishistic disorder** Sexual attraction and fantasies involving objects or nongenital body parts	Disorder is uncommon but fetishistic behavior is not; occurs almost exclusively in males	May rub or smell object and use it in sexual activities; some collect fetish items
	Transvestic disorder Intense sexual arousal from cross-dressing	Fewer than 3% of men report cross-dressing; extremely rare in women	May be aroused by fantasies of being a woman; may masturbate when wearing female clothes
Nonconsenting people	**Exhibitionistic disorder** Urges, acts, or fantasies that involve exposing the genitals to a stranger	Mostly men; best estimates are 2% to 4% of men	May expose to prepubertal children, adults, or both; in general, sexual contact is not sought
	Voyeuristic disorder Urges, acts, or fantasies that involve observing an unsuspecting person disrobing or engaging in sexual activity	Behavior may occur in up to 39% of men; 12% of men and 4% of women may have this disorder	Most common of unlawful sexual behaviors
	Frotteuristic disorder Urges, acts, or fantasies that involve touching or rubbing against a nonconsenting person	Primarily in men; exact figures not available; up to 30% of men may have engaged in frotteuristic acts	Some freely admit behavior but feel no distress or impairment
	Pedophilic disorder Urges, acts, or fantasies that involve sexual contact with a prepubescent child	May occur in up to 3% to 5% of men; rare in women	May access child pornography repeatedly; appears to be a chronic condition
Pain or humiliation	**Sexual sadism disorder** Urges, fantasies, or acts that involve inflicting physical or psychological suffering	Prevalence estimates of sexual sadism range from 2% to 30%; common in sexually motivated homicides	Extensive use of pornography with themes of pain and suffering; sadism may be a chronic condition
	Sexual masochism disorder Sexual urges, fantasies, or acts that involve being humiliated, bound, or made to suffer	2.2% of men; 1.3% of women; up to 18.5% report masochistic fantasies	May extensively use pornography with themes of bondage, being humiliated, or being beaten; may be part of sadomasochistic groups

[a] Paraphilias are diagnosed as a disorder only if the urges cause clinically significant distress/impairment or are acted on with nonconsenting others.

[b] The prevalence of paraphilic disorders is difficult to determine because paraphilic activity is often concealed.

Based on data from Ahlers et al. (2011); APA (2022); Krueger (2010a, 2010b)

Although paraphilic disorders are relatively rare, the prevalence of paraphilias among the general population and in cross-cultural samples is more common. In fact, one third of the participants in one survey in Canada reported engaging in a paraphilic practice or having paraphilic fantasies involving masochism, fetishism, or voyeurism (Joyal & Carpentier, 2016). In an online survey of college students at six different universities in Italy, 51 percent of men and 42 percent of women reported at least one paraphilic behavior. Men were most likely to report engaging in voyeurism, exhibitionism, sadism, and frotteurism, while women had a higher prevalence of fetishism and masochism (Castellini et al., 2018). In a community sample of German men, 62.4 percent reported at least one paraphilia. The most common were voyeurism (38.7 percent), fetishism (35.7 percent), sadism (24.8 percent), masochism (18.5 percent), and frotteurism (15 percent). Less common paraphilias were pedophilia (10.4 percent), transvestism (7.4 percent), and exhibitionism (4.1 percent). Most of the men who reported paraphilias found them to be intensely sexually arousing. In only 1.7 percent of cases did the respondents report distress over their behavior (Ahlers et al., 2011).

In addition to the paraphilic disorders we will be discussing, the DSM-5-TR lists "other specified paraphilic disorders," including intense sexual arousal associated with behaviors such as making obscene telephone calls (telephone scatalogia) and sexual urges involving corpses (necrophilia), animals (zoophilia), urine (urophilia), or feces (coprophilia).

Paraphilic Disorders Involving Nonhuman Objects

This category includes two forms of paraphilic disorders: fetishistic disorder, which involves attraction or arousal related to a nonliving object (the fetish), and transvestic disorder, which involves cross-dressing for sexual arousal.

Fetishistic Disorder

Case Study Mr. D. met his wife at a local church and was strongly attracted to her because of her strong religious convictions. When they dated, they occasionally kissed but never had any other sexual contact. Although he loved his wife very much, he was unable to have sexual intercourse with her after their marriage because he could not obtain an erection. However, he had fantasies involving an apron and was able to get an erection and engage in intercourse while wearing an apron. Mrs. D. was distressed by this discovery but accepted it because she wanted children. Although using the apron allowed them to consummate their marriage, Mrs. D. was concerned about what she considered to be a sexual perversion. Mr. D. also became distressed about his inability to function sexually without the apron.

Fetishistic disorder occurs when there is an extremely strong sexual attraction to or fantasies involving inanimate objects, such as shoes or undergarments, or a specific focus on nongenital body parts such as the feet or toes (Ventriglio et al., 2019). As you saw in the case of Mr. D., the fetish is often used as a sexual stimulus during masturbation or sexual intercourse. Many individuals who report having a sexual fetish do not report impairment or distress, and thus do not qualify as having a fetishistic disorder (APA, 2022).

Many heterosexual males find the sight of female undergarments sexually arousing and stimulating; this does not constitute a fetish. An interest in such inanimate objects as panties, stockings, bras, and shoes becomes a sexual fetish when the person is often sexually aroused to the point of erection in the presence of the fetish item, needs the item for sexual arousal during intercourse, chooses sexual partners on the basis of their having the item, or collects the item. To qualify as a fetishistic disorder, the behavior must also cause the individual significant distress or cause harm to others. In many cases the fetish item is enough by itself for complete sexual satisfaction through masturbation, and the person does not seek contact with a partner. Common fetishes include aprons, shoes, undergarments, and leather or latex items. Sexual arousal to fetish items was reported in 35.7 percent of the previously mentioned sample of German men (Ahlers et al., 2011).

Transvestic Disorder

Case Study An 11-year-old boy reported having an interest in women's clothes since the age of 8. He often stole items of female clothing and felt sexually aroused when wearing them. At the age of 9, he began to get erections while dressed in the clothing, and this resulted in ejaculation. He reported thinking about wearing female clothing nearly the entire day for the previous 3 years and reported the urges to be uncontrollable. He also felt guilty and worried about being caught (Anupama et al., 2016).

Transvestic disorder occurs when intense sexual arousal is associated with fantasies, urges, or behaviors involving cross-dressing (wearing clothes appropriate to a different gender). This disorder should not be confused with having a transgender identity, whereby the individual psychologically identifies with and dresses in accordance with cultural norms for the opposite gender. Although some transgender people and some lesbians and gay men cross-dress, most people who cross-dress are exclusively heterosexual. For a diagnosis of transvestic disorder, the cross-dressing must cause significant distress or impairment in important areas of functioning, as presented in the previous case study.

The prevalence of transvestic disorder is not known. However, transvestic behavior was reported in 7.4 percent of the aforementioned sample of German men (Ahlers et al., 2011). Men who cross-dress often report using pornography, being easily sexually aroused, and engaging in frequent masturbation (Langstrom & Zucker, 2005). Men with a transvestic paraphilia often wear feminine garments or undergarments during masturbation or sexual intercourse with their partners. Some men with this paraphilia are considered to have *autogynephilia*; that is, they become sexually aroused by thoughts or images of themselves as female. For some individuals, the arousal through cross-dressing may diminish over time and is replaced by feelings of contentment or comfort when cross-dressing (APA, 2022).

Paraphilic Disorders Involving Nonconsenting Persons

This category of disorders involves persistent and powerful sexual fantasies about unsuspecting strangers or acquaintances. The targets are nonconsenting in that they do not choose to be the objects of the attention or sexual behavior.

Cross-Dressing Behavior or Transvestic Disorder?

Not all transvestites have a transvestic disorder. Some simply enjoy the activity of cross-dressing and do not experience the intense sexual fantasies, urges, or behaviors associated with transvestic disorder. Here men are participating in the Hartjesdag (Day of Hearts), an annual cross-dressing carnival held in the Netherlands.

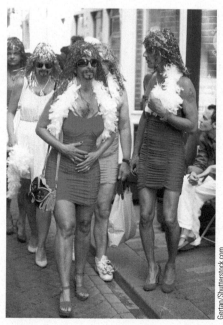

Gertan/Shutterstock.com

Exhibitionistic Disorder

Case Study   A woman reported that she received two pictures of an unknown man's penis on her phone....."I declined the image, instinctively, and another image appeared, at which point I realized someone nearby must be sending them, and that concerned me. I felt violated. It was a very unpleasant thing to have forced upon my screen. I was also worried about who else might have been a recipient. It might have been a child, someone more vulnerable than me." (Bell, 2015)

Exhibitionistic disorder is characterized by urges, acts, or fantasies that involve recurrent episodes of exposing one's genitals to a stranger, often with the intent of shocking or impressing the unsuspecting target. In some cases, exhibitionistic disorder is diagnosed when a person acts on exhibitionistic urges, and thereby harms an unconsenting person such as occurred in the "cyber-flashing" incident in the case study. In other situations, the person seeks treatment because the urges are emotionally distressing or result in impairment in important areas of life functioning (APA, 2022). The prevalence of the disorder is estimated to range from 3.1 percent to 4.1 percent (Ahlers et al., 2011; Långström & Seto, 2006).

Exhibitionistic disorder most commonly occurs in men; their targets are usually women. The act may involve exposing a limp penis or masturbating an erect penis. Exhibitionists generally desire no further contact with their targets but hope to produce a reaction such as surprise or sexual arousal. Most individuals with the disorder are in their 20s—far from being the "dirty old men" of popular myth. Individuals with this paraphilia report lower satisfaction in life, a high level of sexual arousability, and pornography use (Ahlers et al., 2011). Although sexting is common, it is exhibitionism only if it is done by the sender for the purpose of intense sexual arousal.

Voyeuristic Disorder

Case Study   A 26-year-old woman phoned the police when she saw a man looking through her window. The police found the man hiding in the bushes with his pants unzipped and his underwear in his back pocket. He admitted masturbating while watching the woman. The man was arrested for voyeurism. (Burton, 2016)

Voyeuristic disorder is characterized by urges, acts, or fantasies that involve observing an unsuspecting person who is naked, disrobing, or engaging in sexual activity. The disorder is diagnosed only in those who are age 18 or older and only when the individual has acted on voyeuristic urges or is distressed by or has experienced impairment in life functioning due to voyeuristic behavior (APA, 2022). "Peeping," as voyeurism is sometimes termed, is considered aberrant when it violates the rights of others, is done in socially unacceptable circumstances, or is preferred to coitus.

Voyeurism is like exhibitionism in that sexual contact is not the goal; viewing an undressed body is the primary motive. Most people who engage in voyeurism are not interested in looking at their spouses or partners; an overwhelming number of voyeuristic acts involve strangers, as discussed in the case study. Observation alone produces sexual arousal and excitement, and the individual often masturbates during this surreptitious activity. Because the act is repetitive and violates the privacy rights of unsuspecting

Did You Know?

The practice of "sexting" (the sharing of sexually explicit videos or messages on electronic devices) is common among young adults. In one study, a large number of respondents reported sending (38 percent) or receiving (42 percent) sexual messages, while reciprocal sexting was most common (48 percent). Nonconsensual forwarding of a sexual text had affected 15 percent of the respondents, primarily women.
Source: Mori et al., 2020

targets, arrest is predictable when a witness or a target notifies the police. It is estimated that the lifetime prevalence of voyeuristic disorder may be as high as 12 percent in males and 4 percent in females (APA, 2022). Voyeuristic behavior, including adolescent sexual curiosity, is much more common.

Frotteuristic Disorder

Case Study   The 25-year-old man would board trains, stand near unsuspecting women, select a target, and rub his genitals against her body. If no resistance was encountered, he would take this as a positive sign and continue rubbing until orgasm and ejaculation occurred.
On weekends, he would begin by watching pornographic movies and then spend the entire day riding trains and engaging in genital rubbing. He was distressed by this behavior but felt unable to control his urges. (Kalra, 2013)

Physical contact is the primary motive in **frotteuristic disorder**, which is characterized by recurrent and intense sexual urges, acts, or fantasies that involve touching or rubbing against a nonconsenting person. The inappropriate behaviors of the young man in the case study are consistent with the behaviors exhibited by those with this disorder. The touching, not the coercive nature of the act, is the sexually exciting feature. A frotteuristic disorder diagnosis requires that the person has acted on or is markedly distressed by the frotteuristic urges.

Although up to 30 percent of males in the general population may have engaged in some form of frotteuristic behavior, the prevalence of frotteuristic disorder is difficult to determine (Brannon & Bienenfeld, 2013). It may be much more common than thought because the behavior may go unnoticed, be ignored, or be overlooked because it is presumed to be accidental. In a study involving undergraduate students attending an urban university, a high number reported being targets of acts of frotteurism; these incidents were most frequently associated with using public transportation. The affected students reported feelings of being violated and, in some cases, ongoing psychological distress (Clark et al., 2014).

Pedophilic Disorder

Case Study   I'm a pedophile, so I'm sexually attracted to children. I think small girls are just the most wonderful people, and in fantasy or some imaginary world, I'd like to be sexual with them. . . . I identify as a "celibate pedophile." I'm sexually attracted to young girls, but I would never, ever, act on it. (Tsoulis-Reay, 2016)

Pedophilic disorder involves an adult obtaining erotic gratification through urges, acts, or fantasies that involve prepubescent or early pubescent children, generally children under age 13. For the diagnosis, the individual must have acted on or be clinically distressed by these urges. In addition, a person must be at least 16 years of age to be diagnosed with this disorder and at least 5 years older than the child (APA, 2022). People with this disorder may prey upon children within or outside of their families and may be attracted only to children, or to both children and adults. Additionally, they may be attracted only to boys, only to girls, or to children of both genders. People with pedophilia report an early age of onset of an ongoing attraction to children, with approximately 35 percent reporting attractions to pubescent children. Many report having experienced a "romantic involvement" with a child (Martijn et al., 2020).

Individuals with pedophilia frequently use child pornography for sexual gratification. In fact, many men with pedophilic urges acknowledge accessing child pornography but, as with the man in the case study, claim they have never attempted to approach a child in a sexual manner (Berlin & Sawyer, 2012). The actual prevalence of pedophilic disorder is not known, but it is estimated that up to 3 percent to 5 percent of men may have pedophilic urges; it is rare in women (Brannon & Bienenfeld, 2013; Seto, 2012). In one online sample, 6 percent of men and 2 percent of women indicated some interest in having sex with a child—if they would not be caught or punished. These individuals also indicated a greater likelihood of engaging in antisocial behaviors and were more likely to report dysfunctional childhoods (Wurtele et al., 2014).

Pedophilia is usually considered a lifelong condition, although the intensity of urges may decrease with age (Mokros & Habermeyer, 2016). For this reason, pedophilia is the only paraphilic disorder that does not include the diagnostic option for a therapist to specify "in remission" when a client no longer meets the criteria for the disorder. Among pedophiles, the rate of recidivism is particularly high among men who have sexual interest only in children (Eher et al., 2016).

Unfortunately, sexual abuse of children is common; it most frequently affects girls, with girls in their early teens having the highest risk of being molested. It is estimated that by age 17, high-impact sexual abuse (genital touching and actual or attempted vaginal or anal penetration) has affected 15 percent of girls and 6 percent of boys. Strikingly, up to 95 percent of child sexual abuse never comes to the attention of authorities (Martin & Silverstone, 2013). Contrary to the popular view of child molesters as strangers, most people who act on pedophilic urges are relatives, friends, or casual acquaintances of those they prey upon (Lussier et al., 2008).

Although some young survivors of sexual abuse show no overt symptoms, many do experience physical effects such as poor appetite, headaches, or urinary tract infections; additionally, psychological symptoms that include nightmares, difficulty sleeping, decline in school performance, acting out, or sexually focused behavior may occur. Some child survivors show symptoms of posttraumatic stress disorder. The effects of sexual abuse can be lifelong (Hailes et al., 2019). One study of women who were survivors of childhood sexual abuse revealed that they experienced ongoing consequences of the abuse, including a "contaminated identity" characterized by self-loathing, shame, and powerlessness (Phillips & Daniluk, 2004).

Pedophilia can also involve **incest**—sexual contact between individuals who are too closely related to marry legally. The cases of incest most frequently reported to law enforcement agencies involve sexual contact between a father and daughter or stepdaughter. Mother–son incest seems to be rare. Although brother–sister incest is more common, most research has focused on father–daughter incest. This type of incestuous relationship generally begins when the daughter is between 6 and 11 years old. Unlike sex between siblings (which may or may not be exploitive), father–daughter incest is always exploitive. As a result, survivors often feel guilty and powerless.

Psychological symptoms associated with father–daughter incest, such as feeling damaged and ashamed, often continue into adulthood and are reflected in high rates of depression and difficulties with adult sexuality and interpersonal relationships (Stroebel et al., 2012). Research comparing survivors of father–daughter and brother–sister incest found that although there were long-term psychosocial effects for both groups, father–daughter incest produced the most pervasive damage to self-esteem and psychological functioning (Stroebel et al., 2013a). Similarly, women who experienced sister–sister incest reported ongoing psychological distress and strained family relationships (Stroebel et al., 2013b).

Paraphilic Disorders Involving Pain or Humiliation

Case Study From early adolescence, Peter F., a 41-year-old man, had fantasies of being mistreated, humiliated, and beaten. He recalls becoming sexually excited when envisioning such actions. As he grew older, he experienced difficulty achieving an orgasm unless his sexual partners inflicted pain during sexual activities. He was obsessed with these masochistic sexual acts, which made it difficult for him to concentrate on other matters. He had been married and divorced three times because of his proclivity for demanding that his wives engage in "sex games" that involved having them hurt him. These games included binding him spread-eagled on his bed and whipping or biting his upper thighs, sticking pins into his legs, and other forms of torture. During these sessions, he could ejaculate.

Although pain and humiliation are not normally associated with sexual arousal, they play a prominent role in paraphilias involving sadism and masochism. In the case above, Peter had a long-standing paraphilia involving the pain and degradation associated with masochism. **Sexual masochism disorder** is characterized by sexual urges, fantasies, or acts that involve being humiliated, bound, or made to suffer. People who engage in sexual masochism report that they do not seek harm or injury but that they find the sensation of utter helplessness appealing. Because of their passive role, masochists are not considered dangerous to others. A sexual masochism disorder diagnosis occurs only if the paraphilia causes distress or impairment in functioning. The prevalence of sexual masochism is unknown, although it appears to be more common than sadism (Weierstall & Giebel, 2016).

Sexual sadism disorder is characterized by sexual arousal associated with urges, fantasies, or acts that involve inflicting physical or psychological suffering on others. Sadistic sexual behavior may include pretend or fantasized infliction of pain; mild to severe cruelty toward partners; or an extremely dangerous, pathological form of sadism that involves mutilation or murder. Estimates regarding the prevalence of sexual sadism range from 5 percent to 20 percent, depending on the definition of sadism employed by the researchers. Some believe that sexual sadism is best seen as a dimensional disorder that can range from mild to severe (Longpré et al., 2018). As with other paraphilic disorders, the DSM-5-TR specifies that to receive this diagnosis, a person must have acted on the urges with a nonconsenting person or feel markedly distressed by the behavior.

For some people who participate in sexual sadism or masochism, coitus becomes unnecessary; pain or humiliation alone is sufficient to produce sexual pleasure. Some participants engage in both submissive and dominant roles. Their sexual activities may be carefully scripted and involve mutually agreed upon role-playing (Lussier et al., 2008). In one survey of respondents who participate in sadomasochistic activities involving spanking, whipping, and bondage, only 16 percent were exclusively dominant or submissive. Approximately 40 percent had engaged in behaviors that caused minor pain using ice, hot wax, biting, or face slapping. Fewer than 18 percent had engaged in more harmful procedures, such as burning or piercing (Brewslow et al., 1986). However, accidental deaths have been reported with some activities; erotic asphyxiation is particularly dangerous and accounts for about 90 percent of the deaths (Schori et al., 2022).

Many individuals who practice sadomasochism are aware of the tremendous stigma attached to this practice and are secretive about their sexual behavior. They continue with the practices, however, because they find sadomasochistic sexual activities to be more satisfying than "straight" sex (Stiles & Clark, 2011). Sadomasochism appears to be more a recreational activity than an expression of psychopathology for some practitioners, and, as a group, those who practice sadomasochism tend to be extroverted and open to new experiences (De Neef et al., 2019).

Etiology and Treatment of Paraphilic Disorders

We still have much to learn about what causes paraphilias to develop. Investigators have attempted to find genetic, neurohormonal, and brain anomalies that might be associated with paraphilic disorders. Some of the research findings conflict with each other; others need replication and confirmation. Some men may be biologically predisposed to some paraphilias such as pedophilic disorder, as pedophiles have been found to have neurological abnormalities that may influence their sexual preferences (Poeppl et al., 2015). Even if biological factors are found to play a role in the development of paraphilias, psychological factors also contribute in important ways.

In early attempts to explain paraphilic disorders, psychodynamic theorists proposed that these sexual behaviors represent unconscious conflicts that began in early childhood (Schrut, 2005). Castration anxiety in men, for example, is hypothesized to underlie transvestic disorder, fetishistic disorder, exhibitionistic disorder, sexual sadism disorder, and sexual masochism disorder. A man with exhibitionistic disorder, for instance, exposes himself to reassure himself that castration has not occurred. The shock that registers on the faces of others assures him that he still has a penis. A man with sexual sadism disorder may protect himself from castration anxiety by inflicting pain. A man with sexual masochism disorder may engage in self-castration through the acceptance of pain, thereby limiting the power of others to castrate him. The psychodynamic treatment of sexual deviations involves helping the client understand the relationship between the sexual behavior and the unconscious conflicts that produce it.

Research looking into the characteristics of sex offenders has provided insight into early psychosocial variables that may influence their behavior. For example, juvenile sex offenders are more likely to have unusual sexual interests, low self-esteem, and anxiety. Additionally, they are more likely to have early exposure to sex, sexual violence, pornography, or a history of being sexually molested (Seto & Lalumière, 2010). In a confidential study involving self-reported pedophiles and users of child pornography who had not yet been detected or arrested for their actions, participants reported long-standing difficulties regulating their sexual behavior, including high rates of sexual preoccupation and arousal involving a variety of other paraphilias, most commonly voyeurism, sadism, frotteurism, or exhibitionism (Neutze et al., 2012).

Learning theorists stress the importance of early conditioning experiences in the etiology of paraphilias (Brannon & Bienenfeld, 2015). In other words, paraphilias may result from accidental associations between sexual arousal and exposure to certain situations, events, acts, or objects. A young boy may develop a fetish for women's panties after he becomes sexually excited watching girls come down a slide with their underpants exposed. He begins to masturbate to fantasies of girls with their panties showing; this behavior could lead to an underwear fetish. Paraphilias often develop during adolescence when sexual interest and arousal are particularly susceptible to conditioning. Additionally, if an adolescent masturbates while engaged in sexually deviant fantasies, the conditioning may hamper the development of normal sexual patterns.

Behavioral approaches to treating sexual deviations have generally involved one or more of the following elements (Kaplan & Krueger, 2012): (a) weakening or eliminating the sexually inappropriate behaviors through processes such as extinction or aversive conditioning, (b) acquiring or strengthening sexually appropriate behaviors, and (c) developing appropriate social skills. One of the more unique treatments for exhibitionism involves *aversive behavior rehearsal* (Wickramasekera, 1976), in which shame or humiliation is the aversive stimulus. The technique requires that the person exhibit himself in his usual manner to a preselected audience of women. During the exhibiting act, the person must verbalize a conversation between himself and his penis. He must talk about what he is feeling emotionally and physically and must explain his fantasies regarding what he supposes the female observers are thinking about him. One premise of this technique is that exhibitionism often occurs during a state similar to hypnosis, when the exhibitionist's fantasies are extremely active and his judgment is impaired. This method forces him to experience and examine his actions while being fully aware of what he is doing.

The results of behavioral treatments are generally positive, although the majority of research involves single participants rather than group experimental designs. Additionally, many studies incorporate several different behavioral approaches, making it difficult to evaluate specific techniques. In one review of research involving treatment for pedophiles, the results were discouraging—neither psychological nor pharmacological interventions had much effect on reoffending (Långström et al., 2013).

14-5 Rape

Case Study Two former high school football players were convicted of raping a 16-year-old honor student in Steubenville, Ohio. The assaults allegedly took place while the girl was severely intoxicated and sometimes unresponsive. The case garnered national attention when it became apparent that other teenagers at the party sent text messages, made social media posts, and took cell phone pictures and videos of the assaultive behavior but did not intervene. (Macur & Schweber, 2012)

Rape is defined in different ways within the criminal statutes of various states. The latest definition by the U.S. Department of Justice (2012) is as follows: "The penetration, no matter how slight, of the vagina or anus with any body part or object, or oral penetration by a sex organ of another person, without the consent of the victim." This definition recognizes that objects can be used in rape and also that survivors may be incapacitated or unable to give consent because of the use of alcohol or drugs (as was the case of the teenager in the case study). Age is also considered a factor regarding whether or not consent can be given: *Statutory rape* is the legal term referring to prosecutable sexual contact that occurs between an older individual and someone who is younger than the locally defined legal age at which a person is deemed mature enough to consent to sex. Rape is an act surrounded by many myths and misconceptions (refer to Table 14.6).

The sexual harassment and sexual assault of women remain a significant societal concern. The pervasiveness of these oppressive behaviors has been highlighted by the #MeToo social movement, which has raised awareness by encouraging women survivors to speak out. Although rape is not a psychological disorder, we believe that the magnitude and seriousness of problems related to rape in U.S. society warrant a discussion of the topic. Sexual assault and harassment occur with high frequency throughout the United States. The rate of rape or sexual assault increased from 1.6 to 2.7 assaults per 1,000 persons age 12 or older from 2015 to 2018, with the majority of assaults perpetrated against women (Morgan & Oudekerk, 2019). Rape statistics are significantly different for men. Approximately 1 in 71 men have experienced rape; more than one fourth of these rapes occurred at or before age 10. Among male rape survivors, 52.4 percent reported being raped by an acquaintance and 15.1 percent by a stranger (Black et al., 2011). Women and members of racially and ethnically under-represented groups experience a higher burden of sexual violence (Centers for Disease Control and Prevention [CDC], 2022).

According to the Pentagon, there was a 38 percent increase in reports of sexual assault among military personnel between 2016 and 2018, with many incidents involving servicewomen under the age of 24. Over 85 percent of the survivors knew their assailants, and alcohol was involved in 62 percent of the assaults. Nearly 1 percent of military men also reported sexual victimization. Further, about 25 percent of enlistees mentioned that sexual harassment created a psychologically unhealthy environment (Vanden Brook, 2019). In a study of women between the ages of 40 and 60, 19 percent reported a history of sexual harassment at work and 22 percent had been sexually assaulted. Sexual harassment

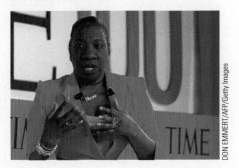
Table 14.6 The Facts About Rape

- Anyone can be raped. Rape happens among all age groups, from infants to elderly women; among all economic classes, from rich to poor; among all racial and ethnic groups; and in heterosexual and same-sex relationships.

- Statistics show that 1 in 4 girls and 1 in 6 boys are sexually assaulted before they reach the age of 18. About 1 in 6 women and 1 in 11 men are raped after turning 18.

- Rape is an act of violence. Rape is used as a way of dominating, humiliating, and terrifying another person.

- Rape is never the fault of the survivor. It has nothing to do with what the survivor wore, where the survivor went, what the survivor did, or whether the survivor is "attractive." Only the person committing the assault is to blame. Rape is painful, humiliating, and hurtful. No one ever asks to be raped.

- You are much more likely to be raped by someone you know than by a stranger. Most rapes happen between people of the same race or ethnicity.

- You have the right to say no to sex, even if you have said yes before. You also have the right to stop having sex at any time. You can be raped by someone you have had sex with before, even your spouse or partner.

- Rape is against the law. Not only is rape always wrong, it's also a crime.

Source: San Francisco Women Against Rape (n.d.).

was associated with higher blood pressure and poorer sleep, and survivors of sexual assault reported more symptoms of depression and anxiety compared to women without this history (Thurston et al., 2019).

Sexual assault is a significant concern among college students. In a report focused on sexual assaults involving 181,752 students from 33 colleges and universities (Cantor et al., 2020), it was found that:

- Among undergraduates, 26 percent of women, 7 percent of men, and 23 percent of transgender or genderqueer students reported nonconsensual physical sexual contact by force or due to inability to provide consent.

- Of nonconsensual penetration, approximately half of the incidents resulted from force and half involved the inability to give consent.

- The vast majority of survivors of nonconsensual penetration reported one or more negative behavioral or emotional symptoms associated with the assault, such as fearfulness, feeling numb or detached, and withdrawal from friends.

- Over three fourths of the rape survivors had consumed alcohol before the nonconsensual contact occurred. One third of this group reported that penetration occurred when they were passed out or asleep. Sixteen percent suspected that they had been given an intoxicating substance without their knowledge or consent.

Are institutions of higher learning doing enough to prevent sexual assaults or provide assistance to those who have been assaulted? Many colleges and universities are addressing the issue by providing information regarding sexual harassment and sexual safety via pamphlets, online modules, and educational films, with a focus on the necessity of both partners clearly communicating affirmative consent prior to sexual activity. Counseling and other support services for sexual assault survivors are also receiving increased emphasis and attention (Howard, 2018). State and federal agencies have also stepped up to hold schools accountable if they do not confront sexual violence on their campuses. California became the first state to pass the "yes means yes" law, which requires "an affirmative, conscious and voluntary agreement to engage in sexual activity." This law, which applies to colleges and universities that receive state aid, highlights the fact that individuals who are drunk, drugged, asleep, or unconscious are unable to give consent.

Effects of Rape

Rape survivors may experience a cluster of emotional reactions known as **rape trauma syndrome**; these reactions include psychological distress, phobic reactions, posttraumatic stress symptoms, or sexual dysfunction. Symptoms may be especially severe among survivors of forceful versus incapacitated assault (Masters et al., 2015). Two phases have been identified in rape trauma syndrome (Cling, 2004; Long et al., 2002):

1. *Acute phase: Disorganization*—During the period immediately following the assault, the rape survivor may have feelings of self-blame, fear, and depression. Survivors may believe they were responsible for the rape (e.g., by not locking the door or by being friendly toward the attacker). They may also have a fear that the attacker will return and that they may again be raped or even killed. They may express these emotional reactions and beliefs directly as anger, fear, rage, anxiety, or depression, or conceal them, appearing amazingly calm. Beneath this exterior, however, are signs of tension, including headaches, irritability, restlessness, sleeplessness, and jumpiness.

2. *Long-term phase: Reorganization*—This second phase may last for several years. Survivors begin to deal directly with their feelings and attempt to reorganize their lives. Fear may continue in the form of posttraumatic stress disorder, especially in situations with reminders of the traumatic incident. Many survivors report one or more sexual dysfunctions as the result of the rape; fear of sex and lack of desire or arousal are most common.

Some rape survivors recover quickly, whereas others report problems years after the attack. Feelings of safety and personal vulnerability may be drastically altered following a rape; survivors may feel unsafe in certain situations, with these feelings sometimes persisting for decades. It is clear that rape has long-lasting consequences and that family, friends, and acquaintances need to exercise patience and understanding as rape survivors go through the process of healing.

Etiology of Rape

The objectification of women, a pervasive characteristic of U.S. culture, is a contributor to sexual aggression. As we mentioned earlier, there has been a dramatic increase in the number of sexual assaults in the military and at U.S. colleges and universities. In research on college sexual assaults, the data from about 5,000 college men from five universities revealed three distinct groups of male perpetrators differing in the probability of committing sexual violence. The first group, which included 88.6 percent of the men surveyed, had a low probability of committing acts of sexual violence but included a small percentage of men who acknowledged using verbally coercive strategies for unwanted sexual contact. The second group, comprised of about 9.8 percent of the men, used anger, verbal coercion, and alcohol to commit sexual violence; this group included the largest number of men who attempted or completed rape, mainly due to the intoxication of the women they preyed upon. The third group included the 1.5 percent of the college men who admitted using or threatening force in perpetrating rape (Brennan et al., 2019). The party culture associated with fraternities appears to increase the risk of sexual acts against women, particularly because fraternity members are more likely to endorse rape-supportive attitudes compared to other college men or sorority women (Seabrook et al., 2018). These data highlight the need to address and change societal norms regarding sexual contact.

Men who are sexually coercive or aggressive share certain characteristics. They tend to:

1. actively create situations in which sexual encounters may occur;
2. misinterpret women's friendliness as provocation or a woman's protests against forced sexual activity as insincere;
3. try to manipulate women into sexual encounters by using alcohol or "date rape drugs";
4. attribute failed attempts at sexual encounters to perceived negative features of the woman, thereby protecting their egos; and/or
5. initiate coitus earlier in life and have more sexual partners than men who are not sexually aggressive (Lussier et al., 2008).

Protesting Rape

The apparent cover-up of an alleged rape involving high school student-athletes in Steubenville, Ohio, garnered national attention. Here activists stand in front of the local county courthouse protesting those in the community who supported the male athletes and criticized the rape survivor.

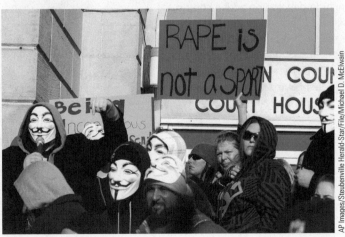

AP Images/Steubenville Herald-Star/File/Michael D. McElwain

Resilience in the Aftermath of Rape

In 1989, while jogging through New York's Central Park, Trisha Meili was raped, sodomized, and beaten so savagely that she lost 75 percent of her blood before she was discovered. At the hospital, doctors believed she would not live, but Meili fought for her life and survived. She became known as the "Central Park Jogger," and her case generated a national debate about rape and violence in society. Similar to many women who have experienced a sexual assault, Meili initially found that she had developed the following beliefs in response to her attack: (a) "I have no control over my life," (b) "The world is an unsafe place," (c) "I am unworthy," and (d) "People are not to be trusted" (Mena, 2012). After years of recovery, she finally wrote a book—*I Am the Central Park Jogger: A Story of Hope and Possibility* (Meili, 2003)—which quickly became a best seller. The book is less about rape and assault than about resilience: the hope, healing, and courage of the human spirit.

Trisha Meili's story exemplifies many of the basic principles that psychologists have discovered about resilience and posttraumatic growth after a rape (Dos Reis et al., 2017; Westphal & Bonanno, 2007). Her story is about positive coping; using personal strengths to move forward after the trauma of sexual assault; and the benefits derived from the support of friends, loved ones, communities, and society at large. Resilience research indicates that the ability to overcome adversity, especially in cases of rape, involves intersecting elements that include regaining control over the environment and events, having positive social support, moving from defining oneself as a "victim" to identifying as a "survivor," and finding a meaningful purpose in life (Hill, 2011). Other suggestions include developing active coping skills (e.g., keeping fit, maintaining a sense of humor) and finding a resilient role model who has recovered from a similar experience (Meichenbaum, 2012).

As Meili describes in her book, supportive social relationships can increase resilience after a sexual assault. Social support from family and friends provides rape survivors with a sense of worth; validation that others love, respect, and value them; and an opportunity to share their thoughts and feelings about the assault in a safe and understanding environment. Unfortunately, rape can alter a person's perception of interpersonal relationships, particularly if the rapist was an acquaintance. This may adversely affect existing social support networks and intimate relationships at a time when the person is most in need. For those who might not have had strong social networks, developing or strengthening supports after a trauma such as rape is imperative.

One of the most potent changes that aided Meili in her healing journey was redefining herself as a survivor rather than as a victim. How a woman defines her identity in relationship to a sexual assault is crucial to recovery. Self-identification as a victim implies helplessness, lack of personal control, and a passive rather than an active stance. Being a survivor, however, acknowledges the trauma but also focuses on one's ability to feel in control and overcome adversity. This cognitive shift in self-definition is all-important in the healing journey.

Finding meaning in life and reestablishing control over one's life can also enhance recovery. Meili, for example, wrote her book to help others overcome a sexual assault. She frequently speaks to groups and organizations about rape recovery and is an active advocate for survivors of rape (Tron, 2019). These activities have given her meaning in life, hope for the future, and the satisfaction of helping others and having a positive influence on society. For rape survivors, other empowerment activities may include pressing charges and testifying against the offender, taking self-defense classes, becoming an activist, and seeking meaning in the experience. In essence, these actions not only foster a sense of control and purpose in life but also include the larger altruistic goal of creating a safer world for others.

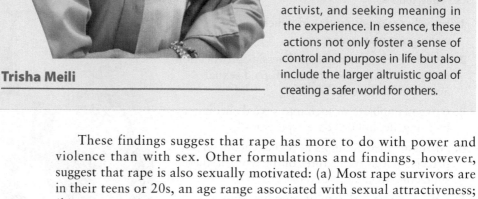

Julia Xanthos/New York Daily News Archive/Getty Images

Trisha Meili

These findings suggest that rape has more to do with power and violence than with sex. Other formulations and findings, however, suggest that rape is also sexually motivated: (a) Most rape survivors are in their teens or 20s, an age range associated with sexual attractiveness; (b) most rapists name sexual motivation as the primary reason for their actions; and (c) many rapists have multiple paraphilias (Lussier et al., 2008). Thus, it appears that sexual motivation plays a role in rape. The effect of pornography and media portrayals of violent sex or sexually aggressive behavior is also of interest to researchers. Exposure to such material may affect sexual attitudes and societal values concerning violence and women and influence patterns of sexual arousal (Altenburger et al., 2016).

Treatment for Rapists

Many people believe that sex offenders are not good candidates for psychiatric treatment or rehabilitation. The most common penalty for rape is imprisonment and, even then, there are high rates of recidivism (repeat offenses) among some sex offenders. Unfortunately, the majority of convicts receive little or no treatment in prison. When intervention occurs, treatment for sexual aggressors (rapists and child abusers) usually incorporates behavioral techniques such as the following (Fedoroff, 2008; Lussier et al., 2008):

1. assessing sexual interests through self-report and measuring erectile responses to different sexual stimuli,

2. reducing deviant interests through aversion therapy (e.g., administering an electric shock when deviant stimuli are presented),

3. reconditioning orgasm or retraining masturbation to increase sexual arousal to appropriate stimuli, and

4. teaching social skills to increase interpersonal competence.

The need for effective treatment is highlighted by sex offenders who desperately want to end their deviant sexual urges, as is demonstrated in the following case.

Case Study James Jenkins was in the county jail after having spent 7.5 years in a Virginia prison for molesting three girls. He was waiting in the cell to be transferred to a high-risk sexual offender facility when he asked a guard for a razor so that he could shave for his court appearance. After receiving the razor, he took out the blade, went into the shower, stuffed an apple in his mouth to muffle his screams, castrated himself, and flushed his testicles down the jail toilet. He says he no longer has sexual urges for young girls. (Rondeaux, 2006)

This case represents an extreme example. However, surgical castration has been used to treat sexual offenders in many European countries, and results indicate that rates of relapse have been low. Rapists, pedophiles, and a sexual murderer who underwent surgical castration all reported a decrease in sexual intercourse, masturbation, and frequency of sexual fantasies. However, some of these men remained sexually active. Chemical castration, which involves the administration of medications that reduce sex drive and sexual activity, is also used with sex offenders. In one randomized clinical trial, chemical castration was found to significantly reduce the risk of men with pedophilic disorder perpetrating child sexual abuse (Landren et al., 2020). However, these drugs appear to reduce sexual urges much more than actual erectile capability (Fedoroff, 2008).

Did You Know?

The Sex Offender Registration and Notification Act (SORNA) requires individuals convicted of sex offenses to register with local authorities and to update their contact information if they move; registration is required for 15 years, 25 years, or life depending on the severity of the offense.

14-6 Contemporary Trends and Future Directions

As you have seen in this chapter, the DSM-5-TR has made a clear distinction between paraphilias and paraphilic disorders. However, many disagree with the notion that sexual fantasies or activities that do not harm others should be labeled disorders. As we mentioned earlier in the chapter, paraphilic sexual fantasies are prevalent in the general population. A working group focused on revisions to the ICD-11 diagnostic system proposed that consensual or solitary sexual activities such as fetishism, transvestism, and sadomasochism should no longer be considered disorders. The working group successfully argued that having these diagnoses served no public health importance, were not associated with distress or dysfunction, led to stigmatization of the individuals practicing these activities, and are "inconsistent with human rights principles endorsed by the United Nations and the World Health Organization" (Moser, 2018). Thus, ICD 11 no longer lists transvestism, fetishism, or sadomasochism as paraphilic disorders. It is quite possible that these behaviors will no longer be classified as disorders in the next revision of the DSM.

Many support the fact that the DSM now clearly acknowledges that most transgender people do not have a mental disorder. A diagnosis of gender dysphoria is made only when someone with a transgender identity experiences clinically significant distress or impairment. This is clearly a move in the right direction. It is critical that we not pathologize normal biological variations or confuse gender nonconformity with mental illness. Indeed, the need for a diagnostic category of gender dysphoria calls into question our bimodal concepts of gender identity, and highlights the need to address the social stigma experienced by individuals who do not conform to societal gender norms. We must also acknowledge that the effects of stigma, prejudice, and societal discrimination on social relationships, health care, employment, and education account for much of the distress associated with gender dysphoria. Unfortunately, the recent laws enacted against gender diverse individuals only increase the mental stress and anguish in this population. The failure of our society to adequately understand transgender issues not only denies transgender people equal opportunity but is also responsible for much of their psychological distress.

There are many indicators that gender dysphoria will eventually be removed as a psychiatric diagnosis. First, there are many parallels between the arguments of advocates and members of the transgender community who oppose the inclusion of gender dysphoria as a mental disorder and those who struggled for years to remove homosexuality as a designated mental disorder (homosexuality was not completely removed from the DSM until 1986). As is true of the gay, lesbian, and bisexual communities, members of the transgender community do not regard their feelings or desires as abnormal. Many hope that future editions of the DSM will go even further in depathologizing transgender identity and acknowledge that the primary reason for any "clinically significant distress" associated with gender dysphoria is discrimination and negative societal reactions. Some argue that "diagnosing gender diverse children just because of who they are and how they express themselves reinforces and institutionalizes cissexism and transphobia in psycho-medical settings—and in society as a whole" (Cabral et al., 2016, p. 405). If there is increased societal openness to and respect for transgender people, there may no longer be a need for a diagnostic category of gender dysphoria.

Another contemporary trend involves the use of virtual reality to treat sexual dysfunctions. Because this technology has been used for anxiety disorders, therapists are beginning to recognize its usefulness in working with clients with sexual disorders, especially when anxiety plays an important etiological role (Lafortune et al., 2020).

Chapter Summary

1 **What are normal sexual behaviors?**

- There is a wide range of normal sexual behavior; what is considered normal is influenced by moral and legal judgments, as well as cultural norms.

2 **What do we know about normal sexual responses and sexual dysfunction?**

- The human sexual response cycle has four stages: the appetitive, arousal, orgasm, and resolution phases. Sexual dysfunctions are disruptions of the normal sexual response cycle. They are fairly common in the general population, and treatment is generally successful.

- The multipath model explains how biological (hormonal variations and medical conditions), psychological (performance anxieties), social (parental upbringing and attitudes), and sociocultural (cultural scripts) factors contribute to sexual dysfunctions.

3 **What causes gender dysphoria, and how is it treated?**

- Gender dysphoria involves distress and impairment in functioning that a transgender individual may experience in reaction to the mismatch between the person's experienced or expressed gender and the gender assigned at birth. Societal misunderstanding of gender diversity, social rejection, bullying, and sexual victimization all increase the risk of gender dysphoria.

- Treatment involves gender-affirming social support and medical interventions such as hormone therapy and gender affirmation surgeries to facilitate a gender transition.

4 **What are paraphilic disorders, what causes them, and how are they treated?**

- Paraphilic disorders occur when a person's sexual arousal and gratification depend on fantasies or behavior involving socially unacceptable objects, situations, or individuals. Diagnosis requires that the individual has acted on these urges with a nonconsenting individual or that the urges produce significant distress. Paraphilias may involve (a) an orientation toward nonhuman objects, (b) repetitive sexual activity with nonconsenting partners, or (c) the association of real or simulated suffering with sexual activity.

- Biological factors such as hormonal or brain abnormalities have been studied as a cause of paraphilic disorders. Psychological factors appear to play a key role in these disorders.

- Treatments are usually behavioral and are aimed at eliminating the disordered sexual behavior while teaching more appropriate behavior.

5 **What factors are associated with rape?**

- The sexual harassment and sexual assault of women remains a significant societal concern. There is particularly high risk for young women in situations involving alcohol.

- Rape survivors experience a variety of emotional reactions and vary in the time needed to recover from their traumatic experience.

Chapter Glossary

assigned gender
the gender to which a child is socially assigned at birth

cisgender
a person's gender identity aligns with the person's sex assigned at birth

delayed ejaculation
persistent delay or inability to ejaculate within the vagina despite adequate excitement and stimulation

dyspareunia
recurrent or persistent pain in the genitals before, during, or after sexual intercourse

erectile disorder
an inability to attain or maintain an erection sufficient for sexual intercourse

exhibitionistic disorder
urges, acts, or fantasies that involve exposing one's genitals to strangers

female orgasmic disorder
sexual dysfunction involving persistent delay or inability to achieve an orgasm with adequate clitoral stimulation

female sexual interest/arousal disorder
sexual dysfunction in women that is characterized by distressing disinterest in sexual activities or inability to attain or maintain physiological or psychological arousal during sexual activity

fetishistic disorder
sexual attraction and fantasies involving inanimate objects

frotteuristic disorder
recurrent and intense sexual urges, acts, or fantasies that involve sexual touching or rubbing against a nonconsenting person

gender dysphoria
distress and impaired functioning resulting from an incongruence between a person's gender identity and assigned gender

gender expression
the way in which gender is manifested, including behavior, clothing, hairstyle, or pronouns used

gender incongruence
state of having a gender identity that does not align with the gender assigned at birth

genito-pelvic pain/penetration disorder
physical pain or discomfort associated with intercourse or penetration

incest
sexual relations between people too closely related to marry legally

male hypoactive sexual desire disorder
sexual dysfunction in men that is characterized by a lack of sexual desire

nonbinary
a gender identity that is not exclusively masculine or feminine

paraphilia
recurring sexual arousal and gratification by means of mental imagery or behavior involving socially unacceptable objects, situations, or individuals

paraphilic disorder
sexual disorder in which the person has either acted on or is severely distressed by recurrent urges or fantasies involving nonhuman objects, nonconsenting individuals, or suffering or humiliation

pedophilic disorder
a disorder in which an adult obtains erotic gratification through urges, acts, or fantasies that involve sexual contact with a prepubescent or early pubescent child

premature (early) ejaculation
ejaculation with minimal sexual stimulation before, during, or within 1 minute after penetration

rape
a form of sexual aggression that involves sexual activity (oral–genital sex, anal intercourse, or vaginal intercourse) performed without a person's consent through the use of force, argument, pressure, alcohol or drugs, or authority

rape trauma syndrome
a two-phase syndrome that rape survivors may experience, involving such emotional reactions as psychological distress, phobic reactions, and sexual dysfunction

sexual dysfunction
a disruption of any part of the normal sexual response cycle that affects sexual desire, arousal, or response

sexual masochism disorder
sexual urges, fantasies, or acts that involve being humiliated, bound, or made to suffer

sexual orientation
sexual identity involving the gender to which a person is physically and emotionally attracted

sexual sadism disorder
sexual urges, fantasies, or acts that involve inflicting physical or psychological suffering on others

transgender
a person's innate psychological gender identification does not correspond with the person's sex assigned at birth

transvestic disorder
intense sexual arousal obtained through cross-dressing (wearing clothes appropriate to a different gender)

vaginismus
involuntary spasms of the outer third of the vaginal wall that prevents or interferes with sexual intercourse

voyeuristic disorder
urges, acts, or fantasies that involve observing an unsuspecting person disrobing or engaging in sexual activity

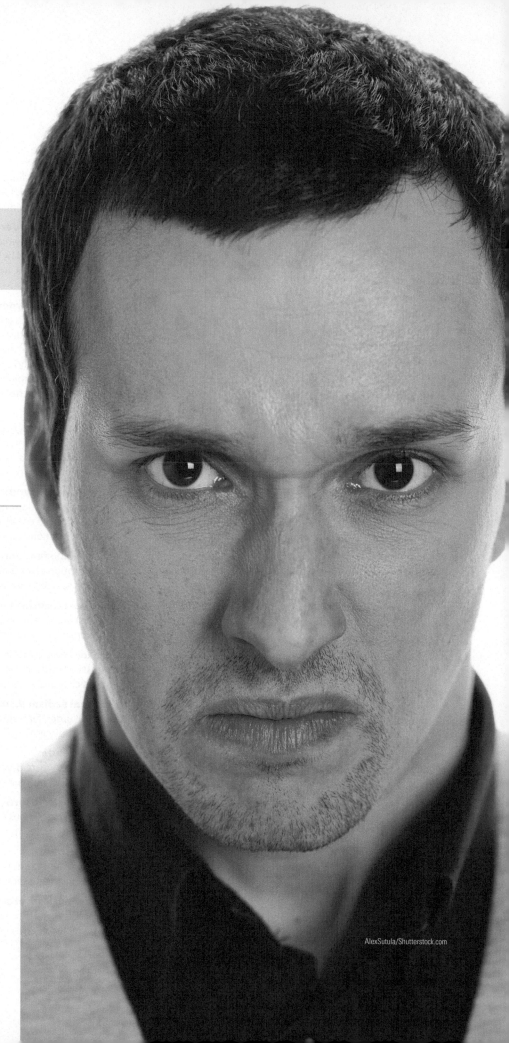

focus Questions

1 Can one's personality be pathological?

2 What traits are associated with personality disorders?

3 How does an antisocial personality develop, and can it be changed?

4 What problems occur with personality assessment?

5 Are there alternative methods of personality assessment?

AlexSutula/Shutterstock.com

15

Personality Psychopathology

Learning Objectives

After studying this chapter, you will be able to . . .

15-1 Compare and contrast the 10 specific personality disorders outlined in the DSM-5-TR.

15-2 Explain how an antisocial personality develops and describe treatment approaches to the disorder.

15-3 Describe the challenges associated with diagnosing personality disorders.

15-4 Explain the DSM-5 alternative method of personality assessment and compare and contrast it with the traditional categorical approach to personality assessment.

Aaron Kopinsky Was Known as a Loner by His Classmates. He seldom participated in social activities, had few friends in his dormitory, and avoided interacting with his roommate. His favorite pastime seemed to be watching TV programs. Few things seemed to interest Aaron; he did not go to movies and had few hobbies or activities that seemed to give him joy. Yet he did not appear lonely. His college major was forestry, so he frequently went on outings that required long stays in the national forest. While his classmates would huddle around a campfire during the evenings for companionship, Aaron preferred to be by himself.

Jennifer Wang, a Project Manager for a Small Technology Start-Up Company, was described by family, friends, and coworkers as extremely compulsive. At team meetings she was demanding, insistent that things be done correctly in a prescribed manner. She frustrated her colleagues when she posted detailed task lists for each project. Team members were expected to use a red marker to check off each task posted on the bulletin board once the job was completed. Jennifer became upset when even the most trivial detail was not completed in accordance with her directions. Everything had to be done flawlessly.

Jordan Mitchell Was "Clubbing" with Friends in San Francisco when he met an attractive sex worker who invited him to a nearby hotel for sex. Despite warnings from his friends to use a condom, he failed to do so. Throughout his life, Jordan was known for being reckless and impulsive. He enjoyed risky and dangerous activities such as racing his car against other willing drivers and discharging his gun into the sky at night. Jordan became bored easily and needed constant excitement. His impulsivity, distractibility, and constant need for change made it difficult for him to hold down a job.

A aron, Jennifer, and Jordan's behaviors, thoughts, and feelings typify how they generally react to life circumstances. Essentially, all three exhibit a consistency in how they perceive the world and respond to situations. These behavioral and mental characteristics make each of them unique and thus form the basis of their personalities. In psychology, *personality* refers to a pattern of recognizable behaviors. Aaron, for example, prefers spending time by himself; he is a loner and avoids almost all social interactions or situations. Jennifer is detail-oriented, perfectionistic, and inflexible. Jordan, in contrast, is impulsive, a thrill seeker, and a risk taker.

Can people's characteristic style of responding to situations prove problematic to themselves or others? Are Aaron, Jennifer, and Jordan's personality patterns pathological? Certainly, social isolation and friendlessness would concern many people, but Aaron does not appear bothered by it. He prefers solitary tasks and situations, and his desire to become a forest ranger appears to be a perfect occupational match for him. Jennifer's compulsivity may be irksome to co-workers, but there are advantages to this **trait**. Although being governed by rules and habits may decrease Jennifer's ability to adapt to unexpected problems or situations, being orderly and attentive to detail is an asset in many situations. On the other hand, Jordan's need for excitement, impulsivity, and risk taking may place both him and others in danger. His personality traits are much more likely to become problematic than are Aaron's or Jennifer's.

15-1 Personality Psychopathology

Most of us are fairly consistent and predictable in our outlook on life and in how we approach people and situations. Additionally, most of us are able to be flexible in how we respond life circumstances. Those of us who are shy, for example, are not necessarily shy in all situations. Individuals with **personality psychopathology**, however, possess rigid patterns of responding that are inflexible, long-standing, and enduring; these dysfunctional personality characteristics are present in nearly all situations.

As you will discover in this chapter, when maladaptive personality characteristics are quite pronounced and the cause of problems for the person or for others, the person may be diagnosed with a **personality disorder**. Specifically, a diagnosis of a personality disorder encompasses enduring personality patterns (involving behavior, thoughts, emotions, and interpersonal functioning) that are (a) extreme and deviate markedly from cultural expectations, (b) inflexible and pervasive across situations, (c) evident in adolescence or early adulthood and stable over time, and (d) associated with distress and impairment (APA, 2022). Although there are often telltale signs of personality psychopathology in childhood, clinicians do not usually consider a personality disorder diagnosis until late adolescence or adulthood when personality development is more complete.

Although people around them may feel frustrated by their rigid personality patterns, people with personality psychopathology usually don't regard themselves as having a problem. They might be described as odd, peculiar, dramatic, or unusual but generally don't seek help or come to the attention of mental health professionals. As a result, the incidence of personality disorders is difficult to determine. The prevalence of personality disorders is estimated to be about 12 percent, which suggests that these disorders are relatively common in the general population (Volkert et al., 2018). Personality disorders are diagnosed in approximately 30 percent of those who receive treatment in hospitals and outpatient clinics (Sansone & Sansone, 2015). Personality disorders are prevalent worldwide but are most common in high-income countries (Winsper et al., 2020).

The DSM-5-TR delineates two distinct methods of diagnosing and classifying personality psychopathology:

1. a categorical diagnostic model, involving 10 specific personality disorder types, which are each qualitatively distinct clinical syndromes and

2. an alternative model, including components of both dimensional and categorical assessment.

We will first review the 10 traditional personality disorders, discuss issues associated with diagnosis, and then examine the alternative system for personality diagnosis that was introduced in the DSM-5.

15-2 Personality Disorders

The 10 specific personality disorders in the DSM-5-TR are grouped into three behavior clusters: (1) odd or eccentric behaviors; (2) dramatic, emotional, or erratic behaviors; or (3) anxious or fearful behaviors (refer to Table 15.1). To diagnose a personality disorder, clinicians use the DSM-5-TR descriptions of the disorder and determine how closely an individual client matches the descriptors for a specific personality category. We will briefly discuss each of the 10 personality disorders and then provide a multipath analysis of the personality disorder that has the greatest impact on society—antisocial personality disorder.

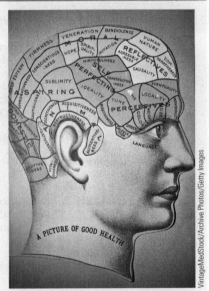

Table 15.1 Personality Disorders

Disorders Chart			
Disorder	**DSM-5-TR Descriptors**	**Gender Differences**	**Prevalence**
Disorders Characterized by Odd or Eccentric Behaviors			
Paranoid personality disorder[a]	Pervasive pattern of mistrust and suspiciousness regarding others' motives	Somewhat more common in males	2.3% to 4.4%
Schizoid personality disorder[a]	Socially isolated, emotionally cold, indifferent to others	Somewhat more common in males	1.3% to 4.9%
Schizotypal personality disorder	Peculiar thoughts and behaviors; poor interpersonal relationships	Slightly more common in males	Up to 3.9%
Disorders Characterized by Dramatic, Emotional, or Erratic Behaviors			
Antisocial personality disorder	Failure to conform to social or legal codes; lack of anxiety and guilt; irresponsible behaviors	Much more common in males	0.6% to 3.6%
Borderline personality disorder	Intense fluctuations in mood, self-image, and interpersonal relationships	More commonly diagnosed in females in clinical samples	1.4% to 5.9%
Histrionic personality disorder[a]	Self-dramatization; exaggerated emotional expression; and seductive, provocative, or attention-seeking behaviors	Mixed findings, but more prevalent in females in clinical settings	0.9% to 1.8%
Narcissistic personality disorder	Exaggerated sense of self-importance; exploitative behavior; lack of empathy	More common in males	1.6% to 6.2%
Disorders Characterized by Anxious or Fearful Behaviors			
Avoidant personality disorder	Pervasive social inhibition; fear of rejection and humiliation	More common in women	2.1% to 5.2%
Dependent personality disorder[a]	Excessive dependence on others; inability to assume responsibilities; submissive	More frequently diagnosed in women in clinical settings	0.4% to 0.6%
Obsessive-compulsive personality disorder	Perfectionism; controlling interpersonal behavior; devotion to details; rigidity	Equally common in men and women	2.4% to 7.9%

Note: Symptoms of personality disorders appear early in life. Personality disorders tend to be stable and to endure over time, although symptoms sometimes remit with age. Prevalence figures and gender differences have varied from study to study.

[a]Not included as a diagnostic category in the DSM Alternative Model for Personality Disorders.

Source: Based on APA, 2022; Volkert et al., 2018

Cluster A: Disorders Characterized by Odd or Eccentric Behaviors

Three personality disorders are included in Cluster A: *paranoid personality*, *schizoid personality*, and *schizotypal personality*. These personality disorders share characteristics, including overlapping environmental and genetic risk factors, which are similar to those found in the schizophrenia spectrum disorders (Esterberg et al., 2010). There is some evidence that individuals with disorders in this grouping have a greater likelihood of having biological relatives with schizophrenia or other psychotic disorders (APA, 2022).

Paranoid Personality Disorder

Case Study Ralph and Ann married after a brief, intense courtship. The first year of their marriage was relatively happy, although Ralph was very domineering, opinionated, and overprotective. Ann had always known that Ralph was a jealous person who demanded a great deal of attention. She was initially flattered that Ralph would become upset when other men flirted with her, believing that his possessiveness demonstrated how much he cared about her. It soon became clear, however, that his jealousy was excessive. For example, when Ann arrived home later than usual, Ralph became agitated and would demand an accounting of her activities. He often doubted her explanations and embarrassed Ann by calling her friends or co-workers to confirm her stories.

As the situation progressively worsened, Ralph began to suspect that Ann was having affairs with other men, so he would leave work early to check on her. Whenever the phone rang, Ralph insisted on answering it himself. Wrong numbers and male callers took on special significance for him; he felt that they must be trying to contact Ann. Ann found it difficult to discuss her concerns with Ralph because he was always quick to take the offensive and seemed unable to understand why his behavior was upsetting her. Ralph persisted in his pathological jealousy and suspiciousness, even after Ann filed for a divorce.

The primary characteristic of **paranoid personality disorder (PPD)** is a "pervasive distrust and suspiciousness of others such that their motives are interpreted as malevolent" (APA, 2022, p. 735). People with PPD exhibit unwarranted suspiciousness, hypersensitivity, and reluctance to trust others because they expect to be exploited or mistreated. As was the case with Ralph, they tend to be rigid in their thinking and preoccupied with unfounded beliefs, such as suspicions about the fidelity of their partners. They may seem aloof and lacking in emotion. People with PPD often interpret others' motives negatively, question people's loyalty or trustworthiness, and bear grudges. These beliefs are extremely resistant to change and result in hostility, social isolation, and difficulties cooperating with others. In clinical and forensic populations, they are likely to have a history of aggressive or stalking behaviors and engage in excessive litigation. The risk of suicide is high among those with this personality pattern (Lee, 2017). The prevalence of PPD is estimated to be about 3 percent in Western countries (Volkert et al., 2018). As you might expect, many people with this disorder fail to seek treatment because of their suspiciousness and mistrust.

Certain social conditions appear to increase the risk of being diagnosed with PPD. For instance, African Americans and people living in poverty are more likely to receive a PPD diagnosis (Lee, 2017). This may occur because people living under oppressed conditions experience everyday discrimination, which understandably leads to suspicion and mistrust, particularly with respect to members of the dominant culture. Thus, to avoid misinterpreting the significance of mistrustful behavior, mental health professionals assessing someone from an oppressed group must take the time to clarify the origins of feelings of wariness, suspiciousness, or defensiveness. It is quite possible that cautious behaviors or attitudes may result from an attempt to cope with aversive social conditions associated with being a member of an underrepresented group, experiences with discrimination, or discomfort or lack of trust in individuals from other cultural groups (Sue et al., 2022).

Causes and Treatment   The heritability of PPD ranges from 21 percent to 50 percent based on twin studies. Thus far, only a few neurobiological studies have identified genetic variations associated with paranoid ideation (Ma et al., 2016). Paranoid personality traits may result from the use of *projection*—a defense mechanism in which unacceptable impulses are denied and attributed to others. In other words, someone with paranoid personality disorder may believe "I am not hostile; they are." From a cognitive-behavioral perspective, individuals with this disorder may filter and interpret the responses of others through a mental schema such as "Other people have hidden motives," which accounts for their suspiciousness (Bhar et al., 2012). In terms of treatment, psychotherapy focuses on helping clients reduce their paranoia so they can function better in daily living. However, due to suspiciousness and difficulty trusting others, it is often difficult for therapists to develop rapport with clients who have PPD.

Schizoid Personality Disorder

The most prominent characteristics of **schizoid personality disorder** include limited interest in social relationships other than first-degree relatives and a restricted range of emotional expressions. People with this disorder have a long history of impairment in social functioning, including social isolation, emotional coldness, a lack of responsiveness to praise or criticism, and indifference to others. They tend to neither desire nor enjoy close friendships and have little interest in sexual relationships. Many live alone, engage in solitary recreational activities, and are described as withdrawn and reclusive (Cook et al., 2020).

People with schizoid personality are perceived by others as peculiar and aloof because of their lack of desire for social connection. They may interact with others in the workplace and similar situations, but their relationships are superficial and frequently awkward (Levi-Belz et al., 2019). In general, individuals with this disorder prefer social isolation and the single life rather than marriage. When they do marry, their spouses are often unhappy due to their lack of affection and reluctance to participate in family activities. Members of different cultures vary in their social behaviors, and diagnosticians must consider the cultural background of individuals who demonstrate schizoid symptoms. The prevalence of this disorder is estimated to be approximately 3 percent in Western countries (Volkert et al., 2018).

Causes and Treatment   The relationship between schizoid personality disorder and schizophrenia spectrum disorders (described in Chapter 12) is unclear. One view is that schizoid personality is a premorbid sign of delusional disorder or schizophrenia (APA, 2022). Some researchers have suggested that schizoid personality disorder is associated with a cold and emotionally impoverished childhood lacking in empathy (Marmar, 1988). Little is known about psychotherapy with individuals with schizoid personality disorder, since few seek treatment. They are most likely to seek therapy if they are experiencing stress or a crisis, but even then, the symptoms of this disorder are difficult to treat (Thylstrup & Hesse, 2009).

Schizotypal Personality Disorder

Case Study A 41-year-old man was referred to a community mental health clinic for help in improving his social skills. He had a lifelong pattern of social isolation, had no real friends, and spent long hours worrying that his angry thoughts about his older brother would cause his brother harm. During one interview, he was distant and distrustful but described in elaborate and often irrelevant detail his rather uneventful and routine daily life. . . . For 2 days he had studied the washing instructions on a new pair of jeans—Did "wash before wearing" mean that the jeans were to be washed before wearing the first time, or did they need, for some reason, to be washed each time before they were worn? . . . He asked the interviewer whether, if he joined the program, he would be required to participate in groups. He said that groups made him very nervous because he felt that if he revealed too much personal information, such as the amount of money that he had in the bank, people would take advantage of him or manipulate him for their own benefit. (Spitzer et al., 1994, pp. 289–290)

People with **schizotypal personality disorder** have odd, eccentric, paranoid, or peculiar thoughts and behaviors and a high degree of discomfort with and reduced capacity for interpersonal relationships (APA, 2022). Many believe they possess magical abilities or special powers (e.g., "I can predict what people will say before they say it"), and some are subject to recurrent illusions (e.g., "I feel that my dead father is watching me"). Speech oddities, such as frequent elaboration, digression, or vagueness in conversation, are often present (Minor & Cohen, 2012). The man in the case study has symptoms that are typical of schizotypal personality disorder: absence of close friends, magical thinking (worrying that his thoughts might harm his brother), conversational oddities, and social anxiety.

In Western countries, approximately 3 percent of adults are estimated to have a schizotypal personality disorder (Volkert et al., 2018). Again, the evaluation of individuals must take into account their cultural milieu. For example, spiritual connection with deceased relatives and hallucinations are common in certain cultures or religions. Schizotypal personality disorder has a relatively stable course, with only a small percentage going on to develop schizophrenia or another psychotic disorder. It is slightly more prevalent in men than women (APA, 2022).

Causes and Treatment Research suggests that people with schizotypal personality disorder have abnormalities in cognitive processing that may explain many of their symptoms. That is, they seem to have an unusual manner of thinking and perceiving, which may lead to social isolation, hypersensitivity, inappropriate emotional responding, and lack of pleasure from social interactions. In fact, many characteristics of schizotypal personality disorder resemble those of schizophrenia, although in less serious form. For example, people with schizophrenia exhibit problems in social functioning and information processing—deficits seen in people with schizotypal personality disorder.

Although some clinicians consider schizotypal personality disorder to be a precursor to schizophrenia, other researchers point out that only certain personality traits associated with schizotypal personality disorder (e.g., social withdrawal, disorganized

Schizotypal Personality Disorder

Army sergeant Bowe Bergdahl was captured and held captive by the Taliban-aligned Haqqani network after he walked away from his army post in a remote region of Afghanistan. He was released after 5 years in captivity but faced court-martial on charges of desertion. Psychiatric evaluation revealed that Bergdahl has schizotypal personality disorder that resulted in the internal, self-critical commentary and fanciful thinking that spurred his unauthorized departure from the army encampment.

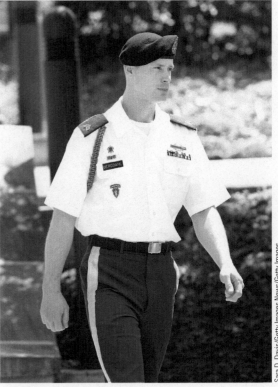

Sara D. Davis/Getty Images News/Getty Images

or paranoid thinking, unusual perceptual experiences) appear to increase the risk of eventual psychotic experiences and a schizophrenia spectrum diagnosis (Schultze-Lutter et al., 2019). Some research has suggested a genetic link between the two disorders (Apthorp et al., 2019). There are also commonalities in brain changes associated with schizophrenia and schizotypal personality disorder, but also some differences (Takayanagi et al., 2020).

Various psychotherapies are used to treat schizotypal personality disorder, such as interpersonal psychotherapy and cognitive-behavioral approaches, as well as group psychotherapy and medication. However, few individuals with schizotypal personality disorder seek therapy.

Cluster B: Disorders Characterized by Dramatic, Emotional, or Erratic Behaviors

The group of disorders in Cluster B, characterized by dramatic, emotional, or erratic behaviors, includes four personality disorders: *antisocial*, *borderline*, *histrionic*, and *narcissistic*.

Antisocial Personality Disorder

Case Study The epitome of a hard-driven, successful businessman, Robert T. seemed to have it all: enormous financial wealth; an apparently healthy marriage; and, despite his reputation as a ruthless corporate raider, high regard from associates for his business acumen. Then, in less than a year, he lost everything. Auditors raised questions about nonstandard accounting practices and inappropriate personal use of funds. Lawsuits against him and his company followed, with the trustees finally demanding his resignation. Robert refused to resign and launched a campaign against his own board of directors, accusing them of pursuing a personal vendetta and of conspiring against him. He hired a private detective to dig up dirt on certain trustees and their families and tried to use that information to intimidate and discredit them. In cases where embarrassing information was lacking, he had no qualms about spreading false rumors. These attempts, however, failed, and Robert was eventually removed from his post. His wife filed for divorce.

It was only after his downfall that the extent of Robert's dishonesty become known. He did not graduate from the Wharton School of Business, as his resume had indicated. He told people that he had been divorced once, but he had been married four times; and his fortune did not come from "old money," but from a series of questionable real estate schemes that left investors holding bad debts, which he referred to as "collateral damage." People who knew him in the past described him as arrogant, deceitful, cunning, and calculating. He disregarded the rights of others, manipulated them, and then discarded them when they served no further use to him. He never expressed regret or remorse for any of his actions.

School records revealed a pattern of juvenile alcohol use, poor grades, frequent lying, and petty theft. At age 14, he was diagnosed with a conduct disorder when school officials became concerned about his fascination with setting fires in the restroom toilets. Nevertheless, the school psychologist described Robert as "very bright, charming, and persuasive."

The primary characteristic of **antisocial personality disorder (APD)** is a "pervasive pattern of disregard for and violation of the rights of others" that has occurred since age 15 (APA, 2022). This diagnosis applies only to individuals age 18 and older. Chronic antisocial behavioral patterns, such as a failure to conform to social or legal codes, a lack of anxiety and guilt, and irresponsible behaviors, are common with APD. People with this disorder may demonstrate little concern about their wrongdoing, which may include lying, manipulating other people, and perpetrating aggressive sexual acts. Relationships with others are superficial and fleeting and involve little loyalty. Those with this disorder seek power over others and often deceive, exploit, and con others for their own needs and purposes. People with APD are prone to engage in unlawful and criminal behavior and have no qualms about violating moral, ethical, or legal codes of conduct.

Robert T. typifies an individual with APD. He exhibits little empathy for others, views them as objects to be manipulated, and has difficulty establishing meaningful and intimate relationships. Robert pushes the boundaries of social convention and often violates moral, legal, and ethical rules for his own personal gain, with little regard for the feelings of others. This characteristic way of handling things is long-standing and was evident early in life. Robert also has a pattern of blaming others; is inflexible in his manner of dealing with life problems; has a callous orientation toward people; and appears to feel no remorse when he attempts to destroy his colleagues through lying, exaggeration, and manipulation.

Antisocial behaviors typically begin early in life, with girls having a later age of onset than boys. Antisocial behaviors in childhood often involve less severe symptoms and may result from peer pressure. Some youth are described as having a time-limited adolescent form of antisocial behavior that does not progress to an APD. Among adults with an APD diagnosis, the course is generally chronic, with 27 percent remitting (i.e., the antisocial behavior subsides), 31 percent demonstrating some degree of improvement, and 42 percent remaining unchanged or worsening. APD is associated with increased mortality, comorbid substance abuse, and other psychiatric conditions. Having a spouse, involvement with the community, and positive family relationships increase the likelihood of remission (Black, 2015).

There are two types of people with APD: those with and those without the characteristic of being callous and unemotional. Those with the callous-unemotional trait (like Robert T.) are often referred to as psychopaths. Individuals in this group tend to be detached from the feelings of others and demonstrate few true emotions or empathy for others. They have low anxiety and are often described as fearless and lacking a conscience or moral compass. The second group, who are sometimes called sociopaths, may also engage in amoral or criminal acts, but—because they have at least some conscience—they also experience tension or stress and are capable of feeling some degree of guilt and shame. At times, their anxiety shows up in the form of nervous tension that results in emotional volatility and unpredictable behavior (Dargis & Koenigs, 2018).

In Western countries, the prevalence of APD (including both "psychopaths" and "sociopaths") is approximately 3 percent (Volkert et al., 2018). In the United States, rates differ by gender; men are three times more likely than women to be diagnosed with the disorder. APD typically has a chronic course, although symptoms may become less evident or remit as the individual grows older (APA, 2022). People with APD are a difficult population to study because they do not voluntarily seek

Neuroscientist Discovers His Own Antisocial Personality

James Fallon, emeritus professor of anatomy, neurobiology, psychiatry, and human behavior, is an expert on "psychopaths" and is well aware of the unique pattern of brain activity associated with psychopathy. When reviewing a set of brain scans from an unrelated study on Alzheimer disease, Fallon noticed one scan in the control group that concerned him—the brain activity pattern seen in "psychopaths." He was surprised to discover that it was a scan of his own brain. His wife, friends, and colleagues were not surprised by the finding, given their observations of his emotional detachment and lack of empathy. Fallon has since attempted to learn and to practice more empathetic behaviors and now considers himself a "prosocial psychopath." He has authored over 300 papers and books, including "The Psychopath Inside: A Neuroscientist's Journey into the Dark Side of the Brain."

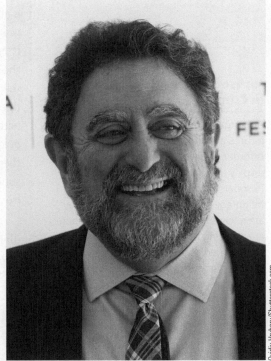

Ovidiu Hrubaru/Shutterstock.com

treatment. Consequently, investigators often locate research participants in prisons, which presumably contain a relatively large proportion of people with the disorder.

The behavior patterns associated with APD are different and distinct from impulse control problems such as pyromania, kleptomania, and intermittent explosive disorder (refer to Table 15.2) and from behaviors involving social protest or criminal lifestyles. Individuals who violate societal laws or conventions by engaging in civil disobedience are not, as a rule, people with APD because they are usually quite capable of forming meaningful interpersonal relationships and experiencing guilt. They may perceive their violations of rules and norms as acts performed for the greater good. Similarly, engaging in criminal behavior does not necessarily reflect a personality disorder. Although many convicted criminals do have antisocial characteristics, many others do not. Instead, they may come from a subculture that encourages and reinforces criminal activity; hence, in perpetrating such acts, they are adhering to group norms and codes of conduct.

We will fully discuss the etiology and treatment for APD later in the chapter when we use APD as an example of how biological, psychological, social, and sociocultural factors interact to produce a personality disorder.

Borderline Personality Disorder

Case Study Dal seems to be unable to maintain a stable sense of self-worth and self-esteem. Her confidence in her ability to "hold on to men" is at a low ebb, having just parted ways with "the love of her life." In the last year alone she confesses to having six "serious relationships"..."No one f***s with me. I stand my ground, you get my meaning?" She admits that she physically assaulted three of her last six boyfriends, hurled things at them, and, amidst uncontrollable rage attacks and temper tantrums, even threatened to kill them.... As she recounts these sad exploits, she alternates between boastful swagger and self-chastising, biting criticism of her own traits and conduct. Her mood swings wildly, in the confines of a single therapy session, between exuberant optimism and unbridled gloom. She sought therapy because she is having intrusive thoughts about killing herself. Her suicidal ideation also manifests in acts of self-injury. (Vaknin, 2012)

Antisocial Personality Disorder in Criminal Populations

Although not all individuals who are incarcerated have an antisocial personality disorder, many people who break the law display many antisocial personality traits. Prisoners who possess these traits have a heightened risk of re-offending once they are released. The participants pictured here are reducing that risk by participating in a class offered as part of a therapeutic work release program in Vanderburgh County, Indiana.

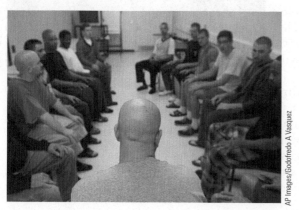

AP Images/Godofredo A Vasquez

Individuals with **borderline personality disorder (BPD)** exhibit an enduring pattern of volatile emotional reactions, instability in interpersonal relationships, poor self-image, and impulsive responding (APA, 2022). They lack a strong sense of self-identity and have a fragile self-concept that is easily disrupted by stress. As with Dal, individuals with BPD also display intense fluctuations in mood; hypersensitivity to social threat; and volatile interactions with family, friends, and sometimes even strangers. They may be quite friendly one day and quite hostile the next (Leichsenring et al., 2023).

People with BPD appear to process information in a way that reinforces their fear of rejection. They not only overreact to rejection but are also suspicious and reactive to acceptance. They expect to be rebuffed when engaging in social interactions, so they become angry when they perceive rejection but also display irritation when accepted. As you might imagine, these actions make it difficult for those with BPD to form stable social

Table 15.2 Impulse Control Disorders

Definitions of some personality disorders include the characteristic of impulsivity. However, there are other mental disorders in which impulse control is a primary characteristic.

1. People with *intermittent explosive disorder*:
   - experience periodic aggressive episodes that result in physical injury or property damage or frequent episodes of lower intensity verbal or physical aggression;
   - display an aggressiveness that is grossly out of proportion to any precipitating stressor or event that may have occurred; and
   - exhibit no signs of general aggressiveness between episodes and may genuinely feel remorse for their actions.

2. People with *kleptomania*:
   - chronically fail to resist impulses to steal;
   - do not need the stolen objects for personal use or monetary value, since they usually have enough money to buy the items and typically discard them, give them away, or surreptitiously return them; and
   - feel irresistible urges and tension before stealing, followed by an intense feeling of relief or gratification after stealing.

3. People with *pyromania*:
   - deliberately set fires;
   - are fascinated by and get intense pleasure or relief from setting the fires, watching things burn, or observing firefighters and their efforts to put out fires; and
   - have fire-setting impulses driven by this fascination rather than by motives involving revenge, sabotage, or financial gains.

Based on APA, 2022

relationships (Liebke et al., 2018). Individuals with this disorder are also likely to engage in behaviors with negative consequences such as binge eating, substance abuse, verbal aggression, or impulsive shopping (Selby & Joiner, 2013).

Individuals with BPD often display poor emotional control and difficulty regulating their emotions, as well as engage in maladaptive rather than adaptive strategies to deal with problems (Southward & Cheavens, 2020). Self-destructive behaviors such as nonsuicidal self-injury (cutting and self-mutilation) frequently occur during periods of high stress or in response to interpersonal conflicts. Further, recurrent suicide attempts and completions are higher among individuals with BPD (Paris, 2019). Sexual difficulties, such as sexual preoccupation and dissatisfaction, are also common (Zanarini et al., 2003). Because of their behavioral excesses, those with BPD have increased risk of chronic illnesses such as cardiovascular disease, diabetes, and obesity (Iacovino et al., 2014).

BPD is one of the most commonly diagnosed personality disorders in both inpatient and outpatient settings (Gunderson et al., 2018). The prevalence of BPD in Western countries is about 2 percent and is more common in women (Volkert et al., 2018). Although the prognosis is often viewed as poor, and up to 5 percent of individuals with BPD die by suicide, some long-term outcome studies indicate a progressive decline in symptoms, with 50 percent to 70 percent achieving remission (Álvarez-Tomás et al., 2019). However, remission or recovery is slow, and individuals with BPD often have high rates of symptom recurrence (Leichsenring et al., 2023).

BPD is a highly stigmatized disorder. In one study involving a mock jury considering a fictitious homicide, the defendant was described as having either a "complex mental health problem"

Comedian Acknowledges Living with Borderline Personality Disorder

Actor Pete Davidson, who is well known for his appearances on *Saturday Night Live* and who is pictured here in the 2020 film *The King of Staten Island*, has shared that he was diagnosed with borderline personality disorder. Davidson, who lost his father in the terrorist attacks on the Twin Towers on September 11, 2001, has also battled ongoing depression.

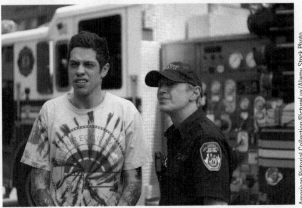

American Pictorial Collection/PictureLux/Alamy Stock Photo

or borderline personality disorder. The BPD description resulted in the defendant being rated as more dangerous and more in need of coercive treatment and segregation (Baker et al., 2021).

Causes and Treatment Difficulty with mood regulation is a central feature of BPD. A biologically based vulnerability to emotional dysregulation may underlie the intense emotional reactivity seen in this disorder. In fact, BPD is now considered a moderately heritable disorder that involves a dysregulation of emotional control (Perez-Rodriguez et al., 2018). This perspective is supported by brain scans. Magnetic resonance imaging (MRI) and positron emission tomography (PET) have revealed structural abnormalities in the prefrontal cortex and limbic regions and an atypical pattern of activation in the amygdala among individuals with BPD (Richter et al., 2014). These brain regions are associated with mood regulation and may reflect the failure of the cortex to dampen the reactivity of the amygdala.

Social factors such as family relationship problems may interact with neurobiological risk factors in the etiology of BPD. In one study, over 93 percent of adolescent patients with BPD symptoms reported at least one type of childhood maltreatment. This percentage was nearly twice as high as those in the comparison group. The most common type of maltreatment reported was sexual abuse and paternal hostility. A biologically vulnerable child raised in a dangerous, invalidating, or rejecting family environment may not develop a strong sense of self; when this occurs, the child may become very sensitive to negative emotions and may be unable to self-soothe when encountering stressful situations. These emotional regulation difficulties may manifest later as BPD (Hope & Chapman, 2019).

According to the cognitive-behavioral perspective, exposure to maladaptive experiences such as abuse or neglect may result in distorted or inaccurate schemas or beliefs about the world (Esmaeilian et al., 2019). Individuals with BPD seem to have three basic assumptions: (1) "The world is dangerous," (2) "I am powerless and vulnerable," and (3) "I am inherently unacceptable." Believing in these assumptions, individuals with BPD become fearful, vigilant, defensive, volatile, and prone to emotional reactivity in interpersonal situations (Bhar et al., 2012).

Cognitive-behavioral therapy can help individuals with BPD identify negative thoughts and replace them with more adaptive cognitions; this approach has been effective in reducing suicidal acts, dysfunctional beliefs, anxiety, and emotional distress (Davidson et al., 2008). Another form of psychotherapy, schema therapy, which combines cognitive-behavioral therapy with psychodynamic techniques, has produced promising results with BPD (Sempértegui et al., 2013); this approach teaches clients to identify and modify maladaptive interpersonal schemas and behaviors.

Dialectical behavior therapy (DBT), developed by Linehan (1993) specifically for clients with BPD, was a major breakthrough in the treatment of BPD and is increasingly viewed as the therapy of choice for this challenging disorder (King et al., 2019; Neacsiu et al., 2014). Averting possible suicidal behaviors, reducing the intensity of emotions, and strengthening the therapist–client relationship are priorities in DBT. Clients are taught skills that address BPD symptoms, including emotional regulation, distress tolerance, and interpersonal effectiveness. The goals of DBT, in descending order of priority, are to address (1) suicidal behaviors, (2) behaviors that interfere with therapy, (3) behaviors that interfere with quality of life, (4) reactive behaviors, (5) posttraumatic stress behaviors, and (6) self-respect behaviors. DBT has proven effective in treating symptoms of BPD, including decreasing suicidal threats and actions.

A number of other therapies such as mentalization-based therapy (strengthening the capacity for interpersonal emotional regulation

Continuum Video Project

Tina: Borderline Personality Disorder

"I kinda get high off of making people as uncomfortable as they make me. It's almost my way of really connecting with myself."

Access the Continuum Video Project in MindTap

Dr. Marsha Linehan: Portrait of Resilience

A 17-year-old girl was institutionalized in a psychiatric facility in Connecticut. Doctors considered her among the most seriously disturbed patients they had ever seen (Carey, 2011). She habitually cut and burned herself and would use any sharp object to slash her arms, legs, and midsection. She expressed a desire to die and made attempts at suicide (Grohol, 2011). Because of these ongoing efforts at self-harm, she was locked in a seclusion room free of any object that she could possibly use to hurt herself. However, this did not prevent her from injuring herself—she constantly and violently banged her head against the floor or walls. She received hours of Freudian analysis; large doses of psychiatric drugs; and, as a last resort, electroconvulsive shock treatments. When she was discharged 2 years later, the doctors believed she had little chance of survival outside of a hospital.

This is the true story of Dr. Marsha Linehan, a world-renowned psychologist who developed a groundbreaking form of psychotherapy called dialectical behavior therapy (DBT)—a highly successful therapeutic approach that focuses on the emotional reactivity and suicidality associated with various mental health conditions, including borderline personality disorder. Linehan is now Professor Emeritus in the Department of Psychology and Director Emeritus of the Behavioral Research and Therapy Clinics at the University of Washington. The mental health community has honored Linehan for her unique professional contributions, and, in 2018, Linehan was featured in a special edition of *Time* magazine highlighting the world's greatest scientists.

Linehan's self-healing journey is truly inspirational and speaks to the courage, inner fortitude, and resilience of the human condition. In her own recovery, Linehan has outlined lessons she learned that involve components of a resilient and peaceful life:

1. *Real change is possible.* According to conventional wisdom, people with personality disorders have great difficulty changing; some people even go so far as to say that very little can be done, especially for those with borderline personality disorder. Yet Linehan is a prime example that change is possible, and her therapeutic approach incorporates the notion that learning new skills and changing behavior ultimately change perceptions and emotions.

2. *Accept life as it is, not as it is supposed to be.* Linehan calls this "radical acceptance" and uses her own recovery as an example. The gulf between who she was and what she wanted to be made her feel hopeless, desperate, and depressed. She despised herself, and her self-harm behaviors symbolized this hatred. Linehan believes that "accepting oneself as one truly is" represents the first step in combating feelings of self-loathing. This self-acceptance eliminates the discrepancy between an unrealistic ideal and the current state of the person and allows realistic and positive views of the self to develop.

3. *A diagnosis of borderline personality disorder or any disorder is not a life sentence.* According to Linehan, receiving a psychiatric diagnosis often fosters a victim mentality that produces helplessness, dependency, and hopelessness. The person begins to believe that little can be done to overcome the disorder. Linehan teaches her clients to think of themselves as survivors, or people who can control their destiny in life and are capable of overcoming challenges. Such a fundamental change in thinking moves clients from a passive to an active stance.

4. *Find faith and meaning in life.* Linehan's religion and belief in God played an important role in her recovery. Her Catholic faith gave her hope and allowed her to experience an epiphany in 1967 that ultimately led her to develop the core principles of DBT. Linehan managed to find the answers to the problems that had haunted her, and she used this insight to guide her work. Since then, Linehan's mission in life has been to help others through the challenges of mental illness.

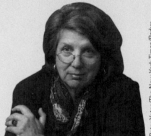

Dr. Marsha Linehan

by increasing the ability to recognize feelings) and schema-focused therapy (identifying self-defeating core themes and maladaptive coping styles arising from unmet childhood needs) have produced some promising results for individuals with BPD (Storebø et al., 2020).

Little research exists on the effectiveness of medications for BPD; in general, use of antidepressants seems to be declining while use of mood stabilizers has been increasing. In general, prescribed medications are used as an adjunct to psychotherapy (Starcevic & Janca, 2018).

Histrionic Personality Disorder

Case Study A 33-year-old real estate agent entered treatment for problems involving severe depression. Her boyfriend had recently told her that she was self-centered and phony. He discovered that she had been dating other men, despite their understanding that neither would go out with others. Once their relationship ended, her boyfriend refused to communicate with her. The woman then angrily called the boyfriend's employer and told him that unless the boyfriend contacted her, she would commit suicide. He never did call, but instead of attempting suicide, she decided to seek psychotherapy.

The woman dressed in a tight and clinging sweater for her first therapy session. Several times during the session she raised her arms, supposedly to fix her hair, in a very seductive manner. Her conversation was animated and intense. When she was describing the breakup with her boyfriend, she was tearful. Later, she raged over the boyfriend's failure to call her. Near the end of the session, she seemed upbeat and cheerful, commenting that the best therapy might be for the therapist to arrange a date for her.

People with **histrionic personality disorder** exhibit a "pervasive pattern of excessive emotionality and attention-seeking" (APA, 2022, p. 754). The term *histrionic* refers to intensely dramatic emotions and behaviors used to draw attention to oneself. Individuals with histrionic personality disorder engage in self-dramatization, exaggerated expression of emotions, and attention-seeking behaviors. The desire for attention may lead to flamboyant acts or flirtatious behaviors.

The real estate agent's behaviors, in isolation, would not warrant a diagnosis of histrionic personality disorder. In combination, however, her self-dramatization, tendency to draw attention to herself via seductive behavior and casual relationships, angry outbursts, manipulative suicidal threats, and lack of genuineness suggest this disorder. Despite superficial warmth and charm, the histrionic person is typically shallow and self-centered. Individuals from some cultures may be very expressive with emotional displays, but the histrionic personality pattern goes well beyond cultural norms. The disorder is relatively rare, with a prevalence between 0.9 percent and 1.8 percent. Gender differences are not evident, although in clinical settings this disorder is diagnosed more frequently in women (APA, 2022).

Causes and Treatment Both biological factors, such as autonomic emotional excitability, and environmental factors, such as histrionic role models or parental reinforcement of a child's attention-seeking behaviors, may be important influences in the development of histrionic personality disorder. The heritability of histrionic personality ranges from 24 percent in the general population to 63 percent among clinical samples (Ma et al., 2016). There is little research on treatment for this disorder. Psychodynamic therapies focus on establishing a therapeutic alliance with the client and determining why the client craves attention (Horowitz, 2001). Cognitive-behavioral therapy targets changing irrational cognitions such as "I should be the center of attention" (Bhar et al., 2012). Therapy focused on helping clients develop self-regulation skills and gain an understanding of themselves and their role in interpersonal difficulties has successfully assisted individuals with histrionic personality disorder to improve their relationships (Babl et al., 2023).

Narcissistic Personality Disorder

Case Study   Roberto was a well-known sociologist at the local community college. He was flamboyant, always seeking attention, and well known for bragging about himself to anyone who would listen. Most people found him superficial and so self-centered that any type of meaningful conversation was nearly impossible. His expertise was in critical race theory, and he had published a few minor articles in professional journals on topics of racism. He saw himself as a great scholar and would often talk about his "accomplishments" to colleagues; Roberto had nominated himself for numerous awards and asked colleagues to write letters on his behalf. Because his accomplishments were considered mediocre by academic standards, Roberto seldom received any of the awards. Nevertheless, he continued to present himself as a renowned pioneer in the field of race relations.

Roberto came for couples counseling at the request of his wife, who was tired of his self-centered behavior. After nearly a year of therapy without significant change in Roberto, his wife filed for divorce.

Similar to many people with **narcissistic personality disorder**, Roberto has a sense of entitlement, exaggerated self-importance, and superiority. He also seems unconcerned with the feelings of others. The characteristics associated with narcissistic personality disorder include a "pervasive pattern of grandiosity (in fantasy or behavior), need for admiration, and lack of empathy" (APA, 2022, p. 761). People with this disorder require constant attention, adulation, and approval and have difficulty accepting personal criticism. When people with high narcissism perceive that someone else is receiving too much attention, they may respond by making personal attacks. They are self-absorbed, preferring to talk about themselves and displaying a lack of interest in others. Many fantasize about or strive for power or influence, and they frequently overestimate their talents and importance (Dashineau et al., 2019).

The prevalence of narcissistic personality disorder is 1.2 percent in Western countries (Volkert et al., 2018), although some estimates are as high as 6 percent (Muir et al., 2021). Up to 75 percent of those who receive this diagnosis are males (Dowgwillo et al., 2019). Narcissistic traits are common among adolescents and do not necessarily imply that a teenager has or will develop a narcissistic personality. Narcissistic characteristics in college students appear to decline after 4 years of college (Lenzenweger, 2023).

Causes and Treatment   The heritability of narcissistic personality disorder ranges from 27 percent in the general population to 77 percent in clinical samples (Ma et al., 2016).

The Challenges of Personality Disorder Diagnosis Reflected in a Fictional Character

Fans of the television show *Always Sunny in Philadelphia* may suspect that Dennis Reynolds, one of the main characters known for his vanity and self-absorption, has narcissistic personality disorder. Some people have also speculated that the character's limited empathy and lack of remorse for amoral actions are consistent with antisocial personality disorder. Many were surprised when he was eventually diagnosed as having borderline personality disorder, emphasizing how overlapping symptoms increase the complexity of personality disorder diagnosis.

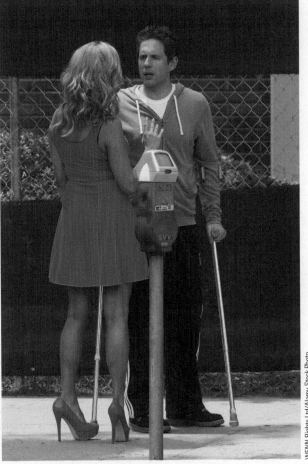

WENN Rights Ltd/Alamy Stock Photo

Brain scans have found differences between healthy controls and those with narcissistic personality disorder. Reduced white matter connectivity between the medial frontal cortex and the ventral striatum may diminish reward sensitivity. To compensate, those with narcissism may continually seek acclaim and admiration from others (Cascio et al., 2015; Chester et al., 2016). Cognitive-behavioral theorists believe cognitive schemas such as "Other people should satisfy my needs" underlie narcissistic characteristics (Bhar et al., 2012).

As with most personality disorders, controlled treatment studies for narcissistic personality disorder are rare; therefore, treatment recommendations are frequently based on clinical experience. Individuals with narcissistic personality who seek treatment are most likely to do so when in a vulnerable state of depression, anxiety, or suicidality. Unfortunately, narcissistic personality disorder is considered very difficult to treat (Muir et al., 2021). Therapists are faced with lack of engagement in therapy, defensiveness, and abrupt termination of therapy (Kacel et al., 2017). Recommended treatments include cognitive-behavioral therapies for borderline personality disorder that are adapted for narcissism (Caligor et al., 2015). Although most treatments have only limited success, some remission of symptoms does occur. Over a 2-year period, about 53 percent of one sample of individuals with narcissistic personality disorder demonstrated some symptom improvement (Vater et al., 2014).

Cluster C: Disorders Characterized by Anxious or Fearful Behaviors

The remaining cluster of personality disorders is characterized by anxious or fearful behaviors. This category includes the *avoidant*, *dependent*, and *obsessive-compulsive* personality disorders.

Avoidant Personality Disorder

Case Study I have moderate to severe avoidant personality disorder.... I feel like I've had this condition my whole life; there just wasn't a name for it yet. I was considered a very shy, sensitive, overly emotional child. My road to diagnosis began a few years ago when I didn't eat for 4 days because I was afraid someone at the grocery store would talk to me.... The fear of being disliked or unwanted is so overwhelming that I'd rather be alone. My daily life involves watching TV or being on the Internet.... I hope to be well enough to go watch a parade, see a movie, or attend a carnival and chat with people whom I know. (Cooper, 2013)

The essential features of **avoidant personality disorder** are a "pervasive pattern of social inhibition, feelings of inadequacy, and hypersensitivity to negative evaluation" (APA, 2022, p. 765). People with avoidant personalities have a lifelong pattern of feeling inferior, depressed, or anxious. As in the case study, fear of rejection and humiliation produce a reluctance to enter into social relationships. People with this disorder tend to have low self-esteem and a strong sense of inadequacy. They avoid social situations and relationships and are often socially inept, shy, and withdrawn. They fear humiliation, are overly sensitive to criticism, blame themselves for things that go wrong, and seem to find little pleasure in life.

Unlike some individuals who avoid others because they lack interest, individuals with avoidant personality disorder crave affection and an active social life. They desire—but fear—social contact, and this ambivalence is reflected in different ways. For example, many people with this disorder engage in intellectual pursuits or are active in the artistic community. Thus, their need for contact and relationships is woven into their activities. A person with avoidant personality disorder may write poems expressing a need for human intimacy or emphasizing the plight of people who are lonely.

In Western countries, the prevalence of avoidant personality disorder is estimated to range between 2.1 percent and 5.2 percent and is somewhat more common in women than men (APA, 2022). As with other personality disorders, avoidant personality disorder is considered to be a chronic and enduring condition. However, some people with avoidant personality disorder show moderate improvement over time, especially those who develop a close, supportive relationship (Kvarstein et al., 2021). Further, studies indicate that in cases where symptoms decrease, individuals become more assertive, less submissive, and more self-assured in social situations (Wright et al., 2013).

Causes and Treatment In one study, the heritability of avoidant personality disorder was 67 percent (Ma et al., 2016). Some researchers believe that avoidant personality disorder is on a continuum with social anxiety disorder, whereas others believe it to be a distinct condition that happens to include the trait of social anxiety. Several research studies have concluded that although they share similarities in symptoms, they are separate disorders (Hemmati et al., 2019).

Avoidant personality results from a complex interaction between early childhood environmental experiences and innate **temperament**. For instance, parental rejection and disapproval, reinforced by rejecting peers, may lead to the development of mental schema such as "I should avoid unpleasant situations at all costs" (Bhar et al., 2012). Other negative thoughts about oneself such as "I am inept," "I am unlovable," or "I don't fit in" result in difficulties making adaptive responses in social situations (Centonze et al., 2021). The reluctance to socialize experienced by people with an avoidant personality may result from excessively high, self-imposed standards for performance in social situations combined with negative beliefs regarding the consequences of poor performance (Rees & Pritchard, 2015). Additionally, people with this disorder are caught in a vicious cycle: Because they are preoccupied with the possibility of rejection, they are constantly alert for signs of negativity or ridicule. Further, because they anticipate being rebuffed, they also avoid social contact. Subsequently, their social skills become deficient, resulting in awkward social interactions. In other words, their very fear of rejection may lead to negative responses from the people they encounter.

Because of this fear of rejection and scrutiny, clients with avoidant personality disorder are often reluctant to disclose personal thoughts and feelings during therapy; therefore, it is essential for the therapist to quickly establish rapport and build a strong therapeutic alliance. A variety of treatment strategies—including cognitive-behavioral, short-term psychodynamic, interpersonal, and acceptance and commitment therapies—have demonstrated some success with avoidant personality disorder (Sørensen et al., 2019).

Dependent Personality Disorder

> **Case Study** Jim was a 56-year-old single man who was living with his 78-year-old widowed mother. When his mother was hospitalized for cancer, Jim decided to consult with a therapist. He was distraught and depressed over his mother's condition and his future. His mother had always taken care of him, and, in his view, she always knew best. Even when he was young, his mother had "worn the pants" in the family. The only time that he was away from his family was during his 6 years of military service. After he was wounded, he spent several months in a Veterans Administration hospital and then went to live with his mother. Because of his service-related injury, Jim was unable to work full time. His mother welcomed him home, and she structured all of his activities.
>
> At one point, Jim met and fell in love with a woman, but his mother disapproved of her. During a confrontation between Jim's mother and his girlfriend, each demanded that Jim make a commitment to her. This was quite traumatic for Jim. His mother finally grabbed him, demanding that Jim tell his girlfriend to leave. Jim tearfully told his girlfriend that he was sorry, but she must go, and she angrily left for good.

Dependent personality disorder is a condition in which an individual displays a "pervasive and excessive need to be taken care of that leads to submissive and clinging behavior and fear of separation" (APA, 2022, p. 768). As we saw in Jim's situation, extreme dependency often interferes with important life decisions and results in depression, helplessness, and suppressed anger. Individuals with dependent personality disorder lack self-confidence and often subordinate their needs to those of the people on whom they depend. Nevertheless, casual observers may fail to recognize or may misinterpret their dependency and inability to make decisions. Friends may describe those with dependent personalities as understanding and tolerant, without realizing that they are fearful of doing anything that might disrupt the friendship. Similarly, individuals with dependent personality disorder may allow their domestic partner to be dominant or abusive for fear that the partner will otherwise leave. Thus, individuals with dependent personality disorder are at high risk of experiencing relationship violence (Loas et al., 2011).

Dependent personality disorder is relatively rare and occurs in about 0.78 percent of the population in Western countries (Volkert et al., 2018). The prevalence by gender is unclear. In clinical and community settings, dependent personality disorder is diagnosed more frequently in women (APA, 2022). The individual's sociocultural environment must be considered before rendering a diagnosis of dependent personality disorder. The socialization process that teaches people to be independent, assertive, and individualistic rather than group oriented does not occur in all cultures. Instead, many cultural groups socialize their children to value interconnected, cross-generational relationships (Sue et al., 2022).

Causes and Treatment Few studies exist on the etiology of dependent personality disorder, and explanations for the condition vary according to theoretical perspective. Genetic studies suggest a 28 percent to 66 percent heritability of a dependent personality trait (Ma et al., 2016). From the psychodynamic perspective, the disorder results from maternal deprivation,

Did You Know?

Personality disorder symptoms were assessed in 214 professional actors. They scored significantly higher in antisocial, narcissistic, histrionic, and borderline traits than a comparative U.S. community sample. For those in the acting profession, characteristics such as low anxiety (antisocial), intense emotions (borderline), grandiosity and need for admiration (narcissistic), and need to be the center of attention (histrionic) can be helpful qualities.

Source: Davison & Furnham, 2018

which causes fixation at the oral stage of development (Marmar, 1988). Behavioral learning theorists believe that dependency develops when a family or social environment rewards dependent behavior. This perspective is supported by research that links dependency with overprotective or authoritarian parenting or having a severe illness in childhood (Disney, 2013). Presumably, these parenting styles prevent the child from developing a sense of autonomy and self-efficacy.

Cognitive theorists attribute dependent personality disorder to the development of distorted beliefs that discourage independence (Loas et al., 2011). They view dependency as more than a matter of being passive and unassertive. Rather, those with dependent personalities have deeply ingrained assumptions that affect their thoughts, perceptions, and behaviors. They regard themselves as inherently inadequate and unable to cope and, therefore, conclude that they need to find someone who can take care of them. Their schema or cognitive framework involves thoughts such as "I need others to help me make decisions or tell me what to do" (Bhar et al., 2012). Different individual and group treatments are used with dependent personality disorder, and, in general, this disorder has more potential to be successfully treated compared to other personality disorders (Perry, 2001).

Obsessive-Compulsive Personality Disorder

Case Study Cecil, a third-year medical student, was referred for therapy by his graduate adviser, who was concerned that Cecil was in danger of being expelled from medical school because of his inability to get along with patients and other students. Cecil often berated patients for failing to follow his advice. On one occasion, he told a patient with a lung condition to stop smoking. When the patient indicated he was unable to stop, Cecil angrily told the patient to go for medical treatment elsewhere—that the medical center had no place for a "weak-willed fool." Cecil's relationships with others were similarly strained. He characterized fellow graduate students as "partygoers" and considered many members of the faculty to be "incompetent old deadwood." The graduate adviser said that the only reason Cecil had not been expelled was because several faculty members thought he was brilliant.

Cecil studied and worked 16 hours a day. He was extremely well read and had an extensive knowledge of medical disorders. Although he was always able to provide a careful and detailed analysis of a patient's condition, it took him a great deal of time to do so. His diagnoses tended to cover every disorder that each patient could conceivably have, with a detailed focus on all possible combinations of symptoms.

Obsessive-compulsive personality disorder (OCPD) involves a "pervasive pattern of preoccupation with orderliness, perfectionism, and mental and interpersonal control, at the expense of flexibility, openness, and efficiency" (APA, 2022, p. 772). The person's preoccupation with details and rules leads to an inability to grasp the big picture. OCPD is associated with high levels of perfectionism and inflexible personal standards (Redden et al., 2023). There is a heightened focus on being in control over aspects of one's own life and one's emotions; additionally, there is a strong devotion to minor details and a need to control other people. Individuals with OCPD lack flexibility, and their rigid behaviors can significantly impair their occupational and social functioning and affect their quality of life (Gadelkarim et al., 2019). As we saw with Cecil,

Creative Genius and Personality Disorder?

Steve Jobs, respected for his innovative work as former CEO of Apple Inc., was reported to have a perfectionistic and volatile management style. His obsessive preoccupation with details led to the development of leading-edge technology but also resulted in a stressful work environment. He was also known for an intense sense of self-importance and arrogance combined with minimal empathy. These traits have led to speculation that Jobs had obsessive-compulsive and/or narcissistic personality disorder.

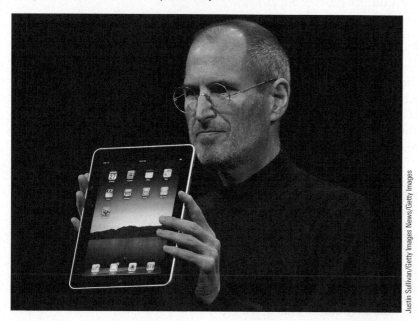

Justin Sullivan/Getty Images News/Getty Images

coworkers may find those with OCPD to be demanding, inflexible, and perfectionistic. In many cases, individuals with OCPD are ineffective on the job, despite devoting long hours to their work.

OCPD is distinct from obsessive-compulsive disorder (OCD), discussed in Chapter 5. The two disorders have similar names, but their clinical manifestations are quite different. Individuals with OCD experience unwanted intrusive thoughts or urges that cause significant distress. On the other hand, OCPD is a pervasive personality and character disturbance. People with OCPD believe their way of functioning is the correct way. They relate to the world through a lens incorporating their own strict standards. Estimates of the prevalence of OCPD range from 2.4 percent to 7.9 percent, and it appears to be equally common in men and women (APA, 2022).

Causes and Treatment Individuals with OCPD have altered activity in parts of the brain that affect rumination, cognitive flexibility, and response switching, a neurological profile that is similar to brain patterns observed among people diagnosed with OCD. This unique pattern of brain functioning accounts for some of the symptoms found in OCPD, such as need for orderliness, inflexibility, and perfectionism (Lei et al., 2020). However, there are distinctive differences in the neurocircuitry associated with the two disorders, which results in different behavioral patterns (Marincowitz et al., 2022). OCPD appears to occur more frequently among family members, which may be due to either genetics or socialization (Blais et al., 2008). Cognitive-behavioral therapy, as well as supportive forms of psychotherapy, has helped some clients with OCPD (Gordon et al., 2016).

The diversity of personality disorders makes it difficult to extensively discuss the etiology and treatment of each. Further, in many cases, we do not have enough knowledge about the disorder to engage in a comprehensive etiological explanation. Yet it is clear that biological, psychological, social, and sociocultural forces influence the development of each personality disorder. In the next section, we use our multipath model to more comprehensively discuss one of the better-researched personality disorders: antisocial personality disorder.

15-3 Multipath Analysis of Antisocial Personality Disorder

Although research on most personality disorders has been quite limited, there is more information about antisocial personality disorder (APD) because APD is prevalent among individuals who are incarcerated for criminal offenses as well as among individuals who are in positions of power (Burkle, 2019).

Thus, there are significant societal consequences associated with this disorder. We use our multipath model to explain how biological, psychological, social, and sociocultural dimensions may interact and contribute to the development of APD, as indicated in Figure 15.1. By focusing on one specific condition, we hope to provide a prototype for understanding the multidimensional development of other personality disorders.

Biological Dimension

The development of APD appears to involve interactions between biological vulnerabilities and environmental adversity. Thus, considerable research has been devoted to trying to uncover the biological and social basis of APD. What has made research difficult is that researchers often combine the two groups of individuals with APD: those who are referred to as "psychopaths" and those who are referred to as "sociopaths" (Dargis & Koenigs, 2018). Interestingly, much of the research conducted is focused on the trait of psychopathy even though it is not a discrete diagnostic category. Only about one third of people with antisocial personality meet the criteria for psychopathy, which include characteristics such as impulsivity, callousness, and a lack of guilt or empathy in addition to antisocial behavior (Abdalla-Filho & Völlm, 2020). Research on antisocial personality is often diluted because of not separating people who have psychopathic traits from the larger group of individuals diagnosed with antisocial personality.

Genetic Influences

Genetic factors are implicated in the development of APD, including behavioral characteristics evident during childhood and adolescence. Support for genetic influences on antisocial behavior comes from

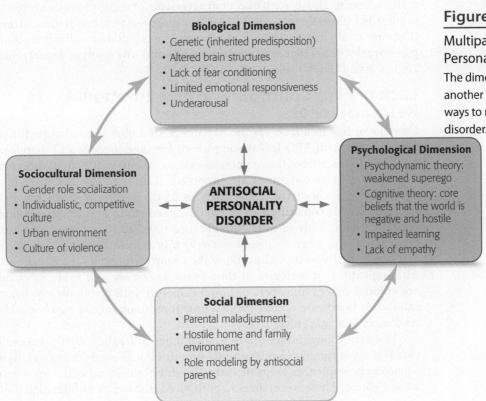

Figure 15.1

Multipath Model of Antisocial Personality Disorder

The dimensions interact with one another and combine in different ways to result in antisocial personality disorder.

Biological Dimension
- Genetic (inherited predisposition)
- Altered brain structures
- Lack of fear conditioning
- Limited emotional responsiveness
- Underarousal

Sociocultural Dimension
- Gender role socialization
- Individualistic, competitive culture
- Urban environment
- Culture of violence

ANTISOCIAL PERSONALITY DISORDER

Psychological Dimension
- Psychodynamic theory: weakened superego
- Cognitive theory: core beliefs that the world is negative and hostile
- Impaired learning
- Lack of empathy

Social Dimension
- Parental maladjustment
- Hostile home and family environment
- Role modeling by antisocial parents

research comparing concordance rates for identical twins with those for fraternal twins. Most studies suggest that identical twins have a higher concordance rate for antisocial tendencies, delinquency, and criminality. In one large twin study, heritability of antisocial traits was estimated to be 51 percent (Rosenström et al., 2017). Further, some children born to biological parents with antisocial personalities but raised by adoptive parents without such a diagnosis still exhibit higher rates of antisocial characteristics (Hyde et al., 2016). Among toddlers ages 14 to 36 months, an early disregard for others (responding to distress from others with anger or aggression) was associated with APD symptoms and psychopathy scores at age 23 years (Rhee et al., 2021).

Neurological Findings

Genetic factors appear to influence structures of the brain involved with characteristics such as fearlessness, anxiety, and empathy. Structural abnormalities have been found in the prefrontal cortex and parts of the limbic system that could explain the characteristic of emotional detachment as well as aggression and impulsivity (Raine, 2018). Much of this research appears to focus on "psychopaths," individuals with APD who exhibit callous-unemotional behavior. Among one group of incarcerated men, neuroimaging revealed reductions in gray matter in specific regions of the prefrontal cortex and temporal lobes—areas associated with empathy, moral reasoning, and prosocial emotions such as guilt and embarrassment. Abnormalities were also found in the nerve pathways linking the posterior cingulate cortex to the medial prefrontal cortex; these areas are associated with learning from rewards and punishment and may explain why people with psychopathic tendencies display atypical responses to positive and negative stimuli (Gregory et al., 2015).

Interestingly, functional magnetic resonance imaging (fMRI) studies have found hypersensitivity to threat (e.g., increased amygdala activity) among individuals with APD who do not possess the callous-unemotional trait, whereas those with the characteristic of callousness exhibited diminished physiological responsivity in response to interpersonal stress (Dotterer et al., 2019). These findings would explain why individuals with psychopathic traits demonstrate fearlessness and low levels of anxiety and are not afraid to take risks.

Lack of Fear Conditioning and Emotional Responsiveness

One line of research involves the hypothesis that biological abnormalities make people with APD less susceptible to fear and anxiety and therefore less likely to learn from their experiences in situations in which punishment or other negative outcomes are involved (Raine, 2018). Because they have less fear about the consequences of their actions, they are less likely to learn to distinguish between appropriate and inappropriate behaviors. One study of over 700,000 men revealed that a low heart rate (associated with lower fear and anxiety) was associated with criminality and psychopathy—especially among the group with the lowest heart rate. Although the vast majority of those who have very low heart rates do not commit crimes (members of bomb dispersal units also have low heart rates), low heart rate is considered a potential biomarker of psychopathic tendencies (Latvala et al., 2015).

In a major longitudinal study, Gao and her colleagues (2010) reasoned that fear conditioning in response to stimuli such as punishment or other negative consequences helps us learn to inhibit antisocial behavior when we are young. These researchers hypothesized that deficient functioning of the amygdala, the part of the brain involved in fear conditioning, might make it difficult for some people to recognize cues that signal threats, making them appear fearless and unconcerned about consequences. Poor fear conditioning would thus predispose individuals to antisocial behavior. Recognizing that this should be detectable early in life, the researchers tested fear conditioning (physiological responses to an unpleasant noise) in children at age 3 using skin conductance measures of fear and arousal. They then probed the association between these findings and adult criminal behavior 20 years later. They found that the research subjects who had criminal records at the time of the follow-up (age 23) had failed to display fear conditioning in early childhood. These findings support the possibility that people with APD never become conditioned to aversive stimuli; thus, they experience little anticipatory anxiety, fail to acquire avoidance behaviors, and consequently have fewer inhibitions about engaging in antisocial behavior.

Similarly, youth exhibiting antisocial behaviors demonstrated diminished reactivity in the amygdala when shown pictures depicting fearful facial expressions, a finding that may partially explain why "psychopaths" lack compassion and demonstrate little emotions toward others (Brouns et al., 2013). In another study using MRI scans, youth scoring high on psychopathic traits were compared with matched controls in their reactions to photos of painful injuries; participants were asked to imagine that the body in the photograph was theirs and, in another condition, that it belonged to someone else. As compared to the healthy controls, the youth with psychopathic traits displayed less activity in the anterior cingulate cortex and amygdala when they were imagining that the injury involved another person. Thus, they appeared to demonstrate lower levels of emotional empathy to the plight of others (Marsh et al., 2013).

Individuals with psychopathic traits appear to have a diminished capacity to experience and identify emotions. They have difficulty distinguishing between emotional facial expressions such as sadness

Risk-Taking and Thrill-Seeking Behaviors

People with low anxiety levels are often thrill seekers. The difference between a risk-taking "psychopath" and an adventurer may largely be a matter of whether the thrill-seeking behaviors are channeled into destructive or constructive acts.

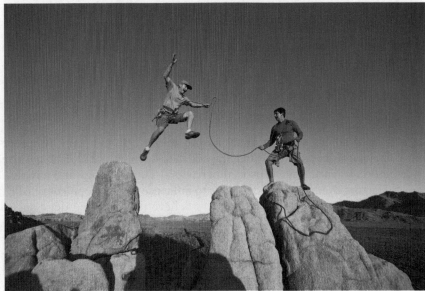

Greg Epperson/Shutterstock.com

and fear, and even have difficulty identifying positive emotions (Kyranides et al., 2022). Further, when listening to emotionally themed music, individuals high in psychopathic characteristics had difficulty identifying any feelings associated with the music (Plate et al., 2023).

Psychological Dimension

Psychological explanations of APD fall into three camps: psychodynamic, cognitive, and learning perspectives.

Psychodynamic Perspectives

According to psychodynamic approaches, faulty superego development may cause those with APD to experience little guilt; they are, therefore, more prone to frequent violations of moral and ethical standards. Thus, the personalities of people with APD are dominated by id impulses that operate primarily from the pleasure principle; they impulsively seek immediate gratification and have minimal regard for others (Millon et al., 2004). People exhibiting antisocial behavior patterns presumably did not adequately identify with their parents and thus did not internalize the morals and values of society. Additionally, frustration, rejection, or inconsistent discipline may have resulted in fixation at an early stage of development.

Cognitive Perspectives

Certain core beliefs, and the ways these beliefs influence behavior, are emphasized in cognitive explanations of APD (Bhar et al., 2012). These core beliefs operate on an unconscious level, occur automatically, and influence emotions and behaviors. Beck and colleagues (1990, p. 361) summarized typical cognitions associated with APD:

- I have to look out for myself.
- Force or cunning is the best way to get things done.
- Lying and cheating are okay as long as you don't get caught.
- I have been unfairly treated and am entitled to get my fair share by whatever means I can.
- Other people are weak and deserve to be taken.
- I should do whatever I can get away with.
- I can get away with things, so I don't need to worry about bad consequences.

These thoughts arise from what Beck and colleagues refer to as a "predatory strategy." Thus, the worldview of those with APD revolves around a need to perceive themselves as strong and independent so they can survive in a competitive, hostile, and unforgiving world.

Learning Perspectives

Learning theories suggest that people with APD (1) have inherent neurobiological characteristics that impede their learning and (2) lack positive role models to encourage prosocial behaviors. Thus, biology and environmental factors combine in unique ways to influence the development of APD.

As we have seen, some researchers believe that learning deficiencies among individuals with APD are caused by the absence of fear or anxiety and by lowered autonomic reactivity. If so, is it possible to improve their learning by increasing their anxiety or arousal ability? In a now classic study, researchers designed two conditions in which those with APD and control participants performed an avoidance-learning task, with electric shock as the unconditioned stimulus (Schachter & Latané, 1964). Under one condition, participants were injected with adrenaline, which presumably increases arousal; under the other, they were injected with a placebo. Those with APD who received the placebo made more errors in avoiding the shocks than did controls; however, after receiving adrenaline, they tended to perform better than controls. These findings imply that those with APD are more able to learn from negative consequences when their anxiety or arousal is increased.

The *kind* of punishment used in avoidance learning is also an important consideration in evaluating learning deficiencies in those with APD. Whereas those with APD may display learning deficits when faced with physical (electric shock) or social (negative verbal feedback) punishments, they learn as well as controls when the punishment is monetary loss (Schmauk, 1970).

Social Dimension

Among the many factors that are implicated in ASD, relationships within the family—the primary agent of socialization—are paramount in the development of antisocial patterns. Some studies have found that adults with the callous-unemotional trait report a childhood history of emotional and physical maltreatment that is particularly severe. Maltreatment during childhood may impair the child's ability to relate to others or learn socially appropriate behaviors. Further, if the child doesn't have positive role models or perceive adults as supportive and caring, they may not learn to understand the feelings of others or to take other people's perspectives into consideration (Dargis & Koenigs, 2018). On the other hand, nurturing parenting can help minimize antisocial traits. In an adoption study, children from mothers with severe antisocial behavior were placed with adoptive mothers. Researchers, who rated these adoptive mothers on the frequency with which they used positive reinforcement during parenting interactions, found there were fewer callous-unemotional behaviors when adoptive mothers provided high levels of positive reinforcement. Thus, providing positive reinforcement appeared to be protective against the genetic expression of traits associated with APD (Hyde et al., 2016).

Sociocultural Dimension

A variety of sociodemographic variables, including gender, social class, and ethnicity, are important in personality development. Determining the relative impact of sociocultural factors on APD, however, is complicated.

Gender

Men are more likely to exhibit characteristics of APD compared to women. Thus, there may be different pathways to developing APD that exist along gender lines. For example, women with APD are more likely to report childhood emotional neglect, sexual abuse, and parental use of substances compared to men with APD. Gender also influences the way APD is expressed. Conventional gender-role socialization by parents may influence antisocial behaviors in children. In many cultural groups, aggressive behavior in boys is accepted or even encouraged, whereas girls are socialized to avoid aggression; this may explain why antisocial patterns involving aggression are more prevalent among men than among women (Alegria et al., 2013).

Whereas men tend to engage in direct acting-out behaviors (e.g., physical aggression), women express themselves in an indirect or

A Successful Psychopath?

Bernard L. Madoff exhibits all the traits of a person with antisocial personality disorder and has often been labeled "a successful psychopath." He lied to family, friends, and investors; manipulated people; experienced feelings of grandiosity; and had a callous disregard for the people that he swindled. A seemingly respected power broker on Wall Street, he is reported to have bilked investors out of some $50 billion. He was convicted on 17 felony counts, and on June 29, 2009, he was sentenced to 150 years in prison.

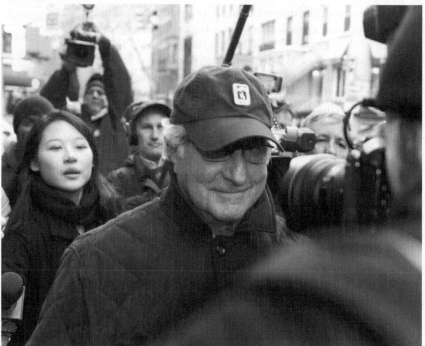

Don Emmert/AFP/Getty Images

passive manner (e.g., spreading rumors or false gossip and rejecting others from their social group), behavior that is referred to as *relational aggression* (Ehlers et al., 2022). Other gender differences exist. Men with APD are more likely to exhibit job problems, violence, and traffic offenses, whereas women with APD are more likely to report relationship and occupational problems, engaging in forgery, and harassing or threatening others (Alegria et al., 2013). As gender roles continue to change, it is possible that antisocial tendencies similar to men will increase among women.

Other Sociocultural Influences

APD occurs much more frequently in urban environments than in rural areas and among people living in poverty. Living in populated, urban neighborhoods increases the risk of exposure to toxins that are associated with neurobiological effects such as lower IQ and antisocial behaviors (Carpenter & Nevin, 2010). Rates of APD appear to be relatively similar across ethnic groups (Ehlers et al., 2022).

Exposure to ethnic-political violence can also result in the development of violent and antisocial behavior. In a study involving Jewish Israeli and Palestinian youth, cumulative exposure to ethnic-political violence during childhood, adolescence, and early adulthood resulted in an increased likelihood of participating in acts such as choking someone, cutting or threating someone with a knife, shooting or threatening someone with a gun, or participating in violent demonstrations. Palestinian youth, the group with the most direct exposure to ethnic-political violence during their formative years, had higher levels of aggressive behaviors and antisocial tendencies. Although the Palestinian youth directed their animosity and dangerous actions toward their perceived enemies, their early exposure to violence appeared to result in increased aggressive tendencies and less remorse over violent encounters (Dubow et al., 2019).

Any assessment of personality functioning must consider ethnic, cultural, and social influences. For example, to be raised in the United States is to be exposed to the standards, beliefs, and values of U.S. society. One dominant value is that of rugged individualism, which involves two assumptions: (a) individualism and independence are viewed as aspects of healthy functioning and (b) people can and should master and control their own lives (Sue et al., 2022). In a capitalistic society, competition and the ability to effectively control the environment are considered pathways to success; achievement is measured by surpassing the attainment of others. In the extreme, this psychological orientation may fuel the manipulative and dominating behaviors of people with APD, resulting in business executives and political figures who are driven by narrow personal interests without concern for broader societal consequences.

Treatment of Antisocial Personality Disorder

APD is not an easy condition to treat because people with the disorder often consider their amoral actions as acceptable and, therefore, believe they have no need to change their behavior or seek treatment. Thus, traditional treatment approaches, which require the genuine cooperation of clients, are often ineffective for those with APD (Koelch et al., 2019). Treatment is most likely to be effective in structured settings in which behavior can be observed and regulated; this provides more opportunities for mental health professionals to assist individuals with APD to recognize how their behavior affects others and to confront their inability to form close relationships. An opportunity to change long-standing patterns of behavior sometimes occurs when individuals with APD are incarcerated, enter inpatient substance abuse programs, or undergo psychiatric hospitalization.

The most effective treatments for APD focus on decreasing deviant activities, combined with opportunities to practice appropriate social skills. Based on the assumption that antisocial behaviors are learned, these treatment programs attempt to modify inappropriate actions by setting rules and enforcing consequences for rule violations; they also teach participants to anticipate consequences of behaviors and practice new ways of interacting with others (Meloy, 2001). Historically, the use of material rewards has been fairly effective in changing antisocial behaviors under controlled conditions. For instance, program participants often earn tokens for prosocial behavior and then exchange the tokens for desired goods or privileges. These behavior modification programs are sometimes used for those at risk of developing APD, such as juvenile offenders with antisocial traits who have limited understanding of the social and interpersonal consequences of their behavior. However, without community and family support for behavioral changes after treatment, youth who have been successful in a structured setting may quickly revert to previous patterns of antisocial behavior.

Treating Antisocial Behaviors

Family members are critically important in the treatment of youth with antisocial personality traits. Here, a therapist celebrates the development of closer connections within this family unit.

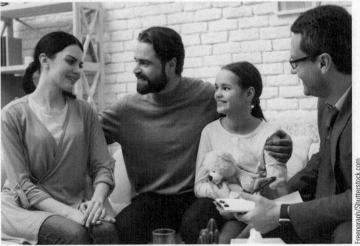

Freeograph/Shutterstock.com

Cognitive approaches are also used in treatment. Because individuals with APD are often influenced by dysfunctional beliefs about themselves, the world, and the future, they have difficulty anticipating possible negative outcomes of their behaviors. Beck et al. (1990) encouraged therapists to build rapport with their clients with APD, and then attempt to guide them away from thinking only in terms of self-interest and immediate gratification and toward broader social concerns. For example, therapists might assist clients to develop a sense of responsibility by helping them understand how their behavior affects others. For one group of individuals with APD and a comorbid substance-use disorder, a brief psychoeducational therapy was helpful in improving both conditions. The manualized program involved (1) identifying thoughts and behaviors related to APD, (2) linking the problematic behaviors to the consequences experienced by the individual and others, (3) discussing how behaviors are related to a dysfunctional belief system, (4) examining how a person's values can support or prevent lifestyle changes, and (5) determining how a person's social network can support or hinder goals for change. In follow-up evaluations, individuals who received this form of treatment had more days of abstinence, were less likely to drop out of treatment, and had higher levels of treatment satisfaction (Thylstrup et al., 2017).

Current treatment options for people with APD are only minimally effective. No evidence-based interventions exist for APD, although promising results have been reported with dialectical behavior therapy, schema-focused therapy, and cognitive-behavioral therapy. However, because APD encompasses a spectrum of characteristics such as psychopathy, it is uncertain which therapies might be effective for those with different symptom profiles (De Wit-De Visser et al., 2023). Although medication is usually used only when there are comorbid conditions such as depression or substance abuse, there have been some promising results with the use of clozapine (an atypical antipsychotic) to reduce impulsive and violent behaviors in a small sample of violent men with APD who were incarcerated in a high-security hospital setting (Brown et al., 2014).

Going Deeper

Sociocultural Considerations in the Assessment of Personality Disorders

In diagnosing a personality disorder, it is important to consider the individual's cultural norms and expectations when determining whether personality traits are maladaptive (APA, 2022). Because culture shapes our habits, customs, values, and personality characteristics, expressions of personality in one culture often differ from those in another culture. Asians in Asia, for example, are more likely to exhibit social constraint and *collectivism*, whereas U.S. Americans are more likely to display assertiveness and individualism (Sue et al., 2022). Japanese people and individuals from India often display overtly dependent, submissive, and socially conforming behaviors, traits that have negative connotations in U.S. society. Does this mean that the people in Japan and India who conform to their country's societal norms have a personality disorder? Of course not. The behaviors of dependence and submissiveness are influenced by cultural values and norms and, thus, would not reflect personality psychopathology. In fact, in these countries, these traits are considered desirable personality characteristics. As you can see, anyone making judgments about personality functioning and disturbance must consider the individual's cultural, ethnic, and social background.

Not surprisingly, there are differences in the prevalence and types of personality disorders between countries. For instance, although obsessive-compulsive personality disorder is one of the most prevalent personality disorders in the United States and Australia, schizotypal personality disorder is the most common disorder in Iceland and avoidant personality disorder is most prevalent in Norway (Sansone & Sansone, 2011). Additionally, low rates of most personality disorders are found in Asian countries (Ryder et al., 2014). What do you think might account for these differences?

15-4 Issues with Diagnosing Personality Psychopathology

Diagnosing personality disorders using the current diagnostic system is challenging for multiple reasons. First, there is poor interrater reliability for the personality disorder categories. Although diagnosticians generally agree on whether a particular client has a personality disorder, there is less consensus regarding the precise type of personality disorder. One of the reasons this occurs is because the different personality disorders have overlapping symptoms. A person who is diagnosed with paranoid personality disorder, for instance, may also have symptoms of and can meet the diagnostic criteria for other personality disorders, such as schizotypal, borderline, narcissistic, avoidant, and obsessive-compulsive personality disorders. Thus, for a specific client, one clinician might diagnose a paranoid personality disorder, whereas another therapist might consider the same set of behaviors and diagnose a borderline personality. The individual might even receive both diagnoses. As you can see, the reliability of the personality disorder categories is a significant concern (Chmielewski et al., 2017).

Second, comorbidity (the presence of other disorders) is high with personality disorders, which also reduces diagnostic accuracy. Up to 35 percent of those with PTSD, 47 percent with panic disorder with agoraphobia or generalized anxiety, 48 percent with social anxiety disorder, and 52 percent with obsessive-compulsive disorder also have a personality disorder (Latas & Milovanovic, 2014). Additionally, disorders such as depression, bipolar disorder, and substance-use disorders often accompany personality disorders. When personality disorders are comorbid with other disorders, the other disorders are more likely to be diagnosed rather than the personality disorder (Westen et al., 2010).

Third, as we discussed in Chapter 4, an exclusive categorical approach has limitations because categorical diagnoses: (1) are based on arbitrary diagnostic thresholds, (2) use an all-or-none method of classification, and (3) do not take into account the continuous nature of personality traits. In reality, we all exhibit some of the traits that characterize personality disorders—for example, suspiciousness, dependency, sensitivity to rejection, or compulsiveness—but not to an extreme degree. We will now discuss an alternative method of determining personality psychopathology that has been proposed as a response to these diagnostic issues.

15-5 Dimensional Personality Assessment and the DSM Alternative Personality Model

In response to the concerns with categorical diagnosis and problems with the reliability and validity of the personality disorder diagnostic categories, the DSM-5 Work Group that was tasked with evaluating personality disorders proposed discarding the traditional categorical system of personality disorders we have reviewed in this chapter. They recommended substituting a dimensional model that would involve looking at personality traits on a continuum; under the proposed alternative model, people with maladaptive and pathological personality traits would receive a personality disorder diagnosis if they displayed a significant degree of impairment in personality functioning. In other words, the clinician would determine if the person had enough of certain traits to qualify as having a personality disorder. The DSM-5 Personality Work Group cited experts in the field of personality who view personality disorders as the extremes of a continuum of normal personality traits. This is the position taken among the authors of ICD 11, the updated version of the International Classification of Disease developed by the World Health Organization; the ICD 11 now uses a dimensional system for personality disorders instead of categorical descriptions (Bach & First, 2018).

The dimensional or trait model considers significant deviations from normal on five key personality dimensions to be the best way to conceptualize personality disorders (Widiger & Crego, 2019). The five major dimensions of personality along which individuals vary are:

- Negative affectivity (as opposed to emotional stability)
- Detachment (as opposed to extraversion)
- Antagonism (as opposed to agreeableness)
- Disinhibition (as opposed to conscientiousness)
- Psychoticism (as opposed to lucidity)

A dimensional approach such as this allows clinicians to consider the degree to which a client possesses specific traits rather than deciding whether or not the client meets the diagnostic criteria for a specific disorder as occurs with a categorical diagnosis. Using a dimensional approach, clinicians can assess clients on particular traits and then rate the extent to which they possess each characteristic. For instance, rather than deciding if a client meets the diagnostic criteria for a schizoid personality disorder, the clinician could instead describe the client as possessing varying degrees of personality traits such as social withdrawal, social detachment, intimacy avoidance, and so forth.

Although the DSM-5 Personality Work Group favored replacing the categorical system with this dimensional, trait-based model, many clinicians expressed concerns about the complete removal of the traditional diagnostic categories for personality disorders. In particular, clinicians opposed the deletion of certain categories because of their high usage and clinical utility. For example, the following are the percentages of clinicians who reported using each of these specific personality categories: borderline (92 percent), antisocial (61 percent), narcissistic (57 percent), and avoidant (51 percent) (Pull, 2013).

In a highly unusual move, the APA Board of Trustees decided to retain the categorical framework of 10 personality disorders in the main text of the DSM-5 and to include an alternative model for personality disorder diagnosis in a separate section of the DSM-5. This alternative model retains some of the categorical diagnoses in a modified form (6 of the 10 traditional personality disorders were retained) but also includes a dimensional classification system based on personality traits. The rationale for including both the traditional and the alternative models of personality disorder diagnosis was to "preserve continuity with current clinical practice, while also introducing a new approach that aims to address numerous shortcomings of the current personality disorders" (APA, 2022, p. 881). Clinicians can choose to use the traditional categorical model or the alternative model when making a personality disorder diagnosis.

The alternative model of personality disorders removed four of the more problematic personality disorders—paranoid, schizoid, histrionic, and dependent. Justification for their removal was based primarily on three lines of evidence:

1. an absence of research on these disorders, making their existence as distinct entities questionable;

2. excessive co-occurrence with other personality disorders, making it difficult to differentiate between the different disorders; and

3. the highly questionable reliability and validity of these four categories.

Does eliminating certain personality types mean there are no longer paranoid, withdrawn, superficially emotional, or dependent persons who qualify as having a personality disorder? The answer is no. The new model allows these traits to be considered in a noncategorical fashion. Table 15.3 outlines the four personality disorders that were removed, contrasting the traditional categorical definitions with how they would be described using the alternative approach.

The DSM-Alternative Personality Model

With the DSM alternative personality model, a diagnosis of personality disorder can be made through two different routes (refer to Figure 15.2):

1. evidence that the client's pattern of personality traits matches characteristics from one of six specific personality disorder types (antisocial, avoidant, borderline, narcissistic, obsessive-compulsive, or schizotypal); or

2. evidence of at least moderate impairment in two key domains of personality functioning (identity, self-direction, empathy, or intimacy) combined with certain specific pathological personality traits.

With both routes, the personality disorder or descriptive personality traits must be maladaptive and result in at least moderate impairment in personal or interpersonal functioning. When using the alternative system to diagnose a personality disorder, clinicians first ask the following questions: Does the person have impairment in personality functioning? If so, how severe is the impairment? To make diagnostic decisions, the clinician begins by carefully assessing four key areas related to personal and interpersonal personality functioning:

- *Identity*: Sense of personal uniqueness, with clear boundaries between oneself and others; capacity to regulate one's emotions; accurate self-appraisal and stable self-esteem

- *Self-direction*: Focus on meaningful goals, using self-reflection and positive standards of behavior

- *Empathy*: Understanding of and tolerance for others' feelings and perspectives; comprehension of the effects of one's behavior on others

- *Intimacy*: Capacity and desire for interpersonal closeness and deep connection with others; respectful interpersonal behavior

Table 15.3 DSM-5 Personality Disorders and Domain-Trait Descriptions

	DSM-5 Categorical Diagnosis	DSM-5 Alternative Trait Description
Paranoid personality disorder	People with paranoid personality disorder: • display unwarranted suspiciousness, hypersensitivity, and reluctance to trust others; and • interpret others' motives as being malevolent, question their loyalty or trustworthiness, persistently bear grudges, or are suspicious of the actions of others.	• The person is described in terms of personality: disorder traits such as *suspiciousness, intimacy avoidance, hostility,* and *unusual beliefs*.
Schizoid personality disorder	People with schizoid personality disorder: • exhibit social isolation, emotional coldness, and indifference to others; • have a long history of impairment of social functioning; • are reclusive and withdrawn; • do not desire or enjoy close relationships, and have few activities that provide pleasure; and • are perceived as peculiar and aloof and therefore inadequate as dating or marital partners due to lack of capacity or desire to form social relationships.	• The person is described in terms of personality disorder traits such as *social withdrawal, social detachment, intimacy avoidance, restricted affectivity,* and *anhedonia*.
Histrionic personality disorder	People with histrionic personality disorder: • engage in self-dramatization, exaggerated expression of emotions, and attention-seeking behaviors; • behave flamboyantly or flirtatiously for attention; • are typically shallow and egocentric, in spite of superficial warmth and charm; and • display emotions well beyond acceptable cultural norms.	• The person is described in terms of personality disorder traits such as *emotional lability* and *histrionism*.
Dependent personality disorder	People with dependent personality disorder: • lack self-confidence and subordinate their needs to those of the people on whom they depend; • are fearful of taking the initiative on most matters; • are afraid of disrupting their relationships with others; • perceive themselves as inherently inadequate and unable to cope; • believe they should find someone who can take care of them; and • often experience feelings of depression, helplessness, and suppressed anger.	• The person is described in terms of personality disorder traits such as *submissiveness, anxiousness,* and *separation insecurity*.

With a DSM categorical diagnosis, the diagnosis is made if the person meets the listed diagnostic criteria. With the alternative trait model, the clinician determines if there is at least moderate impairment in personality functioning in the areas of identity, self-direction, empathy, or intimacy combined with clinical judgment or norm-based assessment that confirms an elevation in pathological personality traits involving 1 of the 5 trait domains or the 25 trait facets.

Source: APA, 2022

The clinician measures personality functioning in each of these areas using the DSM five-point Levels of Personality Functioning Scale. Using this scale and interviews or other assessment tools, the clinician rates the client on the aforementioned personality characteristics of identity, self-direction, empathy, and intimacy; in each area, the rating

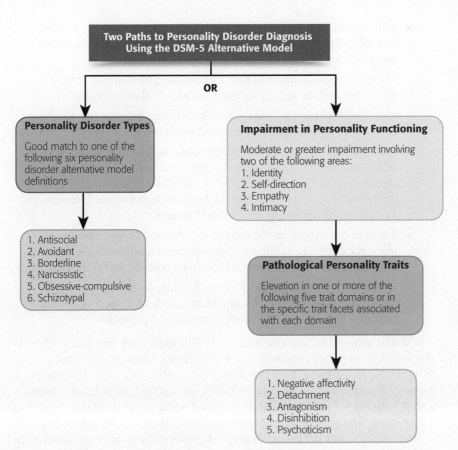

Two Paths to Personality Disorder Diagnosis Using the DSM-5 Alternative Model

OR

Personality Disorder Types

Good match to one of the following six personality disorder alternative model definitions

1. Antisocial
2. Avoidant
3. Borderline
4. Narcissistic
5. Obsessive-compulsive
6. Schizotypal

Impairment in Personality Functioning

Moderate or greater impairment involving two of the following areas:
1. Identity
2. Self-direction
3. Empathy
4. Intimacy

Pathological Personality Traits

Elevation in one or more of the following five trait domains or in the specific trait facets associated with each domain

1. Negative affectivity
2. Detachment
3. Antagonism
4. Disinhibition
5. Psychoticism

indicates if there is *no impairment*, or *mild*, *moderate*, *serious*, or *extreme* impairment.

These four key areas of personal and interpersonal personality functioning are addressed when a clinician uses the alternative model to diagnose someone who meets the description of one of the six personality types retained in the alternative model (antisocial, avoidant, borderline, narcissistic, obsessive-compulsive, or schizotypal). Let's take a diagnosis of antisocial personality disorder using the alternative model as an example (APA, 2022, pp. 884–885):

1. Moderate or greater impairment in personality functioning, manifested by characteristic difficulties in two or more of the following four areas:

   - *Identity*: Egocentrism; self-esteem derived from personal gain, power, or pleasure

   - *Self-direction*: Goal setting based on personal gratification; absence of prosocial internal standards and resultant failure to conform to lawful or culturally normative ethical behavior

   - *Empathy*: Lack of concern for feelings, needs, or suffering of others; lack of remorse after hurting or mistreating another

   - *Intimacy*: Incapacity for mutually intimate relationships, as exploitation is a primary means of relating to others, including by deceit and coercion; use of dominance or intimidation to control others

2. Six or more of the following seven pathological personality traits:

   - *Manipulativeness*: Frequent use of subterfuge to influence or control others; use of seduction, charm, glibness, or ingratiation to achieve one's ends

- *Callousness*: Lack of concern for feelings or problems of others; lack of guilt or remorse about the negative or harmful effects of one's actions on others; aggression; sadism
- *Deceitfulness*: Dishonesty and fraudulence; misrepresentation of self; embellishment or fabrication when relating events
- *Hostility*: Persistent or frequent angry feelings; anger or irritability in response to minor slights and insults; mean, nasty, or vengeful behavior
- *Risk taking*: Engagement in dangerous, risky, and potentially self-damaging activities, unnecessarily and without regard for consequences; boredom proneness and thoughtless initiation of activities to counter boredom; lack of concern for one's limitations and denial of the reality of personal danger
- *Impulsivity*: Acting on the spur of the moment in response to immediate stimuli; acting on a momentary basis without a plan or consideration of outcomes; difficulty establishing and following plans
- *Irresponsibility*: Disregard for—and failure to honor—financial and other obligations or commitments; lack of respect for—and lack of follow-through on—agreements and promises

When clinicians use the alternative model, they not only address the four key areas of personal and interpersonal personality functioning (illustrated in Criteria 1 of the above example), but they also assess a variety of pathological personality traits, including 5 broad trait domains and 25 facets (specific traits) associated with these domains (refer to Table 15.4). The second part of the diagnostic criteria in the above example (Criteria 2) focuses on the pathological personality traits associated with antisocial personality disorder. For each of these traits, the clinician uses clinical judgment or norm-based psychological testing to decide if there is a significant elevation or deviation from the norm in these traits.

Table 15.4 DSM-5 Trait Domains and Related Trait Facets

1. *Negative affectivity* refers to a wide range of negative emotions—such as anxiety, depression, guilt, shame, worry, and so forth—and the behavioral or interpersonal manifestations of those experiences. Emotional stability is the opposite end of this domain. The specific trait facets associated with this domain are:
   - emotional lability, anxiousness, separation insecurity, submissiveness, hostility, perseveration, depressivity, suspiciousness, and restricted emotions.

2. *Detachment* involves withdrawal from others, whether the relationships are with intimate acquaintances or strangers. It includes restricted or limited emotional experiences and expressions, especially hedonic capacity (i.e., an inability to experience pleasure or joys in life). Extraversion is the opposite end of this domain. The specific trait facets associated with this domain are:
   - withdrawal, avoidance of intimacy, lack of pleasure (anhedonia), depressivity, restricted emotions, and suspiciousness.

3. *Antagonism* refers to negative feelings and behaviors toward others and a corresponding exaggerated sense of self-importance and entitlement. Agreeableness is the opposite end of this domain. The specific trait facets associated with this domain are:
   - manipulativeness, deceitfulness, grandiosity, attention seeking, callousness, and hostility.

4. *Disinhibition* involves orientation to the present (including current internal and external stimuli) and seeking immediate gratification. Past learning or future consequences seem minimally important. Conscientiousness is the opposite end of this domain. The specific traits associated with this domain are:
   - irresponsibility, impulsivity, distractibility, risk taking, and lack of rigid perfectionism.

5. *Psychoticism* includes behaviors, perceptions, and thoughts or beliefs considered odd, unusual, or bizarre. Lucidity is the opposite end of this domain. The specific traits associated with this domain are:
   - unusual beliefs and experiences, eccentricity, and cognitive and perceptual dysregulation.

Source: Based on information from APA, 2022

Clinicians can also assess these same aspects of personal and interpersonal personality functioning and pathological traits when working with clients who have another categorical diagnosis; even if a clinician does not believe a client has a personality disorder, assessment of personality traits can provide valuable insight into areas that might interfere with optimal functioning and thus provide guidance for treatment planning.

15-6 Contemporary Trends and Future Directions

Personality disorders are considered to be "enduring," "stable," and of "long duration" (APA, 2022). However, studies raise questions about these descriptions because research data suggest that personality disorders appear to remit (diminish) more often than previously believed (Conway et al., 2017; Paris, 2015). Although many individuals with personality disorders display minimal change or only slow improvement in their maladaptive personality traits, some individuals with personality disorders exhibit rapid symptom remission. In fact, a meta-analysis focused on the stability of personality

Going Deeper

What Personality Traits Best Apply to This Man?

The following case study describes the behavior of a teenager, Roy W. He exhibits some very prominent maladaptive personality traits. After reading the case, consider Roy's personality traits.

What are Roy's most prominent personality characteristics? If you were making a diagnosis, would a categorical or a dimensional perspective be best in attempting to describe and diagnose Roy's condition?

Roy W. is an 18-year-old high school senior who was referred by the court for diagnosis and evaluation after he was arrested for stealing a car, something he had done on several previous occasions. The court agreed with Roy's mother that he needed evaluation and perhaps psychotherapy. The psychologist who interviewed Roy described him as articulate, relaxed, and even witty. He said that stealing was wrong but assured her that he never damaged any of the stolen cars. The last theft occurred because he needed transportation to a beer party (which was located only a mile from his home) and his leg was sore from playing basketball. When the psychologist asked Roy how he got along with young women, he grinned and explained that it is easy to "hustle" them. He then related the following incident.

"About three months ago, I was pulling out of the school parking lot real fast and accidentally sideswiped this other car. The girl who was driving it started to scream at me. God, there was only a small dent on her fender! Anyway, we exchanged names and addresses and I apologized for the accident. When I filled out the accident report later, I said that it was her car that pulled out and hit my car. When she heard about my claim that it was her fault, she had her old man call me. He said that his daughter had witnesses to the accident and that I could be arrested. Bull, he was just trying to bluff me. But I gave him a sob story—about how my parents were ready to get a divorce, how poor we were, and the trouble I would get into if they found out about the accident. I apologized for lying and told him I could fix the dent. Luckily, he never checked with my folks for the real story. Anyway, I went over to look at the girl's car. I really didn't have any idea of how to fix that old heap, so I said I had to wait a couple of weeks to get some tools for the repair job.

"Meanwhile, I started to talk to the girl. Gave her my sob story, told her how nice I thought her folks were. We started to date and I took her out three times. Then one night I laid her. The crummy thing was that she told her folks about it. Can you imagine that? Anyway, her old man called and told me never to get near his precious little thing again. At least I didn't have to fix her old heap. I know I shouldn't lie, but can you blame me? People make such a big deal out of nothing."

disorder diagnoses concluded that about half of individuals with personality disorders will not retain their diagnosis over time (d'Huart et al., 2023). Those with the most rapid symptom improvement have fewer comorbid conditions (Hallquist & Lenzenweger, 2013). Researchers are attempting to discover the reason for the different trajectories for personality disorders. In general, research suggests a less pessimistic outlook for individuals with personality psychopathology than was previously believed.

As you could discern from the description of the DSM alternative model for assessing personality, it is a very complex system. It will be interesting to follow the research arising from this alternative model and to monitor how frequently clinicians use the alternative diagnostic system. The decision to have two parallel diagnostic systems resulted from an impasse that developed between the DSM-5 Work Group, who advocated for the dimensional classification system, and clinicians, who prefer the traditional categorical system. It is difficult to argue against the Work Group recommendations, since research has found that many, if not most, of the traditional personality disorder categories have low reliability and validity. However, since clinicians strongly favored the traditional categorical model and resisted a change to a dimensional system, it remains to be seen if mental health practitioners working outside of research settings will use the alternative methods of diagnosis (though this may change because some clinicians use the ICD 11 for insurance billing). Thus, a major question that remains is whether having two systems to diagnose personality disorders will encourage research into the etiology and treatment of personality disorders or lead to further confusion and more heated debate. Some believe that there are advantages and disadvantages to both systems and that it is time for the diagnosis of personality disorders to "evolve to the next level" (Huprich, 2018). Many hope that that the alternative model of personality disorders will advance research despite the challenges that remain regarding how personality disorders are defined and assessed (Livesley, 2022).

Chapter Summary

1 **Can one's personality be pathological?**

- Personality psychopathology involves inflexible, long-standing personality traits that cause impairment or adaptive failure in the person's everyday life. These traits are usually evident in adolescence and continue into adulthood.

2 **What traits are associated with personality disorders?**

- The DSM lists 10 specific personality disorders associated with notable impairment in social or occupational functioning or significant distress for the person.

- The three personality disorders considered odd or eccentric are paranoid personality disorder (suspiciousness, hypersensitivity, and mistrust), schizoid personality disorder (social isolation and indifference to others), and schizotypal personality disorder (peculiar thoughts and behaviors).

- The four personality disorders considered dramatic, emotional, or erratic are antisocial personality disorder (failure to conform to social or legal codes of conduct), borderline personality disorder (intense mood and self-image fluctuations), histrionic personality disorder (self-dramatization and attention-seeking behaviors), and narcissistic personality disorder (exaggerated sense of self-importance and lack of empathy).

- The three personality disorders involving anxiety and fearfulness are avoidant personality disorder (fear of rejection and humiliation), dependent personality disorder (reliance on others and inability to assume responsibility), and obsessive-compulsive personality disorder (perfectionism and interpersonal control).

3 **How does an antisocial personality develop, and can it be changed?**

- Etiological explanations for antisocial personality disorder focus on genetics and neurobiological factors (e.g., lack of fear conditioning and physiological underarousal); psychological factors (beliefs that the world is hostile); social and family environments (antisocial role models); and sociocultural factors (e.g., gender roles and cultural focus on individualism).

- Traditional treatment approaches are not particularly effective with antisocial personality disorder. Treatment is most effective when it occurs in a setting in which behavior can be closely monitored and controlled.

4 **What problems occur with personality assessment?**

- There is poor interrater reliability with the personality disorder categories.

- Diagnosis is complicated by the fact that comorbidity (the presence of other disorders) is high with personality disorders.

- Categorical diagnoses are based on arbitrary diagnostic thresholds and do not take into account the continuous nature of personality traits.

5 **Are there alternative methods of personality assessment?**

- Increasingly, personality disorders are being viewed in a dimensional manner (e.g., as extremes on a continuum of normal personality traits).

- An alternative DSM-model for personality disorders focuses on determining if there is evidence of significant impairment in personality functioning in key areas of personality development (identity, self-direction, empathy, or intimacy).

- Clinicians also assess 5 trait domains (negative affectivity, detachment, antagonism, disinhibition, and psychoticism) and 25 associated traits to determine if there is evidence of pathological personality traits.

- The alternative model also includes dimensional definitions for six types of personality disorders: schizotypal, borderline, avoidant, narcissistic, obsessive-compulsive, and antisocial.

Chapter Glossary

antisocial personality disorder (APD)
characterized by a failure to conform to social and legal codes, a lack of anxiety and guilt, and irresponsible behaviors

avoidant personality disorder
characterized by a fear of rejection and humiliation and an avoidance of social situations

borderline personality disorder (BPD)
characterized by intense fluctuations in mood, self-image, and interpersonal relationships

dependent personality disorder
characterized by submissive, clinging behavior and an excessive need to be taken care of

histrionic personality disorder
characterized by extreme emotionality and attention seeking

narcissistic personality disorder
characterized by an exaggerated sense of self-importance, an exploitive attitude, and a lack of empathy

obsessive-compulsive personality disorder (OCPD)
characterized by perfectionism, a tendency to be interpersonally controlling, devotion to details, and rigidity

paranoid personality disorder (PPD)
characterized by distrust and suspiciousness regarding the motives of others

personality disorder
the presence of pathological personality traits that are relatively inflexible and long-standing and interfere with interpersonal functioning

personality psychopathology
dysfunctional and maladaptive personality patterns

schizoid personality disorder
characterized by detachment from social relationships and limited emotional expression

schizotypal personality disorder
characterized by peculiar thoughts and behaviors and by poor interpersonal relationships

temperament
innate mental, physical, and emotional traits

trait
a distinguishing quality or characteristic of a person, including a tendency to feel, perceive, behave, or think in a relatively consistent manner

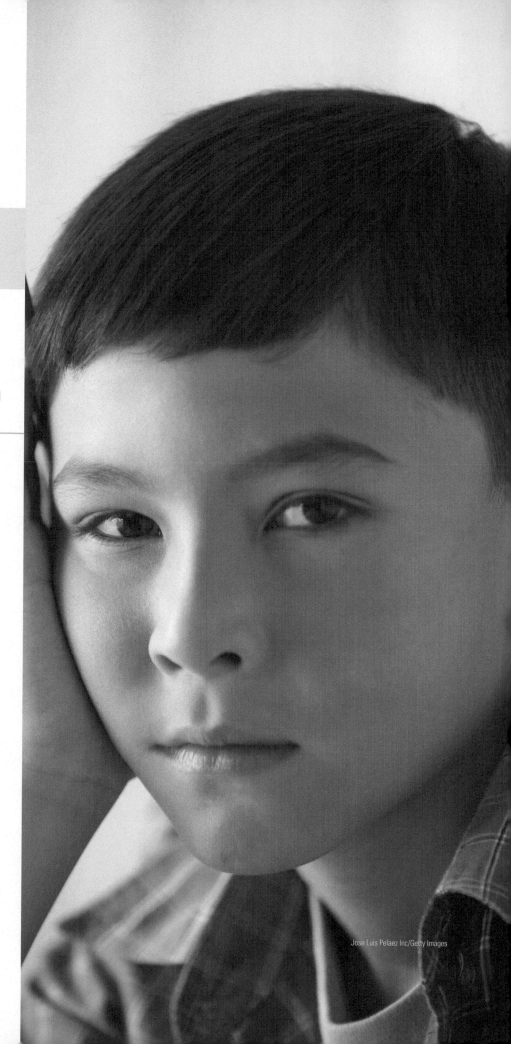

focus
Questions

1 What internalizing disorders occur in childhood and adolescence?

2 What are the characteristics of externalizing disorders?

3 What are neurodevelopmental disorders?

16

Disorders of Childhood and Adolescence

Learning Objectives

After studying this chapter, you will be able to . . .

16-1 Outline the internalizing disorders that may occur in childhood and adolescence.

16-2 Compare and contrast the childhood and adolescent externalizing disorders.

16-3 Summarize key features of each of the neurodevelopmental disorders, and discuss supports and treatments for individuals with these disorders.

Eight-Year-Old Nina cannot tolerate having her parents out of sight. Upon arriving at school, Nina clings to her mother, refusing to leave the car. As her mother walks her to the classroom, Nina cries, screams, and begs her mother not to leave.

Diagnosis: *separation anxiety disorder*

Ten-Year-Old Avery's Parents Are Frustrated by Avery's continuing defiance, constant arguments, and vindictiveness. Today Avery is refusing to come out of his bedroom to greet friends and relatives attending his mother's surprise birthday party. He shouts at his parents, "You can't make me do anything!"

Diagnosis: *oppositional defiant disorder*

Sitting in the Psychologist's Office, the mother explains that ever since he was in preschool, her son Tyler, who is now 10, has disrupted classroom instruction. He has difficulty concentrating, is often reprimanded for talking, and is failing most subjects. Throughout the session, Tyler fidgets in his seat and interrupts his mother.

Diagnosis: *attention-deficit/hyperactivity disorder*

Five-Year-Old Ahmed Sits Apart from the Other Children, spinning the wheels of a toy truck and humming aloud as if to mimic the sound. Ahmed seems to live in a world of his own, interacting with those around him as if they are inanimate objects.

Diagnosis: *autism spectrum disorder*

In this chapter, we discuss psychological disorders occurring in childhood and adolescence. Accurate assessment of mental disorders occurring early in life is not easy; it requires knowledge about normal child development and child **temperament**, as well as psychiatric disorders. Familiarity with **child psychopathology** (how psychological disorders manifest in children and adolescents) is essential because characteristics that signify mental illness in adults (e.g., difficulty with emotional regulation) often occur in normally developing children. Additionally, symptoms of some disorders are quite different in children compared to adults.

Oppositional behavior, anxiety about a parent leaving, or high levels of activity combined with a short attention span are viewed quite differently depending on the age of the child. We would consider these behaviors typical in a 2- or 3-year-old, but they would be of concern in a 10-year-old. Additionally, children differ in their natural temperament; some children are cautious and slow to warm to new situations, whereas others are energetic, strong willed, and intense in their reactions. Further, child mental health professionals are well aware that the prefrontal cortex, the brain region associated with executive functions such as attention, self-control, and perspective taking, continues developing throughout childhood and adolescence, finally maturing during early adulthood.

To determine if a child has an actual disorder, clinicians consider the child's age and developmental level, as well as environmental factors, asking questions such as these:

- Is the child's behavior significantly different from that of other children of the same age?
- Are the symptoms likely to subside as the child matures?
- Are the behaviors present in most contexts or only in particular settings?
- Are the symptoms occurring because adults are expecting too much or too little of the child?

Clinicians are very cautious when making a diagnosis and weigh the effects of "labeling" on a child's future development against the knowledge that untreated disorders can result in ongoing mental distress. Psychiatric disorders are diagnosed only when symptoms cause significant impairment in daily functioning over an extended period.

Childhood disorders are not rare. Face-to-face diagnostic assessment of a representative sample of more than 10,000 U.S. adolescents (ages 13 to 18) found that almost half had already experienced significant mental health concerns. Nearly one third (31.9 percent) reported symptoms of an anxiety disorder, 19.1 percent demonstrated a behavior disorder, and 14 percent had faced symptoms of a depressive or bipolar disorder. Twenty-two percent of the sample reported severe impairment due to their symptoms. Depressive and bipolar disorder symptoms caused the greatest distress. (Refer to Table 16.1 for prevalence, severity, and gender comparisons of specific disorders.) The adolescent girls reported more depression and posttraumatic stress reactions, whereas the boys demonstrated more inattention and hyperactivity; more than 40 percent of those surveyed met diagnostic criteria for more than one disorder (Merikangas et al., 2010). Unfortunately, another comprehensive U.S. national survey of adolescents (ages 12 to 17) conducted in 2021 revealed that of the 5 million adolescents (20.1 percent of youth) who experienced an episode of major depression during the year, only 40.6 percent received treatment; the treatment percentage was only slightly higher (44.2 percent) for those among this group who faced severe impairment in daily functioning during their depression (SAMHSA, 2022).

Among the children and adolescents who do receive treatment, medication is the most frequent intervention. Data from the National Health Interview Survey revealed that an estimated 8.4 percent of youth ages 5 to 17 years take medication for emotional or behavioral difficulties, including 9.8 percent of boys and 7.0 percent of girls; White children were more likely to take medication (11.4 percent) than Black children (5.6 percent) and Hispanic children (4.7 percent) (Zablotsky & Terlizzi, 2020). Critics have expressed outrage over pharmaceutical company practices that encourage doctors to prescribe powerful psychotropic drugs to the newest target group—children and adolescents with state-subsidized insurance such as children in foster care (Osher & Brown, 2014). In fact, children in the welfare system are two to eight times more likely than children in the general population to be prescribed psychotropic medications (Raman et al., 2021).

We begin our discussion with internalizing (i.e., emotions directed inward) and externalizing (i.e., disruptive) disorders. We conclude with a look at childhood disorders involving impaired neurological development. The field of child psychopathology is extensive, so we will address many of the disorders only briefly.

Table 16.1 Lifetime Prevalence of Psychiatric Disorders in Youth Ages 13 to 18

Disorder	Girls (%)	Boys (%)	Percentage with Severe Impairment
Generalized anxiety disorder	3.0	1.5	30
Social phobia	11.2	7.0	14
Specific phobia	22.1	15.7	3
Panic disorder	2.6	2.0	9
Posttraumatic stress disorder	8.0	2.3	30
Depression	15.9	7.7	74
Bipolar disorder	3.3	2.6	89
Attention-deficit/hyperactivity disorder	4.2	13.0	48
Oppositional defiant disorder	11.3	13.9	52
Conduct disorder	5.8	7.9	32

Source: Merikangas et al., 2010

Disorders of Childhood and Adolescence | **605**

16-1 Internalizing Disorders Among Youth

Disorders involving emotional symptoms that are directed inward are referred to as **internalizing disorders**. As with adults, children and adolescents with internalizing disorders often suppress or bottle up their feelings and reactions to trauma, stressors, or negative events. Anxiety and depressive disorders are the most common internalizing disorders. These disorders are prevalent in early life (refer to Table 16.1) and are of particular concern because they often lead to substance abuse and suicide (Cheung et al., 2019).

Anxiety, Trauma, and Stressor-Related Disorders in Early Life

Anxiety, trauma, and stressor-related disorders in childhood or adolescence typically result from a combination of biological predisposition and exposure to environmental influences. Anxiety disorders are one of the most prevalent mental health conditions in childhood and adolescence (Ghandour et al., 2019). Among the 32 percent of adolescents who have experienced an anxiety disorder, specific phobias (19 percent) and social anxiety disorder (9 percent) are most common (Merikangas et al., 2010). Specific phobias often begin in early to middle childhood, whereas social anxiety typically begins in early to middle adolescence (Lijster et al., 2017).

Youth with anxiety disorders experience extreme feelings of worry, discomfort, or fear when facing unfamiliar or anxiety-provoking situations. Early-onset anxiety can significantly affect academic and social functioning and, if untreated, can lead to adult anxiety disorders (Swan et al., 2018). Children who are inhibited and fearful are at higher risk for anxiety symptoms, and overprotective or controlling parenting practices, low parental warmth, or perceived parental rejection can exacerbate the issue (Ryan & Ollendick, 2018). Anxiety disorders associated with childhood include:

- **separation anxiety disorder**—severe distress or worry about leaving home, being alone, or being separated from primary caregivers; and
- **selective mutism**—a consistent failure to speak in certain social situations.

Children with these disorders display exaggerated autonomic responses and are apprehensive in new situations, preferring to stay at home or in other familiar environments. Cognitive-behavioral therapy can be an effective treatment for childhood anxiety disorders. Successful treatment not only reduces the child's anxiety symptoms but can also help alleviate co-occurring behavioral and mood symptoms and reduce stressful interactions within the family (Mahdi et al., 2019).

Attachment Disorders

Infants and children raised in stressful environments that lack predictable parenting and nurturing sometimes demonstrate significant difficulties with emotional attachments and social relationships (Vega et al., 2019). Attachment problems can manifest in the inhibited behaviors seen in *reactive attachment disorder* or the excessive attention-seeking seen in *disinhibited social engagement disorder*. These childhood stressor and trauma-related disorders are diagnosed only when symptoms are apparent before age 5 and when early circumstances prevent the child from forming stable attachments. Situations that can disrupt attachment include frequent changes in primary caregiver, emotional or physical abuse, and environments that are devoid of stimulation or affection.

Children with **reactive attachment disorder (RAD)** appear to have little trust that the adults in their lives will attend to their needs; therefore, they do not readily seek or respond to comfort, attention, or nurturing. Children with RAD often behave in a very inhibited or watchful manner, even with family and caregivers. They appear to use avoidance as a psychological defense and experience difficulty responding to or initiating social or emotional interactions. Children with RAD rarely show positive emotions and may demonstrate irritability, sadness, or fearfulness when interacting with adults (APA, 2022).

Going Deeper

Child Abuse and Neglect

Because the 3-year-old boy had soiled his pants, his mother forced him to sit on the toilet. She told her son that he would not be allowed to get up or eat unless he had a bowel movement. When the son could not comply, the mother pulled him from the toilet seat and lashed his buttocks until they were raw and bleeding.

Child neglect and the physical, emotional, and sexual abuse of children remain a significant problem. In the United States, at least 1 in 7 children were subjected to child neglect or physical or sexual abuse in 2020, including 1,750 who died as a result of their injuries. These distressing statistics are likely an underestimate, since many cases of abuse go unreported, particularly cases of child sexual abuse (CDC, 2022). As seen in Figure 16.1, the majority of deaths from abuse involve children age 3 or younger; in 80 percent of the cases, the perpetrator is one or both parents (U.S. Department of Health and Human Services, 2021).

Why would parents abuse or neglect their own children? We know that multiple factors, including poverty, parental immaturity, and lack of parenting skills, contribute to child maltreatment, and that many adults who abuse were themselves abused as children. Many parents involved in maltreatment are young, high school dropouts, and under severe stress. Many have personality disorders and low tolerance for frustration or abuse alcohol and other substances (Lotto et al., 2023). In the case of child sexual abuse, perpetrators are often friends or other family members, and the parent is often unaware that the abuse occurred.

Childhood physical or sexual abuse can result in a variety of internalized or externalized symptoms during childhood or adolescence, as well as lifelong physical and psychological consequences such as depression, anxiety, eating disorders, PTSD, and suicidality. As you might expect, the more maltreatment or trauma a child encounters, the greater the risk of subsequent psychiatric illness (McCrory et al., 2017).

Many communities offer parent education and support groups for high-risk families, including families who have come to the attention of child protection agencies. There is a particular need for programs to prevent the maltreatment of infants and young children. Interventions such as parent training, individual or family therapy, and substance abuse treatment as well as home visitations have proven effective in reducing child maltreatment (van der Put et al., 2018). Additionally, some promising prevention efforts focus on providing support for new or expectant parents who have themselves been subjected to child abuse; the goal is to help these parents develop the capacity to nurture their own children in a way they were not themselves nurtured, thereby stopping the cycle of intergenerational trauma (Chamberlain et al., 2019).

For Further Consideration

1. How might child maltreatment affect someone's mental health or relationship capacities in adulthood?

2. Why might those who were mistreated as children have an increased risk of becoming abusive themselves?

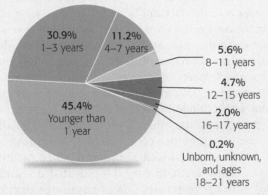

Figure 16.1

Fatalities from Child Abuse or Neglect by Age, 2019

The youngest are the most vulnerable.

Source: U.S. Department of Health & Human Services, 2021

In stark contrast, children with **disinhibited social engagement disorder (DSED)** socialize effortlessly but indiscriminately and readily become superficially "attached" to strangers or casual acquaintances. They often stray away from caregivers as they approach and verbally or physically interact with unknown adults in an overly familiar manner. The children who engage in this behavior appear to be searching for the attention they lacked in early childhood (Minnis, 2018). Children with DSED often have a history of harsh punishment or inconsistent parenting in addition to emotional neglect and limited attachment opportunities (APA, 2022).

The course of attachment disorders depends on the severity of the disruptions in caregiving or childhood adversities, as well as subsequent events in the child's life. Symptoms of these disorders sometimes disappear when children are placed in an alternative setting (e.g., in foster care or the home of a relative) that provides predictable caretaking and

Focus on Resilience

Enhancing Resilience in Youth

Early life experiences influence the development of mental illness. Can modifying a child's environment increase resilience, especially in children who are genetically or environmentally at risk? In other words, are there steps that we can take to decrease the likelihood that a child will develop a mental disorder in childhood or later in life? The answer is yes. Resilience occurs when human adaptive systems are operating optimally—when brain functioning has not been compromised; when children experience social, emotional, and physical security; and when the environment supports their capacity for self-efficacy, emotional regulation, and effective problem solving.

Given the pervasiveness of mental illness, implementing strategies for promoting resilience in the face of adversity is a global priority. 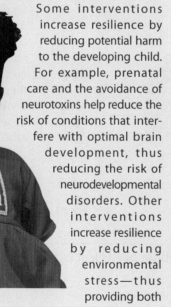 Some interventions increase resilience by reducing potential harm to the developing child. For example, prenatal care and the avoidance of neurotoxins help reduce the risk of conditions that interfere with optimal brain development, thus reducing the risk of neurodevelopmental disorders. Other interventions increase resilience by reducing environmental stress—thus providing both

biological and psychological benefits. For instance, intervening with parents who are experiencing mental illness or engaging in child maltreatment can improve behavioral or emotional outcomes in their children. Similarly, early intervention when children are experiencing behavioral or emotional difficulties can prevent the downward emotional spiral seen with many disorders. With support, children who have been exposed to trauma can experience posttraumatic growth (e.g., increased sense of personal strength or enhanced connection with others) in response to their experiences (Chang et al., 2023).

School experiences that provide children with opportunities to develop competence and engage in healthy social interactions also play a role in enhancing resilience. Close bonds between children and school personnel have the potential to promote positive developmental cascades that increase intellectual and emotional expertise and the ability to cope with adversity—characteristics that extend into adulthood (Fenwick-Smith et al., 2018). Additionally, schools provide youth with opportunities to develop positive attachments and ongoing supportive relationships with positive role models, thereby maximizing the development of interpersonal trust and problem-solving skills (Phillips et al., 2019). Knowing how to solve problems or regulate emotions allows children to reduce biological reactivity in response to stress or adversity. Additionally, promotion of a healthy lifestyle (e.g., ensuring adequate sleep, nutrition, and exercise; monitoring television and computer use) can further support physical and psychological resilience (Sampson et al., 2020). One thing is clear—when their basic physical, social, and emotional needs are met, youth can develop the strengths that allow them not only to overcome adversity but also to flourish.

Kevin Peterson/Getty Images

nurturance (Guyon-Harris et al., 2018). However, issues of mistrust and difficulties with intimate relationships sometimes continue into adulthood. Children who are exposed to prolonged periods of inadequate caregiving are particularly vulnerable to ongoing mental health issues (Guyon-Harris et al., 2019). Once RAD or DSED is identified, therapeutic support focuses on building emotional security. Effective intervention includes providing a stable, nurturing environment and opportunities to develop interpersonal trust and social-relational skills. Fortunately, many children raised under difficult circumstances do not show signs of these disorders.

Posttraumatic Stress Disorder in Early Life

Case Study Several months after witnessing her father seriously injure her mother during a domestic dispute, Jenna remained withdrawn; she spoke little and rarely played with her toys. Although a protection order prevented her father from returning home, Jenna became startled whenever she heard the door open and frequently woke up screaming, "Stop!" She refused to enter the kitchen, the site of the violent assault.

The effects of trauma and resultant posttraumatic stress disorder (PTSD) can be particularly upsetting for the children and adolescents who face recurrent, distressing memories of a shocking experience. The trauma that precipitates PTSD can include threats of or direct experience with death, serious injury, or sexual violation. Witnessing or hearing about trauma experienced by others can also result in PTSD, especially when a primary caregiver or other loved one is involved. Memories of the event may entail (a) distressing dreams, (b) intense physiological or psychological reactions to thoughts or cues associated with the event, (c) episodes of play-acting the event (sometimes without apparent distress), or (d) dissociative reactions in which the child appears to reexperience the trauma or seems unaware of their present surroundings. As with Jenna, the child may cope by attempting to avoid cues associated with the traumatic situation or event.

According to the DSM-5-TR, behavioral evidence of PTSD in youth may include angry, aggressive behavior or temper tantrums; difficulty sleeping or concentrating; and exaggerated startle responses or vigilance for possible threats. Children who experience trauma may appear socially withdrawn, show few positive emotions, or seem disinterested in activities they previously enjoyed (APA, 2022). Lifetime prevalence of PTSD among adolescents is 8 percent for girls and 2.3 percent for boys (Merikangas et al., 2010). Trauma-focused cognitive-behavioral therapies have proven to be effective in treating childhood PTSD (Nixon et al., 2012). Unfortunately, without effective intervention, PTSD symptoms can continue for years and significantly affect the developing brain (Herringa, 2017).

Nonsuicidal Self-Injury

Case Study For the past year, Maria has been secretly cutting her forearms and thighs with a razor blade. She has tried to stop; however, when she feels anxious or depressed, she thinks of the razor blade and the relief she experiences once she feels the cutting. Maria acknowledges that she has difficulty managing her emotions, particularly when she has conflicts with her parents or her friends. She does not understand why she cuts; she just knows it seems to help her cope when she is feeling upset. The more life hurts, the more she cuts.

Nonsuicidal self-injury (NSSI) is a relatively new phenomenon that involves intentionally inflicted, superficial wounds. Those who engage in NSSI cut, burn, stab, hit, or excessively rub themselves to the point of pain and injury but without suicidal intent. As we saw with Maria, intense negative thoughts or emotions and a preoccupation with engaging in self-harm (often accompanied by a desire to resist the impulse to self-injure) frequently precede episodes of self-injury. The DSM-5-TR has included NSSI as a proposed diagnostic condition undergoing further study; for a diagnosis, the individual must display self-injurious behaviors at least 5 or more days over the course of a year (APA, 2022). Approximately, 22 percent of children and adolescents, 39 percent of college students, and 5.5 percent of adults have engaged in NSSI on at least one occasion (Nagy et al., 2023).

Interpersonal difficulties, negative emotions, or a preoccupation with self-harm often occur just before a self-injury episode. Those who self-injure often expect that it will improve their mood and frequently report that the pain produces relief from uncomfortable feelings or a temporary sense of calm and well-being. Those who repeatedly self-injure often have difficulty expressing and regulating their emotions and sometimes use self-harm as a coping strategy to avoid suicidal actions (Kraus et al., 2020). A negative cognitive style and negative self-talk are associated with increased frequency of NSSI and a higher prevalence of suicidal behavior (Wolff et al., 2013).

NSSI tends to begin in early adolescence and peaks in late adolescence or in the early 20s. It is substantially more prevalent among sexual minorities and is somewhat more prevalent in females (APA, 2022). Although adolescent self-harming behavior usually declines during adulthood or resolves spontaneously, underlying mental health issues such as depression, anxiety, or substance use often persist (Borschmann et al., 2017). An effective intervention for adolescents who engage in repeated NSSI is dialectical behavior therapy, which teaches distress tolerance and emotional regulation skills (McCauley et al., 2018).

Mood Disorders in Early Life

Depressive disorders in young people have increased in recent years, particularly among adolescent girls (Mojtabai & Olfson, 2020). Environmental factors are a frequent cause of depression in childhood, whereas genetic and other biological factors exert more influence during adolescence. Children are especially vulnerable to environmental factors because they lack the maturity and skills to deal with stressors. Conditions such as childhood physical or sexual abuse, parental mental or physical illness, or loss of an attachment figure can increase vulnerability to depression (Rosenthal et al., 2013). A recent increase in depression and substance use among Latinx youth appears to be linked to stress associated with changing immigration policies, particularly among youth who know someone who has been picked up and detained by immigration officials—a common occurrence in many Latinx communities (Pinedo, 2020). Further, excessive use of social media is also linked with increases in depression among youth (Zubair et al., 2023).

Adolescents with depression are at high risk of experiencing chronic depressive symptoms, especially if they do not receive treatment (Melvin et al., 2013). Intervention

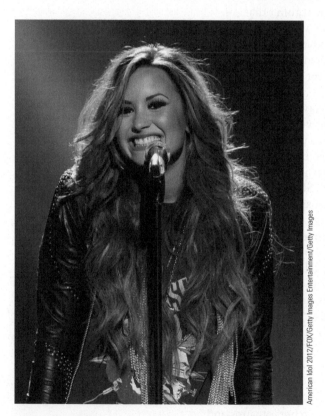

Demi Lovato

Singer and actor Demi Lovato engaged in disordered eating and nonsuicidal self-injury during early adolescence in an effort to cope with her emotions and in response to bullying from classmates. When receiving treatment for these conditions, it was discovered that her mood swings were also related to undiagnosed bipolar disorder.

is important also because of the strong association between depressive disorders and adolescent suicidal ideation and suicide attempts (Nock et al., 2013). Evidence-based treatment for depression in youth includes individual or group cognitive-behavioral therapy and interpersonal therapy. Family therapy also shows promising results (Méndez et al., 2021). Parent participation in therapy appears to increase the likelihood of a positive outcome (Sun et al., 2019).

Using selective serotonin reuptake inhibitors (SSRIs) to treat depressive disorders in youth is a complicated issue because SSRIs have been linked to an increase in suicidality in those younger than age 25. This concern led to a 2004 U.S. Food and Drug Administration (FDA) decision to issue a "black box" warning regarding the use of these medications with this age group. Some practitioners argue that the benefits of using antidepressants outweigh the risk of increased suicidality, especially among youth who are moderately to severely depressed. However, a recent research review concluded that the best-designed studies do, in fact, validate the increased risk of suicidality in youth taking antidepressants and that the black box warning should remain (Spielmans et al., 2020). Best practices support careful monitoring of suicidality in all children and adolescents who are depressed, with particular attention to those taking antidepressants.

Disruptive Mood Dysregulation Disorder

Case Study As an infant and toddler, Thyme was irritable and difficult to please. Temper tantrums, often involving attempts to hit their parents, occurred multiple times daily. Thyme's parents had hoped the behavior would change as Thyme grew older; but at age 8, Thyme is still frequently "grumpy" and has continued temper tantrums in many settings.

Disruptive mood dysregulation disorder (DMDD) is characterized by chronic irritability and severe mood dysregulation, including recurrent temper outbursts triggered by common childhood stressors such as sibling conflict or being denied a request. As we saw with Thyme, anger reactions are extreme in both intensity and duration, and may involve verbal rage or physical aggression toward people and property. According to the DSM-5-TR, DMDD is a depressive disorder; although behavioral symptoms are directed outward, they reflect an irritable, angry, or sad mood state. For a DMDD diagnosis, the child's mood between temper episodes must be irritable or angry most of the day, nearly every day. Further, the outbursts are present in at least two settings and occur at least three times per week for most months over the course of 1 year. Although the behaviors associated with DMDD often begin in early childhood, this diagnosis is not made until a child is at least 6 years of age; additionally, the symptoms must be evident before age 10.

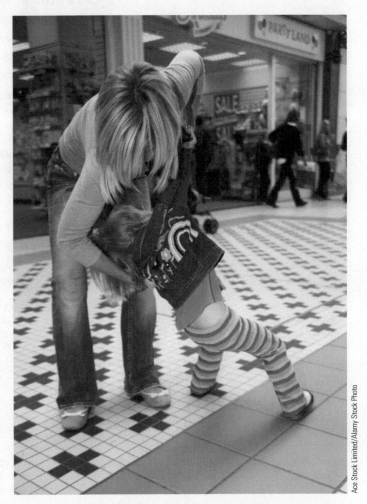

Ace Stock Limited/Alamy Stock Photo

Disruptive Mood Dysregulation Disorder?

Many young children have difficulty regulating their emotions and display occasional temper tantrums. However, persistent irritable or angry behavior that continues beyond the preschool years may eventually result in a diagnosis of disruptive mood dysregulation disorder.

This age requirement ensures that diagnosis is not based on the erratic moods associated with early childhood (e.g., "the terrible 2s") or puberty. The prevalence rates for DMDD have ranged from 0.8 percent to 8.2 percent depending on the age group of the child (APA, 2022).

Many children diagnosed with DMDD have comorbid disorders associated with emotional dysregulation. In fact, there is considerable diagnostic overlap between the symptoms of DMDD and the externalizing behaviors seen in attention-deficit/hyperactivity disorder and oppositional defiant disorder. Additionally, clinicians making a diagnosis of DMDD need to rule out pediatric bipolar disorder, due to the overlapping symptoms involving depression and mood changes (refer to Table 16.2). Differential diagnosis is important because interventions for childhood disorders involving episodes of acting-out behavior are quite different depending on the diagnosis (Bruno et al., 2019).

Pediatric Bipolar Disorder

Case Study Ana was a fairly cooperative, engaging child throughout her early years. However, around her 10th birthday, her behavior changed significantly. At times, she experienced periods of extreme moodiness, depression, and high irritability; on other occasions, she displayed boundless energy and talked incessantly, often moving rapidly from one topic to another as she described different ideas and plans. During her energetic periods, she could go for several weeks with minimal sleep.

Pediatric bipolar disorder (PBD) is a serious disorder that parallels the mood variability, depressive episodes, and significant departure from typical functioning that characterize adult bipolar disorder. Youth with PBD display

Table 16.2 Disruptive Mood Dysregulation Disorder and Pediatric Bipolar Disorder

Disorders Chart				
Disorder	**DSM-5-TR Criteria**	**Prevalence**	**Age of Onset**	**Course**
Disruptive mood dysregulation disorder	• Recurrent episodes of temper, including verbal rage or physical aggression • Anger response that is exaggerated in intensity and duration • Persistent irritable, angry, or sad mood • Behaviors observed in at least two settings over a 12-month period	2.5% to 8.2%; more frequently diagnosed in boys	Diagnosis requires onset before age 10 but is often evident in early childhood (diagnosis is not made after age 18)	May improve with maturity; may evolve into a depressive or anxiety disorder; frequently comorbid with ODD
Pediatric bipolar disorder	• Distinct periods of abnormally elevated mood (i.e., manic or hypomanic episodes) • Periodic mood and behavioral changes (e.g., irritability, depression, increased activity, distractibility, or talkativeness; inflated self-esteem) • Bipolar I or bipolar II is diagnosed based on specific symptoms	Less than 1%; affects boys and girls equally	Onset occurs around age 10 through adolescence, about 5 years later than disruptive mood dysregulation disorder	Poor prognosis; often evolves into a chronic psychiatric disorder

Source: APA, 2022; Brotman et al., 2006; Merikangas et al., 2010; Meyer et al., 2009; Parry et al., 2021

mood changes and distinct periods of elevated energy and activity that may involve diminished need for sleep, distractibility, talkativeness, frequent interrupting, or inflated self-esteem (refer to Table 16.2). In addition to experiencing hypomanic/manic episodes, those with PBD may also display recurring depressive episodes or periods of uncharacteristic irritability that alternate with these energized episodes (Lee, 2016). As was the case with Ana, the behavior represents a change from the child's normal mood or temperament.

In a review of prevalence studies on PBD, the researchers concluded that the disorder is "very rare" in childhood and "rare" in adolescence (Parry et al., 2021). PBD often occurs in families with a history of bipolar illness and is likely to evolve into adult bipolar disorder or another chronic psychiatric disorder (Goldstein, 2012). Unique patterns in the microstructure of the white matter have been found in the brains of youth with this condition compared to healthy volunteers; however, imaging studies also found very similar brain abnormalities in youth diagnosed with DMDD (Linke et al., 2019).

Some experts in the field of bipolar disorder contend that some clinicians give this diagnosis too liberally, without ensuring that the child or adolescent meets full criteria for episodes of hypomania/mania. It was hoped that the addition of the DMDD category to the DSM would allow for greater diagnostic accuracy. Questions have also been raised because the majority of PBD diagnoses occur within the United States where the pharmaceutical industry exerts a strong influence on medical practice (Duffy et al., 2020).

Medications, therapeutic techniques, and psychosocial intervention for PBD are similar to those used with adult bipolar disorder. Lithium and antipsychotic medications are often prescribed as maintenance medications for youth with PBD, a practice that concerns some mental health professionals due to the potential side effects associated with these drugs (Yee et al., 2019). Family-focused therapy and education are important adjunct interventions because family support can be very effective in assisting children and adolescents as they learn and practice effective methods for regulating their mood (Miklowitz et al., 2013). Among adolescents with PBD, dialectical behavior therapy has been effective in reducing suicide attempts among this high-risk population (Goldstein et al., 2023).

16-2 Externalizing Disorders Among Youth

Externalizing disorders (sometimes called *disruptive behavior disorders*) include conditions associated with symptoms that affect others, such as aggressive actions or difficulties with impulse control. Parenting a child with externalizing behaviors can be challenging and can result in negative parent–child interactions, high family stress, and negative feelings about parenting. As you can imagine, these factors can further exacerbate behavioral difficulties. Although early intervention can help interrupt the downward spiral associated with these disorders, diagnosing disruptive behaviors is controversial because it is difficult to distinguish externalizing disorders not only from one another but also from the defiance and noncompliance that occasionally occur in many children and adolescents. Diagnosis of any of

Did You Know?

Bullying can have serious effects on the physical and emotional well-being of children and adolescents. Exposure to bullying during the school years is associated with increased risk of poor mental and physical health and interpersonal difficulties.

Source: Eroglu et al., 2022

the externalizing disorders requires a persistent pattern of behavior that is (a) atypical for the child's culture, gender, age, and developmental level and (b) severe enough to cause distress to the child or to others or negatively affect social or academic functioning. Disorders in this category include oppositional defiant disorder, intermittent explosive disorder, and conduct disorder.

Oppositional Defiant Disorder

> **Case Study** Mark's parents and teachers know that when they ask Mark to do something, it is likely that he will argue and refuse to comply. He has been irritable and oppositional since he was a toddler. Mark's parents have given up trying to enlist cooperation; they vacillate between ignoring Mark's hostile, defiant behavior and threatening punishment. However, they are well aware that when Mark is punished, he finds ways to retaliate.

Oppositional defiant disorder (ODD) is characterized by a persistent pattern of angry, argumentative, or vindictive behavior that continues for at least 6 months. These behaviors are directed toward parents, teachers, and others in authority. At least four symptoms involving short-tempered, resentful, blaming, spiteful, or hostile behaviors must be present. Similar to the response of Mark's parents, caretakers of children with this behavior pattern often do whatever they can to avoid conflict, usually without success. Although youth with ODD often argue, defy adult requests, and blame others, they do not demonstrate the pervasive antisocial behavior or extreme verbal or physical aggression directed toward people, animals, or property that is characteristic of conduct disorder (refer to Table 16.3). ODD is considered mild if symptoms occur only in one setting and severe if the behaviors occur in three or more settings.

Although the symptoms of ODD often resolve, especially with intervention, ODD is associated with interpersonal difficulties in early adulthood (Burke, Rowe, & Boylan, 2014). Additionally, in some cases, youth with ODD begin to demonstrate the more serious rule violations associated with conduct disorder. ODD appears to have two components, one involving negative affect and emotional dysregulation (e.g., angry, irritable mood) and the other involving defiant and oppositional behavior; negative affect predicts future depressive symptoms, whereas oppositional behaviors are more predictive of delinquency and conduct disorder (APA, 2022). Additionally, a large percentage of children with ODD also display inattention and hyperactivity (Vetter et al., 2020).

Intermittent Explosive Disorder

Intermittent explosive disorder (IED) is a "prevalent, persistent, and seriously impairing" disorder that is both underdiagnosed and undertreated (McLaughlin et al., 2012). A diagnosis of IED involves (a) recurrent outbursts of extreme verbal or physical aggression that occur approximately twice weekly for at least 3 months (lower-intensity but high-frequency aggressive outbursts) or (b) three outbursts occurring within a 1-year period that involve damage or injury to people, animals, or property (lower-frequency but high-intensity outbursts) (Coccaro, Lee, &

Table 16.3 Oppositional Defiant, Intermittent Explosive, and Conduct Disorder

Disorders Chart				
Disorder	**DSM-5-TR**	**Prevalence**	**Age of Onset**	**Course**
Oppositional defiant disorder	• Angry, irritable mood • Hostile, defiant, and vindictive behavior • Frequent loss of temper, arguing, and defiance of adult requests • Failure to take responsibility for actions; blaming others • Behaviors continue for at least 6 months	1% to 11%; more common in boys	Childhood	May resolve, or evolve into a conduct disorder or depressive disorder
Intermittent explosive disorder	• Recurrent outbursts of extreme verbal or physical aggression *or* • Three outbursts involving physical injury or damage within 1 year • Outbursts are impulsive or anger based and not premeditated • Outbursts cause marked distress or impairment in interpersonal functioning • Behaviors continue for at least 3 months	One-year prevalence rate of 6.9%	Age 12 is the average age of onset (must be at least age 6 for the diagnosis)	May resolve, but anger episodes often continue into adulthood
Conduct disorder	• Aggression or cruelty to people or animals • Fire setting or destruction of property • Theft or deceit (stealing, "conning" others) • Serious rule violations (truancy, running away) • Behaviors continue for at least 12 months	2% to 10%; more common in boys and in urban settings	Two types: childhood onset and adolescent onset (although onset is rare after age 16)	Poor prognosis with childhood onset; often leads to the criminal behaviors, antisocial acts, and problems in adult adjustment seen in antisocial personality disorder

Source: APA, 2022; Froehlich et al., 2007; McLaughlin et al., 2012; Merikangas et al., 2010; Tynan, 2008, 2010

McCloskey, 2014). The outbursts occur suddenly in response to minor provocation and do not involve premeditation; instead, they are exaggerated angry or impulsive reactions that cause significant distress or impair interpersonal functioning. Unlike the negative mood associated with DMDD, the child's mood is normal between outbursts. A child must be at least 6 years old—an age when children are presumed to have learned to control their aggressive impulses—to receive this diagnosis (APA, 2022).

Not surprisingly, IED is associated with early exposure to familial aggression, violence, and interpersonal trauma (Nickerson et al., 2012). IED may be diagnosed in individuals with attention-deficit/hyperactivity disorder, conduct disorder, or ODD if periodic explosive, aggressive outbursts occur and meet the criteria for IED. A comprehensive study involving 6,483 adolescents found that 63.3 percent of the adolescents interviewed had experienced anger outbursts in which they destroyed property or threatened violence, or behaved violently. In fact, 7.8 percent of the group had displayed behavior that met the criteria for IED (McLaughlin et al., 2012). The impulsive, aggressive outbursts associated with IED sometimes continue into adulthood. As you might expect, adults with IED find that their explosive outbursts interfere with interpersonal relationships, work performance, and ability to sustain employment (Rynar & Coccaro, 2018).

Myth Youth who set fires or engage in shoplifting are likely to develop serious mental disorders such as pyromania or kleptomania.

Reality *Pyromania* (an irresistible impulse to start fires) and *kleptomania* (a compulsion to steal without economic motivation) are very rare impulse-control disorders. Fire-setting during childhood or adolescence often results from stress reactions, poor impulse control, or the antisocial attitudes seen in conduct disorders. However, it is usually distinct from the extreme fascination and arousal associated with fire that occurs in pyromania. Similarly, most youth who engage in shoplifting do so for reasons other than the extreme impulse to steal associated with kleptomania (APA, 2022).

Conduct Disorder

Case Study   Ben, a high school sophomore well known for his ongoing bullying and aggressive behavior, was expelled from school after attempting to stab another student. Two months later, he was arrested for armed robbery and placed in juvenile detention. The adults working with Ben were consistently frustrated by his frequent refusal to comply with behavioral expectations. Additionally, peer relationships at the facility were strained because of Ben's ongoing attempts to intimidate others.

Conduct disorder (CD) is characterized by a persistent pattern of antisocial behavior that reflects dysfunction within the individual (rather than a pattern of behavior accepted within the person's subculture) and includes serious violations of rules and social norms and disregard for the rights of others. Diagnosis of CD requires the presence of at least three different behaviors involving:

(a) deliberate aggression (bullying, physical fights, use of weapons, cruelty to people or animals, aggressive theft, forced sexual contact),

(b) deliberate destruction of property (including malicious fire-setting),

(c) theft or deceit (stealing, forgery, home or car invasion, "conning" others), or

(d) serious violation of rules (staying out at night, truancy, running away).

Deliberate rule violations sometimes begin in early childhood and then continue into adolescence. In many cases, as we saw with Ben, disorderly behavior becomes increasingly serious. Boys with CD are often involved in confrontational aggression (e.g., fighting, aggressive theft), whereas girls are more likely to display truancy, substance abuse, or chronic lying. Approximately 2 percent to 10 percent of youth meet the diagnostic criteria for CD; it is estimated that many of those with childhood-onset CD also display inattention and hyperactivity (APA, 2022).

A subgroup of youth diagnosed with CD have "limited prosocial emotions"—they display minimal guilt or remorse and are consistently unconcerned about the feelings of others, their own wrongdoing, or poor performance at school or work. They are good at manipulating others and may appear superficially polite and friendly when they have something to gain (APA, 2022). Cruelty, aggression, and a pervasive lack of remorse are common characteristics of this subgroup (Viding & McCrory, 2018).

Youth with these callous, unemotional traits are unconcerned about the suffering that they cause or about possible punishment for their behavior. In fact, they show limited neural responsiveness in brain regions associated with empathy when presented with pictures of other people in pain—a reaction that differs significantly from that displayed by children without antisocial traits (Lockwood et al., 2013). In a study using magnetic resonance imaging (MRI), adolescents with CD and callous traits demonstrated strong pleasure responses to video clips of people experiencing pain and distress (Decety et al., 2009). Not surprisingly, individuals with these traits are at

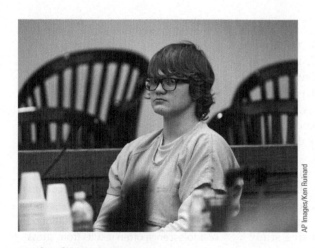

Lack of Remorse

At the age of 14, Jesse Dewitt Osborne, pictured here during a court appearance, killed his father and then drove to an elementary school, where he shot two children and a teacher. He had planned to kill dozens of children. Jesse videoed himself combing his hair before the shooting so that he could "look fabulous." In handing down a life sentence, the judge remarked on Osborn's complete lack of remorse.

high risk for continuing criminal behavior and receiving a diagnosis of anti-social personality disorder in adulthood (Pardini et al., 2018).

The behaviors and criminal acts associated with CD present a significant concern to the public. Some youth advocates endorse widespread screening for CD among young children because early intervention and comprehensive treatment provide a possible means to modify the course of the disorder for some individuals (Hektner et al., 2014).

Etiology of Externalizing Disorders

Externalizing disorders often begin in early childhood. The etiology of these disorders involves an interaction between biological, psychological, social, and sociocultural factors. Among the externalizing disorders, biological factors appear to exert the greatest influence on the development of CD, the disorder we will focus on in this etiological discussion (Figure 16.2).

Biological Dimension

Some of the characteristics seen in some children with conduct disorder show moderate heritability—particularly when there is an absence of protective factors to counteract the impulsive or risk-taking behaviors that lead to adverse outcomes (Salvatore & Dick, 2018). The risk of CD is associated with the genotype "low-activity MAOA" (an allele linked to fear-regulating circuitry in the amygdala), particularly among children who have been subjected to childhood maltreatment (Fergusson et al., 2012). Further, documented abnormalities in brain structures and brain circuits among those with CD may partially explain their lack of empathy as well as deficits in social information processing, reinforcement-based decision making (i.e., the ability to learn from negative consequences), and emotional regulation. Reduced activity of the autonomic nervous system and an associated need for increased stimulation to achieve optimal arousal have also been found in youth with conduct problems (Fairchild et al., 2019).

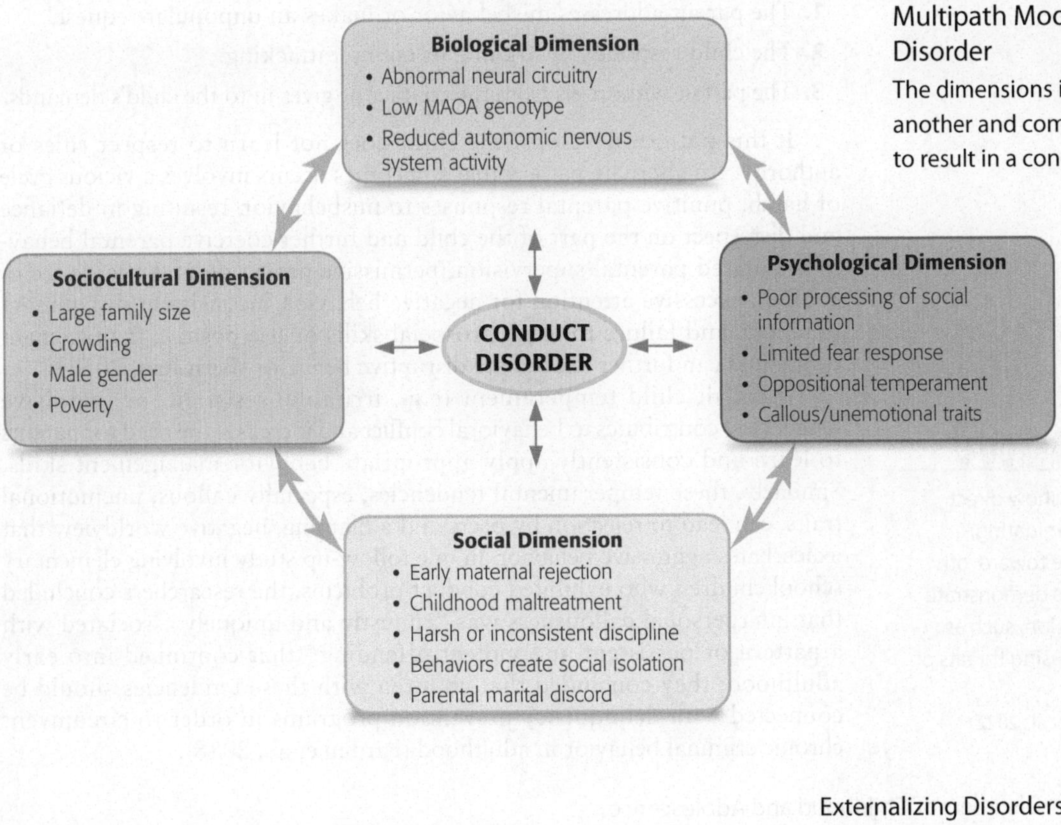

Figure 16.2

Multipath Model of Conduct Disorder

The dimensions interact with one another and combine in different ways to result in a conduct disorder.

Biological Dimension
- Abnormal neural circuitry
- Low MAOA genotype
- Reduced autonomic nervous system activity

Psychological Dimension
- Poor processing of social information
- Limited fear response
- Oppositional temperament
- Callous/unemotional traits

Sociocultural Dimension
- Large family size
- Crowding
- Male gender
- Poverty

Social Dimension
- Early maternal rejection
- Childhood maltreatment
- Harsh or inconsistent discipline
- Behaviors create social isolation
- Parental marital discord

CONDUCT DISORDER

Bullying Without Remorse

Children and adolescents with conduct disorder frequently engage in aggressive behavior and bully other students. Due to the pervasiveness of bullying behaviors, many schools have implemented curricula aimed at encouraging students to take a stand against bullying.

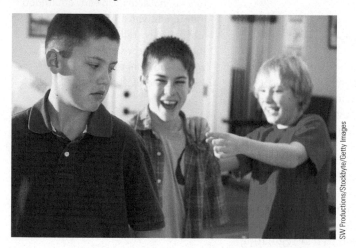

SW Productions/Stockbyte/Getty Images

Psychological, Social, and Sociocultural Dimensions

Both family and social context play a large role in the development of CD. A child's early environment appears to moderate the relationship between individual vulnerability and the age at which antisocial behavior emerges. Youth with CD are sometimes described as morally disengaged; that is, they continue demonstrating socially inappropriate behavior because they believe that societal norms and expectations do not apply to them or they convince themselves that their behavior is acceptable (Zapolski et al., 2016). Parents and teachers have the most success in improving behavior and attitudes such as this during childhood; the potential for a positive outcome decreases in adolescence when peer influences predominate and other youth who violate social norms reinforce these attitudes.

In some cases, disruptive and aggressive behaviors are associated with harsh or inconsistent discipline (Pederson & Fite, 2014). Disruptive behavior may develop when parents respond to typical childhood misbehaviors in a punitive, inconsistent, or impatient manner. Parent–child conflict and power struggles can further intensify inappropriate behaviors. It is not always easy to determine if unsupportive or inconsistent parenting practices are a primary influence on the development of acting-out behaviors in children, or if coercive or erratic parental behaviors are a response to parenting a child with challenging attributes (Georgiou et al., 2023).

Patterson (1986) formulated a classic psychological-behavioral model of disruptive behavior based on the following pattern of parental reaction to misbehavior:

1. The parent addresses misbehavior or makes an unpopular request.
2. The child responds by arguing or counterattacking.
3. The parent withdraws from the conflict or gives in to the child's demands.

If this pattern develops, the child does not learn to respect rules or authority. An alternate pattern that sometimes occurs involves a vicious cycle of harsh, punitive parental responses to misbehavior, resulting in defiance and disrespect on the part of the child and further coercive parental behaviors. Limited parental supervision, permissive parenting and avoidance of conflict, excessive attention for negative behavior, inconsistent disciplinary practices, and failure to teach prosocial skills or use positive management techniques can further exacerbate disruptive behavior (Bernstein, 2012).

Difficult child temperament (e.g., irritable, resistant, or impulsive tendencies) contributes to behavioral conflict and increases the need for parents to learn and consistently apply appropriate behavior management skills. Similarly, these temperamental tendencies, especially callous, unemotional traits, can lead to rejection by peers and a blaming, negative worldview that exacerbates aggressive behavior. In one follow-up study involving elementary school children who exhibited conduct problems, the researchers concluded that interpersonal callousness was "robustly and uniquely associated with a pattern of persistent and violent offending" that continued into early adulthood; they concluded that children with these tendencies should be connected with delinquency prevention programs in order to circumvent chronic criminal behavior in adulthood (Pardini et al., 2018).

Treatment of Externalizing Disorders

Interventions that address the family and social context of behaviors, as well as the child's deficits in psychosocial skills, can significantly improve externalizing behaviors. A well-established intervention is cognitive-behavioral parent education; these programs teach parents to regulate their own emotions, increase positive interactions with their children, establish appropriate rules, and consistently implement consequences for inappropriate behavior. Parent-focused interventions such as this can improve both child behavior and parent mental health (Olthuis et al., 2018). Parent training programs can be particularly effective when they result in increases in positive parent–child interactions and decreases in harsh discipline (Pasalich et al., 2016).

Psychosocial interventions that teach youngsters assertiveness and anger management techniques, and build skills in empathy, communication, social relationships, and problem solving, can also produce marked and durable changes in disruptive behaviors. Mobilizing adult mentors who demonstrate empathy, warmth, and acceptance is another effective intervention. In fact, teachers who develop strong, positive relationships with students with challenging behavior can positively influence behavior, even among youth who display callous and unemotional traits (Baroncelli & Ciucci, 2020).

Although CD is particularly difficult to treat, success is increased when treatment begins before patterns of antisocial behavior are firmly established. Unfortunately, incarceration within juvenile or adult facilities is the one of the most frequent interventions for youth with CD—a practice that often produces additional behavioral or psychological difficulties rather than rehabilitation. Negative outcomes (e.g., adult incarcerations) occur most frequently among African American youth (Abram et al., 2017), perhaps because incarceration at an early age only serves to exacerbate the social inequities associated with systemic racism and diminishes hope for a positive future.

Going Deeper

Are We Overmedicating Children?

Many medications are prescribed to treat childhood disorders, including antidepressants, tranquilizers, stimulants, and antipsychotics. Medication use with children and adolescents has increased dramatically in recent decades. Further, many prescriptions are written by pediatricians and general practitioners rather than mental health specialists such as child psychiatrists (Sultan et al., 2018). Medication use is most successful when parents are aware of the specific symptoms being treated, possible side effects, and the prescriber's plan for monitoring progress; however, this does not always occur. Additionally, controversy continues regarding the overdiagnosis of some childhood disorders, the "quick fix" nature of medication, and the tendency to use medication without first attempting other interventions. For example, despite strong research supporting the effectiveness of psychosocial interventions with ADHD, many children with this diagnosis are treated primarily with drugs. Further, many children who receive an ADHD diagnosis are prescribed antipsychotic medication without a prior trial of a stimulant—the recommended first-line medication for ADHD (Sultan et al., 2019).

Another concern is that many medications prescribed for youth have only been tested on adults; thus, there is insufficient information regarding how these drugs might affect the extensive brain development that occurs throughout childhood and adolescence. Additionally, there is limited evidence supporting the efficacy of medications for many of the disorders for which they are currently being prescribed (Jacobson, 2014). Many agree that we may not yet understand all of the potential adverse effects of the psychotropic medications prescribed for children. For instance, many antipsychotic medications not only cause children or adolescents to gain weight but also significantly increase their risk of developing diabetes (Lee et al., 2018). It is not surprising that many mental health professionals believe that medication should be considered only after comprehensive diagnostic evaluation and prior implementation of alternative interventions.

For Further Consideration

1. How can we determine if medications are prescribed too freely and if their use with children is safe?

2. What can parents do to ensure that adequate assessment and consideration of nonpharmaceutical interventions occur before medication is prescribed?

The majority of juvenile offenders have experienced multiple traumatic events throughout their lives. Therefore, mental health advocates have argued that rehabilitative outcomes would be significantly improved by making transformational changes within the juvenile justice system such as trauma-informed staff training and psychosocial interventions for adjudicated youth (Baetz et al., 2019).

16-3 Neurodevelopmental Disorders

Neurodevelopmental disorders involve impaired development of the brain and central nervous system; symptoms of neurodevelopmental disorders such as difficulties with learning, communication, and behavior become increasingly evident as the child grows and develops. Disorders in this category include tic disorders (such as Tourette disorder), attention-deficit/hyperactivity disorder, autism spectrum disorder, and intellectual and learning disorders (refer to Table 16.4).

Tics and Tourette Disorder

Case Study Singer and Grammy winner Billie Eilish began to display facial and vocal tics as a child and was diagnosed with Tourette disorder at age 11. As a young adult, she continues to experience subtle symptoms involving involuntary flexing of her arm muscles, raising her eyebrows, and clicking her jaw. These tics, which she describes as exhausting, are reduced when she is moving around or engaged in activities such as singing or riding her horse. (Sanchez, 2022)

Table 16.4   Neurodevelopmental Disorders

Disorders Chart			
Disorder	**Characteristics**	**Prevalence**	**Course**
Tic disorder	Involuntary, repetitive movements or vocalizations	0.3% to 0.9%; four times as common in boys	Sometimes persists into adulthood
Attention-deficit/ hyperactivity disorder	Inattention, hyperactivity, and impulsivity	0.1% to 10.2%; twice as common in boys	Some symptoms may persist into adulthood
Autism spectrum disorder	Qualitative impairment in social communication; restricted, stereotyped interests and activities	1% to 2%; three to four times as common in boys	Course depends on severity, presence of intellectual disability, and intervention
Intellectual developmental disability	Mild, moderate, severe, or profound deficits in intellectual functioning and adaptive behavior	1% to 1.6%; more common in boys	Lifelong
Learning disorder	Normal intelligence with significant deficits in basic reading, writing, or math skills	5% to 15%; more common in boys	May improve with intervention or persist into adulthood

Source: APA, 2022; CDC, 2009, 2010b; Knight et al., 2012; Maenner et al., 2023; Robertson, 2010

Tics are recurrent and sudden, involuntary, nonrhythmic motor movements or vocalizations. **Motor tics** involve various physical behaviors, including blinking, grimacing, tapping, jerking the head, flaring the nostrils, and contracting the shoulders. **Vocal tics** include coughing; grunting; throat clearing; sniffling; and sudden, repetitive, and stereotyped outbursts of words. As was the case with Billie Eilish, tics often begin in childhood and can be particularly distressing when peers respond with teasing or ridicule. Short-term suppression of a tic is sometimes possible but often results in subsequent increases in the tic. Many people report feeling tension build before a tic, followed by a sense of relief after the tic occurs. A physician with tics described it this way:

> This urge comes in the form of a sensation . . . a sensation that is somehow incomplete. To complete and resolve the sensation, the tic must be executed, which provides almost instant relief. . . . The relief is very transient. . . . The sensation comes back again, but often more intensely than before. (Turtle & Robertson, 2008, p. 451)

Although tic symptoms frequently begin in early childhood, tics in children are often temporary and disappear without treatment. When a tic has been present for less than a year, a diagnosis of *provisional tic disorder* is given; *chronic motor or vocal tic disorder* refers to tics lasting more than a year (APA, 2022). For those who develop persistent tics, symptoms often peak prior to puberty and decline or disappear during adolescence. Neuroimaging studies suggest that this symptom improvement may be due to compensatory, neuroplastic brain reorganization that allows affected teens to suppress and eventually control their tics (Jackson et al., 2013). Most children with a tic disorder are tic-free or experience only mild tics in adulthood (Ueda & Black, 2021).

Tourette disorder is characterized by multiple motor tics (e.g., blinking, grimacing, shrugging, jerking the head or shoulders) and one or more vocal tics (e.g., repetitive throat clearing, sniffing, or grunting) that are present for at least 1 year, although not necessarily concurrently (APA, 2022). Motor movements involving self-harm (e.g., punching oneself) or **coprolalia** (the involuntary uttering of obscenities or inappropriate remarks) occur in about 10 percent of those with Tourette disorder (Singer, 2005). Up to 83 percent of those with Tourette disorder are diagnosed with at least one additional mental, behavioral, or developmental disorder (CDC, 2023a). Comorbid conditions, including poor anger control, attention-deficit/hyperactivity disorder, obsessive-compulsive disorder, impulsive behavior, and poor social skills, often interfere with quality of life even more than the tics themselves do (Yadegar et al., 2019). In one meta-analysis, transient tic disorders affected almost 3 percent of youth, whereas only 0.77 percent had Tourette syndrome; these disorders are much more common in boys (Knight et al., 2012).

Tic disorders are influenced by a variety of etiological factors. Both chronic tic disorder and Tourette disorder appear to have a genetic basis, with an estimated heritability of 70 percent to 85 percent (APA, 2022). Because Tourette disorder is highly comorbid with obsessive-compulsive disorder, similar neurochemical abnormalities and brain structures are likely involved (Kurlan, 2013). Stress, negative social interactions, anxiety, excitement, or exhaustion can increase the frequency and intensity of tics (Yadegar et al., 2019).

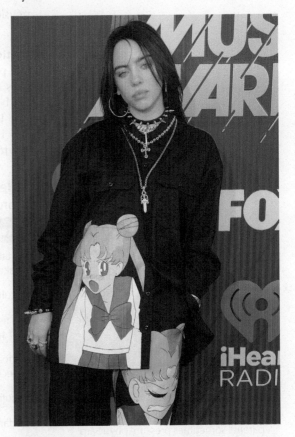

Living with Tourette Disorder

Singer and songwriter Billie Eilish, who has received numerous music awards as well as an Academy Award and a Golden Globe Award, is also known as a social justice advocate who speaks out regarding climate change awareness, reproductive rights and gender equality.

Psychotherapy can help with the distress caused by tic symptoms. Behavioral interventions such as exposure and response prevention (exposing the client to the urge to engage in the tic and teaching habituation to the urge to prevent the tic from occurring) and **habit reversal**, which involves teaching a behavior that is incompatible with the tic, are effective treatments that can be conducted individually or in a small group setting. Virtual behavior intervention programs are also effective in reducing symptoms (Frey & Malaty, 2022). Antipsychotic medications are sometimes used to treat severe tics that have not responded to behavioral techniques (Rothenberger & Roessner, 2019).

Attention-Deficit/Hyperactivity Disorder

Case Study Aries, always on the go as a toddler and preschooler, has had many injuries resulting from continual high activity and risk taking. In kindergarten, Aries talked incessantly and could not stay seated for group work. In first grade, distractibility and off-task behavior persisted despite ongoing efforts to help improve focus. As part of a comprehensive assessment, Aries underwent a psychological evaluation and a complete physical examination.

Attention-deficit/hyperactivity disorder (ADHD) is characterized by attentional problems or impulsive, hyperactive behaviors that are atypical for the child's age and developmental level. As was true for Aries, the symptoms often become increasingly apparent once children enter school. According to the DSM-5-TR, an ADHD diagnosis requires that symptoms (refer to Table 16.5) begin before age 12, persist for at least 6 months, and interfere with social or academic functioning. Individuals with ADHD can have

Table 16.5 Characteristics of Attention-Deficit/Hyperactivity Disorder

Inattention	Hyperactivity and Impulsivity
Poor attention to detail; careless mistakes	Fidgeting
Difficulty sustaining attention	Restlessness
Does not appear to be listening when spoken to	Excessive movement
Poor follow-through with instructions or specific tasks	Excessive loudness
Difficulty organizing tasks	Excessive talking
Avoidance of sustained mental effort	Blurting out answers
Misplacing of important objects	Difficulty waiting for a turn
Distractibility	Interruption of or intrusion on others
Forgetfulness	Impatience

Note: With ADHD, these characteristics occur more frequently than would be expected based on age, gender, and developmental level. A diagnosis of ADHD requires the presence of at least six characteristics involving inattention or hyperactivity/impulsivity. The characteristics must be evident before age 12; be present in at least two settings; persist for at least 6 months; and interfere with social, academic, or work functioning.

Source: APA, 2022

problems involving (a) inattention, (b) hyperactivity and impulsivity, or (c) a combination of these characteristics. Symptoms of hyperactivity and impulsivity involve a mixture of excessive movement and a tendency to act without considering the consequences. Inattention often takes the form of distractibility and intense focus on irrelevant environmental stimuli—symptoms associated with poor regulation of attentional processes.

ADHD can be difficult to diagnose, especially in early childhood, when limited attention, impulsive actions, and high levels of energy are common. Diagnosis relies on observations and input from parents, school personnel, and others knowledgeable about the child's behaviors. To receive a diagnosis of ADHD, a child must display symptoms in at least two settings (APA, 2022).

Hyperactive can be a confusing term because many people use the word in everyday conversation to describe all highly energetic children. The professional who is assessing the child must determine whether the behaviors of concern are (a) typical for the child's age, gender, and overall level of development; (b) a normal temperamental variant involving higher than average energy and impulsivity; or (c) an actual disorder involving significantly atypical behaviors that interfere with day-to-day functioning in multiple settings. Diagnosis can be challenging because ADHD involves varied symptoms (i.e., inattention, impulsivity, and hyperactivity), each with different trajectories of development and treatment options (Musser & Raiker, 2019).

ADHD is the most frequently diagnosed mental disorder in preschool and school-age children. Boys are more than twice as likely as girls to receive an ADHD diagnosis (Bitsko et al., 2022). Data from the 2016 to 2019 survey years of National Survey of Children's Health indicated that 9.8 percent of children ages 3 to 17—approximately 6 million children and adolescents—had received an ADHD diagnosis (Danielson et al., 2022). Although symptoms of ADHD often improve in late adolescence, follow-up studies suggest that approximately 30 percent of those diagnosed with ADHD experience continued symptoms of inattention, disorganization, or impulsive actions in adulthood (Barbaresi et al., 2013).

ADHD is associated with both behavioral and academic problems. Children with ADHD have the most difficulty in situations that are unstructured or involve insufficient stimulation or tedious activities that require sustained attention (Kooistra et al., 2010). The characteristic of inattentiveness, particularly when combined with the excitability, impatience, and difficulty with emotional regulation seen in many children with ADHD, can significantly impair peer relationships and interfere with optimal academic functioning (Bunford et al., 2014). Disorders that often co-occur with ADHD include autism spectrum disorder, oppositional defiant disorder, and conduct disorder (Elwin et al., 2020). Youth with ADHD also have a high risk of smoking and using alcohol and illicit drugs (Gold et al., 2014).

Etiology

Symptoms of ADHD result from multiple etiological factors. ADHD is an early-onset disorder with clear biological as well as psychological, social, and sociocultural etiology.

Biological Dimension ADHD is a highly heritable disorder, with up to 80 percent of symptoms explainable by genetic factors (Grimm et al., 2020). The exact nature of genetic transmission

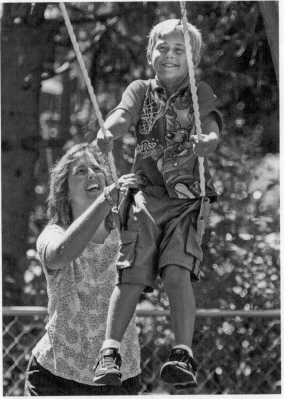

AP Images/George Widman

Interventions for Attention-Deficit/Hyperactivity Disorder

This 6-year-old boy is enrolled in a study called Project Achieve, in which parents and teachers are taught strategies to help minimize problem behaviors. New research finds that providing more structure throughout a child's day can offer a nondrug alternative to help children with attention-deficit/hyperactivity disorder.

is unclear because scientists have not yet identified any specific genes that strongly link to ADHD symptoms. Researchers are now turning to polygenetic risk scores in search of gene combinations or epigenetic changes produced by gene × environment interactions that are connected to ADHD symptoms. Using this approach, scientists have identified epigenetic biomarkers involving several risk genes linked to ADHD (Mooney et al., 2020).

Different hypotheses regarding neurological mechanisms that produce ADHD symptoms include the following:

- *Functional abnormalities in frontal brain regions associated with executive function, attention, and inhibition of responses*: Reduced inhibitory mechanisms in the prefrontal cortex can affect impulsivity, organization, and attentional processes. Fortunately, these frontal lobe variations involving networks associated with sustained attention appear to normalize as children with ADHD grow older (Yasumura et al., 2019).

- *Brain structure and circuitry irregularities in regions such as the accumbens, amygdala, caudate, hippocampus, and putamen*: In a study using the largest dataset available, neuroimaging has confirmed smaller volumes in these subcortical brain structures in children with ADHD as compared to controls. The largest difference was found for the amygdala, which may explain the emotional regulation difficulties often seen in children with ADHD. In adolescence, the only difference in brain volume involved the hippocampus, and by adulthood, no differences were found between the ADHD group and the control group. The researchers concluded that ADHD appears to result from delays in brain maturation (Hoogman et al., 2017). Further, neuroimaging of drug-naïve children (children who have never taken medication for their ADHD) revealed reduced brain connectivity in regions associated with attentional skills and inhibitory control deficits (Chen, Huang, et al., 2019). Additionally, some children with ADHD show slower development of the cerebrum, particularly prefrontal regions associated with attention and motor planning and subcortical areas (Shaw et al., 2007; Wang, Zuo, et al., 2020). These delays (and subsequent catching up) in neurological development may explain why many children with ADHD eventually outgrow their disorder.

- *Reductions in neurotransmitters (such as dopamine and GABA) that affect signal flow to and from the frontal lobes*: Reductions in these neurotransmitters are associated with difficulty inhibiting behavioral impulses. Many medications used to treat ADHD target these neurotransmitters (Faraone, 2018).

Although ADHD is a highly heritable disorder, it is estimated that environmental factors account for between 10 percent and 40 percent of the variance (Sciberras et al., 2017). Some of the other biological factors implicated in the development of ADHD include prematurity, perinatal oxygen deprivation, and very low birth weight (Franz et al., 2018); exposure to PCB (a banned chemical compound that can still be found in air, food, and water) or lead (Nilsen & Tulve, 2020); and maternal smoking or drug or alcohol use during pregnancy (Han et al., 2015).

Psychological, Social, and Sociocultural Dimensions Many psychological, social, and sociocultural factors are associated with ADHD. Sociocultural and social adversity, including family stress, severe marital discord, poverty, family conflicts, paternal criminality, maternal mental disorder, and foster care placement, have been associated with ADHD (Weissenberger et al., 2017). Further, children who are inattentive, hyperactive, or impulsive often encounter negative reactions from parents and rejection from peers. This interpersonal conflict may result in psychological reactions (e.g., depression, low self-esteem, rebelliousness) and lack of opportunities to socialize with peers—factors that further exacerbate symptoms (Ward, Sibley, et al., 2019). Some argue that differing cultural and regional expectations regarding activity levels, inattentiveness, and academic achievement can explain regional differences in ADHD diagnosis (Figure 16.3). Similarly, parenting practices that encourage exercise and outdoor activity or routines that help prevent children from getting overtired or overaroused are associated with reduced risk of ADHD symptoms (Parens & Johnston, 2009).

Treatment

Stimulant medications such as methylphenidate (Ritalin) have been used to treat ADHD for decades and appear to have short-term effectiveness for some individuals. Although approximately 30 percent of those with ADHD experience significant side effects or do not improve, stimulants are the primary medications used to treat ADHD (Gold et al., 2014). Stimulants work by normalizing neurotransmitter functioning and increasing neurological activation in the frontal cortex, thereby increasing attention and reducing impulsivity. Stimulants can produce side effects such as increased heart rate and blood pressure and decreased appetite. Additionally, researchers continue to debate the long-term efficacy of stimulant use and at what point medication intervention should be discontinued (Pliszka, 2019). Due to the frequency of misuse and diversion (i.e., giving, selling, or trading) of prescribed short-acting stimulant medications, physicians are educating patients and their parents about medication safety and are prescribing versions of the medication that are less likely to be abused (Manning, 2013).

The first nonstimulant medication for ADHD received FDA approval in 2021. This medication, Qelbree (viloxazine), works by increasing serotonin, norepinephrine, and dopamine. The randomized, double-blind, placebo-controlled studies that have been conducted thus far suggest that this innovative

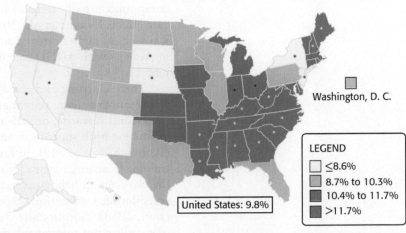

Washington, D. C.

LEGEND
☐ ≤8.6%
☐ 8.7% to 10.3%
☐ 10.4% to 11.7%
☐ >11.7%

United States: 9.8%

*Indicates the state estimate has a statistically significant difference (*p* < .05) from the estimate for the rest of the country.

Figure 16.3

Percent of Youth (Ages 3 to 17) Ever Diagnosed with Attention-Deficit/Hyperactivity Disorder by State, Based on National Survey of Children's Health, 2016 to 2019

The prevalence of parent-reported diagnosis of attention-deficit/hyperactivity disorder (ADHD) varies significantly from state to state and across geographic regions. The percentage of children diagnosed is highest in southern states such as Louisiana (16.3 percent) and lowest in western states such as California (6.1 percent). What might account for the variability in ADHD diagnoses from state to state and region to region?

Source: Danielson et al., 2022

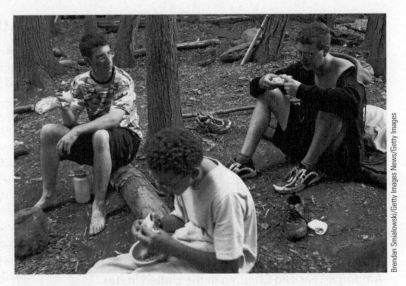

Interventions for Older Youth with Attention-Deficit/Hyperactivity Disorder

Students eat while camping out at the Center for Attention and Related Disorders camp in Connecticut. The 4-week camp matches one instructor with every two campers and provides structure, discipline, and social supports that are helpful for children who have attention-deficit/hyperactivity disorder (ADHD) and similar disorders.

compound rapidly reduces both hyperactivity and inattention with few side effects (Nasser et al., 2020). It does have a boxed warning: "In clinical studies, higher rates of suicidal thoughts and behaviors were reported in patients with ADHD treated with Qelbree than in patients treated with placebo."

There is strong and consistent evidence that behavioral and psychosocial treatments (e.g., parent education, classroom management strategies, behavioral rewards, or self-management training) are highly effective in producing both short-term and long-term reductions in ADHD symptoms (Wolraich et al., 2019). In fact, many experts argue that parent behavior training (teaching parents to use effective disciplinary practices to deal with the challenging behaviors associated with ADHD) should be used before considering medication, especially with preschool-age children (Lange et al., 2018). Additionally, modifying the environment or social context (e.g., allowing movement or ensuring that schoolwork is sufficiently challenging) can enhance feelings of competence, motivation, and self-efficacy for youth with ADHD (Gallichan & Curle, 2008). Simply providing opportunities for moderate exercise can improve attention and reduce impulsivity and hyperactivity (Ludyga et al., 2017).

Interventions are most successful when services are coordinated and when the child's unique characteristics and social and family circumstances are considered. Depending upon the child's needs, support for the child might involve psychoeducation, parent/family therapy, and behavioral or environmental interventions in the home or classroom. Some researchers have proposed that symptom severity should guide treatment decisions, with interventions ranging from environmental modifications for mild symptoms to intensive, combined treatment (e.g., behavior management, parenting strategies, medication) for severe ADHD symptoms. Medications would be considered only if the psychological and environmental interventions proved ineffective (Young et al., 2020).

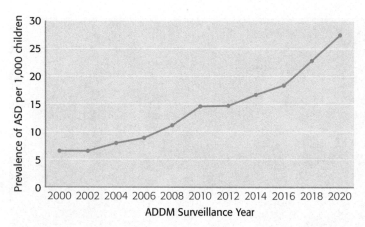

Figure 16.4

Changes in the Prevalence of Autism Spectrum Disorder Among 8-Year-Old Children in the United States, 2002–2020

The prevalence of autism spectrum disorder among 8-year-old children in the United States has dramatically increased over the past two decades. What might account for such significant increases?

Source: Maenner et al., 2023

Autism Spectrum Disorder

Autism spectrum disorder (ASD) is characterized by significant impairment in social communication skills and by the display of stereotyped interests and behaviors. ASD is designated a spectrum disorder because the symptoms vary significantly, occurring along a continuum from mild to severe and affecting each person in different ways. The prevalence of ASD has been increasing at an alarming rate over the past two decades (refer to Figure 16.4); although these increases may have resulted from expanded awareness of the disorder, many experts believe that a variety of environmental influences are involved. According to an ongoing surveillance study involving precise monitoring of ASD prevalence based on the medical and school records of 8-year-olds in 11 selected states, data collected in 2020 suggest that ASD affects approximately 1 out of 36 children in the United States, with significant variations in prevalence between the states—the highest rate was found in California, and the lowest rate was in Maryland (Maenner et al., 2023). The survey revealed that ASD occurs 3.8 times more frequently in boys compared to girls. Overall, ASD prevalence per 1,000 children was highest among Asian or Pacific Islanders (33.4), followed by Hispanic Americans (31.6), African Americans (29.3), and American Indian/Alaska Natives (26.5). Lower rates were found among children of European descent (24.3) and children of two or more races (22.9).

Surprisingly, almost 30 percent of the parents in one study reported that their child was receiving no treatment beyond school-based special educational services; a large number of the parents indicated that they were unable to obtain desired professional care for their child (Xu et al., 2019). A particular concern is the extended delay in ASD diagnosis that occurs for African American children, with a delay of almost 3 years between parents expressing concerns and an ASD diagnosis—long after the window of time during which early intervention has the greatest potential for reducing autistic symptoms and long-term intellectual impairment (Constantino et al., 2020).

As you will see, parenting a child with ASD can be quite challenging. Further, many individuals who have symptoms on the autism spectrum have co-occurring disorders and display a variety of complex symptoms that interfere with day-to-day living (Xu et al., 2019).

Symptoms of Autism Spectrum Disorder

Case Study   Until about 18 months of age, Amy showed normal development—smiling, laughing, babbling, waving to her parents, and playing peekaboo. By age 2, she was withdrawn and spoke no words except meaningless phrases from songs. She now spends much of her time rocking back and forth. The only thing that captures her attention is watching animated characters singing and dancing across the television screen.

Case Study   Danny B. wants chicken and potatoes. He asks for it once, twice . . . ten times. . . . His mother patiently explains that she is fixing spaghetti. "Mom," he asks in a monotone, "why can't we have chicken and potatoes?" If Danny were a toddler, his behavior would be nothing unusual. But Danny is 20 years old. "That's really what life with autism is like," says his mom. "I have to keep laughing. Otherwise, I would cry." (Kantrowitz & Scelfo, 2006, p. 47)

At the beginning of this chapter, we introduced Ahmed, a young child with ASD who spends much of his time humming and spinning the wheels of his toys. The cases of Ahmed, Amy, and Danny give us a glimpse into how ASD presents early in life and in adulthood. In 1943, Leo Kanner, a child psychiatrist, identified a triad of behaviors that have come to define the essential features of ASD: extreme isolation and problems relating to people, a need for sameness, and significant difficulties with communication. Kanner called the syndrome infantile autism, from the Greek autos ("self"), to reflect the profound aloneness and detachment of these children. At its core, ASD involves pervasive deficits in social communication.

ASD is diagnosed when a trained professional documents persistent evidence of all of the following characteristics (APA, 2022):

1. Deficits in social communication and social interaction

   - *Atypical social-emotional reciprocity*: Interest in social interaction may be limited or totally lacking. For example, there may be no acknowledgment of parents or other family members.

Milder symptoms in older children or adults may include failure to understand the back and forth of typical conversations, resulting in one-sided domination of conversation focused on narrow self-interests.

- *Atypical nonverbal communication*: There may be little to no eye contact and an absence of meaningful gestures or facial expressions. Milder symptoms may include unusual nonverbal communication (e.g., pushing people aside as if they were objects) or poor social boundaries involving intrusive behaviors or awkward interactions.

- *Difficulties developing and maintaining relationships*: There may be a lack of interest in others or a failure to recognize people's identity or emotions, including treating people as objects or failing to seek physical or emotional contact from caretakers. Those with milder symptoms may have no interest in imaginative play, may be socially inept, or may have difficulty adjusting their behavior to the social context.

2. Repetitive behavior or restricted interests or activities involving at least two of the following:

- *Repetitive speech, movement, or use of objects*: Rhythmic, repetitive, apparently purposeless movements may occur, including banging the head, flapping the arms, rocking the body, spinning objects, whirling in circles, or rhythmically moving fingers. Those with ASD sometimes repetitively stack or spin objects or move them from side to side. There may be repetitive use of language, including **echolalia** (echoing what is heard); incessant repetition of sounds, words, phrases, or nonsensical word combinations; or repetitive, one-sided conversations involving topics of fixated interest.

- *Intense focus on rituals or routines and strong resistance to change*: Common rituals may involve lining up or dropping objects or insistence on the same foods, order of events, or routines. Even small changes in routine can produce agitation and extreme reactions.

- *Intense fixations or restricted interests*: This may involve fascination with certain objects or a repetitive focus on a narrow range of interests.

- *Atypical sensory reactivity*: There may be a lack of reactivity (e.g., apparent indifference to pain, heat, or cold), overreactivity to sensory input (e.g., aversion to touch or certain sounds), or an unusual focus on sensory aspects of objects (e.g., licking or smelling objects or exhibiting an intense interest in moving objects).

The symptoms seen in ASD are not simply developmental delays but represent differences in development that cause impairment in everyday functioning. ASD symptoms range from mild to severe, and there is wide variation in the characteristics displayed by individuals with ASD. Table 16.6 summarizes the range of symptoms found in ASD.

Identical Twins with Autism Spectrum Disorder

These identical twin boys were both diagnosed with autism spectrum disorder before their second birthday. However, the twins are at opposite ends of the autism spectrum. John, on the left, does not yet speak and engages in many repetitive behaviors such as hand-flapping. In contrast, Sam, on the right, possesses a wealth of information on specific topics such as trains, space, and maps. Sam's greatest struggles involve social interactions, especially with other children.

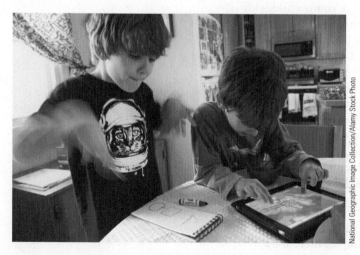

National Geographic Image Collection/Alamy Stock Photo

ASD often occurs in combination with other physical or intellectual conditions. For example, children with ASD have immune system dysregulation and higher rates of food, respiratory, and skin allergies than comparison children (Xu et al., 2018). About 38 percent of children with ASD have an intellectual disability, while nearly 39 percent fall into the average or above average range of intelligence (Maenner et al., 2023). Some individuals with ASD who demonstrate below-average intellectual functioning exhibit *splinter skills*—that is, they do exceptionally well on isolated tasks such as drawing, puzzle construction, musical ability, or rote memory but perform poorly on tasks requiring language skills and symbolic thinking. These children (or adults) are referred to as **autistic savants**. Their remarkable abilities appear to be due to factors such as obsessional focus on specific topics, heightened sensitivity to detail, an aptitude for organizing information, and unique technical interests or mathematical abilities. These qualities are also present in other individuals with ASD, but not to the degree found in autistic savants (Hughes et al., 2018).

Diagnosis of ASD can be complicated. In fact, while some children diagnosed with ASD show "differences" very early in life (refer to Table 16.7), many do not receive an ASD diagnosis until age 4 or later. Unfortunately, many of the early indicators of ASD are so subtle (e.g., limited eye gaze) that they are not easily detectible. For this reason, the American Academy of Pediatrics recommends that health care providers screen all children between 18 and 24 months of age for symptoms of ASD (Estes et al., 2019). When there is a concern that a child might have ASD, typical evaluation procedures include autism screening inventories, observations by medical professionals, parent interviews, developmental histories, communication assessment, and psychological testing. Parent reports and observations are an important part of the diagnostic process. Unfortunately, only about two thirds of the diagnostic evaluations for autism spectrum disorder are made with a high degree of certainty using our current methods of assessment (Dawson, 2023).

Table 16.6 Continuum of Symptoms Associated with Autism Spectrum Disorder

Level of Impairment	Social Communication	Restricted Interests and Repetitive Behaviors
Severe (requires very substantial support)	Minimal or absent communication or response to attempts at social interaction	Ongoing repetitive behaviors; intense preoccupation with rituals; extreme distress upon interference with rituals
Moderate (requires substantial support)	Evident difficulties with social communication; noticeably atypical interactions	Fixated interests and frequent repetitive behaviors and rituals that significantly interfere with functioning
Mild[a] (requires support)	Atypical social interactions; difficulty initiating or responding to social communication	Repetitive behaviors and fixated interests that cause some interference with everyday functioning
Not severe enough for ASD diagnosis	Some atypical behaviors and mild deficits in social communication that do not limit or impair everyday functioning	Ritualized behavior, odd mannerisms, or excessive preoccupations that do not interfere with daily functioning
Variation of normal	Social isolation and awkwardness	Odd preoccupations or mannerisms

[a]Those who demonstrate milder symptoms are sometimes referred to as having high-functioning autism.

Source: Adapted from APA, 2022

Table 16.7 Early Warnings Signs of Possible Autism Spectrum Disorder

Age	Concern
6 to 12 months	• Limited or no eye contact • Minimal or no smiling or joyful responses to people or reciprocal sharing of sounds • Limited or atypical babbling or communicating by pointing, reaching or waving • Limited response when someone speaks to the child
9 to 12 months	• Emerging repetitive behaviors such as spinning or lining up objects • Atypical play behavior or unusual visual or tactile focus on toys
12 to 18 months	• Not using any words • No use of gestures such as pointing • Lack of pretend play • Limited attention to interpersonal interaction
15 to 24 months	• Limited, atypical, or no use of meaningful two-word phrases
Any age	• Parental or caregiver concerns about the possibility of ASD • Loss of previously acquired skills, including reduced frequency or loss of social behaviors or communication skills

Source: Adapted from Zwaigenbaum et al., 2019

Given the importance of early detection and intervention, the U.S. Food and Drug Administration (FDA) has authorized the marketing of the Cognoa ASD Diagnosis Aid, a machine learning–based medical device that health care providers can use to evaluate children who are 18 months to 5 years of age when there is concern of possible symptoms of autism. This system, which relies on uploaded video images of the child as well as data from family, caregivers, and health care providers, yields a conclusion of "Positive for ASD" or "Negative for ASD," unless the system determines that there is insufficient information for the algorithm to make a diagnosis. Preliminary results suggest that the device was able to make a timely and accurate diagnosis in about one third of the children evaluated; in many of the remaining cases, there was insufficient data for the algorithm to confirm or rule out an ASD diagnosis (Megerian et al., 2022).

Eye-tracking technology has also shown some success in detecting decreases in eye contact between 2 and 24 months of age among infants at high risk of ASD. In contrast to the normally developing children who showed progressive increases in eye contact, those who were later diagnosed with ASD showed progressive declines in eye gaze, with the most rapid declines occurring among those who developed the most severe symptoms. The fact that these differences were evident as early as 2 months of age has generated optimism about the possibility of earlier diagnosis. In one study, an eye-tracking measure that quantifies social engagement was found to be as accurate as clinical experts in diagnosing autism in children between the ages of 16 and 30 months. The device has the advantage of being a quick, objective, and relatively inexpensive means to screen for the disorder. Although this appears to be a promising objective screening tool, further research is needed to determine if its accuracy is replicated in other studies (Jones et al., 2023).

These findings are very significant because eye contact is essential for learning and for normal social development. Early diagnosis and intervention might be able to halt or slow down the cascade of biological and psychological symptoms of ASD that begin in early life. In fact, gaze modification programs have demonstrated promising results in increasing attention to eyes and faces among young children with symptoms of ASD (Wang et al., 2020).

Diagnosis may also be delayed among the subgroup of children with ASD who initially have a period of apparently normal social and intellectual development followed by a marked deterioration in skills beginning around 12 months of age or even later. Children with this pattern of regression (referred to as *regressive autism*) often develop more severe symptoms compared to children with ASD without this pattern. Some researchers believe that this regressive onset pattern occurs much more frequently than is realized and that this trajectory is the "rule rather than the exception" (Ozonoff & Iosif, 2019).

Etiology

A great deal of research has focused on the causes of ASD, with the hope of developing early diagnostic procedures and interventions that can prevent, halt, or reverse symptoms. ASD is unique not only because symptoms sometimes appear following a period of relatively normal development but also because intense, early intervention has reversed progression and even eliminated the disorder in some children.

Biological Influences on Autism Spectrum Disorder ASD is considered to be a highly heritable neurodevelopmental disorder in which biological factors play the most critical role (Hu, Devlin, & Debski, 2019). Just as

Going Deeper

Eliminating the Asperger's Diagnosis: Why the Uproar?

I have Asperger's (diagnosed) and my brother has classic autism. I can read and write, I've got a degree, and I can dress myself in the morning. My brother, however, possesses no communication skills and has bowel problems. He is a man in his 20s who is trapped with the mind of a two-year-old. He needs help with every aspect of his life. It doesn't do me any good or him any good by you trying to merge what we've got into one condition. (David, 2010)

Beginning in 1994, Asperger syndrome (named after Austrian pediatrician Hans Asperger) was the DSM diagnosis given to many individuals on the mild end of the autism spectrum—those with average to above-average cognitive skills, intense focus on narrow interests, and poor social skills. The group tasked with revising the autism section of the DSM-5 concluded that the awkwardness in social communication, interpersonal relationship difficulties, desire for sameness, and narrow interests seen in Asperger syndrome could easily be incorporated into the new autism spectrum disorder (ASD) diagnosis. Asperger syndrome was eliminated as a separate diagnostic category. Experts who supported maintaining the Asperger category with modifications in diagnostic criteria—including unique features not previously identified, such as socially insensitive communication; verbose, one-sided conversations pertaining to areas of restricted interests; and

difficulty with practical use of language—were disappointed with the DSM-5 revision (Hosseini & Molla, 2020).

This decision to eliminate Asperger syndrome also generated strong reactions from individuals with the Asperger diagnosis who embrace their uniqueness and who have found social connections within the Asperger community. Like the young man with milder autistic symptoms who is quoted here, they argued that Asperger's syndrome is distinct from ASD. Many further argued that autistic characteristics, particularly the mild Asperger symptoms, should be embraced as a normal variation in human functioning and that this "neurodiversity" should not even constitute a disorder (Hughes, 2020). Heated debate also ensued following the publication of research detailing Hans Asperger's ties to Nazi-era race hygiene policies and the Nazi eugenics movement (Czech, 2018).

For Further Consideration

1. Do individuals previously diagnosed with Asperger's have a point—that they are significantly different from those diagnosed with ASD and that including them on the very broad ASD spectrum creates stigma?

2. Should the milder differences seen in those with high-functioning autism be considered a product of "neurodiversity" and a normal human variation rather than a disorder?

there are a variety of characteristics associated with ASD, it is presumed that multiple factors influence the development of autism spectrum symptoms. Biological researchers are, therefore, approaching the etiology of ASD from a variety of perspectives, including documenting biological processes involved in the development of the disorder; confirming genetic and environmental risk factors; and, most important, elucidating gene × environment interactions. There have been unprecedented advances in genome-wide searches for genes and risk alleles associated with ASD, including spontaneous mutations that occur prior to conception or during early prenatal development (Wisniowiecka-Kowalnik & Nowakowska, 2019). Despite the increase in research on biological influences, no specific biomarkers for ASD have yet been identified (Hirota & King, 2023).

Concordance rates for ASD are much higher for monozygotic twins (ranging from 62 percent to 75 percent) than for dizygotic twins (ranging from 5 percent to 40 percent) (Colvert et al., 2015). Comparisons of monozygotic twins with and without ASD have identified the presence of environmentally driven epigenetic alterations in the twin with ASD, changes associated with specific behavioral traits, and the expression of genes affecting fetal brain development (Wong et al., 2014).

Siblings of individuals with ASD have a much higher prevalence of ASD (over 10 percent) compared to the rest of the population (Sandin et al., 2014). Furthermore, some of the siblings who do not develop ASD show autistic-like traits involving atypical social development and communication patterns (de Zeeuw et al., 2017). Taken together, twin and family studies clearly indicate a strong genetic influence on ASD. However, because monozygotic concordance is less than 100 percent and the degree of impairment varies markedly among monozygotic twin pairs with ASD, other factors are etiologically significant as well.

Although the exact mechanisms by which genetic defects translate into impaired brain functioning are not known, research has linked ASD with numerous neurological findings, including:

- abnormal development of the frontal and temporal lobes, amygdala, and cingulate regions of the brain and altered functional connections between the parts of the brain related to social cognition and emotional processing (Donovan & Basson, 2017);
- reduced gaze toward the eye regions of faces, especially neutral faces, combined with elevated activity in the amygdala in response to human faces (Hadjikhani et al., 2018); and
- atypical responsiveness within the sensory-limbic systems of the brain resulting in sensory overreactivity or atypical negative responses to sensory stimuli (Green et al., 2019).

Ongoing research has also focused on the much higher rate of mitochondrial dysfunction found in children with ASD. Mitochondrial dysfunction affects the energy-producing capacity of cells, a process that is critically important to neural development; some biomarkers of mitochondrial dysfunction correlate with the severity of autistic symptoms, especially in children with a history of developmental regression (Castora, 2019).

A groundbreaking study involving careful analysis of the postmortem brains of children with ASD (ages 2 to 15) yielded important insight into the neurological processes underlying autism spectrum symptoms. The researchers found evidence of patchy areas of disrupted neuronal development that occurred during the normal cell-layering process in all six layers of the cortex; these abnormalities were most prevalent in the early-developing layers of the frontal and temporal cortex, areas associated with social-emotional communication skills. These findings suggest that brain abnormalities associated with ASD begin when the brain is forming during neonatal development. The fact that the pathology was in patches may explain why some children can recover from ASD; early intervention may assist the brain to effectively "rewire" and compensate for the early abnormalities (Stoner et al., 2014). A more recent study looking at postmortem tissue samples of individuals with ASD found epigenetic changes in genes associated with the immune system and the regulation of neurons and biochemical communication processes within the brain (Wong et al., 2019).

Children who develop ASD appear to have an innate vulnerability that is triggered by environmental factors. Prematurity, parental age, congenital rubella infection, as well as exposure to air pollution and pesticides are all associated with the development of ASD (Bölte et al., 2019). Why might environmental toxins cause ASD in some children and not others? A partial answer to this question may come from research showing that children with ASD and typically developing children appear to metabolize toxins differently (Mordaunt et al., 2019). It is unclear if differential exposure to environmental toxins or other variables account for the demographic variance in ASD across the United States (Lyall et al., 2017).

Most researchers agree that ASD is a heterogeneous disorder with multiple causes. Fortunately, biological researchers and experts in the field of ASD are working together to search for interventions that produce documentable biological changes; they are encouraged by the neuroplasticity seen in some children who have received intensive, early intervention.

Other Etiological Influences on Autism Spectrum Disorder Early psychological theories pointed to deviant parent–child interactions as the cause of autism. In fact, Kanner (1943), who named the syndrome, originally concluded that unresponsive parenting was responsible for the development of autistic symptoms, describing parents of children with autism as cold, humorless perfectionists. However, Kanner eventually began to recognize that autism is innate and reassessed his position. It is now widely agreed that biological factors are the primary cause of ASD.

From a psychological perspective, ASD affects the way a child interacts with the world, which in turn affects how others interact with the child. Many children with ASD seldom make eye contact and seem disinterested in socially connecting with others; instead, they prefer to be alone, do not engage in play, and ignore parental efforts at interaction. As you might imagine, all of these characteristics blunt the development of social skills, further interfering with normal neurological and psychological development. This lack of reciprocal social interaction may also result in family members reducing their attempts to maintain social connection, which then adds to the child's isolation. Additionally, behavioral characteristics associated with ASD often create stress and affect interactions within the family, particularly when parents have limited respite from the day-to-day demands of caregiving (Crowell et al., 2019).

Searching for Early Indicators of Autism Spectrum Disorder

Researchers are using a variety of technologies to track eye gaze and brain reactions in infants who are at high risk for autism spectrum disorder, especially those who have siblings with the disorder. These technologies are allowing researchers to document differences between children who develop normally and those who begin to display autistic symptoms.

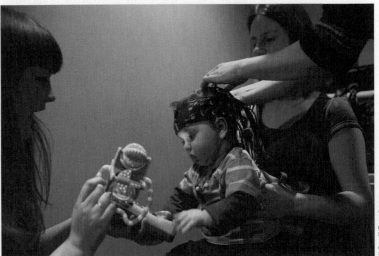

Oli Scarff/Getty Images

Did You Know?

In a large multisite case-control study, children born less than 18 months or more than 60 months after the birth of a sibling had an increased likelihood of developing autism compared to children born between those intervals. Other developmental disabilities did not show this birth spacing effect.

Source: Schieve et al., 2018

Intervention and Treatment

The prognosis for a child with ASD is difficult to predict. Many children diagnosed with ASD retain their diagnosis and require support throughout their lifetime. However, early intervention appears to make a difference. In one study that followed the development of children with ASD who received some type of early intervention, about 75 percent showed improvement in intellectual and communication skills as well as decreases in disruptive behavior; 14 percent no longer met the criteria for ASD at the end of the study (Solomon et al., 2018). In general, those with higher cognitive-adaptive functioning fare better than those who have intellectual disability and behaviors that significantly interfere with social interactions. Although autistic symptoms persist for most people with this diagnosis, comprehensive training and integration into society improve outcome and quality of life. Nearly 20 percent of individuals with ASD exhibit good or very good adaptive behavior, and a growing number of young adults diagnosed with ASD are entering college. Although social awkwardness, restrictive interests, or atypical behaviors often persist, many adults with milder autistic symptoms are self-sufficient, are successfully employed, and function reasonably well (Posar & Visconti, 2019).

Although no medication has been effective in alleviating the core symptoms of ASD, youth with ASD are often given multiple medications in an effort to decrease their anxiety, repetitive behaviors, and hyperactivity. In general, evidence regarding the use of medications in youth with ASD is lacking. Only two medications—the antipsychotics risperidone and aripiprazole—have received FDA approval for the treatment of behavioral symptoms associated with ASD; these drugs require close monitoring for both short-term and long-term side effects (Goel et al., 2018). Some preliminary randomized controlled studies have found that administration of **oxytocin**, a naturally occurring hormone that affects social bonding, can increase social functioning skills in children with ASD (Parker et al., 2017). Thus far, oxytocin is the only biological intervention to address a core symptom of ASD (social communication) rather than the behavioral challenges associated with the disorder. At this point, the findings concerning the effectiveness of oxytocin should be considered mixed (Sikich et al., 2021).

Comprehensive treatment programs have enabled many children with ASD to develop functional skills. The components of effective programs include improving reciprocal social interaction, developing communication skills through imitation, reinforcing behavioral improvement, and social skills training. Parents play a pivotal role in these interventions by learning to allow their child to take the lead in communication and then making it a priority to respond whenever the child attempts to interact. In this manner, parents serve as important coaches and co-therapists using strategies that have the potential to facilitate growth in their child (Crowell et al., 2019). Because of the behavioral, communication, and social impairments associated with ASD, specialized programs often include:

- a high degree of structure through elements such as predictable routine, activity schedules, and clear physical boundaries to minimize distractions;
- intensive, systematically planned, developmentally appropriate educational activities;
- parent education and coaching regarding behavior management and enhancing communication and social interaction at home; and
- opportunities to practice learned skills in new environments, including contact with typically developing peers.

These strategies, combined with opportunities for exposure to normal childhood experiences, are designed to enhance neuroplastic rewiring of connections within the child's brain (Landa, 2018). Many experts in the field emphasize the importance of providing children diagnosed with ASD multiple opportunities to play and communicate with other children in normal social contexts. Training age-level peers in strategies for interacting with children with ASD has been effective in promoting social interaction (Rodda & Estes, 2018).

Pivotal response treatment (PRT), a play-based, child-initiated therapeutic approach, focuses on reducing self-stimulating behaviors and developing communication and social skills by targeting "pivotal behaviors" such as motivation, responding to social cues, and initiating social interaction. The PRT approach also uses natural reinforcers—items of interest to the child rather than contrived rewards. PRT, which has been extensively validated for use with young children, is now used as an early intervention with infants at high risk of ASD (Gengoux et al., 2019). Given the complexity and high variability of symptoms associated with ASD, treatment approaches are most effective when they are individualized and take into account the individual child's skill level, interests, and social-communication strengths.

Intellectual Developmental Disorder

Intellectual developmental disorder (IDD) is characterized by significant limitations in intellectual functioning and adaptive behaviors, including:

- significantly below-average general intellectual functioning (ordinarily interpreted as an IQ score of 70 or less on an individually administered IQ test) and
- deficiencies in **adaptive behavior** (e.g., self-care; understanding of health and safety issues; ability to live, work, or plan leisure activities and use community resources; functional use of academic skills) that are greater than would be expected based on age or cultural background.

IDD is diagnosed only when low intelligence is accompanied by impaired adaptive functioning and the onset of these limitations occurred during the developmental period. Psychologists have traditionally identified four distinct categories of IDD based on IQ score ranges and adaptive behaviors. These categories are (a) *mild* (IQ score 50–55 to 70), (b) *moderate* (IQ score 35–40 to 50–55), (c) *severe* (IQ score 20–25 to 35–40), and (d) *profound* (IQ score below 20–25). Table 16.8 summarizes functional characteristics associated with each of these categories. Social, vocational, and adaptive behaviors can vary significantly not only between categories but also within a given category.

Table 16.8 Adaptive Characteristics Associated with Intellectual Developmental Disorder

Level	Approximate IQ Range	Characteristics
Mild	50–55 to 70	Daily living and social interactions skills are mildly affected; adaptive difficulties involve conceptual and academic understanding; the individual may need assistance with job skills or independent living; the individual may marry and raise children
Moderate	35–40 to 50–55	The individual may have functional self-care skills and the ability to communicate basic needs; the individual may read a few basic words; lifelong support and supervision are required (e.g., supervised meal preparation, sheltered work)
Severe	20–25 to 35–40	The individual may recognize familiar people; communication skills are limited; lifelong support is required
Profound	Below 20–25	Characteristics are similar to those of severe intellectual disability, with even more extensive care needs

The American Association on Intellectual and Developmental Disabilities (2020) asserts that although IQ scores may be used to approximate intellectual functioning for diagnostic purposes, it is much more important to focus on adaptive skills and the nature of psychosocial supports that are needed to maximize functioning. We know that the effects of IDD are variable and that individuals with mild or moderate IDD often function independently or semi-independently in adulthood. Additionally, with support and intervention, those with more severe IDD can make cognitive and social gains and have improved life satisfaction. Approximately 1 percent of children in the United States have an IDD, including many who have coexisting conditions such as ASD or a seizure disorder (Zablotsky et al., 2019).

Etiology of Intellectual Developmental Disorder

The etiology of IDD differs, to some extent, depending on the level of intellectual impairment. Mild IDD is often idiopathic (having no known cause), whereas more pronounced IDD is often associated with genetic factors, brain abnormalities, or brain injury. Although a variety of biological factors are implicated in IDD, psychological, social, and sociocultural factors also play a role in intellectual development and adaptive functioning.

Genetic Factors In up to 80 percent of cases of IDD, the underlying cause is unknown. It is believed that genetic factors that have not yet been identified are responsible for many of these cases; in particular, researchers are focused on genes that affect learning and memory. Also, given the higher prevalence of IDD in males, it is not surprising that researchers have discovered that many of the genes suspected of contributing to IDD are located on the X chromosome (Ibarluzea et al., 2020).

Genetic factors that exert an influence on IDD include both *normal genetic variation* and *genetic abnormalities*. IDD caused by normal genetic variation reflects the fact that in a normal distribution of any trait (such as intelligence), some individuals fall in the lower range. The normal range of intelligence is considered to lie between the IQ scores of 70 and 130. Some individuals with IDD have an IQ that falls at or slightly below the lower end of this normal range (70 or slightly lower); most of the individuals in this group are otherwise physically and emotionally healthy and have no specific physiological anomalies associated with their cognitive and adaptive difficulties.

The genetic abnormalities associated with IDD include chromosomal variations, as well as conditions resulting from the inheritance of a single gene. Many individuals with genetically based IDD have significant cognitive impairment. The most common inherited form of IDD is **fragile X syndrome**, a condition resulting in limited production of proteins required for brain development. Fragile X syndrome results in mild to severe IDD. Females generally have less impairment; males are prone to having communication and social difficulties, including anxious, inattentive, fearful, or aggressive behaviors. Autistic symptoms occur in many individuals with fragile X syndrome, and it is associated with both challenging behavior and difficulties in daily living skills (Usher et al., 2020).

Down syndrome (DS) is the most common and most easily recognized chromosomal disorder resulting in IDD. In the vast majority (95 percent) of cases, an extra copy of chromosome 21 originates during gamete development (involving either the egg or the sperm); this extra chromosome (trisomy 21) alters the course of development and produces the physical and cognitive characteristics associated with the condition. DS occurs once in approximately every 772 live births. The chance of an egg containing an extra copy of chromosome 21 increases significantly with increasing maternal age. However, because most pregnancies occur in women younger than age 35, over half of the babies born with Down Syndrome have a mother in this younger age group (National Down Syndrome Society, 2023).

Distinctive physical characteristics associated with DS include a single crease across the palm of the hand, slanted eyes, a protruding tongue, and a raspy voice. The majority of individuals with DS have mild to moderate IDD; however, minimal intellectual impairment or severe impairment is also possible. With support, many adults with DS have jobs and live semi-independently. Although medical intervention has improved health outcomes and increased life expectancy, those with DS now have a significantly increased risk of experiencing dementia and early-onset Alzheimer disease (National Down Syndrome Society, 2020).

Prenatal screening for DS is performed through several noninvasive techniques that involve analysis of blood samples (e.g., cell-free fetal DNA analysis) and ultrasound imaging. If the screening results indicate a strong likelihood that a fetus has DS, several diagnostic procedures that involve withdrawal of amniotic fluid from the fetal sac are available to confirm chromosomal abnormalities associated with DS; these procedures, which identify DS with almost 100 percent accuracy, involve some risk for both mother and fetus, so they are employed only when prior screening suggests a high likelihood that the fetus has DS (Gray & Wilkins-Haug, 2018). There are regional and cultural differences in the use of genetic screening and decisions regarding termination of pregnancy—a very personal choice that is affected by factors such as religion and the availability of the financial resources and social support systems that would be necessary to parent a child with special needs (Lou et al., 2018).

Nongenetic Biological Factors IDD can result from a variety of environmental influences during the prenatal (from conception to birth), perinatal (just prior to and during the birth process), or postnatal (after birth) period. Many of the circumstances that can cause ID (as well as other neurodevelopmental disorders) are preventable or controllable (refer to Table 16.9). During the prenatal period, the developing fetus is susceptible to viruses and infections (e.g., tuberculosis or German measles), drugs and alcohol, radiation, and poor nutrition. Some risk factors can cause IDD both prenatally and after birth unless steps are taken to alleviate the condition. For example, iodine deficiency either during pregnancy or during early infancy can impair intellectual development (Darnton-Hill, 2017).

Phenylketonuria (PKU), an inherited condition affecting metabolism of a specific amino acid, can also have either prenatal or postnatal effects; if pregnant women with PKU ingest protein or artificial sweeteners, the resultant buildup of the amino acid phenylalanine can cause significant intellectual impairment in a developing fetus. A special diet can prevent this from occurring. Fortunately, IDD resulting from PKU has almost disappeared in most developed countries due to preventive dietary measures taken by mothers with PKU combined with PKU screening for all newborns, and the implementation of dietary restrictions for any infants who have PKU (Kelly et al., 2016).

Table 16.9 Preventable or Controllable Causes of Neurodevelopmental Disorders

Prenatal (Before Birth)
Severe maternal malnutrition
Alcohol or illicit drugs; prescription medications
Iodine or folic acid deficiency[a]
Maternal infections such as rubella[a] or syphilis
Toxoplasma parasites (from cat feces, undercooked meats, or unwashed produce)
Exposure to radiation
Blood incompatibility (Rh factor)
Maternal chronic disease (heart or kidney disease, diabetes)
Untreated phenylketonuria

Perinatal (Just Before or During Birth)
Severe prematurity[a]
Birth trauma
Asphyxia (lack of oxygen)

Infancy and Childhood
Untreated phenylketonuria
Nutritional deficiencies[a]
Iodine deficiency
Severe lack of stimulation
Chronic lead exposure[a]
Other environmental toxins[a]
Brain infections (e.g., meningitis and encephalitis)
Head injury

[a]These factors have also been implicated in the etiology of autism spectrum disorder.

Source: Adapted from the EPA, 2023; World Health Organization, 2011

Any amount of alcohol intake during pregnancy can affect embryonic and fetal development. Although there is a continuum of detrimental neurological and behavioral effects resulting from alcohol consumption (referred to as **fetal alcohol spectrum effects**), children who have **fetal alcohol syndrome (FAS)** have incurred the greatest neurological damage. A proposed DSM-diagnosis, *neurobehavioral disorder associated with prenatal alcohol exposure*, encompasses the impairment in neurocognitive, behavioral, and adaptive functioning associated with prenatal alcohol exposure; this diagnosis would include children with FAS and those with fetal alcohol spectrum effects (APA, 2022). A comprehensive study of first-grade students in four communities across the United States found the prevalence of fetal alcohol spectrum effects was much higher than previously estimated—ranging from 1.5 percent to 5 percent of the children using a conservative approach and 3.1 percent to 9.9 percent using broader definitions. The fetal alcohol spectrum effects observed by the researchers included restricted growth and facial abnormalities as well as cognitive, behavioral, and attentional difficulties (May et al., 2018).

The most common perinatal birth conditions associated with ID are prematurity and low birth weight. Although most premature infants develop normally, some have neurological problems resulting in learning disorders and IDD (Ream & Lehwald, 2018). During the postnatal period, factors such as head injuries, brain infections, tumors, and prolonged malnutrition can cause brain damage and consequent IDD. Exposure to environmental toxins is an increasing concern. Lead, a well-known neurotoxin found in aging water systems and lead-based paint in older homes, is associated with both IDD and hyperactivity (Santa Maria et al., 2019).

Psychological, Social, and Sociocultural Dimensions Psychological, social, and sociocultural factors can affect both intellectual and adaptive functioning. A child's genetic background interacts with environmental factors. For example, children from socioeconomically advantaged homes often attend well-funded schools and are exposed to enriching activities throughout childhood, thereby enhancing cognitive development. In contrast, crowded living conditions, lack of adequate health care, poor nutrition, and inadequate educational opportunities place children living in poverty at an intellectual disadvantage and can influence whether they reach their full potential. Similarly, children raised by parents who have mild IDD may begin their lives with less intellectual stimulation and learning opportunities, further contributing to a generational pattern of lower intellectual functioning. Additionally, the long-term effects of prematurity appear to be moderated by sociocultural factors such as socioeconomic status and parenting style; supportive parenting or increased socioeconomic resources can enhance ultimate cognitive functioning (D'Onofrio et al., 2013).

An enriching and encouraging home environment, as well as ongoing educational intervention focused on targeted cognitive,

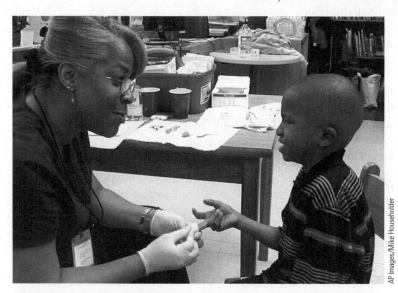

Testing for Neurotoxic Levels of Lead

Exposure to heavy metals such as lead can have toxic effects on the developing brains of infants and children, a concern that emerged after it was determined that approximately 100,000 residents of Flint, Michigan, were exposed to elevated levels of lead that had leached into the city's water supply. Here, a 7-year-old boy receives a blood test at one of the free clinics initiated by the local health department in their effort to detect which children had lead poisoning.

Risks of Substance Use in Pregnancy

It is now common knowledge that alcohol and other drugs can affect a developing fetus. Pregnant women are advised to avoid alcohol throughout pregnancy in order to prevent the physical and cognitive abnormalities associated with fetal alcohol syndrome, the leading cause of preventable intellectual disability (May et al., 2018). Use of tobacco, marijuana, cocaine, heroin, or methamphetamine can also lead to neurodevelopmental disorders (Guille & Auila, 2019). The specific effects on the child depend on the timing (i.e., the stage of fetal development), as well as the type and amount of substance used. Of course, in utero substance exposure is often associated with other prenatal and childhood risk factors, such as poor nutrition; limited prenatal care; a chaotic home environment; and abuse, neglect, or other stressors that can affect brain development (Chu et al., 2020).

Medical professionals continue to debate the advantages, the disadvantages, and the ethics of toxicology screening to detect substance use in pregnant women and newborn infants. Although proponents of screening argue that early detection allows for early intervention to lessen the lifelong consequences of prenatal neurological damage, others are cautious—particularly in states where there are laws or policies requiring mandatory child protection reporting of women who may be endangering their unborn or newborn child. One of the biggest concerns about policies that would allow for widespread screening is that they would cause women using substances to avoid prenatal care—a decision that could have significant negative consequences for both the mother and the unborn child (Polak et al., 2019).

For Further Consideration

1. What do you think are the advantages and disadvantages of widespread screening for prenatal substance abuse?

2. What do you think are the dangers of criminalizing substance use in pregnancy?

3. Do you believe that most young adults are sufficiently aware of the dangers of substance use during pregnancy? What ideas do you have for improving educational efforts in this area?

academic, self-care, social, and problem-solving skills, can have a strong and positive influence on the development of children with IDD (Novak & Morgan, 2019). Coping strategies and the use of outside resources when raising a child with IDD are often influenced by sociocultural context.

Learning Disorders

A **learning disorder (LD)** is diagnosed when the development of basic math, reading, or writing skills is substantially lower than would be expected based on the person's chronological age, educational background, and intellectual ability. Learning disorders primarily interfere with academic achievement and daily living activities that require reading, writing, or math skills. As with any testing, when an assessment for a LD is conducted, care is taken to ensure that testing procedures and test interpretation consider the child's linguistic and cultural background. Specific learning disorders include **dyslexia** (significant difficulties with accuracy or fluency of reading), **dyscalculia** (significant difficulties in understanding quantities, number symbols, or basic arithmetic calculations), and disorders of written expression. Among school-age children, the prevalence of LD is estimated to range between 5 percent and 15 percent (APA, 2022).

Approximately 7.3 million students in the United States received specialized educational services in 2022; one third of this group was diagnosed with a LD (Irwin, 2023). Many children with learning disorders, especially boys, have concurrent disorders such as ADHD (Butterworth & Kovas, 2013). Some individuals continue to cope with severe academic deficits in adulthood. Adults with a severe LD may experience problems with employment, so it is beneficial when their career choice capitalizes on their abilities and strengths.

Did You Know?

Only a small percentage of the 80,000 chemicals used in the United States in 2020 had been tested for neurotoxicity in children.

Source: National Resources Defense Council, 2020

Little is currently known about the precise causes of LD. Some children with a LD appear to have slower brain maturation and eventually catch up academically. However, others have lifelong differences in neurological processing of information related to basic academic skills. Etiological possibilities for chronic LD include many of the same biological explanations for IDD and ADHD (refer to Table 16.9). Additionally, LD tends to run in families, suggesting a genetic component (Fletcher & Grigorenko, 2017).

Support for Individuals with Neurodevelopmental Disorders

Many neurodevelopmental disorders produce lifelong disability; therefore, the goal of intervention is to build skills and develop each individual's potential to the fullest extent possible. For those with moderate to severe IDD or ASD, such support often begins in infancy and extends across the life span. In the case of ASD, early intervention can result in moderate to significant improvement (Rogers et al., 2019). For children with ADHD, LD, mild IDD, or mild ASD, support may occur primarily in the school setting. Interventions for LD and mild IDD typically involve remedial interventions targeting the area of academic difficulty, whereas supports for ASD and more severe intellectual impairment are more comprehensive.

Support in Childhood

When ASD or IDD is identified early, children often participate in individualized home-based or school-based programs focused on decreasing inappropriate behaviors and maximizing overall skill development. Parent involvement is an integral part of early intervention programs; parents can help reduce maladaptive behaviors, as well as enhance cognitive, social, and communication development (Rogers et al., 2019). School services are individualized to meet the needs of the child and to maximize learning opportunities, including skills needed for independent or semi-independent living. Unfortunately, rates of improvement often decrease once adolescents with ASD begin to age out of school programs following high school graduation, or at age 21 for those with more significant impairment (Laxman et al., 2019).

Support in Adulthood

A number of programs are available for young adults with moderate neurodevelopmental disabilities to learn vocational skills or to participate in work opportunities in a specialized setting. These programs focus on specific job skills, social skills for interacting with co-workers and supervisors, and completing work-related tasks with speed and quality. There is a clear need for more support for those with mild IDD or ASD as they make the transition from high school to out-of-school activities, especially for those who are unable to maintain employment without support (Chan et al., 2018).

Institutionalization of adults with neurodevelopmental disorders is rare. Many adults with special needs live with family members; others live independently or semi-independently within the

Work Opportunities for Individuals with Neurodevelopmental Disorders

Many people with Down syndrome and other neurodevelopmental disorders can function well in a supportive work environment. Here a baker's assistant is proudly displaying fresh bread.

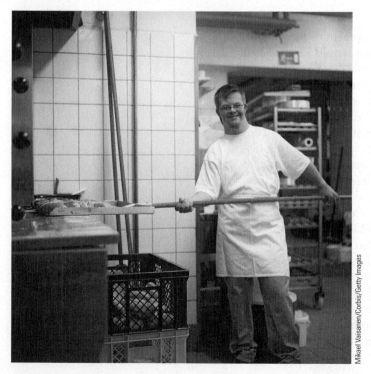

Mikael Vaisanen/Corbis/Getty Images

community. The idea is to provide the least restrictive environment possible—that is, as much independence and personal choice as is safe and practical. Although group arrangements vary considerably from setting to setting, most living arrangements provide opportunities for residents to socialize and to develop independent living skills. Many assisted-living environments promote social interaction with the larger community and continue to support the development of personal competence and independence.

16-4 Contemporary Trends and Future Directions

Exposure to environmental neurotoxins and other factors associated with the development of neurodevelopmental disorders remain a significant concern. For instances, pollution in the environment is associated with structural changes in the brain and impaired cognitive development in children, which can impact academic performance and lifelong learning. Long-term exposure to pollution has been linked to increased risk of childhood disorders such as ASD and ADHD. Children living in lower income households have an increased risk of exposure to pollution since they are more likely to live near factories and major roads, and they experience greater indoor pollution (Mathiarasan & Hüls, 2021). Many environmental and child health advocacy groups continue to highlight the need to enact and enforce legislation to minimize these influences, which disproportionately impact families living in poverty and communities of color (Chesney & Duderstadt, 2022).

Researchers and child advocates have also prioritized adverse childhood experiences (ACEs) and how negative early experiences, particularly in the absence of social support, can produce toxic stress that adversely affects biological, psychological, and social functioning (refer to Figure 16.5).

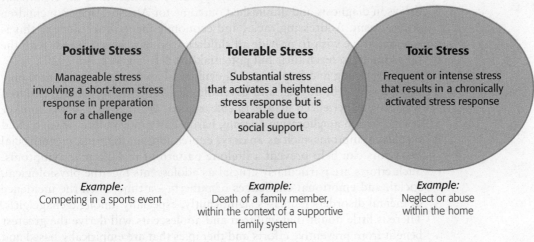

Positive Stress

Manageable stress involving a short-term stress response in preparation for a challenge

Example:
Competing in a sports event

Tolerable Stress

Substantial stress that activates a heightened stress response but is bearable due to social support

Example:
Death of a family member, within the context of a supportive family system

Toxic Stress

Frequent or intense stress that results in a chronically activated stress response

Example:
Neglect or abuse within the home

Figure 16.5

Differentiating Between Positive, Tolerable, and Toxic Stress
When a child's environment lacks the emotional support needed to counteract the effects of frequent or intensely stressful events, the result is toxic stress. This prolonged activation of the stress response system can produce long-term emotional, psychological, and physical consequences.

Long-Term Impact of Emotional Distress

In 2018, presidential policies aimed at deterring future illegal immigration resulted in hundreds of infants and children being abruptly separated from their families. Many mental health professionals have expressed concern that the sudden and prolonged trauma of separation will have long-lasting emotional impacts on the children.

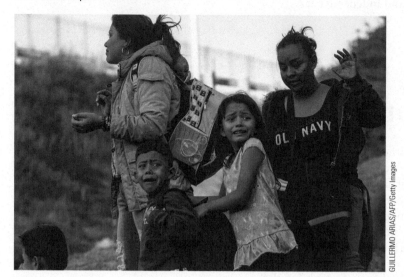

GUILLERMO ARIAS/AFP/Getty Images

Throughout this chapter, we have discussed how ACEs such as neglect, maltreatment, inconsistent parenting, bullying, and domestic violence can affect children on multiple levels. Such experiences can exert lifelong influences on biological processes through the expression of genes or heightened sensitivity of the stress response system. They can also significantly affect emotional processing and emotional regulation (Gladieux et al., 2023). As you have seen throughout this text, many adult mental disorders are rooted in a stressful childhood. Thus, preventing experiences that initiate a negative cascade of events that affect mental health continues to be a high priority.

Mental health professionals continue to search for interventions that minimize the effects of biological, psychological, social, or sociocultural adversity. Recently, there has been a focus on intervening in families where children are exposed to parents or primary caretakers who express contempt or extreme frustration toward the children in their care (Suh & Luthar, 2020). Researchers are also emphasizing that we cannot overlook ACEs such as racism or violence that arise within socioeconomically oppressed neighborhoods or groups, particularly communities of color. Some Indigenous communities are focusing on reversing the downward trajectory associated with ACEs by embracing a holistic healing conceptual framework (Rides at the Door & Shaw, 2023). Child health advocates are also investigating how sociocultural adversity affects the prognosis of youth with neurodevelopmental disabilities. For example, factors associated with systemic racism (e.g., families experiencing discrimination and bias in medical care, limited availability of specialists in communities of color) appear to contribute to the significant delays in diagnosis and diminished outcome for African American children with autism. Addressing racial and economic inequalities such as this is essential if we wish to provide all children who have special needs with the opportunity to reach their full potential (Broder-Fingert et al., 2020).

Developing and implementing evidence-based interventions that promote resilient biological and psychological functioning among children who have experienced maltreatment, trauma, or other stressors is another crucial step in ameliorating ongoing harm. Early intervention when a child displays symptoms such as anxiety, depression, inattention, or antisocial behaviors can help prevent a lifelong pattern of maladaptive symptoms. Such efforts are particularly crucial as adolescents face the physiological, social, and emotional challenges of puberty—a time when the incidence of mental disorders increases significantly, especially among teenage girls. There is little doubt that children and adolescents will derive the greatest benefit from preventive efforts and therapies that are empirically based and carefully tailored to their gender, developmental level, and specific mental health needs as well as the specific requirements of the family system within which they are being raised.

Chapter Summary

1 What internalizing disorders occur in childhood and adolescence?

- Anxiety disorders are the most common internalizing disorders in youth.
- Trauma- and stressor-related disorders include posttraumatic stress disorder and attachment disorders.
- Nonsuicidal self-injury is most likely to emerge during early adolescence.
- Depressive and bipolar disorders can occur in childhood but are more prevalent during adolescence.
- Disruptive mood dysregulation disorder involves negative moods and exaggerated responses to anger.

2 What are the characteristics of externalizing disorders?

- Oppositional defiant disorder involves a pattern of hostile, defiant behavior toward authority figures.
- Intermittent explosive disorder involves either high-frequency/low-intensity aggressive outbursts or low-frequency/high-intensity outbursts.
- Conduct disorders involve serious antisocial behaviors and violations of the rights of others.

3 What are neurodevelopmental disorders, and what are their characteristics?

- Motor and vocal tic disorders and Tourette disorder involve involuntary repetitive movements or vocalizations.
- Attention-deficit/hyperactivity disorder is characterized by inattention, hyperactivity, and impulsivity.
- Autism spectrum disorder involves impairment in social communication and restricted, stereotyped interests and activities.
- Intellectual developmental disability involves limitations in intellectual functioning and adaptive behaviors.
- Learning disorders involve basic reading, writing, or math skills that are substantially below expectations based on age, intelligence, and educational experiences.

Chapter Glossary

adaptive behavior
performance on tasks of daily living, including academic skills, self-care, and the ability to work or live independently

attention-deficit/hyperactivity disorder (ADHD)
childhood-onset disorder characterized by persistent attentional problems and/or impulsive, hyperactive behaviors

autism spectrum disorder (ASD)
a disorder characterized by a continuum of impairment in social communication and restricted, stereotyped interests and activities

autistic savant
an individual with autism spectrum disorder who performs exceptionally well on certain tasks

child psychopathology
the emotional and behavioral manifestation of psychological disorders in children and adolescents

conduct disorder (CD)
a persistent pattern of behavior that violates the rights of others, including aggression, serious rule violations, and illegal behavior

coprolalia
involuntary utterance of obscenities or inappropriate remarks

disinhibited social engagement disorder (DSED)
a trauma-related attachment disorder characterized by indiscriminate, superficial attachments and desperation for interpersonal contact

disruptive mood dysregulation disorder (DMDD)
a childhood disorder involving chronic irritability and significantly exaggerated anger reactions

Down syndrome (DS)
a chromosomal disorder (most frequently involving an extra copy of chromosome 21) that causes physical and neurological abnormalities

dyscalculia
a condition involving difficulties in understanding mathematical skills or concepts

dyslexia
a condition involving significant difficulties with reading skills

echolalia
repetition of vocalizations made by another person

externalizing disorders
disruptive behavior disorders associated with symptoms that disturb others

fetal alcohol spectrum effects
a continuum of detrimental neurological and behavioral effects resulting from maternal alcohol consumption during pregnancy

fetal alcohol syndrome (FAS)
a condition resulting from maternal alcohol consumption during gestation that involves central nervous system dysfunction and altered brain development

fragile X syndrome
an inherited condition involving limited production of proteins required for brain development resulting in mild to severe intellectual disability

habit reversal
a therapeutic technique in which a client is taught to substitute new behaviors for habitual behaviors such as a tic

intellectual developmental disability (IDD)
a disorder characterized by limitations in intellectual functioning and adaptive behaviors

intermittent explosive disorder (IED)
a condition involving frequent lower-intensity outbursts or low-frequency, high-intensity outbursts of extreme verbal or physical aggression

internalizing disorders
conditions involving emotional symptoms directed inward

learning disorder (LD)
an academic disability characterized by reading, writing, or math skills that are substantially below levels that would be expected based on the person's age, intellectual ability, and educational background

motor tic
a tic involving physical behaviors such as eye blinking, facial grimacing, or head jerking

neurodevelopmental disorders
conditions involving impaired development of the brain and central nervous system that are evident early in a child's life

nonsuicidal self-injury (NSSI)
self-harm intended to provide relief from negative feelings or to induce a positive mood state

oppositional defiant disorder (ODD)
a childhood disorder characterized by negativistic, argumentative, and hostile behavior patterns

oxytocin
a powerful hormone that affects social bonding

pediatric bipolar disorder (PBD)
a childhood disorder involving depressive and energized episodes similar to the mood swings seen in adult bipolar disorder

reactive attachment disorder (RAD)
a trauma-related disorder characterized by inhibited, avoidant social behaviors and reluctance to seek or respond to attention or nurturing

selective mutism
consistent failure to speak in certain situations

separation anxiety disorder
severe distress about leaving home, being alone, or being separated from a parent

temperament
innate mental, physical, and emotional traits

tic
an involuntary, repetitive movement or vocalization

Tourette disorder
a condition characterized by multiple motor tics and one or more vocal tics

vocal tic
an audible tic such as coughing, grunting, throat clearing, sniffling, or making sudden, vocal outbursts

1 What are the criteria used to judge insanity, and what is the difference between insanity and incompetency to stand trial?

2 Under what conditions can a person be involuntarily committed for inpatient psychiatric treatment?

3 What rights do the mentally ill have with respect to treatment and care?

4 What legal and ethical issues guide treatment practices?

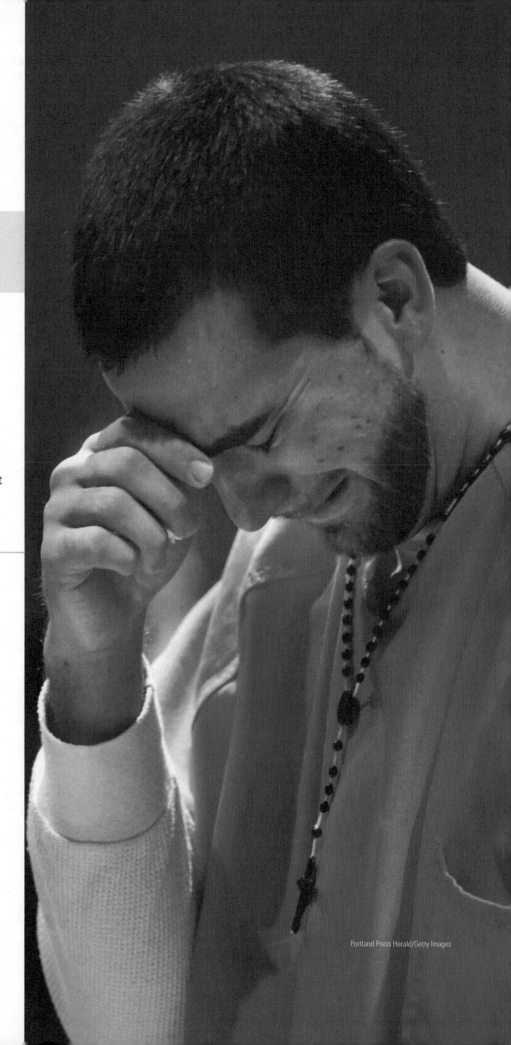

Portland Press Herald/Getty Images

17

Law and Ethical Clinical Practice

Learning Objectives

After studying this chapter, you will be able to . . .

17-1 Discuss the criteria used to judge insanity, and explain the difference between being insane and being incompetent to stand trial.

17-2 Describe the conditions under which a person can be involuntarily committed to an inpatient psychiatric facility.

17-3 Explain the rights people with mental illness have with respect to treatment and care.

17-4 Describe the legal and ethical issues associated with psychotherapy, and explain why it is important for therapists to develop cultural competence.

On July 20, 2012, 24-Year-Old James Eagan Holmes, described as a shy, intelligent man who had recently been a promising graduate student working toward his doctorate in neuroscience at the University of Colorado, committed a horrendous act. Wearing black tactical clothing with a helmet and a gas mask, Holmes set off tear gas grenades during a screening of the movie *The Dark Knight Rises* at a theater in Aurora, Colorado. Then, using a variety of firearms, he killed 12 people and wounded 70 others. He was arrested without resistance outside the theater. During his first court appearance, his recently dyed, red-orange hair was disheveled and he appeared dazed and unaware of his surroundings.

In the opening arguments of his trial, on April 27, 2015, his defense attorney claimed that Holmes committed the massacre during the "throes of a psychotic episode" and that he should be found "not guilty by reason of insanity." The prosecution, however, argued that Holmes meticulously planned the massacre, purchasing firearms, ammunition, explosive chemicals, tear gas, and body armor over several months so he could carry out what he described to his former girlfriend as his "evil plan to kill people" (Gurman, 2015).

Many Unanswered Questions

Colorado theater shooting suspect James Holmes, seen here in his first court appearance, faced charges of murdering 12 people and wounding 70 others. He entered a plea of "not guilty by reason of insanity." This case raised questions about the confidentiality of therapist–client communication and the duty to warn the public about a potentially life-threatening situation.

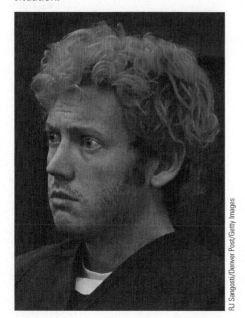

RJ Sangosti/Denver Post/Getty Images

The case of James Holmes raises several important issues that will be covered in this chapter. First, what is the insanity defense, and does it apply to Holmes? Was he so mentally disturbed that he was unable to tell right from wrong? How did the mental health professionals who evaluated him determine his mental state, and what criteria did they use to decide if he was sane or insane at the time of the shooting? Second, prior to withdrawing from his PhD program and prior to the shootings, Holmes met with three mental health professionals at the University of Colorado. Are the conversations he had during these meetings and records from these sessions protected by physician–patient privilege? In other words, is this information admissible as evidence in court proceedings, especially if Holmes does not waive his right to confidentiality? Under what circumstances can privilege and confidentiality be broken? Third, one of those professionals, the psychiatrist, had reportedly been worried about some threatening and homicidal statements made by Holmes during their sessions, such as stating that if he let her know his thoughts in detail, she would "lock him up" (Phillips, 2018). Did she have a duty and obligation to warn others about his threats? Dr. Richard Martinez, a forensic psychiatrist and professor at the University of Colorado School of Medicine, stated, "At the moment you determine that there is a credible threat . . . the duty to warn is triggered" (Sallinger, 2012). However, did the duty to warn apply in this situation? Courts, society, and mental health professionals continue to struggle with these complex issues.

Psychologists and other mental health professionals often participate in the legal system and must deal with the multiple questions posed here. In the past, psychologists primarily evaluated mental competency in criminal cases such as those of James Holmes. Now, determining whether someone is sane or insane is only a small part of the role they play in the judicial system. Psychologists also give expert opinions on topics such as child custody, neuropsychological functioning, traumatic injury, and suicide (Table 17.1). The American Psychological Association has even taken on the role of *amicus curiae* (friend of the court), acting in an advisory capacity by filing briefs summarizing social or psychological research that may help inform legal decisions. Not only do mental health professionals influence decisions in the legal system, mental health laws passed at local, state, and federal levels also affect the practice of therapy.

In this chapter, we cover many topics where psychology and the law intersect. We begin by examining some of the issues related to criminal and civil commitment. We then look at patients' rights, including repercussions of deinstitutionalization. We conclude by examining the legal and ethical parameters of the therapist–client relationship and cultural competence in treatment.

17-1 Criminal Commitment

A basic premise of criminal law is that we exercise free will and are capable of choices. If we do something illegal, we are responsible for our actions and should experience the consequences of our poor judgment. This might result in **criminal commitment** which is the incarceration (imprisonment) of an individual who has been charged with or found guilty of a crime. However, criminal law recognizes that some people lack the ability to discern the ramifications of their actions or to assist in their own defense because they are mentally disturbed. Although they may be technically guilty of a crime, their mental state at the time of the offense might exempt them from legal responsibility. Additionally, they might be mentally incapable of participating

Table 17.1 The Intersection of Psychology and the Law

The expertise of psychologists is often sought in the legal system. A few of these roles and activities are included here.

Psychological Evaluations in Child Protection Matters	Evaluation for Child Custody in Divorce Proceedings
• Attempt to determine whether abuse or neglect has occurred, whether a child is at risk for harm, and what corrective action, if any, should occur	• Provide expertise to help courts and social services agencies determine the best interests of the child • Offer opinions on child well-being, parenting plans, and termination of parental rights in custody cases

Civil Commitment Determination	Protection of Client Rights
• Become involved in the civil commitment of an individual or the discharge of a person who has been so confined • Determine whether the person is at risk of harm to self or others, is too mentally disturbed to practice self-care, or lacks the appropriate resources for care if left alone	• Become involved in seeing that clients are not grievously wronged by the loss of their civil liberties on the grounds of mental health treatment • Advise on the right to receive treatment, to refuse treatment, and to live in the least restrictive environment

Profiling of Criminals	Assessment of Dangerousness
• Work with law enforcement officials in developing profiles of serial killers, mass murderers, or other offenders	• Assess the potential for suicide and homicide, child endangerment, civil commitment, and so on

Filing of Amicus Briefs	Jury Selection
• Use psychological science to help inform the court as to social science research that is relevant to pending litigation • Act as a friend of the court by filing professional opinions based on area of expertise	• Aid attorneys in determining whether prospective jurors might favor one side of a case or the other • Use psychological knowledge in an attempt to screen out individuals who might be biased against clients

Determination of Sanity or Insanity	Testimony in Malpractice Suits
• At the request of a judge, prosecution, or defense, determine the sanity or insanity of someone accused of a crime • Present findings to the judge or in front of a jury	• Testify in a civil suit on whether another therapist failed to follow the standards of the profession and is thus guilty of negligence or malpractice • Determine whether the client bringing the suit incurred psychological harm or damage as a result of the clinician's actions

Determination of Competency to Stand Trial	Determination of Repressed, Recovered, or False Memories
• Determine whether an individual is mentally competent or sufficiently rational to stand trial and to aid in their defense	• Determine the accuracy and validity of repressed memories—claims by adults that they have recovered memories of childhood abuse

in criminal proceedings against them. We will now explore the landmark cases and public policies that have influenced how criminal law is applied to individuals who are seriously mentally ill. Standards arising from these cases and some other important guidelines are summarized in Figure 17.1.

Competency to Stand Trial

Case Study On June 5, 2002, Brian David Mitchell kidnapped 14-year-old Elizabeth Smart at knifepoint from her Salt Lake City, Utah, home. The incident set off a massive search effort and evoked intense media coverage. Smart was rescued 9 months later after enduring a horrendous experience that included a forced polygamous "marriage," rape, and constant threats to her life. Mitchell, a former street preacher, was arrested for the crime, but claimed that God had commanded him to abduct Smart, to enter into a celestial marriage, and to form a religious society of younger females.

Despite his capture and arrest, Mitchell's trial did not begin until November 2010—almost 9 years later. The delays occurred because in three separate court hearings, Mitchell was judged "mentally incapable of assisting in his own defense." In the courtroom he sang hymns and screamed at the judge to "forsake those robes and kneel in the dust." His behavior was so bizarre that he was banished from the courtroom several times. As a result, the judge ordered that Mitchell be hospitalized until he was capable of understanding the proceedings. Mitchell refused to participate in psychiatric treatment or to take antipsychotic medication. Finally, following a series of hearings and review of conflicting opinions from various experts who evaluated Mitchell, a federal judge ruled that Mitchell was competent to stand trial. At the trial, the jury rejected his insanity defense and found him guilty. On May 25, 2011, Mitchell was sentenced to life imprisonment without the possibility of parole.

Most court-appointed psychiatrists and psychologists who examined Mitchell declared him not competent to stand trial, although a few believed he was manipulating the system and feigning psychosis. A determination of **competency to stand trial** is based on a defendant's mental state at the time of psychiatric examination after arrest and before trial. It has nothing to do with the issue of criminal responsibility, which refers to an

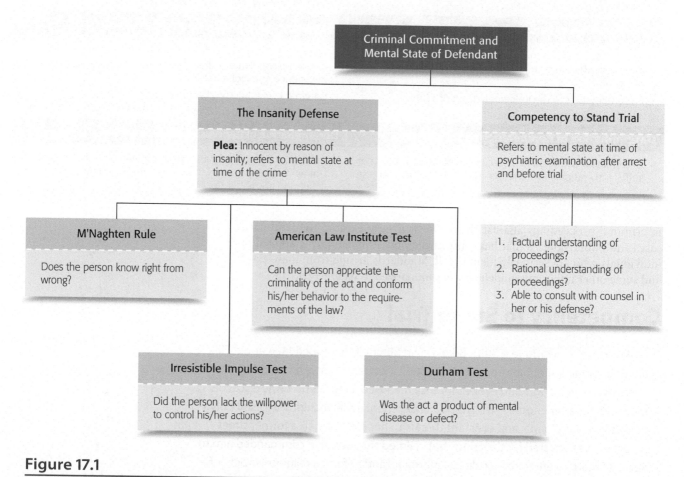

Figure 17.1

Legal Standards That Address the Mental State of the Defendant individual's mental state at the time of the offense. Federal law states that an accused person cannot stand trial unless three criteria are satisfied (Gillis et al., 2016):

- The defendant must have a factual understanding of the proceedings.
- The defendant must have a rational understanding of the proceedings.
- The defendant must be able to rationally consult with counsel in presenting their defense.

These criteria suggest that a defendant who is severely psychotic, for example, could not stand trial because a serious impairment exists. The goal is to protect and preserve the civil rights of people who are mentally disturbed by ensuring that all defendants understand the nature of any legal proceedings. But being judged incompetent to stand trial may have unfair negative consequences as well. A person may be held in custody for an extended period of time, denied the chance to post bail, and isolated from friends and family—all without having been found guilty of a crime.

Such a miscarriage of justice was the focus of a U.S. Supreme Court ruling in the 1972 case of *Jackson v. Indiana*. In that case, a man with an intellectual disability and brain damage who was deaf and unable to speak was charged with robbery. However, he was found incompetent to stand trial and was incarcerated indefinitely—which in his case probably meant for life, because of the severity and unchanging nature of his disabilities. In other words, it was unlikely that he would ever be judged competent to stand trial on the robbery charges, and thus faced the prospect of lifelong incarceration. His lawyers filed a petition to have him released on the basis of deprivation of **due process**—the legal checks and balances that are guaranteed to everyone, such as the right to receive a fair trial, the right to face one's accusers, the right to present evidence, and the right to have counsel.

The U.S. Supreme Court ruled that a defendant cannot be confined indefinitely solely on the grounds of incompetency. After a reasonable time, a determination must be made as to whether the person is likely or unlikely to regain competency in the foreseeable future. If experts conclude that competency is unlikely, the officials in charge must either release the individual or initiate civil commitment procedures. This is a significant ruling because many people remain in jail awaiting a competency hearing or are committed to prison hospitals because of incompetency determinations. It is estimated, for instance, that up to 60,000 people in the United States are evaluated each year for competency to stand trial, and as many as 25 percent are determined to be incompetent (Chen et al., 2017). The *Jackson v. Indiana* decision prompted federal competency hearings in the previously mentioned case of Brian David Mitchell because he could not be held indefinitely without a trial; additionally, prosecutors pushed for the final competency hearing because they did not want the statute of limitations on the charges to expire.

Legal Precedents Regarding the Insanity Defense

The **insanity defense** is a legal argument used by defendants who admit they have committed a crime but plead not guilty because they were mentally disturbed at the time of the crime. The insanity plea recognizes that under specific circumstances, people may not be held accountable for their behavior. As we saw in the case of James Holmes and Brian David Mitchell, defense strategies sometimes involve such a contention—that the defendants are not guilty because they were insane (not of sound mind) at the time of the crime.

In the United States, a number of different standards have been used as legal tests of insanity. One of the earliest is the M'Naghten rule. In 1843, Daniel M'Naghten, a mentally disturbed woodcutter from Glasgow, Scotland, claimed that he was commanded by God to kill the British prime minister, Sir Robert Peel. He killed a lesser minister by mistake and was placed on trial, where it became obvious that M'Naghten was quite delusional. Out of this incident emerged the **M'Naghten rule**, popularly known as the "right–wrong" test, which holds that people can be acquitted of a crime if, at the time of the act, they (a) had such defective reasoning that they did not know what they were doing or (b) were unable to comprehend that the act was wrong. The M'Naghten rule has been criticized for being a cognitive test (knowledge of right or wrong) that does not consider motivation or other factors. Further, it is often difficult to evaluate or determine a defendant's awareness or comprehension at the time of the crime.

The second major precedent associated with the insanity defense is the **irresistible impulse test**. In essence, this doctrine says that defendants are not criminally responsible if they lacked the willpower to control their behaviors. Combined with the M'Naghten rule, this test broadened the criteria for using the insanity defense. In other words, a not guilty by reason of insanity verdict could be obtained if a jury determined that the defendant did not understand that their actions were wrong *or* if the actions resulted from an irresistible impulse to commit the acts. Criticisms of the irresistible impulse defense revolve around what constitutes an irresistible impulse. When, for example, is a person *unable* to exert control (irresistible impulse) rather than *choosing* not to exert control (unresisted impulse)? Is a man who rapes a woman unable to resist his impulses, or is he choosing not to exert control? Neither the mental health profession nor the legal profession has answered this question satisfactorily.

Legal understandings of the insanity plea were further expanded in the case of *Durham v. United States* (1954), when a U.S. Court of Appeals for the District of Columbia Circuit broadened the M'Naghten rule with the so-called product test, or **Durham standard**. This standard maintains that an accused person should not be considered criminally responsible if their unlawful act was the *product* of a mental disease or defect. The intent of the ruling was to (a) give the greatest possible weight to expert evaluation and testimony and (b) allow mental health professionals to define mental illness.

The Durham standard also has its drawbacks. The term *product* is vague and difficult to define. Additionally, if the task of defining mental illness is left to mental health professionals, it becomes necessary to consider definitions of mental illness on a case-by-case basis. In many situations, relying on psychiatric testimony serves only to confuse the issues, because both the prosecution and the defense bring in psychiatric experts, who often present conflicting opinions. What we know from cases such as those of James Holmes and Brian David Mitchell is that expert testimony can vary significantly.

In 1962, the American Law Institute *Model Penal Code* provided guidelines to help jurors determine the validity of the insanity defense. The guidelines combine features from the previous standards (Sec. 401, p. 66):

1. A person is not responsible for criminal conduct if at the time of such conduct as a result of mental disease or defect he lacks substantial capacity either to appreciate the criminality of his conduct or to conform his conduct to the requirements of the law.

2. As used in the Article, the terms "mental disease or defect" do not include an abnormality manifested by repeated criminal or otherwise antisocial conduct.

Did You Know?

Hawaii requires several independent forensic evaluations when the insanity defense is used. Clinicians who evaluate the same defendant for insanity often reach different conclusions. It is not surprising that juries reached a unanimous decision regarding insanity in only 55 percent of cases, according to a review of 165 defendants and 483 evaluations in Hawaii.

Source: Gowensmith et al., 2013

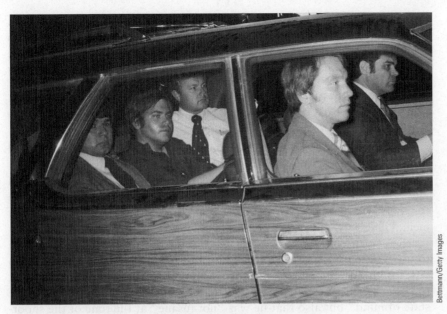

Public Outrage over Acquittal Based on Insanity

John Hinckley, Jr. (center), was charged with the attempted murder of President Ronald Reagan. His acquittal by reason of insanity created a furor among the U.S. public over use of the insanity defense. The outrage led Congress to pass the Insanity Defense Reform Act.

This second point was included to eliminate the insanity defense option for the many criminals diagnosed with an antisocial personality disorder who make a clear decision to violate the law.

In some jurisdictions, the concept of **diminished capacity** has also been incorporated into the American Law Institute standard. Diminished capacity is the absence of a *specific intent* to commit the offense as a result of mental impairment. For example, a person under the influence of drugs or alcohol may commit a crime without premeditation or intent; a person who is grieving over the death of a loved one may harm the person responsible for the death. Although diminished capacity is primarily used to guide the sentencing and disposition of defendants, it is sometimes introduced in the trial phase with the hope that the defendant will be convicted of a lesser charge.

Such was the case in the trial of Dan White, a San Francisco supervisor who killed Mayor George Moscone and Supervisor Harvey Milk on November 27, 1978. White blamed both individuals for his political demise. During the trial, his attorney used the now-famous "Twinkie defense" (White gorged himself on junk food such as Twinkies, chips, and soda) as a partial explanation for his client's actions. White's attorney attempted to convince the jury that the high sugar content of the junk food affected White's cognitive and emotional state and was partially to blame for his actions. White was convicted only of voluntary manslaughter and was sentenced to less than 8 years in jail. Of course, the citizens of San Francisco were outraged by the verdict and never forgave White. Facing constant public condemnation, he died by suicide after his release.

Insanity Defense Reform

Perhaps no trial has challenged the use of the insanity plea more than the case of John W. Hinckley, Jr., who attempted to assassinate President Ronald Reagan. The jury's verdict that he was not guilty by reason of insanity outraged the public, as well as some legal and mental health professionals. Many were concerned that the criteria for the insanity defense were too broadly interpreted, and calls for reforms were rampant. Hinckley's release and move into his mother's home in 2016 reignited this controversy (Wilbur, 2019).

As a result of the public outcry, Congress passed the Insanity Defense Reform Act of 1984, which based the definition of insanity totally on the individual's ability to understand what they did. In the wake of the Hinckley verdict, some states adopted alternative pleas, such as "culpable and mentally disabled," "mentally disabled, but neither culpable nor innocent," and "guilty, but mentally ill." These pleas are attempts to separate mental illness from insanity. Such pleas allow jurors to hold defendants responsible for their crimes while also ensuring that they receive treatment for their mental illness.

Despite attempts at reform, however, states and municipalities continue to use different tests of insanity, with varying outcomes. Under Colorado law, for instance, prosecutors in the Aurora theater shooting were required to prove beyond a reasonable doubt not only that Holmes had "a culpable state of mind" but also that he was "not insane" at the time of the shooting. In other words, the prosecution needed to convince jurors that Holmes understood right from wrong and that he acted with intent, deliberately taking actions that he knew would kill people. Only then could jurors find him guilty. The jury did, in fact, reject the insanity defense and found Holmes guilty on 165 counts of murder and attempted murder, for which he will remain in prison without the possibility of parole.

Contemporary Views on the Insanity Defense

The concept of "not guilty by reason of insanity" continues to provoke controversy among legal scholars, mental health practitioners, and the general public. Most defendants who use this defense have a long history of severe mental illness. James Holmes is an exception to this pattern. Another well-known exception is Andrea Yates, who, on June 30, 2001, waited for her husband to leave for work, filled the bathtub to the very top, and proceeded to drown her five children (ages 7 months to 7 years). After killing her children, she carried them to a bedroom, laid them out next to one another, and covered them with a sheet. She then contacted 911. Afterward, she called her husband and stated, "You need to come home. . . . It's time. I did it." When asked what she meant, Yates responded, "It's the children . . . all of them." When the police arrived, Yates calmly explained how she had killed her five young children.

The case of Andrea Yates shocked the nation. How could a mother possibly commit such an unthinkable act? Her actions were especially heinous because she murdered her five children in such a methodical manner. During Yates's trial, the prosecution asked for the death penalty, but the defense contended that because Yates committed the murders while experiencing severe postpartum depression and postpartum psychosis, she was legally insane and should not be held accountable for her actions. The jury, however, found her guilty. An appellate court subsequently overturned the verdict. During the second trial, another Texas jury found her not guilty by reason of insanity; she has since been confined to a mental hospital. In Yates's case, she had experienced only one previous psychotic breakdown, following the birth of her fourth child. Andrea Yates still resides in a state mental hospital and, according to her attorney, is aware of and emotionally distressed by her actions (ABC, 2018).

Determination of guilt when someone who has an ongoing mental illness commits a serious crime can be especially complicated, as demonstrated in the following case.

Case Study On February 12, 2008, 39-year-old David Tarloff used a meat cleaver to savagely attack and murder Kathryn Faughey, PhD, during an attempted robbery. The intended target of the theft was her colleague, Kent Shinbach, MD, a 70-year-old psychiatrist. Seventeen years earlier, Dr. Shinbach had evaluated and recommended involuntary hospitalization for Tarloff—the first of Tarloff's many hospitalizations. Although Tarloff had not seen Shinbach for years, he tracked down Shinbach's office address after concluding that he "must be rich." Tarloff's plan was to demand $40,000 from Dr. Shinbach so that he could "rescue" his mother from a nursing home and move her to Hawaii, where he could take care of her in a villa that he would rent with the stolen money.

When Tarloff entered the office suite, he unexpectedly encountered Dr. Faughey and brutally attacked and killed her. When Dr. Shinbach heard Faughey's screams and attempted to come to her aid, he was also viciously assaulted. Ignoring Dr. Shinbach's serious injuries, Tarloff demanded money. Dr. Shinbach testified in court that Tarloff abruptly left when the doctor asked him, "Haven't you done enough harm this evening? Why don't you just leave?" After the attack, Tarloff reportedly threw his bloody clothes away and bought a change of clothing. A few days later, following his arrest, Tarloff said he was sorry for killing "that woman" but did not express concern about the serious injuries sustained by Dr. Shinbach; instead, he told detectives that the doctor was "a liar."

During various court appearances, Mr. Tarloff rocked back and forth and appeared to be disoriented. According to his attorneys, Tarloff claimed that he had seen God's eye in tables and floors and that God had approved of his plan to demand money from the psychiatrist. The lawyers explained that Tarloff had been a "normal," well-liked high school student but that he had changed drastically after his first semester of college at Syracuse University. Soon afterward, he was diagnosed with schizophrenia. On numerous occasions over the next 20 years, he was involuntarily hospitalized due to the severity of his mental illness. (McKinley, 2014)

Tarloff's attorneys called the incident "an insane plan by an insane man who was legally insane when it happened" and argued that the jury should find him "not guilty by reason of mental disease or defect." Jury members needed to decide if Tarloff knew right from wrong during his attack. Did his delusions diminish his capacity to understand that his behavior was unlawful?

It took three separate trials before a jury was able to reach a verdict. The first trial, which began in the fall of 2008, was delayed when Tarloff adamantly refused to leave his cell during jury selection. This behavior raised questions about Tarloff's competency to stand trial and led the judge to request that Tarloff receive a mental health evaluation. Based on assessment by two psychiatrists, the judge concluded that Tarloff was not competent to stand trial and ordered him to remain in a secure psychiatric facility until competency was established. Almost 2 years later, it was determined that Tarloff's mental condition had sufficiently stabilized to allow him to understand the proceedings and to assist in his own defense. During the second trial, after 10 days of heated deliberation, the judge conceded

Myth The insanity defense is often used because defendants who are found not guilty by reason of insanity spend less time in custody (jail, mental health facility, or prison) than those who are convicted.

Reality As a rule, defendants found not guilty by reason of insanity spend as much if not more time in custody than those who are convicted. They often face a lifetime of judicial oversight even after their release (Douzenis, 2016). Further, the plea is infrequently used and seldom successful. It may be used with even less frequency now that the Supreme Court has ruled that states have the right to bar the use of the insanity defense (Chung & Hurley, 2020).

that the jury was hopelessly deadlocked; some of the jurors were unable to agree to a guilty verdict, explaining that Tarloff's mental illness clouded his ability to determine right from wrong.

A verdict was finally reached during the third trial. On March 28, 2014, after deliberating for 7 hours, the jurors found Tarloff guilty on all counts, including murder. Some jurors explained that although they recognized that Tarloff has a severe mental illness, they believed that he knew that what he did was wrong. One juror explained: "I believe he's sick to a certain degree but not sick enough to not know right from wrong." Another stated that she had no choice but to find him guilty because of the narrow criteria associated with the insanity defense and voiced her opinion that another choice should have been available to allow him to receive the mental health treatment he needs, the option to acknowledge that he was "an obviously mentally ill person who knows right from wrong" (McKinley, 2014). The delays in the Tarloff case were due to the severity of his mental illness and the complexities of the case rather than any deliberate attempt to manipulate or exploit the legal system. However, as we saw with the Mitchell case, deliberate delays sometimes occur.

Further, some defendants attempt to feign insanity; fortunately, those who fake are seldom successful. Confessed Hillside Strangler Kenneth Bianchi, for example, attempted to fake mental illness as mitigation for his part in raping, torturing, and murdering a number of girls and young women in the late 1970s. Wanting to use the insanity plea to get a reduced sentence, Bianchi tried to convince psychiatrists that he suffered from dissociative identity disorder. Psychologist and hypnosis expert Dr. Martin Orne exposed his scheme as a fake. The jury concluded that Bianchi was guilty of murder and sentenced him to life in prison without parole.

In reality, less than 1 percent of defendants use an insanity defense and, even then, in only a small percentage of cases is the defense successful (Kois et al., 2013). For instance, on February 24, 2015, a Texas jury rejected the insanity defense and convicted Eddie Ray Routh of murder in the shooting deaths of former Marine Chad Littlefield and Chris Kyle, former Navy SEAL and author of *American Sniper*. The jurors concluded that, despite his severe mental illness, Routh failed to meet the legal threshold for insanity—mental illness so severe he was unable to distinguish right from wrong (Keneally, 2015). Many of the cases discussed in this chapter are the exceptions to the rule; however, they are presented to help demonstrate the ways in which psychopathology and the law intersect. These cases also received significant media attention and helped construct popular opinion about the insanity defense.

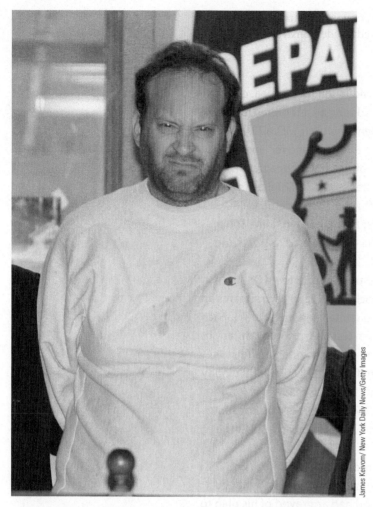

James Keivom/ New York Daily News/Getty Images

Not Guilty by Reason of Mental Disease or Defect?

David Tarloff, who has a longstanding history of schizophrenia, savagely murdered a psychologist and brutally attacked a 70-year-old psychiatrist. Here is a photo taken of Tarloff soon after his arrest. Although his defense attorney argued that he was insane at the time of the murders, on March 28, 2014, a jury found Tarloff guilty on all charges, including murder.

In the limited number of cases where the insanity defense is successfully employed, the defendants usually have past hospitalizations, delusions or paranoia, a previous diagnosis of a serious mental illness, and few victims were involved. When children or a large number of victims are affected by the crime, the chances for a successful insanity defense diminish dramatically. The number of individuals killed and injured by James Holmes in the Aurora shootings may explain why the prosecutors refused to accept a guilty plea in exchange for allowing him to avoid the possibility of receiving the death penalty (Elliott & Banda, 2013).

17-2 Civil Commitment

Case Study She was known as BL ("Bag Lady"). By night, she slept on any number of park benches and storefronts in downtown Oakland, California. By day, she could be seen pushing a shopping cart full of boxes, extra clothing, and garbage, which she collected from numerous trash containers. According to her sister, the woman had lived this way for nearly 10 years, without complaint from local merchants.

Over the previous 6 months, however, BL's behavior had become increasingly disruptive. She had always talked to herself, but recently she had begun shouting and screaming at anyone who approached her. Her use of profanity was graphic, and it was rumored that she urinated in front of local stores. Although she never physically assaulted anyone, her menacing behavior frightened many pedestrians, customers, and shopkeepers. Local law enforcement officials occasionally detained her for short periods, but she always returned to her familiar haunts. Finally, her sister and several merchants requested that the city take action to commit her for inpatient psychiatric treatment.

Action is required when people who are severely disturbed behave in a manner that poses a threat to themselves or others. The government has *parens patriae* ("father of the country" or "power of the state") authority, which is the power to commit disturbed individuals for their own best interest. **Civil commitment** is the name of this action; it is the involuntary confinement of individuals judged to be a danger to themselves or others, even though they have not committed a crime. Thus, the commitment of a person in acute distress is purportedly a form of protective confinement and demonstration of concern for the psychological and physical well-being of that person or others. Civil commitment often involves situations such as potential suicide, threatened violence, destruction of property, or a loss of impulse control. Factors relevant to civil commitment are outlined in Figure 17.2.

Mental health professionals working with individuals who have serious mental illness are increasingly encouraging their clients to consider a *psychiatric advance directive*. Similar to medical advance directives, this paperwork allows people with chronic and serious mental illness to plan ahead regarding their treatment preferences in the event of an incapacitating mental health crisis (Easter et al., 2020). A psychiatric advance directive not only specifies intervention preferences but may also include the appointment of a temporary health care proxy with decision-making authority.

Did You Know?

Each state has its own statute that defines civil incompetency or incapacity. Thus, practicing mental health professionals need to be acutely aware of how the states in which they practice define these concepts.

Source: Demakis, 2013

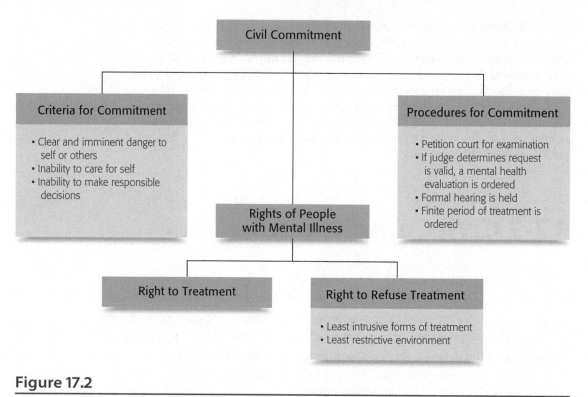

Figure 17.2

Factors in the Civil Commitment of a Nonconsenting Person

It is best when civil commitment can be avoided because it has many potentially negative consequences. It may cause major interruption in the person's life, loss of self-esteem, and dependency on others. It may also cause loss or restriction of civil liberties—a point that becomes even more glaring if the person has committed no crime. In the case study, for example, BL had committed no criminal offense, although she had violated many social norms. But under what circumstances should someone be confined to a mental hospital?

Criteria for Commitment

States vary in the criteria used to commit a person, but there are certain general standards. It is not enough that a person is mentally ill; one or more of these additional conditions must exist before involuntary hospitalization is considered (Corey et al., 2018).

- *Individuals present a clear and imminent danger to themselves or others.* An example is someone who is displaying suicidal or unsafe behavior (such as walking out on a busy freeway) that places the individual in immediate danger. Threats to harm someone else or behavior viewed as assaultive or destructive are also grounds for commitment.

- *Individuals are unable to care for themselves or do not have the social network to provide for such care.* Most civil commitments are based primarily on this criterion. The details vary, but states generally specify an inability to provide sufficient food (the person is malnourished, food is unavailable, and the person has no feasible plan to obtain it), clothing (attire is not appropriate for the climate, and the person has no plans for obtaining other attire), or shelter (the person has no permanent residence, insufficient protection from climatic conditions, and no logical plans for obtaining adequate housing).

- *Individuals are unable to make responsible decisions about appropriate treatments and hospitalization.* This involves an inability to follow through with needed treatment. As a result, the person's well-being is jeopardized and there is a strong chance of further deterioration in functioning.

- *Individuals are in an unmanageable state of fright or panic.* Such people may behave impulsively or feel that they are on the brink of losing control of their behavior.

In the past, commitments could be obtained solely on the basis of mental illness and a person's need for treatment, which was often determined arbitrarily. Increasingly, the courts have narrowed the focus of civil commitment procedures and now concentrate primarily on whether people present a danger to themselves or others. How is this potential danger determined? Many people would not consider BL a danger to herself or others. Some, however, might believe that she *could* become assaultive to others or injurious to herself. Are trained mental health professionals able to accurately make such predictions? We'll now turn to that question.

Assessing Dangerousness

Mental health professionals have difficulty predicting whether someone, even a person they know well such as a client, will commit dangerous acts. Civil commitments are often based on a determination of the person's potential for doing harm to self or others. This criterion can be problematic, particularly when the evaluation is based on a single interview by a mental health professional. The difficulty in predicting potential dangerousness involves four key factors:

1. *The rarer something is, the more difficult it is to predict.* As a group, people with mental illness are not dangerous. Although some evidence suggests that individuals with severe psychotic disorders may have slightly higher rates of violent behavior (Rozel & Mulvey, 2017), the risk is not considered a major concern.

2. *Violence is as much a function of the context in which it occurs as it is of the person's characteristics.* Although it is theoretically possible for a psychologist to accurately assess an individual's personality and mental status, we have little idea about the situations in which people find themselves. A meek and mild person, for example, may display uncontrollable rage when confronted with the tragic death of a loved one.

3. *The best predictor of dangerousness is often past criminal conduct or a history of violence, aggression, or substance abuse.* However, evaluators may be unaware of past history, or official records may be ruled irrelevant or inadmissible by mental health commissions and the courts.

4. *The definition of dangerousness is itself unclear.* Most of us would agree that murder, rape, torture, and physical assaults are dangerous. But are we confining our definition to physical harm only? What about psychological abuse or destruction of property? And what if the individual has access to or attempts to obtain firearms?

Did You Know?

On April 16, 2007, Seung-Hui Cho used two semiautomatic handguns to kill 27 Virginia Tech students and 5 faculty members before killing himself with a shot to his head. There was evidence that Cho was potentially dangerous: (a) He was involved in three stalking incidents on the campus; (b) professors said he was menacing and his writings were often intimidating, obscene, and violent; and (c) a mental health professional believed he was a danger to others. However, Cho was not committed and was legally able to obtain the semiautomatic pistols he used in the massacre.

Predicting Dangerousness and Profiling Serial Killers and Mass Shooters

Seung-Hui Cho (the Virginia Tech shooter), Jeffrey Dahmer (killer of 17 men and boys), and Eric Harris and Dylan Klebold (the Columbine High School killers) were all either serial killers or mass murderers. Were there signs that these individuals were potentially dangerous? Jeffrey Dahmer tortured animals as a small boy and was arrested in 1988 for molesting a child. There is evidence to suggest that Cho was a deeply disturbed young man who harbored great resentment and anger. Harris and Klebold's Internet activity seemed to foretell their proclivity toward violence. In all three situations, there was no intervention despite their potentially dangerous thoughts and behaviors.

Lest we be too harsh on psychologists and law enforcement officials, it is important to realize that few serial killers or mass shooters willingly share their violent fantasies. Furthermore, it is difficult to predict and intervene due to:

1. the lack of one-to-one correspondence between danger signs and possible violence,

2. the fact that violent behavior often results from many variables, and

3. the recognition that incarceration—either criminal or civil—cannot occur on the basis of potential danger alone.

Nevertheless, tragic experiences with mass murderers and serial killers have led mental health practitioners and law enforcement officials to create profiles to help predict dangerous acts. Let's consider the profile developed to help identify serial killers.

Profile of Serial Killers

Although there is much conjecture in the public regarding serial killers, much of it is inaccurate. The FBI published a document about mass shooters and shared the following conclusions (Silver et al., 2018):

■ The 63 active shooters in the study could not be easily identified by demographic information, so there is no one "profile" of a shooter. The majority of adult shooters had no history of violence.

■ The mass shooters had multiple stressors the year preceding the attack. However, the FBI recognizes that most people face similar stressors.

■ Although 62 percent of the sample had mental health symptoms such as depression, anxiety, or paranoia and had a history of acting in an abusive, bullying, or oppressive manner, only 25 percent of the shooters had a psychiatric diagnosis. The FBI notes that because of the prevalence of mental disorders in the general population, a diagnosed mental disorder is not a good predictor for violence of any kind and that "declarations that all active shooters must simply be mentally ill are misleading and unhelpful."

■ School peers and teachers had observed concerning behaviors in the adolescent shooters, whereas domestic partners were most likely to notice behavior changes in the adult shooters.

■ The most common shooter grievance involved interpersonal or employment conflicts. Other motivating factors for the killings included sexual fantasies, anger, thrill, financial gain, and attention.

■ Ninety-four percent of the shooters were male.

■ The majority of the mass shooters were European American (63 percent), followed by African American (16 percent), Asian (10 percent), Latinx (6 percent), Middle Eastern (3 percent), and Native American (2 percent).

The American Psychological Association supports the conclusion that it is difficult to profile serial killers or mass murderers. With respect to perpetrators of mass shootings, it concludes: "In making predictions about the risk for mass shootings, there is no consistent psychological profile or set of warning signs that can be used reliably to identify such individuals in the general population" (Cornell & Guerra, 2013). The American Psychological Association (2019a) has also spoken out against a proposal aimed at using technology to detect when people with mental illnesses are about to become violent, stating, "Research consistently shows a weak link between mental illness and mass shootings. Furthermore, there is no science showing that technology can accurately predict violent behavior in anyone, and no data that if this were possible, such information would somehow solve our nation's gun violence crisis."

For Further Consideration

1. Should we be doing more to develop profiles of mass murderers or serial killers?

2. Why do you think some politicians promote the false belief that there is a strong link between mental illness and mass shootings?

3. Is there a risk that such inaccurate portrayals will unfairly stigmatize individuals living with mental illness?

4. What do you think are possible solutions to address the epidemic of gun violence within the United States?

Extreme Risk Protection Orders

When there is concern that a person is behaving erratically and has the potential to harm themselves or others, 21 states and the District of Columbia allow police, family, or concerned community members to submit a court petition requesting that the person in crisis be temporarily denied access to firearms. These "red flag laws" allow courts to review the available evidence and make a decision regarding whether to issue an *extreme risk protection order*, a civil order that temporarily prohibits an individual determined to be a danger to self or others from purchasing and possessing firearms (John Hopkins School of Public Health, 2023). Those interested in preventing suicides or mass shootings wholeheartedly support these laws aimed at ensuring public safety. However, gun rights advocates argue that any seizure of guns represents a violation of the second amendment. Further, some civil rights advocates contend that some state laws provide insufficient due process protections.

Procedures in Civil Commitment

In many cases, people deemed to be in need of protective confinement agree to *voluntary commitment* to a period of hospitalization. This process is fairly straightforward, and many believe that it is the preferred avenue for ensuring a positive treatment outcome. *Involuntary commitment* proceedings occur only when there is a need for treatment due to concern about potential self-harm or harm to others and the person does not consent to hospitalization.

Involuntary commitment can be a temporary emergency action or may involve a longer period of detention that is determined at a formal hearing. Although states vary in their processes and standards, all recognize that cases arise in which a person is so severely disturbed that an immediate detention is required (Yeung et al., 2019). Thus, commitment policies recognize that in-depth hearings cannot occur immediately and that delaying commitment could result in adverse consequences for the person or other individuals. Thus, they allow for temporary detention prior to a full hearing.

Formal civil commitment proceedings usually occur within several days of temporary detention and follow a similar process, regardless of the state in which they occur. First, a concerned person such as a family member, therapist, or physician petitions the court for an examination of the person. If the judge believes there is reasonable cause for this action, a mental health evaluation is ordered. In most cases, the examiners are physicians or mental health professionals who testify regarding their findings concerning the person's mental state and any potential dangers. The person is allowed to speak on their own behalf and is represented by counsel. Family members, friends, or therapists may also testify. If it is determined that the person must remain hospitalized, a finite period is usually specified. Some states, however, allow indefinite commitment subject to periodic review and assessment.

When to Intervene?

On February 14, 2018, a 19-year-old gunman brought a semiautomatic rifle to Marjory Stoneman Douglas High School in Parkland, Florida, and killed 17 students and faculty members. This deadly mass shooting, perpetrated by someone who had legally purchased a weapon despite his long history of threatening and unpredictable behavior, prompted many of the survivors to become outspoken advocates for gun violence prevention measures. High school classmates are pictured here on the 1-year anniversary of the shooting.

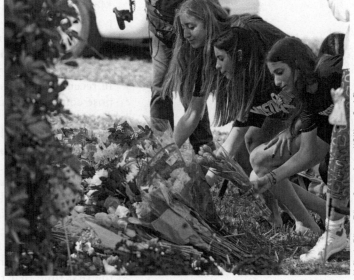

McClatchy-Tribune/Tribune Content Agency LLC/Alamy Stock Photo

A Tragic Case of Failure to Predict Dangerousness

Convicted serial killer Jeffrey Dahmer killed 17 men and boys over a period of many years. Besides torturing many of his victims, Dahmer admitted to dismembering and devouring their bodies. Although previously convicted of sexual molestation, no one had predicted that he was capable of murder. Unsuccessful in his attempt to use the insanity plea, Dahmer was found guilty in 1994 and imprisoned. Another inmate subsequently killed him.

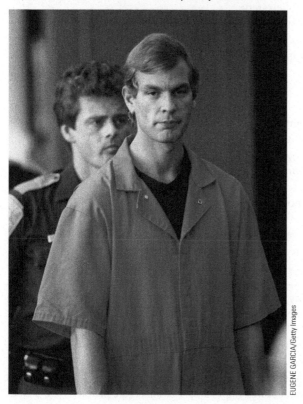

EUGENE GARCIA/Getty Images

Protection Against Involuntary Commitment

Due process procedures are important to ensure that involuntary commitment does not violate a person's civil rights. Some have even argued that criminals are accorded more rights than people who are mentally ill. For example, people accused of a crime are considered innocent until proven guilty in a court of law. They have the opportunity to post bail (assuming they have the financial means to do so) and are incarcerated only after a jury trial. In other words, they are detained only if a crime has been committed, not simply because there is a possibility or even a high probability of danger. Yet people who are mentally ill may be confined to a treatment facility without a jury trial and without having committed a crime; commitment occurs based on a judgment that they *might* do harm to themselves or others.

Some professionals claim that people who are mentally ill are incapable of determining their own treatment needs, and that, once civil confinement occurs and they receive treatment, they will be grateful for the treatment they received. If people resist hospitalization, they are purportedly irrational, which is deemed a symptom of their mental disorder. Critics do not accept this reasoning. They point out that civil commitment is for the benefit of those initiating commitment procedures (society), not for the individual. These concerns have prompted and heightened sensitivity toward patient welfare and rights, resulting in a trend toward restricting the powers of the state over the individual.

17-3 Rights of the Mentally Ill

Many people in the United States are concerned about the balance of power between the state and our citizens. The U.S. Constitution guarantees certain rights such as trial by jury, legal representation, and protection against self-incrimination. The mental health profession has great power, which may be used wittingly or unwittingly to abridge individual freedom. In recent decades, some courts have ruled that commitment for any purpose constitutes a major deprivation of liberty that requires due process protection.

Until 1979, the level of proof required for civil commitments varied from state to state. In a case that set a legal precedent, a Texas man claimed that he was denied due process because the jury that committed him was instructed to use a lower standard than "beyond a reasonable doubt" (a high degree of certainty). The appellate court agreed with the man, but when the case finally reached the Supreme Court in April 1979 (*Addington v. Texas*), the Court ruled that the state must provide only "clear and convincing evidence" (a medium degree of certainty) that a person is mentally ill and potentially dangerous before that person can be committed. This ruling represented the first time that the Supreme Court considered any aspect of the civil commitment process.

Client Disclosures of Violence to Therapists

The patient, a 60-year-old woman, has just attempted suicide by overdosing on a medication. Plagued with guilt, she told the resident psychiatrist that she had just killed two people and had buried them near her house. She gave the names of the people and exactly where the bodies were located (Doting, 2022).

Basic to a therapeutic relationship is the belief that whatever a client discloses is kept private. However, confidentiality and privilege are not absolute. While most states require or allow mental health professionals to report clients they believe to be a danger to themselves or others, no "duty to warn" requirements exist for Nevada, North Dakota, North Carolina, or Maine (National Conference of State Legislatures, 2022). The *Tarasoff* ruling also makes it clear that when clients disclose a potential to harm identifiable third parties, therapists have an obligation to take actions to ward off the danger. The duty to warn principle applies to *future threats of harm*. But what are the legal obligations of therapists who hear from clients that they have committed a *past crime*? What if clients disclose that they have assaulted, raped, or even killed someone?

These questions deal with legal issues as well as moral and ethical concerns. Unfortunately, the law is not clear on this matter. The prevailing consensus is that mental health professionals are not legally required to breach confidentiality when clients inform them that they have committed past crimes.

But how often do therapists hear confessions from their clients about past criminal conduct? The answer is that such confessions do occur. In one survey, many therapists reported occasions when clients mentioned that they had committed violent crimes and were never caught. Out of a sample of 162 doctoral-level psychologists (Walfish et al., 2010), the percentage of therapists who had heard about various past crimes included the following:

- Murder: 13 percent
- Sexual assault/rape: 33 percent
- Physical assault: 69 percent

In therapy, clients are likely to reveal very intimate secrets about their past, including feelings, thoughts, and actions. Thus, therapists need to be prepared to respond in an appropriate manner, carefully weighing any legal, moral, and therapeutic issues associated with the situation.

For Further Consideration

1. Do you believe that therapists should be required to report a past crime such as murder?

2. Can the *Tarasoff* ruling be interpreted to allow therapists latitude in reporting past crimes? How?

3. If you were a therapist and heard a murder confession, how do you think it would affect you and the therapeutic relationship?

Another wide-reaching ruling occurred in 1975 when a U.S. district court issued a landmark decision in the case of *Dixon v. Weinberger*. The ruling established the right of individuals to be treated in the **least restrictive environment** possible. This means that people have a right to the least restrictive alternative to freedom that is appropriate to their condition. Only individuals who are dangerous or who cannot adequately care for themselves are committed to hospitals. Those who can function acceptably should be given alternative choices, such as halfway houses and other shelters.

Right to Treatment

One of the primary justifications for commitment is that treatment improves a person's mental condition and increases the likelihood of a safe return to the community. However, is it acceptable to confine a person involuntarily and not provide therapy—the means for release from the inpatient psychiatric setting? Several cases have raised this problem as a constitutional issue. Together, they have determined that people with mental illness who have been involuntarily committed have a **right to treatment**—a right to receive therapy that would improve their condition.

In 1966, in a lawsuit brought against St. Elizabeth's Hospital in Washington, DC (*Rouse v. Cameron*), the DC Circuit Court held that (a) the right to treatment is a constitutional right, and (b) failure to provide treatment cannot be justified by lack of resources. In the Alabama federal case of *Wyatt v. Stickney* (1972), Judge Frank Johnson specified standards of adequate treatment, such as staff–patient ratios, therapeutic environmental conditions, and professional consensus about appropriate treatment. The court also made it clear that people with mental illness cannot be forced to work or to engage in work-related activities aimed at maintaining the facility in which they live. Thus, the previously common practice of having patients scrub floors, wash laundry, and cook or serve food was declared unconstitutional. Moreover, patients who volunteer to perform tasks must be paid at least the minimum wage instead of merely receiving tokens or special privileges. This landmark decision ensured treatment beyond custodial care and protection against neglect and abuse.

Another important case (tried in a U.S. district court in Florida and affirmed by the U.S. Supreme Court that same year), *O'Connor v. Donaldson* (1975), also had a major impact on the right to treatment issue. It involved Kenneth Donaldson, who at age 49 was committed for a period of 20 years to the Florida State Hospital in Chattahoochee on petition by his father. He was found to be mentally ill, unable to care for himself, easily manipulated, and dangerous. Throughout his confinement, Donaldson petitioned for release, but Dr. O'Connor, the hospital superintendent, determined that Donaldson was "too mentally ill." Finally, Donaldson threatened a lawsuit and was reluctantly discharged by the hospital after 14 years of confinement. He then sued both O'Connor and the hospital, winning an award of $20,000. The monetary award is insignificant compared with the relevance of the ruling. Again, the U.S. Supreme Court reaffirmed a patient's right to treatment. It ruled that Donaldson did not receive appropriate treatment and said that the state cannot detain nondangerous citizens who are capable of caring for themselves or who have the support of friends or family. Further, the court ruled that physicians, as well as psychiatric facilities, are liable for improper confinements.

One major dilemma in all cases of court-ordered treatment is determining what constitutes treatment. Treatment can range from rest and relaxation to psychosurgery, medication, and aversion therapy. Mental health professionals believe that they are in the best position to make treatment recommendations and evaluate treatment outcomes, a position supported by the case of *Youngberg v. Romeo* (1982). The court ruled that Nicholas Romeo, a boy with a significant intellectual disability, had a constitutional right to "reasonable care and safety," and it deferred judgment to the mental health professional as to what constitutes appropriate therapy.

Right to Refuse Treatment

The right to refuse treatment is a complicated issue. As you may recall, Brian David Mitchell, the man who kidnapped Elizabeth Smart, was declared mentally incompetent to stand trial, yet for 8 years he steadfastly refused to take antipsychotic medication; this placed him in a position of being indefinitely unable to participate in a trial involving the multiple charges he faced. His attorneys supported his right to refuse treatment and fought government officials on this point. It was only after a federal judge became convinced that Mitchell was manipulating the system that Mitchell was judged competent to stand trial, allowing the trial to proceed. Although it may be easy for us to surmise the reasons that Mitchell's attorneys supported his refusal of treatment, should defendants who are mentally ill have the option of refusing interventions that could restore their mental competency? Medical patients frequently refuse medical treatment on religious grounds or because the treatment would only prolong a terminal illness. Should people with mental illness have a similar right to refuse treatment?

Proponents of the right to refuse treatment argue that many forms of treatment, such as medication or electroconvulsive therapy, may have long-term side effects, as discussed in previous chapters. They also point out that involuntary treatment is generally much less effective than treatment that is accepted voluntarily. People forced into treatment seem to resist it, thereby nullifying the potentially beneficial effects.

The issue of the right to refuse treatment has been addressed by the courts. The case of *Rennie v. Klein* (1978) involved several state hospitals in New Jersey that had a policy of forcibly medicating patients in nonemergency situations. The court ruled that people have a constitutional right to refuse treatment (psychotropic medication) and to have an opportunity for a due process hearing if professionals believe forced treatment is essential to a patient's well-being. In another related case, *Rogers v. Okin* (1979), a Massachusetts court supported these guidelines. Both cases made the point that psychotropic medication was often used to control behavior or as a substitute for treatment. Further, the decisions noted that drugs might actually inhibit recovery.

Courts have frequently supported the right to refuse treatment and have extended the principle of the least restrictive alternative doctrine to include the least intrusive forms of treatment. Generally, psychotherapy is considered less intrusive than biologically based therapies (e.g., electroconvulsive therapy and medication). Although this compromise may appear reasonable, other problems present themselves. First, how do we define *intrusive treatment*? Second, if patients are allowed to refuse certain forms of treatment and if the hospital does not have alternatives for them, what options do they have? These questions remain unanswered.

The right to refuse treatment occasionally poses ironies. For example, a U.S. Supreme Court ruling (*Ford v. Wainwright* [1986]) concluded that the government cannot execute someone who is incompetent. Why would someone agree to take medication only to be executed? Some courts have ordered prisoners to take medication based on the assumption that doing so will improve their mental condition. In June 2003, however, the U.S. Supreme Court (*Sell v. United States*) placed strict limits on the ability of the government to forcibly medicate defendants who are mentally ill to make them competent to stand trial. Such actions must, according to the court ruling, be in the "best interest of the defendant." Thus, there must be other reasons for treatment, such as reducing self-injury or danger to others. In the absence of safety issues, the government can seek involuntary treatment only under "limited circumstances." That is, the treatment must be medically appropriate, have no competency-impairing side effects, and be the least intrusive means available. In most cases, defendants who are found incompetent to stand trial appear to willingly accept treatment (Landis, 2012). In one study, over three quarters of those with severe mental illnesses who were found to be incompetent to stand trial were restored to competency after being involuntarily medicated (Herbel & Stelmach, 2007).

Deinstitutionalization

Governmental trends such as the policy of deinstitutionalization can also influence access to treatment, especially for those with severe mental illness. **Deinstitutionalization** involved the shifting of responsibility for the care of those who are severely mentally ill from large central institutions to agencies within local communities. When originally formulated in the 1960s and 1970s, many mental health professionals supported this approach. Rather than relying on institutions, the Community Mental Health Act of 1963 was designed to provide funding for mental health centers throughout the United States, allowing treatment in local communities. Since its inception, the number of state-run mental hospitals has declined dramatically with a resultant 90 percent reduction in the availability of psychiatric beds (Smith, 2013).

The impetus behind deinstitutionalization came from several quarters. First, there was (and still is) a feeling that large hospitals mainly provide custodial care, that they produce little benefit, and that they may even impede improvement. Court cases discussed earlier (*Wyatt v. Stickney* and *O'Connor v. Donaldson*) exposed the fact that many mental hospitals do little more than warehouse patients. Confinement in a psychiatric facility can also foster dependency, promote helplessness, and lower self-sufficiency. The longer people are hospitalized, the more likely they are to remain hospitalized or to be readmitted once released.

Second, beginning in the 1970s, the issue of patient rights began to receive increased attention. Mental health professionals became very concerned about keeping people confined against their will and began to discharge patients soon after their mental competency improved. It was believed that **mainstreaming**—integrating people with mental illness back into the community—could be accomplished by providing local outpatient or transition services such as group homes, board-and-care facilities, or halfway houses. In addition, advances in psychopharmacology made it more likely that improvement would continue once patients were discharged.

Third, state hospitals were often overcrowded and inadequately staffed due to insufficient funding. Given these overcrowded conditions, mental health administrators viewed the deinstitutionalization movement favorably and supported the rapid release of patients back into communities. Similarly, state authorities welcomed the trend, especially because it reduced the cost of staffing and maintaining large facilities.

Beyond Deinstitutionalization

Case Study Walter is a 54-year-old DC resident with schizophrenia who lives on the streets. He describes days filled with long walks and prayer. He usually avoids homeless shelters, worried about his safety. His fears are justified. On one occasion when he stayed at a shelter, a group of men sneaked in some alcohol, got drunk, and beat Walter so badly that his jaw was broken. (Mukherjee, 2013)

What has been the impact of deinstitutionalization on people with mental illness? Unfortunately, the goals of the Community Mental Health Act were not achieved. Many of the proposed community mental health centers were never developed or their funding has been inadequate. Although institutionalized patients were released, many communities did not have the resources to offer treatment (Friedman, 2003). Critics believe that deinstitutionalization policies have allowed states to relinquish their responsibility to care for people who are unable to care for themselves.

The experiences of people such as Walter highlight the human cost and tragedy of deinstitutionalization policies. Sadly, many of our existing community programs are woefully inadequate in delivering needed services. Further, the plight of people with severe mental illness continues to worsen due to economic pressures facing local governments as well as cuts in mental health funding at the federal level. The personal toll of inadequate mental health services is immense. It is becoming apparent that many people with severe mental illness are not receiving any treatment. Stories such as Walter's are all too common in communities throughout the United States. Many people with serious mental illness live on the streets under harsh conditions, where they are prone to violent victimization. Others live in nursing homes, board-and-care homes, or group residences. The quality of care in many of these places is marginal, resulting in deterioration in functioning or periodic hospitalization. Additionally, there are alarming indications that deinstitutionalization resulted in many untreated individuals ending up in the criminal justice system. According to statistics from the U.S. Bureau of Justice, approximately 14 percent of prisoners residing in state and federal prisons in 2018 had severe mental illness, with a much higher rate (26 percent) among those incarcerated in local jails. Many large urban jail systems consider themselves to be among the largest psychiatric facilities in the nation (Lyon, 2019).

Many of the problems that have occurred since the deinstitutionalization movement appear to be the result of inadequate community resources for meeting the needs of people with chronic mental illness. Further, many individuals living with severe mental illness often lack family or friends to help them access outpatient psychiatric treatment and live safely within the community. They often struggle to obtain employment and adequate shelter. Even when an individual living with a serious mental illness agrees to treatment, it is not always possible to find needed services.

Insufficient Resources

Case Study   On November 20, 2019, a 15-year-old boy was transported by ambulance after an episode at school in which he became extremely agitated and destructive and began removing his clothing. He was evaluated and eventually placed in an emergency department isolation room, where he became increasingly depressed while he and his family waited for days before a bed opened in a youth psychiatric unit within his insurance network. (Hlavinka, 2020)

As is evident from this case study, the national shortage of acute-care facilities can result in a longer road to recovery for those in need of intervention. Sometimes the barrier to emergency psychiatric hospital admission is an administrative hurdle such as waiting for an insurance company to authorize services. However, a much more common obstacle is the critical shortage of psychiatric beds. This scarcity is forcing patients with severe psychiatric symptoms to be held in emergency departments, hospitals, and jails while they wait for treatment. Courts sometimes intervene, especially when those accused of crimes experience long waits for a competency hearing or are judged incompetent to stand trial yet remain in jail, where it is unlikely that their competency will be restored without treatment (Felthous & Bloom, 2018).

In many states, the majority of psychiatric beds are already occupied by individuals living with a severe mental illness who require long-term supervision, including those with prolonged court-ordered stays. Given this shortage, hospital emergency departments, designed to triage physical health emergencies, find themselves overwhelmed with providing longer-term care

A Mental Health Advocate in the Judicial System

Judge Steven Leifman, who served as chairman of the Florida Supreme Court's Task Force on Substance Abuse and Mental Health Issues in the Courts, is admired for his support for diversion programs that provide individuals with mental illness opportunities to receive treatment rather than be housed in jails or prisons.

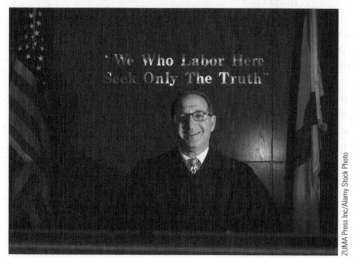

ZUMA Press Inc/Alamy Stock Photo

to individuals experiencing a mental health crisis who are waiting for a bed in a psychiatric facility. Further, some psychiatric facilities focus only on short-term intervention, which may not allow sufficient time for a patient to stabilize before being discharged.

Untreated Mental Illness

It is difficult to estimate how many individuals living with severe and untreated mental illness are among the ranks of the homeless. We do know that homelessness in the United States, especially in large urban areas, is increasing at an alarming pace. Although it is difficult to determine exactly how many unsheltered people are in need of mental health services, it has been estimated that 45 percent of the U.S. adults who are homeless have a mental disorder. with 25 percent being seriously mentally ill (Tarr, 2018). One of the challenges facing communities is how to address the needs of homeless individuals (and others) who have a clear need for mental health services but do not believe they require treatment. Many of the people living with mental illness who end up in jail or on the street have refused treatment. Frequently, friends or family are unsure how to proceed when they realize a loved one's condition is deteriorating, yet they are unable to convince the person to engage in treatment.

Some states and local communities have responded to this need by enacting laws that focus on ensuring treatment for individuals who are displaying dangerous or self-harming behavior. These legal statutes allow courts to order people who meet specified criteria into assisted outpatient treatment

The Downside of Deinstitutionalization

Homelessness has become a significant societal concern, especially in cities. Many believe that deinstitutionalization policies and lack of comprehensive community mental health services have contributed to this problem.

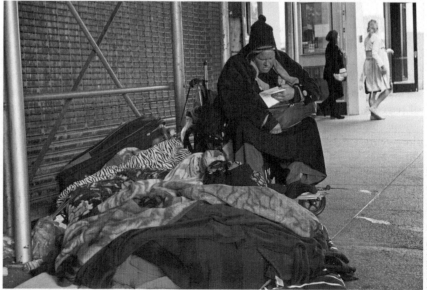

Janine Wiedel Photolibrary/Alamy Stock Photo

(AOT), also known as involuntary outpatient commitment. Remaining in the community is conditioned upon participating in recommended treatment. AOT orders can increase adherence to treatment recommendations and thus improve overall functioning. In locations where AOT is working well, court orders allow for interventions, including psychiatric treatment, case management, supported employment, and housing. Ideally, comprehensive community mental health services are readily available and easy to access when an AOT order is issued. A reliable means of accessing services is important not only for those court-ordered into treatment but also for people voluntarily seeking intensive treatment (Swartz et al., 2017).

We already know that the need for AOT is reduced when community behavioral health systems offer integrated services focused on continuity of care and coordinated treatment of physical, mental, and substance abuse conditions. However, more studies are required before we can reach a clear conclusion regarding the effectiveness of the AOT model. Successful implementation relies on the availability of adequately financed, quality treatment options. Further, given the variability in implementation of AOT orders across the nation, it is essential to have a means of ensuring that individuals ordered into treatment have access to successful interventions. Thus, researchers continue to focus on answering this question: "Under what circumstance are AOT orders most effective?" (Kisely et al., 2017).

Improving Community Care

Police are often called to intervene when someone living with a mental illness experiences a psychotic episode. Unfortunately, a lack of understanding of psychiatric symptoms can accelerate the situation. African Americans, especially those experiencing a mental health crisis, are especially vulnerable to challenging interactions with the police and deadly use of force (Rice, 2020). In order to better respond to individuals experiencing a mental health emergency, many communities have developed crisis intervention teams (CIT) consisting of specially trained police officers and other first responders who partner with mental health and addiction professionals. In some areas, a youth version of the CIT allows for a developmentally appropriate crisis response (Kubiak et al., 2019). Ideally, CIT training is combined with preventive mental health efforts within the community, thereby reducing the need for emergency responses to psychiatric crises (Watson & Compton, 2019). Further, sensitizing police officers and other first responders to the issues of *systemic racism* and *implicit bias* may help prevent tragic events involving individuals from communities of color.

The availability of high-quality and comprehensive community mental health and crisis services can reduce homelessness and contact with the police. It can also decrease the revolving door of hospital readmission; even when inpatient treatment succeeds in stabilizing patients, relapse is likely to occur if there are inadequate services available upon discharge. Full recovery requires comprehensive community-based treatment that includes supports such as therapy, skills training, peer counseling, visiting nurses, and methods for ensuring medication compliance.

Program of Assertive Community Treatment

Some individuals with an AOT order or who have been discharged from a hospital now have the option of an effective evidence-based intervention—Program of Assertive Community Treatment (PACT). This team-based service model provides comprehensive individualized, round-the-clock supportive outreach services. Rather than being forced to navigate a variety of systems and agencies, PACT brings the services to the client, thereby reducing the possibility of relapse or deterioration in functioning.

The multidisciplinary PACT team focuses on decreasing symptoms, thus increasing independent functioning and reducing the need for acute care such as hospitalization. When a client is stabilized, the PACT programs focus on skill development (self-care, money management, vocational training, etc.) that will assist with the client's recovery. The PACT model also provides education and support to family members.

Mental Illness and the Criminal Justice System

Case Study Keaton Farris, who had been diagnosed with bipolar disorder several years previously, was found dead in his isolation cell in a small jail in Washington State; he was naked, dehydrated, and malnourished. Farris, who had been arrested for cashing a stolen check, had been in custody for 18 days, being shuttled from jail to jail. As 25-year-old Farris awaited a mental health evaluation to determine his competency to stand trial, his symptoms became more severe. After Farris caused his jail cell to flood by placing his pillow in the toilet, officers shut off all water, but then failed to provide Farris with sufficient fluid in the days following the shutoff.

The new jail chief has since provided employees with mental health training and has ensured that mentally ill inmates have access to health care, face-to-face security checks, and competency evaluations within a reasonable period of time. (Jenkins, 2019)

Since deinstitutionalization, the criminalization of those with severe mental illness has become a national concern. Individuals living with mental illness frequently come into contact with the criminal justice system, often for minor offenses. In some communities, severely mentally ill people have more contact with the police and other first responders than with mental health

Mental Health Court

A judge, overseeing a mental health court proceeding, joins a probation officer in applauding a young woman who has come before the court to give an update on her efforts to make positive changes in her life.

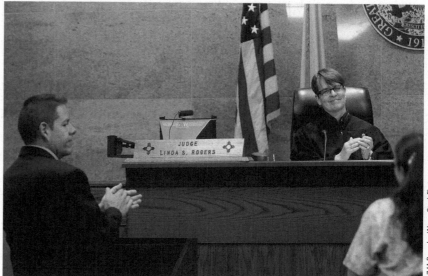

professionals (Dempsey et al., 2019). In many cases, offenders waiting for competency evaluations remain in county jail without the necessary treatment for restoring mental health and stability. The stress of incarceration often aggravates the symptoms of illness and leads to a decline in functioning, sometimes with tragic consequences, as we saw in the case of Keaton Farris. This problem has been exasperated by federal and state reductions in funding for community-based mental health assessment and treatment.

Each year over 2 million people with severe mental health issues are booked into jail. It costs about $31,000 per year to house these individuals, an amount that is two to three times the cost of incarcerating a person without a mental disorder. Ironically, receiving treatment at a community mental health clinic would cost substantially less (approximately one third the amount) compared to incarceration (Giliberti, 2015). Compounding the problem, many mentally ill inmates are unable to access funding for treatment because, according to federal law, anyone jailed following conviction of a crime is no longer eligible for Medicaid or Medicare medical benefits. Additionally, there is often a delay in reinstating benefits after someone is released from jail or prison. Unfortunately, untreated mental illness frequently results in reoffending and a revolving door into the criminal justice system.

The solution, however, is complex and requires much more than a return to the old institutions of the 1950s. Instead, what we need is easily accessible community-based treatment facilities and outpatient resources geared to meet the comprehensive treatment needs of those with severe mental illness. In order to address the issue of warehousing individuals with mental illness within the criminal justice system, some localities have initiated significant changes for individuals whose mental illness is a factor in a pending nonviolent criminal offense. Recognizing that mental health symptoms worsen when a person remains in jail because they are unable to post bail or are waiting for a competency evaluation, these communities have created mental health courts as a more humane and cost-effective alternative to the typical criminal justice process. The goal is to ensure reasonable accountability for criminal acts and to prevent reoffending by connecting the accused to resources for treatment (Loong et al., 2019). At the national level, the Stepping Up initiative is a data-driven framework that aims to assist counties throughout the United States to develop systems which provide treatment rather than incarceration for people with mental illness. The coalition supporting the initiative includes mental health and criminal justice organizations that have joined together to encourage communities to find solutions and initiate effective reforms.

17-4 Ethical Guidelines for Mental Health Professionals

Each mental health profession is guided not only by legal rulings but also by an enforceable code of ethics for its members. For psychologists, the ethical code covers issues such as professional competence, human relations, privacy and confidentiality, record keeping, and continuing education requirements. All psychologists are expected to be aware of these guidelines. Being unaware of or misinterpreting these codes is not a defense against a charge of unethical conduct (American Psychological Association, 2017a). Of particular importance are the legal and ethical issues pertaining to the therapist–client relationship.

Did You Know?

On June 15, 2013, Ethan Couch lost control of his Ford pickup and rammed into two vehicles, killing four people and injuring four others. Couch had three times the legal limit of alcohol in his system. A psychologist hired by the defense testified that Couch suffered from "affluenza" and that he behaved in an irresponsible manner because his family set no boundaries and gave him everything he wanted. Surprisingly, the judge accepted the psychologist's argument and placed Couch on probation with treatment rather than the jail term sought by the prosecution. Couch was subsequently sentenced to 720 days in jail when he broke the conditions of his probation. Is it ethical for a psychologist to use an unrecognized syndrome (such as "affluenza") as a mitigating factor?

Source: Cardona, 2018

The Therapist–Client Relationship

> **Case Study** A psychiatrist was working with a client named Mary, who had five personalities. He was especially concerned with "Sam," who sometimes demonstrated extreme violence—forcefully throwing chairs and other objects and making threats to injure staff members. During one session, Sam made a threat toward a specific individual—the owner of a grocery store where the client lived. He stated, "I'll kill that guy. You know I will. I've already made a plan and bought a gun. I'm going to shoot him tonight when he gets off work" (Norko, 2008, p. 144). Later, the psychiatric resident sitting in on the case asked the psychiatrist if they should inform the police about Sam's threat. The psychiatrist expressed reluctance, believing such a move would undo the work that they accomplished in therapy.

Was the psychiatrist right in his decision? Did he have an obligation to protect the possible victim? The therapist–client relationship involves a number of legal, moral, and ethical issues such as these. We will discuss how they affect cases such as this complex case of dissociative identity disorder. Three common ethical concerns involve issues of confidentiality and privileged communication, the therapist's duty to warn others of a risk posed by a client, and the therapist's obligation to avoid sexual intimacies with clients.

Confidentiality and Privileged Communication

Basic to the therapist–patient relationship is the premise that therapy involves a deeply personal association in which clients have a right to expect that what they say is kept private. Therapists believe that therapy cannot be effective unless clients trust their therapists and are certain that what they share is confidential. Without this guarantee, clients may not be completely open with their thoughts and may subsequently obtain less benefit from therapy. **Confidentiality** is an ethical standard that protects clients from disclosure of information without their consent. Confidentiality, however, is an ethical, not a legal, obligation. **Privileged communication**, a narrower legal concept, protects privacy and prevents the disclosure of confidential communications without a client's permission (Corey et al., 2018).

Our society recognizes how important certain confidential relationships are and protects them by law. The relationships covered by privileged-communication statutes are spousal, attorney–client, pastor–congregant, and therapist–client relationships. Psychiatric practices are regulated in all 50 states and the District of Columbia, and most of those jurisdictions have privileged-communication statutes. The Health Information Portability and Accountability Act (HIPAA) further enhanced privacy protections for individuals who seek mental health evaluation or treatment, including protection of therapist records such as notes taken during therapy. An important aspect of the privacy concept is that the holder of the privilege is the client, not the therapist. In other words, if a client waives this privilege, the therapist has no grounds for withholding information.

The issue of confidentiality and privileged communication has become more complex in recent years. Proposed bills and laws in a number of states have included provisions such as criminalizing gender-affirming care for transgender adolescents; requiring school personnel to reveal the gender identity of transgender youth to parents; defining gender-affirming care as "child abuse"; criminalizing medical personnel who provide gender-affirming care; and allowing civil action to be taken against parents and physicians for supporting gender-affirming treatment (Kraschel et al., 2022). Such legislation also impacts patient confidentiality and the professional ethics of therapists (American Psychological Association, 2022). For instance, laws that define gender-affirming care as "child abuse" require mandatory reporting by professionals who become aware that a child is receiving gender-affirming treatment.

Exemptions from Privileged Communication   Although states vary considerably, they all recognize certain situations in which privileged communications can be divulged. Corey and associates (2018) summarized these conditions:

- In situations that deal with civil or criminal commitment or competency to stand trial, the client has the right to request that privileged information be shared.

- Disclosure can also be made when a client who has been in therapy introduces their mental condition as a claim or defense in a civil action.

- When the client is a minor or a dependent elderly person and information leads the therapist to believe that the individual has been a victim of a crime (e.g., incest, rape, or abuse), the therapist must provide such information to the appropriate protective services agency.

- When the therapist has reason to believe that a client presents a danger to themselves (such as a high risk of suicide) or may potentially harm someone else, the therapist must act to ward off the danger.

As you can see, exemptions from privilege involve a variety of complex situations and decisions. Let's examine one of the important exceptions—the duty to warn.

The Duty to Warn

Case Study   In 1968, Prosenjit Poddar—a graduate student from India studying at the University of California, Berkeley—sought therapy from the student health services for depression. Poddar was apparently upset over what he perceived to be a rebuff from another student, Tatiana Tarasoff, whom he claimed to love. During the course of treatment, Poddar informed his therapist that he intended to purchase a gun and kill Tarasoff. Judging Poddar to be dangerous, the psychologist breached the confidentiality of the professional relationship by informing the campus police. The police detained Poddar briefly but freed him because he agreed to stay away from Tarasoff. On October 27, 1969, Poddar went to Tarasoff's home and killed her, first wounding her with a gun and then stabbing her repeatedly with a knife. In the subsequent lawsuit filed by Tarasoff's family, the California Supreme Court made a landmark ruling in 1976 that established what is popularly known as the *duty to warn*—the court ruled that the therapist should have warned not only the police but also the intended victim.

The therapist had informed the campus police, hoping that they would detain Poddar, which they did, but only briefly. The therapist also notified his supervisor, the director of the psychiatric clinic, about Poddar's

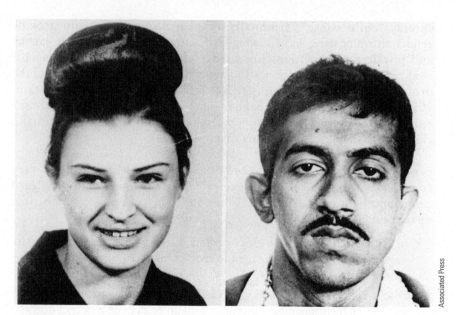

Associated Press

A Duty to Warn

Tatiana Tarasoff, a college student, was stabbed to death in 1969 by Prosenjit Poddar, a graduate student at the University of California, Berkeley. Although Poddar's therapist notified the police about threats made by Poddar, the California Supreme Court ruled that the therapist should have also warned Tarasoff.

comments because he was extremely concerned that Poddar was dangerous and likely to carry out his threat to harm Tarasoff. Surely the therapist had done all that could be reasonably expected. Not so, ruled the California Supreme Court (*Tarasoff v. the Board of Regents of the University of California* [1976]). In the **Tarasoff ruling**, the court stated that when a therapist determines, according to the standards of the mental health profession, that a client presents a serious danger to another individual, the therapist is obligated to warn the intended victim. The court went on to say that protective privilege ends where public peril begins. In general, courts have ruled that therapists have a responsibility to protect the public from dangerous acts of violent clients, and they have held therapists accountable for (a) failing to predict dangerousness, (b) failing to warn potential victims, (c) failing to initiate commitment proceedings for dangerous individuals, and (d) prematurely discharging dangerous patients from a hospital. However, some courts have ruled that although confidentiality can be broken by the duty to warn, it does not cover additional breaches such as judicial testimony regarding threatening statements made by a client (Beckman & Mobbs, 2016).

Although most states have statues consistent with the *Tarasoff* ruling, state differences do exist (refer to Figure 17.3). For example, in response to the James Holmes theater shooting in Aurora, Colorado, the governor of Colorado signed House Bill 14-1271 on April 7, 2014, which extends the duty to warn to include not only specifically identified individual targets but also includes threats to entities such as buildings or specific locations where people might be endangered. Under this law, if there is a perceived danger, Colorado mental health professionals must notify the people responsible for the locations or entities, as well as law enforcement, or take other steps such as initiating commitment proceedings.

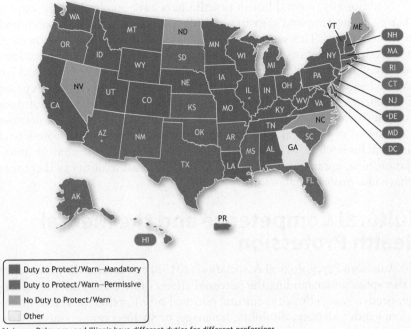

Figure 17.3

Duty to Warn
Most states have laws that either require or permit mental health professionals to disclose information about clients who may become violent. In some states, the duty to warn about possible danger is mandatory. In other states, "permissive" laws allow a therapist to break confidentiality under specific circumstances.

Source: National Conference of State Legislators (2022).

Duty to Protect/Warn—Mandatory
Duty to Protect/Warn—Permissive
No Duty to Protect/Warn
Other

*Arizona, Delaware, and Illinois have different duties for different professions.

Criticism of the Duty to Warn   The *Tarasoff* ruling seems to place the therapist in the unenviable role of being a double agent. Therapists have ethical and legal obligations to their clients, but they also have a legal responsibility to society. These obligations sometimes not only conflict with one another, but they can also be quite ambiguous. State courts are frequently forced to clarify the implications and uncertainties of the duty to warn.

When the *Tarasoff* ruling came out, Siegel (1979) loudly criticized it, stating that the outcome was a hollow victory for individual parties and was devastating for the mental health professions. He reasoned that if confidentiality had been an absolute policy applied to all situations, then Poddar might have continued his treatment, thus ultimately saving Tarasoff's life. In other words, he wondered if the requirement to notify the authorities led to an escalation of events that resulted in Tatiana Tarasoff's death. Other mental health professionals have echoed this sentiment in one form or another (Modak et al., 2016). Hostile clients with pent-up emotions may be less likely to act out or become violent if allowed to vent their feelings. The irony, according to critics, is that the duty to warn may actually be counterproductive to its intent to protect potential victims.

Sexual Relationships with Clients

According to the ethical code for psychologists, sexual intimacies are prohibited with current clients, the relatives or partners of current clients, or former clients for a minimum of 2 years after termination of therapy. Even after 2 years, sexual intimacy with a former client would not be acceptable "except in the most unusual circumstances" (American Psychological Association, 2017b). Unfortunately, such contact does occur—the most common civil complaint related to psychotherapy involves sexual intimacies between a therapist and a current or former client (Corey et al., 2018).

Traditionally, mental health practitioners have emphasized the importance of separating and creating boundaries between their personal and professional lives. This separation is emphasized because therapists need to be objective and because becoming emotionally involved with a client may interfere with therapy. A therapist who is personally involved with a client may be less confrontational, may fulfill their own needs at the expense of the client's, and may unintentionally exploit the client because of their position (Corey et al., 2018). Although some people question the premise that a social or personal relationship interferes with therapy, professional codes make it clear that personal relations, especially sexual intimate relationships, are inappropriate. Fortunately, the vast majority of therapists behave in a professional manner.

Cultural Competence and the Mental Health Profession

The American Psychological Association (2017b) emphasizes the importance of therapists understanding the potential effects of diversity issues involving age, gender, race, ethnicity, culture, national origin, religion, sexual orientation, gender identity, disability, language, or socioeconomic status. Most mental health professionals agree that psychological theories, definitions of mental disorders, and contemporary approaches to therapy are culture bound; that is, they are based on the highly individualistic values of middle- to upper-class European Americans. Unfortunately, services offered to clients from diverse backgrounds often fail to consider the clients' life experiences. Further, inadequate cultural competence not only results in poor sensitivity and understanding of client needs but may result in discriminatory practices toward underrepresented populations. These concerns apply not only to those from underrepresented racial/ethnic groups but also to other marginalized groups such as women, the LGBTQIA+ community, individuals with disabilities, and older adults.

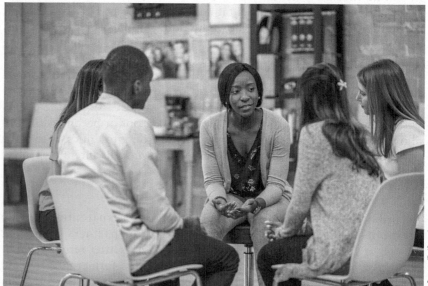

Changing Demographics and Therapy

Therapists often participate in multicultural training in preparation for work with clients from a variety of cultural backgrounds. Here graduate students discuss their personal experiences during a diversity training activity.

FatCamera/E+/Getty Images

Using Positive Psychology to Build Soldier Resilience: An Ethical Dilemma?

Throughout this text, we have extolled the virtues of positive psychology and a strength-based approach to viewing the human condition. Positive psychology has made many contributions to our understanding of resilience and the protective factors that may help safeguard against mental disorders. Positive psychology prompts us to focus on factors that enhance mental health, to value prevention and resilience, and to embrace assets and strengths. But can the basic tenets and principles of positive psychology be misused and misapplied? If so, would that not raise moral and ethical questions?

Such is the case with an intervention that created a major controversy within the psychological community—the Comprehensive Soldier Fitness (CSF) program implemented by the U.S. Army (Cornum et al., 2011; Harms et al., 2013). Using research findings and principles derived from positive psychology, the U.S. Army embarked on an effort to increase the psychological strength and positive performance of soldiers and to reduce any maladaptive responses to military trauma and demands. The goal is to increase soldiers' resilience as they face threat of injury or death, sleep deprivation, separation from family and friends, extreme climates, and the trauma of taking the lives of enemy combatants. Such an undertaking is especially important during times of war.

For example, during the wars in Iraq and Afghanistan, approximately 70 percent of soldiers were exposed to traumatic events. This exposure resulted in high rates of posttraumatic stress disorder, alcohol abuse, suicide, and depression (Cornum et al., 2011).

The CSF training develops psychological resilience in soldiers using an evidence-based approach that strengthens emotional, social, family, and spiritual fitness to ward off the stresses of military life and combat. Just as physical training focuses on physical preparedness for military combat, CSF increases the mental fitness of soldiers by strengthening

S-F/Shutterstock.com

their psychological assets and preparing them to participate in high-risk actions such as going on patrols, killing or injuring their enemies, and interrogating captives (Cornum et al., 2011). Preliminary evidence suggests that the CSF program is effective (Algoe & Fredrickson, 2011; Cacioppo et al., 2011; Tedeschi & McNally, 2011), although questions have been raised regarding the adequacy of the research design in these studies (Eidelson & Soldz, 2012; Sagalyn, 2012). The CSF training has continued and is now known as the Ready and Resilient (R2) program (Lampkin, 2019).

On the surface, the CSF program appears to have very worthy goals—providing the best care possible for those who serve in the military. Yet a number of psychologists have raised serious moral and ethical objections to the use of positive psychology in the CSF program. They assert that the basic premise of the program is flawed and misguided (Eidelson et al., 2011; Krueger, 2011; Phipps, 2011). Among their objections are the following:

- The use of positive psychology in the military operates under the assumption that war is unavoidable and that, as a result, it is the patriotic duty of psychologists to help the military make our men and women more resilient in combat. Critics vehemently question this assumption, and instead advocate for the use of positive psychology principles to reduce conflict between nations, to prevent war, and to promote peace.

- War is horrific and exposes combatants to gruesome sights and situations. Reactions of distress or repugnance are natural, healthy, and humane responses. To train soldiers to experience less distress when encountering or perpetuating death, destruction, and inhumane acts is a frightening prospect. To teach soldiers, for example, to feel better about killing is morally and ethically questionable.

- Psychologists who use positive psychology to help the military are deceiving themselves. The CSF client is the U.S. Army, not the individual soldier. The U.S. Army demands discipline, efficiency, and obedience, and attempts to standardize behavior. It is naive to think that the CSF program would put soldiers' psychological needs ahead of the goals of the U.S. Army.

Is it appropriate for psychologists to lend their considerable expertise in human behavior to military purposes if the outcome involves objectionable goals? We must remember that psychological science can be used for any number of purposes, both good and bad.

In a historic move, the American Psychological Association (2003) adopted guidelines related to multicultural understanding with respect to education, training, research, practice, and organizational structure. These comprehensive guidelines emphasize the importance of culturally sensitive work with racially and ethnically underrepresented groups and make it clear that service providers need to become aware of how their own cultural and life experiences, attitudes, values, and biases have influenced them. The guidelines also emphasize the importance of incorporating cultural and environmental factors throughout diagnosis and treatment, and the value of respecting traditional healing approaches that are intrinsic to a client's culture. Finally, therapists are encouraged to learn more about cultural issues and seek consultation when confronted with culture-specific problems. The guidelines call for cultural competence and emphasize that if therapists ignore the racial and cultural backgrounds of their clients or have inadequate training in working with a culturally diverse population, the result may be biased or discriminatory treatment.

Mental health professionals who provide culturally appropriate treatment strive toward attaining three goals (Sue et al., 2022):

1. becoming aware of and dealing with biases, stereotypes, and assumptions that may affect their assessment and treatment practices;

2. understanding the values and worldviews of clients from different backgrounds and cultures; and

3. developing appropriate intervention strategies that take into account the social, cultural, historical, and environmental factors that influence clients from diverse backgrounds.

Fortunately, in an effort to improve the assessment and treatment of diverse populations, the DSM now has an increased focus on how multicultural factors can influence the development of mental disorders. This increased cultural sensitivity should lead to improvements in both diagnosis and intervention with individuals from a wide variety of cultural groups.

Chapter Summary

1 **What are the criteria used to judge insanity, and what is the difference between being insane and being incompetent to stand trial?**

- People can be acquitted of a crime using an insanity defense if they (a) did not know right from wrong (M'Naghten rule), (b) were unable to control their behavior (irresistible impulse), or (c) acted out of a mental disease or defect (Durham standard). The American Law Institute guidelines attempt to define insanity by combining aspects of these three standards.

- Competency to stand trial refers to defendants' mental state (whether they can rationally aid attorneys in their own defense) at the time they are evaluated, not at the time of the offense.

2 **Under what conditions can a person be involuntarily committed for inpatient psychiatric treatment?**

- People who have committed no crime can be confined against their will if it can be shown that they (a) present a clear and imminent danger to themselves or others, (b) are unable to care for themselves, (c) are unable to make responsible decisions about appropriate treatment and hospitalization, or (d) are in an unmanageable mental state.

3 **What rights do the mentally ill have with respect to treatment and care?**

- Court rulings have established that individuals living with mental illness have the right to receive treatment and the right to refuse treatment.

- Deinstitutionalization, the shifting of responsibility for the care of the mentally ill from large central institutions to agencies within the local community, has led to concerns about the adequacy of community services for many people with severe mental illness.

4 **What legal and ethical issues guide treatment practices?**

- Confidentiality and privileged communication are crucial to the therapist–client relationship. Exceptions involve (a) civil or criminal commitment and determinations of competency to stand trial, (b) a client's involvement in court actions in which their mental condition is introduced, (c) concern that child abuse or elder abuse has occurred, and (d) a client who poses a danger to himself or herself or to others.

- The *Tarasoff* decision makes therapists responsible for warning a potential victim in order to avoid liability.

- Sexual misconduct by therapists is considered to be one of the most serious of all ethical violations.

- It is important to consider diversity involving factors such as culture, ethnicity, and gender in therapy. Adequate training and expertise in multicultural psychology is important for therapists treating members of marginalized groups.

Chapter Glossary

civil commitment
the involuntary confinement of individuals judged to be a danger to themselves or others, even though they have not committed a crime

competency to stand trial
a judgment that a defendant has a factual and rational understanding of the criminal proceedings and can rationally consult with counsel in presenting a defense

confidentiality
an ethical standard that protects clients from disclosure of information without their consent

criminal commitment
the incarceration of an individual for having committed a crime

deinstitutionalization
the shifting of responsibility for the care of people with mental illness from large central institutions to agencies within local communities

diminished capacity
a law standard allowing a defendant to be convicted of a lesser offense due to mental impairment

due process
the constitutional guarantee of fair treatment within the judicial system

Durham standard
a test of legal insanity also known as the *product test*—an accused person is not responsible if the unlawful act was the product of a mental disease or defect

insanity defense
the legal argument used by defendants who admit that they have committed a crime but plead not guilty because they were mentally disturbed at the time of the offense

irresistible impulse test
a doctrine that contends that a defendant is not criminally responsible if they lacked the willpower to control their behavior

least restrictive environment
the least restrictive alternative to freedom that is appropriate to a person's condition

mainstreaming
integrating people with mental illness back into the community

M'Naghten rule
a test of legal insanity that inquires whether the accused knew right from wrong when the crime was committed

privileged communication
a therapist's legal obligation to protect a client's privacy and to prevent the disclosure of confidential communications without the client's permission

right to treatment
the concept that people with mental illness who have been involuntarily committed have a right to receive therapy for their condition

***Tarasoff* ruling**
a California Supreme Court decision that obligates mental health professionals to break confidentiality when their clients pose a clear and imminent danger to another person

Glossary

abstinence restraint from the use of alcohol, drugs, or other addictive substances

acculturative stress the psychological, physical, and social pressures experienced by individuals who are adapting to a new culture

acute stress disorder (ASD) a condition characterized by flashbacks, hypervigilance, and avoidance symptoms that last up to 1 month after exposure to a traumatic stressor

adaptive behavior performance on tasks of daily living, including academic skills, self-care, and the ability to work or live independently

addiction compulsive drug-seeking behavior and a loss of control over drug use

adjustment disorder a condition involving reactions to life stressors that are disproportionate to the severity or intensity of the event or situation

adrenal gland a gland that releases sex hormones and other hormones, such as cortisol, in response to stress

advance directive written health care instructions specifying the treatments a person is willing to have or not have if unable to make decisions because of mental or physical incapacity

agoraphobia an intense fear of being in public places where escape or help may not be readily available

alcoholism a condition in which the individual is dependent on alcohol and has difficulty controlling drinking

alcohol poisoning potentially life-threatening, toxic effects resulting from rapidly consuming alcohol or ingesting a large quantity of alcohol

allele each of two or more alternative forms of a gene responsible for a specific trait

alleles the gene pair responsible for a specific trait

alogia lack of meaningful speech

Alzheimer disease dementia involving memory loss and other declines in cognitive and adaptive functioning

amygdala the brain structure involved with physiological reactivity and emotional memories

analogue study an investigation that attempts to replicate or simulate, under controlled conditions, a situation that occurs in real life

anhedonia inability to experience pleasure from previously enjoyed activities

anorexia nervosa an eating disorder characterized by low body weight, an intense fear of becoming obese, and body image distortion

anosognosia a lack of awareness of or insight into one's own mental dysfunction

antipsychotic medication medicine developed to counteract symptoms of psychosis

anxiety an anticipatory emotion that produces bodily reactions that prepare us for "fight or flight"

anxiety disorder fear or anxiety symptoms that interfere with an individual's day-to-day functioning

anxiety sensitivity a trait involving fear of physiological changes within the body

anxiolytics a class of medications that reduce anxiety

anxious distress symptoms of motor tension, difficulty relaxing, pervasive worries, or feelings that something catastrophic will occur

asociality minimal interest in social relationships

asthma a chronic inflammatory disease of the airways in the lungs

asymptomatic without symptoms

assigned gender the gender to which a child is socially assigned at birth

atherosclerosis a condition involving the progressive thickening and hardening of the walls of arteries

due to an accumulation of fats and cholesterol along their inner lining

attention-deficit/hyperactivity disorder (ADHD) childhood-onset disorder characterized by persistent attentional problems and/or impulsive, hyperactive behaviors

attenuated psychosis syndrome a condition being researched that involves distressing or disabling early signs of delusions, hallucinations, or disorganized speech that emerged or became progressively worse over the previous year; reality testing remains fairly intact

attributional style a characteristic way of explaining why a positive or negative event occurred

atypical antipsychotics newer antipsychotic medications that are less likely to produce the side effects associated with first-generation antipsychotics

aura a visual or physical sensation (e.g., tingling of an extremity or flashes of light) that precedes a migraine headache

autism spectrum disorder (ASD) a disorder characterized by a continuum of impairment in social communication and restricted, stereotyped interests and activities

autistic savant an individual with autism spectrum disorder who performs exceptionally well on certain tasks

autonomic nervous system (ANS) a system that coordinates basic physiological functions and regulates physical responses associated with emotional reactions

avoidant personality disorder characterized by a fear of rejection and humiliation and an avoidance of social situations

avolition lack of motivation; an inability to take action or become goal oriented

axon an extension on the neuron cell body that sends signals to other neurons, muscles, and glands

antisocial personality disorder (APD) characterized by a failure to conform to social and legal codes, a lack of anxiety and guilt, and irresponsible behaviors

base rate the rate of natural occurrence of a phenomenon in the population studied

behavioral inhibition shyness

behavioral models models of psychopathology concerned with the role of learning in the development of behavior

behavioral undercontrol a personality trait associated with rebelliousness, novelty seeking, risk taking, and impulsivity

beta-amyloid plaques clumps of beta-amyloid proteins found in the spaces between neurons

binge-eating disorder (BED) an eating disorder that involves the consumption of large amounts of food over a short period of time with accompanying feelings of loss of control and distress over the excess eating

binge drinking episodic intake of five or more alcoholic beverages for men or four or more drinks for women

binge eating rapid consumption of large quantities of food

biofeedback training a physiological and behavioral approach in which an individual receives information regarding particular autonomic functions and is rewarded for influencing those functions in a desired direction

biological viewpoint the belief that mental disorders have a physical or physiological basis

biological vulnerability genetic or physiological susceptibility

biopsychosocial model the perspective suggesting that interactions between biological, psychological, and social factors cause mental disorders

bipolar I disorder a diagnosis that involves at least one manic episode that has impaired social or occupational functioning; the person may or may not experience depression or psychotic symptoms

bipolar II disorder a diagnosis that involves at least one major depressive episode and at least one hypomanic episode

blood pressure the measurement of the force of blood against the walls of the arteries

body dysmorphic disorder (BDD) a condition involving a preoccupation with a perceived physical defect or excessive concern over a slight physical defect

body mass index (BMI) an estimate of body fat calculated on the basis of a person's height and weight

borderline personality disorder (BPD) characterized by intense fluctuations in mood, self-image, and interpersonal relationships

brain pathology a dysfunction or disease of the brain

brief psychotic disorder a condition characterized by psychotic episodes with a duration of at least 1 day but less than 1 month

bulimia nervosa an eating disorder in which episodes involving rapid consumption of large quantities of food and a loss of control over eating are followed by purging, excessive exercise, or fasting in an attempt to compensate for binges

cardiovascular pertaining to the heart and blood vessels

case study an intensive study of one individual that relies on clinical data, such as observations, psychological tests, and historical and biographical information

catatonia a condition characterized by marked disturbance in motor activity ranging from extreme excitement to motoric immobility

cathartic method a therapeutic use of verbal expression to release pent-up emotional conflicts

caudate nuclei the deep brain structure that stores and processes memories and signals when something is amiss

cerebral contusion bruising of the brain, often resulting from a blow that causes the brain to forcefully strike the skull

cerebral cortex the outermost layers of brain tissue; covers the cerebrum

cerebral laceration an open head injury in which brain tissue is torn, pierced, or ruptured

cerebrum the largest part of the brain, consisting of the right and left hemisphere

child psychopathology the emotional and behavioral manifestation of psychological disorders in children and adolescents

chronic traumatic encephalopathy (CTE) a progressive, degenerative condition involving brain damage resulting from multiple episodes of head trauma

circadian rhythm an internal clock or daily cycle of internal biological rhythms that influence various bodily processes such as body temperature and sleep–wake cycles

circadian rhythm sleep disorder sleep disturbance due to a disrupted sleep–wake cycle

cisgender a person's gender identity aligns with the person's sex assigned at birth

civil commitment the involuntary confinement of individuals judged to be a danger to themselves or others, even though they have not committed a crime

classical conditioning a process in which responses to new stimuli are learned through association

cluster headache excruciating stabbing or burning sensations located in the eye or cheek

co-rumination extensively discussing negative feelings or events with peers or others

cognitive models explanations based on the assumption that thoughts mediate an individual's emotional state or behavior in response to a stimulus

cognitive restructuring a cognitive strategy that attempts to alter unrealistic thoughts that are believed to be responsible for fears and anxiety

cognitive symptoms symptoms of schizophrenia associated with problems with attention, memory, and developing a plan of action

comorbid existing simultaneously with another condition

competency to stand trial a judgment that a defendant has a factual and rational understanding of the criminal proceedings and can rationally consult with counsel in presenting a defense

compulsion the need to perform acts or mental tasks to reduce anxiety

concordance rate the degree of similarity between twins or family members with respect to a trait or disorder

concussion trauma-induced changes in brain functioning, typically caused by a blow to the head

conditioned response (CR) in classical conditioning, a learned response to a previously neutral stimulus that has acquired some of the properties of another stimulus with which it has been paired

conditioned stimulus (CS) in classical conditioning, a previously neutral stimulus that has acquired some of the properties of another stimulus with which it has been paired

conduct disorder (CD) a persistent pattern of behavior that violates the rights of others, including aggression, serious rule violations, and illegal behavior

confidentiality an ethical standard that protects clients from disclosure of information without their consent

controlled drinking consuming no more than a predetermined amount of alcohol

coprolalia involuntary utterance of obscenities or inappropriate remarks

coronary vascular disease (CVD) a disease process involving the narrowing of cardiac arteries, resulting in the restriction or partial blockage of the flow of blood and oxygen to the heart

correlation the extent to which variations in one variable are accompanied by increases or decreases in a second variable

cortisol a hormone released by the adrenal glands in response to stress

couples therapy a treatment aimed at helping couples understand and clarify their communications, role relationships, unfulfilled needs, and unrealistic or unmet expectations

criminal commitment the incarceration of an individual for having committed a crime

critical periods a specific time in early development during which there is heightened sensitivity to environmental influences or experiences

cross-cutting measure assesses common symptoms that are not specific to one disorder

cultural relativism the idea that a person's beliefs, values, and behaviors are affected by the culture within which that person lives

cultural universality the assumption that a fixed set of mental disorders exists whose manifestations and symptoms are similar across cultures

culture the configuration of shared values, beliefs, attitudes, and behaviors that is transmitted from one generation to another by members of a particular group

cyclothymic disorder a condition involving milder hypomanic symptoms that are consistently interspersed with milder depressed moods for at least 2 years

comorbidity co-occurrence of two or more disorders in the same person

defense mechanism in psychoanalytic theory, an ego-protection strategy that shelters the individual from anxiety, operates unconsciously, and distorts reality

deficit model an early attempt to explain differences in minority groups that contended differences are the result of "cultural deprivation"

deinstitutionalization the shifting of responsibility for the care of people with mental illness from large central institutions to agencies within local communities

delayed ejaculation persistent delay or inability to ejaculate within the vagina despite adequate excitement and stimulation

delirium an acute state of confusion involving diminished awareness, disorientation, and impaired attentional skills

delirium tremens life-threatening withdrawal symptoms that can result from chronic alcohol use

delusion a false belief that is firmly and consistently held

delusional disorder persistent delusions without other unusual or odd behaviors; tactile and olfactory hallucinations related to the delusional theme may be present

dementia condition with symptoms involving deterioration in cognition and independent functioning

dementia with Lewy bodies (DLB) dementia involving visual hallucinations, cognitive fluctuations, and atypical movements

dendrite a short, rootlike structure on the neuron cell body that receives signals from other neurons

dependent personality disorder characterized by submissive, clinging behavior and an excessive need to be taken care of

dependent variable a variable that is expected to change when an independent variable is manipulated in a psychological experiment

depersonalization/derealization disorder (DDD) a dissociative condition characterized by feelings of unreality concerning the self and the environment

depressant a substance that causes a slowing of responses and generalized depression of the central nervous system

depression a mood state characterized by sadness or despair, feelings of worthlessness, and withdrawal from others

detoxification the phase of alcohol or drug treatment during which the body is purged of intoxicating substances

diastolic pressure the arterial force exerted when the heart is relaxed and the ventricles of the heart are filling with blood

diminished capacity a law standard allowing a defendant to be convicted of a lesser offense due to mental impairment

diminished emotional expression reduced display of observable verbal and nonverbal behaviors that communicate internal emotions

disconfirmatory evidence information that contradicts a delusional belief

discrimination unjust or prejudicial treatment toward a person based on the person's actual or perceived membership in a certain group

disinhibited social engagement disorder (DSED) a trauma-related attachment disorder characterized by indiscriminate, superficial attachments and desperation for interpersonal contact

disordered eating physically or psychologically unhealthy eating behavior such as chronic overeating or dieting

disruptive mood dysregulation disorder (DMDD) a childhood disorder involving **chronic irritability** and significantly exaggerated anger reactions

dissociation a psychological coping mechanism characterized by a sense of disconnection from traumatic circumstances

dissociative amnesia a psychologically based sudden loss of important personal information or recall of events

dissociative amnesia with fugue an episode involving complete loss of memory of one's life and identity, unexpected travel to a new location, or assumption of a new identity

dissociative anesthetic a substance that produces a dreamlike detachment

dissociative disorders a group of disorders, including dissociative amnesia, dissociative identity disorder, and depersonalization/derealization disorder, all of which involve some sort of dissociation, or separation, of a part of the person's consciousness, memory, or identity

dissociative identity disorder (DID) a condition in which two or more relatively independent personality states appear to exist in one person, including experiences of possession

dopamine hypothesis the suggestion that schizophrenia may result from excess dopamine activity at certain synaptic sites

double-blind design an experimental design in which neither those helping with the experiment nor the participants are aware of experimental conditions

Down syndrome (DS) a chromosomal disorder (most frequently involving an extra copy of chromosome 21) that causes physical and neurological abnormalities

dream analysis a psychoanalytic technique focused on interpreting the hidden meanings of dreams

drug–drug interactions when the effect of a medication is changed, enhanced, or diminished when taken with another drug, including herbal substances

due process the constitutional guarantee of fair treatment within the judicial system

Durham standard a test of legal insanity also known as the product test—an accused person is not responsible if the unlawful act was the product of a mental disease or defect

dyscalculia a condition involving difficulties in understanding mathematical skills or concepts

dyslexia a condition involving significant difficulties with reading skills

dyspareunia recurrent or persistent pain in the genitals before, during, or after sexual intercourse

dyssomnias disorders involving abnormalities in the quality, amount, or timing of sleep

echolalia repetition of vocalizations made by another person

elevated blood pressure a condition believed to be a precursor to hypertension, stroke, and heart disease, characterized by systolic blood pressure of 120 to 129 mm Hg and diastolic pressure less than 80 mm Hg

elevated mood a mood state involving exaggerated feelings of confidence, energy, and well-being

emotional lability unstable and rapidly changing emotions and mood

empowerment increasing one's sense of personal strength and self-worth

endophenotypes measurable characteristics (neurochemical, endocrinological, neuroanatomical, cognitive, or neuropsychological) that can give clues regarding the specific genes involved in disorders

enteric nervous system (ENS) an independent neural system involved with digestion; capable of signaling the brain regarding stress and other emotions

epidemiological research the study of the prevalence and distribution of mental disorders in a population

epigenetics a field of biological research focused on understanding how environmental factors influence gene expression

epinephrine a hormone released by the adrenal glands in response to physical or mental stress; also known as *adrenaline*

erectile disorder an inability to attain or maintain an erection sufficient for sexual intercourse

etiological model model developed to explain the cause of a disorder

etiology the cause or causes for a condition

euphoria an exceptionally elevated mood; exaggerated feeling of well-being

evidence-based practice treatment decisions based on best current research combined with clinician judgment and client characteristics and needs

evidence-based therapies treatment techniques that have strong research support

excoriation (skin-picking) disorder distressing and recurrent compulsive picking of the skin resulting in skin lesions

executive functioning mental processes that involve the planning, organizing, and attention required to meet short-term and long-term goals

exhibitionistic disorder urges, acts, or fantasies that involve exposing one's genitals to strangers

existential approach a set of philosophical attitudes that focus on human alienation, the individual in the context of the human condition, and personal responsibility to others as well as to oneself

exorcism a practice used to cast evil spirits out of an afflicted person's body

expansive mood a mood in which a person may feel extremely confident or self-important and behave impulsively

experimental hypothesis a prediction concerning how an independent variable will affect a dependent variable in an experiment

experiment a technique of scientific inquiry in which a prediction is made about two variables; the independent variable is then manipulated in a controlled situation, and changes in the dependent variable are measured

exposure therapy a treatment approach based on extinction principles that involves gradual or rapid exposure to feared objects or situations

expressed emotion (EE) a negative communication pattern found among some relatives of individuals with schizophrenia

externalizing disorders disruptive behavior disorders associated with symptoms that disturb others

external validity the degree to which findings of a particular study can be generalized to other groups or conditions

extinction the decrease or cessation of a behavior due to the gradual weakening of a classically or operantly conditioned response

extrapyramidal symptoms side effects such as restlessness, involuntary movements, and muscular tension produced by antipsychotic medications

eye movement desensitization and reprocessing a therapy for PTSD involving visualization of the traumatic experience combined with rapid, rhythmic eye movements

factitious disorder a condition in which a person deliberately induces or simulates symptoms of physical or mental illness with no apparent incentive other than attention

factitious disorder imposed on another a pattern of falsification or production of physical or psychological symptoms in another individual

factitious disorder imposed on self symptoms of illness are deliberately induced, simulated, or exaggerated, with no apparent external incentive

family systems model an explanation that assumes that the family is an interdependent system and that mental disorders reflect processes occurring within the family system

fear an intense emotion experienced in response to a threatening situation

fear extinction the elimination of conditioned fear responses associated with a trauma

female orgasmic disorder sexual dysfunction involving persistent delay or inability to achieve an orgasm with adequate clitoral stimulation

female sexual interest/arousal disorder sexual dysfunction in women

that is characterized by distressing disinterest in sexual activities or inability to attain or maintain physiological or psychological arousal during sexual activity

fetal alcohol spectrum effects a continuum of detrimental neurological and behavioral effects resulting from maternal alcohol consumption during pregnancy

fetal alcohol syndrome (FAS) a condition resulting from maternal alcohol consumption during gestation that involves central nervous system dysfunction and altered brain development

fetishistic disorder sexual attraction and fantasies involving inanimate objects

field study an investigative technique in which behaviors and events are observed and recorded in their natural environment

first-generation antipsychotics a group of medications originally developed to combat psychotic symptoms by reducing dopamine levels in the brain; also called *conventional* or *typical antipsychotics*

flight of ideas rapidly changing or disjointed thoughts

flooding a technique that involves inducing a high anxiety level through continued actual or imagined exposure to a fear-arousing situation

fragile X syndrome an inherited condition involving limited production of proteins required for brain development resulting in mild to severe intellectual disability

free association a psychoanalytic therapeutic technique in which clients are asked to say whatever comes to mind for the purpose of revealing their unconscious thoughts

frontotemporal lobar degeneration (FTLD) dementia involving degeneration in the frontal and temporal lobes of the brain causing declines in language, behavior, or motor skills

frotteuristic disorder recurrent and intense sexual urges, acts, or fantasies that involve sexual touching or rubbing against a nonconsenting person

functional imaging procedures that provide data regarding

physiological and biochemical processes occurring within the brain

functional neurological symptom disorder (FNSD) a condition involving sensory or motor impairment suggestive of a neurological disorder but with no underlying medical cause

GABA gamma-aminobutyric acid, an inhibitory neurotransmitter involved in inducing sleep and relaxation

gateway drug a substance that leads to the use of additional substances that are even more lethal

gender dysphoria distress and impaired functioning resulting from an incongruence between a person's gender identity and assigned gender

gender expression the way in which gender is manifested, including behavior, clothing, hairstyle, or pronouns used

gender incongruence state of having a gender identity that does not align with the gender assigned at birth

gene expression the process by which heritable information in a gene is translated into a specialized function within a cell; although the DNA within the cell does not change, epigenetic changes can be passed on to new cells during cell division and can be inherited

generalized anxiety disorder (GAD) a condition characterized by persistent, high levels of anxiety and excessive worry over many life circumstances

genes segments of DNA coded with information needed for the biological inheritance of various traits

genetic linkage studies studies that attempt to determine whether a disorder follows a genetic pattern

genetic mutation an alteration in a gene that changes the instructions within the gene; some mutations result in biological dysfunction

genito-pelvic pain/penetration disorder physical pain or discomfort associated with intercourse or penetration

genome the complete set of DNA in a cell; the human genome consists of approximately 30,000 genes located in the nucleus of every cell

genotype a person's genetic makeup

glia the cells that support and protect neurons

grandiosity an overvaluation of one's significance or importance

gray matter brain tissue comprised of the cell bodies of neurons and glia

group therapy a form of therapy that involves the simultaneous treatment of two or more clients and may involve more than one therapist

habit reversal a therapeutic technique in which a client is taught to substitute new behaviors for habitual behaviors such as a tic

hallucination a sensory experience (such as an image, sound, smell, or taste) that seems real but that does not exist outside of the mind

hallucinogen a substance that induces perceptual distortions and heightens sensory awareness

heavy drinking chronic alcohol intake of more than two drinks per day for men and more than one drink per day for women

hemorrhagic stroke a stroke involving leakage of blood into the brain

heredity the genetic transmission of personal characteristics

heterogeneous different or diverse

hippocampus the brain structure involved with the formation, organization, and storing of emotionally relevant memories

histrionic personality disorder characterized by extreme emotionality and attention seeking

hoarding disorder a condition involving congested living conditions due to the accumulation of possessions and distress over the thought of discarding them

homeostasis the ability to maintain internal equilibrium by adjusting physiological processes

hormones regulatory chemicals that influence various physiological activities, such as metabolism, digestion, growth, and mood

humanism a philosophical movement that emphasizes human welfare and the worth and uniqueness of the individual

humanistic perspective the optimistic viewpoint that people are born with the ability to fulfill their potential and that mental distress results from disharmony between a person's potential and self-concept

Huntington disease a genetic disease characterized by involuntary twitching movements and eventual dementia

hypersomnolence (excessive sleepiness) disorder a condition involving difficulty waking up after sleeping and excessive daytime sleepiness or prolonged unrefreshing sleep

hypertension a chronic condition characterized by a systolic blood pressure of 130 mm Hg or higher or a diastolic pressure of 80 mm Hg or higher

hyperthermia significantly elevated body temperature

hypervigilance a state of ongoing anxiety in which the person is constantly tense and alert for threats

hypnotics a class of medications that induce sleep

hypomania a milder form of mania involving increased levels of activity and goal-directed behaviors combined with an elevated, expansive, or irritable mood

hypothalamic-pituitary-adrenal (HPA) axis a system activated under conditions of stress or emotional arousal

hypothalamus the brain structure that regulates bodily drives, such as hunger, thirst, and sexual response, and body conditions, such as body temperature and circadian rhythms

hypothesis a tentative explanation for certain facts or observations

hysteria an outdated term referring to excessive or uncontrollable emotion, sometimes resulting in somatic symptoms (such as blindness or paralysis) that have no apparent physical cause

iatrogenic disorder a condition unintentionally produced by a therapist's actions and treatment strategies

iatrogenic effects unintended effects of an intervention—such as an unintended change in behavior resulting from a medication or a psychological technique used in treatment

illness anxiety disorder persistent health anxiety and/or concern that one has an undetected physical illness, even when the person has only mild or no physical symptoms

implicit bias unconscious assumptions about or stereotyping of members of a specific group

impulsivity a tendency to act quickly without careful thought

incest sexual relations between people too closely related to marry legally

incidence the number of new cases of a disorder that appear in an identified population within a specified time period

independent variable a variable or condition that an experimenter manipulates to determine its effect on a dependent variable

inferiority model an early attempt to explain differences in minority groups that contended racial and ethnic minorities are somehow inferior to the majority population

insanity defense the legal argument used by defendants who admit that they have committed a crime but plead not guilty because they were mentally disturbed at the time of the offense

insomnia disorder chronic difficulty falling asleep or remaining asleep

intellectual developmental disability (IDD) a disorder characterized by limitations in intellectual functioning and adaptive behaviors

intermittent explosive disorder (IED) a condition involving frequent lower-intensity outbursts or low-frequency, high-intensity outbursts of extreme verbal or physical aggression

internalized racism unconscious belief and acceptance of the dominant culture's negative portrayal of one's own racial group

internalizing disorders conditions involving emotional symptoms directed inward

internal validity the degree to which changes in the dependent variable are due solely to the effect of changes in the independent variable

interoceptive conditioning when internal bodily sensations of fear and anxiety that have preceded panic attacks serve as signals for new panic attacks

intoxication a condition involving problem behaviors or psychological changes that occur with excessive substance use

intrapsychic psychological processes occurring within the mind

irresistible impulse test a doctrine that contends that a defendant is not criminally responsible if they lacked the willpower to control their behavior

ischemic stroke a stroke due to reduced blood supply caused by a clot or severe narrowing of the arteries supplying blood to the brain

learned helplessness a learned belief that one is helpless and unable to affect outcomes

learning disorder (LD) an academic disability characterized by reading, writing, or math skills that are substantially below levels that would be expected based on the person's age, intellectual ability, and educational background

least restrictive environment the least restrictive alternative to freedom that is appropriate to a person's condition

lethality the capability of causing death

lifetime prevalence the percentage of people in the population who have had a disorder at some point in their lives

limbic system a group of deep brain structures associated with emotions, decision making, and memory formation

localized amnesia lack of memory for a specific event or events

longitudinal research a research method that involves observing, assessing, or evaluating a group of people over a long period of time

loosening of associations continual shifting from topic to topic without any apparent logical or meaningful connection between thoughts

mainstreaming integrating people with mental illness back into the community

major depressive disorder (MDD) a condition diagnosed if someone (without a history of hypomania/mania) experiences a depressive episode involving severe depressive symptoms that have negatively affected functioning most of the day, nearly every day, for at least 2 full weeks

major depressive episode a period involving severe depressive symptoms that have impaired functioning for at least 2 full weeks

major neurocognitive disorder a condition involving significant decline in independent living skills and in one or more areas of cognitive functioning

male hypoactive sexual desire disorder sexual dysfunction in men that is characterized by a lack of sexual desire

malingering feigning illness for an external purpose

managed health care the industrialization of health care, whereby large organizations in the private sector control the delivery of services

mania a mental state characterized by very exaggerated activity and emotions, including euphoria, excessive excitement, or irritability that result in impairment in social or occupational functioning

MDD with a seasonal pattern major depressive episodes that occur seasonally more than nonseasonally; at least two seasonal episodes of severe depression have occurred and ended at a predictable time of year

medically induced coma a deliberately induced state of deep sedation that allows the brain to rest and heal

mental disorder psychological symptoms or behavioral patterns that reflect an underlying psychobiological dysfunction; are associated with distress or disability; and are not merely an expectable response to common stressors or losses

mental health professional health care practitioners (such as psychologists, psychiatrists, psychiatric nurses, social workers, and mental health counselors) whose services focus on improving mental health or treating mental illness

mental illness a mental health condition that negatively affects a person's emotions, thinking, behavior, relationships with others, or overall functioning

meta-analysis a statistical method in which researchers combine and analyze the results from numerous studies focused on the same or similar phenomena

metabolic syndrome a medical condition associated with obesity, diabetes, high cholesterol, and hypertension

microaggression subtle comments or actions that intentionally or unintentionally insult or invalidate members of socially marginalized groups

migraine headache moderate to severe head pain resulting from abnormal brain activity affecting the cranial blood vessels and nerves

mild neurocognitive disorder a condition involving a modest decline in at least one major cognitive area

mindfulness nonjudgmental awareness of thoughts, feelings, physical sensations, and the environment

mixed features concurrent hypomanic/manic and depressive symptoms

model an analogy used by scientists, usually to describe or explain a phenomenon or process they cannot directly observe

modeling the process of learning by observing models and later imitating them

modeling therapy a treatment procedure involving observation of an unfearful individual successfully interacting with a phobic object or situation

moderate drinking a lower-risk pattern of alcohol intake (no more than one or two drinks per day)

mood an emotional state or prevailing frame of mind

moral treatment movement a crusade to institute more humane treatment for people with mental illness

motivational enhancement therapy a therapeutic approach that addresses ambivalence and helps clients consider the advantages and disadvantages of changing their behavior

motor tic a tic involving physical behaviors such as eye blinking, facial grimacing, or head jerking

multicultural model a contemporary view that emphasizes the importance of considering a person's cultural background and related experiences

multipath model a model that provides an organizational framework for understanding the numerous influences on the development of mental disorders, the complexity of their interacting components, and the need to view disorders from a holistic framework

multiple-baseline study a single-participant experimental design in which baselines on two or more behaviors or the same behavior in two or more settings are obtained prior to intervention

muscle dysmorphia a belief that one's body is too small or insufficiently muscular

myelination the process by which myelin sheaths increase the efficiency of signal transmission between nerve cells

myelin white, fatty material that surrounds and insulates axons

M'Naghten rule a test of legal insanity that inquires whether the accused knew right from wrong when the crime was committed

narcissistic personality disorder characterized by an exaggerated sense of self-importance, an exploitive attitude, and a lack of empathy

negative appraisal interpreting events as threatening

negative reinforcement increasing the frequency or magnitude of a behavior by removing something aversive

negative symptoms symptoms of schizophrenia associated with an inability or decreased ability to initiate actions or speech, express emotions, or feel pleasure

neural circuits a signal-relaying network of interconnected neurons

neural stem cells uncommitted cells that can be stimulated to form new neurons and glia

neurocognitive disorder a disorder that occurs when brain dysfunction affects thinking processes, memory, consciousness, or perception

neurodegeneration declining brain functioning due to progressive loss of brain structure, neurochemical abnormalities, or the death of neurons

neurodevelopmental disorders conditions involving impaired development of the brain and central nervous system that are evident early in a child's life

neurofibrillary tangles twisted fibers of tau protein found inside nerve cells

neurogenesis the birth and growth of new neurons

neuron a nerve cell that transmits messages throughout the body

neuropeptides small molecules that can directly and indirectly influence a variety of hormones and neurotransmitters

neuroplasticity the process by which the brain changes to compensate for injury or to adapt to environmental changes

neurotransmitter any of a group of chemicals that help transmit messages between neurons

nightmare disorder a condition involving frightening dreams that produce awakening

nonbinary a gender identity that is not exclusively masculine or feminine

nonsuicidal self-injury (NSSI) self-harm intended to provide relief from negative feelings or to induce a positive mood state

normal blood pressure the normal amount of force exerted by blood against the artery walls; systolic pressure is less than 120 mm Hg and diastolic pressure is less than 80 mm Hg

obesity a condition involving a body mass index (BMI) greater than 30

observational learning theory the theory that suggests an individual can acquire new behaviors by watching other people perform them

obsession an intrusive, repetitive thought or image that produces anxiety

obsessive-compulsive disorder (OCD) a condition characterized by intrusive, repetitive anxiety-producing thoughts or a strong need to perform acts or dwell on thoughts to reduce anxiety

obsessive-compulsive personality disorder (OCPD) characterized by perfectionism, a tendency to be interpersonally controlling, devotion to details, and rigidity

obstructive sleep apnea (OSA) a breathing-related sleep disorder involving partial or complete upper-airway obstruction

operant behavior voluntary and controllable behavior, such as walking or thinking, that "operates" on an individual's environment

operant conditioning the theory of learning that holds that behaviors are controlled by the consequences that follow them

operational definition a concrete description of the variables that are being studied

opioid a painkilling agent that depresses the central nervous system, such as heroin and prescription pain relievers

oppositional defiant disorder (ODD) a childhood disorder characterized by negativistic, argumentative, and hostile behavior patterns

optimal human functioning qualities such as subjective well-being, optimism, self-determinism, resilience, hope, courage, and ability to manage stress

orbitofrontal cortex the brain region associated with planning and decision making

other specified feeding or eating disorders a seriously disturbed eating pattern that does not fully meet criteria for another eating disorder diagnosis

oxytocin a powerful hormone that affects social bonding

panic attack an episode of intense fear accompanied by symptoms such as a pounding heart, trembling, shortness of breath, and fear of losing control or dying

panic disorder a condition involving recurrent, unexpected panic attacks with apprehension over future attacks or behavioral changes to avoid attacks

paranoid ideation suspiciousness about the actions or motives of others

paranoid personality disorder (PPD) characterized by distrust and suspiciousness regarding the motives of others

paraphilia recurring sexual arousal and gratification by means of mental imagery or behavior involving socially unacceptable objects, situations, or individuals

paraphilic disorder sexual disorder in which the person has either acted on or is severely distressed by recurrent urges or fantasies involving nonhuman objects, non-consenting individuals, or suffering or humiliation

parasomnias sleep abnormalities occurring during sleep or in the sleep–wake transition

Parkinson disease a progressive disorder characterized by poorly controlled motor movements that are sometimes accompanied by cognitive decline and psychiatric symptoms

pediatric bipolar disorder (PBD) a childhood disorder involving depressive and energized episodes similar to the mood swings seen in adult bipolar disorder

pedophilic disorder a disorder in which an adult obtains erotic gratification through urges, acts, or fantasies that involve sexual contact with a prepubescent or early pubescent child

penetrance the proportion of individuals carrying a specific variant of a gene (allele or genotype) who also express the associated trait (phenotype)

persecutory delusions beliefs of being targeted by others

persistent depressive disorder (PDD) a condition involving chronic depressive symptoms that are present most of the day for more days than not during a 2-year period with no more than 2 months symptom-free

personality disorder the presence of pathological personality traits that are relatively inflexible and long-standing and interfere with interpersonal functioning

personality psychopathology dysfunctional and maladaptive personality patterns

personalized medicine the use of a person's genetic profile to guide decisions about prevention and treatment of disease and mental disorders

phenotype observable physical and behavioral characteristics resulting from the interaction between the genotype and the environment

phobia a strong, persistent, and exaggerated fear of a specific object or situation

physiological dependence a state of adaptation that occurs after chronic exposure to a substance; can result in craving and withdrawal symptoms

pituitary gland the gland that stimulates hormones associated with growth, sexual and reproductive development, metabolism, and stress responses

placebo an ineffectual or sham treatment, such as an inactive substance, used as a control in an experimental study

placebo effect improvement produced by expectations of a positive treatment outcome

plaque sticky material (composed of fat, cholesterol, and other substances) that builds up on the walls of veins or arteries

pleasure principle the impulsive, pleasure-seeking aspect of our being, from which the id operates

polymorphic variation a common DNA mutation of a gene

polymorphism a common DNA mutation or variation of a gene

positive psychology the philosophical and scientific study of positive human functioning focused on the strengths and assets of individuals, families, and communities

positive reinforcement desirable actions or rewards that increase the likelihood that a particular behavior will occur

positive symptoms symptoms of schizophrenia that involve unusual thoughts or perceptions, such as delusions, hallucinations, disordered thinking, or atypical behavior

possession the replacement of a person's sense of personal identity with a supernatural spirit or power

posttraumatic stress disorder (PTSD) a condition characterized by flashbacks, hypervigilance, avoidance, and other symptoms that last for more than 1 month and that occur as a result of exposure to extreme trauma

predisposition a susceptibility to certain symptoms or disorders

prefrontal cortex the outer layer of the prefrontal lobe responsible for inhibiting instinctive responses and performing complex cognitive behavior such as managing attention, behavior, and emotions

prefrontal lobotomy a surgical procedure in which the frontal lobes are disconnected from the remainder of the brain

prejudice a biased, preconceived judgment about a person or group based on supposed characteristics of the group

premature (early) ejaculation ejaculation with minimal sexual stimulation before, during, or within 1 minute after penetration

premenstrual dysphoric disorder (PMDD) a condition involving distressing and disruptive symptoms of depression, irritability, and tension that occur the week before menstruation

premorbid before the onset of major symptoms

pressured speech rapid; frenzied; or loud, disjointed communication

prevalence the percentage of individuals in a targeted population who have a particular disorder during a specific period of time

privileged communication a therapist's legal obligation to protect a client's privacy and to prevent the disclosure of confidential communications without the client's permission

prodromal phase early signs of illness have developed but are not sufficiently apparent for diagnosis

prognosis prediction of the probable outcome of a disorder, including the chances of full recovery

projective personality test testing involving responses to ambiguous stimuli, such as inkblots, pictures, or incomplete sentences

prolonged exposure therapy an approach incorporating sustained imaginary and real-life exposure to trauma-related cues

prolonged grief disorder clinically significant grief symptoms over the loss of a loved one that last more than a year for adults and more than 6 months for children and adolescents

protective factors conditions or attributes that lessen or eliminate the risk of a negative psychological or social outcome

provisional diagnosis an initial diagnosis based on currently available information

psychache a term created to describe the unbearable psychological hurt, pain, and anguish associated with suicide

psychiatric epidemiology the study of the prevalence of mental illness in a society

psychoactive substance a substance that alters mood, thought processes, and/or other psychological states

psychoanalysis therapy aimed at helping clients uncover repressed material, achieve insight into inner motivations and desires, and resolve childhood conflicts that affect current relationships

psychodiagnosis assessment and description of an individual's psychological symptoms, including inferences about possible causes for the psychological distress

psychodynamic model a model of psychopathology concerned with unconscious conflicts

psychogenic originating from psychological causes

psychological assessment the process of gathering information and drawing conclusions about an individual's traits, skills, abilities, and emotional functioning

psychological autopsy the systematic examination of existing information after a person's death for the purpose of understanding and explaining the person's behavior before death

psychological flexibility the ability to mentally and emotionally adapt to situational demands

psychological resilience the capacity to effectively adapt to and bounce back from stress, trauma, and other adversities

psychological viewpoint the belief that mental disorders are caused by psychological and emotional factors rather than biological influences

psychopathology the study of the symptoms, causes, and treatments of mental disorders

psychopharmacology the study of the effects of medications on thoughts, emotions, and behaviors

psychophysiological disorder any physical disorder that has a strong psychological basis or component

psychosexual stages in psychodynamic theory, the sequence of stages—oral, anal, phallic, latency, and genital—through which human personality develops

psychosis a condition involving loss of contact with or a distorted view of reality, including disorganized thinking, false beliefs, or seeing or hearing things that are not there

psychotherapy a program of systematic intervention aimed at improving a client's behavioral, emotional, or cognitive symptoms

psychotic symptoms the loss of contact with reality that may involve disorganized thinking, false beliefs, or seeing or hearing things that are not there

psychotropic medications drugs that treat or manage psychiatric symptoms by influencing brain activity associated with emotions and behavior

purge to rid the body of unwanted calories by means such as self-induced vomiting or misuse of laxatives, diuretics, or other medications

racism subtle or direct prejudice, discrimination, or systemic oppression against an individual or group based on their race or ethnicity

rape a form of sexual aggression that involves sexual activity (oral–genital sex, anal intercourse, or vaginal intercourse) performed without a person's consent through the use of force, argument, pressure, alcohol or drugs, or authority

rape trauma syndrome a two-phase syndrome that rape survivors may experience, involving such emotional reactions as psychological distress, phobic reactions, and sexual dysfunction

rapid cycling the occurrence of four or more mood episodes per year

reactive attachment disorder (RAD) a trauma-related disorder characterized by inhibited, avoidant social behaviors and reluctance to seek or respond to attention or nurturing

reality principle an awareness of the demands of the environment and of the need to adjust behavior to meet these demands, from which the ego operates

reappraisal minimizing negative responses by looking at a situation from various perspectives

recovery movement the perspective that with appropriate treatment and support those with mental illness can improve and live satisfying lives despite any lingering symptoms of illness

reinforcer anything that increases the frequency or magnitude of a behavior

relapse a return to drug or alcohol use after a period of abstinence

relaxation training a therapeutic technique in which a person acquires the ability to relax the muscles of the body in almost any circumstance

reliability the degree to which a measure or procedure yields the same results repeatedly

remission a significant improvement in the symptoms of a disorder

remit diminish or disappear

REM sleep behavior disorder a condition involving dream-related vocalizations and motor behavior that occur during REM sleep

repressed memory a memory of a traumatic event has been repressed and is, therefore, unavailable for recall

resilience the ability to recover from stress or adversity

resistance during psychoanalysis, a process in which the client unconsciously attempts to impede the analysis by preventing the exposure of repressed material

response prevention a treatment in which an individual is prevented from performing a compulsive behavior

restricted affect severely diminished or limited emotional responsiveness

reuptake the reabsorption of a neurotransmitter after an impulse has been transmitted across the synapse

right to treatment the concept that people with mental illness who have been involuntarily committed have a right to receive therapy for their condition

rumination repeatedly thinking about concerns or details of past events

schema a mental framework for organizing and interpreting information

schizoaffective disorder a condition involving the existence of symptoms of schizophrenia and either major depressive or manic symptoms

schizoid personality disorder characterized by detachment from social relationships and limited emotional expression

schizophrenia a disorder characterized by severely impaired cognitive processes, disordered thinking and behaviors, and social withdrawal

schizophrenia spectrum a group of disorders that range in severity and that have similar clinical features, including some degree of reality distortion

schizophreniform disorder psychotic episodes with a duration of at least 1 month but less than 6 months

schizotypal personality disorder characterized by peculiar thoughts and behaviors and by poor interpersonal relationships

scientific method a method of inquiry that provides for the systematic collection of data, controlled observation, and the testing of hypotheses

sedatives a class of drugs that have a calming or sedating effect

selective amnesia an inability to remember certain details of an event

selective mutism consistent failure to speak in certain situations

self-actualization an inherent tendency to strive toward the realization of one's full potential

self-efficacy a belief in one's ability to succeed

self-schema a stable set of beliefs and assumptions about the self that are based on the person's experiences, values, and perceived capabilities

self-stigma acceptance of prejudice and discrimination based on internalized negative societal beliefs or stereotypes

separation anxiety disorder severe distress about leaving home, being alone, or being separated from a parent

serotonin a neurotransmitter associated with mood, sleep, appetite, and impulsive behavior

sexual dysfunction a disruption of any part of the normal sexual response cycle that affects sexual desire, arousal, or response

sexual masochism disorder sexual urges, fantasies, or acts that involve being humiliated, bound, or made to suffer

sexual orientation sexual identity involving the gender to which a person is physically and emotionally attracted

sexual sadism disorder sexual urges, fantasies, or acts that involve inflicting physical or psychological suffering on others

single-blind design an experimental design in which only the participants are unaware of the purpose of the research

single-participant experiment an experiment performed on a single individual in which some aspect of the person's behavior is used as a control or baseline for comparison with future behaviors

sleep inertia significant grogginess and impaired alertness after sleeping or napping

sleep terrors episodes of intense fear that occur during deep sleep

social anxiety disorder (SAD) an intense fear of being scrutinized in social or performance situations

social stigma a negative societal belief about a group, including the view that the group is somehow different from other members of society

sociocultural influences factors such as gender, sexual orientation, spirituality, religion, socioeconomic status, race/ethnicity, and culture that can exert an effect on mental health

somatic symptom and related disorders a broad grouping of psychological disorders that involve physical symptoms or anxiety over illness, including somatic symptom disorder, illness anxiety disorder, functional neurological symptom disorder, and factitious disorder

somatic symptom disorder (SSD) a condition involving a pattern of distressing thoughts regarding the seriousness of one's physical symptoms combined with excessive time and concern devoted to worrying about these symptoms

somatic symptom disorder with predominant pain a condition involving excessive anxiety or persistent concerns over severe or lingering pain

somatic symptoms physical or bodily symptoms

specific phobia an extreme fear of a specific object (such as snakes) or situation (such as being in an enclosed place)

specifier specific features associated with a diagnostic category

spirituality the belief in an animating life force or energy beyond what we can perceive with our senses

standardization sample the comparison group on which test norms are based

standardization the use of identical procedures in the administration of tests

statistical significance the likelihood that a research finding is not due to chance alone

stereotype an oversimplified, often inaccurate, image or idea about a group of people

stimulant a substance that energizes the central nervous system

stressor a difficult life circumstance or event that places a physical or psychological demand on a person

stress the internal psychological or physiological response to a stressor

striatum the region within the basal ganglia associated with movement planning, goal-directed action, memory, and decision making

stroke a sudden halting of blood flow to a portion of the brain, leading to brain damage

structural imaging procedures that allow for visualization of brain anatomy

substance-use disorder a condition in which cognitive, behavioral, and physiological symptoms contribute to the continued use of alcohol or drugs despite significant substance-related problems

substance abuse a pattern of excessive or harmful use of any substance for mood-altering purposes

subtype mutually exclusive subgrouping within a diagnosis

suicidal ideation thoughts about suicide

suicide the intentional, direct, and conscious taking of one's own life

suicidologist a professional who studies the manifestation, dynamics, and prevention of suicide

sympathetic nervous system the part of the nervous system that automatically performs functions such as increasing heart rate, constricting blood vessels, and raising blood pressure

synapse a tiny gap that exists between the axon of the sending neuron and the dendrites of the receiving neuron

syndrome certain symptoms that tend to occur regularly in clusters

synergistic effect the result of chemicals (or substances) interacting to multiply one another's effects

systematic desensitization a treatment technique involving repeated exposure to a feared stimulus while a client is in a competing emotional or physiological state such as relaxation

systematized amnesia loss of memory for certain categories of information

systemic racism deeply imbedded societal policies and structures that disadvantage certain racial groups

systolic pressure the force on blood vessels when the heart contracts

tarantism a form of mass hysteria prevalent during the Middle Ages; characterized by wild raving, jumping, dancing, and convulsing

Tarasoff **ruling** a California Supreme Court decision that obligates mental health professionals to break confidentiality when their clients pose a clear and imminent danger to another person

temperament innate mental, physical, and emotional traits

tension headache head pain produced by prolonged contraction of the scalp and neck muscles, resulting in constriction of the blood vessels and steady pain

theory a group of principles and hypotheses that together explain some aspect of a particular area of inquiry

theory of mind the ability to recognize that others have emotions, beliefs, and desires that may be different from one's own

tic an involuntary, repetitive movement or vocalization

tolerance decreases in the effects of a substance that occur after chronic use

Tourette disorder a condition characterized by multiple motor tics and one or more vocal tics

trait a distinguishing quality or characteristic of a person, including a tendency to feel, perceive, behave, or think in a relatively consistent manner

transference the process by which a client undergoing psychoanalysis reenacts early conflicts by applying to the analyst feelings and attitudes that the person has toward significant others

transgender a person's innate psychological gender identification does not correspond with the person's sex assigned at birth

transient ischemic attack (TIA) a "mini-stroke" resulting from temporary blockage of arteries

transvestic disorder intense sexual arousal obtained through cross-dressing (wearing clothes appropriate to a different gender)

trauma-focused cognitive-behavioral therapy a therapeutic approach that helps clients identify and challenge dysfunctional cognitions about a traumatic event

traumatic brain injury (TBI) a physical wound or internal injury to the brain

treatment-resistant depression a depressive episode that has not improved despite an adequate trial of antidepressant medication or other traditional forms of treatment

treatment plan a proposed course of therapy, developed collaboratively by a therapist and client, that addresses the client's most distressing mental health symptoms

trephining a surgical method from the Stone Age in which part of the skull was chipped away to provide an opening through which an evil spirit could escape

trichotillomania recurrent and compulsive hair pulling that results in hair loss and causes significant distress

unconditioned response (UCR) in classical conditioning, the unlearned response made to an unconditioned stimulus

unconditioned stimulus (UCS) in classical conditioning, the stimulus that elicits an unconditioned response

universal shamanic tradition the set of beliefs and practices from non-Western Indigenous traditions that assume that special healers are blessed with powers to act as messengers between the human and spirit worlds

vaginismus involuntary spasms of the outer third of the vaginal wall that prevents or interferes with *sexual interco*urse

vagus nerve a nerve that creates a mind–body pathway from the brain through the digestive tract to the abdomen; regulates autonomic nervous system processes and body reactivity

validity the extent to which a test or procedure actually measures what it was designed to measure

vascular dementia progressive mental deterioration associated with impaired blood flow to the brain

vascular neurocognitive disorder a condition involving cognitive impairment due to reduced blood flow to the brain

vocal tic an audible tic such as coughing, grunting, throat clearing, sniffling, or making sudden, vocal outbursts

voyeuristic disorder urges, acts, or fantasies that involve observing an unsuspecting person disrobing or engaging in sexual activity

white matter brain tissue comprised of myelinated nerve pathways

withdrawal the adverse physical and psychological symptoms that occur after reducing or ceasing intake of a substance

References

Aas, M., Etain, B., Bellivier, F., Henry, C., Lagerberg, T., Ringen, A., . . . Melle, I. (2014). Additive effects of childhood abuse and cannabis abuse on clinical expressions of bipolar disorders. *Psychological Medicine, 44*(8), 1653–1662.

ABC. (2018). Where is Andrea Yates now? A peek inside her life in a state mental hospital. https://abc13.com/1980992/

Abdalla-Filho, E., & Völlm, B. (2020). Does every psychopath have an antisocial personality disorder? *Revista Brasileira de Psiquiatria (Sao Paulo, Brazil: 1999), 42*(3), 241–242. https://doi.org/10.1590/1516-4446-2019-0762

Abdel-Hamid, I. A., & Ali, O. I. (2018). Delayed ejaculation: Pathophysiology, diagnosis, and treatment. *World Journal of Men's Health, 36,* 22–40.

Abdurrachid, N., & Gama Marques, J. (2022). Munchausen syndrome by proxy (MSBP): A review regarding perpetrators of factitious disorder imposed on another (FDIA). *CNS Spectrums, 27*(1), 16–26.

Abouzaid, S., Tian, H., Zhou, H., Kahler, K. H., Harris, M., & Kim, E. (2014). Economic burden associated with extrapyramidal symptoms in a Medicaid population with schizophrenia. *Community Mental Health Journal, 50,* 51–58.

Abram, K. M., Azores-Gococo, N. M., Emanuel, K. M., Aaby, D. A., Welty, L. J., Hershfield, J. A., . . . Teplin, L. A. (2017). Sex and racial/ethnic differences in positive outcomes in delinquent youth after detention: A 12-year longitudinal study. *JAMA Pediatrics, 171*(2), 123–132.

Accordini, S., Calcian, L., Johannessen, A., Portas, L., Benediktsdóttir, B., Bertelsen, R. J., . . . Ageing Lungs in European Cohorts (ALEC) Study. (2018). A three-generation study on the association of tobacco smoking with asthma. *International Journal of Epidemiology, 47*(4), 1106–1117.

Acevedo, N. (2018). Suicide rates spike in Puerto Rico, five months after Maria. https://www.nbcnews.com/storyline/puerto-rico-crisis/suicide-rates-spike-puerto-rico-five-months-after-maria-n849666

Achilles, M. R., Anderson, M., Li, S. H., Subotic-Kerry, M., Parker, B., & O'Dea, B. (2020). Adherence to e-mental health among youth: Considerations for intervention development and research design. *Digital Health, 6,* 2055207620926064. https://doi.org/10.1177/2055207620926064

Achtyes, E., Simmons, A., Skabeev, A., Levy, N., Jiang, Y., Marcy, P., & Weiden, P. J. (2018). Patient preferences concerning the efficacy and side-effect profile of schizophrenia medications: A survey of patients living with schizophrenia. *BMC Psychiatry, 18*(1), 292.

Acosta, J. R., Librenza-Garcia, D., Watts, D., Francisco, A. P., Zórtea, F., Raffa, B., . . . Passos, I. C. (2020). Bullying and psychotic symptoms in youth with bipolar disorder. *Journal of Affective Disorders, 265,* 603–610.

Adams, L. B., Gottfredson, N., Lightfoot, A. F., Corbie-Smith, G., Golin, C., & Powell, W. (2019). Factor analysis of the CES-D 12 among a community sample of black men. *American Journal of Men's Health, 13*(2), 1557988319834105. https://doi.org/10.1177/1557988319834105

Adigun, M., Liu, L., & Vashi, P. (2015). Pharmacologic management of acute and chronic panic disorder. *US Pharmacist, 40*(11), 24–30.

Adigun, T. (2022). Young women are subtly flaunting their abs and protruding hip bones on social media: Why body checking is the latest dangerous trend to look out for. https://news.yahoo.com/what-is-body-checking-trend-140008310.html

Adler, A. (1929/1964). *Social interest: A challenge to mankind.* New York: Capricorn Books.

Adriaanse, M., van Domburgh, L., Hoek, H. W., Susser, E., Doreleijers, T. A., & Veling, W. (2015). Prevalence, impact and cultural context of psychotic experiences among ethnic minority youth. *Psychological Medicine, 45*(3), 637–646.

Afzal, S., Tybjaerg-Hansen, A., Jensen, G. B., & Nordestgaard, B. G. (2016). Change in body mass index associated with lowest mortality in Denmark, 1976–2013. *JAMA, 315*(18), 1989–1996.

Agabio, R., Pisanu, C., Gessa, G. L., & Franconi, F. (2017). Sex differences in alcohol use disorder. *Current Medicinal Chemistry, 24*(24), 2661–2670.

Agam-Bitton, R., Abu Ahmad, W., & Golan, M. (2018). Girls-only vs. mixed-gender groups in the delivery of a universal wellness programme among adolescents: A cluster-randomized controlled trial. *PLOS One, 13*(6), e0198872. https://doi.org/10.1371/journal.pone.0198872

Aghaei, M., Ghorbani, N., Rostami, R., & Mahdavi, A. (2015). Comparison of anger management, anxiety and perceived stress in patients with cancer and coronary heart disease (CHD). *Journal of Medicine and Life, 8*(4), 97–101.

Agimi, Y., Marion, D., Schwab, K., & Stout, K. (2021). Estimates of long-term disability among US service members with traumatic brain injuries. *The Journal of Head Trauma Rehabilitation, 36*(1), 1–9. https://doi.org/10.1097/HTR.0000000000000573

Ahlers, C. J., Schaefer, G. A., Mundt, I. A., Roll, S., Englert, H., Willich, S. N., & Beier, K. M. (2011). How unusual are the contents of paraphilias? Paraphilia-associated sexual arousal patterns in a community-based sample of men. *Journal of Sexual Medicine, 8*, 1362–1370.

Ahlich, E., Choquette, E. M., & Rancourt, D. (2019). Body talk, athletic identity, and eating disorder symptoms in men. *Psychology of Men and Masculinities, 20*(3), 347–355.

Ahmed, I., Cook, T., Genen, L., & Schwartz, R. A. (2014). Body dysmorphic disorder. http://emedicine.medscape.com/article/291182-overview#aw2aab6b2b3

Åhs, F., Rosén, J., Kastrati, G., Fredrikson, M., Agren, T., & Lundström, J. N. (2018). Biological preparedness and resistance to extinction of skin conductance responses conditioned to fear relevant animal pictures: A systematic review. *Neuroscience and Biobehavioral Reviews, 95*, 430–437.

Akbar, M., Egli, M., Cho, Y. E., Song, B. J., & Noronha, A. (2018). Medications for alcohol use disorders: An overview. *Pharmacology and Therapeutics, 185*, 64–85.

Akinaga, M. (2013). Japanese Actroid robots—Latest human robots. http://wordsinjapanese.com/japaneseactroid-robot-latest-human-robots.php

Akinhanmi, M. O., Biernacka, J. M., Strakowski, S. M., McElroy, S. L., Balls Berry, J. E., Merikangas, K. R., . . . Frye, M. A. (2018). Racial disparities in bipolar disorder treatment and research: A call to action. *Bipolar Disorders, 20*(6), 506–514.

Alam, R., Abdolmaleky, H. M., & Zhou, J. R. (2017). Microbiome, inflammation, epigenetic alterations, and mental diseases. *American Journal of Medical Genetics, 174*(6), 651–660.

Al Saif, F., & Al Khalili, Y. (2020). *Shared psychotic disorder.* StatPearls Publishing.

Albert, M. A., Glynn, R. G., & Buring, J. (2010, November 15). Women with high job strain have 40 percent increased risk of heart disease. Presented at the Annual Meetings of the American Heart Association, Chicago.

Albuquerque, J., & Tulk, S. (2019). Physician suicide. *Canadian Medical Association Journal, 191*(18), E505. https://doi.org/10.1503/cmaj.181687

Alcantara, C., & Gone, J. P. (2014). Multicultural issues in the clinical interview and diagnostic process. In F. T. L. Leong, L. Comas-Diaz, G. C. Nagayama Hall, V. C. McLoyd, & J. E. Trimble (Eds.), *APA handbook of multicultural psychology. Vol. 2: Applications and training* (pp. 153–163). Washington, DC: APA.

Alduhishy, M. (2018). The overprescription of antidepressants and its impact on the elderly in Australia. *Trends in Psychiatry and Psychotherapy, 40*(3), 241–243.

Aleaziz, H. (2020). The government's own experts say separating immigrant families during the coronavirus pandemic will add to their mental trauma. https://www.buzzfeednews.com/article/hamedaleaziz/government-experts-opppose-separating-immigrant-families

Alegria, A. A., Blanco, C., Petry, N. M., Skodol, A. E., Liu, S. M., Grant, B., & Hasin, D. (2013). Sex differences in antisocial personality disorder: Results from the National Epidemiological Survey on Alcohol and Related Conditions. *Personality Disorders, 4*, 214–222.

Alegría, M., Fortuna, L. R., Lin, J. Y., Norris, F. H., Gao, S., Takeuchi, D. T., . . . Valentine, A. (2013). Prevalence, risk, and correlates of posttraumatic stress disorder across ethnic and racial minority groups in the United States. *Medical Care, 51*(12), 1114–1123.

Alexander, F. G., & Selesnick, S. T. (1966). *The history of psychiatry.* New York: Harper & Row.

Algoe, S. B., & Fredrickson, B. L. (2011). Emotional fitness and the movement of affective science from lab to field. *American Psychologist, 66*, 35–42.

Alif, A., Nelson, B. S., Stefancic, A., Ahmed, R., & Okazaki, S. (2020).

Documentation status and psychological distress among New York City community college students. *Cultural Diversity and Ethnic Minority Psychology, 26*(1), 11–21.

Allen, A. M., Wang, Y., Chae, D. H., Price, M. M., Powell, W., Steed, T. C., . . . Woods-Giscombe, C. L. (2019). Racial discrimination, the superwoman schema, and allostatic load: Exploring an integrative stress-coping model among African American women. *Annals of the New York Academy of Sciences, 1457*(1), 104–127.

Allen, J., Rasmus, S. M., Fok, C., Charles, B., Henry, D., & Qungasvik Team. (2018). Multi-level cultural intervention for the prevention of suicide and alcohol use risk with Alaska native youth: A nonrandomized comparison of treatment intensity. *Prevention Science, 19*(2), 174–185.

Allen, S. (2016). Dr. Drew leads the Hillary Clinton health truthers. *The Daily Beast.* http://www.thedailybeast.com/articles/2016/08/18/dr-drew-leads-the-clinton-health-truthers.html

Alloy, L. B., Olino, T., Freed, R. D., & Nusslock, R. (2016). Role of reward sensitivity and processing in major depressive and bipolar spectrum disorders. *Behavior Therapy, 47*(5), 600–621.

Allport, L., Song, M., Leung, C. W., McGlumphy, K. C., & Hasson, R. E. (2019). Influence of parent stressors on adolescent obesity in African American youth. *Journal of Obesity, 1316765.* https://doi.org/10.1155/2019/1316765

Almazan, A. N., & Keuroghlian, A. S. (2021). Association between gender-affirming surgeries and mental health outcomes. *JAMA Surgery, 156*(7), 611–618.

Alnæs, D., Kaufmann, T., van der Meer, D., Córdova-Palomera, A., Rokicki, J., Moberget, T., . . . Karolinska Schizophrenia Project Consortium. (2019). Brain heterogeneity in schizophrenia and its association with polygenic risk. *JAMA Psychiatry, 76*(7), 739–748.

Aloi, M., Rania, M., Carbone, E. A., Calabrò, G., Caroleo, M., Carcione, A., . . . Segura-Garcia, C. (2020). The role of self-monitoring metacognition sub-function and negative urgency related to binge severity. *European Eating Disorders Review, 28*(5), 580–586. https://doi.org/10.1002/erv.2742

Alonso, J., Serrano-Blanco, A., & Forero, C. G. (2019). Translational research in psychiatry: The Research Domain Criteria Project (RDoC). Investigación traslacional en psiquiatría: el marco Research Domain Criteria (RDoC). *Revista de Psiquiatria y Salud Mental, 12*(3), 187–195. https://doi.org/10.1016/j.rpsm.2018.04.002

Alonzo, R., Hussain, J., Stranges, S., & Anderson, K. K. (2021). Interplay between social media use, sleep quality, and mental health in youth: A systematic review. *Sleep Medicine Reviews, 56*, 101414. https://doi.org/10.1016/j.smrv.2020.101414

Altenburger, L. E., Carotta, C. L., Bonomi, A. E., & Synder, A. (2017). Sexist attitudes among emerging adult women readers of fifty shades fiction. *Archives of Sexual Behavior, 46*(2), 455–464.

Alvarez-Jimenez, M., O'Donoghue, B., Thompson, A., Gleeson, J. F., Bendall, S., Gonzalez-Blanch, C., . . . McGorry, P. D. (2016). Beyond clinical remission in first episode psychosis: Thoughts on antipsychotic maintenance vs. guided discontinuation in the functional recovery era. *CNS Drugs, 30*(5), 357–368.

Álvarez-Tomás, I., Ruiz, J., Guilera, G., & Bados, A. (2019). Long-term clinical and functional course of borderline personality disorder: A meta-analysis of prospective studies. *European Psychiatry, 56*, 75–83.

Alves, N. D., Correia, J. S., Patrício, P., Mateus-Pinheiro, A., Machado-Santos, A. R., Loureiro-Campos, E., . . . Pinto, L. (2017). Adult hippocampal neuroplasticity triggers susceptibility to recurrent depression. *Translational Psychiatry, 7*(3), e1058. https://doi.org/10.1038/tp.2017.29

Alvy, L. M. (2013). Do lesbian women have a better body image? Comparisons with heterosexual women and model of lesbian-specific factors. *Body Image, 11*, 524–534.

Alzheimer's Association. (2023a). Alzheimer's disease facts and figures. *Alzheimer's & Dementia: The Journal of the Alzheimer's Association, 19*(4), 1598–1695. https://doi.org/10.1002/alz.13016

Alzheimer's Association. (2023b). Navigating treatment options. https://www.alz.org/alzheimers-dementia/treatments

Alzheimer's Association. (2023c). Types of dementia. https://www.alz.org/alzheimers-dementia/what-is-dementia/types-of-dementia/

Alzheimer's Disease International. (2023). Dementia statistics. https://www.alzint.org/about/dementia-facts-figures/dementia-statistics/

Alzheimer's Research Association. (2023). Alzheimer's. https://www.alzra.org/alzheimers/facts-and-figures

Amadeo, K. (2020). Deinstitutionalization, its causes, effects, pros and cons. https://www.thebalance.com/deinstitutionalization-3306067

Amador, X. (2006). Percentage of patients with schizophrenia who were unaware of these signs and symptoms of their illness. http://mentalillnesspolicy.org/medical/lack-of-insight-schizophrenia.pdf

Amaducci, A., Aldy, K., Campleman, S. L., Li, S., Meyn, A., Abston, S., . . . Toxicology Investigators Consortium Fentalog Study Group (2023). Naloxone use in novel potent opioid and fentanyl overdoses in emergency department patients. *JAMA Network Open, 6*(8), e2331264. https://doi.org/10.1001/jamanetworkopen.2023.31264

American Academy of Neurology. (2020). AAN position: Sports concussion. https://www.aan.com/policy-and-guidelines/policy/position-statements/sports-concussion/

American Association on Intellectual and Developmental Disabilities. (2020). FAQ on intellectual disability. https://www.aaidd.org/intellectual-disability/definition/faqs-on-intellectual-disability

American College Health Association (ACHA). (2019). *National College Health Assessment II: Reference group executive summary spring 2019.* Silver Spring, MD: Author.

American College Health Association (ACHA). (2021). *National College Health Assessment III, fall 2021.* Silver Spring, MD: Author.

American College Health Association (ACHA). (2022). *National College Health Assessment III: Reference group executive summary fall 2021.* Silver Spring, MD: Author.

American Foundation for Suicide Prevention. (2020). Suicide statistics. https://afsp.org/about-suicide/suicide-statistics/

American Parkinson Disease Association. (2023). New laboratory tests for Parkinson's disease. https://www.apdaparkinson.org/article/new-laboratory-tests-for-parkinsons-disease/

American Psychiatric Association. (2022). *Diagnostic and statistical manual of mental disorders* (5th ed., text rev.). https://doi.org/10.1176/appi.books.9780890425787

American Psychological Association. (2003). Guidelines on multicultural education, training, research, practice, and organizational change for psychologists. *American Psychologist, 58*, 377–402.

American Psychological Association. (2015). Guidelines for psychological practice with transgender and gender nonconforming people. *American Psychologist, 70*, 832–864.

American Psychological Association. (2017a). APA ethical principles of psychologists and code of conduct. https://www.apa.org/ethics/code/

American Psychological Association. (2017b). Multicultural guidelines: An ecological approach to context, identity, and intersectionality. http://www.apa.org/about/policy/multicultural-guidelines.pdf

American Psychological Association. (2018). APA guidelines for psychological practice with girls and women. http://www.apa.org/about/policy/psychological-practice-girls-women.pdf

American Psychological Association. (2019). APA statement on proposal that federal government use technology to predict who will become violent. https://www.apa.org/news/press/releases/2019/09/technology-violence-prevention

American Psychological Association. (2020a). Gender and stress. https://www.apa.org/news/press/releases/stress/2010/gender-stress

American Psychological Association. (2020b). Stress in America 2020: Stress in the time of COVID-19, volume one. https://www.apa.org/news/press/releases/stress/2020/report#

American Psychological Association. (2020c). Stress in America 2020: Stress in the time of COVID-19, volume two. https://www.apa.org/news/press/releases/stress/2020/infographics-june

American Psychological Association. (2022). APA president condemns Texas governor's directive to report parents of transgender minors. https://www.apa.org/news/press/releases/2022/02/report-parents-transgender-children

American Stroke Association. (2023). About stroke. https://www.stroke.org/en/about-stroke/

Amir, L., Voracek, M., Yousef, S., Galadari, A., Yammahi, S., Sadeghi, M.-R., . . . Dervic, K. (2013). Suicidal behavior and attitudes among medical students in the United Arab Emirates. *Crisis, 34*, 116–123.

Andersen, C. H. (2020). 12 Celebs airbrushed to look bigger and less muscular. https://www.shape.com/celebrities/celebrity-photos/12-celebs-airbrushed-look-bigger-and-less-muscular

Anderson, D., Laforge, J., Ross, M. M., Vanlangendonck, R., Hasoon, J., Viswanath, O., . . . & Urits, I. (2022). Male sexual dysfunction. *Health Psychology Research, 10*(3), 37533. https://doi.org/10.52965/001c.37533

Anderson, K. N., & Bradley, A. J. (2013). Sleep disturbance in mental health problems and neurodegenerative disease. *Nature and Science of Sleep, 5*, 61–75.

Anderson, K. N., Swedo, E. A., Trinh, E., Ray, C. M., Krause, K. H., Verlenden, J. V., . . . Holditch Niolon, P. (2022). Adverse childhood experiences during the COVID-19 pandemic and associations with poor mental health and suicidal behaviors among high school students: Adolescent Behaviors and Experiences Survey. United States, January–June 2021. *MMWR: Morbidity and Mortality Weekly Report, 71*(41), 1301–1305. https://doi.org/10.15585/mmwr.mm7141a2

Anderson, K. W., Taylor, S., & McLean, P. H. (1996). Panic disorder associated with blood-injury reactivity: The necessity of establishing functional relationships among maladaptive behaviors. *Behavior Therapy, 27*, 463–472.

Anderson, P. (2018). Physicians experience highest suicide rate of any profession. https://www.medscape.com/viewarticle/896257

Anderson, S. E., Gooze, R. A., Lemeshow, S., & Whitaker, R. C. (2012). Quality of early maternal-child relationship and risk of adolescent obesity. *Pediatrics, 129*, 132–140.

Andrews, G., Cuijpers, P., Craske, M. G., McEvoy, P., & Titov, N. (2010). Computer therapy for the anxiety and depressive disorders is effective, acceptable and practical health care: A meta-analysis. *PLOS One, 5*, e13196.

Anglin, D. M., Ereshefsky, S., Klaunig, M. J., Bridgwater, M. A., Niendam, T. A., Ellman, L. M., . . . van der Ven, E. (2021). From womb to neighborhood: A racial analysis of social determinants of psychosis in the United States. *The American Journal of Psychiatry, 178*(7), 599–610.

Ani, C., Reading, R., Lynn, R., Forlee, S., & Garralda, E. (2013). Incidence and 12-month outcome of non-transient childhood conversion disorder in the U.K. and Ireland. *British Journal of Psychiatry, 202*, 413–418.

Anorexia Nervosa and Associated Disorders. (2014). Eating disorder statistics. http://www.anad.org/get-information/about-eating-disorders/eating-disorders-statistics

Antonsen, A. N., Zdaniuk, B., Yule, M., & Brotto, L. A. (2020). Ace and aro: Understanding differences in romantic attractions among persons identifying as asexual. *Archives of Sexual Behavior.* https://doi-org.ezproxy.library.wwu.edu/10.1007/s10508-019-01600-1

Antypa, N., Serretti, A., & Rujescu, D. (2013). Serotonergic genes and suicide: A systematic review. *European Neuropsychopharmacology, 23*, 1125–1142.

Anupama, M., Gangadhar, K. H., Shetty, V. B., & Dip, P. B. (2016). Transvestism as a symptom: A case series. *Indian Journal of Psychological Medicine, 38*, 78–80.

Anxiety and Depression Association of America. (2020). Screening for obsessive-compulsive disorder (OCD). https://adaa.org/screening-obsessive-compulsive-disorder-ocd

APA Presidential Task Force on Evidence-Based Practice. (2006). Evidence-based practice in psychology. *American Psychologist, 61*, 271–285.

Aparicio-Martinez, P., Perea-Moreno, A. J., Martinez-Jimenez, M. P., Redel-Macías, M. D., Pagliari, C., & Vaquero-Abellan, M. (2019). Social media, thin-ideal, body dissatisfaction and disordered eating attitudes: An exploratory analysis. *International Journal of Environmental Research and Public Health, 16*(21), 4177. https://doi.org/10.3390/ijerph16214177

Apostolou, M., & Khalil, M. (2019). Aggressive and humiliating sexual play: Occurrence rates and discordance between the sexes. *Archives of Sexual Behavior, 48*, 2187–2200.

Apthorp, D., Bolbecker, A. R., Bartolomeo, L. A., O'Donnell, B. F., & Hetrick, W. P. (2019). Postural sway abnormalities in schizotypal personality disorder. *Schizophrenia Bulletin, 45*(3), 512–521.

Aquila, I., Sacco, M. A., Gratteri, S., Sirianni, M., De Fazio, P., & Ricci, P. (2018). The "social-mobile autopsy": The evolution of psychological autopsy with new technologies in forensic investigations on suicide. *Legal Medicine, 32*, 79–82.

Arcelus, J., Haslam, M., Farrow, C., & Meyer, C. (2013). The role of interpersonal functioning in the maintenance of eating psychopathology: A systematic review and testable model. *Clinical Psychology Review, 33*, 156–167.

Ardakani, A., Monroe-Lord, L., Wakefield, D., & Castor, C. (2023). Parenting styles, food parenting practices, family meals, and weight status of African American families. *International Journal of Environmental Research and Public Health, 20*(2), 1382. https://doi.org/10.3390/ijerph20021382

Arditte Hall, K. A., Quinn, M. E., Vanderlind, W. M., & Joormann, J. (2019). Comparing cognitive styles in social anxiety and major depressive disorders: An examination of rumination, worry, and reappraisal. *The British Journal of Clinical Psychology, 58*(2), 231–244.

Arkin, D. (2018). News coverage of high-profile suicides sparks debate about journalism ethics. https://www.nbcnews.com/news/us-news/news-coverage-high-profile-suicides-sparks-debate-about-journalism-ethics-n881566

Arns, M., Loo, S. K., Sterman, M. B., Heinrich, H., Kuntsi, J., Asherson, P., . . . Brandeis, D. (2016). Editorial perspective: How should child psychologists and psychiatrists interpret FDA device approval? Caveat emptor. *Journal of Child Psychology and Psychiatry, and Allied Disciplines, 57*(5), 656–658.

Aroke, E. N., Joseph, P. V., Roy, A., Overstreet, D. S., Tollefsbol, T. O., Vance, D. E., & Goodin, B. R. (2019). Could epigenetics help explain racial disparities in chronic pain? *Journal of Pain Research, 12*, 701–710.

Aron, N. R. (2017). The murder of this 20-year-old Berkeley coed changed the laws around psychology forever. https://timeline.com/tanya-tarasoff-notify-law-7d43951cb004

Arseneault, L., Cannon, M., Fisher, H. L., Polanczyk, G., Moffitt, T. E., & Caspi, A. (2011). Childhood trauma and children's emerging psychotic symptoms: A genetically sensitive longitudinal cohort study. *American Journal of Psychiatry, 168*, 65–72.

Arya, D., Khan, T., Margolius, A. J., & Fernandez, H. H. (2019). Tardive dyskinesia: Treatment update. *Current Neurology and Neuroscience Reports, 19*(9), 69. https://doi.org/10.1007/s11910-019-0976-1

Asarnow, J. R., Hughes, J. L., Babeva, K. N., & Sugar, C. A. (2017). Cognitive-behavioral family treatment for suicide attempt prevention: A randomized controlled trial. *Journal of the American Academy of Child and Adolescent Psychiatry, 56*(6), 506–514.

Asarnow, L. D., & Manber, R. (2019). Cognitive behavioral therapy for insomnia in depression. *Sleep Medicine Clinics, 14*(2), 177–184.

Ashina, S., Mitsikostas, D. D., Lee, M. J., Yamani, N., Wang, S. J., Messina, R., . . . Lipton, R. B. (2021). Tension-type headache. *Nature Reviews: Disease Primers, 7*(1), 24. https://doi.org/10.1038/s41572-021-00257-2

Askarova, S., Umbayev, B., Masoud, A. R., Kaiyrlykyzy, A., Safarova, Y., Tsoy, A., . . . Kushugulova, A. (2020). The links between the gut microbiome, aging, modern lifestyle and Alzheimer's disease. *Frontiers in Cellular and Infection Microbiology, 10*, 104. https://doi.org/10.3389/fcimb.2020.00104

Askew, A. J., Peterson, C. B., Crow, S. J., Mitchell, J. E., Halmi, K. A., Agras, W. S., & Haynos, A. F. (2020). Not all body image constructs are created equal: Predicting eating disorder outcomes from preoccupation, dissatisfaction, and overvaluation. *The International Journal of Eating Disorders, 53*(6), 954–963. https://doi.org/10.1002/eat.23277

Asmundson, G. J. G., & Taylor, S. (2020). How health anxiety influences responses to viral outbreaks like COVID-19: What all decision makers, health authorities, and health care professionals need to know. *Journal of Anxiety Disorder, 71*, 1–2.

Associated Press. (1998, August 14). Psychiatrist is sued over multiple bad personalities. *Seattle Post Intelligencer*, p. A12.

Associated Press. (2007, January 26). Man loses memory, wanders for 25 days. www.msnbc.msn.com/id/16829260/print/1/display-mode/1098

Associated Press. (2015). Settlement reached in Northern California teen suicide. http://www.msn.com/en-us/news/crime/settlement-reached-in-northern-california-teen-suicide/ar-AAaqb58

Association for Frontotemporal Degeneration. (2023). What is FTD? https://www.theaftd.org/what-is-ftd/faqs/

Association for Psychological Science. (2007, March 2). Genes and stressed-out parents lead to shy kids. *Science Daily*. http://www.sciencedaily.com/releases/2007/03/070302111100.htm

Auerbach, R. P., Mortier, P., Bruffaerts, R., Alonso, J., Benjet, C., Cuijpers, P., . . . Kessler, R. C. (2018). WHO World Mental Health Surveys International College Student Project: Prevalence and distribution of mental disorders. *Journal of Abnormal Psychology, 127*, 623–638.

Aust, J., & Bradshaw, T. (2017). Mindfulness interventions for psychosis: A systematic review of the literature. *Journal of Psychiatric and Mental Health Nursing, 24*(1), 69–83.

Axelsen, T. M., & Woldbye, D. (2018). Gene therapy for Parkinson's disease, an update. *Journal of Parkinson's Disease, 8*(2), 195–215.

Axelsson, E., Hesser, H., Andersson, E., Ljótsson, B., & Hedman-Lagerlöf, E. (2020). Mediators of treatment effect in minimal-contact cognitive behaviour therapy for severe health anxiety: A theory-driven analysis based on a randomised controlled trial. *Journal of Anxiety Disorders, 69*, 102172. https://doi.org/10.1016/j.janxdis.2019.102172

Ayers, J. W., Poliak, A., Dredze, M., Leas, E. C., Zhu, Z., Kelley, J. B., . . . Smith, D. M. (2023). Comparing physician and artificial intelligence chatbot responses to patient questions posted to a public social media forum. *JAMA Internal Medicine, 183*(6), 589–596. https://doi.org/10.1001/jamainternmed.2023.1838

Ayllon, T., Haughton, E., & Hughes, H. B. (1965). Interpretation of symptoms: Fact or fiction.

Behaviour Research and Therapy, 3, 1–7.

Azorin, J. M., Belzeaux, R., Kaladjian, A., Adida, M., Hantouche, E., Lancrenon, S., & Fakra, E. (2013). Risks associated with gender differences in bipolar I disorder. *Journal of Affective Disorders,* 151(3), 1033–1040.

Babl, A., Gómez Penedo, J. M., Berger, T., Schneider, N., Sachse, R., & Kramer, U. (2023). Change processes in psychotherapy for patients presenting with histrionic personality disorder. *Clinical Psychology & Psychotherapy,* 30(1), 64–72. https://doi.org/10.1002/cpp.2769

Bach, B., & First, M. B. (2018). Application of the ICD-11 classification of personality disorders. *BMC Psychiatry,* 18(1), 351. https://doi.org/10.1186/s12888-018-1908-3

Bachi, K., Mani, V., Jeyachandran, D., Fayad, Z. A., Goldstein, R. Z., & Alia-Klein, N. (2017). Vascular disease in cocaine addiction. *Atherosclerosis,* 262, 154–162.

Bachmann, S. (2018). Epidemiology of suicide and the psychiatric perspective. *International Journal of Environmental Research and Public Health,* 15(7), 1425. https://doi.org/10.3390/ijerph15071425

Baetz, C. L., Surko, M., Moaveni, M., McNair, F., Bart, A., Workman, S., . . . Horwitz, S. M. (2019). Impact of a trauma-informed intervention for youth and staff on rates of violence in juvenile detention settings. *Journal of Interpersonal Violence,* 886260519857163. https://doi.org/10.1177/0886260519857163

Bagarić, B., Jokić-Begić, N., & Sangster Jokić, C. (2022). The nocebo effect: A review of contemporary experimental research. *International Journal of Behavioral Medicine,* 29(3), 255–265.

Bagge, C. L., Glenn, C. R., & Lee, H.-J. (2013). Quantifying the impact of recent negative life events on suicide attempts. *Journal of Abnormal Psychology,* 122, 359–368.

Bahji, A., Hawken, E. R., Sepehry, A. A., Cabrera, C. A., & Vazquez, G. (2019). ECT beyond unipolar major depression: Systematic review and meta-analysis of electroconvulsive therapy in bipolar depression. *Acta Psychiatrica Scandinavica,* 139(3), 214–226.

Bahrampour, T. (2013, June 3). Baby boomers are killing themselves at an alarming rate, raising question: Why? http://www.washingtonpost.com/local/baby-boomers-are-killing-themselves-at-an-alarming-rate-begging-question-why/2013/06/03/d98acc7a-c41f-11e2-8c3b-0b5e9247e-8ca_print.html

Baker, J., Edwards, I., & Beazley, P. (2021). Juror decision-making regarding a defendant diagnosed with borderline personality disorder. *Psychiatry, Psychology, and Law: An Interdisciplinary Journal of the Australian and New Zealand Association of Psychiatry, Psychology and Law,* 29(4), 516–534. https://doi.org/10.1080

Baker, J. H., Higgins Neyland, M. K., Thornton, L. M., Runfola, C. D., Larsson, H., . . . Bulik, C. (2019). Body dissatisfaction in adolescent boys. *Developmental Psychology,* 55(7), 1566–1578.

Bakker, A., Spinhoven, P., Van Balkom, A. J. L. M., & Van Dyck, R. (2002). Relevance of assessment of cognitions during panic attacks in the treatment of panic disorder. *Psychotherapy and Psychosomatics,* 71, 158–162.

Balazs, J., Miklosi, M., Kereszteny, A., Hoven, C. W., Carli, V., Wasserman, C., . . . Wasserman, D. (2013). Adolescent subthreshold-depression and anxiety: Psychopathology, functional impairment and increased suicide risk. *Journal of Child Psychology and Psychiatry,* 54, 670–677.

Baldessarini, R. J., Vázquez, G. H., & Tondo, L. (2020). Bipolar depression: A major unsolved challenge. *International Journal of Bipolar Disorders,* 8(1), 1. https://doi.org/10.1186/s40345-019-0160-1

Baldwin, G. T., Breiding, M. J., & Dawn Comstock, R. (2018). Epidemiology of sports concussion in the United States. *Handbook of Clinical Neurology,* 158, 63–74.

Baldwin, J. R., Arseneault, L., Odgers, C., Belsky, D. W., Matthews, T., Ambler, A., . . . Danese, A. (2016). Childhood bullying victimization and overweight in young adulthood: A cohort study. *Psychosomatic Medicine,* 78(9), 1094–1103.

Ball, N., Teo, W. P., Chandra, S., & Chapman, J. (2019). Parkinson's disease and the environment. *Frontiers in Neurology,* 10, 218. https://doi.org/10.3389/fneur.2019.00218

Ballard, E. D., Cwik, M., Van Eck, K., Goldstein, M., Alfes, C., Wilson, M. E., . . . Wilcox, H. C. (2017). Identification of at-risk youth by suicide screening in a pediatric emergency department. *Prevention Science,* 18, 174–182.

Ballenger, J. C., Davidson, J. R. T., Lecrubier, Y., Nutt, D. J., Borkovec, T. D., Rickels, K., . . . Wittchen, H. U. (2000). Consensus statement on generalized anxiety disorder from the International Consensus Group on depression and anxiety. *Journal of Clinical Psychiatry,* 62, 53–58.

Ballew, L., Morgan, Y., & Lippmann, S. (2003). Intravenous diazepam for dissociative disorder: Memory lost and found. *Psychosomatics,* 44, 346–349.

Balon, R. (2017). Burden of sexual dysfunction. *Journal of Sex and Marital Therapy,* 43, 49–55.

Bandura, A. (1982). Self-efficacy mechanism in human agency. *American Psychologist,* 37, 122–147.

Bandura, A. (1997). *Self-efficacy: The exercise of self-control.* New York: Freeman.

Bandura, A., & Rosenthal, T. L. (1966). Vicarious classical conditioning as a function of arousal level. *Journal of Personality and Social Psychology,* 13, 173–199.

Banks, D. E., & Zapolski, T. C. B. (2017). Impulsivity and problem drinking in college: Examining the mediating role of sex-related alcohol expectancies and alcohol use at sex. *Substance Use & Misuse,* 52(8), 992–1002. https://doi.org/10.1080/10826084.2016.1268629

Banks, D. E., Winningham, R. D., Wu, W., & Zapolski, T. (2019). Examination of the indirect effect of alcohol expectancies on ethnic identity and adolescent drinking outcomes. *American Journal of Orthopsychiatry,* 89(5), 600–608.

Banks, E., Yazidjoglou, A., Brown, S., Nguyen, M., Martin, M., Beckwith, K., . . . Joshy, G. (2023).

Electronic cigarettes and health outcomes: Umbrella and systematic review of the global evidence. *The Medical Journal of Australia, 218*(6), 267–275. https://doi.org/10.5694/mja2.51890

Bao, S., Qiao, M., Lu, Y., & Jiang, Y. (2022). Neuroimaging mechanism of cognitive behavioral therapy in pain management. *Pain Research & Management, 2022,* 6266619. https://doi.org/10.1155/2022/6266619

Barakat, S., McLean, S. A., Bryant, E., Le, A., Marks, P., National Eating Disorder Research Consortium, . . . Maguire, S. (2023). Risk factors for eating disorders: Findings from a rapid review. *Journal of Eating Disorders, 11*(1), 8. https://doi.org/10.1186/s40337-022-00717-4

Barak-Corren, Y., Castro, V. M., Javitt, S., Hoffnagle, A. G., Dai, Y., Perlis, R. H., . . . Reis, B. Y. (2017). Predicting suicidal behavior from longitudinal electronic health records. *The American Journal of Psychiatry, 174*(2), 154–162.

Barbano, A. C., van der Mei, W. F., deRoon-Cassini, T. A., Grauer, E., Lowe, S. R., Matsuoka, Y. J., . . . International Consortium to Prevent PTSD. (2019). Differentiating PTSD from anxiety and depression: Lessons from the ICD-11 PTSD diagnostic criteria. *Depression and Anxiety, 36*(6), 490–498.

Barbaresi, W. J., Colligan, R. C., Weaver, A. L., Voigt, R. G., Killian, J. M., & Katusic, S. K. (2013). Mortality, ADHD, and psychosocial adversity in adults with childhood ADHD: A prospective study. *Pediatrics, 131,* 637–644.

Barker, R. A., & Björklund, A. (2023). Restorative cell and gene therapies for Parkinson's disease. *Handbook of Clinical Neurology, 193,* 211–226. https://doi.org/10.1016/B978-0-323-85555-6.00012-6

Barker, V., Bois, C., Johnstone, E. C., Owens, D. G., Whalley, H. C., McIntosh, A. M., & Lawrie, S. M. (2016). Childhood adversity and cortical thickness and surface area in a population at familial high risk of schizophrenia.

Psychological Medicine, 46(4), 891–896.

Barker, V., Bois, C., Neilson, E., Johnstone, E. C., Owens, D., Whalley, H. C., . . . Lawrie, S. M. (2016). Childhood adversity and hippocampal and amygdala volumes in a population at familial high risk of schizophrenia. *Schizophrenia Research, 175*(1–3), 42–47.

Barlow, D. H., Farchione, T. J., Bullis, J. R., Gallagher, M. W., Murray-Latin, H., Sauer-Zavala, S., . . . Cassiello-Robbins, C. (2017). The unified protocol for transdiagnostic treatment of emotional disorders compared with diagnosis-specific protocols for anxiety disorders: A randomized clinical trial. *JAMA Psychiatry, 74*(9), 875–884.

Barnett, J. H., McDougall, F., Xu, M. K., Croudace, T. J., Richards, M., & Jones, P. B. (2012). Childhood cognitive function and adult psychopathology: Associations with psychotic and non-psychotic symptoms in the general population. *British Journal of Psychiatry, 201,* 124–130.

Baroncelli, A., & Ciucci, E. (2020). Bidirectional effects between callous-unemotional traits and student-teacher relationship quality among middle school students. *Journal of Abnormal Child Psychology, 48*(2), 277–288.

Baroud, E., Hourani, R., & Talih, F. (2019). Brain imaging in new onset psychiatric presentations. *Innovations in Clinical Neuroscience, 16,* 21–26.

Barsky, E. E., Giancola, L. M., Baxi, S. N., & Gaffin, J. M. (2018). A practical approach to severe asthma in children. *Annals of the American Thoracic Society, 15*(4), 399–408.

Barsness, R. E. (2020). Therapeutic practices in relational psychoanalysis: A qualitative study. *Psychoanalytic Psychology.* https://doi.org/10.1037/pap0000319

Bartik, W., Maple, M., Edwards, H., & Kiernan, M. (2013). Adolescent survivors after suicide: Australian young people's bereavement narratives. *Crisis, 34,* 211–217.

Bartoli, F., Carrà, G., Crocamo, C., & Clerici, M. (2015). From DSM-IV to DSM-5 alcohol use

disorder: An overview of epidemiological data. *Addictive Behavior, 41,* 46–50.

Baruth, M., Sharpe, P. A., Magwood, G., Wilcox, S., & Schlaff, R. A. (2015). Body size perceptions among overweight and obese African American women. *Ethnicity and Disease, 25*(4), 391–398.

Barzilay, R., Patrick, A., Calkins, M. E., Moore, T. M., Wolf, D. H., Benton, T. D., . . . Gur, R. E. (2019). Obsessive-compulsive symptomatology in community youth: Typical development or a red flag for psychopathology? *Journal of the American Academy of Child and Adolescent Psychiatry, 58*(2), 277–286.

Baslet, G., & Hill, J. (2011). Case report: Brief mindfulness-based psychotherapeutic intervention during inpatient hospitalization in a patient with conversion and dissociation. *Clinical Case Studies, 10,* 95–109.

Bassetti, C., Adamantidis, A., Burdakov, D., Han, F., Gay, S., Kallweit, U., . . . Dauvilliers, Y. (2019). Narcolepsy—Clinical spectrum, aetiopathophysiology, diagnosis and treatment. *Nature Reviews: Neurology, 15*(9), 519–539.

Bassetti, C., & Aldrich, M. S. (1997). Idiopathic hypersomnia: A series of 42 patients. *Brain, 120,* 1423–1435.

Battiste, N., & Effron, L. (2012). EDNOS: Deadliest eating disorder is quietly the most common. http://news.yahoo.com/ednos-deadliest-eating-disorder-quietly-most-common-204016641—abc-news-health.html

Bauer, S., Bili, S., Reetz, C., Ozer, F., Becker, K., Eschenbeck, H., ProHEAD Consortium. (2019). Efficacy and cost-effectiveness of Internet-based selective eating disorder prevention: Study protocol for a randomized controlled trial within the ProHEAD Consortium. *Trials, 20*(1), 91. https://doi.org/10.1186/s13063-018-3161-y

Baumgartner, J. C., & Radley. D. C. (2023, March 13). Overdose deaths declined but remained near record levels during the first nine months of 2022 as states cope with synthetic opioids. *To the Point* [blog], Commonwealth Fund. https://doi.org/10.26099/b912-4124

Baur, E., Forsman, M., Santtila, P., Johansson, A., Sandnabba, K., & Långström, N. (2016). Paraphilic sexual interests and sexually coercive behavior: A population-based twin study. *Archives of Sexual Behavior*, 45, 1163–1172.

Bayless, S. J., & Harvey, A. J. (2017). Testing alcohol myopia theory: Examining the effects of alcohol intoxication on simultaneous central and peripheral attention. *Perception*, 46(1), 90–99.

Beard, C., Moitra, E., Weisberg, R., & Keller, M. (2010). Characteristics and predictors of social phobia course in a longitudinal study of primary-care patients. *Depression and Anxiety*, 27(9), 839–845.

Beauchamp, G. A., Ho, M. L., & Yin, S. (2014). Variation in suicide occurrence by day and during major American holidays. *Journal of Emergency Medicine*, 46, 776–781.

Beck, A. T. (1976). *Cognitive therapy and emotional disorders*. New York: International Universities Press.

Beck, A. T., Freeman, A. F., & Associates. (1990). *Cognitive therapy of personality disorders*. New York: Guilford Press.

Beck, A. T., Grant, P. M., Huh, G. A., Perivoliotis, D., & Chang, N. A. (2013). Dysfunctional attitudes and expectancies in deficit syndrome schizophrenia. *Schizophrenia Bulletin*, 39, 43–51.

Beck, A. T., Steer, R. A., & Brown, G. K. (1996). *Manual for the Beck Depression Inventory-II*. San Antonio, TX: Psychological Corporation.

Becker, A. E. (2004). Television, disordered eating, and young women in Fiji: Negotiating body image and identity during rapid social change. *Cultural Medical Psychiatry*, 28, 533–559.

Becker, A. E., Burwell, R. A., Herzog, D. B., Hamburg, P., & Gilman, S. E. (2002). Eating behaviours and attitudes following prolonged exposure to television among ethnic Fijian adolescent girls. *British Journal of Psychiatry*, 180, 509–514.

Becker, B., Scheele, D., Moessner, R., Maier, W., & Hurlemann, R. (2013). Deciphering the neural signature of conversion blindness. *American Journal of Psychiatry*, 170, 121.

Beckman, M., & Mobbs, K. E. (2016). Threatening statements and the therapist-client privilege. *Journal of the American Academy of Psychiatry and the Law*, 44, 392–394.

Begemann, M., Thompson, I. A., Veling, W., Gangadin, S. S., Geraets, C., van't Hag, E., . . . Sommer, I. (2020). To continue or not to continue? Antipsychotic medication maintenance versus dose-reduction/discontinuation in first episode psychosis: HAMLETT, a pragmatic multicenter single-blind randomized controlled trial. *Trials*, 21(1), 147. https://doi.org/10.1186/s13063-019-3822-5

Beheshti, N. (2020). 10 eye-opening statistics on the mental health impact of the coronavirus pandemic. https://www.forbes.com/sites/nazbeheshti/2020/05/28/10-eye-opening-statistics-on-the-mental-health-impact-of-the-coronavirus-pandemic/#2845fc832df0

Bell, I. H., Marx, W., Nguyen, K., Grace, S., Gleeson, J., & Alvarez-Jimenez, M. (2023). The effect of psychological treatment on repetitive negative thinking in youth depression and anxiety: A meta-analysis and meta-regression. *Psychological Medicine*, 53(1), 6–16.

Bell, S. (2015). Police investigate "first cyber-flashing" case. http://www.bbc.com/news/technology-33889225

Bellack, A. S. (2006). Scientific and consumer models of recovery in schizophrenia: Concordance, contrasts, and implications. *Schizophrenia Bulletin*, 32, 432–442.

Bello, N. T., & Yeomans, B. L. (2018). Safety of pharmacotherapy options for bulimia nervosa and binge eating disorder. *Expert Opinion on Drug Safety*, 17(1), 17–23.

Belluck, P. (2010, June 20). Hallucinations in hospital pose risk to elderly. *New York Times*. http://www.nytimes.com

Belsky, D. W., Moffitt, T. E., Baker, T. B., Biddle, A. K., Evans, J. P., Harrington, H., . . . Caspi, A. (2013). Polygenic risk and the developmental progression to heavy, persistent smoking and nicotine dependence: Evidence from a 4-decade longitudinal study. *JAMA Psychiatry*, 70, 534–542.

Benard, V., Vaiva, G., Masson, M., & Geoffroy, P. A. (2016). Lithium and suicide prevention in bipolar disorder. *L'Encephale*, 42(3), 234–241.

Benatti, B., Arici, C., Altamura, A. C., & Dell'Osso, B. (2019). Shared obsessive-compulsive disorder: An Italian case report. *The Journal of Nervous and Mental Disease*, 207(4), 311–313.

Bender, L. (1938). A visual motor gestalt test and its clinical use. *Research Monographs of the American Orthopsychiatric Association*, 3(11), 176.

Benjamin, E. J., Muntner, P., Alonso, A., Bittencourt, M. S., Callaway, C. W., Carson, A. P., . . . American Heart Association Council on Epidemiology and Prevention Statistics Committee and Stroke Statistics Subcommittee. (2019). Heart disease and stroke statistics—2019 update: A report from the American Heart Association. *Circulation*, 139(10), e56–e528.

Bennett, J., Greene, G., & Schwartz-Barcott, D. (2013). Perceptions of emotional eating behavior. A qualitative study of college students. *Appetite*, 60, 187–192.

Benowitz, N. L. (2010). Nicotine addiction. *New England Journal of Medicine*, 362, 2295–2303.

Benton, D., & Young, H. A. (2017). Reducing calorie intake may not help you lose body weight. *Perspectives on Psychological Science*, 12, 703–714.

Ben-Zeev, D., Kaiser, S. M., Brenner, C. J., Begale, M., Duffecy, J., & Mohr, D. C. (2013). Development and usability testing of FOCUS: A smartphone system for self-management of schizophrenia. *Psychiatric Rehabilitation Journal*. Advance online publication. doi:10.1037/prj0000019

Beresin, E. (2019). Why are we denying purple hearts to veterans with PTSD? https://www.psychologytoday

.com/us/blog/inside-out-outside -in/201902/why-are-we-denying -purple-hearts-veterans-ptsd

Berg, H., Ma, Y., Rueter, A., Kaczkurkin, A., Burton, P. C., DeYoung, C. G., . . . Lissek, S. M. (2020). Salience and central executive networks track overgeneralization of conditioned fear in post-traumatic stress disorder. *Psychological Medicine*, 1–10. https://doi.org/10.1017 /S0033291720001166

Berg, K. C., Crosby, R. D., Cao, L., Peterson, C. B., Engel, S. G., Mitchell, J. E., & Wonderlich, S. A. (2013). Facets of negative affect prior to and following binge-only, purge-only, and binge/purge events in women with bulimia nervosa. *Journal of Abnormal Psychology*, 122, 111–118.

Berg, S. (2023). AMA: Use of BMI alone is an imperfect clinical measure. https://www.ama-assn.org /delivering-care/public-health/ama-use -bmi-alone-imperfect-clinical -measure

Bergemann, N., Parzer, P., Jaggy, S., Auler, B., Mundt, C., & Maier-Braunleder, S. (2008). Estrogen and comprehension of metaphoric speech in women suffering from schizophrenia: Results of a double-blind, placebo-controlled trial. *Schizophrenia Bulletin, 34*, 1172–1181.

Berger, W., Mendlowicz, M. V., Marques-Portella, C., Kinrys, G., Fontenelle, L. F., Marmar, C. R., & Figueira, I. (2009). Pharmacologic alternatives to antidepressants in posttraumatic stress disorder: A systematic review. *Progress in Neuropsychopharmacology and Biological Psychiatry, 33*, 169–180.

Bergold, S., Christiansen, H., & Steinmayr, R. (2019). Interrater agreement and discrepancy when assessing problem behaviors, social-emotional skills, and developmental status of kindergarten children. *Journal of Clinical Psychology, 75*, 2210–2232.

Berlim, M. T., & Turecki, G. (2007). Definition, assessment, and staging of treatment-resistant refractory major depression: A review of current concepts and methods. *Canadian Journal of Psychiatry, 52*, 46–54.

Berlin, F. S., & Sawyer, D. (2012). Potential consequences of accessing child pornography over the Internet and who is accessing it. *Sexual Addiction and Compulsivity, 19*, 30–40.

Bernstein, E. B. (2012). Conduct disorder. http://emedicine.medscape. com/article/918213-overview

Bertholet, N., Faouzi, M., Studer, J., Daeppen, J. B., & Gmel, G. (2013). Perception of tobacco, cannabis, and alcohol use of others is associated with one's own use. *Addiction Science and Clinical Practice, 8*, 15. doi:10.1186/1940-0640-8-15

Bertron, J. L., Seto, M., & Lindsley, C. W. (2018). DARK classics in chemical neuroscience: Phencyclidine (PCP). *ACS Chemical Neuroscience, 9*(10), 2459–2474.

Beseler, C. L., Taylor, L. A., Kraemer, D. T., & Leeman, R. F. (2012). A latent class analysis of DSM-IV alcohol use disorder criteria and binge drinking in undergraduates. *Alcoholism: Clinical and Experimental Research, 36*, 153–161.

Betts, S. S., Adise, S., Hayati Rezvan, P., Marshall, A. T., Kan, E., Johnson, D. L., & Sowell, E. R. (2023). Socioeconomic adversity and weight gain during the COVID-19 pandemic. *JAMA Pediatrics, 177*(10), 1102–1105. https://doi.org/10.1001/ jamapediatrics.2023.2823

Bewernick, B. H., Urbach, A. S., Bröder, A., Kayser, S., & Schlaepfer, T. E. (2017). Walking away from depression-motor activity increases ratings of mood and incentive drive in patients with major depression. *Psychiatry Research, 247*, 68–72.

Bhalla, R. N. (2013). Schizophreniform disorder. http:// emedicine.medscape.com /article/2008351-overview

Bhalla, R. N., & Ahmed, I. (2011). Schizophreniform disorder. http:// emedicine.medscape.com /article/2008351-overview

Bhar, S. S., Beck, A. T., & Butler, A. C. (2012). Beliefs and personality disorders: An overview of the Personality Beliefs Questionnaire. *Journal of Clinical Psychology, 68*, 88–100.

Bhat, N. V., Baker, M. J., & Jain, V. B. (2019). Anxiety disorders.

https://emedicine.medscape.com /article/286227-overview

Bhattacharyya, S., Schoeler, T., Di Forti, M., Murray, R., Cullen, A. E., & Colizzi, M. (2023). Stressful life events and relapse of psychosis: Analysis of causal association in a 2-year prospective observational cohort of individuals with first-episode psychosis in the UK. *The Lancet: Psychiatry, 10*(6), 414–425. https://doi.org/10.1016 /S2215-0366(23)00110-4

Bighelli, I., Castellazzi, M., Cipriani, A., Girlanda, F., Guaiana, G., Koesters, M., . . . Barbui, C. (2018). Antidepressants versus placebo for panic disorder in adults. *The Cochrane Database of Systematic Reviews*, 4(4), CD010676. https:// doi.org/10.1002/14651858. CD010676.pub2

Birch, J. (2019). Could social media and diet trends be contributing to a little-known eating disorder? https:// www.washingtonpost.com/lifestyle /wellness/could-social-medias -healthy-food-focus-be-contributing -to-a-little-known-eating-disorder

Biswas, J., Gangadhar, B. N., & Keshavan, M. (2016). Cross cultural variations in psychiatrists' perception of mental illness: A tool for teaching culture in psychiatry. *Asian Journal of Psychiatry, 23*, 1–7.

Bitsko, R. H., Claussen, A. H., Lichstein, J., Black, L. I., Jones, S. E., Danielson, M. L., . . . Contributor. (2022). Mental health surveillance among children: United States, 2013–2019. *MMWR Supplements, 71*(2), 1–42. https://doi.org/10.15585/mmwr .su7102a1

Bjornsson, A. S., Sibrava, N. J., Beard, C., Moitra, E., Weisberg, R. B., Benítez, C., & Keller, M. B. (2014). Two-year course of generalized anxiety disorder, social anxiety disorder, and panic disorder with agoraphobia in a sample of Latino adults. *Journal of Consulting and Clinical Psychology, 82*, 1186–1192.

Black, D. L., Cawthon, B., Robert, T., Moser, F., Caplan, Y. H., & Cone, E. J. (2009). Multiple drug ingestion by ecstasy abusers in the United

States. *Journal of Analytical Toxicology, 33,* 143–147.

Black, D. W. (2015). The natural history of antisocial personality disorder. *Canadian Journal of Psychiatry, 60*(7), 309–314.

Black, M. C., Basile, K. C., Breiding, M. J., Smith, S. G., Walters, M. L., Merrick, M. T., . . . Stevens, M. R. (2011). *The National Intimate Partner and Sexual Violence Survey (NISVS): 2010 summary report.* Atlanta, GA: National Center for Injury Prevention and Control, Centers for Disease Control and Prevention.

Blais, M. A., Smallwood, P., Groves, J. E., & Rivas-Vazquez, R. A. (2008). Personality and personality disorders. In T. A. Stern, J. F. Rosenbaum, M. Fava, J. Biederman, & S. L. Rauch (Eds.), *Massachusetts General Hospital comprehensive clinical psychiatry.* Philadelphia: Elsevier Mosby.

Blais, R. K., Tirone, V., Orlowska, D., Lofgreen, A., Klassen, B., Held, P., Stevens, N., & Zalta, A. K. (2021). Self-reported PTSD symptoms and social support in U.S. military service members and veterans: A meta-analysis. *European Journal of Psychotraumatology, 12*(1), 1851078. https://doi.org/10.1080/20008198.2020.1851078

Blake, M. J., & Allen, N. B. (2020). Prevention of internalizing disorders and suicide via adolescent sleep interventions. *Current Opinion in Psychology, 34,* 37–42.

Blanco-Vieira, T., Hoexter, M. Q., Batistuzzo, M. C., Alvarenga, P., Szejko, N., Fumo, A. M. T., . . . do Rosário, M. C. (2021). Association between obsessive-compulsive symptom dimensions in mothers and psychopathology in their children. *Frontiers in Psychiatry, 12,* 674261. https://doi.org/10.3389/fpsyt.2021.674261

Blase, K., Vermetten, E., Lehrer, P., & Gevirtz, R. (2021). Neurophysiological approach by self-control of your stress-related autonomic nervous system with depression, stress and anxiety patients. *International Journal of Environmental Research and Public Health, 18*(7),

3329. https://doi.org/10.3390/ijerph18073329

Bleidorn, W., Arslan, R. C., Denissen, J. J., Rentfrow, P. J., Gebauer, J. E., Potter, J., & Gosling, S. D. (2016). Age and gender differences in self-esteem—A cross-cultural window. *Journal of Personality and Social Psychology, 111,* 396–410.

Blokland, G., Del Re, E. C., Mesholam-Gately, R. I., Jovich, J., Trampush, J. W., Keshavan, M. S., . . . Petryshen, T. L. (2018). The Genetics of Endophenotypes of Neurofunction to Understand Schizophrenia (GENUS) consortium: A collaborative cognitive and neuroimaging genetics project. *Schizophrenia Research, 195,* 306–317. https://doi.org/10.1016/j.schres.2017.09.024

Blumberger, D. M., Vila-Rodriguez, F., Thorpe, K. E., Feffer, K., Noda, Y., Giacobbe, P., . . . Downar, J. (2018). Effectiveness of theta burst versus high-frequency repetitive transcranial magnetic stimulation in patients with depression (THREE-D): A randomised non-inferiority trial. *Lancet (London, England), 391*(10131), 1683–1692.

Blume, H. K., Brockman, L. N., & Breuner, C. C. (2012). Biofeedback therapy for pediatric headache: Factors associated with response. *Headache, 52,* 1377–1386.

Bobevski, I., Clarke, D. M., & Meadows, G. (2016). Health anxiety and its relationship to disability and service use: Findings from a large epidemiological survey. *Psychosomatic Medicine, 78*(1), 13–25.

Bochukova, E. G., Huang, N., Keogh, J., Henning, E., Purmann, C., Blaszczyk, K., . . . Farooqui, I. S. (2010). Large, rare chromosomal deletions associated with severe early-onset obesity. *Nature, 463,* 666–669.

Bock, M. A. (2007). The impact of social-behavioral learning strategy training on the social interaction skills of four students with Asperger syndrome. *Focus on Autism and Other Developmental Disabilities, 22,* 88–95.

Boeding, S. E., Paprocki, C. M., Baucom, J. S., Abramowitz, M. C.,

Wheaton, M. L. E., & Fischer, M. S. (2013). Let me check that for you: Symptom accommodation in romantic partners of adults with obsessive compulsive disorder. *Behaviour Research and Therapy, 51,* 316–322.

Boehmer, U., Bowen, D. J., & Bauer, G. R. (2007). Overweight and obesity in sexual-minority women: Evidence from population-based data. *American Journal of Public Health, 29,* 1134–1140.

Bogers, J. P. A. M., Hambarian, G., Walburgh Schmidt, N., Vermeulen, J. M., & de Haan, L. (2023). Risk factors for psychotic relapse after dose reduction or discontinuation of antipsychotics in patients with chronic schizophrenia. A meta-analysis of randomized controlled trials. *Schizophrenia Bulletin, 49*(1), 11–23. https://doi.org/10.1093/schbul/sbac138

Bohm, M. K., Liu, Y., Esser, M. B., Mesnick, J. B., Lu, H., Pan, Y., & Greenlund, K. J. (2021). Binge drinking among adults, by select characteristics and state: United States, 2018. *MMWR: Morbidity and Mortality Weekly Report, 70*(41), 1441–1446. https://doi.org/10.15585/mmwr.mm7041a2

Bohman, H., Jonsson, U., Päären, A., von Knorring, L., Olsson, G., & von Knorring, A. L. (2012). Prognostic significance of functional somatic symptoms in adolescence: A 15-year community-based follow-up study of adolescents with depression compared with healthy peers. *BMC Psychiatry, 12,* 90. doi:10.1186/1471-244X-12-90

Bohnert, A., & Ilgen, M. A. (2019). Understanding links among opioid use, overdose, and suicide. *New England Journal of Medicine, 380,* 71–79.

Bohnert, K. M., Ilgen, M. A., Louzon, S., McCarthy, J. F., & Katz, I. R. (2017). Substance use disorders and the risk of suicide mortality among men and women in the U.S. Veterans Health Administration. *Addiction, 112,* 1193–1201.

Bokszczanin, A. (2008). Parental support, family conflict, and overprotectiveness: Predicting PTSD symptom levels of adolescents 28 months after a natural disaster. *Anxiety, Stress, and Coping, 21*, 325–335.

Bollu, P. C. (2019). Normal sleep, sleep physiology, and sleep deprivation. https://emedicine.medscape.com/article/1188226-overview

Bolsinger, J., Seifritz, E., Kleim, B., & Manoliu, A. (2018). Neuroimaging correlates of resilience to traumatic events—A comprehensive review. *Frontiers in Psychiatry, 9*, 693. https://doi.org/10.3389/fpsyt.2018.00693

Bölte, S., Girdler, S., & Marschik, P. B. (2019). The contribution of environmental exposure to the etiology of autism spectrum disorder. *Cellular and Molecular Life Sciences, 76*(7), 1275–1297.

Boniel-Nissim, M., & Latzer, Y. (2016). The characteristics of pro-ANA community. In Y. Latzer & D. Stein (Eds.), *Bio-psycho-social contributions to understanding eating disorders* (pp. 155–167). Berlin: Springer International Publishing.

Borschmann, R., Becker, D., Coffey, C., Spry, E., Moreno-Betancur, M., Moran, P., & Patton, G. C. (2017). 20-year outcomes in adolescents who self-harm: A population-based cohort study. *The Lancet: Child & Adolescent Health, 1*(3), 195–202. https://doi.org/10.1016/S2352-4642(17)30007-X

Bošković, A., & Rando, O. J. (2018). Transgenerational epigenetic inheritance. *Annual Review of Genetics, 52*, 21–41.

Bossio, J. A., Basson, R., Driscoll, M., Correia, S., & Brotto, L. A. (2018). Mindfulness-based group therapy for men with situational erectile dysfunction: A mixed-methods feasibility analysis and pilot study. *Journal of Sexual Medicine, 15*, 1478–1490.

Bottini, S., Polizzi, C., Vizgaitis, A., Ellenberg, S., & Krantweiss, A. (2019). When measures diverge: The intersection of psychometric instruments and clinical judgment in multimodal adult attention-deficit/hyperactivity disorder assessment. *Professional Psychology: Research and Practice, 50*, 353–363.

Bowlby, J. (1969). *Attachment.* New York: Basic Books.

Boyd, D. (2017). Christopher had 323 doctor visits and 13 major surgeries: Here's why his mom was arrested. https://www.star-telegram.com/news/local/dallas/article188865169.html#storylink=cpy

Boyd, J. E., Lanius, R. A., & McKinnon, M. C. (2018). Mindfulness-based treatments for posttraumatic stress disorder: A review of the treatment literature and neurobiological evidence. *Journal of Psychiatry and Neuroscience, 43*(1), 7–25.

Boyington, J. E. A., Carter-Edwards, L., Piehl, M., Hutson, J., Langdon, D., & McManus, S. (2008). Cultural attitudes toward weight, diet, and physical activity among overweight African American girls. *Preventing Chronic Disease, 5*, 1–9.

Bozzatello, P., Rocca, P., Mantelli, E., & Bellino, S. (2019). Polyunsaturated fatty acids: What is their role in treatment of psychiatric disorders? *International Journal of Molecular Sciences, 20*(21), 5257. https://doi.org/10.3390/ijms20215257

Braden, A., Flatt S. W., Boutelle, K. N., Strong, D., Sherwood, N. E., & Rock, C. L. (2016). Emotional eating is associated with weight loss success among adults enrolled in a weight loss program. *Journal of Behavioral Medicine, 39*, 727–732.

Bradford, J. M. W., & de Amorim Levin, G. V. (2020). Vicarious trauma and PTSD in forensic mental health professionals. *Journal of the American Academy of Psychiatry and the Law, 48*(3), 315–318.

Brady, J. E., & Li, G. (2014). Trends in alcohol and other drugs detected in fatally injured drivers in the United States, 1999–2010. *American Journal of Epidemiology, 179*, 692–699.

Braff, T. L., & Tamminga, C. A. (2017). Endophenotypes, epigenetics, polygenicity and more: Irv Gottesman's dynamic legacy. *Schizophrenia Bulletin, 43*, 10–16.

Brand, B. L., Myrick, A. C., Loewenstein, R. J., Classen, C. C., Lanius, R., McNary, S. W., & Putnam, F. W. (2012). A survey of practices and recommended treatment interventions among expert therapists treating patients with dissociative identity disorder and dissociative disorder not otherwise specified. *Psychological Trauma: Theory, Research, Practice, and Policy, 4*, 490–500.

Brand, B. L., Schielke, H. J., Putnam, K. T., Putnam, F. W., Loewenstein, R. J., Myrick, A., . . . Lanius, R. A. (2019). An online educational program for individuals with dissociative disorders and their clinicians: 1-year and 2-year follow-up. *Journal of Traumatic Stress, 32*(1), 156–166.

Brand, M., Eggers, C., Reinhold, N., Fujiwara, E., Kessler, J., Heiss, W.-D., & Markowitsch, H. J. (2009). Functional brain imaging in 14 patients with dissociative amnesia reveals right inferolateral prefrontal hypometabolism. *Psychiatry Research: Neuroimaging, 174*, 32–39.

Brander, G., Rydell, M., Kuja-Halkola, R., Fernández de la Cruz, L., Lichtenstein, P., Serlachius, E., . . . Mataix-Cols, D. (2016). Association of perinatal risk factors with obsessive-compulsive disorder: A population-based birth cohort, sibling control study. *JAMA Psychiatry, 73*(11), 1135–1144.

Brannigan, G. G., Decker, S. L., & Madsen, D. H. (2004). *Innovative features of the Bender-Gestalt II and expanded guidelines for the use of the Global Scoring System* (Bender Visual-Motor Gestalt Test, 2nd ed., Assessment Service Bulletin No. 1). Itasca, IL: Riverside.

Brannon, G. E., & Bienenfeld, D. (2012). Schizoaffective disorder. http://emedicine.medscape.com/article/294763-overview

Brannon, G. E., & Bienenfeld, D. (2013). History and mental status examination. http://emedicine.medscape.com/article/293402-overview

Brannon, G. E., & Bienenfeld, D. (2015). Paraphilic disorders. http://emedicine.medscape.com/article/291419-overview?src=refgatesrc1#a4

Brannon, G. E., & Bienenfeld, D. (2016). Schizoaffective disorder. https://emedicine.medscape.com/article/294763-overview#a5

Bränström, R., & Pachankis, J. E. (2018). Sexual orientation disparities in the co-occurrence of substance use and psychological distress: A national population-based study (2008–2015). *Social Psychiatry and Psychiatric Epidemiology, 53*(4), 403–412.

Breakstone, J., Smith, M., & Wineburg, S. Rapaport, A., Carle, J., Garland, M., & Saavedrak, A. (2019). *Students' civic online reasoning: A national portrait.* Stanford, CA: Stanford History Education Group.

Breese-McCoy, S. J. (2011). Postpartum depression: An essential overview for the practitioner. *Southern Medical Journal, 104,* 128–132.

Brennan, C. L., Swartout, K. M., Goodnight, B. L., Cook, S. L., Parrott, D. J., Thompson, M. P., . . . Leone, R. M. (2019). Evidence for multiple classes of sexually-violent college men. *Psychology of Violence, 9*(1), 48–55.

Bresnahan, M., Begg, M. D., Brown, A., Schaefer, C., Sohler, N., Insel B., . . . Susser, E. (2007). Race and risk of schizophrenia in a US birth cohort: Another example of health disparity? *International Journal of Epidemiology, 36,* 751–758.

Breuer, J., & Freud, S. (1957). *Studies in hysteria.* New York: Basic Books. (Original work published 1895)

Brewslow, N., Evans, L., & Langley, J. (1986). Comparisons among heterosexual, bisexual, and homosexual male sadomasochists. *Journal of Homosexuality, 13,* 83–107.

Breyer, B. N., Cohen, B. E., Bertenthal, D., Rosen, R. C., Neylan, T. C., & Seal, K. H. (2014). Sexual dysfunction in male Iraq and Afghanistan war veterans: Association with posttraumatic stress disorder and other combat-related mental health disorders: A population-based cohort study. *Journal of Sexual Medicine, 11,* 75–83.

Brezing, C. A., & Levin, F. R. (2018). The current state of pharmacological treatments for cannabis use disorder and withdrawal. *Neuropsychopharmacology, 43*(1), 173–194.

Bridge, J. A., Horowitz, L. M., Fontanella, C. A., Sheftall, A. H., Greenhouse, J., Kelleher, K. J., & Campo, J. V. (2018). Age-related racial disparity in suicide rates among US youths from 2001 through 2015. *JAMA Pediatrics, 172*(7), 697–699.

Brière, F. N., Rohde, P., Shaw, H., & Stice, E. (2014). Moderators of two indicated cognitive-behavioral depression prevention approaches for adolescents in a school-based effectiveness trial. *Behavior Research & Therapy, 53,* 55–62.

Briguglio, M., Vitale, J. A., Galentino, R., Banfi, G., Zanaboni Dina, C., Bona, A., . . . Glick, I. D. (2020). Healthy eating, physical activity, and sleep hygiene (HEPAS) as the winning triad for sustaining physical and mental health in patients at risk for or with neuropsychiatric disorders: Considerations for clinical practice. *Neuropsychiatric Disease and Treatment, 16,* 55–70.

Briken, P., Matthiesen, S., Pietras, L., Wiessner, C., Klein, V., Reed, G. M., & Dekker, A. (2020). Estimating the prevalence of sexual dysfunction using the new ICD-11 guidelines. *Deutsches Arzteblatt International, 117*(39), 653–658. https://doi.org/10.3238/arztebl.2020.0653

Briken, P., Wiessner, C., Štulhofer, A., Klein, V., Fuß, J., Reed, G. M., & Dekker, A. (2022). Who feels affected by "out of control" sexual behavior? Prevalence and correlates of indicators for ICD-11 compulsive sexual behavior disorder in the German Health and Sexuality Survey (GeSiD). *Journal of Behavioral Addictions, 11*(3), 900–911. https://doi.org/10.1556/2006.2022.00060

Broder-Fingert, S., Mateo, C., & Zuckerman, K. E. (2020). Structural racism and autism. *Pediatrics,* e2020015420. https://doi.org/10.1542/peds.2020-015420

Brody, G. H., Yu, T., Chen, E., & Miller, G. E. (2020). Persistence of skin-deep resilience in African American adults. *Health Psychology.* https://doi.org/10.1037/hea0000945

Broeren, S., Lester, K. J., Muris, P., & Field, A. P. (2011). They are afraid of the animal, so therefore I am too: Influence of peer modeling on fear beliefs and approach–avoidance behaviors towards animals in typically developing children. *Behaviour Research and Therapy, 49,* 50–57.

Broniatowski, D. A., Jamison, A. M., Qi, S., AlKulaib, L., Chen, T., Benton, A., . . . Dredze, M. (2018). Weaponized health communication: Twitter bots and Russian trolls amplify the vaccine debate *American Journal of Public Health, 108,* 1378–1384.

Broniatowski, D. A., Quinn, S. C., Dredze, M., & Jamison, A. M. (2020). Vaccine communication as weaponized identity politics. *American Journal of Public Health, 110*(5), 617–618.

Brooks, J. R., Hong, J. H., Madubata, I. J., Odafe, M. O., Cheref, S., & Walker, R. L. (2020). The moderating effect of dispositional forgiveness on perceived racial discrimination and depression for African American adults. *Cultural Diversity and Ethnic Minority Psychology.* https://doi.org/10.1037/cdp0000385

Brooks, S., Prince, A., Stahl, D., Campbell, C., & Treasure, J. (2011). A systematic review and meta-analysis of cognitive bias to food stimuli in people with disordered eating behavior. *Clinical Psychology Review, 31,* 37–51.

Brotman, M. A., Schmajuk, M., Rich, B. A., Dickstein, D. P., Guyer, A. E., Costello, E. J., . . . Leibenluft, E. (2006). Prevalence, clinical correlates, and longitudinal course of severe mood dysregulation in children. *Biological Psychiatry, 60,* 991–997.

Brotto, L., Atallah, S., Johnson-Agbakwu, C., Rosenbaum, T., Abdo, C., Byers, E. S., . . . Wylie, K. (2016). Psychological and interpersonal dimensions of sexual function and dysfunction. *The Journal of Sexual Medicine, 13*(4), 538–571.

Brotto, L. A., Chivers, M. L., Millman, R. D., & Albert, A. (2016). Mindfulness-based sex therapy improves genital-subjective arousal concordance in women with sexual desire/arousal difficulties. *Archives of Sexual Behavior, 45*(8), 1907–1921.

Brouns, B. H., de Wied, M. A., Keijsers, L., Branje, S., van Goozen, S. H., & Meeus, W. H. (2013). Concurrent and prospective effects of psychopathic traits on affective and cognitive empathy in a community sample of late adolescents. *Journal of Child Psychology and Psychiatry, 54,* 969–976.

Brown, D., Larkin, F., Sengupta, S., Romero-Ureclay, J. L., Ross, C. C., Gupta, N., . . . Das, M. (2014). Clozapine: An effective treatment for seriously violent and psychopathic men with antisocial personality disorder in a UK high-security hospital. *CNS Spectrums, 3,* 1–12.

Brown, J., Blackshaw, E., Stahl, D., Fennelly, L., McKeague, L., Sclare, I., & Michelson, D. (2019). School-based early intervention for anxiety and depression in older adolescents: A feasibility randomised controlled trial of a self-referral stress management workshop programme ("DISCOVER"). *Journal of Adolescence, 71,* 150–161.

Brown, R. J., & Lewis-Fernández, R. (2011). Culture and conversion disorder: Implications for DSM-5. *Psychiatry: Interpersonal and Biological Processes, 74,* 187–206.

Browne, B. (2011). Sinister secrets in the sky. http://coto2.wordpress.com/2011/02/05/sinister-secrets-in-the-ky-and-morgellons-disease

Browne, D. (2018). Music's fentanyl crisis: Inside the drug that killed Prince and Tom Petty. https://www.rollingstone.com/music/music-features/musics-fentanyl-crisis-inside-the-drug-that-killed-prince-and-tom-petty-666019/

Brownley, K. A., Berkman, N. D., Peat, C. M., Lohr, K. N., Cullen, K. E., Bann, C. M., & Bulik, C. M. (2016). Binge-eating disorder in adults: A systematic review and meta-analysis. *Annals of Internal Medicine, 165*(6), 409–420. https://doi.org/10.7326/M15-2455

Bruch, M. A., & Heimberg, R. G. (1994). Differences in perceptions of parental and personal characteristics between generalized and nongeneralized social phobics. *Journal of Anxiety Disorders, 8,* 155–168.

Brunner, E. J., Shipley, M. J., Britton, A. R., Stansfeld, S. A., Heuschmann, P. U., Rudd, A. G., . . . Kivimaki, M. (2014). Depressive disorder, coronary heart disease, and stroke: Dose-response and

reverse causation effects in the Whitehall II cohort study. *European Journal of Preventive Cardiology, 21,* 340–346.

Bruno, A., Celebre, L., Torre, G., Pandolfo, G., Mento, C., Cedro, C., . . . Muscatello, M. (2019). Focus on disruptive mood dysregulation disorder: A review of the literature. *Psychiatry Research, 279,* 323–330.

Bruno, R., Matthews, A. J., Topp, L., Degenhardt, L., Gomez, R., & Dunn, M. (2009). Can the severity of dependence scale be usefully applied to "Ecstasy"? *Neuropsychobiology, 60,* 137–147.

Brunwasser, S. M., & Gillham, J. E. (2018). Identifying moderators of response to the Penn Resiliency Program: A synthesis study. *Prevention Science, 19*(Suppl 1), 38–48. https://doi.org/10.1007/s11121-015-0627-y

Bryan, C. J., & Clemans, T. A. (2013). Repetitive traumatic brain injury, psychological symptoms, and suicide risk. *JAMA Psychiatry, 15,* 1–6.

Bryant, K. (2001, February 20). Eating disorders: In their own words. *Atlanta Journal-Constitution,* p. B4.

Bryant, R. A. (2013). An update of acute stress disorder. *PTSD Research Quarterly, 24,* 1–7.

Bryant, R. A. (2019). Post-traumatic stress disorder: A state-of-the-art review of evidence and challenges. *World Psychiatry, 18*(3), 259–269.

Bryant, R. A., & Das, P. (2012). The neural circuitry of conversion disorder and its recovery. *Journal of Abnormal Psychology, 121,* 289–296.

Buckingham-Howes, S., Armstrong, B., Pejsa-Reitz, M. C., Wang, Y., Witherspoon, D. O., Hager, E. R., & Black, M. M. (2018). BMI and disordered eating in urban, African American, adolescent girls: The mediating role of body dissatisfaction. *Eating Behaviors, 29,* 59–63.

Buckman, J., Underwood, A., Clarke, K., Saunders, R., Hollon, S. D., Fearon, P., & Pilling, S. (2018). Risk factors for relapse and recurrence of depression in adults and how they operate: A four-phase systematic review

and meta-synthesis. *Clinical Psychology Review, 64,* 13–38.

Budenz, A., Purtle, J., Klassen, A., Yom-Tav, E., Yudell, M., & Massey, P. (2019). The case of a mass shooting and violence-related mental illness stigma on Twitter. *Stigma and Health, 4,* 411–420.

Buetow, S., & Zawaly, K. (2022). Rethinking researcher bias in health research. *Journal of Evaluation in Clinical Practice, 28*(5), 843–846.

Bulik, C. M., Blake, L., & Austin, J. (2019). Genetics of eating disorders: What the clinician needs to know. *The Psychiatric Clinics of North America, 42*(1), 59–73.

Bunford, N., Evans, S. W., & Langberg, J. M. (2014). Emotion dysregulation is associated with social impairment among young adolescents with ADHD. *Journal of Attention Disorders.* doi:10.1177/1087054714527793

Bunney, B. G., Li, J. Z., Walsh, D. M., Stein, R., Vawter, M. P., Cartagena, P., . . . Bunney, W. E. (2015). Circadian dysregulation of clock genes: Clues to rapid treatments in major depressive disorder. *Molecular Psychiatry, 20*(1), 48–55.

Burke, J. D., Rowe, R., & Boylan, K. (2014). Functional outcomes of child and adolescent oppositional defiant disorder symptoms in young adult men. *Journal of Child Psychology and Psychiatry, 55,* 264–272.

Burke, S. M., Menks, W. M., Cohen-Kettenis, P. T., Klink, D. T., & Bakker, J. (2014). Click-evoked otoacoustic emissions in children and adolescents with gender identity disorder. *Archives of Sexual Behavior.* http://dare.ubvu.vu.nl/bitstream/handle/1871/51287/chapter_2.pdf?sequence56

Burkle, F. M. (2019). Character disorders among autocratic world leaders and the impact on health security, human rights, and humanitarian care. *Prehospital and Disaster Medicine, 34,* 2–7.

Burnes, T. R., Dexter, M. M., Richmond, K., Singh, A. A., & Cherrington, A. (2016). The experiences of transgender survivors of trauma who undergo social and medical transition. *Traumatology, 22,* 75–84.

Burri, A. (2013). Bringing sex research into the 21st century: Genetic and epigenetic approaches on female sexual function. *Journal of Sex Research, 50*, 318–328.

Burrows, R. D., Slavec, J. J., Nangle, D. W., & O'Grady, A. C. (2013). ERP, medication, and brief hospitalization in the treatment of an adolescent with severe BDD. *Clinical Case Studies, 12*, 3–21.

Burstein, M., & Ginsburg, G. S. (2010). The effect of parental modeling of anxious behaviors and cognitions in school-aged children: An experimental pilot study. *Behaviour Research and Therapy, 48*, 506–515.

Burton, C., McGorm, K., Weller, D., & Sharpe, M. (2010). Depression and anxiety in patients repeatedly referred to secondary care with medically unexplained symptoms: A case-control study. *Psychological Medicine, 41*(3), 555–563.

Burton, L. (2016). Police catch suspected Redmond voyeur with pants unzipped. http://www.seattlepi.com/local/crime/article/Police-catch-suspected-Redmond-voyeur-with-pants-10058286.php

Buster, J. E. (2013). Managing female sexual dysfunction. *Fertility and Sterility, 100*, 905–915.

Butcher, J. N. (2010). Personality assessment from the nineteenth to the early twenty-first century: Past achievements and contemporary challenges. *Annual Review of Clinical Psychology, 6*, 1–20.

Butt, J. H., Dalsgaard, S., Torp-Pedersen, C., Køber, L., Gislason, G. H., Kruuse, C., & Fosbøl, E. L. (2017). Beta-blockers for exams identify students at high risk of psychiatric morbidity. *Journal of Child and Adolescent Psychopharmacology, 27*(3), 266–273.

Butterworth, B., & Kovas, Y. (2013). Understanding neurocognitive developmental disorders can improve education for all. *Science, 340*(6130), 300. doi:10.1126/science.1231022

Button, S., Thornton, A., Lee, S. Shakespeare, J., & Ayers, S. (2017). Seeking help for perinatal psychological distress: A meta-synthesis of women's experiences. *British Journal of General Practice, 67*(663), e692–e699.

Butz, C., Iske, C., Truba, N., & Trott, K. (2019). Treatment of functional gait abnormality in a rehabilitation setting: Emphasizing the physical interventions for treating the whole child. *Innovations in Clinical Neuroscience, 16*(7–8), 18–21.

Byrd, A. S., Toth, A. T., & Stanford, F. C. (2018). Racial disparities in obesity treatment. *Current Obesity Reports, 7*(2), 130–138.

Cabral, M., Suess, A., Ehrt, J., Seehole, T. J., Wong, J. (2016). Removal of gender incongruence of childhood diagnostic category: A human rights perspective. *Lancet Psychiatry, 3*, 405–406.

Cacabelos, R. (2020). Pharmacogenomics of cognitive dysfunction and neuropsychiatric disorders in dementia. *International Journal of Molecular Sciences, 21*(9), 3059. https://doi.org/10.3390/ijms21093059

Cacciatore, J., & Francis, A. (2022). DSM-5-TR turns normal grief into a mental disorder. *The Lancet: Psychiatry, 9*(7), e32. https://doi.org/10.1016/S2215-0366(22)00150-X

Cachelin, F. M., Gil-Rivas, V., Palmer, B., Vela, A., Phimphasone, P., de Hernandez, B. U., & Tapp, H. (2019). Randomized controlled trial of a culturally-adapted program for Latinas with binge eating. *Psychological Services, 16*(3), 504–512.

Cacioppo, J. T., Reis, H. T., & Zautra, A. J. (2011). The value of social fitness with an application to the military. *American Psychologist, 66*, 43–51.

Cai, Y., Liu, P., Zhou, X., Yuan, J., & Chen, Q. (2023). Probiotics therapy show significant improvement in obesity and neurobehavioral disorders symptoms. *Frontiers in Cellular and Infection Microbiology, 13*, 1178399. https://doi.org/10.3389/fcimb.2023.1178399

Caldwell, B. (2019). Why therapists stopped creating no-harm contracts. https://www.simplepractice.com/blog/why-therapists-stopped-creating-no-harm-contracts/

Caligor, E., Levy, K. N., & Yeomans, F. E. (2015). Narcissistic personality disorder: Diagnostic and clinical challenges. *American Journal of Psychiatry, 172*(5), 415–422.

Calik, M. W. (2016). Treatments for obstructive sleep apnea. *Journal of Clinical Outcomes Management, 23*, 181–192.

Calzo, J. P., Blashill, A. J., Brown, T. A., & Argenal, R. L. (2017). Eating disorders and disordered weight and shape control behaviors in sexual minority populations. *Current Psychiatry Reports, 19*(8), 49. https://doi.org/10.1007/s11920-017-0801-y

Camerer, C. F., Dreber, A., Holzmeister, F., Ho, T.-H., Huber, J., Johannesson, M., . . . Wu, H. (2018). Evaluating the replicability of social science experiments in *Nature* and *Science* between 2010 and 2015. *Nature Human Behaviour, 2*, 637–644.

Canan, F., & North, C. S. (2019). Dissociation and disasters: A systematic review. *World Journal of Psychiatry, 9*(6), 83–98.

Canavera, K. E., Ollendick, T. H., May, J. T. E., & Pincus, D. B. (2010). Clinical correlates of comorbid obsessive-compulsive disorder and depression in youth. *Child Psychiatry and Human Development, 41*, 583–594.

Cantor, D., Fisher, B., Chibnall, S., Harps, S., Townsend, R., Thomas, G., . . . Madden, K. (2020). *Report on the AAU Campus Climate Survey on Sexual Assault and Sexual Misconduct (Revised)*. Rockville, MD: Westat.

Cao, J., Wei, J., Fritzsche, K., Toussaint, A. C., Li, T., Jiang, Y., . . . Leonhart, R. (2020). Prevalence of DSM-5 somatic symptom disorder in Chinese outpatients from general hospital care. *General Hospital Psychiatry, 62*, 63–71.

Cao, K. X., Ma, M. L., Wang, C. Z., Iqbal, J., Si, J. J., Xue, Y. X., & Yang, J. L. (2021). TMS-EEG: An emerging tool to study the neurophysiologic biomarkers of psychiatric disorders. *Neuropharmacology, 197*, 108574. https://doi.org/10.1016/j.neuropharm.2021.108574

Capizzi, A., Woo, J., & Verduzco-Gutierrez, M. (2020). Traumatic brain injury: An overview of epidemiology, pathophysiology, and medical management. *The Medical Clinics* of North America, 104(2), 213–238. https://doi.org/10.1016/j.mcna.2019.11.001

Cardno, A. G., & Owen, M. J. (2014, February 24). Genetic relationships between schizophrenia, bipolar disorder, and schizoaffective disorder. *Schizophrenia Bulletin*, 40, 504–515.

Cardona, C. (2018). A history of Texas "affluenza teen" Ethan Couch and his family's troubles with the law. https://www.dallasnews.com/news/crime/2018/08/22/a-history-of-texas-affluenza-teen-ethan-couch-and-his-family-s-troubles-with-the-law/

Carey, B. (2011, June 23). Expert on mental illness reveals her own fight. *New York Times*. https://www.nytimes.com/2011/06/23/health/23lives.html

Carey, B. (2017). The true story behind Sybil and her multiple personalities. https://www.cbc.ca/books/the-true-story-behind-sybil-and-her-multiple-personalities-1

Carey, K. B., Scott-Sheldon, L., Carey, M. P., & DeMartini, K. S. (2007). Individual-level interventions to reduce college student drinking: A meta-analytic review. *Addictive Behaviors*, 32, 2469–2494.

Carlier, N., Marshe, V. S., Cmorejova, J., Davis, C., & Müller, D. J. (2015). Genetic similarities between compulsive overeating and addiction phenotypes: A case for "food addiction"? *Current Psychiatry Reports*, 17(12), 96. https://doi.org/10.1007/s11920-015-0634-5

Carlton, C., Banks, M., & Sundararajan, S. (2018). Oral contraceptives and ischemic stroke risk. *Stroke*, 49(4), e157–e159.

Carmi, L., Alyagon, U., Barnea-Ygael, N., Zohar, J., Dar, R., & Zangen, A. (2018). Clinical and electrophysiological outcomes of deep TMS over the medial prefrontal and anterior cingulate cortices in OCD patients. *Brain Stimulation*, 11(1), 158–165.

Carpenter, D. O., & Nevin, R. (2010). Environmental causes of violence. *Physiology and Behavior*, 99(2), 260–268.

Carr, F. (2018). Astronaut Scott Kelly now has different DNA than his identical twin brother after one year in space. *Time*.

https://time.com/5201064/scott-kelly-mark-nasa-dna-study/

Carr, M. (2017). Nightmares may signal increased risk of suicide. https://www.scientificamerican.com/article/nightmares-may-signal-increased-risk-of-suicide/

Carroll, J. E., Irwin, M. R., Seeman, T. E., Diez-Roux, A. V., Prather, A. A., Olmstead, R., . . . Redline, S. (2019). Obstructive sleep apnea, nighttime arousals, and leukocyte telomere length: The Multi-Ethnic Study of Atherosclerosis. *Sleep*, 42(7), zsz089. https://doi.org/10.1093/sleep/zsz089

Carroll, K. M., Nich, C., Petry, N. M., Eagan, D. A., Shi, J. M., & Ball, S. A. (2016). A randomized factorial trial of disulfiram and contingency management to enhance cognitive behavioral therapy for cocaine dependence. *Drug and Alcohol Dependence*, 160, 135–142.

Carter, D. J. (2018). Case study: A transactional analysis model for a single mother and her adult child with bipolar disorder. *Clinical Case Studies*, 17, 296–310.

Carter, L., Read, J., Pyle, M., & Morrison, A. P. (2019). Are causal beliefs associated with stigma? A test of the impact of biogenetic versus psychosocial explanations on stigma and internalized stigma in people experiencing psychosis. *Stigma and Health*, 4, 170–178.

Cartwright, S. (1851, May). Report on the diseases and physical peculiarities of the Negro race. *DeBow's Review*, 11, 64–69.

Carvalheira, A., Træen, B., & Štulhofer, A. (2014). Correlates of men's sexual interest: A cross-cultural study. *Journal of Sexual Medicine*, 11, 154–164.

Carvalho, A. C., & Rodrigues, D. L. (2022). Sexuality, sexual behavior, and relationships of asexual individuals: Differences between aromantic and romantic orientation. *Archives of Sexual Behavior*, 51(4), 2159–2168.

Carvalho, J., Veríssimo, A., & Nobre, P. J. (2013). Cognitive and emotional determinants characterizing women with persistent genital arousal disorder. *Journal of Sexual Medicine*, 10, 1549–1558.

Cascio, C. N., Konrath, S. H., & Falk, E. B. (2015). Narcissists' social pain seen only in the brain. *Social Cognitive and Affective Neuroscience*, 10(3), 335–341.

Caseras, X., Murphy, K., Lawrence, N. S., Fuentes-Claramonte, P., Watts, J., Jones, D. K., & Phillips, M. L. (2015). Emotion regulation deficits in euthymic bipolar I versus bipolar II disorder: A functional and diffusion-tensor imaging study. *Bipolar Disorders*, 17(5), 461–470.

Casey, D. E. (2006). Implications of the CATIE trial on treatment: Extrapyramidal symptoms. *CNS Spectrums*, 11, 25–31.

Cass, S. P. (2017). Alzheimer's disease and exercise: A literature review. *Current Sports Medicine Reports*, 16(1), 19–22.

Cassidy, F. (2010). Insight in bipolar disorder: Relationship to episode subtypes and symptom dimensions. *Journal of Neuropsychiatric Disease and Treatment*, 6, 627–631.

Castaneda, R. (2019). How virtual reality can help treat chronic pain. https://health.usnews.com/health-care/patient-advice/articles/2019-01-14/how-virtual-reality-can-help-treat-chronic-pain

Castelli, J. (2009). The unspeakable. https://mental-health-matters.com/the-unspeakable/

Castellini, G., Rellini, A. H., Appignanesi, C., Pinucci, I., Fattorini, M., Grano, E., . . . Ricca, V. (2018). Deviance or normalcy? The relationship among paraphilic thoughts and behaviors, hypersexuality, and psychopathology in a sample of university students. *Journal of Sexual Medicine*, 15, 1322–1335.

Castelnuovo, G. (2010). Empirically supported treatments in psychotherapy: Towards an evidence-based or evidence-biased psychology in clinical settings? *Frontiers in Psychology*, 1, 27. doi:10.3389/fpsyg.2010.00027

Castora, F. J. (2019). Mitochondrial function and abnormalities implicated in the pathogenesis of ASD. *Progress in Neuro-Psychopharmacology and Biological Psychiatry*, 92, 83–108. https://doi.org/10.1016/j.pnpbp.2018.12.015

Catapan, S. C., Oliveira, W. F., & Rotta, T. M. (2019). Clown therapy in the hospital setting: A review of the literature. *Ciencia & Saude Coletiva, 24*(9), 3417–3429. https://doi.org/10.1590/1413-81232018249.22832017

Cather, C. (2005). Functional cognitive-behavioural therapy: A brief, individual treatment for functional impairments resulting from psychotic symptoms in schizophrenia. *Canadian Journal of Psychiatry, 50*, 258–263.

Caulley, L., Kohlert, S., Gandy, H., Olds, J., & Bromwich, M. (2018). When symptoms don't fit: A case series of conversion disorder in the pediatric otolaryngology practice. *Journal of Otolaryngology—Head and Neck Surgery, 47*(1), 39. https://doi.org/10.1186/s40463-018-0286-7

Cavedini, P., Zorzi, C., Piccinni, M., Cavallini, M. C., & Bellodi, L. (2010). Executive dysfunctions in obsessive-compulsive patients and unaffected relatives: Searching for a new intermediate phenotype. *Biological Psychiatry, 67*, 1178–1184.

Cayouette, A., Thibaudeau, É., Cellard, C., Roy, M. A., & Achim, A. M. (2023). Associations between theory of mind and clinical symptoms in recent onset schizophrenia spectrum disorders. *Frontiers in Psychiatry, 14*, 1044682. https://doi.org/10.3389/fpsyt.2023.1044682

Cea, D. M. (2019). Supporting survivors of suicide loss. https://ct.counseling.org/2019/10/supporting-survivors-of-suicide-loss/

Cechnicki, A., Bielańska, A., Hanuszkiewicz, I., & Daren, A. (2013). The predictive validity of expressed emotions (EE) in schizophrenia. A 20-year prospective study. *Journal of Psychiatric Research, 47*(2), 208–214.

Cedillo, Y. E., Lomax, R. O., Fernandez, J. R., & Moellering, D. R. (2020). Physiological significance of discrimination on stress markers, obesity, and LDL oxidation among a European American and African American cohort of females. *International Journal of Behavioral Medicine, 27*(2), 213–224.

Cella, M., Preti, A., Edwards, C., Dow, T., & Wykes, T. (2017). Cognitive remediation for negative symptoms of schizophrenia: A network meta-analysis. *Clinical Psychology Review, 52*, 43–51.

Cénat, J. M., Dalexis, R. D., Darius, W. P., Kogan, C. S., & Guerrier, M. (2023). Prevalence of current PTSD symptoms among a sample of Black individuals aged 15 to 40 in Canada: The major role of everyday racial discrimination, racial microaggresions, and internalized racism. *Canadian Journal of Psychiatry, 68*(3), 178–186.

Centers for Disease Control and Prevention (CDC). (2009). Prevalence of autism spectrum disorders—Autism and Developmental Disabilities Monitoring Network, United States, 2006. http://www.cdc.gov/mmwr/preview/mmwrhtml/ss5810a1.htm

Centers for Disease Control and Prevention (CDC). (2011). CDC investigation of unexplained dermopathy. http://www.cdc.gov/unexplained-dermopathy

Centers for Disease Control and Prevention (CDC). (2018). Youth Risk Behavior Survey: Data summary and trends report 2007–2017. https://www.cdc.gov/features/dsyouthmonitoring/index.html

Centers for Disease Control and Prevention (CDC). (2019). Risk and protective factors for suicide. https://www.cdc.gov/violenceprevention/suicide/riskprotectivefactors.html

Centers for Disease Control and Prevention (CDC). (2020). Summary health statistics: National Health Interview Survey: 2018. Table A-15a. https://www.cdc.gov/nchs/nhis/shs/tables.htm

Centers for Disease Control and Prevention (CDC). (2021). Hypertension cascade: Hypertension prevalence, treatment and control estimates among US adults aged 18 years and older applying the criteria from the American College of Cardiology and American Heart Association's 2017 Hypertension Guideline—NHANES 2015–2018. Atlanta, GA: U.S. Department of Health and Human Services.

Centers for Disease Control and Prevention (CDC). (2022a). Adult obesity facts. https://www.cdc.gov/obesity/data/adult.html

Centers for Disease Control and Prevention (CDC). (2022b). Fast facts: Preventing child abuse & neglect. https://www.cdc.gov/violenceprevention/childabuse-andneglect/fastfact.html

Centers for Disease Control and Prevention (CDC). (2022c). Fast facts: Preventing sexual violence. https://www.cdc.gov/violenceprevention/sexualviolence/fastfact.html

Centers for Disease Control and Prevention (CDC). (2022d). Heart disease facts. https://www.cdc.gov/heartdisease/facts.htm

Centers for Disease Control and Prevention (CDC). (2022e). Most recent asthma data. https://www.cdc.gov/asthma/most_recent_national_asthma_data.htm

Centers for Disease Control and Prevention (CDC). (2022f). Most recent national asthma data. https://www.cdc.gov/asthma/most_recent_national_asthma_data.htm

Centers for Disease Control and Prevention (CDC). (2022g). Prevalence of childhood obesity in the United States. https://www.cdc.gov/obesity/data/childhood.html

Centers for Disease Control and Prevention (CDC). (2022h). Prevention strategies. https://www.cdc.gov/suicide/prevention/index.html

Centers for Disease Control and Prevention (CDC). (2023a). Adult obesity prevalence maps. https://www.cdc.gov/obesity/data/prevalence-maps.html

Centers for Disease Control and Prevention (CDC). (2023b). Data & statistics on Tourette syndrome. https://www.cdc.gov/ncbddd/tourette/data.html

Centers for Disease Control and Prevention (CDC). (2023c). Death rate maps & graphs. https://www.cdc.gov/drugoverdose/deaths/2020.html

Centers for Disease Control and Prevention (CDC). (2023d). Disparities in suicide. https://www.cdc.gov/suicide/facts/disparities-in-suicide.html

Centers for Disease Control and Prevention (CDC). (2023e). Facts about hypertension. https://www.cdc.gov/bloodpressure/facts.htm

Centers for Disease Control and Prevention (CDC). (2023f). Facts about suicide. https://www.cdc.gov/suicide/facts/index.html

Centers for Disease Control and Prevention (CDC). (2023g). Stroke facts. https://www.cdc.gov/stroke/facts.htm

Centers for Disease Control and Prevention (CDC). (2023h). Suicide rates by state. https://www.cdc.gov/suicide/suicide-rates-by-state.html

Centonze, A., Popolo, R., MacBeth, A., & Dimaggio, G. (2021). Building the alliance and using experiential techniques in the early phases of psychotherapy for avoidant personality disorder. *Journal of Clinical Psychology*, 77(5), 1219–1232.

Chadda, R. K., & Gupta, A. (2019). Looking into biological markers of suicidal behaviours. *The Indian Journal of Medical Research*, 150(4), 328–331.

Chalder, M., Elgar, F. J., & Bennett, P. (2006). Drinking and motivations to drink among adolescent children of parents with alcohol problems. *Alcohol and Alcoholism*, 41, 107–113.

Chamberlain, C., Ralph, N., Hokke, S., Clark, Y., Gee, G., Stansfield, C., . . . Healing the Past by Nurturing the Future Group. (2019). Healing the past by nurturing the future: A qualitative systematic review and meta-synthesis of pregnancy, birth and early postpartum experiences and views of parents with a history of childhood maltreatment. *PLOS One*, 14(12), e0225441. https://doi.org/10.1371/journal.pone.0225441

Chambliss, C. H. (2000). *Psychotherapy and managed care: Reconciling research and reality*. Boston: Allyn & Bacon.

Champion, H. R., Holcomb, J. B., & Young, L. A. (2009). Injuries from explosions. *Journal of Trauma*, 66, 1468–1476.

Chan, J. S. Y., Yan, J. H., & Payne, V. G. (2013). The impact of obesity and exercise on cognitive aging. *Frontiers in Aging Neuroscience*, 5, 97. doi:10.3389/fnagi.2013.00097

Chan, W., Smith, L. E., Hong, J., Greenberg, J. S., Lounds Taylor, J., & Mailick, M. R. (2018). Factors associated with sustained community employment among adults with autism and co-occurring intellectual disability. *Autism: The International Journal of Research and Practice*, 22(7), 794–803.

Chand, S. P., Kuckel, D. P., & Huecker, M. R. (2020). Cognitive behavior therapy (CBT). In *StatPearls*. StatPearls Publishing.

Chandler, J., Sisso, I., & Shapiro, D. (2020). Participant carelessness and fraud: Consequences for clinical research and potential solutions. *Journal of Abnormal Psychology*, 129, 49–55.

Chaney, M. P., Filmore, J. M., & Goodrich, K. M. (2011). No more sitting on the sidelines: Practical strategies for working with LGBT clients on issues of heterosexism and transphobia, coming out and bullying. *Counseling Today*, 53, 34–37.

Chang, W. C., Ming Hui, C. L., Yan Wong, G. H., Wa Chan, S. K., Ming Lee, E. H., & Hai Chen, E. Y. (2013). Symptomatic remission and cognitive impairment in first-episode schizophrenia: A prospective 3-year follow-up study. *Journal of Clinical Psychiatry*, 74(11), e1046–e1053.

Chang, Y., Yoon, S., Maguire-Jack, K., & Lee, J. (2022). Family-, school-, and neighborhood-level predictors of resilience for adolescents with a history of maltreatment. *Children (Basel, Switzerland)*, 10(1), 1. https://doi.org/10.3390/children10010001

Chapman, C., Gilger, K., & Chestnutt, A. (2010). The challenge of eating disorders on a college campus. *Counseling Today*, 53, 44–45.

Charernboon, T. (2020). Negative and neutral valences of affective theory of mind are more impaired than positive valence in clinically stable schizophrenia patients. *Psychiatry Investigation*, 17(5), 460–464. https://doi.org/10.30773/pi.2020.0040

Charland, L. C. (2007). Benevolent theory: Moral treatment at the York Retreat. *History of Psychiatry*, 18, 61–80.

Chartier, K., & Caetano, R. (2010). Ethnicity and health disparities in alcohol research. *Alcohol Research and Health*, 33(1/2), 152–160. http://pubs.niaaa.nih.gov/publications/arh40/152-160.pdf

Chechko, N., Stickel, S., Kellermann, T., Kirner, A., Habel, U., Fernández, G., . . . Kohn, N. (2018). Progressively analogous evidence of covert face recognition from functional magnetic resonance imaging and skin conductance responses studies involving a patient with dissociative amnesia. *European Journal of Neuroscience*, 48(3), 1964–1975.

Chee, C. L., Shorty, G., & Robinson Kurpius, S. E. (2019). Academic stress of Native American undergraduates: The role of ethnic identity, cultural congruity, and self-beliefs. *Journal of Diversity in Higher Education*, 12(1), 65–73.

Chen, A. (2019). The FDA approved a new ketamine depression drug—Here's what's next. https://www.theverge.com/2019/3/11/18260297/esketamine-fda-approval-depression-ketamine-clinic-science-health

Chen, C., Hsie, K., & Harris, A. (2017). Is it medically appropriate to involuntarily treat mentally incompetent defendants in a correctional facility? *Journal of Legal Medicine*, 37, 1–2.

Chen, P. A., Cheong, J. H., Jolly, E., Elhence, H., Wager, T. D., & Chang, L. J. (2019). Socially transmitted placebo effects. *Nature Human Behaviour*, 3, 1295–1305.

Chen, P., Li, X. H., Su, Z., Tang, Y. L., Ma, Y., Ng, C. H., & Xiang, Y. T. (2022). Characteristics of global retractions of schizophrenia-related publications: A bibliometric analysis. *Frontiers in Psychiatry*, 13, 937330. https://doi.org/10.3389/fpsyt.2022.937330

Chen, X., Zhang, G., Liang, Z., Zhang, M., Way, N., Yoshikawa, H., . . . Deng, H. (2014). The association between 5-HTTLPR gene polymorphism and behavioral inhibition in Chinese toddlers. *Developmental Psychobiology*, 56(7), 1601–1608. https://doi.org/10.1002/dev.21253

Chen, Y., Huang, X., Wu, M., Li, K., Hu, X., Jiang, P., . . . Gong, Q. (2019). Disrupted brain functional networks in drug-naïve children with attention deficit hyperactivity disorder assessed using graph theory analysis. *Human Brain Mapping*, 40(17), 4877–4887.

Cheng, Y., Xu, J., Nie, B., Luo, C., Yang, T., Li, H., . . . Xu, X. (2013). Abnormal resting-state activities and functional connectivities of the anterior and the posterior cortexes in medication-naïve patients with obsessive-compulsive disorder. *PLOS One, 8,* e67478.

Chentsova-Dutton, Y. E., Tsai, J. L., & Gotlib, I. H. (2010). Further evidence for the cultural norm hypothesis: Positive emotion in depressed and control European American and Asian American Women. *Cultural Diversity and Ethnic Minority Diversity, 16,* 284–295.

Cheong, E. V., Sinnott, C., Dahly, D., & Kearney, P. M. (2017). Adverse childhood experiences (ACEs) and later-life depression: Perceived social support as a potential protective factor. *BMJ Open, 7*(9), e013228. https://doi.org/10.1136/bmjopen-2016-013228

Cherian, A. V., Math, S. B., Kandavel, T., & Reddy, Y. C. (2014). A 5-year prospective follow-up study of patients with obsessive-compulsive disorder treated with serotonin reuptake inhibitors. *Journal of Affective Disorders, 154,* 387–394.

Chesney, M. L., & Duderstadt, K. (2022). Children's rights, environmental justice, and environmental health policy in the United States. *Journal of Pediatric Health Care: Official Publication of National Association of Pediatric Nurse Associates & Practitioners, 36*(1), 3–11. https://doi.org/10.1016/j.pedhc.2021.08.006

Chester, D. S., Lynam, D. R., Powell, D. K., & DeWall, C. N. (2016). Narcissism is associated with weakened frontostriatal connectivity: A DTI study. *Social Cognitive and Affective Neuroscience, 11*(7), 1036–1040.

Cheung, A. H., Cook, S., Kozloff, N., Chee, J. N., Mann, R. E., & Boak, A. (2019). Substance use and internalizing symptoms among high school students and access to health care services: Results from a population-based study. *Canadian Journal of Public Health, 110*(1), 85–92.

Chierigo, F., Capogrosso, P., Dehò, F., Pozzi, E., Schifano, N., Belladelli, F., . . . Salonia, A. (2019). Long-term follow-up after penile prosthesis implantation—Survival and quality of life outcomes.
Journal of Sexual Medicine, 16, 1827–1833.

Chmielewski, M., Ruggero, C. J., Kotov, R., Liu, K., & Krueger, R. F. (2017). Comparing the dependability and associations with functioning of the DSM–5 Section III trait model of personality pathology and the DSM–5 Section II personality disorder model. *Personality Disorders: Theory, Research, and Treatment, 8*(3), 228–236.

Cho, G., Betensky, R. A., & Chang, V. W. (2023). Internet usage and the prospective risk of dementia: A population-based cohort study. *Journal of the American Geriatrics Society, 71*(8), 2419–2429. https://doi.org/10.1111/jgs.18394

Chodzen, G., Hidalgo, M. A., Chen, D., & Garofalo, R. (2019). Minority stress factors associated with depression and anxiety among transgender and gender-nonconforming youth. *The Journal of Adolescent Health, 64*(4), 467–471.

Choi, K. R., Seng, J. S., Briggs, E. C., Munro-Kramer, M. L., Graham-Bermann, S. A., Lee, R. C., & Ford, J. D. (2017). The dissociative subtype of posttraumatic stress disorder (PTSD) among adolescents: Co-occurring PTSD, depersonalization/derealization, and other dissociation symptoms. *Journal of the American Academy of Child and Adolescent Psychiatry, 56*(12), 1062–1072.

Choi, K. W., Stein, M. B., Dunn, E. C., Koenen, K. C., & Smoller, J. W. (2019). Genomics and psychological resilience: A research agenda. *Molecular Psychiatry, 24*(12), 1770–1778.

Chopik, W. J., & O'Brien, E. (2017). Happy you, healthy me? Having a happy partner is independently associated with better health in oneself. *Health Psychology, 36*(1), 21–30.

Chopra, S., & Bienenfeld, D. (2011). Delusional disorder. http://emedicine.medscape.com/article/292991-overview

Choukas-Bradley, S., Nesi, J., Widman, L., & Higgins, M. K. (2019). Camera-ready: Young women's appearance-related social media consciousness. *Psychology*
of Popular Media Culture, 8(4), 473–481.

Christakis, N. A., & Fowler, J. H. (2007). The spread of obesity in a large social network over 32 years. *New England Journal of Medicine, 357,* 370–379.

Christiansen, D. M. (2016). Examining sex and gender differences in anxiety disorders. In F. Duburno (Ed.), *A fresh look at anxiety disorders.* https://www.intechopen.com/books/a-fresh-look-at-anxiety-disorders/examining-sex-and-gender-differences-in-anxiety-disorders

Christiansen, D. M., & Berke, E. T. (2020). Gender- and sex-based contributors to sex differences in PTSD. *Current Psychiatry Reports, 22*(4), 19. https://doi.org/10.1007/s11920-020-1140-y

Chu, E. K., Smith, L. M., Derauf, C., Newman, E., Neal, C. R., Arria, A. M., . . . Lester, B. M. (2020). Behavior problems during early childhood in children with prenatal methamphetamine exposure. *Pediatrics, 146*(6), e20190270. https://doi.org/10.1542/peds.2019-0270

Chung, A., & Hurley, L. (2020). U.S. Supreme Court lets states bar insanity defense. https://www.reuters.com/article/us-usa-court-insanity-idUSKBN21A2E6

Chung, Y., Haut, K. M., He, G., van Erp, T., McEwen, S., Addington, J., . . . North American Prodrome Longitudinal Study (NAPLS) Consortium. (2017). Ventricular enlargement and progressive reduction of cortical gray matter are linked in prodromal youth who develop psychosis. *Schizophrenia Research, 189,* 169–174.

Cicero, D. C., Kerns, J. G., & McCarthy, D. M. (2010). The Aberrant Salience Inventory: A new measure of psychosis proneness. *Psychological Assessment, 22,* 688–701.

Cipriani, A., Zhou, X., Del Giovane, C., Hetrick, S. E., Qin, B., Whittington, C., . . . Xie, P. (2016). Comparative efficacy and tolerability of antidepressants for major depressive disorder in children and adolescents: A network meta-analysis. *Lancet*, *388*, 881–890.

Cisewski, D. H., Santos, C., Koyfman, A., & Long, B. (2019). Approach to buprenorphine use for opioid withdrawal treatment in the emergency setting. *The American Journal of Emergency Medicine, 37*(1), 143–150.

Clark, M., Gosnell, M., Witherspoon, J., Huck, J., Hager, M., Junkin, D., . . . Robinson, T. L. (1984, December 3). A slow death of the mind. *Newsweek, 104*(22), 56–62.

Clark, R. (2006). Perceived racism and vascular reactivity in black college women: Moderating effects of seeking social support. *Health Psychology, 25*, 20–25.

Clark, S. K., Jeglic, E. L., Calkins, C., & Tatar, J. R. (2014). More than a nuisance: The prevalence and consequences of frotteurism and exhibitionism. *Sexual Abuse: A Journal of Research and Treatment, 28*, 3–19.

Clarke, K., Cooper, P., & Creswell, C. (2013). The parental overprotection scale: Associations with child and parental anxiety. *Journal of Affective Disorders, 151*(2), 618–624.

Clement, A., Wiborg, O., & Asuni, A. A. (2020). Steps towards developing effective treatments for neuropsychiatric disturbances in Alzheimer's disease: Insights from preclinical models, clinical data, and future directions. *Frontiers in Aging Neuroscience, 12*, 56. https://doi.org/10.3389/fnagi.2020.00056

Cliffe, C., Shetty, H., Himmerich, H., Schmidt, U., Stewart, R., & Dutta, R. (2020). Suicide attempts requiring hospitalization in patients with eating disorders: A retrospective cohort study. *The International Journal of Eating Disorders, 53*(5), 458–465.

Cling, B. J. (2004). Rape and rape trauma syndrome. In B. J. Cling (Ed.), *Sexualized violence against women and children: A psychology and law perspective* (pp. 13–37). New York: Guilford Press.

Cloud, J. (2010, February 13). The DSM: How psychiatrists define "disordered." *Time.* http://www.time.com/time/health

/article/0,8599,1964196,00.html?xid=rsstopstories#ixzz0fRfQE5B9

Cloud, J. (2011, January 15). The troubled life of Jared Loughner. *Time.* http://www.time.com

Cohen, N. (2009, July 28). A Rorschach cheat sheet on Wikipedia? *New York Times.*

Cohen, R., Newton-John, T., & Slater, A. (2018). "Selfie"-objectification: The role of selfies in self-objectification and disordered eating in young women. *Computers in Human Behavior, 79*, 68–74.

Cohen, Z. E., & Appelbaum, P. S. (2016). Experience and opinions of forensic psychiatrists regarding PTSD in criminal cases. *The Journal of the American Academy of Psychiatry and the Law, 44*(1), 41–52.

Coleman, D., Feigelman, W., & Rosen, Z. (2020). Association of high traditional masculinity and risk of suicide death: Secondary analysis of the Add Health Study. *JAMA Psychiatry, 77*, 435–437.

Coleman, D., Kaplan, M. S., & Casey, J. T. (2011). The social nature of male suicide: A new analytical model. *International Journal of Men's Health, 10*, 240–252.

Coleman, E., Radix, A. E., Bouman, W. P., Brown, G. R., de Vries, A. L. C., Deutsch, M. B., . . . Arcelus, J. (2022). Standards of care for the health of transgender and gender diverse people, version 8. *International Journal of Transgender Health, 23*(Suppl 1), S1–S259. https://doi.org/10.1080/26895269.2022.2100644

Collardeau, F., Corbyn, B., Abramowitz, J., Janssen, P. A., Woody, S., & Fairbrother, N. (2019). Maternal unwanted and intrusive thoughts of infant-related harm, obsessive-compulsive disorder and depression in the perinatal period: Study protocol. *BMC Psychiatry, 19*(1), 94. https://doi.org/10.1186/s12888-019-2067-x

Collins, E. (2019, February 28). Gun control: Gabby Giffords' activism is symbolic of the Democratic Party's shift on guns. *USA Today.* https://www.usatoday.com/story/news/politics/2019/02/28/gabby

-giffords-gun-control-advocate/2931938002/

Collins, J. (2013, April 26). SC woman pleads guilty, mentally ill in 4 slayings. http://news.yahoo.com/sc-woman-pleads-guilty-mentally-ill-4-slayings-191300209.html

Collins, L. M., & Coles, M. E. (2018). A preliminary investigation of pathways to inflated responsibility beliefs in children with obsessive compulsive disorder. *Behavioural and Cognitive Psychotherapy, 46*(3), 374–379.

Collip, D., Wigman, J. T. W., Lin, A., Nelson, B., Oorschot, M., Vollebergh, W. A. M., . . . Yung, A. R. (2013). Dynamic association between interpersonal functioning and positive symptom dimensions of psychosis over time: A longitudinal study of healthy adolescents. *Schizophrenia Bulletin, 39*, 179–185.

Coltheart, M., Langdon, R., & McKay, R. (2007). Schizophrenia and monothematic delusions. *Schizophrenia Bulletin, 33*, 642–647.

Colvert, E., Tick, B., McEwen, F., Stewart, C., Curran, S. R., Woodhouse, E., . . . Bolton, P. (2015). Heritability of autism spectrum disorder in a UK population-based twin sample. *JAMA Psychiatry, 72*(5), 415–423.

Conejero, I., Olié, E., Courtet, P., & Calati, R. (2018). Suicide in older adults: Current perspectives. *Clinical Interventions in Aging, 13*, 691–699.

Conner, K. R., & Bagge, C. L. (2019). Suicidal behavior: Links between alcohol use disorder and acute use of alcohol. *Alcohol Research: Current Reviews, 40*(1), arcr.v40.1.02. https://doi.org/10.35946/arcr.v40.1.02

Connolly, M. D., Zervos, M. J., Barone, C. J., Johnson, C. C., & Joseph, C. L. (2016). The mental health of transgender youth: Advances in understanding. *Journal of Adolescent Health, 59*, 489–495.

Conoley, C. W., & Scheel, M. J. (2018). *Goal focused positive psychotherapy: A strengths based approach*. New York: Oxford University Press.

Constantino, J. N., Abbacchi, A. M., Saulnier, C., Klaiman, C., Mandell, D. S., Zhang, Y., . . . Geschwind, D. H. (2020). Timing of the diagnosis of autism in African American children. *Pediatrics*, e20193629. https://doi.org/10.1542/peds.2019-3629

Conway, C. C., Hipwell, A. E., & Stepp, S. D. (2017). Seven-year course of borderline personality disorder features: Borderline pathology is as unstable as depression during adolescence. *Clinical Psychological Science*, 5(4), 742–749.

Conway, C. R., Chibnall, J. T., Gebara, M. A., Price, J. L., Snyder, A. Z., Mintun, M. A., . . . Sheline, Y. I. (2013). Association of cerebral metabolic activity changes with vagus nerve stimulation antidepressant response in treatment-resistant depression. *Brain Stimulation*, 6, 788–797.

Cook, M. L., Zhang, Y., & Constantino, J. N. (2020). On the continuity between autistic and schizoid personality disorder trait burden: A prospective study in adolescence. *The Journal of Nervous and Mental Disease*, 208(2), 94–100.

Cooper, D. (2013). First person: Avoidant personality disorder often means hiding from the world. https://drugtreatmentnewsweekly.wordpress.com/2013/05/03/first-person-avoidant-personality-disorder-often-means-hiding-from-the-world/

Cope, L. M., Munier, E. C., Trucco, E. M., Hardee, J. E., Burmeister, M., Zucker, R. A., & Heitzeg, M. M. (2017). Effects of the serotonin transporter gene, sensitivity of response to alcohol, and parental monitoring on risk for problem alcohol use. *Alcohol (Fayetteville, N.Y.)*, 59, 7–16.

Copeland, W. E., Wolke, D., Angold, A., & Costello, E. J. (2013). Adult psychiatric outcomes of bullying and being bullied by peers in childhood and adolescence. *JAMA Psychiatry*, 70, 419–426.

Coppersmith, G., Leary, R., Crutchley, P., & Fine, A. (2018). Natural language processing of social media as screening for suicide risk. *Biomedical Informatics Insights*, 10, 1178222618792860. https://doi.org/10.1177/1178222618792860

Corey, G. (2017). *Theory and practice of counseling and psychotherapy* (10th ed.). Stamford, CT: Cengage.

Corey, G., Corey, M. S., & Corey, C. (2018). *Issues and ethics in the helping professions*. Stamford, CT: Cengage.

Cornell, C. (2017). Abilify: America's once best-selling drug now offers a classic tale of big pharma greed. https://www.legalreader.com/abilify-americas-best-selling-drug-now-offers-classic-tale-big-pharma-greed/

Cornell, D., & Guerra, N. G. (2013). Gun violence: Prediction, prevention, and policy. http://www.apa.org/pubs/info/reports/gun-violence-prevention.aspx?item52

Cornic, F., Consoli, A., & Cohen, D. (2007). Catatonia in children and adolescents. *Psychiatric Annals*, 37, 19–26.

Cornum, R., Matthews, M. D., & Seligman, M. E. P. (2011). Comprehensive Soldier Fitness: Building resilience in a challenging institutional context. *American Psychologist*, 66, 4–9.

Correll, C. U., Galling, B., Pawar, A., Krivko, A., Bonetto, C., Ruggeri, M., . . . Kane, J. M. (2018). Comparison of early intervention services vs treatment as usual for early-phase psychosis: A systematic review, meta-analysis, and meta-regression. *JAMA Psychiatry*, 75(6), 555–565.

Cortés-Cortés J., Fernández, R., Teijeiro N., Gómez-Gil, E., Esteva, I., Almaraz M. C., . . . Pásaro, E. (2017). Genotypes and haplotypes of the estrogen receptor gene (ESR1) are associated with female-to-male gender dysphoria. *Journal of Sexual Medicine*, 14, 464–472.

Cortina, L. M., & Kubiak, S. P. (2006). Gender and posttraumatic stress: Sexual violence as an explanation for women's increased risk. *Journal of Abnormal Psychology*, 115, 753–759.

Cosgrove, L., & Krimsky, S. (2012). A comparison of DSM-IV and DSM-5 panel members' financial associations with industry: A pernicious problem persists. *PLOS Medicine*, 9(3), e1001190. doi:10.1371/journal.pmed.1001190

Costandache, G. I., Munteanu, O., Salaru, A., Oroian, B., & Cozmin, M. (2023). An overview of the treatment of eating disorders in adults and adolescents: Pharmacology and psychotherapy. *Postepy Psychiatrii Neurologii*, 32(1), 40–48. https://doi.org/10.5114/ppn.2023.127237

Cota, M. R., Moses, A. D., Jikaria, N. R., Bittner, K. C., Diaz-Arrastia, R. R., Latour, L. L., & Turtzo, L. C. (2019). Discordance between documented criteria and documented diagnosis of traumatic brain injury in the emergency department. *Journal of Neurotrauma*, 36(8), 1335–1342.

Cottler, L. B., Leung, K. S., & Abdallah, B. (2009). Test–re-test reliability of DSM-IV adopted criteria for 3,4-methylenedioxy-methamphetamine (MDMA) abuse and dependence: A cross-national study. *Addiction*, 104, 1679–1690.

Cougle, J. R., Mueller, N. E., McDermott, K. A., Wilver, N. L., Carlton, C. N., & Okey, S. A. (2020). Text message safety behavior reduction for social anxiety: A randomized controlled trial. *Journal of Consulting and Clinical Psychology*, 88(5), 445–454.

Cousins, N. (1979). *Anatomy of an illness*. New York: Norton.

Couturier, J., Isserlin, L., Norris, M., Spettigue, W., Brouwers, M., Kimber, M., . . . Pilon, D. (2020). Canadian practice guidelines for the treatment of children and adolescents with eating disorders. *Journal of Eating Disorders*, 8, 4. https://doi.org/10.1186/s40337-020-0277-8

Cowley, G., & Underwood, A. (1997, May 26). Why Ebonie can't breathe. *Newsweek*, 58–63.

Craig, K. D., Holmes, C., Hudspith, M., Moor, G., Moosa-Mitha, M., Varcoe, C., & Wallace, B. (2020). Pain in persons who are marginalized by social conditions. *Pain*, 161(2), 261–265.

Craigmyle, N. A. (2013). The beneficial effects of meditation: Contribution of the anterior cingulate and locus coeruleus. *Frontiers in Psychology, 4*, 731. doi:10.3389/fpsyg.2013.00731

Cramer, R. J., Judah, M. R., Badger, N. L., Holley, A. M., Judd, S., Peterson, M., . . . Foss, J. J. (2022). Suicide on college campuses: A public health framework and case illustration. *Journal of American College Health, 70*(1), 1–8. https://doi.org/10.1080/07448481.2020.1739053

Cropley, V. L., Klauser, P., Lenroot, R. K., Bruggemann, J., Sundram, S., Bousman, C., . . . Zalesky, A. (2017). Accelerated gray and white matter deterioration with age in schizophrenia. *American Journal of Psychiatry, 174*(3), 286–295.

Crow, S. J., Peterson, C. B., Swanson, S. A., Raymond, N. C., Specker, S., Eckert, E. D., & Mitchell, J. E. (2009). Increased mortality in bulimia nervosa and other eating disorders. *American Journal of Psychiatry, 166*, 1342–1346.

Crowell, J. A., Keluskar, J., & Gorecki, A. (2019). Parenting behavior and the development of children with autism spectrum disorder. *Comprehensive Psychiatry, 90*, 21–29.

Crowell-Williamson, G. A., Fruhbauerova, M., DeCou, C. R., & Comtois, K. A. (2019). Perceived burdensomeness, bullying, and suicidal ideation in suicidal military personnel. *Journal of Clinical Psychology, 75*, 2147–2159.

Crowley, N. A., Dao, N. C., Magee, S. N., Bourcier, A. J., & Lowery-Gionta, E. G. (2019). Animal models of alcohol use disorder and the brain: From casual drinking to dependence. *Translational Issues in Psychological Science, 5*(3), 222–242.

Csipke, E., & Horne, O. (2007). Pro-eating disorder websites: Users' opinions. *European Eating Disorders Review, 15*, 196–206.

Csonka, B., & Hevesi, K. (2022). Do pornography use and masturbation play a role in erectile dysfunction and relationship satisfaction in men? *International Journal of Impotence Research, 35*(6), 548–557. https://doi.org/10.1038/s41443-022-00596-y

Cuperfain, A. B., Furqan, Z., Sinyor, M., Mulsant, B. H., Shulman, K., Kurdyak, P., & Zaheer, J. (2022). A qualitative analysis of suicide notes to understand suicidality in older adults. *The American Journal of Geriatric Psychiatry: Official Journal of the American Association for Geriatric Psychiatry, 30*(12), 1330–1338.

Czech, H. (2018). Hans Asperger, national socialism, and "race hygiene" in Nazi-era Vienna. *Molecular Autism, 9*, 29. https://doi.org/10.1186/s13229-018-0208-6

D'Amico, E. J., Parast, L., Shadel, W. G., Meredith, L. S., Seelam, R., & Stein, B. D. (2018). Brief motivational interviewing intervention to reduce alcohol and marijuana use for at-risk adolescents in primary care. *Journal of Consulting and Clinical Psychology, 86*(9), 775–786.

d'Huart, D., Seker, S., Bürgin, D., Birkhölzer, M., Boonmann, C., Schmid, M., & Schmeck, K. (2023). The stability of personality disorders and personality disorder criteria: A systematic review and meta-analysis. *Clinical Psychology Review, 102*, 102284. https://doi.org/10.1016/j.cpr.2023.102284

D'Onofrio, B. M., Class, Q. A., Rickert, M. E., Larsson, H., Långström, N., & Lichtenstein, P. (2013). Preterm birth and mortality and morbidity: A population-based quasi-experimental study. *JAMA Psychiatry, 70*, 1231–1240.

D'Souza, D. C., Ganesh, S., Cortes-Briones, J., Campbell, M. H., & Emmanuel, M. K. (2020, October). Characterizing psychosis-relevant phenomena and cognitive function in a unique population with isolated, chronic and very heavy cannabis exposure. *Psychological Medicine, 50*(14), 2452–2459. doi: 10.1017/S0033291719002721

Dahlenburg, S. C., Gleaves, D. H., & Hutchinson, A. D. (2019). Anorexia nervosa and perfectionism: A meta-analysis. *The International Journal of Eating Disorders, 52*(3), 219–229.

Dahlhamer, J., Lucas, J., Zelaya, C., Nahin, R., Mackey, S., DeBar, L., . . . Helmick, C. (2018). Prevalence of chronic pain and high-impact chronic pain among adults: United States, 2016. *MMWR. Morbidity and Mortality Weekly Report, 67*(36), 1001–1006.

Dai, Y. X., Chen, M. H., & Chen, T. J. (2016). Low prevalence of the use of the Chinese term for "psychiatry" in the names of community psychiatry clinics: A nationwide study in Taiwan. *International Journal of Social Psychiatry, 62*, 601–607.

Dalenberg, C. J., Brand, B. L., Gleaves, D. H., Dorahy, M. J., Loewenstein, R. J., Cardeña, E., . . . Spiegel, D. (2012). Evaluation of the evidence for the trauma and fantasy models of dissociation. *Psychological Bulletin, 138*(3), 550–588. doi:10.1037/a0027447

Dalles, S. K., Liu, P. J., & Ubel, P. A. (2019). Don't count calorie labeling out: Calorie counts on the left side of menu items lead to lower calorie food choices. *Journal of Consumer Psychology, 29*, 60–69.

Dambrauskiene, K., Adomaitiene, V., Zalinkevicius, R., Jariene, G., Vilkas, V., Rybakova, I., & Dunderiene, L. (2019). Can suicide attempt be related to problem drinking: Cohort study. *Alcohol and Alcoholism, 54*, 104–111.

Dams-O'Conner, K., Martens, M. P., & Anderson, D. A. (2006). Alcohol-related consequences among women who want to lose weight. *Eating Behaviors, 7*, 188–195.

Danielson, M. L., Bitsko, R. H., Ghandour, R. M., Holbrook, J. R., Kogan, M. D., & Blumberg, S. J. (2018). Prevalence of parent-reported ADHD diagnosis and associated treatment among U.S. children and adolescents, 2016. *Journal of Clinical Child and Adolescent Psychology: The Official Journal for the Society of Clinical Child and Adolescent Psychology, American Psychological Association, Division 53, 47*(2), 199–212. https://doi.org/10.1080/15374416.2017.1417860

Danielson, M. L., Holbrook, J. R., Bitsko, R. H., Newsome, K., Charania, S. N., McCord, R. F., Kogan, M. D., & Blumberg, S. J. (2022). State-Level Estimates of the Prevalence of Parent-Reported ADHD Diagnosis and Treatment Among U.S. Children and Adolescents, 2016 to 2019. *Journal of Attention Disorders, 26*(13), 1685–1697. https://doi.org/10.1177/10870547221099961

Dantchev, S., Zammit, S., & Wolke, D. (2018). Sibling bullying in middle childhood and psychotic disorder at 18 years: A prospective cohort study. *Psychological Medicine, 48*(14), 2321–2328.

Dao, J. (2011, December 1). After duty, dogs suffer like soldiers. *New York Times.* http://www.nytimes.com

Dardick, H. (2004, February 13). Psychiatric patient tells of ordeal in treatment. *Chicago Tribune,* p. 1.

Dargis, M., & Koenigs, M. (2018). Two subtypes of psychopathic criminals differ in negative affect and history of childhood abuse. *Psychological Trauma: Theory, Research, Practice and Policy, 10*(4), 444–451.

Drapalski, A. L., Lucksted, A., Brown, C. H., & Fang, L. J. (2021). Outcomes of ending self-stigma, a group intervention to reduce internalized stigma, among individuals with serious mental illness. *Psychiatric Services, 72*(2), 136–142.

Darnton-Hill, I. (2017). Iodine in pregnancy and lactation. https://www.who.int/elena/titles/bbc/iodine_pregnancy/en/

Dashineau, S. C., Edershile, E. A., Simms, L. J., & Wright, A. (2019). Pathological narcissism and psychosocial functioning. *Personality Disorders, 10*(5), 473–478.

Daskalakis, N. P., Rijal, C. M., King, C., Huckins, L. M., & Ressler, K. J. (2018). Recent genetics and epigenetics approaches to PTSD. *Current Psychiatry Reports, 20*(5), 30. https://doi.org/10.1007/s11920-018-0898-7

Das-Munshi, J., Bécares, L., Boydell, J. E., Dewey, M. E., Morgan, C., Stansfeld, S. A., & Prince, M. J. (2012). Ethnic density as a buffer for psychotic experiences: Findings from a national survey (EMPIRIC). *British Journal of Psychiatry, 201,* 282–290.

Datar, A., & Nicosia, N. (2018). Assessing social contagion in body mass index, overweight, and obesity using a natural experiment. *JAMA Pediatrics, 172*(3), 239–246.

Datar, A., Nicosia, N., Mahler, A., Prados, M. J., & Ghosh-Dastidar, M. (2023). Association of place with adolescent obesity. *JAMA Pediatrics, 177*(8), 847–855. https://doi.org/10.1001/jamapediatrics.2023.1329

Davenport, K., Hardy, G., Tai, S., & Mansell, W. (2019). Individual experiences of psychological-based interventions for bipolar disorder: A systematic review and thematic synthesis. *Psychology and Psychotherapy, 92*(4), 499–522.

Davico, C., Amianto, F., Gaiotti, F., Lasorsa, C., Peloso, A., Bosia, C., . . . Vitiello, B. (2019). Clinical and personality characteristics of adolescents with anorexia nervosa with or without non-suicidal self-injurious behavior. *Comprehensive Psychiatry, 94,* 152115. https://doi.org/10.1016/j.comppsych.2019.152115

David. (2010). Child psychology research blog: Autism and Asperger's in the DSM-V. Thoughts on clinical utility. https://www.childpsych.org/autism-and-aspergers-in-the-dsm-v-going-beyond-the-politics.html

Davidson, K., Norrie, J., & Palmer, S. (2008). The effectiveness of cognitive behavior therapy for borderline personality disorder: Results from the borderline personality disorder study of cognitive therapy (BOSCOT) trial. *Journal of Personality Disorders, 20,* 450– 465.

Davidson, L. (2016). The recovery movement: Implications for mental health care and enabling people to participate fully in life. *Health Affairs, 35,* 1091–1097.

Davidson, M. (2018). The debate regarding maintenance treatment with antipsychotic drugs in schizophrenia. *Dialogues in Clinical Neuroscience, 20*(3), 215–221.

Davis, M. A., Lin, L. A., Liu, H., & Sites, B. D. (2017). Prescription opioid use among adults with mental health disorders in the United States. *Journal of the American Board of Family Medicine, 30*(4), 407–417.

Davis, M. P., Digwood, G., Mehta, Z., & McPherson, M. L. (2020). Tapering opioids: A comprehensive qualitative review. *Annals of Palliative Medicine, 9*(2), 586–610.

Davis, R. F., 3rd, & Kiang, L. (2016). Religious identity, religious participation, and psychological well-being in Asian American adolescents. *Journal of Youth and Adolescence, 45*(3), 532–546.

Davison, M., & Furnham, A. (2018). The personality disorder profile of professional actors. *Psychology of Popular Media Culture, 7*(1), 33–46.

Dawson, G. (2023). Could an eye-tracking test aid clinicians in making an autism diagnosis? New findings and a look to the future. *JAMA, 330*(9), 815–817. https://doi.org/10.1001/jama.2023.3092

de Boer, J. N., Brederoo, S. G., Voppel, A. E., & Sommer, I. (2020). Anomalies in language as a biomarker for schizophrenia. *Current Opinion in Psychiatry, 33*(3), 212–218.

De Geus, E. J. C., Kupper, N., Boomsma, D. I., & Snieder, H. (2007). Bivariate genetic modeling of cardiovascular stress reactivity: Does stress uncover genetic variance? *Psychosomatic Medicine, 69,* 356–364.

de Jonge, P., Roest, A. M., Lim, C. C., Florescu, S. E., Bromet, E. J., Stein, D. J., . . . Scott, K. M. (2016). Cross-national epidemiology of panic disorder and panic attacks in the world mental health surveys. *Depression and Anxiety, 33*(12), 1155–1177.

De Leo, D., Milner, A., Fleischmann, A., Bertolote, J., Collings, S., Amadeo, S., . . . Wang, X. (2013). Suicidal behaviors across different areas of the world. *Crisis, 34,* 156–163.

De Martino, E. (2005). *The land of remorse: A study of southern Italian tarantism* (translated by D. L. Zinn with an introduction by V. Crapanzano). London: Free Association Books.

de Miranda Neto, A. A., de Moura, D., Ribeiro, I. B., Khan, A., Singh, S., da Ponte Neto, A. M., . . . de Moura, E. (2020). Efficacy and safety of endoscopic sleeve gastroplasty at mid term in the management of overweight and obese patients: A systematic review and meta-analysis. *Obesity Surgery, 30*(5), 1971–1987.

De Neef, N., Coppens, V., Huys, W., & Morrens, M. (2019). Bondage: Discipline, dominance-submission and sadomasochism (BDSM) from an integrative biopsychosocial perspective. A systematic review. *Sexual Medicine, 7*(2), 129–144. https://doi.org/10.1016/j.esxm .2019.02.002

de Rossi, P. (2010). *Unbearable lightness: A story of loss and gain.* Chicago: Atria.

De Sanctis, V., Soliman, N., Soliman, A. T., Elsedfy, H., Di Maio, S., El Kholy, M., & Fiscina, B. (2017). Caffeinated energy drink consumption among adolescents and potential health consequences associated with their use: A significant public health hazard. *Acta Biomedica: Atenei Parmensis, 88*(2), 222–231.

De Smet, M. M., Meganck, R., De Geest, R., Norman, U. A., Truijens, F., & Desmet, M. (2020). What "good outcome" means to patients: Understanding recovery and improvement in psychotherapy for major depression from a mixed-methods perspective. *Journal of Counseling Psychology, 67*(1), 25–39.

De Vries, Y., Roest, A., De Jonge, P., Cuijpers, P., Munafò, M., & Bastiaansen, J. (2018). The cumulative effect of reporting and citation biases on the apparent efficacy of treatments: The case of depression. *Psychological Medicine, 48*, 2453–2455.

De Wit-De Visser, B., Rijckmans, M., Vermunt, J. K., & van Dam, A. (2023). Pathways to antisocial behavior: A framework to improve diagnostics and tailor therapeutic interventions. *Frontiers in Psychology, 14*, 993090. https://doi .org/10.3389/fpsyg.2023.993090

De Young, K. P., Zander, M., & Anderson, D. A. (2014). Beliefs about the emotional consequences of eating and binge eating frequency. *Eating Behaviors, 15*, 31–36.

de Zeeuw, E. L., van Beijsterveldt, C., Hoekstra, R. A., Bartels, M., &

Boomsma, D. I. (2017). The etiology of autistic traits in preschoolers: A population-based twin study. *Journal of Child Psychology and Psychiatry, and Allied Disciplines, 58*(8), 893–901.

DeAngelis, T. (2019). The legacy of trauma. *APA Monitor.* https:// www.apa.org/monitor/2019/02 /legacy-trauma

Decety, J., Michalska, K. J., Akitsuki, Y., & Lahey, B. B. (2009). Atypical empathic responses in adolescents with aggressive conduct disorder: A functional MRI investigation. *Biological Psychology, 80*, 203–211.

DeCou, C. R., Comtois, K. A., & Landes, S. J. (2019). Dialectical behavior therapy is effective for the treatment of suicidal behavior: A meta-analysis. *Behavior Therapy, 50*(1), 60–72.

Degnan, K. A., & Fox, N. A. (2007). Behavioral inhibition and anxiety disorders: Multiple levels of a resilience process. *Development and Psychopathology, 19*, 729–746.

DeJong, C., Aguilar, T., Tseng, C. W., Lin, G. A., Boscardin, W. J., & Dudley, R. A. (2016). Pharmaceutical industry-sponsored meals and physician prescribing patterns for Medicare beneficiaries. *JAMA Internal Medicine, 176*, 1114–1122.

Delaney, A. J., Crane, J. W., Holmes, N. M., Fam, J., & Westbrook, R. F. (2018). Baclofen acts in the central amygdala to reduce synaptic transmission and impair context fear conditioning. *Scientific Reports, 8*(1), 1–11.

DeLany, J. P., Jakicic, J. M., Lowery, J. B., Hames, K. C., Kelley, D. E., & Goodpaster, B. H. (2013, December 19). African American women exhibit similar adherence to intervention but lose less weight due to lower energy requirements. *International Journal of Obesity.* doi:10.1038/ ijo.2013.240

DeLisi, M., Drury, A. J., & Elbert, M. J. (2019). The etiology of antisocial personality disorder: The differential roles of adverse childhood experiences and childhood psychopathology. *Comprehensive Psychiatry, 92*, 1–6.

Demakis, D. J. (2013). State statutory definitions of civil incompetency/ incapacity: Issues for psychologists. *Psychology, Public Policy, and Law, 19*, 331–342.

Demmler, J. C., Brophy, S. T., Marchant, A., John, A., & Tan, J. (2020). Shining the light on eating disorders, incidence, prognosis and profiling of patients in primary and secondary care: National data linkage study. *The British Journal of Psychiatry, 216*(2), 105–112.

Dempsey, C., Quanbeck, C., Bush, C., & Kruger, K. (2019). Decriminalizing mental illness: Specialized policing responses. *CNS Spectrums,* 1–15. doi:10.1017 /S1092852919001640

den Boer, C., Dries, L., Terluin, B., van der Wouden, J. C., Blankenstein, A. H., van Wilgen, C. P., . . . van der Horst, H. E. (2019). Central sensitization in chronic pain and medically unexplained symptom research: A systematic review of definitions, operationalizations and measurement instruments. *Journal of Psychosomatic Research, 117*, 32–40.

Denney, J. T. (2010). Family and household formations and suicide in the United States. *Journal of Marriage and Family, 72*, 202–213.

Denney, J. T., Rogers, R. G., Krueger, P. M., & Wadsworth, T. (2009). Adult suicide mortality in the United States: Marital status, family size, socioeconomic status, and differences by sex. *Social Science Quarterly, 90*, 1167–1185.

Desai, G., & Chaturvedi, S. K. (2017). Idioms of distress. *Journal of Neurosciences in Rural Practice, 8*(1), S94–S97. https:// doi.org/10.4103/jnrp.jnrp_235_17

Desmond, S., Price, J., Hallinan, C., & Smith, D. (1989). Black and white adolescents' perceptions of their weight. *Journal of School Health, 59*, 353–358.

DeStefano, F., & Shimabukuro, T. T. (2020). The MMR vaccine and autism. *Annual Review of Virology, 6*, 585–600.

Detka, J., Kurek, A., Basta-Kaim, A., Kubera, M., Lasoń, W., & Budziszewska, B. (2013). Neuroendocrine link between stress, depression and diabetes.

Pharmacological Reports, 65, 1591–1600.

DeVille, D. C., Kuplicki, R., Stewart, J. L., Tulsa 1000 Investigators, Aupperle, R. L., Bodurka, J., . . . Khalsa, S. S. (2020). Diminished responses to bodily threat and blunted interoception in suicide attempters. *eLife, 9,* e51593. https://doi.org/10.7554 /eLife.51593

Dewald-Kaufmann, J., de Bruin, E., & Michael, G. (2019). Cognitive behavioral therapy for insomnia (CBT-i) in school-aged children and adolescents. *Sleep Medicine Clinics, 14*(2), 155–165.

Deyama, S., & Duman, R. S. (2020). Neurotrophic mechanisms underlying the rapid and sustained antidepressant actions of ketamine. *Pharmacology, Biochemistry, and Behavior, 188,* 172837. https://doi.org/10.1016 /j.pbb.2019.172837

Di Forti, M., Quattrone, D., Freeman, T. P., Tripoli, G., Gayer-Anderson, C., Quigley, H., . . . EU-GEI WP2 Group. (2019). The contribution of cannabis use to variation in the incidence of psychotic disorder across Europe (EU-GEI): A multicentre case-control study. *The Lancet: Psychiatry, 6*(5), 427–436.

di Giacomo, E., Krausz, M., Colmegna, F., Aspesi, F., & Clerici, M. (2018). Estimating the risk of attempted suicide among sexual minority youths: A systematic review and meta-analysis. *JAMA Pediatrics, 172,* 1145–1152.

Diaconescu, A. O., Hauke, D. J., & Borgwardt, S. (2019). Models of persecutory delusions: A mechanistic insight into the early stages of psychosis. *Molecular Psychiatry, 24*(9), 1258–1267.

Dickenson, J. A., Gleason, N., Coleman, E., & Miner, M. H. (2018). Prevalence of distress associated with difficulty controlling sexual urges, feelings, and behaviors in the United States. *JAMA Network Open, 1*(7), e184468. https://doi.org/10.1001 /jamanetworkopen.2018.4468

Dickerman, A. L., & Jiménez, X. F. (2023). Psychosocial and psychodynamic considerations informing factitious disorder. *Psychodynamic Psychiatry, 51*(1),

98–113. https://doi.org/10.1521 /pdps.2023.51.1.98

Dickinson, D., Zaidman, S. R., Giangrande, E. J., Eisenberg, D. P., Gregory, M. D., & Berman, K. F. (2020). Distinct polygenic score profiles in schizophrenia subgroups with different trajectories of cognitive development. *American Journal of Psychiatry, 177*(4), 298–307.

DiClemente, C. C., Corno, C. M., Graydon, M. M., Wiprovnick, A. E., & Knoblach, D. J. (2017). Motivational interviewing, enhancement, and brief interventions over the last decade: A review of reviews of efficacy and effectiveness. *Psychology of Addictive Behaviors: Journal of the Society of Psychologists in Addictive Behaviors, 31*(8), 862–887. https://doi.org/10.1037 /adb0000318

Diflorio, A., & Jones, I. (2010). Is sex important? Gender differences in bipolar disorder. *International Review of Psychiatry, 22,* 437–452.

Difrancesco, S., Lamers, F., Riese, H., Merikangas, K. R., Beekman, A., van Hemert, A. M., . . . Penninx, B. (2019). Sleep, circadian rhythm, and physical activity patterns in depressive and anxiety disorders: A 2-week ambulatory assessment study. *Depression and Anxiety, 36*(10), 975–986.

DiFranza, J. R., Savageau, J. A., Fletcher, K., Pbert, L., O'Loughlin, J., McNeill, A. D., . . . Wellman, R. J. (2007). Susceptibility to nicotine dependence: The Development and Assessment of Nicotine Dependence in Youth 2 study. *Pediatrics, 120,* 974–983.

Diles, K. (2013). My story. https:// www.save.org/index.cfm ?fuseaction5home.viewPage &page_id584B187C2-D156 -503D-6B56FA19D6126E5B &previewMode5true&r51

Dilks, S., Tasker, F., & Wren, B. (2010). Managing the impact of psychosis: A grounded theory exploration of recovery processes in psychosis. *British Journal of Clinical Psychology, 49,* 87–107.

Ding, K., Chang, G. A., & Southerland, R. (2009). Age of inhalant first time use and its association to

the use of other drugs. *Journal of Drug Education, 39,* 261–272.

Disney K. L. (2013). Dependent personality disorder: A critical review. *Clinical Psychology Review, 33*(8), 1184–1196.

Doane, L. D., & Zeiders, K. H. (2013). Contextual moderators of momentary cortisol and negative affect in adolescents' daily lives. *Journal of Adolescent Health, 54,* 536–542.

Dobrescu, S. R., Dinkler, L., Gillberg, C., Råstam, M., Gillberg, C., & Wentz, E. (2020). Anorexia nervosa: 30-year outcome. *The British Journal of Psychiatry, 216*(2), 97–104.

Dominguez, M. D. G., Saka, M. C., Lieb, R., Wittchan, H.-U., & Van Os, J. (2010). Early expression of negative/disorganized symptoms predicting psychotic experiences and subsequent clinical psychosis: A 10-year study. *American Journal of Psychiatry, 167,* 1075–1082.

Dondé, C., Moirand, R., & Carre, A. (2018). Behavioral activation programs: A tool for treating depression efficiently. *L'Encephale, 44*(1), 59–66.

Donker, T., Cornelisz, I., van Klaveren, C., van Straten, A., Carlbring, P., Cuijpers, P., & van Gelder, J. L. (2019). Effectiveness of self-guided app-based virtual reality cognitive behavior therapy for acrophobia: A randomized clinical trial. *JAMA Psychiatry, 76*(7), 682–690.

Donkor, E. S. (2018). Stroke in the 21st century: A snapshot of the burden, epidemiology, and quality of life. *Stroke Research and Treatment, 2018,* 3238165. https://doi .org/10.1155/2018/3238165

Donnelly, M. (2015). Bruce Jenner reveals to Diane Sawyer: "Yes, I am a woman." http://www.msn .com/en-us/tv/news/bruce-jenner -reveals-to-diane-sawyer-%E2 %80%98yes-i-am-a-woman %E2%80%99/ar-BBiEgXM

Donovan, A. P., & Basson, M. A. (2017). The neuroanatomy of autism—A developmental perspective. *Journal of Anatomy, 230*(1), 4–15.

Donovan, M. H., & Tecott, L. H. (2013). Serotonin and the regulation of mammalian energy balance. *Frontiers in Neuroscience.* doi:10.3389/fnins.2013.00036

Dorahy, M. J., Shannon, C., Seagar, L., Corr, M., Stewart, K., Hanna, D., . . . Middleton, W. (2009). Auditory hallucinations in dissociative identity disorder and schizophrenia with and without a childhood trauma history: Similarities and differences. *Journal of Nervous and Mental Disease, 197,* 892–898.

Döring, N., Daneback, K., Shaughnessy, K., Grov, C., & Byers, E. S. (2017). Online sexual activity experiences among college students: A four-country comparison. *Archives of Sexual Behavior, 46*(6), 1641–1652.

Doroszkiewicz, J., Groblewska, M., & Mroczko, B. (2021). The role of gut microbiota and gut-brain interplay in selected diseases of the central nervous system. *International Journal of Molecular Sciences, 22*(18), 10028. https://doi.org/10.3390/ijms221810028

Dos Reis, M. J., Lopes, M., & Osis, M. (2017). "It's much worse than dying": The experiences of female victims of sexual violence. *Journal of Clinical Nursing, 26*(15–16), 2353–2361.

Doting, R. (2022). A psychiatric patient confesses to murder: Now what? https://www.medscape.com/viewarticle/974470?

Dotterer, H. L., Waller, R., Shaw, D. S., Plass, J., Brang, D., Forbes, E. E., & Hyde, L. W. (2019). Antisocial behavior with callous-unemotional traits is associated with widespread disruptions to white matter structural connectivity among low-income, urban males. *NeuroImage. Clinical, 23,* 101836. https://doi.org/10.1016/j.nicl.2019.101836

Doughty, O. J., Lawrence, V. A., Al-Mousawi, A., Ashaye, K., & Done, D. J. (2009). Overinclusive thought and loosening of associations are not unique to schizophrenia and are produced in Alzheimer's dementia. *Cognitive Neuropsychiatry, 14,* 149–164.

Douzenis, A. (2016). The importance of the patients deemed not guilty by reason of insanity for the psychiatric reform. *Psychiatriki, 27*(3), 165–168.

Dovey, D. (2015). Deemed "too skinny to treat," anorexic woman goes public for help. http://www.msn.com/en-us/health/medical/deemed-too-skinny-to-treat-anorexic-woman-goes-public-for-help/ar-BBk4Gbp

Dowgwillo, E. A., Pincus, A. L., & Lenzenweger, M. F. (2019). A parallel process latent growth model of narcissistic personality disorder symptoms and normal personality traits. *Personality Disorders, 10*(3), 257–266.

Downey, R., III, Gold, P. M., Rowley, J. A., Wickramasinghe, H., Sharma, S., Talavera, F., . . . Mosenifar, Z. (2013). Obstructive sleep apnea. http://emedicine.medscape.com/article/295807-overview#a0156

Drapeau, C. W., Lockman, J. D., Moore, M. M., & Cerel, J. (2019). Predictors of posttraumatic growth in adults bereaved by suicide. *Crisis, 40*(3), 196–202.

Dreher, D. E. (2013). Abnormal psychology in the Renaissance. In T. G. Plante (Ed.), *Abnormal psychology across the ages. Vol. I: History and conceptualizations* (pp. 33–50). Santa Barbara, CA: Praeger/ABC-CLIO.

Dreier, H. (2020). Trust and consequences. https://www.msn.com/en-us/news/us/trust-and-consequences/ar-BB102nlj?li=BBnb7Kz

Drum, D. J., Brownson, C., Denmark, A. B., & Smith, S. E. (2009). New data on the nature of suicidal crisis in college students: Shifting the paradigm. *Professional Psychology: Research and Practice, 40,* 213–222.

D'Souza, D. C., Ganesh, S., Cortes-Briones, J., Campbell, M. H., & Emmanuel, M. K. (2020). Characterizing psychosis-relevant phenomena and cognitive function in a unique population with isolated, chronic and very heavy cannabis exposure. *Psychological Medicine, 50*(14), 2452–2459. https://doi.org/10.1017/S0033291719002721

Dubow, E. F., Huesmann, L. R., Boxer, P., Smith, C., Landau, S. F., Dvir Gvirsman, S., & Shikaki, K. (2019). Serious violent behavior and antisocial outcomes as consequences of exposure to ethnic-political conflict and violence among Israeli and Palestinian youth. *Aggressive Behavior, 45*(3), 287–299.

Dudley, R., Siitarinen, J., James, I., & Dodson, G. (2009). What do people with psychosis think caused their psychosis? A Q methodology study. *Behavioural and Cognitive Psychotherapy, 37,* 11–24.

Dudley, R., Taylor, P., Wickham, S., & Hutton, P. (2016). Psychosis, delusions and the "jumping to conclusions" reasoning bias: A systematic review and meta-analysis. *Schizophrenia Bulletin, 42*(3), 652–665.

Duffy, A., Carlson, G., Dubicka, B., & Hillegers, M. (2020). Prepubertal bipolar disorder: Origins and current status of the controversy. *International Journal of Bipolar Disorders, 8*(1), 18. https://doi.org/10.1186/s40345-020-00185-2

Dugré, J. R., Bitar, N., Dumais, A., & Potvin, S. (2019). Limbic hyperactivity in response to emotionally neutral stimuli in schizophrenia: A neuroimaging meta-analysis of the hypervigilant mind. *The American Journal of Psychiatry, 176*(12), 1021–1029.

Dunham, D. (2012). "Skinny doesn't sell" so disturbing trend has models airbrushed to look fatter. http://www.blisstree.com/2012/08/23/beauty-shopping/

Dunlap, S. (2019). Butte psychiatrist with troubled past faces new suit alleging negligence. https://mtstandard.com/news/local/butte-psychiatrist-with-troubled-past-faces-new-suit-alleging-negligence/article

Dunlop, B. W., Still, S., LoParo, D., Aponte-Rivera, V., Johnson, B. N., Schneider, R. L., . . . Craighead W. E. (2020). Somatic symptoms in treatment-naïve Hispanic and non-Hispanic patients with major depression. *Depression and Anxiety, 37,* 156–165.

Dunn, B. D., Widnall, E., Warbrick, L., Warner, F., Reed, N., Price, A., . . . Kuyken, W. (2023). Preliminary clinical and cost effectiveness of augmented depression therapy versus cognitive behavioural therapy for the treatment of anhedonic depression (ADepT):

A single-centre, open-label, parallel-group, pilot, randomised, controlled trial. *EClinical-Medicine*, 61, 102084. https://doi.org/10.1016/j.eclinm.2023.102084

Dunn, E. C., Soare T. W., Zhu, Y., Simpkin, A. J., Suderman, M. J., Klengel, T., . . . Relton, C. L. (2019). Sensitive periods for the effect of childhood adversity on DNA methylation: Results from a prospective, longitudinal study. *Biological Psychiatry*, 85, 838–849.

Dunne, L., Perich, T., & Meade, T. (2019). The relationship between social support and personal recovery in bipolar disorder. *Psychiatric Rehabilitation Journal*, 42(1), 100–103.

Durkheim, É. (1951). *Suicide*. New York: Free Press. (Original work published 1897)

Durso, L. E., Latner, J. D., White, M. A., Masheb, R. M., Blomquist, K. K., Morgan, P. T., & Grilo, C. M. (2012). Internalized weight bias in obese patients with binge eating disorder: Associations with eating disturbances and psychological functioning. *International Journal of Eating Disorders*, 45, 423–427.

Durwood, L., McLaughlin, K. A., & Olson, K. R. (2017). Mental health and self-worth in socially transitioned transgender youth. *Journal of the American Academy of Child and Adolescent Psychiatry*, 56(2), 116–123.

Dworkin, A. (2009, November 11). After stroke, Portland woman's brain on the rebound [Blog post]. http://www.oregonlive.com/health/index.ssf/2009/11/after_stroke_portland_womans_b.html

Dworkin, E. R., DeCou, C. R., & Fitzpatrick, S. (2020). Associations between sexual assault and suicidal thoughts and behavior: A meta-analysis. *Psychological Trauma: Theory, Research, Practice, and Policy*, 14(7), 1208–1211.

Dworkin, E. R., Jaffe, A. E., Bedard-Gilligan, M., & Fitzpatrick, S. (2023). PTSD in the year following sexual assault: A meta-analysis of prospective studies. *Trauma, Violence & Abuse*, 24(2), 497–514. https://doi.org/10.1177/15248380211032213

Dworkin, E. R., Wanklyn, S., Stasiewicz, P. R., & Coffey, S. F. (2018). PTSD symptom presentation among people with alcohol and drug use disorders: Comparisons by substance of abuse. *Addictive Behaviors*, 76, 188–194.

Dwulit, A. D., & Rzymski, P. (2019). The potential associations of pornography use with sexual dysfunctions: An integrative literature review of observational studies. *Journal of Clinical Medicine*, 8, 914. https://doi.org/10.3390/jcm8070914

Dye, L., Boyle, N. B., Champ, C., & Lawton, C. (2017). The relationship between obesity and cognitive health and decline. *Proceedings of the Nutrition Society*, 76(4), 443–454.

Easter, M. M., Swanson, J. W., Robertson, A. G., Moser, L. L., & Swartz, M. S. (2020, February 4). Impact of psychiatric advance directive facilitation on mental health consumers: Empowerment, treatment attitudes and the role of peer support specialists. *Journal of Mental Health*, 1–9.

Eberhart, N. K. (2011). Maladaptive schemas and depression: Tests of stress generation and diathesis-stress models. *Journal of Social and Clinical Psychology*, 30, 75–104.

Economou, A., Pavlou, D., Beratis, I., Andronas, N., Papadimitriou, E., Papageorgiou, S. G., & Yannis, G. (2020). Predictors of accidents in people with mild cognitive impairment, mild dementia due to Alzheimer's disease and healthy controls in simulated driving. *International Journal of Geriatric Psychiatry*, 35(8), 859–869.

Eddy, K. T., Tabri, N., Thomas, J. J., Murray, H. B., Keshaviah, A., Hastings, E., . . . Franko, D. L. (2017). Recovery from anorexia nervosa and bulimia nervosa at 22-year follow-up. *The Journal of Clinical Psychiatry*, 78(2), 184–189.

Edenberg, H. J., & McClintick, J. N. (2018). Alcohol dehydrogenases, aldehyde dehydrogenases, and alcohol use disorders: A critical review. *Alcoholism, Clinical and Experimental Research*, 42(12), 2281–2297.

Edens, J. F., Davis, K. M., Fernandez Smith, K., & Guy, L. S. (2013). No sympathy for the devil: Attributing psychopathic traits to capital murderers also predicts support for executing them. *Personality Disorders*, 4, 175–181.

Editorial Team. (2017, February 23). How does Parkinson's disease develop? ParkinsonsDisease.net. https://parkinsonsdisease.net/basics/pathophysiology-what-is-it/

Edmonds, E. C., Martin, A. S., Palmer, B. W., Eyler, L. T., Rana, B. K., & Jeste, D. V. (2018). Positive mental health in schizophrenia and healthy comparison groups: Relationships with overall health and biomarkers. *Aging & Mental Health*, 22(3), 354–362.

Edvardsen, J., Torgersen, S., Røysamb, E., Lygren, S., Skre, I., Onstad, S., & Oien, P. A. (2008). Heritability of bipolar spectrum disorders: Unity or heterogeneity? *Journal of Affective Disorders*, 106, 229–240.

Efrati, S., Hadanny, A., Daphna-Tekoah, S., Bechor, Y., Tiberg, K., Pik, N., . . . Lev-Wiesel, R. (2018). Recovery of repressed memories in fibromyalgia patients treated with hyperbaric oxygen—Case series presentation and suggested bio-psycho-social mechanism. *Frontiers in Psychology*, 9, 848. https://doi.org/10.3389/fpsyg.2018.00848

Eftekhari, A., Ruzek, J. I., Crowley, J. J., Rosen, C. S., Greenbaum, M. A., & Karlin, B. E. (2013). Effectiveness of national implementation of prolonged exposure therapy in Veterans Affairs care. *JAMA Psychiatry*, 70, 949–955.

Egan, S. J., Laidlaw, K., & Starkstein, S. (2015). Cognitive behaviour therapy for depression and anxiety in Parkinson's disease. *Journal of Parkinson's Disease*, 5(3), 443–451.

Eher, R., Olver, M. E., Heurix, I., Schilling, F., & Rettenberger, M. (2016). Predicting reoffense in pedophilic child molesters by clinical diagnoses and risk assessment. *Law and Human Behavior*, 39, 571–580.

Ehlers, C. L., Schuckit, M. A., Hesselbrock, V., Gilder, D. A., Wills, D., & Bucholz, K. (2022). The clinical course of antisocial behaviors in men and women of three racial groups. *Journal of Psychiatric Research*, 151, 319–327.

Eidelman, P., Gershon, A., Kaplan, K., McGlinchey, E., & Harvey, A. G. (2012). Social support and social strain in inter-episode bipolar disorder. *Bipolar Disorders*, 14, 628–640.

Eidelman, P., Talbot, L. S., Gruber, J., & Harvey, A. G. (2010). Sleep, illness course, and concurrent symptoms in inter-episode bipolar disorder. *Journal of Behavior Therapy and Experimental Psychiatry*, 41, 145–149.

Eidelson, R., & Soldz, S. (2012). Does Comprehensive Soldier Fitness work? CSF research fails the test. http://www.ethicalpsychology.org/Eidelson-&-Soldz-CSF_Research_Fails_the_Test.pdf

Eidelson, R., Pilisuk, M., & Soldz, S. (2011). The dark side of Comprehensive Soldier Fitness. *American Psychologist*, 66, 643–644.

Eisenberg, M. E., & Neumark-Sztainer, D. (2010). Friends' dieting and disordered eating behaviors among adolescents five years later: Findings from Project EAT. *Journal of Adolescent Health*, 47, 67–73.

Eisenberg, N., Spinrad, T. L., & Knafo-Noam, A. (2015). Prosocial development. In M. Lamb (Vol. Ed.) & R. M. Lerner (Series Ed.), *Handbook of child psychology and developmental science: Vol. 3. Socioemotional processes* (7th ed., pp. 610–656). New York: Wiley.

Eisenberg, N., Spinrad, T. L., Taylor, Z. E., & Liew, J. (2019). Relations of inhibition and emotion-related parenting to young children's prosocial and vicariously induced distress behavior. *Child Development*, 90(3), 846–858.

Eisenlohr-Moul, T. A., Girdler, S. S., Schmalenberger, K. M., Dawson, D. N., Surana, P., Johnson, J. L., & Rubinow, D. R. (2017). Toward the reliable diagnosis of DSM-5 premenstrual dysphoric disorder: The Carolina Premenstrual Assessment Scoring System (C-PASS). *The American Journal of Psychiatry*, 174(1), 51–59.

Eisma, M. C., & Tamminga, A. (2022). COVID-19, natural, and unnatural bereavement: Comprehensive comparisons of loss circumstances and grief severity. *European Journal of Psychotraumatology*, 13(1), 2062998. https://doi.org/10.1080/20008198.2022.2062998

Elder, G. A., Ehrlich, M. E., & Gandy, S. (2019). Relationship of traumatic brain injury to chronic mental health problems and dementia in military veterans. *Neuroscience Letters*, 707, 134294. https://doi.org/10.1016/j.neulet.2019.134294

El-Hamd, M. A., Saleh, R., & Majzoub, A. (2019). Premature ejaculation: An update on definition and pathophysiology. *Asian Journal of Andrology*, 21(5), 425–432. https://doi.org/10.4103/aja.aja_122_18

Ellard, K. K., Bernstein, E. E., Hearing, C., Baek, J. H., Sylvia, L. G., Nierenberg, A. A., . . . Deckersbach, T. (2017). Transdiagnostic treatment of bipolar disorder and comorbid anxiety using the Unified Protocol for Emotional Disorders: A pilot feasibility and acceptability trial. *Journal of Affective Disorders*, 219, 209–221.

Elliott, D., & Banda, P. S. (2013). Prosecutors not ready to agree to Holmes plea. http://bigstory.ap.org/article/prosecutors-not-ready-agree-holmes-plea

Ellis, A. (1997). The evolution of Albert Ellis and rational emotive behavior therapy. In J. K. Zeig (Ed.), *The evolution of psychotherapy: The third conference.* New York: Brunner/Mazel.

Ellis, A. (2008). Rational emotive behavior therapy. In R. J. Corsini & D. Wedding (Eds.), *Current psychotherapies* (8th ed., pp. 187–222). Belmont, CA: Brooks/Cole.

Ellis, D. M., & Hudson, J. L. (2010). The metacognitive model of generalized anxiety disorder in children and adolescents. *Clinical Child and Family Psychology Review*, 13, 151–163.

El-Wakeel, L. M., Fouad, F. A., Saleem, M. D., & Saber-Khalaf, M. (2020). Efficacy and tolerability of sildenafil/L-arginine combination relative to sildenafil alone in patients with organic erectile dysfunction. *Andrology*, 8(1), 143–147. https://doi.org/10.1111/andr.12671

Elwin, M., Elvin, T., & Larsson, J. O. (2020). Symptoms and level of functioning related to comorbidity in children and adolescents with ADHD: A cross-sectional registry study. *Child and Adolescent Psychiatry and Mental Health*, 14, 30. https://doi.org/10.1186/s13034-020-00336-4

Elwyn, T. S., Ahmed, I., & Feldman, M. D. (2019). Factitious disorder imposed on self. https://emedicine.medscape.com/article/291304-overview#a5

English, S., & Vallis, M. (2023). Moving beyond eat less, move more using willpower: Reframing obesity as a chronic disease impact of the 2020 Canadian obesity guidelines reframed narrative on perceptions of self and the patient-provider relationship. *Clinical Obesity*, e12615. Advance online publication. https://doi.org/10.1111/cob.12615

Eom, E., Restaino, S., Perkins, A. M., Neveln, N., & Harrington, J. W. (2015). Sexual harassment in middle and high school children and effects on physical and mental health. *Clinical Pediatrics*, 54(5), 430–438.

Epel, E. S., & Prather, A. A. (2018). Stress, telomeres, and psychopathology: Toward a deeper understanding of a triad of early aging. *Annual Review of Clinical Psychology*, 14, 371–397.

Epperson, C. N., Steiner, M., Hartlage, S. A., Eriksson, E., Schmidt, P. J., Jones, I., & Yonkers, K. A. (2012). Premenstrual dysphoric disorder: Evidence for a new category for DSM-5. *American Journal of Psychiatry*, 169, 465–475.

Erdely, S. R. (2004, March). What women sacrifice to be thin. *Redbook*, 202(3), 114–120.

Erickson, E. H. (1968). *Identity: Youth and crisis.* New York: Norton.

Eroglu, Y., Peker, A., & Cengiz, S. (2022). Cyber victimization and well-being in adolescents: The sequential mediation role of forgiveness and coping with cyberbullying. *Frontiers in Psychology*, 13, 819049. https://doi.org/10.3389/fpsyg.2022.819049

Esmaeilian, N., Dehghani, M., Koster, E., & Hoorelbeke, K. (2019). Early maladaptive schemas and borderline personality disorder features in a nonclinical sample: A network analysis. *Clinical Psychology and Psychotherapy, 26*(3), 388–398.

Espay, A. J., Aybek, S., Carson, A., Edwards, M. J., Goldstein, L. H., Hallett, M., . . . Morgante, F. (2018). Current concepts in diagnosis and treatment of functional neurological disorders. *JAMA Neurology, 75*(9), 1132–1141. https://doi.org/10.1001/jamaneurol.2018.1264

Ester. (2013). Ester's story. https://www.save.org/ester

Esterberg, M. L., Goulding, S. M., & Walker, E. L. (2010). Cluster A personality disorders: Schizotypal, schizoid and paranoid personality disorders in childhood and adolescence. *Journal of Psychopathology and Behavioral Assessment, 32*, 515–528.

Estes, A., St John, T., & Dager, S. R. (2019). What to tell a parent who worries a young child has autism. *JAMA Psychiatry.* https://doi.org/10.1001/jamapsychiatry.2019.1234

Everitt, B. J., & Robbins, T. W. (2016). Drug addiction: Updating actions to habits to compulsions ten years on. *Annual Review of Psychology, 67*, 23–50.

Ewing, C. P. (1998, February). Indictment fuels repressed-memory debate. *APA Monitor*, p. 52.

Fadus, M. C., Squeglia, L. M., Valadez, E. A., Tomko, R. L., Bryant, B. E., & Gray, K. M. (2019). Adolescent substance use disorder treatment: An update on evidence-based strategies. *Current Psychiatry Reports, 21*(10), 96. https://doi.org/10.1007/s11920-019-1086-0

Fairburn, C. G., Cooper, Z., Doll, H. A., Norman, P., & O'Connor, M. (2000). The natural course of bulimia nervosa and binge eating disorder in young women. *Archives of General Psychiatry, 57*, 659–665.

Fairchild, G., Hawes, D. J., Frick, P. J., Copeland, W. E., Odgers, C. L., Franke, B., . . . De Brito, S. A. (2019). Conduct disorder. Nature reviews. *Disease Primers, 5*(1), 43. https://doi.org/10.1038/s41572-019-0095-y

Falcon, R. (2022). These are the most depressed cities data shows. https://thehill.com/homenews/nexstar_media_wire/3624879-these-are-americas-most-depressed-cities-data-shows/

Fallon, E. A., Harris, B. S., & Johnson, P. (2014). Prevalence of body dissatisfaction among a United States adult sample. *Eating Behaviors, 15*, 151–158.

Faraone, S. V. (2018). The pharmacology of amphetamine and methylphenidate: Relevance to the neurobiology of attention-deficit/hyperactivity disorder and other psychiatric comorbidities. *Neuroscience and Biobehavioral Reviews, 87*, 255–270.

Farchione, T. J., Fairholme, C. P., Ellard, K. K., Boisseau, C. L., Thompson-Hollands, J., Carl, J. R., . . . Barlow, D. H. (2012). Unified protocol for transdiagnostic treatment of emotional disorders: A randomized controlled trial. *Behavior Therapy, 43*, 666–678.

Faulk, C., & Dolinoy, D. C. (2011). Timing is everything: The when and how of environmentally induced changes in the epigenome of animals. *Epigenetics, 6*, 791–797.

Fava, G. A., & Rafanelli, C. (2019). Iatrogenic factors in psychopathology. *Psychotherapy and Psychosomatics, 88*, 129–140.

Favrod, J., Nguyen, A., Fankhauser, C., Ismailaj, A., Hasler, J. D., Ringuet, A., . . . Bonsack, C. (2015). Positive Emotions Program for Schizophrenia (PEPS): A pilot intervention to reduce anhedonia and apathy. *BMC Psychiatry, 15*, 231. https://doi.org/10.1186/s12888-015-0610-y

Fedoroff, J. P. (2008). Treatment of paraphilic sexual disorders. In D. Rowland & L. Incrocci (Eds.), *Handbook of sexual and gender identity disorders* (pp. 563–586). Hoboken, NJ: Wiley.

Fehling, K. B., & Selby, E. A. (2021). Suicide in DSM-5: Current evidence for the proposed suicide behavior disorder and other possible improvements. *Frontiers in Psychiatry, 11*, 499980. https://doi.org/10.3389/fpsyt.2020.499980

Feinberg, A. (2019). Trump's mental state is deteriorating dangerously due to impeachment with potentially "catastrophic outcomes," psychiatrists urgently warn Congress. https://www.independent.co.uk/news/world/americas/us-politics/trump-mental-state-impeachment-psychiatrist-petition-congress-a9232386.html

Feinstein B. A. (2020). Response to Commentaries: Toward a unifying framework for understanding and improving sexual and gender minority mental health. *Archives of Sexual Behavior, 49*(7), 2295–2300.

Feinstein, J. S., Adolphs, R., Damasio, A., & Tranel, D. (2011). The human amygdala and the induction and experience of fear. *Current Biology, 21*, 1–5.

Feinstein, J. S., Duff, M. C., & Tranela, D. (2010). Sustained experience of emotion after loss of memory in patients with amnesia. *Proceedings of the National Academy of Sciences, 107*, 7674–7679.

Felthous, A. R., & Bloom, J. D. (2018). Jail-based competency restoration. *Journal of the American Academy of Psychiatry and Law, 46*, 364–372.

Fenton, M. C., Keyes, K. M., Martins, S. S., & Hasin, D. S. (2010). The role of a prescription in anxiety medication use, abuse, and dependence. *American Journal of Psychiatry, 167*, 1247–1253.

Fentz, H. N., Hoffart, A., Jensen, M. B., Arendt, M., O'Toole, M. S., Rosenberg, N. K., & Hougaard, E. (2013). Mechanisms of change in cognitive behaviour therapy for panic disorder: The role of panic self-efficacy and catastrophic misinterpretations. *Behaviour Research and Therapy, 51*(9), 579–587.

Fenwick-Smith, A., Dahlberg, E. E., & Thompson, S. C. (2018). Systematic review of resilience-enhancing, universal, primary school-based mental health promotion programs. *BMC Psychology, 6*(1), 30. https://doi.org/10.1186/s40359-018-0242-3

Fergusson, D. M., Boden, J. M., Horwood, L. J., Miller, A., & Kennedy, M. A. (2012). Moderating role of the MAOA genotype in antisocial behaviour. *British Journal of Psychiatry, 200*, 116–123.

Ferrarelli, F., & Phillips, M. L. (2021). Examining and modulating neural circuits in psychiatric disorders with transcranial magnetic stimulation and electroencephalography: Present practices and future developments. *The American Journal of Psychiatry*, *178*(5), 400–413.

Fernandez, C. A., Choi, K. W., Marshall, B., Vicente, B., Saldivia, S., Kohn, R., . . . Buka, S. L. (2020). Assessing the relationship between psychosocial stressors and psychiatric resilience among Chilean disaster survivors. *The British Journal of Psychiatry*, 1–8. https://doi.org/10.1192/bjp.2020.88

Fernández-Álvarez, J., Di Lernia, D., & Riva, G. (2020). Virtual reality for anxiety disorders: Rethinking a field in expansion. *Advances in Experimental Medicine and Biology*, *1191*, 389–414.

Fernández-Cabana, M., García-Caballero, A., Alves-Pérez, M. T., García-García, M. J., & Mateos, R. (2013). Suicidal traits in Marilyn Monroe's Fragments. *Crisis*, *34*, 124–130.

Ferrier-Auerbach, A. G., & Martens, M. P. (2009). Perceived incompetence moderates the relationship between maladaptive perfectionism and disordered eating. *Eating Disorders*, *17*, 333–344.

Fesharaki-Zadeh A. (2019). Chronic traumatic encephalopathy: A brief overview. *Frontiers in Neurology*, *10*, 713. https://doi.org/10.3389/fneur.2019.00713

Field, A. E., Sonneville, K. R., Crosby, R. D., Swanson, S. A., Eddy, K. T., Camargo, C. A., Jr., . . . Micali, N. (2014). Prospective associations of concerns about physique and the development of obesity, binge drinking, and drug use among adolescent boys and young adult men. *JAMA Pediatrics*, *168*, 34–39.

Field, A. P., Ball, J. E., Kawycz, N. J., & Moore, H. (2007). Parent-child relationships and verbal information pathway to fear in children: Two preliminary experiments. *Behavioural and Cognitive Psychotherapy*, *35*, 473–486.

Fiery, M. F., Martz, D. M., Webb, R. M., & Curtin, L. (2016). A preliminary investigation of racial differences in body talk in age-diverse U.S. adults. *Eating Behaviors*, *21*, 232–235.

Figurasin, R., & Maguire, N. J. (2022). 3,4-Methylenedioxymethamphetamine toxicity. In *StatPearls*. StatPearls Publishing.

Fineberg, N. A., Menchón, J. M., Hall, N., Dell'Osso, B., Brand, M., Potenza, M. N., . . . Zohar, J. (2022). Advances in problematic usage of the internet research: A narrative review by experts from the European network for problematic usage of the internet. *Comprehensive Psychiatry*, *118*, 152346. https://doi.org/10.1016/j.comppsych.2022.152346

Fink, D. S., Santaella-Tenorio, J., & Keyes, K. M. (2018). Increase in suicides the months after the death of Robin Williams in the US. *PLOS One*, *13*(2), e0191405. https://doi.org/10.1371/journal.pone.0191405

Fisher, H. L., Jones, P. B., Fearon, P., Craig, T. K., Dazzan, P., Morgan, K., . . . Morgan, C. (2010). The varying impact of type, timing and frequency of exposure to childhood adversity on its association with adult psychotic disorder. *Psychological Medicine*, *40*, 1967–1978.

Fisher, K. A., & Marwaha, R. (2020). *Paraphilia*. StatPearls [Internet]. Treasure Island, FL: StatPearls Publishing. https://www.ncbi.nlm.nih.gov/books/NBK554425/

Fitzgerald, P. B., Hoy, K. E., Elliot, D., McQueen, S., Wambeek, L. E., Chen, L., . . . Daskalakis, Z. J. (2018). A pilot study of the comparative efficacy of 100 Hz magnetic seizure therapy and electroconvulsive therapy in persistent depression. *Depression and Anxiety*, *35*(5), 393–401

Fitzpatrick, O. M., Whelen, M. L., Falkenström, F., & Strunk, D. R. (2020). Who benefits the most from cognitive change in cognitive therapy of depression? A study of interpersonal factors. *Journal of Consulting and Clinical Psychology*, *88*(2), 128–136

Fitzsimmons-Craft, E. E., Chan, W. W., Smith, A. C., Firebaugh, M. L., Fowler, L. A., Topooco, N., . . . Jacobson, N. C. (2022). Effectiveness of a chatbot for eating disorders prevention: A randomized clinical trial. *The International Journal of Eating Disorders*, *55*(3), 343–353.

Flegal, K. M., Kit, B. K., Orpana, H., & Graubard, B. I. (2013). Association of all-cause mortality with overweight and obesity using standard body mass index categories: A systematic review and meta-analysis. *Journal of the American Medical Association*, *309*, 71–82.

Fleming, T. M., Gillham, B., Bavin, L. M., Stasiak, K., Lewycka, S., Moore, J., . . . Merry, S. N. (2019). SPARX-R computerized therapy among adolescents in youth offenders' program: Step-wise cohort study. *Internet Interventions*, *18*, 100287. https://doi.org/10.1016/j.invent.2019.100287

Fleming, T. M., Stasiak, K., Moselen, E., Hermansson-Webb, E., Shepherd, M., Lucassen, M., . . . Merry, S. N. (2019). Revising computerized therapy for wider appeal among adolescents: Youth perspectives on a revised version of SPARX. *Frontiers in Psychiatry*, *10*, 802. https://doi.org/10.3389/fpsyt.2019.00802

Fletcher, J. M., & Grigorenko, E. L. (2017). Neuropsychology of learning disabilities: The past and the future. *Journal of the International Neuropsychological Society*, *23*(9–10), 930–940.

Flores-Cordero, J. A., Pérez-Pérez, A., Jiménez-Cortegana, C., Alba, G., Flores-Barragán, A., & Sánchez-Margalet, V. (2022). Obesity as a risk factor for dementia and Alzheimer's disease: The role of leptin. *International Journal of Molecular Sciences*, *23*(9), 5202. https://doi.org/10.3390/ijms23095202

Florio, L., Lassi, D. L. S., de Azevedo-Marques Perico, C., Vignoli, N. G., Torales, J., Ventriglio, A., & Castaldelli-Maia, J. M. (2022). Food addiction: A comprehensive review. *The Journal of Nervous and Mental Disease*, *210*(11), 874–879.

Foa, E. B., & Kozak, M. J. (1995). DSM-IV field trial: Obsessive-compulsive disorder. *American Journal of Psychiatry*, *152*, 90–96.

Foa, E., Gillihan, S., & Bryant, R. (2013). Challenges and successes in dissemination of evidence-based treatments for posttraumatic stress: Lessons learned from prolonged exposure therapy for PTSD. *Psychological Science in the Public Interest, 14*, 65–111.

Fonte, C., Smania, N., Pedrinolla, A., Munari, D., Gandolfi, M., Picelli, A., . . . Venturelli, M. (2019). Comparison between physical and cognitive treatment in patients with MCI and Alzheimer's disease. *Aging, 11*(10), 3138–3155. https://doi.org/10.18632/aging.101970

Foote, B., & Van Orden, K. (2016). Adapting dialectical behavior therapy for the treatment of dissociative identity disorder. *American Journal of Psychotherapy, 70*(4), 343–364.

Ford, H., Fraser, C. L., Solly, E., Clough, M., Fielding, J., White, O., & Van Der Walt, A. (2022). Hallucinogenic persisting perception disorder: A case series and review of the literature. *Frontiers in Neurology, 13*, 878609. https://doi.org/10.3389/fneur.2022.878609

Foreman, M., Hare, L., York, K., Balakrishnan, K., Sánchez, F. J., Harte, F., . . . Harley, V. R. (2019). Genetic link between gender dysphoria and sex hormone signaling. *The Journal of Clinical Endocrinology and Metabolism, 104*(2), 390–396.

Forneris, C. A., Nussbaumer-Streit, B., Morgan, L. C., Greenblatt, A., Van Noord, M. G., Gaynes, B. N., . . . Gartlehner, G. (2019). Psychological therapies for preventing seasonal affective disorder. *The Cochrane Database of Systematic Reviews, 5*(5), CD011270. https://doi.org/10.1002/14651858.CD011270.pub3

Forrester, S. N., Gallo, J. J., Whitfield, K. E., & Thorpe, R. J. (2019). A framework of minority stress: From physiological manifestations to cognitive outcomes. *The Gerontologist, 59*(6), 1017–1023.

Forstner, A. J., Awasthi, S., Wolf, C., Maron, E., Erhardt, A., Czamara, . . . Schumacher, J. (2021). Genome-wide association study of panic disorder reveals genetic overlap with neuroticism and depression. *Molecular Psychiatry, 26*(8), 4179–4190.

Forsyth, J. K., Ellman, L. M., Tanskanen, A., Mustonen, U., Huttunen, M. O., Suvisaari, J., & Cannon, T. D. (2013). Genetic risk for schizophrenia, obstetric complications, and adolescent school outcome: Evidence for gene-environment interaction. *Schizophrenia Bulletin, 39*, 1067–1076.

Fortgang, R. G., Hultman, C. M., & Cannon, T. D. (2016). Coping styles in twins discordant for schizophrenia, bipolar disorder, and depression. *Clinical Psychological Science: A Journal of the Association for Psychological Science, 4*(2), 216–228.

Fosha, D. (2018). The introduction to commentaries on sociocultural identity, trauma treatment, and AEDP through the lens of bilingualism in the case of "Rosa." *Pragmatic Case Studies in Psychotherapy, 14*, 115–130.

Fossos-Wong, N., Litt, D. M., King, K. M., Kilmer, J. R., Fairlie, A. M., Larimer, M. E., . . . Lewis, M. A. (2022). Behavioral willingness, descriptive normative perceptions, and prescription stimulant misuse among young adults 18–20. *Substance Use & Misuse, 57*(2), 287–294. https://doi.org/10.1080/10826084.2021.2003403

Fountoulakis, K. N., Kontis, D., Gonda, X., & Yatham, L. N. (2013). A systematic review of the evidence on the treatment of rapid cycling bipolar disorder. *Bipolar Disorder, 15*, 115–137.

Fox, N. A., Henderson, H. A., Marshall, P. J., Nichols, K. E., & Ghera, M. M. (2005). Behavioral inhibition: Linking biology and behavior within a developmental framework. *Annual Review of Psychology, 56*, 235–262.

Francalanza, K., Raila, H., & Rodriguez, C. I. (2021). Could written imaginal exposure be helpful for hoarding disorder? A case series. *Journal of Obsessive-Compulsive and Related Disorders, 29*. https://doi.org/10.1016/j.jocrd.2021.100637

Frances, A. (2013). The new crisis in confidence in psychiatric diagnosis. *Annals of Internal Medicine, 159*, 221–222.

Francis, A. (2014). Teen trying experimental treatment for narcolepsy. http://news.ninemsn.com.au /world/2014/01/07/14/17/teen-trying -experimental-treatment-for -narcolepsy

Franco, M. (2014). Man loses fear of spiders with chunk of his brain. http://www.cnet.com/news/man -loses-fear-of-spiders-with-chunk -of-his-brain

Frangou, S. (2019). Neuroimaging markers of risk, disease expression, and resilience to bipolar disorder. *Current Psychiatry Reports, 21*(7), 52. https://doi.org/10.1007/s11920-019-1039-7

Franklin, G., Carson, A. J., & Welch, K. A. (2016). Cognitive behavioural therapy for depression: Systematic review of imaging studies. *Acta Neuropsychiatrica, 28*(2), 61–74.

Franklin, J. C., Huang, X., & Bastidas, D. (2019). Virtual reality suicide: Development of a translational approach for studying suicide causes. *Behaviour Research and Therapy, 120*, 103360. https://doi.org/10.1016/j.brat.2018.12.013

Franko, D. L., Thompson-Brenner, H., Thompson, D. R., Boisseau, C. L., Davis, A., Forbush, K. T., . . . Wilson, G. T. (2012). Racial/ethnic differences in adults in randomized clinical trials of binge eating disorder. *Journal of Consulting and Clinical Psychology, 80*, 186–195.

Franz, A. P., Bolat, G. U., Bolat, H., Matijasevich, A., Santos, I. S., Silveira, R. C., . . . Moreira-Maia, C. R. (2018). Attention-deficit /hyperactivity disorder and very preterm/very low birth weight: A meta-analysis. *Pediatrics, 141*(1), e20171645. https://doi.org/10.1542/peds.2017-1645

Frederick, C. B., Snellman, K., & Putnam, R. D. (2014). Increasing socioeconomic disparities in adolescent obesity. *Proceedings of the National Academy of Sciences, 111*, 1338–1342.

Fredrickson, B. L. (2013). Learning to self-generate positive emotions. In D. Hermans, B. Rimé, & B. Mesquita (Eds.), *Changing emotions*. London: Psychology Press.

Freedman, R., Lewis, D. A., Michels, R., Pine, D. S., Schultz, S. K., Tamminga, C. A., . . . Yager, J. (2013). The initial field trials of DSM-5: New blooms and old thorns. *American Journal of Psychiatry, 170*, 1–5.

Freis, S. D., & Gurung, R. A. R. (2013). A Facebook analysis of helping behavior in online bullying. *Psychology of Popular Media Culture, 2*, 11–19.

Freud, S. (1938). The psychopathology of everyday life. In A. B. Brill (Ed.), *The basic writings of Sigmund Freud*. New York: Modern Library.

Freud, S. (1949). *An outline of psychoanalysis*. New York: Norton.

Frey, J., & Malaty, I. A. (2022). Tourette syndrome treatment updates: A review and discussion of the current and upcoming literature. *Current Neurology and Neuroscience Reports, 22*(2), 123–142. https://doi.org/10.1007/s11910-022-01177-8

Frey, W. H. (2018). The US will become "minority white" in 2045, Census projects. https://www.brookings.edu/blog/the-avenue/2018/03/14/the-us-will-become-minority-white-in-2045-census-projects/

Frick, A., Engman, J., Alaie, I., Björkstrand, J., Gingnell, M., Larsson, E. M., . . . Furmark, T. (2020). Neuroimaging, genetic, clinical, and demographic predictors of treatment response in patients with social anxiety disorder. *Journal of Affective Disorders, 261*, 230–237.

Friedman, M. B. (2003). Keeping the promise of community mental health. https://web.archive.org/web/20040623200438/http://mhawestchester.org/advocates/opromise81303.asp

Friedman, R. A., & Michels, R. (2013). How should the psychiatric profession respond to the recent mass killings? *American Journal of Psychiatry, 170*, 455–458.

Friedman, S. (2007). *Just for boys*. Vancouver, BC: Salah Books.

Friedrich, A., Claßen, M., & Schlarb, A. A. (2018). Sleep better, feel better? Effects of a CBT-I and HT-I sleep training on mental health, quality of life and stress coping in university students: A randomized pilot controlled trial. *BMC Psychiatry, 18*(1), 268.

https://doi.org/10.1186/s12888-018-1860-2

Friedrich, A., & Schlarb, A. A. (2018). Let's talk about sleep: A systematic review of psychological interventions to improve sleep in college students. *Journal of Sleep Research, 27*(1), 4–22.

Froehlich, T. E., Lanphear, B. P., Epstein, J. N., Barbaresi, W. J., Katusic, S. K., & Kahn, R. S. (2007). Prevalence and treatment of ADHD in a national sample of U.S. children. *Archives of Pediatrics and Adolescent Medicine, 161*, 857–864.

Frojd, S., Ranta, K., Kaltiala-Heino, R., & Marttunen, M. (2011). Associations of social phobia and general anxiety with alcohol and drug use in a community sample of adolescents. *Alcohol and Alcoholism, 46*(2), 192–199.

Frühauf, S., Gerger, H., Schmidt, H. M., Munder, T., & Barth, J. (2013). Efficacy of psychological interventions for sexual dysfunction: A systematic review and meta-analysis. *Archives of Sexual Behavior, 42*, 915–933.

Fryar, C. D., Carroll, M. D., Gu, Q., Afful, J., & Ogden, C. L. (2021). Anthropometric reference data for children and adults: United States, 2015–2018. National Center for Health Statistics. *Vital Health Statistics, 3*(46).

Fryar, C. D., Kruszon-Moran, D., Gu, Q., & Ogden, C. L. (2018). Mean body weight, height, waist circumference, and body mass index among adults: United States, 1999–2000 through 2015–2016. *National Health Statistics Reports*, (122), 1–16.

Frye, L. A., & Spates, C. R. (2012). Prolonged exposure, mindfulness, and emotion regulation for the treatment of PTSD. *Clinical Case Studies, 11*, 184–200.

Fullana, M. A., Mataix-Cols, D., Caspi, A., Harrington, H., Grisham, J. R., Moffitt, T. E., Poulton, R. (2009). Obsessions and compulsions in the community: Prevalence, interference, help-seeking, developmental stability, and co-occurring psychiatric conditions. *American Journal of Psychiatry, 166*, 329–336.

Fuller-Thompson, E. (2012). Evidence supporting an

independent association between childhood physical abuse and lifetime suicidal ideation. *Suicide and Life-Threatening Behavior*, 279–291.

Fusetti, V., Re, L., Pigni, A., Tallarita, A., Cilluffo, S., Caraceni, A. T., & Lusignani, M. (2022). Clown therapy for procedural pain in children: A systematic review and meta-analysis. *European Journal of Pediatrics, 181*(6), 2215–2225. https://doi.org/10.1007/s00431-022-04440-9

Gadelkarim, W., Shahper, S., Reid, J., Wikramanayake, M., Kaur, S., Kolli, S., . . . Fineberg, N. A. (2019). Overlap of obsessive-compulsive personality disorder and autism spectrum disorder traits among OCD outpatients: An exploratory study. *International Journal of Psychiatry in Clinical Practice, 23*(4), 297–306.

Gainer, D., Alam, S., Alam, H., & Redding, H. (2020). A flash of hope: Eye movement desensitization and reprocessing (EMDR) therapy. *Innovations in Clinical Neuroscience, 17*(7–9), 12–20.

Galea, S., Ahern, J., Resnick, H., Kilpatrick, D., Bucuvalas, M., Gold, J., & Vlahov, D. (2002). Psychological sequelae of the September 11 terrorist attacks in New York City. *New England Journal of Medicine, 346*, 982–987.

Gallagher, M. G., Naragon-Gainey, K., & Brown, T. A. (2014). Perceived control is a transdiagnostic predictor of cognitive-behavior therapy outcome for anxiety disorders. *Cognitive Therapy and Research, 38*, 10–22.

Gallagher, M. W., Long, L. J., & Phillips, C. A. (2020). Hope, optimism, self-efficacy, and posttraumatic stress disorder: A meta-analytic review of the protective effects of positive expectancies. *Journal of Clinical Psychology, 76*(3), 329–355.

Gallegos, M. I., Zaring-Hinkle, B., Wang, N., & Bray, J. H. (2020). Detachment, peer pressure, and age of first substance use as gateways to later substance use. *Drug and Alcohol Dependence*. https://doi.org/10.1016/j.drugalcdep.2020.108352

Gallichan, D. J., & Curle, C. (2008). Fitting square pegs into round holes: The challenge of coping with attention-deficit hyperactivity disorder. *Clinical Child Psychology and Psychiatry, 13,* 343–363.

Galmiche, M., Déchelotte, P., Lambert, G., & Tavolacci, M. P. (2019). Prevalence of eating disorders over the 2000–2018 period: A systematic literature review. *The American Journal of Clinical Nutrition, 109*(5), 1402–1413.

Gao, Y., Raine, A., Venables, P. H., Dawson, M. E., & Mednick, S. A. (2010). Association of poor childhood fear conditioning and adult crime. *American Journal of Psychiatry, 167,* 56–60.

Gara, M. A., Vega, W. A., Arndt, S., Escamilla, M., Fleck, D. E., Lawson, W. B., . . . Strakowski, S. M. (2012). Influence of patient race and ethnicity on clinical assessment in patients with affective disorders. *Archives of General Psychiatry, 69,* 593–600.

Garcia, E., Johnston, J., McConnell, R., Palinkas, L., & Eckel, S. P. (2023). California's early transition to electric vehicles: Observed health and air quality co-benefits. *The Science of the Total Environment, 867,* 161761. https://doi.org/10.1016/j.scitotenv.2023.161761

Garcia, M. A., Downer, B., Chiu, C. T., Saenz, J. L., Rote, S., & Wong, R. (2019). Racial/ethnic and nativity differences in cognitive life expectancies among older adults in the United States. *The Gerontologist, 59*(2), 281–289.

Garcia-Toro, M., Rubio, J. M., Gili, M., Roca, M., Jin, C. J., Liu, S. M., . . . Blanco, C. (2013). Persistence of chronic major depression: A national prospective study. *Journal of Affective Disorders, 151,* 306–312.

Garcini, L. M., Chen, M. A., Brown, R., LeRoy, A. S., Cano, M. A., Peek, K., & Fagundes, C. (2020). "Abrazame que ayuda" (hug me, it helps): Social support and the effect of perceived discrimination on depression among US- and foreign-born Latinxs in the USA. *Journal of Racial and Ethnic Health Disparities, 7*(3), 481–487.

Gardener, H., Wright, C. B., Dong, C., Cheung, K., DeRosa, J., Nannery, M., . . . Sacco, R. L. (2016). Ideal cardiovascular health and cognitive aging in the Northern Manhattan Study. *Journal of the American Heart Association, 5,* e002731.

Garey, L., Zvolensky, M. J., & Spada, M. M. (2020). Third wave cognitive and behavioral processes and therapies for addictive behaviors: An introduction to the special issue. *Addictive Behaviors, 108,* 106465. https://doi.org/10.1016/j.addbeh.2020.106465

Garmendia, C. A., Nassar Gorra, L., Rodriguez, A. L., Trepka, M. J., Veledar, E., & Madhivanan, P. (2019). Evaluation of the inclusion of studies identified by the FDA as having falsified data in the results of meta-analyses: The example of the apixaban trials. *JAMA Internal Medicine, 179,* 582–584.

Garrett, M., & Silva, R. (2003). Auditory hallucinations, source monitoring, and the belief that "voices" are real. *Schizophrenia Bulletin, 29,* 445–451.

Gates, P. J., Sabioni, P., Copeland, J., Le Foll, B., & Gowing, L. (2016). Psychosocial interventions for cannabis use disorder. *The Cochrane Database of Systematic Reviews, 2016*(5), CD005336. https://doi.org/10.1002/14651858.CD005336.pub4

Gauvin, G., Labelle, R., Daigle, M., Breton, J. J., & Houle, J. (2019). Coping, social support, and suicide attempts among homeless adolescents. *Crisis, 40,* 390–399.

Gaynor, K., Ward, T., Garety, P., & Peters, E. (2013). The role of safety-seeking behaviours in maintaining threat appraisals in psychosis. *Behaviour Research and Therapy, 51,* 75–81.

Geddes, J. R., & Miklowitz, D. J. (2013). Treatment of bipolar disorder. *Lancet, 381,* 1672–1682.

Gelauff, J., Stone, J., Edwards, M., & Carson, A. (2014). The prognosis of functional (psychogenic) motor symptoms: A systematic review. *Journal of Neurology, Neurosurgery, and Psychiatry, 85,* 220–226

Gelaye, B., Do, N., Avila, S., Carlos Velez, J., Zhong, Q. Y., Sanchez, S. E., . . . Williams, M. A. (2016). Childhood abuse, intimate partner violence and risk of migraine among pregnant women: An epidemiologic study. *Headache, 56*(6), 976–986.

Gelfo, F. (2019). Does experience enhance cognitive flexibility? An overview of the evidence provided by the Environmental Enrichment Studies. *Frontiers in Behavioral Neuroscience, 13,* 150. https://doi.org/10.3389/fnbeh.2019.00150

Gengoux, G. W., Abrams, D. A., Schuck, R., Millan, M. E., Libove, R., Ardel, C. M., . . . Hardan, A. Y. (2019). A pivotal response treatment package for children with autism spectrum disorder: An RCT. *Pediatrics, 144*(3), e20190178. https://doi.org/10.1542/peds.2019-0178

Gentile, J. P., Dillon, K. S., & Gillig, P. M. (2013). Psychotherapy and pharmacotherapy for patients with dissociative identity disorder. *Innovations in Clinical Neuroscience, 10,* 22–29.

George, M. G., Tong, X., & Bowman, B. A. (2017). Prevalence of cardiovascular risk factors and strokes in younger adults. *JAMA Neurology, 74*(6), 695–703.

Georgiou, G., Demetriou, C. A., Colins, O. F., Roetman, P. J., & Fanti, K. A. (2023). Psychopathic traits and parental practices in Greek-Cypriot community and Dutch clinical referred samples. *Research on Child and Adolescent Psychopathology.* https://doi.org/10.1007/s10802-023-01060-1

Gerbasi, M. E., Richards, L. K., Thomas, J. J., Agnew-Blais, J. C., Thompson-Brenner, H., Gilman, S. E., & Becker, A. E. (2014). Globalization and eating disorder risk: Peer influence, perceived social norms, and adolescent disordered eating in Fiji. *The International Journal of Eating Disorders, 47*(7), 727–737.

Gerhard, T., Stroup, T. S., Correll, C. U., Setoguchi, S., Strom, B. L., Huang, C., . . . Olfson, M. (2020). Mortality risk of antipsychotic augmentation for adult depression. *PLOS One, 15*(9), e0239206. https://doi.org/10.1371/journal.pone.0239206

Gerson, R., & Rappaport, N. (2013). Traumatic stress and posttraumatic stress disorder in youth: Recent research findings on clinical impact, assessment, and treatment. *Journal of Adolescent Health, 52*, 137–143.

Ghaemi, N. (2016). Is psychoanalyzing our politicians fair game? http://www.medscape.com/viewarticle/867320?src=wnl_edit_tpal

Ghaemi, S. N. (2010). Levels of evidence. *Psychiatric Times, 27*, 1–4.

Ghandour, R. M., Sherman, L. J., Vladutiu, C. J., Ali, M. M., Lynch, S. E., Bitsko, R. H., & Blumberg, S. J. (2019). Prevalence and treatment of depression, anxiety, and conduct problems in US children. *The Journal of Pediatrics, 206*, 256–267.

Gharaibeh, N. (2009). Dissociative identity disorder: Time to remove it from DSM-V? *Current Psychiatry, 8*, 30–37.

Gianaros, P. J., & Jennings, J. R. (2018). Host in the machine: A neurobiological perspective on psychological stress and cardiovascular disease. *The American Psychologist, 73*(8), 1031–1044.

Giannakopoulou, O., Lin, K., Meng, X., Su, M. H., Kuo, P. H., Peterson, R. E., . . . 23andMe Research Team, China Kadoorie Biobank Collaborative Group, and Major Depressive Disorder Working Group of the Psychiatric Genomics Consortium. (2021). The genetic architecture of depression in individuals of East Asian ancestry: A genome-wide association study. *JAMA Psychiatry, 78*(11), 1258–1269.

Giel, K. E., Bulik, C. M., Fernandez-Aranda, F., Hay, P., Keski-Rahkonen, A., Schag, K., Schmidt, U., & Zipfel, S. (2022). Binge eating disorder. *Nature Reviews: Disease Primers, 8*(1), 16. https://doi.org/10.1038/s41572-022-00344-y

Giesbrecht, T., Lynn, S. J., Lilienfeld, S. O., & Merckelbach, H. (2008). Cognitive processes in dissociation: An analysis of core theoretical assumptions. *Psychological Bulletin, 134*, 617–647.

Gil, S., & Weinberg, M. (2015). Coping strategies and internal resources of dispositional optimism and mastery as predictors of traumatic exposure and of PTSD symptoms: A prospective study. *Psychological Trauma: Theory, Research, Practice and Policy, 7*(4), 405–411

Giliberti, M. (2015). Treatment, not jail: It's time to step up. https://www.nami.org/Blogs/From-the-Executive-Director/May-2015/Treatment,-Not-Jail-It%E2%80%99s-Time-to-Step-Up

Gill, G., Dumlao, N., Singh, G., Susaimanickam, B., & Korenis, P. (2023). Dissociative amnesia with fugue in a middle-aged man. *The Primary Care Companion for CNS Disorders, 25*(2), 22cr03306. https://doi.org/10.4088/PCC.22cr03306

Gill, K. R. (2019). Why twins don't have identical fingerprints. https://www.healthline.com/health/do-identical-twins-have-the-same-fingerprints

Gillan, C. M., Kalanthroff, E., Evans, M., Weingarden, H. M., Jacoby, R. J., . . . Simpson, H. B. (2019). Comparison of the association between goal-directed planning and self-reported compulsivity vs obsessive-compulsive disorder diagnosis. *JAMA Psychiatry, 9*, 1–10. doi:10.1001/jamapsychiatry.2019.2998

Gillig, P. M. (2013). Psychogenic nonepileptic seizures. *Innovations in Clinical Neuroscience, 10*, 15–18.

Gillis, A., Holoyda, B., Newman, W. J., Wilson, M. D., & Xiong, G. L. (2016). Characteristics of misdemeanants treated for competency restoration. *The Journal of the American Academy of Psychiatry and the Law, 44*(4), 442–450.

Ginzburg, K., & Solomon, Z. (2010). Trajectories of stress reactions and somatization symptoms among war veterans: A 20-year longitudinal study. *Psychological Medicine, 41*, 353–362.

Giotakos O. (2022). Fake news in the age of COVID-19: evolutional and psychobiological considerations. *Psychiatrike = Psychiatriki, 33*(3), 183–186.

Gladieux, M., Gimness, N., Rodriguez, B., & Liu, J. (2023). Adverse childhood experiences (ACEs) and environmental exposures on neurocognitive outcomes in children: Empirical evidence, potential mechanisms, and implications. *Toxics, 11*(3), 259. https://doi.org/10.3390/toxics11030259

Glasner-Edwards, S., Mooney, L. J., Marinelli-Casey, P., Hillhouse, M.,

Ang, A., & Rawson, R. A. (2010). Psychopathology in methamphetamine-dependent adults 3 years after treatment. *Drug and Alcohol Review, 29*, 12–20.

Gmeiner, M. S., & Warschburger, P. (2022). Simply too much: the extent to which weight bias internalization results in a higher risk of eating disorders and psychosocial problems. *Eating and Weight Disorders : EWD, 27*(1), 317–324. https://doi.org/10.1007/s40519-021-01170-z

Gobbi, G., Atkin, T., Zytynski, T., Wang, S., Askari, S., Boruff, J., . . . Mayo, N. (2019). Association of cannabis use in adolescence and risk of depression, anxiety, and suicidality in young adulthood: A systematic review and meta-analysis. *JAMA Psychiatry, 76*(4), 426–434.

Goel, R., Hong, J. S., Findling, R. L., & Ji, N. Y. (2018). An update on pharmacotherapy of autism spectrum disorder in children and adolescents. *International Review of Psychiatry (Abingdon, England), 30*(1), 78–95.

Goff, D. C. (1993). Reply to Dr. Armstrong. *Journal of Nervous and Mental Disease, 181*, 604–605.

Goff, D. C., & Simms, C. A. (1993). Has multiple personality disorder remained consistent over time? *Journal of Nervous and Mental Disease, 181*, 595–600.

Goggin, B. (2019). Inside Facebook's suicide algorithm. https://www.businessinsider.com/facebook-is-using-ai-to-try-to-predict-if-youre-suicidal-2018-12

Gold, M. S., Blum, K., Oscar-Berman, M., & Braverman, E. R. (2014). Low dopamine function in attention deficit/ hyperactivity disorder: Should genotyping signify early diagnosis in children? *Postgraduate Medicine, 126*, 153–177.

Goldberg, C. (2009). The mental status exam (MSE). http://meded.ucsd.edu/clinicalmed/mental.htm

Goldberg, D. (2006). The aetiology of depression. *Psychological Medicine, 36*, 1341–1347.

Goldfein, J. A., Devlin, M. J., & Spitzer, R. L. (2000). Cognitive behavioral therapy for the treatment of binge eating disorder: What constitutes success? *American Journal of Psychiatry, 157*, 1051–1056.

Goldin, P. R., Thurston, M., Allende, S., Moodie, C., Dixon, M. L., Heimberg, R. G., & Gross, J. J. (2021). Evaluation of cognitive behavioral therapy vs mindfulness meditation in brain changes during reappraisal and acceptance among patients with social anxiety disorder: A randomized clinical trial. *JAMA Psychiatry*, 78(10), 1134–1142.

Goldstein, B. I. (2012). Recent progress in understanding pediatric bipolar disorder. *Archives of Pediatrics and Adolescent Medicine*, 166, 362–371.

Goldstein, D. M., & Hall, K. (2015). Mass hysteria in Le Roy, New York: How brain experts materialized truth and outscienced environmental inquiry. *American Ethnologist*. https://www.colorado.edu/faculty/hall-kira/sites/default/files/attached-files/goldstein-hall-2015-mass_hysteria_in_le_roy_new_york.pdf

Goldstein, G., & Beers, S. (2004). *Comprehensive handbook of psychological assessment, intellectual and neuropsychological assessment* (Vol. 1). New York: John Wiley.

Goldstein, I., Kim, N. N., Clayton, A. H., DeRogatis, L. R., Giraldi, A., Parish, S. J., . . . Worsley, R. (2017). Hypoactive sexual desire disorder: International Society for the Study of Women's Sexual Health (ISSWSH) Expert Consensus Panel review. *Mayo Clinic Proceedings*, 92(1), 114–128. https://doi.org/10.1016/j.mayocp.2016.09.018

Goldstein, T. R., Merranko, J., Rode, N., Sylvester, R., Hotkowski, N., Fersch-Podrat, R., . . . Birmaher, B. (2023). Dialectical behavior therapy for adolescents with bipolar disorder: A randomized clinical trial. *JAMA Psychiatry*, e233399. Advance online publication. https://doi.org/10.1001

Gonçalves-Pinho, M., Bragança, M., & Freitas, A. (2020). Psychotic disorders hospitalizations associated with cannabis abuse or dependence: A nationwide big data analysis. *International Journal of Methods in Psychiatric Research*, 29(1), e1813. https://doi.org/10.1002/mpr.1813

Goode, R. W., Webster, C. K., & Gwira, R. E. (2022). A review of binge-eating disorder in Black women: Treatment recommendations and implications for healthcare providers. *Current Psychiatry Reports*, 24(12), 757–766.

Goodwin, G. M., Aaronson, S. T., Alvarez, O., Arden, P. C., Baker, A., Bennett, J. C., . . . Malievskaia, E. (2022). Single-dose psilocybin for a treatment-resistant episode of major depression. *New England Journal of Medicine*, 387(18), 1637–1648. https://doi.org/10.1056/NEJMoa2206443

Goodwin, G. M., Price, J., De Bodinat, C., & Laredo, J. (2017). Emotional blunting with antidepressant treatments: A survey among depressed patients. *Journal of Affective Disorders*, 221, 31–35.

Goossen, B., van der Starre, J., & van der Heiden, C. (2019). A review of neuroimaging studies in generalized anxiety disorder: "So where do we stand?" *Journal of Neural Transmission*, 126(9), 1203–1216.

Gordon, A., Davis, P. J., Patterson, S., Pepping, C. A., Scott, J. G., Salter, K., & Connell, M. (2018). A randomized waitlist control community study of social cognition and interaction training for people with schizophrenia. *The British Journal of Clinical Psychology*, 57(1), 116–130.

Gordon, O. M., Salkovskis, P. M., & Bream, V. (2016). The impact of obsessive compulsive personality disorder on cognitive behaviour therapy for obsessive compulsive disorder. *Behavioural and Cognitive Psychotherapy*, 44(4), 444–459.

Gorka, S. M., Young, C. B., Klumpp, H., Kennedy, A. E., Francis, J., Ajilore, O., . . . Phan, K. L. (2019). Emotion-based brain mechanisms and predictors for SSRI and CBT treatment of anxiety and depression: A randomized trial. *Neuropsychopharmacology*, 44(9), 1639–1648.

Gottesman, I. I. (1978). Schizophrenia and genetics: Where are we? Are you sure? In L. C. Wynne, R. L. Cromwell, & S. Matthysse (Eds.), *The nature of schizophrenia: New approaches to research and treatment* (pp. 59–69). New York: Wiley.

Gottesman, I. I. (1991). *Schizophrenia genesis*. New York: Freeman.

Gottesman, I. I., & Gould, T. D. (2003). The endophenotype concept in psychiatry: Etymology and strategic intentions. *The American Journal of Psychiatry*, 160(4), 636–645.

Gottschalk, M. G., & Domschke, K. (2017). Genetics of generalized anxiety disorder and related traits. *Dialogues in Clinical Neuroscience*, 19(2), 159–168.

Goulding, E. H., Dopke, C. A., Rossom, R., Jonathan, G., Mohr, D., & Kwasny, M. J. (2023). Effects of a smartphone-based self-management intervention for individuals with bipolar disorder on relapse, symptom burden, and quality of life: A randomized clinical trial. *JAMA Psychiatry*, 80(2), 109–118.

Gourgouvelis, J., Yielder, P., Clarke, S. T., Behbahani, H., & Murphy, B. A. (2018). Exercise leads to better clinical outcomes in those receiving medication plus cognitive behavioral therapy for major depressive disorder. *Frontiers in Psychiatry*, 9, 37. https://doi.org/10.3389/fpsyt.2018.00037

Goveas, J. S., & Shear, M. K. (2020). Grief and the COVID-19 pandemic in older adults. *The American Journal of Geriatric Psychiatry: Official Journal of the American Association for Geriatric Psychiatry*, 28(10), 1119–1125.

Gow, M. L., Tee, M., Garnett, S. P., Baur, L. A., Aldwell, K., Thomas, S., . . . Jebeile, H. (2020). Pediatric obesity treatment, self-esteem, and body image: A systematic review with meta-analysis. *Pediatric Obesity*, 15(3), e12600. https://doi.org/10.1111/ijpo.12600

Gowensmith, W. N., Murrie, D. C., & Boccaccini, M. T. (2013). How reliable are forensic evaluations of legal sanity? *Law and Human Behavior*, 37, 98–106.

Grabski, B., Kasparek, K., Müldner-Nieckowski, Ł., & Iniewicz, G. (2019). Sexual quality of life in homosexual and bisexual men: The relative role of minority stress. *The Journal of Sexual Medicine*, 16(6), 860–871.

Grácio, J., Gonçalves-Pereira, M., & Leff, J. (2018). Key elements of a family intervention for schizophrenia: A qualitative analysis of an RCT. *Family Process, 57*(1), 100–112.

Graf, W. D., Nagel, S. K., Epstein, L. G., Miller, G., Nass, R., & Larriviere, D. (2013). Pediatric neuroenhancement: Ethical, legal, social, and neurodevelopmental implications. *Neurology, 80*, 1251–1260.

Graham, R. (2012). Mass hysteria in upstate New York. https://slate.com/human-interest/2012/01/mass-hysteria-in-upstate-new-york-why-lori-brownell-and-13-other-teenage-girls-are-showing-tourettes-like-symptoms.html

Granieri, A., Guglielmucci, F., Costanzo, A., Caretti, V., & Schimmenti, A. (2018). Trauma-related dissociation is linked with maladaptive personality functioning. *Frontiers in Psychiatry, 9*, 206. https://doi.org/10.3389/fpsyt.2018.00206

Grant, J. E., & Chamberlain, S. R. (2016). Trichotillomania. *The American Journal of Psychiatry, 173*(9), 868–874.

Gravina, G., Milano, W., Nebbiai, G., Piccione, C., & Capasso, A. (2018). Medical complications in anorexia and bulimia nervosa. *Endocrine, Metabolic and Immune Disorders Drug Targets, 18*(5), 477–488.

Gray, B. (2008). Hidden demons: A personal account of hearing voices and the alternative of the hearing voices movement. *Schizophrenia Bulletin, 34*, 1006–1007.

Gray, D., Coon, H., McGlade, E., Callor, W. B., Byrd, J., Viskochil, J., . . . McMahon, W. M. (2014). Comparative analysis of suicide, accidental, and undetermined cause of death classification. *Suicide and Life-Threatening Behavior, 44*, 304–316.

Gray, K. J., & Wilkins-Haug, L. E. (2018). Have we done our last amniocentesis? Updates on cell-free DNA for Down syndrome screening. *Pediatric Radiology, 48*(4), 461–470.

Green, A. A., & Kinchen, E. V. (2021). The effects of mindfulness meditation on stress and burnout in nurses. *Journal of Holistic Nursing, 39*(4), 356–368.

Green, S. A., Hernandez, L., Lawrence, K. E., Liu, J., Tsang, T.,

Yeargin, J., . . . Bookheimer, S. Y. (2019). Distinct patterns of neural habituation and generalization in children and adolescents with autism with low and high sensory overresponsivity. *The American Journal of Psychiatry, 176*(12), 1010–1020.

Green, S., Moll, J., Deakin, J. F., Hulleman, J., & Zahn, R. (2013). Proneness to decreased negative emotions in major depressive disorder when blaming others rather than oneself. *Psychopathology, 46*, 34–44.

Greenbaum, Z. (2020). Should practicing psychologists use dating apps? https://www.apa.org/news/apa/2020/01/psychologists-dating-apps

Greenberg, J. L., Phillips, K. A., Steketee, G., Hoeppner, S. S., & Wilhelm, S. (2019). Predictors of response to cognitive-behavioral therapy for body dysmorphic disorder. *Behavior Therapy, 50*(4), 839–849.

Greenberg, W. M. (2010). Obsessive-compulsive disorder. http://emedicine.medscape.com/article/287681-print

Greenberger, E., Chen, C., Tally, S. R., & Dong, Q. (2000). Family, peer, and individual correlates of depressive symptomatology among U.S. and Chinese adolescents. *Journal of Consulting and Clinical Psychology, 68*, 209–219.

Greenwood, T. A. (2017). Positive traits in the bipolar spectrum: The space between madness and genius. *Molecular Neuropsychiatry, 2*(4), 198–212.

Gregory, R. J., & Jindal, S. (2006). Factitious disorder on an inpatient psychiatry ward. *American Journal of Orthopsychiatry, 76*, 31–36.

Gregory, S., Blair, R. J., Ffytche, D., Simmons, A., Kumari, V., Hodgins, S., & Blackwood, N. (2015). Punishment and psychopathy: A case-control functional MRI investigation of reinforcement learning in violent antisocial personality disordered men. *The Lancet. Psychiatry, 2*(2), 153–160.

Grekin, E. R., & Sher, K. J. (2006). Alcohol dependence symptoms among college freshmen: Prevalence, stability and person-environment interactions.

Experimental and Clinical Psychopharmacology, 14, 329–338.

Gressier, F., Calati, R., Balestri, M., Marsano, A., Alberti, S., Antypa, N., & Serretti, A. (2013). The 5-HTTLPR polymorphism and posttraumatic stress disorder: A meta-analysis. *Journal of Traumatic Stress, 26*, 645–653.

Griffith, J. D., Mitchell, S., Hart, C. L., Adams, L. T., & Gu, L. L. (2013). Pornography actresses: An assessment of the damaged goods hypothesis. *Journal of Sex Research, 50*, 621–632.

Griffiths, S., Murray, S. B., Krug, I., & McLean, S. A. (2018). The contribution of social media to body dissatisfaction, eating disorder symptoms, and anabolic steroid use among sexual minority men. *Cyberpsychology, Behavior and Social Networking, 21*(3), 149–156.

Grimm, O., Kranz, T. M., & Reif, A. (2020). Genetics of ADHD: What should the clinician know? *Current Psychiatry Reports, 22*(4), 18. https://doi.org/10.1007/s11920-020-1141-x

Grimminck, R. (2015). 10 famous cases of dissociative identity disorder. https://listverse.com/2015/03/16/10-famous-cases-of-dissociative-identity-disorder/

Grisanzio, K. A., Goldstein-Piekarski, A. N., Wang, M. Y., Rashed Ahmed, A. P., Samara, Z., & Williams, L. M. (2018). Transdiagnostic symptom clusters and associations with brain, behavior, and daily function in mood, anxiety, and trauma disorders. *JAMA Psychiatry, 75*, 201–209.

Groenewold, N. A., Opmeer, E. M., de Jonge, P., Aleman, A., & Costafreda, S. G. (2013). Emotional valence modulates brain functional abnormalities in depression: Evidence from a meta-analysis of fMRI studies. *Neuroscience and Biobehavioral Reviews, 37*, 152–163.

Grohol, J. (2011, June 27). Marsha Linehan acknowledges her own struggle with borderline personality disorder [Blog post]. http://psychcentral.com/blog/archives/2011/06/27/marsha-linehan-acknowledges-her-own-struggle-with-borderline-personality-disorder

Grohol, J. M. (2018). Psychology secrets: Most psychology studies are college student biased. https://psychcentral.com/blog/psychology-secrets-most-psychology-studies-are-college-student-biased/

Gross, E., & Brubaker, L. (2022). Dyspareunia in women. *JAMA, 327*(18), 1817–1818.

Grossman, N. L., Ortega, V. E., King, T. S., Bleecker, E. R., Ampleford, E. A., Bacharier, L. B., . . . Israel, E. (2019). Exacerbation-prone asthma in the context of race and ancestry in Asthma Clinical Research Network trials. *The Journal of Allergy and Clinical Immunology, 144*(6), 1524–1533.

Groth, G. G., Longo, L. M., & Martin, J. L. (2017). Social media and college student risk behaviors: A mini-review. *Addictive Behaviors, 65,* 87–91.

Groth-Marnat, G., & Wright, A. J. (2016). *Handbook of psychological assessment* (6th ed.). Hoboken, NJ: John Wiley.

Grotto, L., Atallah, S., Johnson-Agbakwu, C., Rosenbaum, T., Abdo, C., Byers, E. S., . . . Wylie, K. (2016). Psychological and interpersonal dimensions of sexual function and dysfunction. *The Journal of Sexual Medicine, 13*(4), 538–571.

Gruenwald, I., Lauterbach, R., Gartman, I., Aharoni, S., & Lowenstein, L. (2020). Female sexual orgasmic dysfunction and genital sensation deficiency. *Journal of Sexual Medicine, 17,* 273–278.

Guerri, C., & Pascual, M. (2019). Impact of neuroimmune activation induced by alcohol or drug abuse on adolescent brain development. *International Journal of Developmental Neuroscience, 77,* 89–98.

Guille, C., & Aujla, R. (2019). Developmental consequences of prenatal substance use in children and adolescents. *Journal of Child and Adolescent Psychopharmacology, 29*(7), 479–486. https://doi.org/10.1089/cap.2018.0177

Gul, M., & Diri, M. A. (2019). YouTube as a source of information about premature ejaculation treatment. *Journal of Sexual Medicine, 16,* 1734–1740.

Gulbas, L., Szlyk, H., & Zayas, L. H. (2019). Evaluating the interpersonal-psychological theory of suicide among Latina adolescents using qualitative comparative analysis. *Qualitative Psychology, 6*(3), 297–311.

Gullo, M. J., Matveeva, M., Feeney, G. F., Young, R. M., & Connor, J. P. (2017). Social cognitive predictors of treatment outcome in cannabis dependence. *Drug and Alcohol Dependence, 170,* 74–81.

Guloksuz, S., Pries, L. K., Delespaul, P., Kenis, G., Luykx, J. J., Lin, B. D., . . . van Os, J. (2019). Examining the independent and joint effects of molecular genetic liability and environmental exposures in schizophrenia: Results from the EUGEI study. *World Psychiatry, 18*(2), 173–182.

Gunderson, J. G., Herpertz, S. C., Skodol, A. E., Torgersen, S., & Zanarini, M. C. (2018). Borderline personality disorder. *Nature Reviews: Disease Primers, 4,* 18029.

Guo, L., Gu, L., Peng, Y., Gao, Y., Mei, L., Kang, Q., . . . Chen, J. (2022). Online media exposure and weight and fitness management app use correlate with disordered eating symptoms: Evidence from the mainland of China. *Journal of Eating Disorders, 10*(1), 58. https://doi.org/10.1186/s40337-022-00577-y

Guo, Q., Li, C., & Wang, J. (2017). Updated review on the clinical use of repetitive transcranial magnetic stimulation in psychiatric disorders. *Neuroscience Bulletin, 33*(6), 747–756. https://doi.org/10.1007/s12264-017-0185-3

Gurman, A. S., Lebow, J. L., & Snyder, D. K. (Eds.). (2015). *Clinical handbook of couple therapy* (5th ed.). New York: Guilford Press.

Gurman, S. (2015). Prosecutor: 2 exams found James Holmes to be sane. http://news.yahoo.com/prosecutor-2-exams-found-james-193435617.html

Guyll, M., Cutrona, C., Burzette, R., & Russell, D. (2010). Hostility, relationship quality, and health among African American couples. *Journal of Consulting and Clinical Psychology, 78,* 646–654.

Guyon-Harris, K. L., Humphreys, K. L., Fox, N. A., Nelson, C. A., & Zeanah, C. H. (2018). Course of disinhibited social engagement disorder from early childhood to early adolescence. *Journal of the American Academy of Child and Adolescent Psychiatry, 57*(5), 329–335.

Guyon-Harris, K. L., Humphreys, K. L., Miron, D., Gleason, M. M., Nelson, C. A., Fox, N. A., & Zeanah, C. H. (2019). Disinhibited social engagement disorder in early childhood predicts reduced competence in early childhood predicts reduced competence in early adolescence. *Journal of Abnormal Child Psychology, 47*(10), 1735–1745.

Haagsma, J. A., Ringburg, A. N., van Lieshout, E. M., van Beeck, E. F., Patka, P., Schipper, I. B., & Polinder, S. (2012). Prevalence rate, predictors and long-term course of probable posttraumatic stress disorder after major trauma: A prospective cohort study. *BMC Psychiatry, 12,* 236. doi:10.1186/1471-244X-12-236

Habel, M. A., Leichliter, J. S., Dittus, P. J., Spicknall, I. H., & Aral, S. O. (2018). Heterosexual anal and oral sex in adolescents and adults in the United States, 2011–2015. *Sexually Transmitted Diseases, 45,* 775–782.

Hadjikhani, N., Åsberg Johnels, J., Lassalle, A., Zürcher, N. R., Hippolyte, L., Gillberg, C., . . . Ben-Ari, Y. (2018). Bumetanide for autism: More eye contact, less amygdala activation. *Scientific Reports, 8*(1), 3602. https://doi.org/10.1038/s41598-018-21958-x

Hadland, S. E., Rivera-Aguirre, A., Marshall, B., & Cerdá, M. (2019). Association of pharmaceutical industry marketing of opioid products with mortality from opioid-related overdoses. *JAMA Network Open, 2*(1), e186007. https://doi.org/10.1001/jamanetworkopen.2018.6007

Hafner, M., Stepanek, M., Taylor, J., Troxel, W. M., & van Stolk, C. (2017). Why sleep matters—The economic costs of insufficient sleep: A cross-country comparative analysis. *Rand Health Quarterly*, 6(4), 11.

Haggarty, S. J., Karmacharya, R., & Perlis, R. H. (2020). Advances toward precision medicine for bipolar disorder: Mechanisms & molecules. *Molecular Psychiatry*. https://doi.org/10.1038/s41380-020-0831-4

Haijma, S. V., Van Haren, N., Cahn, W., Koolschijn, P. C., Hulshoff Pol, H. E., & Kahn, R. S. (2013). Brain volumes in schizophrenia: A meta-analysis in over 18,000 subjects. *Schizophrenia Bulletin*, 39, 1129–1138.

Hailes, H. P., Yu, R., Danese, A., & Fazel, S. (2019). Long-term outcomes of childhood sexual abuse: An umbrella review. *The Lancet: Psychiatry*, 6(10), 830–839. https://doi.org/10.1016/S2215-0366(19)30286-X

Haines, J. (2023). *The most depressed states in the U.S.* https://www.usnews.com/news/best-states/articles/2023-05-04/the-most-depressed-states-in-the-u-s

Hakimi, D., Bryant-Davis, T., Ullman, S. E., & Gobin, R. L. (2018). Relationship between negative social reactions to sexual assault disclosure and mental health outcomes of Black and White female survivors. *Psychological Trauma: Theory, Research, Practice and Policy*, 10(3), 270–275.

Hale, J. M., Schneider, D. C., Mehta, N. K., & Myrskylä, M. (2020). Cognitive impairment in the U.S.: Lifetime risk, age at onset, and years impaired. *SSM—Population Health*, 11, 100577. https://doi.org/10.1016/j.ssmph.2020.100577

Haley, J. (1963). *Strategies of psychotherapy*. New York: Grune & Stratton.

Haley, J. (1987). *Problem-solving therapy* (2nd ed.). New York: Jossey-Bass.

Haley, J. (2003, October 31). Defendant's wife testifies about his multiple personas. *Bellingham Herald*, p. B4.

Hall, G. C. N., Ibaraki, A. Y., Huang, E. R., Marti, C. N., & Stice, E. (2016). A meta-analysis of cultural adaptations of psychological interventions. *Behavior Therapy*, 47, 993–1014

Hall, G. C. N., & Yee, A. (2014). Evidence-based practice. In F. T. L. Leong, L. Comas-Diaz, G. C. N. Hall, V. McLoyd, & J. Trimble (Eds.), *APA handbook of multicultural psychology. Vol. 2: Applications and training* (pp. 59–79). Washington, DC: American Psychological Association.

Hallak, J. E. C., Crippa, J. A. S., & Zuardi, A. W. (2000). Treatment of koro with citalopram. *Journal of Clinical Psychology*, 61, 951–952.

Hallett, M., Aybek, S., Dworetzky, B. A., McWhirter, L., Staab, J. P., & Stone, J. (2022). Functional neurological disorder: New subtypes and shared mechanisms. *The Lancet: Neurology*, 21(6), 537–550.

Hallquist, M. N., & Lenzenweger, M. F. (2013). Identifying latent trajectories of personality disorder symptom change: Growth mixture modeling in the longitudinal study of personality disorders. *Journal of Abnormal Psychology*, 122, 138–155.

Hamilton, J. E., Heads, A. M., Meyer, T. D., Desai, P. V., Okusaga, O. O., & Cho, R. Y. (2018). Ethnic differences in the diagnosis of schizophrenia and mood disorders during admission to an academic safety-net psychiatric hospital. *Psychiatry Research*, 267, 160–167.

Hammoud, N., & Jimenez-Shahed, J. (2019). Chronic neurologic effects of alcohol. *Clinics in Liver Disease*, 23(1), 141–155.

Hampl, S. E., Hassink, S. G., Skinner, A. C., Armstrong, S. C., Barlow, S. E., Bolling, C. F., . . . Okechukwu, K. (2023). Clinical practice guideline for the evaluation and treatment of children and adolescents with obesity. *Pediatrics*, 151(2), e2022060640. https://doi.org/10.1542/peds.2022-060640

Han, J. Y., Kwon, H. J., Ha, M., Paik, K. C., Lim, M. H., Gyu Lee, S., . . . Kim, E. J. (2015). The effects of prenatal exposure to alcohol and environmental tobacco smoke on risk for ADHD: A large population-based study. *Psychiatry Research*, 225(1–2), 164–168.

Han, K. M., De Berardis, D., Fornaro, M., & Kim, Y. K. (2019). Differentiating between bipolar and unipolar depression in functional and structural MRI studies. *Progress in Neuro-Psychopharmacology and Biological Psychiatry*, 91, 20–27.

Han, Y. J., Roy, S., Siau, A. M. P. L., & Majid, A. (2022). Binge-eating and sodium bicarbonate: A potent combination for gastric rupture in adults-two case reports and a review of literature. *Journal of Eating Disorders*, 10(1), 157. https://doi.org/10.1186/s40337-022-00677-9

Hancock, N., Smith-Merry, J., Jessup, G., Wayland, S., & Kokany, A. (2018). Understanding the ups and downs of living well: The voices of people experiencing early mental health recovery. *BMC Psychiatry*, 18(1), 121. https://doi.org/10.1186/s12888-018-1703-1

Handford, C. M., Rapee, R. M., & Fardouly, J. (2018). The influence of maternal modeling on body image concerns and eating disturbances in preadolescent girls. *Behaviour Research and Therapy*, 100, 17–23.

Hanrahan, F., Field, A. P., Jones, F. W., & Davey, G. C. (2013). A meta-analysis of cognitive therapy for worry in generalized anxiety disorder. *Clinical Psychology Review*, 33, 120–132.

Hargreaves, D. A., & Tiggemann, M. (2009). Muscular ideal media images and men's body image: Social comparison processing and individual vulnerability. *Psychology of Men and Masculinity*, 10, 109–119.

Hariton, E., & Locascio, J. J. (2018). Randomised controlled trials—The gold standard for effectiveness research: Study design: Randomised controlled trials. *BJOG*, 125, 1716.

Harms, P. D., Herian, M. N., Krasikova, D. V., Vanhove, A., & Lester, P. B. (2013). The Comprehensive Soldier and Family Fitness Program evaluation report #4: Evaluation of resilience training and mental and behavioral health outcomes. https://digitalcommons.unl.edu/cgi/viewcontent.cgi?article=1009&context=pdharms

Harned, M. S., Wilks, C. R., Schmidt, S. C., & Coyle, T. N. (2018). Improving functional outcomes in women with borderline personality disorder and PTSD by changing PTSD severity and post-traumatic cognitions. *Behaviour Research and Therapy, 103*, 53–61.

Harrer, M., Adam, S. H., Messner, E. M., Baumeister, H., Cuijpers, P., Bruffaerts, R., . . . Ebert, D. D. (2020). Prevention of eating disorders at universities: A systematic review and meta-analysis. *The International Journal of Eating Disorders, 53*(6), 813–833. https://doi.org/10.1002/eat.23224

Harris, E. A., Gormezano, A. M., & van Anders, S. M. (2022). Gender inequities in household labor predict lower sexual desire in women partnered with men. *Archives of Sexual Behavior, 51*(8), 3847–3870.

Harris, J. C. (2010). Asylum at Saint-Rémy. *Archives of General Psychiatry, 67*, 666.

Harrison, N. A., Johnston, K., Corno, F., Casey, S. J., Friedner, K., Humphreys, K., . . . Kopelman, M. D. (2017). Psychogenic amnesia: Syndromes, outcome, and patterns of retrograde amnesia. *Brain, 140*(9), 2498–2510.

Harvard Health. (2019). Headache: When to worry, what to do. https://www.health.harvard.edu/pain/headache-when-to-worry-what-to-do

Harvey, A. G., Soehner, A. M., Kaplan, K. A., Hein, K., Lee, J., Kanady, J., . . . Buysse, D. J. (2014). Treating insomnia improves mood state, sleep, and functioning in bipolar disorder: A pilot randomized controlled trial. *Journal of Consulting and Clinical Psychology, 83*(3), 564–577.

Harvey, A. G., Soehner, A. M., Kaplan, K. A., Hein, K., Lee, J., Kanady, J., . . . Buysse, D. J. (2015). Treating insomnia improves mood state, sleep, and functioning in bipolar disorder: A pilot randomized controlled trial. *Journal of Consulting and Clinical Psychology, 83*(3), 564–577.

Hasanović, M., Kuldija, A., Pajević, I., Jakovljević, M., & Hasanović, M. (2021). Gambling disorder as an addictive disorder and creative psychopharmacotherapy. *Psychiatria Danubina, 33*(Suppl 4), 1118–1129.

Hasin, D. S., Sarvet, A. L., Meyers, J. L., Saha, T. D., Ruan, W. J., Stohl, M., . . . Grant, B. F. (2018). Epidemiology of adult DSM-5 Major depressive disorder and its specifiers in the United States. *JAMA Psychiatry, 75*(4), 336–346.

Hattingh, C. J., Ipser, J., Tromp, S. A., Syal, S., Lochner, C., Brooks, S. J., & Stein, D. J. (2013). Functional magnetic resonance imaging during emotion recognition in social anxiety disorder: An activation likelihood meta-analysis. *Frontiers in Human Neuroscience, 6*, 347. doi:10.3389/fnhum.2012.00347

Hatzenbuehler, M. L. (2011). The social environment and suicide attempts in lesbian, gay, and bisexual youth. *Pediatrics, 127*, 896–903.

Hawley, K. J., Winter Plumb, E. I., & Conoley, C. W. (2020). Goal-focused positive psychotherapy in action: A case study. *Journal of Clinical Psychology, 76*, 1217–1225.

Hawley, L. L., Niederkrotenthaler, T., Zaheer, R., Schaffer, A., Redelmeier, D. A., Levitt, A. J., . . . Sinyor, M. (2023). Is the narrative the message? The relationship between suicide-related narratives in media reports and subsequent suicides. *The Australian and New Zealand Journal of Psychiatry, 57*(5), 758–766. https://doi.org/10.1177/00048674221117072

Hay, P. (2020). Current approach to eating disorders: A clinical update. *Internal Medicine Journal, 50*(1), 24–29. https://doi.org/10.1111/imj.14691

Hayashi, K., Kawachi, I., Ohira, T., Kondo, K., Shirai, K., & Kondo, N. (2016). Laughter is the best medicine? A cross-sectional study of cardiovascular disease among older Japanese adults. *Journal of Epidemiology, 26*(10), 546–552.

Hayley, S., & Litteljohn, D. (2013). Neuroplasticity and the next wave of antidepressant strategies. *Frontiers in Cellular Neuroscience, 7*, 218. doi:10.3389/fncel.2013

Hearld, K. R., Budhwani, H., & Chavez-Yenter, D. (2015). Panic attacks in minority Americans: The effects of alcohol abuse, tobacco smoking, and discrimination. *Journal of Affective Disorders, 174*, 106–112.

Hebert, K. K., Cummins, S. E., Hernández, S., Tedeschi, G. J., & Zhu, S. (2011). Current major depression among smokers using a state quitline. *American Journal of Preventive Medicine, 40*, 47–53.

Heesacker, M., Perez, C., Quinn, M. S., & Benton, S. (2019). Computer-assisted psychological assessment and psychotherapy for collegians. *Journal of Clinical Psychology, 76*(6), 952–972. https://doi:10.1002/jclp.22854.

Heinssen, R. K., & Cuthbert, B. N. (2001). Barrier to relationship formation in schizophrenia: Implications for treatment, social recovery, and translational research. *Psychiatry, 64*, 126–132.

Heinz, A. J., Wu, J., Witkiewitz, K., Epstein, D. H., & Preston, K. L. (2009). Marriage and relationship closeness as predictors of cocaine and heroin use. *Addictive Behavior, 34*, 258–263.

Hektner, J. M., August, G. J., Bloomquist, M. L., Lee, S., & Klimes-Dougan, B. (2014). A 10-year randomized controlled trial of the Early Risers conduct problems preventive intervention: Effects on externalizing and internalizing in late high school. *Journal of Consulting and Clinical Psychology, 82*, 355–360.

Heldman, C., Cooper, R., Narayanan, S., Somandepalli, K., Burrows, E., Christensen, S., . . . Virgo, J. (2020). See Jane 2020 report. https://seejane.org/wp-content/uploads/2020-film-historic-gender-parity-in-family-films-report-4.20.pdf

Hemmati, A., Mirghaed, S. R., Rahmani, F., & Komasi, S. (2019). The differential profile of social anxiety disorder (SAD) and avoidant personality disorder (APD) on the basis of criterion B of the DSM-5-AMPD in a college sample. *The Malaysian Journal of Medical Sciences, 26*(5), 74–87.

Henningsen, P. (2018). Management of somatic symptom disorder. *Dialogues in Clinical Neuroscience, 20*(1), 23–31. https://doi.org/10.1016/j.jpsychores.2020.110111

Henssler, J., Heinz, A., Brandt, L., & Bschor, T. (2019). Antidepressant withdrawal and rebound phenomena. *Deutsches Arzteblatt International, 116*(20), 355–361.

Henssler, J., Müller, M., Carreira, H., Bschor, T., Heinz, A., & Baethge, C. (2021). Controlled drinking-non-abstinent versus abstinent treatment goals in alcohol use disorder: A systematic review, meta-analysis and meta-regression. *Addiction (Abingdon, England), 116*(8), 1973–1987. https://doi.org/10.1111/add.15329

Hepp, U., Stulz, N., Unger-Köppel, J., & Ajdacic-Gross, V. (2012). Methods of suicide used by children and adolescents. *European Child and Adolescent Psychiatry, 21*, 67–73.

Herbel, B. L., & Stelmach, H. (2007). Involuntary medication treatment for competency restoration of 22 defendants with delusional disorder. *Journal of the American Academy of Psychiatry and Law, 35*, 47–59.

Herhaus, B., Ullmann, E., Chrousos, G., & Petrowski, K. (2020). High/low cortisol reactivity and food intake in people with obesity and healthy weight. *Translational Psychiatry, 10*(1), 40. https://doi.org/10.1038/s41398-020-0729-6

Herle, M., Stavola, B., Hübel, C., Abdulkadir, M., Ferreira, D. S., Loos, R., . . . Micali, N. (2020). A longitudinal study of eating behaviours in childhood and later eating disorder behaviours and diagnoses. *The British Journal of Psychiatry, 216*(2), 113–119.

Herpertz-Dahlmann, B. (2021). Intensive treatments in adolescent anorexia nervosa. *Nutrients, 13*(4), 1265. https://doi.org/10.3390/nu13041265

Herringa, R. J. (2017). Trauma, PTSD, and the developing brain. *Current Psychiatry Reports, 19*(10), 69. https://doi.org/10.1007/s11920-017-0825-3

Herringa, R. J., Birn, R. M., Ruttle, P. L., Burghy, C. A., Stodola, D. E., Davidson, R. J., &

Essex, M. J. (2013). Childhood maltreatment is associated with altered fear circuitry and increased internalizing symptoms by late adolescence. *Proceedings of the National Academy of Science of the United States of America, 110*, 19119–19124.

Herrnstein, R. J., & Murray, C. (1994). *The bell curve: Intelligence and class structure in American life.* New York: Free Press.

Hicken, M. T., Lee, H., & Hing, A. K. (2018). The weight of racism: Vigilance and racial inequalities in weight-related measures. *Social Science & Medicine (1982), 199*, 157–166.

Hicks, T. V., Leitenberg, H., Barlow, D. H., & Gorman, K. M. (2005). Physical, mental, and social catastrophic cognitions as prognostic factors in cognitive-behavioral and pharmacological treatments for panic disorder. *Journal of Consulting and Clinical Psychology, 73*, 506–514.

Higbee, F. (2016). Is Hillary Clinton sick and is it mental or physical? http://unclesamsmisguidedchildren.com/hillary-clinton-sick-mental-physical/

Hilbert, A., Bishop, M. E., Stein, R. I., Tanofsky-Kraff, M., Swenson, A. K., Welch, R. R., & Wilfley, D. E. (2012). Long-term efficacy of psychological treatments for binge eating disorder. *British Journal of Psychiatry, 200*, 232–237.

Hilditch, C. J., & McHill, A. W. (2019). Sleep inertia: Current insights. *Nature and Science of Sleep, 11*, 155–165.

Hill, J. K. (2011). *Victims of Crime Research Digest, issue no. 2.* http://www.justice.gc.ca/eng/pi/rs/rep-rap/rd-rr/rd09_2-rr09_2/p1.html

Hill, L. K., Hoggard, L. S., Richmond, A. S., Gray, D. L., Williams, D. P., & Thayer, J. F. (2017). Examining the association between perceived discrimination and heart rate variability in African Americans. *Cultural Diversity and Ethnic Minority Psychology, 23*(1), 5–14.

Hiller, R. M., Lovato, N., Gradisar, M., Oliver, M., & Slater, A. (2014). Trying to fall asleep while catastrophising: What sleep-disordered adolescents think and feel. *Sleep Medicine, 15*, 96–103.

Hiller, W., Leibbrand, R., Rief, W., & Fichter, M. M. (2002). Predictors of course and outcome in hypochondriasis after cognitive-behavioral treatment. *Psychotherapy and Psychosomatics, 71*, 318–327.

Hill, K. P., Gold, M. S., Nemeroff, C. B., McDonald, W., Grzenda, A., Widge, A. S., Rodriguez, C., Kraguljac, N. V., Krystal, J. H., & Carpenter, L. L. (2022). Risks and benefits of cannabis and cannabinoids in psychiatry. *The American Journal of Psychiatry, 179*(2), 98–109.

Hilliard-Boone, T., Firminger, K., Dutta, T., Cowans, T., DePatie, H., Maurer, M., . . . Powell, W. (2022). Stakeholder-driven principles for advancing equity through shared measurement. *Health Services Research, 57*(Suppl 2), 291–303.

Himmerich, H., Bentley, J., Kan, C., & Treasure, J. (2019). Genetic risk factors for eating disorders: An update and insights into pathophysiology. *Therapeutic Advances in Psychopharmacology, 9*, 2045125318814734. https://doi.org/10.1177/2045125318814734

Hinojosa-Marqués, L., Domínguez-Martínez, T., Kwapil, T. R., & Barrantes-Vidal, N. (2019). Ecological validity of expressed emotion in early psychosis. *Frontiers in Psychiatry, 10*, 854.

Hirota, T., & King, B. H. (2023). Autism spectrum disorder: A review. *JAMA, 329*(2), 157–168. https://doi.org/10.1001/jama.2022.23661

Hirsch, C. R., Beale, S., Grey, N., & Liness, S. (2019). Approaching cognitive behavior therapy for generalized anxiety disorder from a cognitive process perspective. *Frontiers in Psychiatry, 10*, 796. https://doi.org/10.3389/fpsyt.2019.00796

Hjorthøj, C., Compton, W., Starzer, M., Nordholm, D., Einstein, E., Erlangsen, A., . . . Han, B. (2023). Association between cannabis use disorder and schizophrenia stronger in young males than in females. *Psychological Medicine*, 1–7. Advance online publication. https://doi.org/10.1017/S0033291723000880

Hjorthøj, C., Posselt, C. M., & Nordentoft, M. (2021). Development over time of the population-attributable risk fraction for cannabis use disorder in schizophrenia in Denmark. *JAMA Psychiatry, 78*(9), 1013–1019.

Hlavinka, E. (2020). Teenager in psych crisis waits 25 days in ED for admission. https://www.medpagetoday.com/special-reports/exclusives/84236

Ho, C., & Adcock, L. (2017). *Short-term psychodynamic psychotherapy for the treatment of mental illness: A review of clinical effectiveness and guidelines.* Ottawa: CADTH

Hodgekins, J., Lower, R., Wilson, J., Cole, H., Ugochukwu, U., Maxwell, S., & Fowler, D. (2018). Clinician-rated and self-reported psychotic-like experiences in individuals accessing a specialist Youth Mental Health Service. *The British Journal of Clinical Psychology, 57*(3), 367–381.

Hofmann, S. G., & Gómez, A. F. (2017). Mindfulness-based interventions for anxiety and depression. *The Psychiatric Clinics of North America, 40*(4), 739–749.

Hogue, J. V., Rosen, N. O., Bockaj, A., Impett, E. A., & Muise, A. (2019). Sexual communal motivation in couples coping with low sexual interest/arousal: Associations with sexual well-being and sexual goals. *PLOS One, 14*(7), e0219768. https://doi.org/10.1371/journal.pone.0219768

Holdaway, A. S., Luebbe, A. M., & Becker, S. P. (2018). Rumination in relation to suicide risk, ideation, and attempts: Exacerbation by poor sleep quality? *Journal of Affective Disorders, 236*, 6–13.

Holland, K. M., Vivolo-Kantor, A. M., Logan, J. E., & Leemis, R. W. (2017). Antecedents of suicide among youth aged 11–15: A multistate mixed methods analysis. *Journal of Youth and Adolescence, 46*(7), 1598–1610.

Hollander, A. C., Dal, H., Lewis, G., Magnusson, C., Kirkbride, J. B., & Dalman, C. (2016). Refugee migration and risk of schizophrenia and other non-affective psychoses: Cohort study of 1.3 million people in Sweden. *British Medical Journal, 352*, i1030. https://doi.org/10.1136/bmj.i1030

Hollender, M. H. (1980). The case of Anna O.: A reformulation. *American Journal of Psychiatry, 137*, 797–800.

Hollon, S. D., Cohen, Z. D., Singla, D. R., & Andrews, P. W. (2019). Recent developments in the treatment of depression. *Behavior Therapy, 50*(2), 257–269.

Hollstein, T., Ando, T., Basolo, A., Krakoff, J., Votruba, S. B., & Piaggi, P. (2019). Metabolic response to fasting predicts weight gain during low-protein overfeeding in lean men: Further evidence for spendthrift and thrifty metabolic phenotypes. *The American Journal of Clinical Nutrition, 110*(3), 593–604.

Holmes, S. C., Gonzalez, A., Allen, P. A., & Johnson, D. M. (2019). Utilizing group acceptance and commitment therapy (ACT) to address chronic pain, coping, and functioning for patients with Chiari malformation: A case example. *Professional Psychology: Research and Practice, 50*(5), 296–306.

Holth, J., Patel, T., & Holtzman, D. M. (2017). Sleep in Alzheimer's disease—Beyond amyloid. *Neurobiology of Sleep and Circadian Rhythms, 2*, 4–14.

Holt-Lunstad, J., Robles, T. F., & Sbarra, D. A. (2017). Advancing social connection as a public health priority in the United States. *The American Psychologist, 72*(6), 517–530.

Hölzel, B. K., Hoge, E. A., Greve, D. N., Gard, T., Creswell, J. D., Brown, K. W., . . . Lazar, S. W. (2013). Neural mechanisms of symptom improvements in generalized anxiety disorder following mindfulness training. *NeuroImage Clinical, 2*, 448–458.

Hoogman, M., Bralten, J., Hibar, D. P., Mennes, M., Zwiers, M. P., Schweren, L., . . . Franke, B. (2017). Subcortical brain volume differences in participants with attention deficit hyperactivity disorder in children and adults: A cross-sectional mega-analysis. *The Lancet: Psychiatry, 4*(4), 310–319.

Hoorelbeke, K., Van den Bergh, N., Wichers, M., & Koster, E. (2019). Between vulnerability and resilience: A network analysis of fluctuations in cognitive risk and protective factors following remission from depression. *Behaviour Research and Therapy, 116*, 1–9.

Hope, N. H., & Chapman, A. L. (2019). Difficulties regulating emotions mediates the associations of parental psychological control and emotion invalidation with borderline personality features. *Personality Disorders, 10*(3), 267–274.

Horowitz, M. J. (2001). Histrionic personality disorder. In G. O. Gabbard (Ed.), *Treatment of psychiatric disorders* (pp. 2293–2307). Washington, DC: American Psychiatric Press.

Horton, S. E., Hughes, J. L., King, J. D., Kennard, B. D., Westers, N. J., Mayes, T. L., & Stewart, S. M. (2016). Preliminary examination of the interpersonal psychological theory of suicide in an adolescent clinical sample. *Journal of Abnormal Child Psychology, 44*(6), 1133–1144.

Hosseini, S. A., & Molla, M. (2020). *Asperger syndrome.* Treasure Island, FL: StatPearls Publishing.

Hosseinichimeh, N., Wittenborn, A. K., Rick, J., Jalali, M. S., & Rahmandad, H. (2018). Modeling and estimating the feedback mechanisms among depression, rumination, and stressors in adolescents. *PLOS One, 13*(9), e0204389. https://doi.org/10.1371/journal.pone.0204389

Howard, B. (2018). How colleges handle sexual assault in the #MeToo Era. https://www.usnews.com/education/best-colleges/articles/2018-10-01/how-colleges-handle-sexual-assault-in-the-metoo-era

Howard, L. M., Heron, K. E., MacIntyre, R. I., Myers, T. A., & Everhart, R. S. (2017). Is use of social networking sites associated with young women's body dissatisfaction and disordered eating? A look at black–white racial differences. *Body Image, 23*, 109–113.

Howard, M. O., Perron, B. E., Sacco, P., Ilgen, M., Vaughn, M.

G., Garland, E., & Freedentahl, S. (2010). Suicide ideation and attempts among inhalant users: Results from the National Epidemiologic Survey on Alcohol and Related Conditions. *Suicide and Life-Threatening Behavior, 40,* 276–286.

Howard, M. O., Perron, B. E., Vaughn, M. G., Bender, K. A., & Garland, E. (2010). Inhalant use, inhalant-use disorders, and anti-social behavior: Findings from the National Epidemiologic Survey on Alcohol and Related Conditions (NESARC). *Journal of Studies on Alcohol and Drugs, 71,* 201–209.

Howman, M., Walters, K., Rosenthal, J., Ajjawi, R., & Buszewicz, M. (2016). "You kind of want to fix it don't you?" Exploring general practice trainees' experiences of managing patients with medically unexplained symptoms. *BMC Medical Education, 16,* 27. https://doi.org/10.1186/s12909-015-0523-y

Hoyer, J., Burmann, I., Kieseler, M. L., Vollrath, F., Hellrung, L., Arelin, K., . . . Sacher, J. (2013). Menstrual cycle phase modulates emotional conflict processing in women with and without premenstrual syndrome (PMS)—A pilot study. *PLOS One, 8,* e59780. https://doi:10.1371/journal.pone.0059780

Hoyt, L. T., Niu, L., Pachucki, M. C., & Chaku, N. (2020). Timing of puberty in boys and girls: Implications for population health. *SSM—Population Health, 10,* 100549. https://doi.org/10.1016/j.ssmph.2020.100549

Hsu, L., Woody, S. R., Lee, H. J., Peng, Y., Zhou, X., & Ryder, A. G. (2012). Social anxiety among East Asians in North America: East Asian socialization or the challenge of acculturation? *Cultural Diversity and Ethnic Minority Diversity, 18,* 181–191.

Hu, G., Liu, D., Tong, H., Huang, W., Hu, Y., & Huang, Y. (2019). Lipoprotein- associated phospholipase A2 activity and mass as independent risk factor of stroke: A meta-analysis. *BioMed Research International, 2019,* 8642784. https://doi.org/10.1155/2019/8642784

Hu, V. W., Devlin, C. A., & Debski, J. J. (2019). ASD phenotype-genotype associations in concordant and discordant monozygotic and dizygotic twins stratified by severity of autistic traits. *International Journal of Molecular Sciences, 20*(15), 3804. https://doi.org/10.3390/ijms20153804

Hu, Y. H., Chen, K., Chang, I. C., & Shen, C. C. (2020). Critical predictors for the early detection of conversion from unipolar major depressive disorder to bipolar disorder: Nationwide population-based retrospective cohort study. *JMIR Medical Informatics, 8*(4), e14278. https://doi.org/10.2196/14278

Hueston, C. M., Cryan, J. F., & Nolan, Y. M. (2017). Stress and adolescent hippocampal neurogenesis: Diet and exercise as cognitive modulators. *Translational Psychiatry, 7*(4), e1081. https://doi.org/10.1038/tp.2017.48

Huff, C. (2021). How psychologists can help patients with injection fear. *Monitor on Psychology, 52.* https://www.apa.org/monitor/2021/06/injection-fear

Huffman, J. C., DuBois, C. M., Healy, B. C., Boehm, J. K., Kashdan, T. B., Celano, C. M., . . . Lyubomirsky, S. (2014). Feasibility and utility of positive psychology exercises for suicidal inpatients. *General Hospital Psychiatry, 36,* 88–94.

Hughes, E. (2021). "I'm supposed to be thick": Managing body image anxieties among Black American women. *Journal of Black Studies, 52*(3), 310–330. https://doi.org/10.1177/0021934720972440

Hughes, J. A. (2020). Does the heterogeneity of autism undermine the neurodiversity paradigm? *Bioethics.* https://doi.org/10.1111/bioe.12780

Hughes, J. E. A., Ward, J., Gruffydd, E., Baron-Cohen, S., Smith, P., Allison, C., & Simner, J. (2018). Savant syndrome has a distinct psychological profile in autism. *Molecular Autism, 9,* 53. https://doi.org/10.1186/s13229-018-0237-1

Hughes, S. H. (2015, April 10). I have a mental illness, and I am

more than the same single story. http://www.huffingtonpost.com/stephanie-mitchell-hughes/i-have-a-mental-illness-a_b_7030224.html?ncid=txtlnkusaolp00000592

Hughes, V. (2012). Roots of post-trauma resilience sought in genetics and brain changes. http://www.scientificamerican.com/article.cfm? id5roots-post-trauma-resilience-sought-genetics-brain-changes

Hukic, D. S., Frisén, L., Backlund, L., Lavebratt, C., Landén, M., Träskman-Bendz, L., . . . Ösby, U. (2013). Cognitive manic symptoms in bipolar disorder associated with polymorphisms in the DAOA and COMT genes. *PLOS One, 8*(7), e67450. https://doi.org/10.1371/journal.pone.0067450

Humphreys, C. L., Rubin, J. S., Knudson, R. M., & Stiles, W. B. (2005). The assimilation of anger in a case of dissociative identity disorder. *Counselling Psychology Quarterly, 18,* 121–132.

Humphreys, K. L., Gleason, M. M., Drury, S. S., Miron, D., Nelson, C. A., 3rd, Fox, N. A., & Zeanah, C. H. (2015). Effects of institutional rearing and foster care on psychopathology at age 12 years in Romania: follow-up of an open, randomised controlled trial. *The lancet. Psychiatry, 2*(7), 625–634.

Hunsley, J. (2007). Addressing key challenges in evidence-based practice in psychology. *Professional Psychology: Research and Practice, 38,* 113–121.

Hunter, E. C. M., Salkovskis, P. M., & David, A. S. (2014). Attributions, appraisals and attention for symptoms in depersonalisation disorder. *Behaviour Research and Therapy, 53,* 20–29.

Huntjens, R., Rijkeboer, M. M., & Arntz, A. (2019). Schema therapy for dissociative identity disorder (DID): Further explanation about the rationale and study protocol. *European Journal of Psychotraumatology, 10*(1), 1684629. https://doi.org/10.1080/20008198.2019.1684629

Huprich, S. K. (2018). Moving beyond categories and dimensions in personality pathology assessment and diagnosis. *The British Journal of Psychiatry, 213*(6), 685–689.

Huq, N., Stein, G. L., & Gonzalez, L. M. (2016). Acculturation conflict among Latino youth: Discrimination, ethnic identity, and depressive symptoms. *Cultural Diversity and Ethnic Minority Psychology, 22*(3), 377–385.

Hussong, A. M., Jones, D. J., Stein, G. L., Baucom, D. H., & Boeding, S. (2011). An internalizing pathway to alcohol use and disorder. *Psychology of Addictive Behaviors, 25*, 390–404.

Hviid, A., Hansen, J. V., Frisch, M., & Melbye, M. (2019). Measles, mumps, rubella vaccination and autism: A nationwide cohort study. *Annals of Internal Medicine, 170*(8), 513–520.

Hwang, J. Y., Aromolaran, K. A., & Zukin, R. S. (2017). The emerging field of epigenetics in neurodegeneration and neuroprotection. *Nature Reviews. Neuroscience, 18*(6), 347–361.

Hyde, L. W., Waller, R., Trentacosta, C. J., Shaw, D. S., Neiderhiser, J. M., Ganiban, J. M., . . . Leve, L. D. (2016). Heritable and nonheritable pathways to early callous-unemotional behaviors. *The American Journal of Psychiatry, 173*(9), 903–910.

Hylwa, S. A., & Ronkainen, S. D. (2018). Delusional infestation versus Morgellons disease. *Clinics in Dermatology, 36*(6), 714–718.

Iacovino, J. M., Powers, A. D., & Oltmanns, T. F. (2014). Impulsivity mediates the association between borderline personality pathology and body mass index. *Personality and Individual Differences, 56*, 100–104.

Iancu, I., Sarel, A., Avital, A., Abdo, B., Joubran, S., & Ram, E. (2011). Shyness and social phobia in Israeli Jewish vs Arab students. *Comprehensive Psychiatry, 52*, 708–714.

Ibarluzea, N., Hoz, A. B., Villate, O., Llano, I., Ocio, I., Martí, I., . . . Tejada, M. I. (2020). Targeted next-generation sequencing in patients with suggestive X-linked intellectual disability. *Genes, 11*(1), 51. https://doi.org/10.3390/genes11010051

Imai, H., Tajika, A., Chen, P., Pompoli, A., & Furukawa, T. A. (2016). Psychological therapies versus pharmacological interventions for panic disorder with or without agoraphobia in adults. *The Cochrane Database of Systematic Reviews, 10*(10), CD011170. https://doi.org/10.1002/14651858.CD011170.pub2

Imuta, K., Scarf, D., Pharo, H., & Hayne, H. (2013). Drawing a close to the use of human figure drawings as a projective measure of intelligence. *PLOS One, 8*(3), e58991. https://doi.org/10.1371/journal.pone.0058991

Innamorati, M., Taradel, R., & Foschi, R. (2019). Between sacred and profane: Possession, psychopathology, and the Catholic Church. *History of Psychology, 22*, 1–16.

Inoue-Choi, M., Liao, L. M., Reyes-Guzman, C., Hartge, P., Caporaso, N., & Freedman, N. D. (2017). Association of long-term, low-intensity smoking with all-cause and cause-specific mortality in the National Institutes of Health-AARP Diet and Health Study. *JAMA Internal Medicine, 177*(1), 87–95.

Inslicht, S. S., Niles, A. N., Metzler, T. J., Lipshitz, S. L., Otte, C., Milad, M. R., . . . Neylan, T. C. (2022). Randomized controlled experimental study of hydrocortisone and D-cycloserine effects on fear extinction in PTSD. *Neuropsychopharmacology, 47*(11), 1945–1952.

Iob, E., & Steptoe, A. (2019). Cardiovascular disease and hair cortisol: A novel biomarker of chronic stress. *Current Cardiology Reports, 21*(10), 116. https://doi.org/10.1007/s11886-019-1208-7

Iorfino, F., Marangoni, C., Cui, L., Hermens, D. F., Hickie, I. B., & Merikangas, K. R. (2021). Familial aggregation of anxiety disorder subtypes and anxious temperament in the NIMH family study of affective spectrum disorders. *Journal of Affective Disorders, 281*, 751–758.

Irwin, V., Wang, K., Tezil, T., Zhang, J., Filbey, A., Jung, J., . . . Parker, S. (2023). *Report on the condition of education, 2023 (NCES 2023-144): U.S. Department of Education.* Washington, DC: National Center for Education Statistics. https://nces.ed.gov/pubsearch/pubsinfo.asp?pubid=2023144.

Isaac, M., Elias, B., Katz, L. Y., Belik, S. L., Deane, F. P., Enns, M. W., . . . Swampy Cree Suicide Prevention Team (12 members). (2009). Gatekeeper training as a preventative intervention for suicide: A systematic review. *La Revue Canadienne de Psychiatrie, 54*, 260–268.

Isaacs, J. Y., Smith, M. M., Sherry, S. B., Seno, M., Moore, M. L., & Stewart, S. H. (2022). Alcohol use and death by suicide: A meta-analysis of 33 studies. *Suicide & Life-Threatening Behavior, 52*(4), 600–614.

IsHak, W. W., Rasyidi, E., Saah, T., Vasa, M., Ettekal, A., & Fan, A. (2010). Factitious disorder case series with variations of psychological and physical symptoms. *Primary Psychiatry, 17*, 40–43.

Iverson, G. L., Luoto, T. M., Karhunen, P. J., & Castellani, R. J. (2019). Mild chronic traumatic encephalopathy neuropathology in people with no known participation in contact sports or history of repetitive neurotrauma. *Journal of Neuropathology and Experimental Neurology, 78*(7), 615–625.

Iyadurai, L., Blackwell, S. E., Meiser-Stedman, R., Watson, P. C., Bonsall, M. B., Geddes, J. R., . . . Holmes, E. A. (2018). Preventing intrusive memories after trauma via a brief intervention involving Tetris computer game play in the emergency department: A proof-of-concept randomized controlled trial. *Molecular Psychiatry, 23*(3), 674–682.

Jaberi, N., Faramarzi, E., Farahbakhsh, M., Ostadarahimi, A., Asghari Jafarabadi, M., & Fakhari, A. (2020). Prevalence of metabolic syndrome in schizophrenia patients treated with antipsychotic medications. *Caspian Journal of Internal Medicine, 11*(3), 310–314. https://doi.org/10.22088/cjim.11.3.310

Jackson, K. M., Janssen, T., Barnett, N. P., Rogers, M. L., Hayes, K. L.,

& Sargent, J. (2018). Exposure to alcohol content in movies and initiation of early drinking milestones. *Alcoholism, Clinical and Experimental Research*, 42(1), 184–194.

Jackson, S. E., Beeken, R. J., & Wardle, J. (2015). Obesity, perceived weight discrimination, and psychological well- being in older adults in England. *Obesity*. doi:0.1002/oby.21052

Jackson, S. R., Parkinson, A., Manfredi, V., Millon, G., Hollis, C., & Jackson, G. M. (2013). Motor excitability is reduced prior to voluntary movements in children and adolescents with Tourette syndrome. *Journal of Neuropsychology*, 7, 29–44.

Jackson, W. T., & Starling, A. J. (2019). Concussion evaluation and management. *Medical Clinics of North America*, 103(2), 251–261.

Jacob, J. A., & Kuruvilla, A. (2018). Quality of life and explanatory models of illness in patients with schizophrenia. *Indian Journal of Psychological Medicine*, 40(4), 328–334.

Jacobs, T., Geysemans, B., Van Hal, G., Glazemakers, I., Fog-Poulsen, K., Vermandel, A., De Wachter, S., & De Win, G. (2021). Associations between online pornography consumption and sexual dysfunction in young men: Multivariate analysis based on an international web-based survey. *JMIR Public Health and Surveillance*, 7(10), e32542.

Jacobsen, D. P., Nielsen, M. B., Einarsen, S., & Gjerstad, J. (2018). Negative social acts and pain: Evidence of a workplace bullying and 5-HTT genotype interaction. *Scandinavian Journal of Work, Environment and Health*, 44(3), 283–290.

Jacobson, R. (2014). Should children take antipsychotic drugs? *Scientific American*. http://www .scientificamerican.com/article /should-children-take-antipsychotic -drugs

Jaderek, I., & Lew-Starowicz, M. (2019). A systematic review on mindfulness meditation-based interventions for sexual dysfunctions. *Journal of Sexual Medicine*, 16, 1581–1596.

Jaffe, J., Robinson, L., & Segal, J. (2013). Coping with suicidal thoughts: The first steps. http://beta.help guide.org /mental/suicide_help.htm

Jafferany, M., Khalid, Z., McDonald, K. A., & Shelley, A. J. (2018). Psychological aspects of factitious disorder. *The Primary Care Companion for CNS Disorders*, 20(1), 17nr02229. https://doi.org /10.4088/PCC.17nr02229

Jagielska, G., & Kacperska, I. (2017). Outcome, comorbidity and prognosis in anorexia nervosa. *Psychiatria Polska*, 51(2), 205–218.

Jaisoorya, T. S., Janardhan Reddy, Y. C., Nair, B. S., Rani, A., Menon, P. G., Revamma, M., . . . Thennarasu, K. (2017). Prevalence and correlates of obsessive-compulsive disorder and subthreshold obsessive-compulsive disorder among college students in Kerala, India. *Indian Journal of Psychiatry*, 59(1), 56–62.

James, H., & O'Shea, S. (2014). Porn causing erectile dysfunction in young men. http://globalnews.ca /news/1232726/porn-causing-erectile -dysfunction-in-young-men/

Janiri, D., Doucet, G. E., Pompili, M., Sani, G., Luna, B., Brent, D. A., & Frangou, S. (2020). Risk and protective factors for childhood suicidality: A US population-based study. *The Lancet Psychiatry*, 7, 317–326.

Janssen, M., Heerkens, Y., Kuijer, W., van der Heijden, B., & Engels, J. (2018). Effects of mindfulness-based stress reduction on employees' mental health: A systematic review. *PLOS One*, 13(1), e0191332. https://doi.org/10.1371 /journal.pone.0191332

Janus, S. S., & Janus, C. L. (1993). *The Janus report on sexual behavior*. New York: Wiley.

Jardin, C., Mayorga, N. A., Bakhshaie, J., Garey, L., Viana, A. G., Sharp, C., . . . Zvolensky, M. J. (2018). Clarifying the relation of acculturative stress and anxiety/ depressive symptoms: The role of anxiety sensitivity among Hispanic college students. *Cultural Diversity and Ethnic Minority Psychology*, 24(2), 221–230.

Jarvis, G. E., Kirmayer, L. J., Gómez-Carrillo, A., Aggarwal, N. K., & Lewis-Fernández, R. (2020).

Update on the Cultural Formulation Interview. *Focus (American Psychiatric Publishing)*, 18, 40–46.

Jefsen, O. H., Erlangsen, A., Nordentoft, M., & Hjorthøj, C. (2023). Cannabis use disorder and subsequent risk of psychotic and nonpsychotic unipolar depression and bipolar disorder. *JAMA Psychiatry*, 80(8), 803–810.

Jelicic, M. (2018). Testing claims of crime-related amnesia. *Frontiers in Psychiatry*, 9, 617. https://doi .org/10.3389/fpsyt.2018.00617

Jenike, M. A. (2001). A forty-five-year-old woman with obsessive-compulsive disorder. *Journal of the American Medical Association*, 285, 2121–2128.

Jenkins, A. (2019). After dehydration death, grieving father and new jail chief forge surprising bond. https://www.nwnewsnetwork.org /post/after-dehydration-death -grieving-father-and-new-jail-chief -forge-surprising-bond

Jenkins, T. A., Nguyen, J. C., Polglaze, K. E., & Bertrand, P. P. (2016). Influence of tryptophan and serotonin on mood and cognition with a possible role of the gut-brain axis. *Nutrients*, 8(1), 56. https:// doi.org/10.3390/nu8010056

Jennings, J. R., Pardini, D. A., & Matthews, K. A. (2017). Heart rate, health, and hurtful behavior. *Psychophysiology*, 54(3), 399–408.

Jepson, J. A. (2013). Teach them to be self-aware. *Schizophrenia Bulletin*, 39, 483–484.

Ji, E., Lejuste, F., Sarrazin, S., & Houenou, J. (2019). From the microscope to the magnet: Disconnection in schizophrenia and bipolar disorder. *Neuroscience and Biobehavioral Reviews*, 98, 47–57.

Jia, J., Zhao, T., Liu, Z., Liang, Y., Li, F., Li, Y., . . . Cummings, J. (2023). Association between healthy lifestyle and memory decline in older adults: 10 year, population based, prospective cohort study. *BMJ (Clinical research ed.)*, 380, e072691. https://doi.org/10.1136/ bmj-2022-072691

Jiang, T., Osadchiy, V., Mills, J. N., & Eleswarapu, S. V. (2020). Is it all in my head? Self-reported psychogenic erectile dysfunction and depression are common among young men seeking advice on social media. *Urology, 142,* 133–140.

Jiann, B.-P., Su, C.-C., & Tsai, J.-Y. (2013). Is female sexual function related to the male partners' erectile function? *Journal of Sexual Medicine, 10,* 420–429.

Jiménez, L., Hidalgo, V., Baena, S., León, A., & Lorence, B. (2019). Effectiveness of structural–strategic family therapy in the treatment of adolescents with mental health problems and their families. *International Journal of Environmental Research and Public Health, 16*(7), 1255. https://doi.org/10.3390/ijerph16071255

John Hopkins School of Public Health. (2020). Extreme risk protection orders: State laws at a glance. https://americanhealth.jhu.edu/sites/default/files/inline-files/GENERAL_StateLawTable_v5.1_0.pdf

John Hopkins School of Public Health. (2023). Extreme risk protection orders. https://americanhealth.jhu.edu/implementERPO

Johnco, C. J., Magson, N. R., Fardouly, J., Oar, E. L., Forbes, M. K., Richardson, C., & Rapee, R. M. (2021). The role of parenting behaviors in the bidirectional and intergenerational transmission of depression and anxiety between parents and early adolescent youth. *Depression and Anxiety, 38*(12), 1256–1266.

Johns, L. C., Cannon, M., Singleton, N., Murray, R. M., Farrell, M., Brugha, T., . . . Metzer, H. (2004). Prevalence and correlates of self-reported psychotic symptoms in the British population. *British Journal of Psychiatry, 185,* 298–305.

Johnson, B., Leibowitz, S., Chavez, A., & Herbert, S. E. (2019). Risk versus resiliency: Addressing depression in lesbian, gay, bisexual, and transgender youth. *Child and Adolescent Psychiatric Clinics of North America, 28*(3), 509–521.

Johnson, D. W., & Johnson, F. P. (2003). *Joining together.* Boston: Allyn & Bacon.

Johnson, J. G., Cohen, P., Kasen, S., & Brook, J. S. (2006). Dissociative disorders among adults in the community, impaired functioning, and Axis I and II comorbidity. *Journal of Psychiatric Research, 40,* 131–140.

Johnson, V. C., Kryski, K. R., Sheikh, H. I., Smith, H. J., Singh, S. M., & Hayden, E. P. (2016). The serotonin transporter promoter polymorphism moderates the continuity of behavioral inhibition in early childhood. *Development and Psychopathology, 28*(4pt1), 1103–1116.

Johnston, L. D., Miech, R. A., O'Malley, P. M., Bachman, J. G., Schulenberg, J. E., & Patrick, M. E. (2020). *Monitoring the Future national survey results on drug use, 1975–2019: Overview, key findings on adolescent drug use.* Ann Arbor: Institute for Social Research, University of Michigan.

Joiner, T. E., Van Orden, K. A., Witte, T. K., Selby, E. A., Ribeiro, J. D., Lewis, R., & Rudd, M. D. (2009). Main predictions of the interpersonal-psychology theory of suicidal behavior: Empirical tests in two samples of young adults. *Journal of Abnormal Psychology, 118,* 634–646.

Jones, G., Keuthen, N., & Greenberg, E. (2018). Assessment and treatment of trichotillomania (hair pulling disorder) and excoriation (skin picking) disorder. *Clinics in Dermatology, 36*(6), 728–736.

Jones, W., Klaiman, C., Richardson, S., Aoki, C., Smith, C., Minjarez, M., Bernier, R., . . . Klin, A. (2023). Eye-tracking-based measurement of social visual engagement compared with expert clinical diagnosis of autism. *JAMA, 330*(9), 854–865. https://doi.org/10.1001/jama.2023.13295

Jordan, C. J., & Xi, Z. X. (2018). Discovery and development of varenicline for smoking cessation. *Expert Opinion on Drug Discovery, 13*(7), 671–683.

Joseph, A. W., Ishii, L., Joseph, S. S., Smith, J. I., Su, P., Bater, K., . . . Ishii, M. (2017). Prevalence of body dysmorphic disorder and surgeon diagnostic accuracy in facial plastic and oculoplastic surgery clinics. *JAMA Facial Plastic Surgery, 19*(4), 269–274.

Joyal, C. C., & Carpentier, J. (2016). The prevalence of paraphilic interests and behaviors in the general population: A provincial survey. *Journal of Sex Research.* https://doi.org:/10.1080/00224499.2016.1139034

Ju, Y. E., McLeland, J. S., Toedebusch, C. D., Xiong, C., Fagan, A. M., Duntley, S. P., . . . Holtzman, D. M. (2013). Sleep quality and preclinical Alzheimer disease. *JAMA Neurology, 70*(5), 587–593.

Juang, L. P., Syed, M., Cookston, J. T., Wang, Y., & Kim, S. Y. (2012). Acculturation-based and everyday family conflict in Chinese American families. *New Directions for Child and Adolescent Development, 2012*(135), 13–34.

Jung, H. J., Shin, I. S., & Lee, J. E. (2019). Olfactory function in mild cognitive impairment and Alzheimer's disease: A meta-analysis. *The Laryngoscope, 129*(2), 362–369.

Jung, J. S., Park, S. J., Kim, E. Y., Na, K. S., Kim, Y. J., & Kim, K. G. (2019). Prediction models for high risk of suicide in Korean adolescents using machine learning techniques. *PLOS One, 14*(6), e0217639. https://doi.org/10.1371/journal.pone.0217639

Jurin, T., & Biglbauer, S. (2018). Anxiety sensitivity as a predictor of panic disorder symptoms: A prospective 3-year study. *Anxiety, Stress, and Coping, 31*(4), 365–374.

Juruena, M. F., Bocharova, M., Agustini, B., & Young, A. H. (2018). Atypical depression and non-atypical depression: Is HPA axis function a biomarker? A systematic review. *Journal of Affective Disorders, 233,* 45–67.

Just, M. A., Pan, L., Cherkassky, V. L., McMakin, D. L., Cha, C., Nock, M. K., & Brent, D. (2017). Machine learning of neural representations of suicide and emotion concepts identifies suicidal youth. *Nature Human Behaviour, 1,* 911–919.

Kacel, E. L., Ennis, N., & Pereira, D. B. (2017). Narcissistic personality disorder in clinical health psychology practice: Case studies of comorbid psychological distress and life-limiting illness. *Behavioral Medicine, 43*(3), 156–164.

Kachaner, A., Lemogne, C., Dave, J., Ranque, B., de Broucker, T., & Meppiel, E. (2022). Somatic symptom disorder in patients with post-COVID-19 neurological symptoms: A preliminary report from the somatic study (Somatic Symptom Disorder Triggered by COVID-19). *Journal of Neurology, Neurosurgery, and Psychiatry*. Advance online publication. https://doi.org/10.1136/jnnp-2021-327899

Kailas, M., Lu, H. M. S., Rothman, E. F., & Safer, J. D. (2017). Prevalence and types of gender-affirming surgery among a sample of transgender endocrinology patients prior to state expansion of insurance coverage. *Endocrine Practice: Official Journal of the American College of Endocrinology and the American Association of Clinical Endocrinologists, 23*(7), 780–786. https://doi.org/10.4158/EP161727.OR

Kalogeraki, L., & Michopoulos, I. (2017). Hoarding disorder in DSM-5: Clinical description and cognitive approach. *Psychiatriki, 28*(2), 131–141.

Kalra, G. (2013). The depressive façade in a case of compulsive sex behavior with frottage. *Indian Journal of Psychiatry, 55*, 183–186.

Kamal, R. M., van Noorden, M. S., Franzek, E., Dijkstra, B. A., Loonen, A. J., & De Jong, C. A. (2016). The neurobiological mechanisms of gamma-hydroxybutyrate dependence and withdrawal and their clinical relevance: A review. *Neuropsychobiology, 73*(2), 65–80.

Kamarck, T. W., Muldoon, M. F., Shiffman, S. S., & Sutton-Tyrrell, K. (2007). Experiences of demand and control during daily life are predictors of carotid progression among healthy men. *Health Psychology, 26*, 324–332.

Kane, A. E., & Sinclair, D. A. (2019). Epigenetic changes during aging and their reprogramming potential. *Critical Reviews in Biochemistry and Molecular Biology, 54*(1), 61–83.

Kane, J. M., Robinson, D. G., Schooler, N. R., Mueser, K. T., Penn, D. L., Rosenheck, R. A., . . . Heinssen, R. K. (2016). Comprehensive versus usual community care for first-episode psychosis: 2-year outcomes from the NIMH RAISE Early Treatment Program. *American Journal of Psychiatry, 173*(4), 362–372.

Kane, W. (2019). Anxiety "epidemic" brewing on college campuses, researchers find. https://news.berkeley.edu/2019/04/18/anxiety-epidemic-brewing-on-college-campuses-researchers-find/

Kang, L., Li, Y., Hu, S., Chen, M., Yang, C., Yang, B. X., . . . Liu, Z. (2020). The mental health of medical workers in Wuhan, China dealing with the 2019 novel coronavirus. *The Lancet: Psychiatry, 7*(3), e14. https://doi.org/10.1016/S2215-0366(20)30047-X

Kanner, L. (1943). Autistic disturbances of affective content. *Nervous Child, 2*, 217–240.

Kanter, J. W., Puspitasari, A. J., Santos, M. M., & Nagy, G. A. (2012). Behavioural activation: History, evidence and promise. *British Journal of Psychiatry, 200*, 361–363.

Kantrowitz, B., & Scelfo, J. (2006, November 27). What happens when they grow up? *Newsweek*, pp. 47–53.

Kao, Y. C., Lien, Y. J., Chang, H. A., Tzeng, N. S., Yeh, C. B., & Loh, C. H. (2017). Stigma resistance in stable schizophrenia: The relative contributions of stereotype endorsement, self-reflection, self-esteem, and coping styles. *Canadian Journal of Psychiatry, 62*(10), 735–744.

Kaplan, M. S., & Krueger, R. B. (2012). Cognitive-behavioral treatment of the paraphilias. *Israel Journal of Psychiatry and Related Sciences, 49*, 291–296.

Kaplan, M. S., McFarland, B. H., Huguet, N., Conner, K., Caetano, R., Giesbrecht, N., & Nolte, K. B. (2012). Acute alcohol intoxication and suicide: A gender-stratified analysis of the National Violent Death Reporting System. *Injury Prevention, 19*, 38–43.

Karcher, N. R., Hua, J., & Kerns, J. G. (2019). Probabilistic category learning and striatal functional activation in psychosis risk. *Schizophrenia Bulletin, 45*(2), 396–404.

Karra, E., O'Daly, O. G., Choudhury, A. I., Yousseif, A., Millership, S., & Neary, M. T., . . . Batterham, R. L. (2013). A link between FTO, ghrelin, and impaired brain food-cue responsivity. *Journal of Clinical Investigation, 123*, 3539–3551.

Kasen S., Wickramaratne, P., & Gameroff, M. J. (2013, May 29). Religiosity and longitudinal change in psychosocial functioning in adult offspring of depressed parents at high risk for major depression. *Depression and Anxiety*. https:/doi.org/10.1002/da.22131

Kashdan, T. B., Ferssizidis, P., Farmer, A. S., Adams, L. M., & McKnight, P. E. (2013). Failure to capitalize on sharing good news with romantic partners: Exploring positivity deficits of socially anxious people with self-reports, partner-reports, and behavioral observations. *Behaviour Research and Therapy, 51*, 656–668.

Kashdan, T. B., & Rottenberg, J. (2010). Psychological flexibility as a fundamental aspect of health. *Clinical Psychology Review, 30*, 865–878.

Kate, M. A., Hopwood, T., & Jamieson, G. (2020). The prevalence of dissociative disorders and dissociative experiences in college populations: A meta-analysis of 98 studies. *Journal of Trauma and Dissociation, 21*(1), 16–61.

Katz, T. C., Bui, T. H., Worhach, J., Bogut, G., & Tomczak, K. K. (2022). Touretic OCD: Current understanding and treatment challenges of a unique endophenotype. *Frontiers in Psychiatry, 13*, 929526. https://doi.org/10.3389/fpsyt.2022.929526

Kaye, S., Darke, S., & Duflou, J. (2009). Methylenedioxymethamphetamine (MDMA)–related fatalities in Australia: Demographics, circumstances, toxicology and major organ pathology. *Drug and Alcohol Dependence, 104*, 254–261.

Kaye, W. H., & Bulik, C. M. (2021). Treatment of patients with anorexia nervosa in the USA crisis in care. *JAMA Psychiatry, 78*(6), 591–592.

Kaynak, O., Meyers, K., Caldeira, K. M., Vincent, K. B., Winters, K. C., & Arria, A. M. (2013). Relationships among parental monitoring and sensation seeking on the development of substance use disorder among college students. *Addictive Behavior, 38,* 1457–1463.

Kaysen, D. L., Bedard-Gilligan, M. A., & Saxon, A. J. (2019). Use of prolonged exposure and sertraline in the treatment of posttraumatic stress disorder for veterans. *JAMA Psychiatry, 76*(2), 109–110.

Kaywan, P., Ahmed, K., Ibaida, A., Miao, Y., & Gu, B. (2023). Early detection of depression using a conversational AI bot: A nonclinical trial. *PLOS One, 18*(2), e0279743. https://doi.org/10.1371/journal.pone.0279743

Kazda, L., Bell, K., Thomas, R., McGeechan, K., Sims, R., & Barratt, A. (2021). Overdiagnosis of attention-deficit/hyperactivity disorder in children and adolescents: A systematic scoping review. *JAMA network open, 4*(4), e215335. https://doi.org/10.1001/jamanetworkopen.2021.5335

Kazdin, A. E. (2019). Single-case experimental designs. Evaluating interventions in research and clinical practice. *Behaviour Research and Therapy, 117,* 3–17.

Kean, C. (2011). Battling with the life instinct: The paradox of the self and suicidal behavior in psychosis. *Schizophrenia Bulletin, 37,* 4–7.

Keding, T. J., Heyn, S. A., Russell, J. D., Zhu, X., Cisler, J., McLaughlin, K. A., & Herringa, R. J. (2021). Differential patterns of delayed emotion circuit maturation in abused girls with and without internalizing psychopathology. *The American Journal of Psychiatry, 178*(11), 1026–1036.

Keefe, R. S. E., Cañadas, E., Farlow, D., & Etkin, A. (2022). Digital intervention for cognitive deficits in major depression: A randomized controlled trial to assess efficacy and safety in adults. *The American Journal of Psychiatry, 179*(7), 482–489.

Keel, P. K., Forney, K. J., Brown, T. A., & Heatherton, T. F. (2013). Influence of college peers on disordered eating in women and men at 10-year follow-up. *Journal of Abnormal Psychology, 122,* 105–110.

Kelleher, I., Keeley, H., Corcoran, P., Ramsay, H., Wasserman, C., Carli, V., . . . Cannon, M. (2013). Childhood trauma and psychosis in a prospective cohort study: Cause, effect, and directionality. *American Journal of Psychiatry, 170,* 734–741.

Keller, N. E., Hennings, A. C., & Dunsmoor, J. E. (2020). Behavioral and neural processes in counterconditioning: Past and future directions. *Behaviour Research and Therapy, 125,* 103532. https://doi.org/10.1016/j.brat.2019.103532

Kelly, J. F., Bergman, B., Hoeppner, B. B., Vilsaint, C., & White, W. L. (2017). Prevalence and pathways of recovery from drug and alcohol problems in the United States population: Implications for practice, research, and policy. *Drug and Alcohol Dependence, 181,* 162–169.

Kelly, J. F., Humphreys, K., & Ferri, M. (2020). Alcoholics Anonymous and other 12-step programs for alcohol use disorder. *The Cochrane Database of Systematic Reviews, 3*(3), CD012880. https://doi.org/10.1002/14651858.CD012880.pub2

Kelly, N., Makarem, D. C., & Wasserstein, M. P. (2016). Screening of newborns for disorders with high benefit-risk ratios should be mandatory. *The Journal of Law, Medicine and Ethics, 44*(2), 231–240.

Keltner, N. G., & Dowben, J. S. (2007). Psychobiological substrates of posttraumatic stress disorder: Part 1. *Perspectives in Psychiatric Care, 43,* 97–101.

Kendler, K. S., Ohlsson, H., Sundquist, J., & Sundquist, K. (2020). The rearing environment and risk for major depression: A Swedish National high-risk home-reared and adopted-away co-sibling control study. *The American Journal of Psychiatry, 177*(5), 447–453.

Kendler, K. S., & Prescott, C. A. (2006). *Genes, environment, and psychopathology: Understanding the causes of psychiatric and substance use disorders.* New York: Guilford Press.

Kendzor, D. E., Businelle, M. S., Reitzel, L. R., Castro, Y., Vidrine, J. I., Mazas, C. A., . . . Wetter, D. W. (2014). The influence of discrimination on smoking cessation among Latinos. *Drug and Alcohol Dependence, 136,* 143–148.

Keneally, M. (2015). "American Sniper" trial: Eddie Ray Routh found guilty in double murder case. http://abcnews.go.com/US/american-sniper-tri-al-guilty-verdict-reached-double-murder/story?id=29199422

Kenneally, L. B., Szűcs, A., Szántó, K., & Dombrovski, A. Y. (2019). Familial and social transmission of suicidal behavior in older adults. *Journal of Affective Disorders, 245,* 589–596.

Kerr, W. C., Kaplan, M. S., Huguet, N., Caetano, R., Giesbrecht, N., & McFarland, B. H. (2017). Economic recession, alcohol, and suicide rates: Comparative effects of poverty, foreclosure, and job loss. *American Journal of Preventive Medicine, 52*(4), 469–475.

Kerr, Z. Y., Chandran, A., Nedimyer, A. K., Arakkal, A., Pierpoint, L. A., & Zuckerman, S. L. (2019). Concussion incidence and trends in 20 high school sports. *Pediatrics, 144*(5), e20192180. https://doi.org/10.1542/peds.2019-2180

Kessler, R. C., Akiskal, H. S., Ames, M., Birnbaum, H., Greenberg, P., Hirschfeld, R. M., . . . Wang, P. S. (2006). Prevalence and effects of mood disorders on work performance in a nationally representative sample of U.S. workers. *American Journal of Psychiatry, 163,* 1561–1568.

Kessler, R. C., Bossarte, R. M., Luedtke, A. Zaslavsky, A. M., & Zubizarreta, J. R. (2020). Suicide prediction models: A critical review of recent research with recommendations for the way forward. *Molecular Psychiatry, 25,* 168–179.

Kessler, R. C., Chiu, W. T., Demler, O., & Walters, E. E. (2005). Prevalence, severity, and comorbidity of 12-month DSM-IV disorders in the National Co-morbidity Survey Replication. *Archives of General Psychiatry, 62,* 617–627.

Ketter, T. A. (2010). Diagnostic features, prevalence, and impact of bipolar disorder. *Journal of Clinical Psychiatry, 71,* e14.

Khambaty, M., & Parikh, R. M. (2017). Cultural aspects of anxiety disorders in India. *Dialogues in Clinical Neuroscience, 19*(2), 117–126.

Khan, S., Lovell, K., Lunat, F., Masood, Y., Shah, S., Tomenson, B., & Husain, N. (2019). Culturally-adapted cognitive behavioural therapy based intervention for maternal depression: A mixed-methods feasibility study. *BMC Women's Health, 19*(1), 21. https://doi.org/10.1186 /s12905-019-0712-7

Khurana, A., Bleakley, A., Ellithorpe, M. E., Hennessy, M., Jamieson, P. E., & Weitz, I. (2019). Media violence exposure and aggression in adolescents: A risk and resilience perspective. *Aggressive Behavior, 45*(1), 70–81.

Kidd, T., Hamer, M., & Steptoe, A. (2011). Examining the association between adult attachment style and cortisol responses to acute stress. *Psychoneuroendocrinology, 36,* 771–779.

Kidger, J. (2011). The association between bankruptcy and hospital-presenting attempted suicide: A record linkage study. *Suicide and Life-Threatening Behavior, 41,* 676–684.

Kiely, E., & Robertson, L. (2016). How to spot fake news. https:// www.factcheck.org/2016/11/how -to-spot-fake-news/

Kilgore, K. (2015). Clinical psychologists diagnose Donald Trump— And it isn't pretty, especially for his supporters. http://www .inquisitr.com/2595334/clinical -psychologists-diagnose-donald -trump-and-it-isnt-pretty -especially-for-his-supporters /#WKjkhgXVcsLz0I1p.99

Kilmer, E. D., Villarreal, C., Janis, B. M., Callahan, J. L., Ruggero, C. J., Kilmer, J. N., . . . Cox, R. J. (2019). Differential early termination is tied to client race/ethnicity

status. *Practice Innovations, 4*(2), 88–98.

Kim, H. J., Park, E., Storr, C. L., Tran, K., & Juon, H. S. (2015). Depression among Asian-American adults in the community: Systematic review and meta-analysis. *PLOS One, 10*(6), e0127760. https://doi.org/10.1371 /journal.pone.0127760

Kim, J. H., & Duffy, J. F. (2018). Circadian rhythm sleep-wake disorders in older adults. *Sleep Medicine Clinics, 13*(1), 39–50.

Kim, K. M. (2020). What makes adolescents psychologically distressed? Life events as risk factors for depression and suicide. *European Child and Adolescent Psychiatry.* https://doi.org/10.1007/s00787 -020-01520-9

Kim, S., Kwon, S. H., Kam, T. I., Panicker, N., Karuppagounder, S. S., Lee, S., . . . Ko, H. S. (2019). Transneuronal propagation of pathologic α-synuclein from the gut to the brain models Parkinson's disease. *Neuron, 103*(4), 627–641.

Kimble, M., Sripad, A., Fowler, R., Sobolewski, S., & Fleming, K. (2018). Negative world views after trauma: Neurophysiological evidence for negative expectancies. *Psychological Trauma: Theory, Research, Practice and Policy, 10*(5), 576–584.

Kimbrel, N. A., Ashley-Koch, A. E., Qin, X. J., Lindquist, J. H., Garrett, M. E., Dennis, M. F., . . . Million Veteran Program Suicide Exemplar Workgroup, the International Suicide Genetics Consortium, the Veterans Affairs Mid-Atlantic Mental Illness Research, Education, and Clinical Center Workgroup, and the Veterans Affairs Million Veteran Program. (2023). Identification of novel, replicable genetic risk loci for suicidal thoughts and behaviors among US military veterans. *JAMA Psychiatry, 80*(2), 135–145.

King, A. M., Rizvi, S. L., & Selby, E. A. (2019). Emotional experiences of clients with borderline personality disorder in dialectical behavior therapy: An empirical investigation of in-session affect. *Personality Disorders, 10*(5), 468–472.

King, N. J., Eleonora, G., & Ollendick, T. H. (1998). Etiology

of childhood phobias: Current status of Rachman's three pathways theory. *Behavior Research and Therapy, 36,* 297–309.

Kingsbury, M., Hammond, N. G., Johnstone, F., & Colman, I. (2022). Suicidality among sexual minority and transgender adolescents: A nationally representative population-based study of youth in Canada. *CMAJ: Canadian Medical Association Journal (Journal de l'Association Medicale Canadienne), 194*(22), E767–E774. https://doi.org/10.1503/cmaj .212054

Kinsey, A. C., Pomeroy, W. B., & Martin, C. E. (1948). *Sexual behavior in the human male.* Philadelphia: Saunders.

Kinsey, A. C., Pomeroy, W. B., Martin, C. E., & Gebhard, P. H. (1953). *Sexual behavior in the human female.* Philadelphia: Saunders.

Kirkbride, J. B., Hameed, Y., Ankireddypalli, G., Ioannidis, K., Crane, C. M., Nasir, M., . . . Jones, P. B. (2017). The epidemiology of first-episode psychosis in early intervention in psychosis services: Findings from the Social Epidemiology of Psychoses in East Anglia (SEPEA) Study. *American Journal of Psychiatry, 174*(2), 143–153.

Kirouac, M., Kruger, E., Wilson, A. D., Hallgren, K. A., & Witkiewitz, K. (2019). Consumption outcomes in clinical trials of alcohol use disorder treatment: Consideration of standard drink misestimation. *American Journal of Drug and Alcohol Abuse, 45*(5), 451–459.

Kirwan, E., & Fortune, D. G. (2020). Exploding head syndrome, chronotype, parasomnias and mental health in young adults. *Journal of Sleep Research, 30*(2), e13044. https://doi.org/10.1111 /jsr.13044

Kisely, S. R., Campbell, L. A., & O'Reilly, R. (2017). Compulsory community and involuntary outpatient treatment for people with severe mental disorders. *The Cochrane Database of Systematic Reviews.* https://doi .org/10.1002/14651858 .CD004408.pub5

Kivipelto, M., Mangialasche, F., & Ngandu, T. (2018). Lifestyle interventions to prevent cognitive impairment, dementia and Alzheimer disease. *Nature Reviews: Neurology, 14*(11), 653–666.

Klauke, B., Deckert, J., Reif, A., Pauli, P., & Domschke, K. (2010). Life events in panic disorder—An update on "candidate stressors." *Depression and Anxiety, 27*, 716–730.

Klauser, P., Baker, S. T., Cropley, V. L., Bousman, C., Fornito, A., Cocchi, L., . . . Zalesky, A. (2017). White matter disruptions in schizophrenia are spatially widespread and topologically converge on brain network hubs. *Schizophrenia Bulletin, 43*(2), 425–435.

Kleeman, J. (2011, February 25). Sick note: Faking illness online. *Guardian.* http://www.guardian-news.com

Kleim, B., Grey, N., Wild, J., Nussbeck, F. W., Stott, R., Hackmann, A., . . . Ehlers, A. (2013). Cognitive change predicts symptom reduction with cognitive therapy for posttraumatic stress disorder. *Journal of Consulting and Clinical Psychology, 81*, 383–393.

Klimas, J., Fairgrieve, C., Tobin, H., Field, C. A., O'Gorman, C. S., Glynn, L. G., . . . Cullen, W. (2018). Psychosocial interventions to reduce alcohol consumption in concurrent problem alcohol and illicit drug users. *The Cochrane Database of Systematic Reviews, 12*(12), CD009269. https://doi.org/10.1002/14651858.CD009269.pub4

Kline, T. J. (2005). *Psychological testing: A practical approach to design and evaluation.* Thousand Oaks, CA: Sage.

Klopfer, B., & Davidson, H. (1962). *The Rorschach technique.* New York: Harcourt, Brace & World.

Kluft, R. P. (1987). Dr. Kluft replies. *American Journal of Psychiatry, 144*, 125.

Klumpp, H., Keutmann, M. K., Fitzgerald, D. A., Shankman, S. A., & Phan, K. L. (2014). Resting state amygdala-prefrontal connectivity predicts symptom change after cognitive behavioral therapy in generalized social anxiety disorder. *Biology of Mood and Anxiety Disorders, 4*(1), 14.

Knight, T., Steeves, T., Day, L., Lowerison, M., Jette., N, & Pringsheim, T. (2012). Prevalence of tic disorders: A systematic review and meta-analysis. *Pediatric Neurology, 47*, 77–90.

Koelch, M. G., Döpfner, M., Freitag, C. M., Dulz, B., & Rösler, M. (2019). Conduct disorder and antisocial personality disorders: Challenges for treatment in adolescence and young adulthood. *Fortschritte der Neurologie-Psychiatrie, 87*(11), 634–637. https://doi.org/10.1055/a-0984-5929

Koffer, R., Drewelies, J., Almeida, D. M., Conroy, D. E., Pincus, A. L., Gerstorf, D., & Ram, N. (2019). The role of general and daily control beliefs for affective stressor-reactivity across adulthood and old age. *The Journals of Gerontology. Series B, Psychological Sciences and Social Sciences, 74*(2), 242–253.

Kohler, J. (2001, March 30). Therapists on trial in death of girl, 10. *Washington Post,* p. A19.

Köhler, S., Friedel, E., & Stamm, T. (2017). Rapid cycling in bipolar disorders: Symptoms, background and treatment recommendations. *Fortschritte der Neurologie-Psychiatrie, 85*(4), 199–211.

Köhler-Forsberg, O., Rohde, C., Nierenberg, A. A., & Østergaard, S. D. (2022). Association of lithium treatment with the risk of osteoporosis in patients with bipolar disorder. *JAMA Psychiatry, 79*(5), 454–463.

Kohrt, B. A., Rasmussen, A., Kaiser, B. N., Haroz, E. E., Maharjan, S. M., Mutamba, B. B., . . . Hinton, D. E. (2014). Cultural concepts of distress and psychiatric disorders: Literature review and research recommendations for global mental health epidemiology. *International Journal of Epidemiology, 43*(2), 365–406.

Kois, L., Pearson, J., Chauhan, P., Goni, M., & Saraydarian, L. (2013). Competency to stand trial among female inpatients. *Law and Human Behavior, 37*, 231–240.

Kokkinou, M., Irvine, E. E., Bonsall, D. R., Natesan, S., Wells, L. A., Smith, M., . . . Howes, O. D. (2020). Reproducing the dopamine pathophysiology of schizophrenia and approaches to ameliorate it: A translational imaging study with ketamine. *Molecular Psychiatry, 26*(6), 2562–2576. https://doi.org/10.1038/s41380-020-0740-6

Kolar, D. R., Rodriguez, D. L., Chams, M. M., & Hoek, H. W. (2016). Epidemiology of eating disorders in Latin America: A systematic review and meta-analysis. *Current Opinion in Psychiatry, 29*(6), 363–371.

Kolata, G. (2023). New obesity drugs come with a side effect of shaming. https://news.yahoo.com/obesity-drugs-come-side-effect-115136988.html

Kolp, H., Wilder, S., Andersen, C., Johnson, E., Horvath, S., Gidycz, C. A., & Shorey, R. (2020). Gender minority stress, sleep disturbance, and sexual victimization in transgender and gender nonconforming adults. *Journal of Homosexuality, 76*, 688–698.

Komasi, S., Hemmati, A., Rezaei, F., Rahmani, K., Miettunen, J., Amianto, F., & Hopwood, C. J. (2022). Comparison of the relative sensitivity of two dimensional personality models to the psychopathological symptoms: The section III DSM-5 maladaptive traits versus affective temperaments. *BMCP Psychiatry, 22*(1), 503. https://doi.org/10.1186/s12888-022-04156-y

Kondo, K., Noonan, K. M., Freeman, M., Ayers, C., Morasco, B. J., & Kansagara, D. (2019). Efficacy of biofeedback for medical conditions: An evidence map. *Journal of General Internal Medicine, 34*(12), 2883–2893.

Konstantakopoulos, G. (2019). Insight across mental disorders: A multifaceted metacognitive phenomenon. *Psychiatriki, 30*(1), 13–16.

Kooistra, L., Crawford, S., Gibbard, B., Ramage, B., & Kaplan, B. J. (2010). Differentiating attention deficits in children with fetal alcohol spectrum disorder or attention-deficit-hyperactivity disorder. *Developmental Medicine and Child Neurology, 52*, 205–211.

Kopstein, M., & Mohlman, D. J. (2020). HIV-1 encephalopathy

and AIDS dementia complex. *StatPearls*. StatPearls Publishing.

Kosiborod, M. N., Bhatta, M., Davies, M., Deanfield, J. E., Garvey, W. T., Khalid, U., . . . Verma, S. (2023). Semaglutide improves cardiometabolic risk factors in adults with overweight or obesity: Step 1 and 4 exploratory analyses. *Diabetes, Obesity & Metabolism*, 25(2), 468–478. https://doi.org/10.1111/dom.14890

Kosic, A., Lindholm, P., Järvholm, K., Hedman-Lagerlöf, E., & Axelsson, E. (2020). Three decades of increase in health anxiety: Systematic review and meta-analysis of birth cohort changes in university student samples from 1985 to 2017. *Journal of Anxiety Disorders*, 71, 102208.

Kountza, M., Garyfallos, G., Ploumpidis, D., Varsou, E., & Gkiouzepas, I. (2018). The psychiatric comorbidity of anorexia nervosa: A comparative study in a population of French and Greek anorexic patients. *L'Encephale*, 44(5), 429–434.

Kovner, R., Oler, J. A., & Kalin, N. H. (2019). Cortico-limbic interactions mediate adaptive and maladaptive responses relevant to psychopathology. *The American Journal of Psychiatry*, 176(12), 987–999.

Kponee, K. Z., Siegel, M., & Jernigan, D. H. (2014). The use of caffeinated alcoholic beverages among underage drinkers: Results of a national survey. *Addictive Behavior*, 39, 253–258.

Kraepelin, E. (1923). *Textbook of psychiatry* (8th ed.). New York: Macmillan. (Original work published 1883)

Kraines, M. A., Kelberer, L., & Wells, T. T. (2018). Rejection sensitivity, interpersonal rejection, and attention for emotional facial expressions. *Journal of Behavior Therapy and Experimental Psychiatry*, 59, 31–39.

Kramer, A. D., Guillory, J. E., & Hancock, J. T. (2014). Experimental evidence of massive-scale emotional contagion through social networks. *Proceedings of the National Academy of Sciences*, 111(24), 8788–8790.

Krämer, J., Nolte, K., Zupanc, L., Schnitker, S., Roos, A., Göpel, C., . . . Duning, T. (2022). Structured delirium management in the hospital. *Deutsches Arzteblatt International*, 119(11), 188–194. https://doi.org/10.3238/arztebl.m2022.0131

Krantz, T. E., Andrews, N., Petersen, T. R., Dunivan, G. C., Montoya, M., Swanson, N., . . . Komesu, Y. M. (2019). Adverse childhood experiences among gynecology patients with chronic pelvic pain. *Obstetrics and Gynecology*, 134(5), 1087–1095.

Kraschel, K. L., Chen, A., Turban, J. L., & Cohen, I. G. (2022). Legislation restricting gender-affirming care for transgender youth: Politics eclipse healthcare. *Cell Reports: Medicine*, 3(8), 100719. https://doi.org/10.1016/j.xcrm.2022.100719

Kraus, L., Schmid, M., & In-Albon, T. (2020). Anti-suicide function of nonsuicidal self-injury in female inpatient adolescents. *Frontiers in Psychiatry*, 11, 490. https://doi.org/10.3389/fpsyt.2020.00490

Kraus, R. P., & Nicholson, I. R. (1996). AIDS-related obsessive compulsive disorder: Deconditioning based in fluoxetine-induced inhibition of anxiety. *Journal of Behavior Therapy and Experimental Psychiatry*, 27, 51–56.

Krebs, G., Fernández de la Cruz, L., & Mataix-Cols, D. (2017). Recent advances in understanding and managing body dysmorphic disorder. *Evidence-Based Mental Health*, 20(3), 71–75.

Krell-Roesch, J., Syrjanen, J. A., Vassilaki, M., Machulda, M. M., Mielke, M. M., . . . Geda, Y. E. (2019). Quantity and quality of mental activities and the risk of incident mild cognitive impairment. *Neurology*, 93(6), e548–e558.

Kreukels, B. P., & Guillamon, A. (2016). Neuroimaging studies in people with gender incongruence. *International Review of Psychiatry*, 28, 120–128.

Krieg, A., & Xu, Y. (2018). From self-construal to threat appraisal: Understanding cultural differences in social anxiety between Asian Americans and European Americans. *Cultural Diversity and Ethnic Minority Psychology*, 24(4), 477–488

Krieger, H., Young, C. M., Anthenien, A. M., & Neighbors, C. (2018). The epidemiology of binge drinking among college-age individuals in the United States. *Alcohol Research: Current Reviews*, 39(1), 23–30.

Kripke, D. F., Elliott, J. A., Welsh, D. K., & Youngstedt, S. D. (2015). Photoperiodic and circadian bifurcation theories of depression and mania. *F1000Research*, 4, 107. https://doi.org/10.12688/f1000research.6444.1

Krishnan, M., Major, T. J., Topless, R. K., Dewes, O., Yu, L., Thompson, J., . . . Merriman, T. R. (2018). Discordant association of the CREBRF rs373863828 A allele with increased BMI and protection from type 2 diabetes in Maori and Pacific (Polynesian) people living in Aotearoa/New Zealand. *Diabetologia*, 61(7), 1603–1613.

Kroon, J. S., Wohlfarth, T. D., Dieleman, J., Sutterland, A. L., Storosum, J. G., Denys, D., . . . Sturkenboom, M. C. (2013). Incidence rates and risk factors of bipolar disorder in the general population: A population-based cohort study. *Bipolar Disorders*, 15, 306–313.

Krueger, J. (2011). Shock without awe. *American Psychologist*, 66, 642–643.

Krueger, R. B. (2010a). The DSM diagnostic criteria for sexual masochism. *Archives of Sexual Behavior*, 39, 346–356.

Krueger, R. B. (2010b). The DSM diagnostic criteria for sexual sadism. *Archives of Sexual Behavior*, 39, 325–345.

Krupa, M. (2017). The alarming rise of female genital mutilation in America. https://www.cnn.com/2017/05/11/health/female-genital-mutilation-fgm-explainer-trnd/index.html

Krzastek, S. C., Bopp, J., Smith, R. P., & Kovac, J. R. (2019). Recent advances in the understanding and management of erectile dysfunction. *F1000Research*, 8, F1000 Faculty Rev-102. https://doi.org/10.12688/f1000research.16576.1

Krzyzanowski, D. J., Howell, A. J., & Passmore, H.-A. (2019). Predictors and causes of the use of noun-based mental disorder labels. *Stigma and Health, 4*, 86–97.

Ku, H. L., Lin, C. S., Chao, H. T., Tu, P. C., Li, C. T., Cheng, C. M., . . . Hsieh, J. C. (2013). Brain signature characterizing the body-brain-mind axis of transsexuals. *PLOS One, 8*, e70808. https://doi.org/10.1371/journal.pone.0070808

Kuba, K., & Weißflog, G. (2017). Acceptance and commitment therapy in the treatment of chronic disease. *Psychotherapie, 67*(12), 525–536.

Kubiak, S., Shamrova, D., & Comartin, E. (2019). Enhancing knowledge of adolescent mental health among law enforcement: Implementing youth-focused crisis intervention team training. *Evaluation and Program Planning, 73*, 44–52.

Kuehn, K. S., Wagner, A., & Velloza, J. (2019). Estimating the magnitude of the relation between bullying, e-bullying, and suicidal behaviors among United States youth, 2015. *Crisis, 40*(3), 157–165.

Kukla, M., Salyers, M. P., Strasburger, A. M., Johnson-Kwochka, A., Amador, E., & Lysaker, P. H. (2019). Work-focused cognitive behavioral therapy to complement vocational services for people with mental illness: Pilot study outcomes across a 6-month posttreatment follow-up. *Psychiatric Rehabilitation Journal, 42*(4), 366–371.

Kulkarni, G. B., Mathew, T., & Mailankody, P. (2021). Medication overuse headache. *Neurology India, 69*(Supplement), S76–S82. https://doi.org/10.4103/0028-3886.315981

Kumanyika, S. K. (2019). Unraveling common threads in obesity risk among racial/ethnic minority and migrant populations. *Public Health, 172*, 125–134.

Kuntsche, S., & Kuntsche, E. (2016). Parent-based interventions for preventing or reducing adolescent substance use—A systematic literature review. *Clinical Psychology Review, 45*, 89–101.

Kuper, L. E., Lindley, L., & Lopez, X. (2019). Exploring the gender development histories of children and adolescents presenting for gender affirming medical care. *Clinical Practice in Pediatric Psychology, 7*, 217–228.

Kupfer, D. (2013). *Chair of DSM-5 task force discusses future of mental health research*. Arlington, VA: American Psychiatric Association.

Kuramoto, S. J., Runeson, B., Stuart, E. A., Lichtenstein, P., & Wilcox, H. C. (2013). Time to hospitalization for suicide attempt by the timing of parental suicide during offspring early development. *JAMA Psychiatry, 70*, 149–157.

Kuramoto, S., Stuart, E. A., Runeson, B., Lichtenstein, P., Långström, N., & Wilcox, H. C. (2010). Maternal or paternal suicide and offspring's psychiatric and suicide-attempt hospitalization risk. *Pediatrics, 126*, 1026–1032.

Kurlan, R. M. (2013). Treatment of Tourette syndrome. *Neurotherapeutics, 11*, 161–165.

Kurth, T., Winter, A. C., Eliassen, A. H., Dushkes, R., Mukamal, K. J., Rimm, E. B., . . . Rexrode, K. M. (2016). Migraine and risk of cardiovascular disease in women: Prospective cohort study. *BMJ (Clinical Research ed.), 353*, i2610. https://doi.org/10.1136/bmj.i2610

Kusek, K. (2001, May). Could a fear wreak havoc on your life? *Cosmopolitan, 230*(5), 182–184.

Kushida, C. A., Shapiro, C. M., Roth, T., Thorpy, M. J., Corser, B. C., Ajayi, A. O., . . . Dauvilliers, Y. (2022). Once-nightly sodium oxybate (FT218) demonstrated improvement of symptoms in a phase 3 randomized clinical trial in patients with narcolepsy. *Sleep, 45*(6), zsab200. https://doi.org/10.1093/sleep/zsab200

Kuss, D. J. (2013). Internet gaming addiction: Current perspectives. *Psychological Research and Behavior Management, 6*, 125–137.

Kvaale, E. P., Gottdiener, W. H., & Haslam, N. (2013). Biogenic explanations and stigma: A meta-analytic review of associations among lay people. *Social Science & Medicine, 96*, 95–103.

Kvarstein, E. H., Antonsen, B. T., Klungsøyr, O., Pedersen, G., & Wilberg, T. (2021). Avoidant personality disorder and social functioning: A longitudinal, observational study investigating predictors of change in a clinical sample. *Personality Disorders, 12*(6), 594–605. https://doi.org/10.1037/per0000471

Kwon, S., & Han, D. (2019). Discrimination, mental disorders, and suicidal ideation in Latino adults: Decomposing the effects of discrimination. *Journal of Immigrant and Minority Health, 21*(1), 143–150.

Kyranides, M. N., Christofides, D., & Çetin, M. (2022). Difficulties in facial emotion recognition: Taking psychopathic and alexithymic traits into account. *BMC Psychology, 10*(1), 239. https://doi.org/10.1186/s40359-022-00946-x

Kyung-Sook, W., SangSoo, S., Sangjin, S., & Young-Jeon, S. (2018). Marital status integration and suicide: A meta-analysis and meta-regression. *Social Science & Medicine, 197*, 116–126.

Labonté, B., Suderman, M., Maussion, G., Lopez, J. P., Navarro-Sánchez, L., Yerko, V., . . . Turecki, G. (2013). Genome-wide methylation changes in the brains of suicide completers. *American Journal of Psychiatry, 170*, 511–520.

Lafortune, D., Dion, L., & Renaud, P. (2020). Virtual reality and sex therapy: Future directions for clinical research. *Journal of Sex and Marital Therapy, 46*, 1–17.

Laher, S., & Cockcroft, K. (2017). Moving from culturally biased to culturally responsive assessment practices in low-resource, multicultural settings. *Professional Psychology: Research and Practice, 48*, 115–121.

Lam, R. W., Levitt, A. J., Levitan, R. D., Enns, M. W., Morehouse, R., Michalak, E. E., & Tam, E. M. (2006). The CanSAD study: A randomized controlled trial of the effectiveness of light therapy and fluoxetine in patients with winter seasonal affective disorder. *American Journal of Psychiatry, 163*, 805–812.

Lam, R. W., McIntosh, D., Wang, J., Enns, M. W., Kolivakis, T., Michalak, E. E., . . . CANMAT

Depression Work Group. (2016). Canadian Network for Mood and Anxiety Treatments (CANMAT) 2016 clinical guidelines for the management of adults with major depressive disorder: Section 1. Disease burden and principles of care. *Canadian Journal of Psychiatry*, *61*(9), 510–523.

Lambert, C. E., Troister, T., Ramadan, Z., Montemarano, V., Fekken, G. C., & Holden, R. R. (2020). Psychache predicts suicide attempter status change in students starting university. *Suicide and Life-Threatening Behavior*. https://doi.org/10.1111/sltb.1262

Lambiase, M. J., Kubzansky, L. D., & Thurston, R. C. (2014). Prospective study of anxiety and incident stroke. *Stroke*, *45*, 438–443.

Lampert, R. (2016). Mental stress and ventricular arrhythmias. *Current Cardiology Reports*, *18*(12), 118. https://doi.org/10.1007/s11886-016-0798-6

Lampkin, D. R. (2019). The Army's Ready and Resilient (R2) program. https://www.armyupress.army.mil/Journals/NCO-Journal/Archives/2019/April/R2-Program/

Lancaster, V. (2021). Münchausen by Internet. https://www.psychologytoday.com/us/blog/digital-world-real-world/202111/m-nchausen-internet

Landa, R. J. (2018). Efficacy of early interventions for infants and young children with, and at risk for, autism spectrum disorders. *International Review of Psychiatry*, *30*(1), 25–39.

Landau, S. M., Marks, S. M., Mormino, E. C., Rabinovici, G. D., Oh, H., O'Neil, J. P., . . . Jagust, W. J. (2012). Association of lifetime cognitive engagement and low b-amyloid deposition. *Archives of Neurology*, *69*, 623–629.

Landeo-Gutierrez, J., Forno, E., Miller, G. E., & Celedón, J. C. (2020). Exposure to violence, psychosocial stress, and asthma. *American Journal of Respiratory and Critical Care Medicine*, *201*(8), 917–922.

Landeo-Gutierrez, J., Marsland, A. L., Acosta-Pérez, E., Canino, G., & Celedón, J. C. (2020). Exposure to violence, chronic stress, asthma, and bronchodilator response in Puerto Rican children. *Annals of Allergy, Asthma and Immunology*, *124*(6), 626–627

Landgren, V., Malki, K., Bottai, M., Arver, S., & Rahm, C. (2020). Effect of gonadotropin-releasing hormone antagonist on risk of committing child sexual abuse in men with pedophilic disorder: A randomized clinical trial. *JAMA Psychiatry*, *77*(9), 897–905.

Landis, E. E. (2012). Restoration of competency. http://lawandjusticegov.org/psychology-and-law/criminal-competencies/98-restoration-of-competency.html

Lane, M. M., Gamage, E., Travica, N., Dissanayaka, T., Ashtree, D. N., Gauci, S., . . . Marx, W. (2022). Ultra-processed food consumption and mental health: A systematic review and meta-analysis of observational studies. *Nutrients*, *14*(13), 2568. https://doi.org/10.3390/nu14132568

Lange, A. M., Daley, D., Frydenberg, M., Houmann, T., Kristensen, L. J., Rask, C., . . . Thomsen, P. H. (2018). Parent training for preschool ADHD in routine, specialist care: A randomized controlled trial. *Journal of the American Academy of Child and Adolescent Psychiatry*, *57*(8), 593–602.

Lange, S., Meesters, P. D., Stek, M. L., Wunderink, L., Penninx, B., & Rhebergen, D. (2019). Course and predictors of symptomatic remission in late-life schizophrenia: A 5-year follow-up study in a Dutch psychiatric catchment area. *Schizophrenia Research*, *209*, 179–184.

Langlois, C., Potvin, S., Khullar, A., & Tourjman, S. V. (2021). Down and high: Reflections regarding depression and cannabis. *Frontiers in Psychiatry*, *12*, 625158. https://doi.org/10.3389/fpsyt.2021.625158

Långström, N., & Seto, M. C. (2006). Exhibitionistic and voyeuristic behavior in a Swedish national population survey. *Archives of Sexual Behavior*, *35*, 427–435.

Långström, N., & Zucker, K. J. (2005). Transvestic fetishism in the general population: Prevalence and correlates. *Journal of Sex and Marital Therapy*, *31*, 87–95.

Långström, N., Enebrink, P., Laurén, E. M., Lindblom, J., Werkö, S., & Hanson, R. K. (2013). Preventing sexual abusers of children from reoffending: Systematic review of medical and psychological interventions. *British Medical Journal*, *9*, 347:f4630. https://doi.org/10.1136/bmj.f4630

Lanska, D. J. (2018). Jumping Frenchmen, Miryachit, and Latah: Culture-specific hyperstartle-plus syndromes. *Frontiers of Neurology and Neuroscience*, *42*, 122–131.

Lara-Cinisomo, S., Akinbode, T. D., & Wood, J. (2020). A systematic review of somatic symptoms in women with depression or depressive symptoms: Do race or ethnicity matter? *Journal of Women's Health (2002)*, *29*, 1273–1282.

Large, M., Sharma, S., Compton, M. T., Slade, T., & Nielssen, O. (2011). Cannabis use and earlier onset of psychosis: A systematic meta-analysis. *Archives of General Psychiatry*, *68*, 555–561. doi:10.1001/archgenpsychiatry.2011.5

Larkin H. D. (2023). Child asthma tied to specific urban air pollutants. *JAMA*, *329*(5), 363. https://doi.org/10.1001/jama.2022.24493

Larsson, H., Rydén, E., Boman, M., Långström, N., Lichtenstein, P., & Landén, M. (2013). Risk of bipolar disorder and schizophrenia in relatives of people with attention-deficit hyperactivity disorder. *British Journal of Psychiatry*, *203*, 103–106.

Latas, M., & Milovanovic, S. (2014). Personality disorders and anxiety disorders: What is the relationship? *Current Opinion in Psychiatry*, *27*, 57–61.

Lathan, H. S., Kwan, A., Takats, C., Tanner, J. P., Wormer, R., Romero, D., & Jones, H. E. (2023). Ethical considerations and methodological uses of Facebook data in public health research: A systematic review. *Social Science & Medicine (1982)*, *322*, 115807. https://doi.org/10.1016/j.socscimed.2023.115807

Latimer, W., & Zur, J. (2010). Epidemiologic trends of adolescent use of alcohol, tobacco, and other drugs. *Child and Adolescent*

Psychiatric Clinics of North America, 19, 451–464.

Latvala, A., Kuja-Halkola, R., Almqvist, C., Larsson, H., & Lichtenstein, P. (2015). A longitudinal study of resting heart rate and violent criminality in more than 700 000 men. *JAMA Psychiatry*, 72(10), 971–978.

Lau, H. L., Rundek, T., & Ramos, A. R. (2019). Sleep and stroke: New updates on epidemiology, pathophysiology, assessment, and treatment. *Current Sleep Medicine Reports*, 5(2), 71–82.

Lau, J., Burlingham, A., & Quraishi, S. (2021). ECT and somatoform disorder: Case report and literature review. *Progress in Neurology and Psychiatry*, 25, 40–43. https://doi.org/10.1002/pnp.699

Lavakumar, M., Garlow, S. J., & Schwartz, A. C. (2011). A case of returning psychosis. *Current Psychiatry*, 10, 51–57.

Lavelle, M., Healey, P. G., & McCabe, R. (2013). Is nonverbal communication disrupted in interactions involving patients with schizophrenia? *Schizophrenia Bulletin*, 39, 1150–1158.

Lawrence, R. E., Oquendo, M. A., & Stanley, B. (2016). Religion and suicide risk: A systematic review. *Archives of Suicide Research: Official Journal of the International Academy for Suicide Research*, 20(1), 1–21. https://doi.org/10.1080/13811118.2015.1004494

Lawrie, S. M. (2018). Are structural brain changes in schizophrenia related to antipsychotic medication? A narrative review of the evidence from a clinical perspective. *Therapeutic Advances in Psychopharmacology*, 8(11), 319–326.

Laxman, D. J., Taylor, J. L., DaWalt, L. S., Greenberg, J. S., & Mailick, M. R. (2019). Loss in services precedes high school exit for teens with autism spectrum disorder: A longitudinal study. *Autism Research*, 12(6), 911–921.

Lazaridou, A., Kim, J., Cahalan, C. M., Loggia, M. L., Franceschelli, O., Berna, C., . . . Edwards, R. R. (2017). Effects of cognitive-behavioral therapy (CBT) on brain connectivity supporting catastrophizing in fibromyalgia. *The*

Clinical Journal of Pain, 33(3), 215–221.

Leal, W. E., & Jackson, D. B. (2019). The role of energy drink consumption in the intention to initiate marijuana use among adolescents. *Addictive Behaviors*, 93, 240–245.

Leary, P. M. (2003). Conversion disorder in childhood: Diagnosed too late, investigated too much? *Journal of the Royal Society of Medicine*, 96, 436–444.

Lee, C. M., & Hunsley, J. (2015). Evidence-based practice: Separating science from pseudoscience. *Canadian Journal of Psychiatry*, 60, 534–540.

Lee, D. Y., Kim, E., & Choi, M. H. (2015). Technical and clinical aspects of cortisol as a biochemical marker of chronic stress. *BMB Reports*, 48(4), 209–216. https://doi.org/10.5483/bmbrep.2015.48.4.275

Lee, H., Song, D. H., Kwon, J. W., Han, E., Chang, M. J., & Kang, H. Y. (2018). Assessing the risk of type 2 diabetes mellitus among children and adolescents with psychiatric disorders treated with atypical antipsychotics: A population-based nested case-control study. *European Child and Adolescent Psychiatry*, 27(10), 1321–1334.

Lee, R. (2017). Mistrustful and misunderstood: A review of paranoid personality disorder. *Current Behavioral Neuroscience Reports*, 4(2), 151–165. https://doi.org/10.1007/s40473-017-0116-7

Lee, R. D., & Chen, J. (2017). Adverse childhood experiences, mental health, and excessive alcohol use: Examination of race/ethnicity and sex differences. *Child Abuse and Neglect*, 69, 40–48.

Lee, T. (2016). Pediatric bipolar disorder. *Pediatric Annals*, 45(10), e362–e366. https://doi.org/10.3928/19382359-20160920-01

Legge, S. E., Jones, H. J., Kendall, K. M., Pardiñas, A. F., Menzies, G., Bracher-Smith, M., . . . Walters, J. (2019). Association of genetic liability to psychotic experiences with neuropsychotic disorders and traits. *JAMA Psychiatry*, 76(12), 1256–1265. https://doi.org/10.1001/jamapsychiatry.2019.2508

Lehrer, H. M., Goosby, B. J., Dubois, S. K., Laudenslager, M. L., &

Steinhardt, M. A. (2020). Race moderates the association of perceived everyday discrimination and hair cortisol concentration. *Stress (Amsterdam, Netherlands)*, 23(5), 529–537. https://doi.org/10.1080/10253890.2019.1710487

Lei, H., Huang, L., Li, J., Liu, W., Fan, J., Zhang, X., . . . Rao, H. (2020). Altered spontaneous brain activity in obsessive-compulsive personality disorder. *Comprehensive Psychiatry*, 96, 152144. https://doi.org/10.1016/j.comppsych.2019.152144

Leibovich, T., Cohen, N., & Henik, A. (2016). Itsy bitsy spider? Valence and self-relevance predict size estimation. *Biological Psychology*, 121(Part B), 138–145.

Leichsenring, F., Heim, N., Leweke, F., Spitzer, C., Steinert, C., & Kernberg, O. F. (2023). Borderline personality disorder: A review. *JAMA*, 329(8), 670–679.

Lemmens, L., van Bronswijk, S. C., Peeters, F., Arntz, A., Hollon, S. D., & Huibers, M. (2019). Long-term outcomes of acute treatment with cognitive therapy v. interpersonal psychotherapy for adult depression: Follow-up of a randomized controlled trial. *Psychological Medicine*, 49(3), 465–473.

Lemonick, M. D. (2004). In search of sleep. *Time*, 164, 100.

Lenferink, L., Egberts, M. R., Kullberg, M. L., Meentken, M. G., Zimmermann, S., L Mertens, Y., . . . Krause-Utz, A. (2020). Latent classes of DSM-5 acute stress disorder symptoms in children after single-incident trauma: Findings from an international data archive. *European Journal of Psychotraumatology*, 11(1), 1717156. https://doi.org/10.1080/20008198.2020.1717156

Le-Niculescu, H., Roseberry, K., Gill, S. S., Levey, D. F., Phalen, P. L., Mullen, J., . . . Niculescu, A. B. (2021). Precision medicine for mood disorders: Objective assessment, risk prediction, pharmacogenomics, and repurposed drugs. *Molecular Psychiatry*, 26(7), 2776–2804. https://doi.org/10.1038/s41380-021-01061-w

Lenzenweger, M. F. (2023). Narcissistic personality disorder studied the long way: Predicting change in narcissistic pathology during college. *American Journal of Psychotherapy*, 76(1), 15–25. https://doi.org/10.1176/appi .psychotherapy.20220020

Leonardi-Bee, J., Nderi, M., & Britton, J. (2016). Smoking in movies and smoking initiation in adolescents: Systematic review and meta-analysis. *Addiction*, 111(10), 1750–1763.

Lerman, C., & Audrain-McGovern, J. (2010). Reinforcing effects of smoking: More than feeling. *Biological Psychiatry*, 67, 699–701.

Lervolino, A. C., Perroud, N., Fullana, M. A., Guipponi, M., Cherkas, L., Collier, D. A., & Mataix-Cols, D. (2009). Prevalence and heritability of compulsive hoarding: A twin study. *American Journal of Psychiatry*, 166, 1156–1161.

Leschak, C. J., & Eisenberger, N. I. (2019). Two distinct immune pathways linking social relationships with health: Inflammatory and antiviral processes. *Psychosomatic Medicine*, 81(8), 711–719.

Leung, A., Leung, A., Wong, A., & Hon, K. L. (2020). Sleep terrors: An updated review. *Current Pediatric Reviews*, 16, 176–182.

Levi-Belz, Y., Gvion, Y., Levi, U., & Apter, A. (2019). Beyond the mental pain: A case-control study on the contribution of schizoid personality disorder symptoms to medically serious suicide attempts. *Comprehensive Psychiatry*, 90, 102–109.

Levin, J. B., Tatsuoka, C., Cassidy, K. A., Aebi, M. E., & Sajatovic, M. (2015). Trajectories of medication attitudes and adherence behavior change in non-adherent bipolar patients. *Comprehensive Psychiatry*, 58, 29–36.

Levine, M. D., Perkins, K. A., Kalarchian, M. K., Cheng, Y., Houck, P. R., Slane, J. D., & Marcus, M. D. (2010). Bupropion and cognitive behavioral therapy for weight-concerned women smokers. *Archives of Internal Medicine*, 170, 543–550.

Levy, M., Boulle, F., Steinbusch, H. W., van den Hove, D., Kenis, G., & Lanfumey, L. (2018). Neurotrophic factors and neuroplasticity pathways in the pathophysiology and treatment of depression. *Psychopharmacology*, 235(8), 2195–2220. https://doi .org/10.1007/s00213-018-4950-4

Levy, S., & Weitzman, E. R. (2019). Acute mental health symptoms in adolescent marijuana users. *JAMA Pediatrics*, 173, 185–186.

Lewinsohn, P. M., Muñoz, R. F., Youngren, M. A., & Zeiss, A. M. (1994). *Control your depression* (rev. ed.). New York: Fireside.

Lewis, C. R., Tafur, J., Spencer, S., Green, J. M., Harrison, C., Kelmendi, B., . . . Cahn, B. R. (2023). Pilot study suggests DNA methylation of the glucocorticoid receptor gene (NR3C1) is associated with MDMA-assisted therapy treatment response for severe PTSD. *Frontiers in Psychiatry*, 14, 959590. https://doi .org/10.3389/fpsyt.2023.959590

Lewis, G., Duffy, L., Ades, A., Amos, R., Araya, R., Brabyn, S., . . . Lewis, G. (2019). The clinical effectiveness of sertraline in primary care and the role of depression severity and duration (PANDA): A pragmatic, double-blind, placebo-controlled randomised trial. *The Lancet: Psychiatry*, 6(11), 903–914.

Lewis, G., Rice, F., Harold, G. T., Collishaw, S., & Thapar, A. (2011). Investigating environmental links between parent depression and child depressive/anxiety symptoms using an assisted conception design. *Journal of the American Academy of Child and Adolescent Psychiatry*, 50, 451–459.

Lewy Body Dementia Association. (2023). Understanding Lewy body dementias. https://www.lbda.org /go/10-things-you-should-know -about-lbd

Li, X. L., Wei, J., Zhang, X., Meng, Z., & Zhu, W. (2023). Relationship between night-sleep duration and risk for depression among middle-aged and older people: A dose-response meta-analysis. *Frontiers in Physiology*, 14, 1085091. https://doi.org/10.3389/fphys .2023.1085091

Liberman, R. P., Kopelowicz, A., & Young, A. S. (1994). Biobehavioral treatment and rehabilitation of schizophrenia. *Behavior Therapy*, 25, 89–107.

Lie, D. A. (2012). The many faces of depression. http://www.medscape .com/viewarticle/768764

Liebers, D. T., Pirooznia, M., Ganna, A., Bipolar Genome Study (BiGS), & Goes, F. S. (2020). Discriminating bipolar depression from major depressive disorder with polygenic risk scores. *Psychological Medicine*, 51(9), 1451–1458. https://doi.org/10.1017 /S003329172000015X

Liebke, L., Koppe, G., Bungert, M., Thome, J., Hauschild, S., Defiebre, N., . . . Lis, S. (2018). Difficulties with being socially accepted: An experimental study in borderline personality disorder. *Journal of Abnormal Psychology*, 127(7), 670–682.

Lijster, J. M., Dierckx, B., Utens, E. M., Verhulst, F. C., Zieldorff, C., Dieleman, G. C., & Legerstee, J. S. (2017). The age of onset of anxiety disorders. *Canadian Journal of Psychiatry. Revue Canadienne de Psychiatrie*, 62(4), 237–246. https://doi.org/10.1177 /0706743716640757

Lilienfeld, S. O., Lynn, S. J., Kirsch, I., Chaves, J. F., Sarbin, T. R., Ganaway, G. K., & Powell, R. A. (1999). Dissociative identity disorder and the sociocognitive model: Recalling the lessons of the past. *Psychological Bulletin*, 125, 507–523.

Lilly, M. M., Pole, N., Best, S. R., Metzler, T., & Marmar, C. R. (2009). Gender and PTSD: What can we learn from female police officers. *Journal of Anxiety Disorders*, 23, 767–774.

Lima, I., Peckham, A. D., & Johnson, S. L. (2018). Cognitive deficits in bipolar disorders: Implications for emotion. *Clinical Psychology Review*, 59, 126–136.

Lin, C. S., Ku, H. L., Chao, H. T., Tu, P. C., Li, C. T., Cheng, C. M., . . . Hsieh, J. C. (2014). Neural network of body representation differs between transsexuals and cissexuals. *PLOS One*, 9, e85914. https://doi.org/10.1371/journal .pone.0085914

Lin, S. K. (2022). Racial/ethnic differences in the pharmacokinetics of antipsychotics: Focusing on East Asians. *Journal of Personalized Medicine*, 12(9), 1362. https://doi .org/10.3390/jpm12091362

Lin, Z.-B., Deng, J.-H., Huang, L.-L., Shi, H., Liu, J.-M., Bin, O.-Y., & Xie, J.-X. (2018). Penile erectile strength measurement band for differentiation and classification of erectile dysfunction. *National Journal of Andrology, 24,* 520–524.

Lind, M. J., Aggen, S. H., Kirkpatrick, R. M., Kendler, K. S., & Amstadter, A. B. (2015). A longitudinal twin study of insomnia symptoms in adults. *Sleep, 38,* 1423–1430.

Linde, E. S., Varga, T. V., & Clotworthy, A. (2022). Obsessive-compulsive disorder during the COVID-19 pandemic: A systematic review. *Frontiers in Psychiatry, 13,* 806872. https:// doi.org/10.3389/fpsyt.2022 .806872

Lindner, K., Lacefield, K., Dunn, S. T., & Dunn, M. E. (2014). The use of videoconference in the treatment of panic disorder with agoraphobia in a housebound woman: A case study. *Clinical Case Studies, 13,* 146–166.

Lindsey, M. A., Brown, D. R., & Cunningham, M. (2017). Boys do(n't) cry: Addressing the unmet mental health needs of African American boys. *The American Journal of Orthopsychiatry, 87*(4), 377–383.

Lindstrom, C. M., Cann, A., Calhoun, L. G., & Tedeschi, R. G. (2013). The relationship of core belief challenge, rumination, disclosure, and sociocultural elements to posttraumatic growth. *Psychological Trauma: Theory, Research, Practice, and Policy, 5,* 50–55.

Linehan, M. M. (1993). *Cognitive-behavioral treatment of borderline personality disorder.* New York: Guilford Press.

Linehan, M. M. (2020). *Building a life worth living.* New York: Random House.

Linke, J. O., Adleman, N. E., Sarlls, J., Ross, A., Perlstein, S., Frank, H. R., . . . Brotman, M. A. (2019). White matter microstructure in pediatric bipolar disorder and disruptive mood dysregulation disorder. *Journal of the American Academy of Child and Adolescent Psychiatry, 59*(10), 1135–1145. https://doi.org/10.1016/j.jaac .2019.05.035

Linn, V. (2004, June 26). Headache "beast" holds tight grip on sufferers. *Seattle Post-Intelligencer,* p. A1.

Linton, J. (2019, April 29). Child health implications of hostile immigration policies: A medical perspective [Presentation]. Pediatric Academic Societies Meeting, Baltimore, MD. https://www .xcdsystem.com/pas/program/2019/

Liptak, A. (2010, May 17). Extended civil commitment of sex offenders is upheld. *New York Times,* p. A3.

Lipton, R. B., Nicholson, R. A., Reed, M. L., Araujo, A. B., Jaffe, D. H., Faries, D. E., . . . Pearlman, E. M. (2022). Diagnosis, consultation, treatment, and impact of migraine in the US: Results of the OVERCOME (US) study. *Headache, 62*(2), 122–140. https://doi.org/10.1111/head .14259

Liu, J., Chua, J. J., Chong, S. A., Subramaniam, M., & Mahendran, R. (2020). The impact of emotion dysregulation on positive and negative symptoms in schizophrenia spectrum disorders: A systematic review. *Journal of Clinical Psychology, 76*(4), 612–624.

Liu, Y., Wheaton, A. G., Chapman, D. P., Cunningham, T. J., Lu, H., & Croft, J. B. (2016). Prevalence of healthy sleep duration among adults—United States, 2014. *Morbidity and Mortality Weekly Report, 65,* 137–141.

Livesley, W. J. (2022). Progress but no cigar: Comment on Bach and Tracy (2022). *Personality Disorders, 13*(4), 383–386. https://doi .org/10.1037/per000058

Lloret, M. A., Cervera-Ferri, A., Nepomuceno, M., Monllor, P., Esteve, D., & Lloret, A. (2020). Is sleep disruption a cause or consequence of Alzheimer's disease? Reviewing its possible role as a biomarker. *International Journal of Molecular Sciences, 21*(3), 1168.

Lo Buono, V., Lucà Trombetta, M., Palmeri, R., Bonanno, L., Cartella, E., Di Lorenzo, G., . . . Corallo, F. (2021). Subthalamic nucleus deep brain stimulation and impulsivity in Parkinson's disease: A descriptive review. *Acta Neurologica Belgica, 121*(4), 837–847. https://doi.org/10.1007/ s13760-021-01684-4

Loas, G., Cormier, J., & Perez-Diaz, F. (2011). Dependent personality disorder and physical abuse. *Psychiatry Research, 185,* 167–170.

Lochner, C., Roos, A., & Stein, D. J. (2017). Excoriation (skin-picking) disorder: A systematic review of treatment options. *Neuropsychiatric Disease and Treatment, 13,* 1867–1872.

Locke, A. B., Kirst, N., & Shultz, C. G. (2015). Diagnosis and management of generalized anxiety disorder and panic disorder in adults. *American Family Physician, 91*(9), 617–624.

Lockwood, P. L., Sebastian, C. L., McCrory, E. J., Hyde, Z. H., Gu, X., De Brito, S. A., & Viding, E. (2013). Association of callous traits with reduced neural response to others' pain in children with conduct problems. *Current Biology, 23,* 901–905.

Loeffler, L., Radke, S., Habel, U., Ciric, R., Satterthwaite, T. D., Schneider, F., & Derntl, B. (2018). The regulation of positive and negative emotions through instructed causal attributions in lifetime depression—A functional magnetic resonance imaging study. *NeuroImage: Clinical, 20,* 1233–1245.

Loew, T., & Barreda, V. (2020, November 4). Oregon becomes first state to decriminalize small amounts of drugs, including heroin. *USA Today.* https://www .usatoday.com/story/news /politics/elections/2020/11/03 /oregon-decriminalizes -small-amounts-drugs-including -heroin/6156552002/

Loewenstein, R. J. (1994). Diagnosis, epidemiology, clinical course, treatment, and cost effectiveness of treatment for dissociative disorders and MPD: Report submitted to the Clinton Administration Task Force on Health Care Reform. *Dissociation, 7,* 3–11.

Loewenstein, R. J. (2018). Dissociation debates: Everything you know is wrong. *Dialogues in Clinical Neuroscience, 20*(3), 229–242.

Loewenstein, R. J., Frewen, P. A., & Lewis-Fernández, R. (2017). Dissociative disorders. In B. J. Saddock, V. Saddock, & P. Ruiz

(Eds.), *Kaplan and Sadock's comprehensive textbook of psychiatry. Vol 1.* (10th ed., pp. 1866–1952). Philadelphia: Wolters Kluwer/ Lippincott Williams & Wilkens.

Löffler, M., Levine, S. M., Usai, K., Desch, S., Kandić, M., Nees, F., & Flor, H. (2022). Corticostriatal circuits in the transition to chronic back pain: The predictive role of reward learning. *Cell Reports: Medicine, 3*(7), 100677. https:// doi.org/10.1016 /j.xcrm.2022.100677

Loftus, E. F., Garry, M., & Hayne, H. (2008). Repressed and recovered memory. In E. Borgida & S. T. Fiske (Eds.), *Beyond common sense: Psychological science in the courtroom* (pp. 177–194). Malden, MA: Blackwell Publishing.

Logan, J. E., Haileyesus, T., Ertl, A., Rostad, W. L., & Herbst, J. H. (2019). Nonfatal assaults and homicides among adults aged ≥ 60 years—United States, 2002–2016. *Morbidity and Mortality Weekly Report, 68,* 297–302.

Lommen, M. J. J., Engelhard, I. M., Sijbrandij, M., van den Hout, M. A., & Hermans, D. (2013). Pre-trauma individual differences in extinction learning predict posttraumatic stress. *Behaviour Research and Therapy, 51,* 63–67.

Long, D., Long, B., & Koyfman, A. (2017). The emergency medicine management of severe alcohol withdrawal. *The American Journal of Emergency Medicine, 35*(7), 1005–1011.

Long, E. C., Kaneva, R., Vasilev, G., Moeller, F. G., & Vassileva, J. (2020). Neurocognitive and psychiatric markers for addiction: Common vs. specific endophenotypes for heroin and amphetamine dependence. *Current Topics in Medicinal Chemistry, 20*(7), 585–597.

Long, F. Y., Pang, E., & Kee, C. (2002). Pilot study to assess the viability of a rape trauma syndrome questionnaire. *Annals of the Academy of Medicine, 31,* 777–784.

Longpré, N., Guay, J., Knight, R. A., & Benbouriche, M. (2018). Sadistic offender or sexual sadism? Taxometric evidence for a dimensional structure of sexual sadism.

Archives of Sexual Behavior, 47, 403–416.

Loong, D., Bonato, S., Barnsley, J., & Dewa, C. S. (2019). The effectiveness of mental health courts in reducing recidivism and police contact: A systematic review. *Community Mental Health Journal, 55,* 1073–1098.

Lopez, S. J., Pedrotti, J. T., & Snyder, C. R. (2018). *Positive psychology: The scientific and practical explorations of human strengths.* Thousand Oaks, CA: Sage.

Lopez, S. R., Hipke, K. N., Polo, A. J., Jenkins, J. H., Karno, M., Vaughn, C., & Snyder, K. S. (2004). Ethnicity, expressed emotion, attributions, and course of schizophrenia: Family warmth matters. *Journal of Abnormal Psychology, 113,* 428–439.

Lopez-Leon, S., Lopez-Gomez, M. I., Warner, B., & Ruiter-Lopez, L. (2018). Psychotropic medication in children and adolescents in the United States in the year 2004 vs 2014. *Daru: Journal of Faculty of Pharmacy, Tehran University of Medical Sciences, 26*(1), 5–10.

Lorains, F. K., Stout, J. C., Bradshaw, J. L., Dowling, N. A., & Enticott, P. G. (2014). Self-reported impulsivity and inhibitory control in problem gamblers. *Journal of Clinical and Experimental Neuropsychology, 36,* 144–157.

Lotto, C. R., Altafim, E. R. P., & Linhares, M. B. M. (2023). Maternal history of childhood adversities and later negative parenting: A systematic review. *Trauma, Violence & Abuse, 24*(2), 662–683.

Lou, S., Carstensen, K., Petersen, O. B., Nielsen, C. P., Hvidman, L., Lanther, M. R., & Vogel, I. (2018). Termination of pregnancy following a prenatal diagnosis of Down syndrome: A qualitative study of the decision-making process of pregnant couples. *Acta Obstetricia et Gynecologica Scandinavica, 97*(10), 1228–1236.

Lourida, I., Hannon, E., Littlejohns, T. J., Langa, K. M., Hyppönen, E., Kuzma, E., & Llewellyn, D. J. (2019). Association of lifestyle and genetic risk with incidence of dementia. *JAMA, 322*(5), 430–437.

Lövdén, M., Xu, W., & Wangy, H.-X. (2013). Lifestyle change and the prevention of cognitive decline and dementia: What is the evidence? *Current Opinion in Psychiatry, 26,* 239–243.

Löwe, B., Levenson, J., Depping, M., Hüsing, P., Kohlmann, S., Lehmann, M., . . . Weigel, A. (2022). Somatic symptom disorder: A scoping review on the empirical evidence of a new diagnosis. *Psychological Medicine, 52*(4), 632–648. https://doi.org /10.1017/S0033291721004177

Lowery-Gionta, E. G., May, M. D., Taylor, R. M., Bergman, E. M., Etuma, M. T., & Moore, N. L. T. (2019). Modeling trauma to develop treatments for posttraumatic stress. *Translational Issues in Psychological Science, 5,* 243–275.

Loxton, H., Roomaney, R., & Cobb, C. (2018). Students' self-reported fears and the perceived origins thereof. *Journal of Child and Adolescent Mental Health, 30*(3), 183–189.

Lozupone, M., Seripa, D., Stella, E., La Montagna, M., Solfrizzi, V., Quaranta, N., . . . Panza, F. (2017). Innovative biomarkers in psychiatric disorders: A major clinical challenge in psychiatry. *Expert Review of Proteomics, 14,* 809–824.

Lu, C. F., Wu, Y. T., Teng, S., Wang, P. S., Tu, P. C., Su, T. P., . . . Li, C. T. (2019). Genetic predisposition and disease expression of bipolar disorder reflected in shape changes of the anterior limbic network. *Brain Sciences, 9*(9), 240. https:// doi.org/10.3390/brainsci9090240

Lu, J., Li, S., Li, H., Mou, T., Zhou, L., Huang, B., . . . Xu, Y. (2019). Changes in plasma NPY, IL-1β and hypocretin in people who died by suicide. *Neuropsychiatric Disease and Treatment, 15,* 2893–2900.

Lu, Y., & Temple, J. R. (2019). Dangerous weapons or dangerous people? The temporal associations between gun violence and mental health. *Preventive Medicine, 121,* 1–6.

Lubit, R. H., Bonds, C. L., II, & Lucia, M. A. (2013). Sleep disorders. http://emedicine.medscape. com/article/287104-overview

Luca, M., Vecchio, C., Luca, A., & Calandra, C. (2012). Haloperidol augmentation of fluvoxamine in skin picking disorder: A case report. *Journal of Medical Case Reports, 6,* 219–233.

Lucas, M., O'Reilly, E. J., Pan, A., Mirzaei, F., Willett, W. C., Okereke, O. I., & Ascherio, A. (2013, July 2). Coffee, caffeine, and risk of completed suicide: Results from three prospective cohorts of American adults. *World Journal of Biological Psychiatry, 15*(5), 377–386.

Luck, C. C., Patterson, R. R., & Lipp, O. V. (2020). "Prepared" fear or socio-cultural learning? Fear conditioned to guns, snakes, and spiders is eliminated by instructed extinction in a within-participant differential fear conditioning paradigm. *Psychophysiology, 57*(4), e13516. https://doi.org/10.1111/psyp.13516

Ludyga, S., Brand, S., Gerber, M., Weber, P., Brotzmann, M., Habibifar, F., & Pühse, U. (2017). An event-related potential investigation of the acute effects of aerobic and coordinative exercise on inhibitory control in children with ADHD. *Developmental Cognitive Neuroscience, 28,* 21–28.

Luethi, D., & Liechti, M. E. (2020). Designer drugs: Mechanism of action and adverse effects. *Archives of Toxicology, 94*(4), 1085–1133. https://doi.org/10.1007/s00204-020-02693-7

Luft, M. J., Lamy, M., DelBello, M. P., McNamara, R. K., & Strawn, J. R. (2018). Antidepressant-induced activation in children and adolescents: Risk, recognition and management. *Current Problems in Pediatric and Adolescent Health Care, 48*(2), 50–62.

Lui, P. P. (2017). Incorporating meta-emotions in integrative cognitive-affective therapy to treat comorbid bulimia nervosa and substance use disorders in a Latina American. *Clinical Case Studies, 16,* 328–345.

Luo, H., Lou, V., Chen, C., & Chi, I. (2020). The effectiveness of the positive mood and active life program on reducing depressive symptoms in long-term care facilities. *The Gerontologist, 60*(1), 193–204.

Lurie, A. (2011). Obstructive sleep apnea in adults: Epidemiology, clinical presentation, and treatment options. *Advances in Cardiology, 46,* 1–42.

Lussier, P., McCann, K., & Beauregard, E. (2008). The etiology of sexual deviance. In D. Rowland & L. Incrocci (Eds.), *Handbook of sexual and gender identity disorders* (pp. 529–562). Hoboken, NJ: Wiley.

Luta, X., Bagnoud, C., Lambiris, M., Decollogny, A., Eggli, Y., Le Pogam, M. A., . . . Marti, J. (2020). Patterns of benzodiazepine prescription among older adults in Switzerland: A cross-sectional analysis of claims data. *BMJ Open, 10*(1), e031156. https://doi.org/10.1136/bmjopen-2019-031156

Lutrick, K., Clark, R., Nuño, V. L., Bauman, S., & Carvajal, S. (2020). Latinx bullying and depression in children and youth: A systematic review. *Systematic Reviews, 9*(1), 126. https://doi.org/10.1186/s13643-020-01383-w

Lutz, P. E., Mechawar, N., & Turecki, G. (2017). Neuropathology of suicide: Recent findings and future directions. *Molecular Psychiatry, 22*(10), 1395–1412.

Lyall, K., Croen, L., Daniels, J., Fallin, M. D., Ladd-Acosta, C., Lee, B. K., . . . Newschaffer, C. (2017). The changing epidemiology of autism spectrum disorders. *Annual Review of Public Health, 38,* 81–102. https://doi.org/10.1146/annurev-publhealth-031816-044318

Lydecker, J. A., Ivezaj, V., & Grilo, C. M. (2020). Testing the validity and clinical utility of the severity specifiers for binge-eating disorder for predicting treatment outcomes. *Journal of Consulting and Clinical Psychology, 88,* 172–178.

Lyke, M. L. (2004, August 27). Once a "people person," vet couldn't leave home. *Seattle Post-Intelligencer,* p. A8.

Lynch, B. A., Finney Rutten, L. J., Wilson, P. M., Kumar, S., Phelan, S., Jacobson, R. M., . . . Agunwamba, A. (2018). The impact of positive contextual factors on the association between adverse family experiences and obesity in a National Survey of Children. *Preventive Medicine, 116,* 81–86.

Lynn, S. J., Lilienfeld, S. O., Merckelbach, H., Giesbrecht, T., McNally, R. J., Loftus, E. F., . . . Malaktaris, A. (2014). The trauma model of dissociation: Inconvenient truths and stubborn fictions. Comment on Dalenberg et al. (2012). *Psychological Bulletin, 140*(3), 896–910.

Lyons-Ruth, K., Riley, C., Patrick, M., & Hobson, R. P. (2019). Disinhibited attachment behavior among infants of mothers with borderline personality disorder, depression, and no diagnosis. *Personality Disorders, 10*(2), 163–172.

Lysaker, P. H., Pattison, M. L., Leonhardt, B. L., Phelps, S., & Vohs, J. L. (2018). Insight in schizophrenia spectrum disorders: Relationship with behavior, mood and perceived quality of life, underlying causes and emerging treatments. *World Psychiatry, 17*(1), 12–23.

Ma, G., Fan, H., Shen, C., & Wang, W. (2016). Genetic and neuroimaging features of personality disorders: State of the art. *Neuroscience Bulletin, 32*(3), 286–306.

Ma, J., Rosas, L. G., Lv, N., Xiao, L., Snowden, M. B., Venditti, E. M., . . . Lavori, P. W. (2019). Effect of integrated behavioral weight loss treatment and problem-solving therapy on body mass index and depressive symptoms among patients with obesity and depression: The RAINBOW randomized clinical trial. *JAMA, 321*(9), 869–879.

Ma, L., Zhang, Y., Huang, C., & Cui, Z. (2020). Resilience-oriented cognitive behavioral interventions for depressive symptoms in children and adolescents: A meta-analytic review. *Journal of Affective Disorders, 270,* 150–164.

MacCabe, J. H., Wicks, S., Löfving, S., David, A. S., Berndtsson, Å., Gustafsson, J. E., . . . Dalman, C. (2013). Decline in cognitive performance between ages 13 and 18 years and the risk for psychosis in adulthood: A Swedish longitudinal cohort study in males. *JAMA Psychiatry, 70*(3), 261–270.

Mac Donald, C. L., Barber, J., Patterson, J., Johnson, A. M., Dikmen, S., Fann, J. R., & Temkin, N. (2019). Association between

5-year clinical outcome in patients with nonmedically evacuated mild blast traumatic brain injury and clinical measures collected within 7 days postinjury in combat. *JAMA Network Open*, 2(1), e186676. https://doi.org/10.1001/jamanetworkopen.2018.6676

Machover, K. (1949). *Personality projection in the drawing of the human figure: A method of personality investigation*. Springfield, IL: Thomas.

MacIntyre, M. M., Zare, M., & Williams, M. T. (2023). Anxiety-related disorders in the context of racism. *Current Psychiatry Reports*, 25(2), 31–43.

Mackin, D. M., Kotov, R., Perlman, G., Nelson, B. D., Goldstein, B. L., Hajcak, G., & Klein, D. N. (2019). Reward processing and future life stress: Stress generation pathway to depression. *Journal of Abnormal Psychology*, 128(4), 305–314.

Mackin, D. M., Perlman, G., Davila, J., Kotov, R., & Klein, D. N. (2017). Social support buffers the effect of interpersonal life stress on suicidal ideation and self-injury during adolescence. *Psychological Medicine*, 47(6), 1149–1161.

MacQueen, G., Santaguida, P., Keshavarz, H., Jaworska, N., Levine, M., Beyene, J., & Raina, P. (2017). Systematic review of clinical practice guidelines for failed antidepressant treatment response in major depressive disorder, dysthymia, and subthreshold depression in adults. *Canadian Journal of Psychiatry*, 62(1), 11–23.

Macur, J., & Schweber, N. (2012). Rape case unfolds on Web and splits city. http://www.nytimes.com/2012/12/17/sports/high-school-football-rape-case-unfolds-online-and-divides-steubenville-ohio.html?pagewanted5all

Madra, M., Ringel, R., & Margolis, K. G. (2020). Gastrointestinal issues and autism spectrum disorder. *Child and Adolescent Psychiatric Clinics of North America*, 29(3), 501–513. https://doi.org/10.1016/j.chc.2020.02.005

Maenner M. J., Shaw, K. A., Baio, J., Washington, A., Patrick, M., DiRienzo, M., . . . Dietz, P. M. (2020). Prevalence of autism spectrum disorder among children aged 8 years—Autism and Developmental Disabilities Monitoring Network, 11 sites, United States, 2016. *MMWR Surveillance Summary*, 69(No. SS-4), 1–12.

Maenner, M. J., Warren, Z., Williams, A. R., Amoakohene, E., Bakian, A. V., Bilder, D. A., . . . Shaw, K. A. (2023). Prevalence and characteristics of autism spectrum disorder among children aged 8 years: Autism and Developmental Disabilities Monitoring Network, 11 Sites, United States, 2020. *MMWR: Morbidity and Mortality Weekly Report*, 72(No. SS-2), 1–14. http://doi.org/10.15585/mmwr.ss7202a1

Magon, S., Sprenger, T., Otti, A., Papadopoulou, A., Gündel, H., & Noll-Hussong, M. (2018). Cortical thickness alterations in chronic pain disorder: An exploratory MRI study. *Psychosomatic Medicine*, 80(7), 592–598.

Maguen, S., Luxton, D. D., Skopp, N. A., & Madden, E. (2012). Gender differences in traumatic experiences and mental health in active duty soldiers redeployed from Iraq and Afghanistan. *Journal of Psychiatric Research*, 46, 311–316.

Mahdi, M., Jhawar, S., Bennett, S. D., & Shafran, R. (2019). Cognitive behavioral therapy for childhood anxiety disorders: What happens to comorbid mood and behavioral disorders? A systematic review. *Journal of Affective Disorders*, 251, 141–148.

Mahgoub, N., & Hossain, A. (2006). A 28-year-old woman and her 58-year-old mother with a shared psychotic disorder. *Psychiatric Annals*, 36, 306–309.

Mahler, M. (1968). *On human symbiosis and the vicissitudes of individuation*. New York: International University Press.

Mahoney, C. E., Cogswell, A., Koralnik, I. J., & Scammell, T. E. (2019). The neurobiological basis of narcolepsy. *Nature Reviews: Neuroscience*, 20(2), 83–93.

Maijer, K., Begemann, M., Palmen, S., Leucht, S., & Sommer, I. (2018). Auditory hallucinations across the lifespan: A systematic review and meta-analysis. *Psychological Medicine*, 48(6), 879–888.

Majrashi, N. A., Ahearn, T. S., & Waiter, G. D. (2020). Brainstem volume mediates seasonal variation in depressive symptoms: A cross sectional study in the UK Biobank cohort. *Scientific Reports*, 10(1), 3592. https://doi.org/10.1038/s41598-020-60620-3

Makhoul, G. S., Sugrue, L. P., Zamanian, H., Liu, T. X., Rao, V. R., Sellers, K. K., . . . Chang, E. F. (2021). Closed-loop neuromodulation in an individual with treatment-resistant depression. *Nature Medicine*, 27(10), 1696–1700.

Malhi, G. S., Bell, E., Outhred, T., & Berk, M. (2020). Lithium therapy and its interactions. *Australian Prescriber*, 43(3), 91–93.

Malik, A. B. (2013). Neuropsychological evaluation. http://emedicine.medscape.com/article/317596-overview#a30

Malouff, J. M., & Schutte, N. S. (2017). A meta-analysis of the relationship between anxiety and telomere length. *Anxiety, Stress, and Coping*, 30(3), 264–272.

Mangiulli, I., Otgaar, H., Jelicic, M., & Merckelbach, H. (2022). A critical review of case studies on dissociative amnesia. *Clinical Psychological Science*, 10(2), 191–211.

Mann, J. J., Arango, V. A., Avenevoli, S., Brent, D. A., Champagne, F. A., Clayton, P., . . . Wenzel, A. (2009). Candidate endophenotypes for genetic studies of suicidal behavior. *Biological Psychiatry*, 65, 556–563.

Mann, K., & Hermann, D. (2010). Individualized treatment in alcohol-dependent patients. *European Archives of Psychiatry and Clinical Neuroscience*, 2, S116–S120.

Manning, J. S. (2013). Strategies for managing the risks associated with ADHD medications. *Journal of Clinical Psychiatry*, 74, e19. https://doi.org/10.4088/JCP.12077tx2c

Manschreck, T. C., Merrill, A. M., Jabbar, G., Chun, J., & Delisi, L. E. (2012). Frequency of normative word associations in the speech of individuals at familial high-risk for schizophrenia. *Schizophrenia Research*, 140(1–3), 99–103.

Marceaux, J. C., & Melville, C. L. (2011). Twelve-step facilitated versus mapping- enhanced cognitive-behavioral therapy for pathological gambling: A controlled study. *Journal of Gambling Studies, 27,* 171–190.

March, E., & Steele, G. (2020). High esteem and hurting others online: Trait sadism moderates the relationship between self-esteem and Internet trolling. *Cyberpsychology, Behavior and Social Networking, 23*(7), 441–446.

Marchant, A., Hawton, K., Stewart, A., Montgomery, P., Singaravelu, V., Lloyd, K., . . . John, A. (2017). A systematic review of the relationship between internet use, self-harm and suicidal behaviour in young people: The good, the bad and the unknown. *PLOS One, 12*(8), e0181722. https://doi.org/10.1371/journal.pone.0181722

Marcus, M. B. (2017). Ban on super-thin models takes effect in France. https://www.cbsnews.com/news/ban-on-super-thin-models-anorexia-takes-effect-in-france/

Marek, R., Sun, Y., & Sah, P. (2019). Neural circuits for a top-down control of fear and extinction. *Psychopharmacology, 236*(1), 313–320.

Mariani, M. (2018). American exorcism. *The Atlantic.* https://www.theatlantic.com/magazine/archive/2018/12/catholic-exorcisms-on-the-rise/573943/

Marincowitz, C., Lochner, C., & Stein, D. J. (2022). The neurobiology of obsessive-compulsive personality disorder: A systematic review. *CNS Spectrums, 27*(6), 664–675. https://doi.org/10.1017/S1092852921000754

Marjoribanks, J., Brown, J., O'Brien, P. M., & Wyatt, K. (2013). Selective serotonin reuptake inhibitors for premenstrual syndrome. *Cochrane Database of Systematic Reviews, 6,* CD001396. https://doi.org/10.1002/14651858.CD001396.pub3

Markarian, Y., Larson, M. J., Aldea, M. A., Baldwin, S. A., Good, D., Berkeljon, A., . . . McKay, D. (2010). Multiple pathways to functional impairment in obsessive-compulsive disorder. *Clinical Psychology Review, 30,* 78–88.

Marmar, C. R. (1988). Personality disorders. In H. H. Goldman (Ed.), *Review of general psychiatry* (pp. 401–424). Norwalk, CT: Appleton & Lange.

Marquine, M., & Jimenez, D. (2020). Cultural and linguistic proficiency in mental health care: A crucial aspect of professional competence. *International Psychogeriatrics, 32,* 1–3.

Marras, C., Beck, J. C., Bower, J. H., Roberts, E., Ritz, B., Ross, G. W., . . . Parkinson's Foundation P4 Group. (2018). Prevalence of Parkinson's disease across North America. *NPJ Parkinson's Disease, 4,* 21.

Marsh, A. A., Finger, E. C., Fowler, K. A., Adalio, C. J., Jurkowitz, I. T., Schechter, J. C., . . . Blair, R. J. (2013). Empathic responsiveness in amygdala and anterior cingulate cortex in youths with psychopathic traits. *Journal of Child Psychology and Psychiatry, 8,* 900–910.

Marsh, R. J., Dorahy, M. J., Verschuere, B., Butler, C., Middleton, W., & Huntjens, R. (2018). Transfer of episodic self-referential memory across amnesic identities in dissociative identity disorder using the Autobiographical Implicit Association Test. *Journal of Abnormal Psychology, 127*(8), 751–757.

Marshall, S. A., Landau, M. E., Carroll, C. G., Schwieters, B., Llewellyn, A., Liskow, B. I., . . . Bienenfeld, D. (2013). Conversion disorders. http://emedicine.medscape.com/article/287464-overview

Marshe, V. S., Gorbovskaya, I., Kanji, S., Kish, M., & Müller, D. J. (2019). Clinical implications of APOE genotyping for late-onset Alzheimer's disease (LOAD) risk estimation: A review of the literature. *Journal of Neural Transmission (Vienna, Austria: 1996), 126*(1), 65–85. https://doi.org/10.1007/s00702-018-1934-9

Martiadis, V., Pessina, E., Raffone, F., Iniziato, V., Martini, A., & Scognamiglio, P. (2023). Metacognition in schizophrenia: A practical overview of psychometric metacognition assessment tools for researchers and clinicians. *Frontiers in Psychiatry, 14,* 1155321. https://doi.org/10.3389/fpsyt.2023.1155321

Martijn, F. M., Babchishin, K. M., Pullman, L. E., & Seto, M. C. (2020). Sexual attraction and falling in love in persons with pedohebephilia. *Archives of Sexual Behavior, 49*(4), 1305–1318.

Martin, C. G., Cromer, L. D., Deprince, A. P., & Freyd, J. J. (2013). The role of cumulative trauma, betrayal, and appraisals in understanding trauma symptomatology. *Psychological Trauma, 52,* 110–118.

Martin, C., Nolen, H., Podolnick, J., & Wang, R. (2017). Current and emerging therapies in premature ejaculation: Where we are coming from, where we are going. *International Journal of Urology, 24,* 40–50.

Martin, E. B., Jr. (2020). Brief psychotic disorder triggered by fear of coronavirus? https://www.psychiatrictimes.com/view/brief-psychotic-disorder-triggered-fear-coronavirus-small-case-series

Martin, E. K., & Silverstone, P. H. (2013). How much child sexual abuse is "below the surface." *Frontiers in Psychiatry, 4,* 58. https//doi.org/10.3389/fpsyt/2013.00058

Martin, L. A., Neighbors, H. W., & Griffith, D. M. (2013). The experience of symptoms of depression in men vs women: Analysis of the National Comorbidity Survey Replication. *JAMA Psychiatry, 70,* 1100–1106.

Martinez-Taboas, A. (2005). Psychogenic seizures in an espiritismo context: The role of culturally sensitive psychotherapy. *Psychotherapy: Theory, Research, Practice, Training, 42,* 6–13.

Martinou, E., Stefanova, I., Iosif, E., & Angelidi, A. M. (2022). Neurohormonal changes in the gut-brain axis and underlying neuroendocrine mechanisms following bariatric surgery. *International Journal of Molecular Sciences, 23*(6), 3339. https://doi.org/10.3390/ijms23063339

Masataka, N., & Shibasaki, M. (2012). Premenstrual enhancement of snake detection in visual search in healthy women. *Scientific Reports.* http://www.nature.com/srep/2012/120308/srep00307/full/srep00307.html.

Maseroli, E., Scavello, I., Rastrelli, G., Limoncin, E., Cipriani, S., Corona, G., . . . Vignozzi, L. (2018). Outcome of medical and psychosexual interventions for vaginismus: A systematic review and meta-analysis. *Journal of Sexual Medicine, 15,* 1752–1764.

Mason, E. C., Gaston, J. E., Pestell, C. F., & Page, A. C. (2022). A comprehensive group-based cognitive behavioural treatment for blood-injection-injury phobia. *The British Journal of Clinical Psychology, 61*(2), 494–509.

Mason, S. M., Flint, A. J., Field, A. E., Austin, S. B., & Rich-Edwards, J. W. (2013). Abuse victimization in childhood or adolescence and risk of food addiction in adult women. *Obesity, 21,* 775–781.

Masters, N. T., Casey, E., Wells, E. A., & Morrison, D. M. (2013). Sexual scripts among young heterosexually active men and women: Continuity and change. *Journal of Sex Research, 50,* 409–420.

Masters, N. T., Stappenbeck, C. A., Kaysen, D., Kajumulo, K. F., Davis, K. C., George, W. H., . . . Heiman, J. R. (2015). A person-centered approach to examining heterogeneity and subgroups among survivors of sexual assault. *Journal of Abnormal Psychology, 124,* 685–696.

Masters, W. H., & Johnson, V. E. (1966). *Human sexual response.* Boston: Little, Brown.

Masters, W. H., & Johnson, V. E. (1970). *Human sexual inadequacy.* London: Churchill.

Masuda, R. (2019). Multiple emotion regulation in Rorschach color responses. *Rorschachiana, 40,* 112–130.

Mataix-Cols, D., Boman, M., Monzani, B., Rück, C., Serlachius, E., Långström, N., & Lichtenstein, P. (2013). Population-based, multigenerational family clustering study of obsessive-compulsive disorder. *JAMA Psychiatry, 70,* 709–717.

Mataix-Cols, D., Fernández de la Cruz, L., Monzani, B., Rosenfield, D., Andersson, E., Pérez-Vigil, A., . . . Thuras, P. (2017). D-cycloserine augmentation of exposure-based cognitive behavior therapy for anxiety, obsessive-compulsive, and posttraumatic stress disorders: A systematic review and meta-analysis of individual participant data. *JAMA Psychiatry, 74*(5), 501–510.

Mathes, B. M., Kennedy, G. A., Wilver, N. L., Carlton, C. N., & Cougle, J. R. (2019). A multi-method analysis of incompleteness in behavioral treatment of contamination-based OCD. *Behaviour Research and Therapy, 114,* 1–6.

Mathes, B. M., Morabito, D. M., & Schmidt, N. B. (2019). Epidemiological and clinical gender differences in OCD. *Current Psychiatry Reports, 21*(5), 36. https://doi.org/10.1007/s11920-019-1015-2

Mathes, B. M., Norr, A. M., Allan, N. P., Albanese, B. J., & Schmidt, N. B. (2018). Cyberchondria: Overlap with health anxiety and unique relations with impairment, quality of life, and service utilization. *Psychiatry Research, 261,* 204–211.

Mathes, B. M., Quick, A. D., Albanese, B. J., Morabito, D. M., Bedford, C. E., & Schmidt, N. B. (2020). Hostility and suicide risk among veterans: The mediating role of perceived burdensomeness. *Cognitive Therapy and Research, 44,* 636–644.

Mathews, B., & Collin-Vézina, D. (2019). Child sexual abuse: Toward a conceptual model and definition. *Trauma, Violence and Abuse, 20,* 131–148.

Mathiarasan, S., & Hüls, A. (2021). Impact of environmental injustice on children's health-interaction between air pollution and socioeconomic status. *International Journal of Environmental Research and Public Health, 18*(2), 795. https://doi.org/10.3390/ijerph18020795

Mathison, L. A. (2019). Internalized stigma of mental illness: More than a scale. *Stigma and Health, 4,* 165–169.

Matsuzaka, S., & Knapp, M. (2019). Anti-racism and substance use treatment: Addiction does not discriminate, but do we? *Journal of Ethnicity in Substance Abuse,* 1–27.

Matta, A. G., & Carrié, D. (2023). Epidemiology, pathophysiology, diagnosis, and principles of management of takotsubo cardiomyopathy: A review. *Medical Science Monitor: International Medical Journal of Experimental and Clinical Research, 29,* e939020. https://doi.org/10.12659/MSM.939020

Matthews, C. (2017). Anxiety disorder statistics. https://anxietyhub.org/anxiety-disorder-statistics/

May, A. C., Aupperle, R. L., & Stewart, J. L. (2020). Dark times: The role of negative reinforcement in methamphetamine addiction. *Frontiers in Psychiatry, 11,* 114. https://doi.org/10.3389/fpsyt.2020.00114

May, P. A., Chambers, C. D., Kalberg, W. O., Zellner, J., Feldman, H., Buckley, D., . . . Hoyme, H. E. (2018). Prevalence of fetal alcohol spectrum disorders in four US communities. *JAMA, 319*(5), 474–482.

Mayhew, S. L., & Gilbert, P. (2008). Compassionate mind training with people who hear malevolent voices: A case series report. *Clinical Psychology and Psychotherapy, 15,* 113–138.

McAllister, T. W., Flashman, L. A., Maerlender, A., Greenwald, R. M., Beckwith, J. G., Tosteson, T. D., . . . Turco, J. H. (2012). Cognitive effects of one season of head impacts in a cohort of collegiate contact sport athletes. *Neurology, 78*(22), 1777–1784.

McCabe, M. P., & Goldhammer, D. L. (2013). Prevalence of women's sexual desire problems: What criteria do we use? *Archives of Sexual Behavior, 42,* 1073–1078.

McCabe, M. P., Sharlip, I. D., Lewis, R., Atalla, E., Balon, R., Fisher, A. D., & Segraves, R. T. (2016). Incidence and prevalence of sexual dysfunction in women and men: A consensus statement from the Fourth International Consultation on Sexual Medicine 2015. *Journal of Sexual Medicine, 13,* 144–152.

McCabe, R., & Priebe, S. (2004). Explanatory models of illness in schizophrenia: Comparison of four ethnic groups. *British Journal of Psychiatry, 185,* 25–30.

McCabe, S. E., Veliz, P., & Schulenberg, J. E. (2018). How collegiate fraternity and sorority involvement relates to substance use during young adulthood and substance use disorders in early midlife: A national longitudinal study. *The Journal of Adolescent Health: Official Publication of the Society for Adolescent Medicine, 62*(3S), S35–S43. https://doi .org/10.1016/j.jadohealth .2017.09.029

McCann, A. C. (2023). 2023's happiest cities in America. https://wallethub.com/edu /happiest-places-to-live/32619

McCarthy, J. (2021). Record-high 70% in U.S. support same-sex marriage. Retrieved from https:// news.gallup.com/poll/350486/ record-high-support-same-sex -marriage.aspx

McCarthy, S., Thomas, S. L., Bell-ringer, M. E., & Cassidy, R. (2019). Women and gambling-related harm: A narrative literature review and implications for research, policy, and practice. *Harm Reduction Journal, 16*(1), 18. https://doi .org/10.1186/s12954-019-0284-8

McCauley, E., Berk, M. S., Asarnow, J. R., Adrian, M., Cohen, J., Korslund, K., . . . Linehan, M. M. (2018). Efficacy of dialectical behavior therapy for adolescents at high risk for suicide: A randomized clinical trial. *JAMA Psychiatry, 75*(8), 777–785.

McClintock, S. M., Reti, I. M., Carpenter, L. L., McDonald, W. M., Dubin, M., Taylor, S. F., . . . National Network of Depression Centers rTMS Task Group, & American Psychiatric Association Council on Research Task Force on Novel Biomarkers and Treatments. (2018). Consensus recommendations for the clinical application of repetitive transcranial magnetic stimulation (rTMS) in the treatment of depression. *The Journal of Clinical Psychiatry, 79*(1), 16cs10905. https://doi .org/10.4088/JCP.16cs10905

McCloskey, R. J., & Pei, F. (2019). The role of parenting stress in mediating the relationship between neighborhood social cohesion and depression and anxiety among mothers of young children in fragile families. *Journal of Community Psychology, 47*(4), 869–881.

McColgan, P., & Tabrizi, S. J. (2018). Huntington's disease: A clinical review. *European Journal of Neurology, 25*(1), 24–34.

McCool-Myers, M., Theurich, M., Zuelke, A., Knuettel, H., & Apfelbacher, C. (2018). Predictors of female sexual dysfunction: A systematic review and qualitative analysis through gender inequality paradigms. *BMC Women's Health, 18*(1), 108. https://doi. org/10.1186/s12905-018-0602-4

McCracken, L. M., & Larkin, K. T. (1991). Treatment of paruresis with in vivo desensitization: A case report. *Journal of Behavior Therapy and Experimental Psychiatry, 22*, 57–62.

McCrea, M. A., Shah, A., Duma, S., Rowson, S., Harezlak, J., McAllister, T. W., . . . Stemper, B. D. (2021). Opportunities for prevention of concussion and repetitive head impact exposure in college football players: A Concussion Assessment, Research, and Education (CARE) Consortium Study. *JAMA Neurology, 78*(3), 346–350.

McCrory, E. J., Gerin, M. I., & Viding, E. (2017). Annual research review: Childhood maltreatment, latent vulnerability and the shift to preventative psychiatry—The contribution of functional brain imaging. *Journal of Child Psychology and Psychiatry, and Allied Disciplines, 58*(4), 338–357.

McCuen-Wurst, C., Ruggieri, M., & Allison, K. C. (2018). Disordered eating and obesity: Associations between binge-eating disorder, night-eating syndrome, and weight-related comorbidities. *Annals of the New York Academy of Sciences, 1411*(1), 96–105.

McCutcheon, J. C., & Watts, S. J. (2018). An examination of the importance of strain in the cannabis gateway effect. *International Journal of Offender Therapy And Comparative Criminology, 62*(11), 3603–3617.

McDermott, P. A., Watkins, M. W., & Rhoad, A. M. (2013). Whose IQ is it? Assessor bias variance in high-stakes psychological assessment. *Psychological Assessment, 26*, 207–214.

McDonagh, L. K., Stewart, I., Morrison, M. A., & Morrison,

T. G. (2016). Development and psychometric evaluation of the gay male sexual difficulties scale. *Archives of Sexual Behavior, 45*(6), 1299–1315.

McDonald, K. L., Vernberg, E. M., Lochman, J. E., Abel, M. R., Jarrett, M. A., Kassing, F., . . . Qu, L. (2019). Trajectories of tornado-related posttraumatic stress symptoms and pre-exposure predictors in a sample of at-risk youth. *Journal of Consulting and Clinical Psychology, 87*(11), 1003–1018.

McElroy, S. L., Frye, M. A., Hellemann, G., Altshuler, L., Leverich, G. S., Suppes, T., . . . Post, R. M. (2011). Prevalence and correlates of eating disorders in 875 patients with bipolar disorder. *Journal of Affective Disorders, 128*, 191–198.

McEwen, B. S. (2017). Neurobiological and systemic effects of chronic stress. *Chronic Stress (Thousand Oaks, Calif.), 1*, 2470547017692328. https://doi .org/10.1177/2470547017692328

McFarlane, W. R. (2016). Family interventions for schizophrenia and the psychoses: A review. *Family Process, 55*(3), 460–482.

McGovern, C. M., Arcoleo, K., & Melnyk, B. (2019). COPE for asthma: Outcomes of a cognitive behavioral intervention for children with asthma and anxiety. *School Psychology, 34*(6), 665–676.

McGowan, P. O. (2013, September 26). Epigenomic mechanisms of early adversity and HPA dysfunction: Considerations for PTSD research. *Frontiers in Psychiatry, 4*, 110.

McGrath, C. L., Kelley, M. D., Holzheimer, P. E., III, Dunlop, B. W., Craighead, W. E., Franco, R., . . . Mayberg, H. S. (2013). Toward a neuroimaging treatment selection biomarker for major depressive disorder. *JAMA Psychiatry, 70*, 821–829.

McIntosh, V. V. W., Carter, F. A., Bulik, C. M., Frampton, C. M. A., & Joyce, P. R. (2010). Five-year outcome of cognitive behavioral therapy and exposure with response: Prevention for bulimia nervosa. *Psychological Medicine,*

41(5), 1061–1071. doi:10.1017/S0033291710001583

McIntosh, W. L., Spies, E., Stone, D. M., Lokey, C. N., Trudeau, A. T., & Bartholow, B. (2016). Suicide rates by occupational group—17 states, 2012. *Morbidity and Mortality Weekly Report, 65*, 641–645.

McIntyre, R. S., & Calabrese, J. R. (2019). Bipolar depression: The clinical characteristics and unmet needs of a complex disorder. *Current Medical Research and Opinion, 35*(11), 1993–2005.

McKee, A. C., Mez, J., Abdolmohammadi, B., Butler, M., Huber, B. R., Uretsky, M., . . . Alosco, M. L. (2023). Neuropathologic and clinical findings in young contact sport athletes exposed to repetitive head impacts. *JAMA Neurology, 80*(10), 1037–1050. https://doi.org/10.1001/jamaneurol.2023.2907

McKibben, J. B., Bresnick, M. G., Wiechman Askay, S. A., & Fauerbach, J. A. (2008). Acute stress disorder and posttraumatic stress disorder: A prospective study of prevalence, course, and predictors in a sample with major burn injuries. *Journal of Burn Care and Research, 29*, 22–35.

McKinley, J. C., Jr. (2014). Life sentence is imposed in '08 killing of therapist. http://www.nytimes.com/2014/05/03/nyregion/david-tarloff-is-given-life-sentence-for-08-killing-of-psychologist.html?_r50

McLaughlin, K. A., Green, J. G., Hwang, I., Sampson, N. A., Zaslavsky, A. M., & Kessler, R. C. (2012). Intermittent explosive disorder in the National Comorbidity Survey Replication Adolescent Supplement. *Archives of General Psychiatry, 69*, 1131–1139.

McLaughlin, K. A., Weissman, D., & Bitrán, D. (2019). Childhood adversity and neural development: A systematic review. *Annual Review of Developmental Psychology, 1*, 277–312.

McLean, S. A., Paxton, S. J., Wertheim, E. H., & Masters, J. (2015). Photoshopping the selfie: Self photo editing and photo investment are associated with body dissatisfaction in adolescent girls. *The International Journal of Eating Disorders, 48*(8), 1132–1140.

Mealer, M., Jones, J., Newman, J., McFann, K. K., Rothbaum, B., & Moss, M. (2013). The presence of resilience is associated with a healthier psychological profile in intensive care unit (ICU) nurses: Results of a national survey. *International Journal of Nursing Studies, 49*, 292–299.

Meerwijk, E. L., & Sevelius, J. M. (2017). Transgender population size in the United States: A meta-regression of population-based probability samples. *American Journal of Public Health, 107*(2), e1–e8.

Megerian, J. T., Dey, S., Melmed, R. D., Coury, D. L., Lerner, M., Nicholls, C. J., . . . Taraman, S. (2022). Evaluation of an artificial intelligence-based medical device for diagnosis of autism spectrum disorder. *NPJ Digital Medicine, 5*(1), 57. https://doi.org/10.1038/s41746-022-00598-6

Mehler, P. S., Anderson, K., Bauschka, M., Cost, J., & Farooq, A. (2023). Emergency room presentations of people with anorexia nervosa. *Journal of Eating Disorders, 11*(1), 16. https://doi.org/10.1186/s40337-023-00742-x

Mehta, S., & Herath, P. (2019). Mild cognitive impairment. https://emedicine.medscape.com/article/1136393-overview

Meichenbaum, D. (2012). Important facts about resilience: A consideration of research findings about resilience and implications for assessment and treatment. http://www.melissainstitute.org/documents/facts_resilience.pdf

Meili, T. (2003). *I am the Central Park Jogger: A story of hope and possibility*. New York: Scribner.

Meints, S. M., Cortes, A., Morais, C. A., & Edwards, R. R. (2019). Racial and ethnic differences in the experience and treatment of non-cancer pain. *Pain Management, 9*(3), 317–334. https://doi.org/10.2217/pmt-2018-0030

Meiser-Stedman, R., McKinnon, A., Dixon, C., Boyle, A., Smith, P., & Dalgleish, T. (2017). Acute stress disorder and the transition to posttraumatic stress disorder in children and adolescents: Prevalence, course, prognosis, diagnostic suitability, and risk markers. *Depression and Anxiety, 34*(4), 348–355.

Meissner, V. H., Schroeter, L., Köhn, F. M., Kron, M., Zitzmann, M., Arsov, C., . . . Herkommer, K. (2019). Factors associated with low sexual desire in 45-year-old men: Findings from the German Male Sex-Study. *Journal of Sexual Medicine, 16*, 981–991.

Melka, S. E., Lancaster, S. L., Adams, L. J., Howarth, E. A., & Rodriguez, B. F. (2010). Social anxiety across ethnicity: A confirmatory factor analysis of the FNE and SAD. *Journal of Anxiety Disorders, 24*, 680–685.

Mellins, C. A., Walsh, K., Sarvet, A. L., Wall, M., Gilbert, L., Santelli, J. S., . . . Hirsch, J. S. (2017). Sexual assault incidents among college undergraduates: Prevalence and factors associated with risk. *PLOS One, 12*(11), e0186471. https://doi.org/10.1371/journal.pone.0186471

Meloy, J. R. (2001). Antisocial personality disorder. In G. O. Gabbard (Ed.), *Treatment of psychiatric disorders* (pp. 2251–2271). Washington, DC: American Psychiatric Publishing.

Melvin, G. A., Dudley, A. L., Gordon, M. S., Ford, S., Taffe, J., & Tonge, B. J. (2013). What happens to depressed adolescents? A follow-up study into early adulthood. *Journal of Affective Disorders, 151*, 298–305.

Memon, A., Rogers, I., Fitzsimmons, S., Carter, B., Strawbridge, R., Hidalgo-Mazzei, D., & Young, A. (2020). Association between naturally occurring lithium in drinking water and suicide rates: Systematic review and meta-analysis of ecological studies. *British Journal of Psychiatry, 217*(6), 667–678.

Memon, M. A. (2013). Brief psychotic disorder. http://emedicine.medscape.com/article/294416-overview

Mena, A. (2012). Rape trauma syndrome: The journey to healing belongs to everyone. http://www.adkanenough.com/rape-trauma-syndrome.html

Méndez, J., Sánchez-Hernández, Ó., Garber, J., Espada, J. P., & Orgilés, M. (2021). Psychological treatments for depression in adolescents: More than three decades later. *International Journal of Environmental Research and Public Health, 18*(9), 4600. https://doi.org/10.3390/ijerph18094600

Meneguzzo, P., Collantoni, E., Gallicchio, D., Busetto, P., Solmi, M., Santonastaso, P., & Favaro, A. (2018). Eating disorders symptoms in sexual minority women: A systematic review. *European Eating Disorders Review, 26*(4), 275–292.

Menkes, M. W., Armstrong, K., Blackford, J. U., Heckers, S., & Woodward, N. D. (2019). Neuropsychological functioning in early and chronic stages of schizophrenia and psychotic bipolar disorder. *Schizophrenia Research, 206*, 413–419.

Mercer, J. (2013). Deliverance, demonic possession, and mental illness: Some considerations for mental health professionals. *Mental Health, Religion and Culture, 16*, 595–611.

Merikangas, K. R., Akiskal, H. S., Angst, J., Greenberg, P. E., Hirschfeld, R. M., Petukhova, M., & Kessler, R. C. (2007). Lifetime and 12-month prevalence of bipolar spectrum disorder in the National Comorbidity Survey Replication. *Archives of General Psychiatry, 64*, 543–552.

Merikangas, K. R., He, J.-P., Burstein, M., Swanson, S. A., Avenevoli, S., Cui, L., . . . Swendsen, J. (2010). Lifetime prevalence of mental disorders in U.S. adolescents: Results from the National Comorbidity Survey Replication—Adolescent Supplement (NCS-A). *Journal of the Academy of Child and Adolescent Psychiatry, 49*, 980–989.

Merikangas, K. R., Jin, R., He, J.-P., Kessler, R. C., Lee, S., Sampson, N. A., . . . Zarkov, Z. (2011). Prevalence and correlates of bipolar spectrum disorder in the world mental health survey initiative. *Archives of General Psychiatry, 68*, 241–251.

Merritt Hawkins. (2018). The silent shortage: A white paper examining supply, demand and recruitment trends in psychiatry. https://www.hasc.org/sites/main/files/file-attachments/mhawhitepaperpsychiatry.pdf

Merry, S. N., Stasiak, K., Shepherd, M., Frampton, C., Fleming, T., & Lucassen, M. F. G. (2012). The effectiveness of SPARX, a computerized self help intervention for adolescents seeking help for depression: Randomized controlled non-inferiority trial. *British Medical Journal, 344*, e2598. https://doi.org/10.1136/bmj.e2598

Metzger, N. (2013). Battling demons with medical authority: Werewolves, physicians and rationalization. *History of Psychiatry, 24*, 341–355.

Meulepas, J. M., Ronckers, C. M., Smets, A. M., J. B., Nievelstein, J. B., Nievelstein, R. A. J., Gradowska, P., . . . Hauptmann, M. (2019). Radiation exposure from pediatric CT scans and subsequent cancer risk in the Netherlands. *Journal of the National Cancer Institute, 111*(3), 256–263.

Meuret, A. E., Simon, E., Bhaskara, L., & Ritz, T. (2017). Ultra-brief behavioral skills trainings for blood injection injury phobia. *Depression and Anxiety, 34*(12), 1096–1105.

Mewes, R. (2022). Recent developments on psychological factors in medically unexplained symptoms and somatoform disorders. *Frontiers in Public Health, 10*, 1033203. https://doi.org/10.3389/fpubh.2022.1033203

Meyer, B., Keller, A., Müller, B., Wöhlbier, H. G., & Kropp, P. (2018). Progressive muscle relaxation according to Jacobson for migraine prophylaxis: Clinical effectiveness and mode of action. *Schmerz, 32*(4), 250–258.

Meyer, E. C., Szabo, Y. Z., Frankfurt, S. B., Kimbrel, N. A., DeBeer, B. B., & Morissette, S. B. (2019). Predictors of recovery from post-deployment posttraumatic stress disorder symptoms in war veterans: The contributions of psychological flexibility, mindfulness, and self-compassion. *Behaviour Research and Therapy, 114*, 7–14.

Meyer I. H. (2020). Rejection sensitivity and minority stress: A challenge for clinicians and interventionists. *Archives of Sexual Behavior, 49*(7), 2287–2289.

Meyer, S. E., Carlson, G. A., Youngstrom, E., Ronsaville, D. S., Martinez, P. E., Gold, P. W., . . . Radke-Yarrow, M. (2009). Long-term outcomes of youth who manifested the CBCL-pediatric bipolar disorder phenotype during childhood and/or adolescence. *Journal of Affective Disorders, 113*, 227–235.

Mez, J., Daneshvar, D. H., Kiernan, P. T., Abdolmohammadi, B., Alvarez, V. E., Huber, B. R., . . . McKee, A. C. (2017). Clinicopathological evaluation of chronic traumatic encephalopathy in players of American football. *JAMA, 318*(4), 360–370.

Mezulis, A. H., Priess, H. A., & Hyde, J. S. (2011). Rumination mediates the relationship between infant temperament and adolescent depressive symptoms. *Depression Research and Treatment, 487873.*

Michael, K. D., Payne, L. O., & Albright, A. E. (2012). An adaptation of the coping cat program: The successful treatment of a 6-year-old boy with generalized anxiety disorder. *Clinical Case Studies.* https://doi.org/10.1177/1534650112460912

Michl, L. C., McLaughlin, K. A., Shepherd, K., & Nolen-Hoeksema, S. (2013). Rumination as a mechanism linking stressful life events to symptoms of depression and anxiety: Longitudinal evidence in early adolescents and adults. *Journal of Abnormal Psychology, 122*, 339–352.

Middelveen, M. J., Fesler, M. C., & Stricker, R. B. (2018). History of Morgellons disease: From delusion to definition. *Clinical, Cosmetic and Investigational Dermatology, 11*, 71–90.

Midei, A. J., & Matthews, K. A. (2009). Social relationships and negative emotional traits are associated with central adiposity and arterial stiffness in health adolescents. *Health Psychology, 28*, 347–353.

Miech, R. A., Johnston, L. D., Patrick, M. E., O'Malley, P. M., Bachman, J. G., & Schulenberg, J. E. (2023). Monitoring the future national survey results on drug use, 1975–2022: Secondary school students. *Monitoring the Future Monograph Series.* Ann Arbor: Institute for Social Research, University of Michigan. https://

monitoringthefuture.org/results /publications/monographs

Miettunen, J., Tormanen, S., Murray, G. K., Jones, P. B., Maki, P., Ebeling, H., . . . Veijola, J. (2008). Association of cannabis use with prodromal symptoms of psychosis in adolescence. *British Journal of Psychiatry*, 192, 470–471.

Mikkelson, D. (2014). Death of Leelah Alcorn. https://www.snopes.com /fact-check/death-of-leelah-alcorn/

Miklowitz, D. J., Price, J., Holmes, E. A., Rendell, J., Bell, S., Budge, K., . . . Geddes, J. R. (2012). Facilitated integrated mood management for adults with bipolar disorder. *Bipolar Disorders*, 14, 185–197.

Miklowitz, D. J., Schneck, C. D., Singh, M. K., Taylor, D. O., George, E. L., Cosgrove, V. E., . . . Chang, K. D. (2013). Early intervention for symptomatic youth at risk for bipolar disorder: A randomized trial of family-focused therapy. *Journal of American Academy of Child and Adolescent Psychiatry*, 52, 121–131.

Milic, J., Glisic, M., Voortman, T., Borba, L. P., Asllanaj, E., Rojas, L. Z., . . . Franco, O. H. (2018). Menopause, ageing, and alcohol use disorders in women. *Maturitas*, 111, 100–109.

Miller, A. B., Esposito-Smythers, C., Weismoore, J. T., & Renshaw, K. D. (2013). The relation between child maltreatment and adolescent suicidal behavior: A systematic review and critical examination of the literature. *Clinical Child and Family Psychology Review*, 16, 146–172.

Miller, J. (2015). Dredging and projecting the depths of personality: The Thematic Apperception Test and the narratives of the unconscious. *Science in Context*, 28, 9–30.

Miller, J. N., & Black, D. W. (2019). Schizoaffective disorder: A review. *Annals of Clinical Psychiatry: Official Journal of the American Academy of Clinical Psychiatrists*, 31(1), 47–53.

Miller, M. W., Lin, A. P., Wolf, E. J., & Miller, D. R. (2018). Oxidative stress, inflammation, and neuroprogression in chronic PTSD. *Harvard Review of Psychiatry*, 26(2), 57–69.

Miller, M., Swanson, S. A., Azrael, D., Pate, V., & Stürmer, T. (2014). Antidepressant dose, age, and the risk of deliberate self-harm. *JAMA Internal Medicine*, 174, 899–909.

Miller, T. C., & Zwerdling, D. (2010, June 9). With traumatic brain injuries, soldiers face battle for care. http://www.npr.org/templates/story /story.php?storyId5127542820

Millon, T., Grossman, S., Millon, C., Meagher, S., & Ramnath, R. (2004). *Personality disorders in modern life*. Hoboken, NJ: Wiley.

Milojevich, H. M., & Lukowski, A. F. (2016). Sleep and mental health in undergraduate students with generally healthy sleep habits. *PLOS One*, 11, e0156372.

Mineka, S., & Zinbarg, R. (2006). A contemporary learning theory perspective on the etiology of anxiety disorders. *American Psychologist*, 61, 10–26.

Minnis H. (2018). What happens to disinhibited social engagement disorder over time? *Journal of the American Academy of Child and Adolescent Psychiatry*, 57(5), 304–305.

Minor, K. S., & Cohen, A. S. (2012). The role of atypical semantic activation and stress in odd speech: Implications for individuals with psychometrically defined schizotypy. *Journal of Psychiatric Research*, 46, 1231–1236.

Minster, R. L., Hawley, N. L., Su, C. T., Sun, G., Kershaw, E. E., Cheng, H., . . . McGarvey, S. T. (2016). A thrifty variant in CREBRF strongly influences body mass index in Samoans. *Nature Genetics*, 48(9), 1049–1054. https://doi.org/10.1038/ng.3620

Minuchin, S. (1974). *Families and family therapy*. Cambridge, MA: Harvard University Press.

Miralles, I., Granell, C., García-Palacios, A., Castilla, D., González-Pérez, A., Casteleyn, S., & Bretón-López, J. (2020). Enhancing in vivo exposure in the treatment of panic disorder and agoraphobia using location-based technologies: A case study. *Clinical Case Studies*, 19, 143–159.

Misch, M. R., & Raukar, N. P. (2020). Sports medicine update: Concussion. *Emergency Medicine Clinics of North America*, 38(1), 207–222.

Mishra, S., Das, N., Mohapatra, D., & Mishra, B. R. (2022). Mindfulness-based cognitive therapy in depersonalization-derealization disorder: A case report. *Indian Journal of Psychological Medicine*, 44(6), 620–621. https://doi.org /10.1177/02537176211040259

Misra, D. P., Ravindran, V., & Agarwal, V. (2018). Integrity of authorship and peer review practices: Challenges and opportunities for improvement. *Journal of Korean Medical Science*, 33(46), e287. http://doi.org/10.3346 /jkms.2018.33.e287.eCollection

Misselhorn, C., Pompe, U., & Stapleton, M. (2013). Ethical considerations regarding the use of social robots in the fourth age. *GeroPsychology*, 26, 121–133.

Mitchell, J. M. (2022). A psychedelic may soon go to the FDA for approval to treat trauma. *Scientific American*. https://www .scientificamerican.com/article/a -psychedelic-may-soon-go-to-the -fda-for-approval-to-treat-trauma/

Moccia, L., Pettorruso, M., De Crescenzo, F., De Risio, L., di Nuzzo, L., Martinotti, G., . . . Di Nicola, M. (2017). Neural correlates of cognitive control in gambling disorder: A systematic review of fMRI studies. *Neuroscience and Biobehavioral Reviews*, 78, 104–116.

Modak, T., Sarkar, S., & Sagar, R. (2016). The story of Prosenjit Poddar. *Journal of Mental Health and Human Behavior*, 21, 138–140.

Moezzi, M. (2014). Depression and Bipolar Support Alliance: Life unlimited stories. http://www .dbsalliance.org/site/PageServer?- pagename5peer _life_unlimited

Mohajerin, B., Bakhtiyar, M., Olesnycky, O. S., Dolatshahi, B., & Motabi, F. (2019). Application of a transdiagnostic treatment for emotional disorders to body dysmorphic disorder: A randomized controlled trial. *Journal of Affective Disorders*, 245, 637–644.

Mohajerin, B., Lynn, S. J., Bakhtiyari, M., & Dolatshah, B. (2019). Evaluating the unified protocol in the treatment of dissociative identify disorder. *Cognitive and Behavioral Practice*. https://doi.org/10.1016/j.cbpra.2019.07.012

Mohr, D. C., Cox, D., & Merluzzi, N. (2005). Self-injection anxiety training: Successful treatment for patients unable to self-inject injectable medication. *Multiple Sclerosis, 11*, 182–185.

Mohr, J. J., Weiner, J. L., Chopp, R. M., & Wong, S. J. (2009). Effects of client bisexuality on clinical judgment: When is bias most likely to occur? *Journal of Counseling Psychology, 56*, 164–175.

Moise, R. K., Meca, A., Schwartz, S. J., Unger, J. B., Lorenzo-Blanco, E. I., Ángel Cano, M., . . . Lizzi, K. M. (2019). The use of cultural identity in predicting health lifestyle behaviors in Latinx immigrant adolescents. *Cultural Diversity and Ethnic Minority Psychology, 25*(3), 371–378.

Moisse, K., & Davis, L. (2012, January 27). Erin Brockovich launches investigation into tic illness affecting N.Y. teenagers. http://abcnews.go.com/Health/Wellness/erin-brockovich-launches-investigation-tic-illness-affecting-ny/story?id515456672

Mojtabai, R., & Olfson, M. (2020). National trends in mental health care for US adolescents. *JAMA Psychiatry, 77*(7), 1–12.

Mokros, A., & Habermeyer, E. (2016). Regression to the mean mimicking changes in sexual arousal to child stimuli in pedophiles. *Archives of Sexual Behavior, 45*, 1863–1867.

Mollaioli, D., Ciocca, G., Limoncin, E., Di Sante, S., Gravina, G. L., Carosa, E., . . . Jannini, E. A. F. (2020). Lifestyles and sexuality in men and women: The gender perspective in sexual medicine. *Reproductive Biology and Endocrinology: RB&E, 18*(1), 10. https://doi.org/10.1186/s12958-019-0557-9

Möller, H. J. (2016). The relevance of negative symptoms in schizophrenia and how to treat them with psychopharmaceuticals? *Psychiatria Danubina, 28*(4), 435–440.

Molock, S. D., Boyd, R. C., Alvarez, K., Cha, C., Denton, E.-G., Glenn, C. R., . . . Miller, A. B. (2023,

March 13). Culturally responsive assessment of suicidal thoughts and behaviors in youth of color. *American Psychologist*. Advance online publication. https://dx.doi.org/10.1037/amp0001140

Monzani, B., Rijsdijk, F., Cherkas, L., Harris, J., Keuthen, N., & Mataix-Cols, D. (2012). Prevalence and heritability of skin picking in an adult community sample: A twin study. *American Journal of Medical Genetics, 159*, 605–610.

Mooney, M. A., Ryabinin, P., Wilmot, B., Bhatt, P., Mill, J., & Nigg, J. T. (2020). Large epigenome-wide association study of childhood ADHD identifies peripheral DNA methylation associated with disease and polygenic risk burden. *Translational Psychiatry, 10*(1), 8. https://doi.org/10.1038/s41398-020-0710-4

Morales, E., & Norcross, J. C. (2010). Evidence-based practices with ethnic minorities: Strange bedfellows no more. *Journal of Clinical Psychology, 66*, 821–829.

Mordaunt, C. E., Park, B. Y., Bakulski, K. M., Feinberg, J. I., Croen, L. A., Ladd-Acosta, C., . . . Fallin, M. D. (2019). A meta-analysis of two high-risk prospective cohort studies reveals autism-specific transcriptional changes to chromatin, autoimmune, and environmental response genes in umbilical cord blood. *Molecular Autism, 10*, 36. https://doi.org/10.1186/s13229-019-0287-z

Moreau, C., Kågesten, A. E., & Blum, R. W. (2016). Sexual dysfunction among youth: An overlooked sexual health concern. *BMC Public Health, 16*, 1170. https://doi.org/10.1186/s12889-016-3835-x

Moreira, P. S., Marques, P., Soriano-Mas, C., Magalhães, R., Sousa, N., Soares, J. M., & Morgado, P. (2017). The neural correlates of obsessive-compulsive disorder: A multimodal perspective. *Translational Psychiatry, 7*(8), e1224. https://doi.org/10.1038/tp.2017.189

Morgan Consoli, M. L., & Llamas, J. D. (2013). The relationship between Mexican American cultural values and resilience among

Mexican American college students: A mixed methods study. *Journal of Counseling Psychology, 60*, 617–624.

Morgan, R. E., & Oudekerk, B. A. (2019). U.S. Department of Justice Criminal Victimization, 2018. https://www.bjs.gov/content/pub/pdf/cv18.pdf

Morgan, V. A., Di Prinzio, P., Valuri, G., Croft, M., McNeil, T., & Jablensky, A. (2019). Are familial liability for schizophrenia and obstetric complications independently associated with risk of psychotic illness, after adjusting for other environmental stressors in childhood? *The Australian and New Zealand Journal of Psychiatry, 53*(11), 1105–1115.

Morgenthaler, T. I., Auerbach, S., Casey, K. R., Kristo, D., Maganti, R., Ramar, K., . . . Kartje, R. (2018). Position paper for the treatment of nightmare disorder in adults: An American Academy of Sleep Medicine position paper. *Journal of Clinical Sleep Medicine, 14*(6), 1041–1055.

Mori, C., Cooke, J. E., Temple, J. R. Ly, A., Lu, Y., Anderson, N., . . . Madigan, S. (2020). The prevalence of sexting behaviors among emerging adults: A meta-analysis. *Archives of Sexual Behavior, 49*(4), 1103–1119.

Moritz, S., Favrod, J., Andreou, C., Morrison, A. P., Bohn, F., Veckenstedt, R., . . . Karow, A. (2013). Beyond the usual suspects: Positive attitudes towards positive symptoms is associated with medication noncompliance in psychosis. *Schizophrenia Bulletin, 39*, 917–922.

Moritz, S., Purdon, C., Jelinek, L., Chiang, B., & Hauschildt, M. (2018). If it is absurd, then why do you do it? The richer the obsessional experience, the more compelling the compulsion. *Clinical Psychology and Psychotherapy, 25*(2), 210–216.

Moser, C. (2018). Paraphilias and the ICD-11: Progress but still logically inconsistent. *Archives of Sexual Behavior, 47*(4), 825–826.

Moss, A. C., De Silva, D., Cox, S., Notley, C., & Nanda, M. (2020). Measuring the impact of the Capital Card®, a novel form of contingency management, on substance misuse treatment outcomes: A retrospective evaluation. *PLOS One, 15*(3), e0229905. https://doi.org/10.1371/journal.pone.0229905

Mueller, D. R., Khalesi, Z., & Roder, V. (2020). Can cognitive remediation in groups prevent relapses? Results of a 1-year follow-up randomized controlled trial. *The Journal of Nervous and Mental Disease, 208*(5), 362–370.

Mufaddel, A., Osman, O. T., Almugaddam, F., & Jafferany, M. (2013). A review of body dysmorphic disorder and its presentation in different clinical settings. *Primary Care Companion to CNS Disorders, 15*(4), PCC.12r01464. https://doi.org/10.4088/PCC.12r01464

Muhlberger, A., Wiedemann, G., Herrmann, M. J., & Pauli, P. (2006). Phylo- and ontogenetic fears and expectations of danger: Differences between spider- and flight-phobic subjects in cognitive and physiological responses to disorder-specific stimuli. *Journal of Abnormal Psychology, 115*, 580–589.

Muir, O., Weinfeld, J. N., Ruiz, D., Ostrovsky, D., Fiolhais, M., & MacMillan, C. (2021). Mental health clinicians' attitudes toward narcissistic personality disorder. *Personality Disorders, 12*(5), 389–399.

Mukherjee, S. (2013). This town: What it's like being homeless with a mental illness in Washington DC. http://thinkprogress.org/health/2013/08/28/2310961/mentally-homeless-district

Mulkens, S. A. N., de Jong, P. J., & Merckelbach, H. (1996). Disgust and spider phobia. *Journal of Abnormal Psychology, 105*, 464–468.

Müller, T. D., & Tschöp, M. H. (2013). Ghrelin—A key pleiotropic hormone- regulating systemic energy metabolism. *Endocrine Development, 25*, 91–100.

Mulvaney-Day, N., Gibbons, B. J., Alikhan, S., & Karakus, S. M. (2019). Mental Health Parity and Addiction Equity Act and the use of outpatient behavioral health services in the United States, 2005–2016. *American Journal of Public Health, 109*, S190–S196.

Muneer A. (2017). Mixed states in bipolar disorder: Etiology, pathogenesis and treatment. *Chonnam Medical Journal, 53*(1), 1–13.

Munkholm, K. (2019). Caution should be advised when recommending increased use of ECT based on low-quality evidence. *Acta Psychiatrica Scandinavica, 139*(5), 485–486.

Munkholm, K., Paludan-Müller, A. S., & Boesen, K. (2019). Considering the methodological limitations in the evidence base of antidepressants for depression: A reanalysis of a network meta-analysis. *BMJ Open, 9*(6), e024886. https://doi.org/10.1136/bmjopen-2018-024886

Munsey, C. (2010). Medicine or menace? Psychologists' research can inform the growing debate over legalizing marijuana. *APA Monitor, 41*(6), 50.

Munson, S. A., Friedman, E. C., Osterhage, K., Allred, R., Pullmann, M. D., Areán, P. A., Lyon, A. R., & UW ALACRITY Center Researchers (2022). Usability issues in evidence-based psychosocial interventions and implementation strategies: Cross-project analysis. *Journal of Medical Internet Research, 24*(6), e37585. https://doi.org/10.2196/37585

Murata, S., Rezeppa, T., Thoma, B., Marengo, L., Krancevich, K., Chiyka, E., . . . Melhem, N. M. (2021). The psychiatric sequelae of the COVID-19 pandemic in adolescents, adults, and health care workers. *Depression and Anxiety, 38*(2), 233–246.

Muris, P., van Zwol, L., Huijding, J., & Mayer, B. (2010). Mom told me scary things about this animal: Parents installing fear beliefs in their children via the verbal information pathway. *Behaviour Research and Therapy, 48*, 341–346.

Murphy, H., & Perera-Delcourt, R. (2014). "Learning to live with OCD is a little mantra I often repeat": Understanding the lived experience of obsessive- compulsive disorder (OCD) in the contemporary therapeutic context. *Psychology and Psychotherapy, 87*, 111–125.

Murray, C. K., Reynolds, J. C., Schroeder, J. M., Harrison, M. B., Evans, O. M., & Hospenthal, D. R. (2005). Spectrum of care provided at an Echelon II medical unit during Operation Iraqi Freedom. *Military Medicine, 170*, 516–520.

Murray, H. A., & Morgan, H. (1938). *Explorations in personality.* New York: Oxford University Press.

Murrie, B., Lappin, J., Large, M., & Sara, G. (2020). Transition of substance-induced, brief, and atypical psychoses to schizophrenia: A systematic review and meta-analysis. *Schizophrenia Bulletin, 46*(3), 505–516.

Muschalla, B., & Schönborn, F. (2021). Induction of false beliefs and false memories in laboratory studies: A systematic review. *Clinical Psychology & Psychotherapy, 28*(5), 1194–1209.

Muse, K., McManus, F., Hackmann, A., Williams, M., & Williams, M. (2010). Intrusive imagery in severe health anxiety: Prevalence, nature and links with memory and maintenance cycles. *Behaviour Research and Therapy, 48*, 792–798.

Musliner, K. L., & Østergaard, S. D. (2018). Patterns and predictors of conversion to bipolar disorder in 91,587 individuals diagnosed with unipolar depression. *Acta Psychiatrica Scandinavica, 137*(5), 422–432.

Musser, E. D., & Raiker, J. S., Jr. (2019). Attention-deficit/hyperactivity disorder: An integrated developmental psychopathology and Research Domain Criteria (RDoC) approach. *Comprehensive Psychiatry, 90*, 65–72.

Mustelin, L., Lehtokari, V. L., & Keski-Rahkonen, A. (2016). Other specified and unspecified feeding or eating disorders among women in the community. *The International Journal of Eating Disorders, 49*(11), 1010–1017.

Myers, S. G., & Wells, A. (2013). An experimental manipulation of metacognition: A test of the metacognitive model of obsessive-compulsive symptoms. *Behaviour Research and Therapy, 51*, 177–184.

Na, H. R., Kang, E. H., Lee, J. H., & Yu, B. H. (2011). The genetic basis of panic disorder. *Journal of Korean Medical Science*, 26(6), 701–710.

Nademanee, K., Veerakul, G., Nimmannit, S., Chaowakul, V., Bhuripanyo, K., Likittanasombat, K., . . . Tatsanavivat, P. (1997). Arrhythmogenic marker for sudden unexplained death syndrome in Thai men. *Circulation*, 96, 2595–2600.

Naggiar, S. (2012). "Broken heart" syndrome can be triggered by stress, grief. http://vitals.nbcnews.com/_news/2012/09/24/14072649-broken-heart-syndrome-can-be-triggered-by-stress-grief?lite

Nagy, C., Vaillancourt, K., & Turecki, G. (2018). A role for activity-dependent epigenetics in the development and treatment of major depressive disorder. *Genes, Brain, and Behavior*, 17(3), e12446. https://doi.org/10.1111/gbb.12446

Nagy, L. M., Shanahan, M. L., & Seaford, S. P. (2023). Nonsuicidal self-injury and rumination: A meta-analysis. *Journal of Clinical Psychology*, 79(1), 7–27.

Najib, U., Moore, M., & Watson, D. (2019). Unique considerations for special populations in episodic migraine: The underserved. *Current Pain and Headache Reports*, 23(2), 9. https://doi.org/10.1007/s11916-019-0749-1

Nakagami, Y., Ii, T., Russ, T. C., Marques, J. G., Riese, F., Sönmez, E., . . . Akiyama, T. (2017). Taijin kyofusho: A culture-bound diagnosis discussed by Japanese and international early career psychiatrists. *Psychiatry and Clinical Neurosciences*, 71(2), 146.

Nakagawa, A., Mitsuda, D., Sado, M., Abe, T., Fujisawa, D., Kikuchi, T., . . . Ono, Y. (2017). Effectiveness of supplementary cognitive-behavioral therapy for pharmacotherapy-resistant depression: A randomized controlled trial. *The Journal of Clinical Psychiatry*, 78(8), 1126–1135.

Namiki, C., Yamada, M., Yoshida, H., Hanakawa, T., Fukuyama, H., & Murai, T. (2008). Small orbitofrontal traumatic lesions detected by high resolution MRI in a patient with major behavioral changes. *Neurocase*, 14, 474–479.

Nasser, A., Liranso, T., Adewole, T., Fry, N., Hull, J. T., Chowdhry, F., . . . Schwabe, S. (2020). A phase III, randomized, placebo-controlled trial to assess the efficacy and safety of once-daily SPN-812 (viloxazine extended-release) in the treatment of attention-deficit/hyperactivity disorder in school-age children. *Clinical Therapeutics*, 42, 1452–1466.

National Alliance on Mental Illness (NAMI). (2019). Mental health by the numbers. https://www.nami.org/Learn-More/Mental-Health-By-the-Numbers

National Center for Health Statistics. (2020). Household Pulse Survey, 2020. https://www.cdc.gov/nchs/covid19/pulse/mental-health.htm

National Center for Health Statistics. (2023). Percentage of regularly experienced chronic pain for adults aged 18 and over: United States, 2019–2021. National Health Interview Survey. Generated interactively. https://wwwn.cdc.gov/NHISDataQueryTool/SHS_adult/index.html

National Conference of State Legislatures. (2022). Mental health professionals' duty to warn. https://www.ncsl.org/health/mental-health-professionals-duty-to-warn

National Down Syndrome Society. (2020). Down syndrome facts. https://www.ndss.org/about-down-syndrome/down-syndrome-facts/

National Down Syndrome Society. (2023). Facts, myths & truths about Down syndrome. https://ndss.org/myths-truths

National Highway Traffic Safety Administration. (2017). Traffic safety facts 2016 data: Alcohol-impaired driving. U.S. Department of Transportation, Washington, DC. https://crashstats.nhtsa.dot.gov/Api/Public/ViewPublication/812450

National Human Genome Research Institute. (2020). Whole genome association studies. https://www.genome.gov/17516714/2006-release-about-whole-genome-association-studies

National Institute of Mental Health (NIMH). (2009). Anxiety disorders. http://www.nimh.nih.gov/health/publications/anxiety-disorders/nimhanxiety.pdf

National Institute of Mental Health (NIMH). (2014). Eating disorders. http://www.nimh.nih.gov/health/publi-cations/eating-disorders/index.shtml#pub1

National Institute of Mental Health (NIMH). (2016a). Panic disorder: When fear overwhelms. https://www.nimh.nih.gov/health/publica-tions/panic-disorder-when-fear-over-whelms/index.shtml

National Institute of Mental Health (NIMH). (2016b). *Social anxiety disorder: More than just shyness*. https://www.nimh.nih.gov/health/publications/social-anxiety-disorder-more-than-just-shyness

National Institute of Mental Health (NIMH). (2017a). Agoraphobia. https://www.nimh.nih.gov/health/statistics/agoraphobia.shtml

National Institute of Mental Health (NIMH). (2017b). Any anxiety disorder. https://www.nimh.nih.gov/health/statistics/any-anxiety-disorder.shtml

National Institute of Mental Health (NIMH). (2017c). Generalized anxiety disorder. https://www.nimh.nih.gov/health/statistics/generalized-anxiety-disorder.shtml

National Institute of Mental Health (NIMH). (2017d). Obsessive-compulsive disorder. https://www.nimh.nih.gov/health/statistics/obsessive-compulsive-disorder-ocd.shtml

National Institute of Mental Health (NIMH). (2017e). Panic disorder. https://www.nimh.nih.gov/health/statistics/panic-disorder.shtml

National Institute of Mental Health (NIMH). (2017f). Specific phobia. https://www.nimh.nih.gov/health/statistics/specific-phobia.shtml

National Institute of Mental Health (NIMH). (2019). 5 action steps for helping someone in emotional pain. https://www.nimh.nih.gov/health/publications/5-action-steps-for-helping-someone-in-emotional-pain/index.shtml

National Institute on Alcohol and Alcoholism. (2023). Understanding the dangers of alcohol overdose. https://www.niaaa.nih.gov/publications/brochures-and

-fact-sheets/understanding-dangers -of-alcohol-overdose

National Institute on Drug Abuse. (2020). Bath salts. https:// teens.drugabuse.gov/drug-facts/ bath-salts

National Institutes of Health (NIH). (2018). Energy drinks. https:// www.nccih.nih.gov/health/energy -drinks

National Resources Defense Council. (2020). Toxic chemicals. https:// www.nrdc.org/issues/toxic -chemicals

National Sleep Foundation. (2023). How much sleep do you need? https://www.sleepfoundation .org/articles/how-much -sleep-do-we-really-need

National Survey of Sexual Health and Behavior (2023). Key findings. https://nationalsexstudy .indiana.edu/keyfindings/index.html

Naumann, E., Svaldi, J., Wyschka, T., Heinrichs, M., & von Dawans, B. (2018). Stress-induced body dissatisfaction in women with binge eating disorder. *Journal of Abnormal Psychology, 127*(6), 548–558.

Navaneelan, T. (2013). Suicide rates: An overview. http://www.statcan. gc.ca/pub/82-624-x/2012001 /article/11696-eng.htm

Neacsiu, A. D., Lungu, A., Harned, M. S., Rizvi, S. L., & Linehan, M. M. (2014). Impact of dialectical behavior therapy versus community treatment by experts on emotional experience, expression, and acceptance in borderline personality disorder. *Behaviour Research and Therapy, 53*, 47–54.

Neitzke, A. B. (2016). An illness of power: Gender and the social causes of depression. *Culture, Medicine and Psychiatry, 40*(1), 59–73.

Nelson, D. S., Gerras, J. M., McGlumphy, K. C., Shaver, E. R., Gill, A. K., Kanneganti, K., Ajibewa, T. A., & Hasson, R. E. (2018). Racial discrimination and low household education predict higher body mass index in African American youth. *Childhood Obesity, 14*(2), 114–121.

Nelson, J. (2017). Joni Mitchell says battle with rare Morgellons disease makes her feel like she's being "eaten alive." https://people .com/music/joni-mitchell-morgellons -syndrome-mysterious-disease- eaten-alive/

Nemesure, M. D., Park, C., Morris, R. R., Chan, W. W., Fitzsimmons-Craft, E. E., Rackoff, G. N., . . . Jacobson, N. C. (2023). Evaluating change in body image concerns following a single session digital intervention. *Body Image, 44*, 64–68.

Németh, G., Laszlovszky, I., Czobor, P., Szalai, E., Szatmári, B., Harsányi, J., . . . Fleischhacker, W. W. (2017). Cariprazine versus risperidone monotherapy for treatment of predominant negative symptoms in patients with schizophrenia: A randomised, double-blind, controlled trial. *Lancet (London, England), 389*(10074), 1103–1113.

Neng, J. M., & Weck, F. (2014). Attribution of somatic symptoms in hypochondriasis. *Clinical Psychology and Psychotherapy.* https://doi.org/10.1002/cpp.1871

Nestor, P. G., O'Donovan, K., Lapp, H. E., Hasler, V. C., Boodai, S. B., & Hunter, R. (2019). Risk and protective effects of serotonin and BDNF genes on stress-related adult psychiatric symptoms. *Neurobiology of Stress, 11*, 100186. https://doi .org/10.1016/j.ynstr.2019.100186

Neugebauer, R. (1979). Medieval and early modern theories of mental illness. *Archives of General Psychiatry, 36*, 477–483.

Neutze, J., Grundmann, D., Scherner, G., & Beier, K. M. (2012). Undetected and detected child sexual abuse and child pornography offenders. *International Journal of Law and Psychiatry, 35*, 168–175.

Newby, J. M., Mewton, L., & Andrews, G. (2017). Transdiagnostic versus disorder-specific internet-delivered cognitive behaviour therapy for anxiety and depression in primary care. *Journal of Anxiety Disorders, 46*, 25–34.

Newman, C. F. (2010). The case of Gabriel: Treatment with Beckian cognitive therapy. *Journal of Constructivist Psychology, 23*, 25–41.

Nguyen, H., Gabrielson, A. T., & Hellstrom, W. (2017). Erectile dysfunction in young men—A review of the prevalence and risk factors. *Sexual Medicine Reviews, 5*, 508–520.

Nichols, M. P., & Schwartz, R. C. (2005). *The essentials of family therapy.* New York: Allyn & Bacon.

Nicholson, P., O'Hare, A., Power, S., Looby, S., Javadpour, M., Thornton, J., & Brennan, P. (2019). Decreasing incidence of subarachnoid hemorrhage. *Journal of Neurointerventional Surgery, 11*(3), 320–322.

Nickerson, A., Aderka, I. M., Bryant, R. A., & Hofmann, S. G. (2012). The relationship between childhood exposure to trauma and intermittent explosive disorder. *Psychiatry Research, 197*, 128–134.

Niederkrotenthaler, T., & Till, B. (2019). Effects of suicide awareness materials on individuals with recent suicidal ideation or attempt: Online randomised controlled trial. *British Journal of Psychiatry, 1*–8. https://doi.org/10.1192 /bjp.2019.259

Nierenberg, A. A. (2019). Bipolar II disorder is NOT a myth. *Canadian Journal of Psychiatry, 64*(8), 537–540.

Nilsen, F. M., & Tulve, N. S. (2020). A systematic review and meta-analysis examining the interrelationships between chemical and non-chemical stressors and inherent characteristics in children with ADHD. *Environmental Research, 180*, 108884. https://doi.org/10.1016 /j.envres.2019.108884

Nisbett, R. E., Aronson, J., Blair, C., Dickens, W., Flynn, J., Halpern, D. F., & Turkheimer E. (2012). Intelligence: New findings and theoretical developments. *American Psychologist, 67*, 130–159.

Nixon, R., Sterk, J., & Pearce, A. (2012). A randomized trial of cognitive behaviour therapy and cognitive therapy for children with posttraumatic stress disorder following single-incident trauma. *Journal of Abnormal Child Psychology, 40*, 327–337.

Nock, M. K., Green, J. G., Hwang, I., McLaughlin, K. A., Sampson, N. A., Zaslavsky, A. M., & Kessler, R. C. (2013). Prevalence, correlates, and treatment of lifetime suicidal behavior among adolescents: Results from the National Comorbidity Survey Replication Adolescent Supplement. *JAMA Psychiatry, 70,* 300–310.

Nolan, B. J., Zwickl, S., Locke, P., Zajac, J. D., & Cheung, A. S. (2023). Early access to testosterone therapy in transgender and gender-diverse adults seeking masculinization: A randomized clinical trial. *JAMA Network Open, 6*(9), e2331919. https://doi.org/10.1001/jamanetworkopen.2023.31919

Nolen-Hoeksema, S. (2012). Emotion regulation and psychopathology: The role of gender. *Annual Review of Clinical Psychology, 8,* 161–187.

Nolen-Hoeksema, S., Girgus, J. S., & Seligman, M. E. (1992). Predictors and consequences of childhood depressive symptoms: A 5-year longitudinal study. *Journal of Abnormal Psychology, 101,* 405–422.

Nolfi, J. (2021). You'll cry watching Lady Gaga's emotional new music video with Tony Bennet. https://ew.com/music/lady-gaga-tony-bennett-i-get-a-kick-out-of-you-music-video/

Norbye, A. D., Abelsen, B., Førde, O. H., & Ringberg, U. (2022a). The association between health anxiety, physical disease and cardiovascular risk factors in the general population: A cross-sectional analysis from the Tromsø study. Tromsø 7. *BMC Primary Care, 23*(1), 140. https://doi.org/10.1186/s12875-022-01749-0

Norbye, A. D., Abelsen, B., Førde, O. H., & Ringberg, U. (2022b). Distribution of health anxiety in a general adult population and associations with demographic and social network characteristics. *Psychological Medicine, 52*(12), 2255–2262.

Norfleet, M. A. (2002). Responding to society's needs: Prescription privileges for psychologists. *Journal of Clinical Psychology, 58,* 599–610.

Norko, M. A. (2008). Duty to warn and dissociative identity disorder. *American Medical Association Journal of Ethics, 10,* 144–149.

Norton, A. R., & Abbott, M. J. (2016). The efficacy of imagery

rescripting compared to cognitive restructuring for social anxiety disorder. *Journal of Anxiety Disorders, 40,* 18–28.

Noseda, R., Bernstein, C. A., Nir, R. R., Lee, A. J., Fulton, A. B., Bertisch, S. M., . . . Burstein, R. (2016). Migraine photophobia originating in cone-driven retinal pathways. *Brain: A Journal of Neurology, 139*(Pt 7), 1971–1986.

Novak, I., & Morgan, C. (2019). High-risk follow-up: Early intervention and rehabilitation. *Handbook of Clinical Neurology, 162,* 483–510.

Novick, D. M., & Swartz, H. A. (2019). Evidence-based psychotherapies for bipolar disorder. *Focus, 17*(3), 238–248.

Novick, D., Montgomery, W., Treuer, T., Moneta, M. V., & Haro, J. M. (2016). Sex differences in the course of schizophrenia across diverse regions of the world. *Neuropsychiatric Disease and Treatment, 12,* 2927–2939.

Noyes, R., Jr., Stuart, S., Watson, D. B., & Langbehn, D. R. (2006). Distinguishing between hypochondriasis and somatization disorder: A review of the existing literature. *Psychotherapy and Psychosomatics, 75,* 270–281.

Nuevo, R., Chatterji, S., Verdes, E., Naidoo, N., Arango, C., & Ayuso-Mateos, J. L. (2012). The continuum of psychotic symptoms in the general population: A cross-national study. *Schizophrenia Bulletin, 38,* 475–485.

Nunziato, C. A., Egeland, B. M., Gurman, A., & Henry, S. L. (2021). Morgellons disease: The spread of a mass psychogenic illness via the Internet and its implications in hand surgery. *Hand (New York), 16*(6), NP5–NP9. https://doi.org/10.1177/1558944720976648

Nussbaumer-Streit, B., Forneris, C. A., Morgan, L. C., Van Noord, M. G., Gaynes, B. N., Greenblatt, A., . . . Gartlehner, G. (2019). Light therapy for preventing seasonal affective disorder. *The Cochrane Database of Systematic Reviews, 3*(3), CD011269. https://doi.org/10.1002/14651858.CD011269.pub3

Nusslock, R., & Alloy, L. B. (2017). Reward processing and mood-related symptoms: An RDoC and translational neuroscience perspective. *Journal of Affective Disorders, 216,* 3–16. https://doi.org/10.1016/j.jad.2017.02.001

Nutt, D. J., King, L. A., & Phillip, L. D. (2010). Drug harms in the UK: A multicriteria decision analysis. *Lancet, 376*(9752), 1558–1565.

O'Brien, M. P., Gordon, J. L., Bearden, C. E., Lopez, S. R., Kopelowicz, A., & Cannon, T. D. (2006). Positive family environment predicts improvement in symptoms and social functioning among adolescents at imminent risk for onset of psychosis. *Schizophrenia Research, 81,* 269–275.

O'Brien, P. E., Hindle, A., Brennan, L., Skinner, S., Burton, P., Smith, A., . . . Brown, W. (2019). Long-term outcomes after bariatric surgery: A systematic review and meta-analysis of weight loss at 10 or more years for all bariatric procedures and a single-centre review of 20-year outcomes after adjustable gastric banding. *Obesity Surgery, 29*(1), 3–14.

O'Brien, W. H., & Carhart, V. (2011). Functional analysis in behavioral medicine. *European Journal of Psychological Assessment, 27,* 4–16.

O'Connor, E., Fourier, C., Ran, C., Sivakumar, P., Liesecke, F., Southgate, L., . . . Belin, A. C. (2021). Genome-wide association study identifies risk loci for cluster headache. *Annals of Neurology, 90*(2), 193–202. https://doi.org/10.1002/ana.26150

O'Connor, S. M., Culbert, K. M., Mayhall, L. A., Burt, S. A., & Klump, K. L. (2020). Differences in genetic and environmental influences on body weight and shape concerns across pubertal development in females. *Journal of Psychiatric Research, 121,* 39–46.

O'Dea, B., Achilles, M. R., Larsen, M. E., Batterham, P. J., Calear, A. L., & Christensen, H. (2018). The rate of reply and nature of responses to suicide-related posts on Twitter. *Internet Interventions, 13,* 105–107.

O'Donnell, M. L., Agathos, J. A., Metcalf, O., Gibson, K., & Lau, W. (2019). Adjustment disorder: Current developments and future directions. *International Journal of Environmental Research and Public Health*, 16(14), 2537. https://doi.org/10.3390/ijerph16142537

O'Keefe, V. M., & Reger, G. M. (2017). Suicide among American Indian/Alaska Native military service members and veterans. *Psychological Services*, 14(3), 289–294.

O'Neill, A., Wilson, R., Blest-Hopley, G., Annibale, L., Colizzi, M., Brammer, M., . . . Bhattacharyya, S. (2020). Normalization of mediotemporal and prefrontal activity, and mediotemporal-striatal connectivity, may underlie antipsychotic effects of cannabidiol in psychosis. *Psychological Medicine*, 51(4), 596–606. https://doi.org/10.1017/S0033291719003519

O'Sullivan, L. F., Byers, E. S., Brotto, L. A., Majerovich, J. A., & Fletcher, J. (2016). A longitudinal study of problems in sexual functioning and related sexual distress among middle to late adolescents. *Journal of Adolescent Health*, 59, 318–324.

Oakey-Frost, N., Moscardini, E. H., Cowan, T., Cohen, A., & Tucker, R. P. (2023). The temporal dynamics of wish to live, wish to die, and their short-term prospective relationships with suicidal desire. *Behavior Therapy*, 54(3), 584–594.

Oberndorfer, T. A., Frank, G. K., Simmons, A. N., Wagner, A., McCurdy, D., Fudge, J. L., . . . Kaye, W. H. (2013). Altered insula response to sweet taste processing after recovery from anorexia and bulimia nervosa. *American Journal of Psychiatry*, 170, 1143–1151.

Obregon-Cuesta, A. I., Mínguez-Mínguez, L. A., León-Del-Barco, B., Mendo-Lázaro, S., Fernández-Solana, J., González-Bernal, J. J., & González-Santos, J. (2022). Bullying in adolescents: Differences between gender and school year and relationship with academic performance. *International Journal of Environmental Research and Public Health*, 19(15), 9301. https://doi.org/10.3390/ijerph19159301

Oduola, S., Das-Munshi, J., Bourque, F., Gayer-Anderson, C., Tsang, J., Murray, R. M., . . . Morgan, C. (2019). Change in incidence rates for psychosis in different ethnic groups in south London: Findings from the Clinical Record Interactive Search-First Episode Psychosis (CRIS-FEP) study. *Psychological Medicine*, 51(2), 300–309. https://doi.org/10.1017/S0033291719003234

Office on Women's Health. (2022). *Bulimia nervosa*. https://www.womenshealth.gov/mental-health/mental-health-conditions/eating-disorders/bulimia-nervosa

Ogden, J., Gosling, C., Hazelwood, M., & Atkins, E. (2020). Exposure to body diversity images as a buffer against the thin-ideal: An experimental study. *Psychology, Health and Medicine*, 25(10), 1165–1178. https://doi.org/10.1080/13548506.2020.1734219

Oh, H., Stickley, A., Koyanagi, A., Yau, R., & DeVylder, J. E. (2019). Discrimination and suicidality among racial and ethnic minorities in the United States. *Journal of Affective Disorders*, 245, 517–523.

Ohayon, M. M., Dauvilliers, Y., & Reynolds, C. F. (2012). Operational definitions and algorithms for excessive sleepiness in the general population: Implications for DSM-5 nosology. *Archives of General Psychiatry*, 69, 71–79.

Ojalehto, H. J., Abramowitz, J. S., Hellberg, S. N., Buchholz, J. L., & Twohig, M. P. (2020). Adherence to exposure and response prevention as a predictor of improvement in obsessive-compulsive symptom dimensions. *Journal of Anxiety Disorders*, 72, 102210. https://doi.org/10.1016/j.janxdis.2020.102210

Okun, M. L., Mancuso, R. A., Hobel, C. J., Schetter, C. D., & Coussons-Read, M. (2018). Poor sleep quality increases symptoms of depression and anxiety in postpartum women. *Journal of Behavioral Medicine*, 41(5), 703–710.

Olatunji, B. O., Taylor, S., & Zald, D. (2019). Sex differences in the etiology of disgust sensitivity: A preliminary behavioral genetic analysis. *Journal of Anxiety Disorders*, 65, 41–46.

Olsen, Y. (2022). What is addiction? History, terminology, and core concepts. *The Medical Clinics of North America*, 106(1), 1–12. https://doi.org/10.1016/j.mcna.2021.08.001

Olshansky, S. J. (2011). Aging of US presidents. *Journal of the American Medical Association*, 306, 2328–2329.

Olson, J., Schrager, S. M., Belzer, M., Simons, L. K., & Clark, L. F. (2015). Baseline physiologic and psychosocial characteristics of transgender youth seeking care for gender dysphoria. *Journal of Adolescent Health*, 57, 374–380.

Olson, K. R., Durwood, L., DeMeules, M., & McLaughlin, K. A. (2016). Mental health of transgender children who are supported in their identities. *Pediatrics*, 16, 2015–3223.

Olsson, A., Nearing, K. I., & Phelps, E. A. (2007). Learning fears by observing others: The neural systems of social fear transmission. *Scan*, 2, 3–11.

Olthuis, J. V., McGrath, P. J., Cunningham, C. E., Boyle, M. H., Lingley-Pottie, P., Reid, G., . . . Sdao-Jarvie, K. (2018). Distance-delivered parent training for childhood disruptive behavior (Strongest Families™): A randomized controlled trial and economic analysis. *Journal of Abnormal Child Psychology*, 46(8), 1613–1629.

Omura, M., Levett-Jones, T., & Stone, T. E. (2019). Design and evaluation of an assertiveness communication training programme for nursing students. *Journal of Clinical Nursing*, 28(9–10), 1990–1998.

Onega, L. L., Pierce, T. W., & Epperly, L. (2018). Bright light therapy to treat depression in individuals with mild/moderate or severe dementia. *Issues in Mental Health Nursing*, 39(5), 370–373.

Onitsuka, T., Hirano, Y., Nakazawa, T., Ichihashi, K., Miura, K., Inada, K., Mitoma, R., Yasui-Furukori, N., & Hashimoto, R. (2022). Toward recovery in schizophrenia: Current concepts, findings, and future research directions. *Psychiatry and Clinical Neurosciences*, 76(7), 282–291.

Onwordi, E. C., Halff, E. F., Whitehurst, T., Mansur, A., Cotel, M. C., Wells, L., . . . Howes, O. D. (2020). Synaptic density marker SV2A is reduced in schizophrenia patients and unaffected by antipsychotics in rats. *Nature Communications*, 11(1), 246. https://doi.org/10.1038/s41467-019-14122-0

Ooteman, W., Naassila, M., Koeter, M. W., Verheul, R., Schippers, G. M., Houchi, H., . . . van den Brink, W. (2009). Predicting the effect of naltrexone and acamprosate in alcohol-dependent patients using genetic indicators. *Addictive Biology*, 14, 328–337.

Ophuis, R. H., Olij, B. F., Polinder, S., & Haagsma, J. A. (2018). Prevalence of post-traumatic stress disorder, acute stress disorder and depression following violence related injury treated at the emergency department: A systematic review. *BMC Psychiatry*, 18(1), 311. https://doi.org/10.1186/s12888-018-1890-9

Oquendo, M. A. (2016). The Goldwater rule: Why breaking it is unethical and irresponsible. https://www.psychiatry.org/newsroom/apa-blogs/apa-blog/2016/08/the-goldwater-rule

Oransky, M., Burke, E. Z., & Steever, J. (2019). Building professional competency: Training psychologists in gender affirmative care. *Clinical Practice in Pediatric Psychology*, 7, 322–333.

Ordóñez, A. E., Loeb, F. F., Zhou, X., Shora, L., Berman, R. A., Broadnax, D. D., . . . Rapoport, J. L. (2016). Lack of gender-related differences in childhood-onset schizophrenia. *Journal of the American Academy of Child and Adolescent Psychiatry*, 55(9), 792–799.

Ordóñez, A. E., Luscher, Z. I., & Gogtay, N. (2016). Neuroimaging findings from childhood onset schizophrenia patients and their non-psychotic siblings. *Schizophrenia Research*, 173(3), 124–131

Oregon Public Health Division. (2013). Oregon's Death with Dignity Act—2012. http://public.health.oregon.gov/ProviderPartnerResources/EvaluationResearch/DeathwithDignityAct/Documents/year15.pdf

Ortiz, R. M. (2011, October). Physiology of cardiovascular disease: Gender disparities. Presented at the meeting of the American Physiological Society, Jackson, MS.

Osbourne, L. (2001, May 6). Regional disturbances. *New York Times Magazine*. http://www.nytimes.com/2001/05/06/magazine/06LATAH.html?pagewanted5all

Osher, C. N., & Brown, J. (2014). Drug firms have used dangerous tactics to drive sales to treat kids. http://www.denverpost.com/investigations/ci_25561024/drug-firms-have-used-dangerous-tactics-drive-sales

Öst, L. G., Havnen, A., Hansen, B., & Kvale, G. (2015). Cognitive behavioral treatments of obsessive-compulsive disorder. A systematic review and meta-analysis of studies published 1993–2014. *Clinical Psychology Review*, 40, 156–169.

Öst, L.-G. (1992). Blood and injection phobia: Background and cognitive, physiological, and behavioral variables. *Journal of Abnormal Psychology*, 101, 68–74.

Østergaard, T., Lundgren, T., Zettle, R. D., Landrø, N. I., & Haaland, V. Ø. (2020). Psychological flexibility in depression relapse prevention: Processes of change and positive mental health in group-based ACT for residual symptoms. *Frontiers in Psychology*, 11, 528. https://doi.org/10.3389/fpsyg.2020.00528

Otaiku, D. A. I. (2022). Distressing dreams and risk of Parkinson's disease: A population-based cohort study. *EClinicalMedicine*, 48, 101474. https://doi.org/10.1016/j.eclinm.2022.101474

Otgaar, H., Curci, A., Mangiulli, I., Battista, F., Rizzotti, E., & Sartori, G. (2022). A court ruled case on therapy-induced false memories. *Journal of Forensic Sciences*, 67(5), 2122–2129.

Otgaar, H., Howe, M. L., Dodier, O., Lilienfeld, S. O., Loftus, E. F., Lynn, S. J., Merckelbach, H., & Patihis, L. (2021). Belief in unconscious repressed memory persists. *Perspectives on Psychological Science*, 16(2), 454–460.

Otgaar, H., Howe, M. L., & Muris, P. (2017). Maltreatment increases spontaneous false memories but decreases suggestion-induced false memories in children. *The British Journal of Developmental Psychology*, 35(3), 376–391.

Otgaar, H., Howe, M. L., Patihis, L., Merckelbach, H., Lynn, S. J., Lilienfeld, S. O., & Loftus, E. F. (2019). The return of the repressed: The persistent and problematic claims of long-forgotten trauma. *Perspectives on Psychological Science*, 14(6), 1072–1095.

Otiniano-Verissimo, A. D., Gee, G. C., Ford, C. L., & Iguchi, M. Y. (2014). Racial discrimination, gender discrimination, and substance abuse among Latina/os nationwide. *Cultural Diversity and Ethnic Minority Psychology*, 20, 43–51.

Ousdal, O. T., Milde, A. M., Craven, A. R., Ersland, L., Endestad, T., Melinder, A., . . . Hugdahl, K. (2019). Prefrontal glutamate levels predict altered amygdala-prefrontal connectivity in traumatized youths. *Psychological Medicine*, 49(11), 1822–1830.

Owen, R., Gooding, P., Dempsey, R., & Jones, S. (2017). The reciprocal relationship between bipolar disorder and social interaction: A qualitative investigation. *Clinical Psychology and Psychotherapy*, 24(4), 911–918.

Ozonoff, S., & Iosif, A. M. (2019). Changing conceptualizations of regression: What prospective studies reveal about the onset of autism spectrum disorder. *Neuroscience and Biobehavioral Reviews*, 100, 296–304.

Palamar, J. J. (2019). Use of "lean" among electronic dance music party attendees. *American Journal on Addictions*, 28(5), 347–352.

Palamar, J. J., Rutherford, C., & Keyes, K. M. (2019). "Flakka" use among high school seniors in the United States. *Drug and Alcohol Dependence, 196*, 86–90.

Palamar, J. J., & Shearston, J. A. (2018). Nonmedical opioid use in relation to recency of heroin use in a nationally representative sample of adults in the United States. *Journal of Psychoactive Drugs, 50*(2), 159–166.

Palk, A. C., Dalvie, S., de Vries, J., Martin, A. R., & Stein, D. J. (2019). Potential use of clinical polygenic risk scores in psychiatry— Ethical implications and communicating high polygenic risk. *Philosophy, Ethics, and Humanities in Medicine: PEHM, 14*(1), 4. https://doi.org/10.1186/s13010-019-0073-8

Palmisano, M., & Pandey, S. C. (2017). Epigenetic mechanisms of alcoholism and stress-related disorders. *Alcohol (Fayetteville, NY), 60*, 7–18.

Palpacuer, C., Duprez, R., Huneau, A., Locher, C., Boussageon, R., Laviolle, B., & Naudet, F. (2018). Pharmacologically controlled drinking in the treatment of alcohol dependence or alcohol use disorders: A systematic review with direct and network meta-analyses on nalmefene, naltrexone, acamprosate, baclofen and topiramate. *Addiction, 113*(2), 220–237.

Pan, D. (2013). Map: Which states have cut treatment for the mentally ill the most? http://www.mother-jones.com/mojo/2013/04/map-states-cut-treatment-for-mentally-ill

Pan, S., Sun, S., Li, X., Chen, J., Xiong, Y., He, Y., & Pachankis, J. E. (2020). A pilot cultural adaptation of LGB-affirmative CBT for young Chinese sexual minority men's mental and sexual health. *Psychotherapy (Chicago).* https://doi.org/10.1037/pst0000318

Pandey, G. N. (2013). Biological basis of suicide and suicidal behaviour. *Bipolar Disorders, 15*(5), 524–541.

Pani, L., & Keefe, R. (2019). Approaches to attenuated psychosis syndrome treatments: A perspective on the regulatory issues. *Schizophrenia Research. Cognition, 18*, 100155. https://doi.org/10.1016/j.scog.2019.100155

Pankalainen, M. T., Kerola, T. V., & Hintikka, J. J. (2015). Pessimism and the risk for coronary heart disease among middle-aged and older Finnish men and women: A ten-year follow-up study. *BMC Cardiovascular Disorders, 15*, 113. https://doi.org/10.1186/s12872-015-0097-y

Pantoni, M. M., Kim, J. L., Van Alstyne, K. R., & Anagnostaras, S. G. (2022). MDMA and memory, addiction, and depression: Dose-effect analysis. *Psychopharmacology, 239*(3), 935–949. https://doi.org/10.1007/s00213-022-06086-9

Papageorgiou, M., Raza, A., Fraser, S., Nurgali, K., & Apostolopoulos, V. (2019). Methamphetamine and its immune-modulating effects. *Maturitas, 121*, 13–21.

Parasrampuria, S., & Murphy, S. (2022). *Trends in prescription drug spending, 2016–2021.* Washington, DC: U.S. Department of Health and Human Services.

Pardini, D. A., Byrd, A. L., Hawes, S. W., & Docherty, M. (2018). Unique dispositional precursors to early-onset conduct problems and criminal offending in adulthood. *Journal of the American Academy of Child and Adolescent Psychiatry, 57*(8), 583–592.

Parekh, R. (2016). What is gender dysphoria. https://psychiatry.org/patients-families/gender-dysphoria/what-is-gender-dysphoria

Parens, E., & Johnston, J. (2009). Facts, values, and attention-deficit hyperactivity disorder (ADHD): An update on the controversies. *Child and Adolescent Psychiatry and Mental Health, 3*, 1–17.

Paris, J. (2015). The natural history of personality disorders: Recovery and residual symptoms. *Canadian Journal of Psychiatry, 60*(7), 301–302.

Paris, J. (2019). Suicidality in borderline personality disorder. *Medicina (Kaunas, Lithuania), 55*(6), 223. https://doi.org/10.3390/medicina55060223

Paris, J., & Kirmayer, L. J. (2016). The National Institute of Mental Health Research Domain Criteria: A bridge too far. *Journal of Nervous and Mental Disease, 204*, 26–32.

Park, B. Y., Wilson, G., Berger, J., Christman, M., Reina, B., Bishop, F., . . . Doan, A. P. (2016). Is Internet pornography causing sexual dysfunctions? A review with clinical reports. *Behavioral Sciences, 6*(3), 17. https://doi.org/10.3390/bs6030017

Park, C., Brietzke, E., Rosenblat, J. D., Musial, N., Zuckerman, H., Ragguett, R. M., . . . McIntyre, R. S. (2018). Probiotics for the treatment of depressive symptoms: An anti-inflammatory mechanism? *Brain, Behavior, and Immunity, 73*, 115–124.

Park, Y. M., White, A. J., Jackson, C. L., Weinberg, C. R., & Sandler, D. P. (2019). Association of exposure to artificial light at night while sleeping with risk of obesity in women. *JAMA Internal Medicine, 179*(8), 1061–1071. https://doi.org/10.1001

Parker, K. J., Oztan, O., Libove, R. A., Sumiyoshi, R. D., Jackson, L. P., Karhson, D. S., . . . Hardan, A. Y. (2017). Intranasal oxytocin treatment for social deficits and biomarkers of response in children with autism. *Proceedings of the National Academy of Sciences of the United States of America, 114*(30), 8119–8124.

Parkin, S. (2017). How virtual reality is helping heal soldiers with PTSD. http://www.nbcnews.com/mach/features/how-virtual-reality-helping-heal-soldiers-ptsd-n733816

Parkinson's Foundation. (2023). What is Parkinson's? https://www.parkinson.org/understanding-parkinsons

Parra-Cardona, J. R., Bybee, D., Sullivan, C. M., Rodríguez, M. M., Dates, B., Tams, L., & Bernal, G. (2017). Examining the impact of differential cultural adaptation with Latina/o immigrants exposed to adapted parent training interventions. *Journal of Consulting and Clinical Psychology, 85*(1), 58–71.

Parry, P., Allison, S., & Bastiampillai, T. (2021). "Pediatric bipolar disorder" rates are still lower than claimed: A re-examination of eight epidemiological surveys used by an updated meta-analysis. *International Journal of Bipolar Disorders, 9*(1), 21. https://doi.org/10.1186/s40345-021-00225-5

Parsons, J. T., Grov, C., & Kelly, B. C. (2009). Club drug use and dependence among young adults recruited through time-space sampling. *Public Health Reports*, *124*(2), 246–254.

Pasalich, D. S., Witkiewitz, K., McMahon, R. J., Pinderhughes, E. E., & Conduct Problems Prevention Research Group. (2016). Indirect effects of the fast track intervention on conduct disorder symptoms and callous-unemotional traits: Distinct pathways involving discipline and warmth. *Journal of Abnormal Child Psychology*, *44*(3), 587–597.

Pascoe, M. C., & Parker, A. G. (2019). Physical activity and exercise as a universal depression prevention in young people: A narrative review. *Early Intervention in Psychiatry*, *13*(4), 733–739.

Pataki, C., & Johnson, C. (2016). Child sexual abuse. https://reference.medscape.com/article/915841

Patel, M. S., Small, D. S., Harrison, J. D., Fortunato, M. P., Oon, A. L., Rareshide, C., . . . Hilbert, V. (2019). Effectiveness of behaviorally designed gamification interventions with social incentives for increasing physical activity among overweight and obese adults across the United States: The STEP UP randomized clinical trial. *JAMA Internal Medicine*, *179*(12), 1–9.

Patel, R. S., Virani, S., Saeed, H., Nimmagadda, S., Talukdar, J., & Youssef, N. A. (2018). Gender differences and comorbidities in U.S. adults with bipolar disorder. *Brain Sciences*, *8*(9), 168. https://doi.org/10.3390/brainsci8090168

Patel, R., Wilson, R., Jackson, R., Ball, M., Shetty, H., Broadbent, M., . . . Bhattacharyya, S. (2016). Association of cannabis use with hospital admission and antipsychotic treatment failure in first episode psychosis: An observational study. *BMJ Open*, *6*(3), e009888. https://doi.org/10.1136/bmjopen-2015-009888

Patel, S. R. (2019). Obstructive sleep apnea. *Annals of Internal Medicine*, *171*(11), ITC81–ITC96. https://doi.org/10.7326/AITC201912030

Patihis, L., Ho, L. Y., Loftus, E. F., & Herrera, M. E. (2021). Memory experts' beliefs about repressed memory. *Memory (Hove, England)*, *29*(6), 823–828.

Patihis, L., Ho, L. Y., Tingen, I. W., Lilienfeld, S. O., & Loftus, E. F. (2014). Are the "memory wars" over? A scientist-practitioner gap in beliefs about repressed memory. *Psychological Science*, *25*, 519–530.

Patihis, L., & Pendergrast, M. H. (2018). Reports of recovered memories of abuse in therapy in a large age-representative U.S. national sample: Therapy type and decade comparisons. *Clinical Psychological Science*, *6*, 1–19.

Patil, S., Arakeri, G., Patil, S., Ali Baeshen, H., Raj, T., Sarode, S. C., . . . Brennan, P. A. (2020). Are electronic nicotine delivery systems (ENDs) helping cigarette smokers quit? Current evidence. *Journal of Oral Pathology and Medicine*, *49*(3), 181–189.

Patterson, G. R. (1986). Performance models for antisocial boys. *American Psychologist*, *41*, 432–444.

Pazmany, E., Bergeron, S., Van Oudenhove, L., Verhaeghe, J., & Enzlin, P. (2013). Body image and genital self-image in pre-menopausal women with dyspareunia. *Archives of Sexual Behavior*, *42*, 999–1010.

Pearce, L. R., Atanassova, N., Banton, M. C., Bottomley, B., van der Klaauw, A. A., Revelli, J. P., . . . Farooqi, I. S. (2013). KSR2 mutations are associated with obesity, insulin resistance, and impaired cellular fuel oxidation. *Cell*, *155*, 765–777.

Pearl, T. A., Dumkrieger, G., Chong, C. D., Dodick, D. W., & Schwedt, T. J. (2020). Sensory hypersensitivity symptoms in migraine with vs without aura: Results from the American Registry for Migraine Research. *Headache*, *60*(3), 506–514.

Pearlman, A. T., Schvey, N. A., Neyland, M., Solomon, S., Hennigan, K., Schindler, R., . . . Tanofsky-Kraff, M. (2019). Associations between family weight-based teasing, eating pathology, and psychosocial functioning among adolescent military dependents. *International Journal of Environmental Research and Public Health*, *17*(1), 24. https://doi.org/10.3390/ijerph17010024

Pearson, C. M., Pisetsky, E. M., Goldschmidt, A. B., Lavender, J. M., Wonderlich, S. A., Crosby, R. D., . . . Peterson, C. B. (2016). Personality psychopathology differentiates risky behaviors among women with bulimia nervosa. *The International Journal of Eating Disorders*, *49*(7), 681–688.

Pearson, M. L., Selby, J. V., Katz, K. A., Cantrell, V., Braden, C. R., Parise, M. E., . . . Eberhard, M. L. (2012). Clinical, epidemiologic, histopathologic and molecular features of an unexplained dermopathy. *PLOS One*, *7*, 1–23.

Pederson, C. A., & Fite, P. J. (2014). The impact of parenting on the associations between child aggression subtypes and oppositional defiant disorder symptoms. *Child Psychiatry and Human Development*. https://doi.org/10.1007/s10578-014-0441-y

Pedraza, O. (Ed.) (2019). *Clinical cultural neuroscience: An integrative approach to cross-cultural neuropsychology*. New York: Oxford University Press.

Peira, N., Fredrikson, M., & Pourtois, G. (2014). Controlling the emotional heart: Heart rate biofeedback improves cardiac control during emotional reactions. *International Journal of Psychophysiology*, *91*, 225–231.

Peixoto, M. M., & Nobre, P. (2014). Dysfunctional sexual beliefs: A comparative study of heterosexual men and women, gay men, and lesbian women with and without sexual problems. *Journal of Sexual Medicine*, *11*, 2690–2700.

Pellizzer, M. L., Waller, G., & Wade, T. D. (2019). Predictors of outcome in cognitive behavioural therapy for eating disorders: An exploratory study. *Behaviour Research and Therapy*, *116*, 61–68.

Peng, J., Yuan, Y., Zhao, Y., & Ren, H. (2022). Effects of exercise on patients with obstructive sleep apnea: A systematic review and meta-analysis. *International Journal of Environmental Research and Public Health*, *19*(17), 10845. https://doi.org/10.3390/ijerph191710845

Penney, D., Sauvé, G., Mendelson, D., Thibaudeau, É., Moritz, S., &

Lepage, M. (2022). Immediate and sustained outcomes and moderators associated with metacognitive training for psychosis: A systematic review and meta-analysis. *JAMA Psychiatry*, 79(5), 417–429.

Penninx, B. W., Pine, D. S., Holmes, E. A., & Reif, A. (2021). Anxiety disorders. *Lancet*, 397, 914–927.

Perez, D. L., Matin, N., Barsky, A., Costumero-Ramos, V., Makaretz, S. J., Young, S. S., . . . Dickerson, B. C. (2017). Cingulo-insular structural alterations associated with psychogenic symptoms, childhood abuse and PTSD in functional neurological disorders. *Journal of Neurology, Neurosurgery, and Psychiatry*, 88(6), 491–497.

Perez, D. L., Matin, N., Williams, B., Tanev, K., Makris, N., LaFrance, W. C., Jr., & Dickerson, B. C. (2018). Cortical thickness alterations linked to somatoform and psychological dissociation in functional neurological disorders. *Human Brain Mapping*, 39(1), 428–439.

Pérez-Fuentes, G., Olfson, M., Villegas, L., Morcillo, C., Wang, S., & Blanco, C. (2013). Prevalence and correlates of child sexual abuse: A national study. *Comprehensive Psychiatry*, 54(1), 16–27. https://doi.org/10.1016/j.comppsych.2012.05.010

Perez-Rodriguez, M. M., Bulbena-Cabré, A., Bassir Nia, A., Zipursky, G., Goodman, M., & New, A. S. (2018). The neurobiology of borderline personality disorder. *The Psychiatric Clinics of North America*, 41(4), 633–650.

Perich, T. A., Roberts, G., Frankland, A., Sinbandhit, C., Meade, T., Austin, M. P., & Mitchell, P. B. (2017). Clinical characteristics of women with reproductive cycle-associated bipolar disorder symptoms. *The Australian and New Zealand Journal of Psychiatry*, 51(2), 161–167.

Perkins, K. A. (2009). Sex differences in nicotine reinforcement and reward: Influences on the persistence of tobacco smoking. *The Motivational Impact of Nicotine and Its Role in Tobacco Use: Nebraska Symposium on Motivation*, 55, 1–27.

Perlini, C., Donisi, V., & Del Piccolo, L. (2020). From research to clinical practice: A systematic review of the implementation of psychological interventions for chronic headache in adults. *BMC Health Services Research*, 20(1), 459. https://doi.org/10.1186/s12913-020-05172-y

Perlis, R. H., Ostacher, M., Fava, M., Nierenberg, A. A., Sachs, G. S., & Rosenbaum, J. F. (2010). Assuring that double-blind is blind. *American Journal of Psychiatry*, 167, 250–252.

Perona-Garcelán, S., López-Jiménez, A. M., Bellido-Zanin, G., Senín-Calderón, C., Ruiz-Veguilla, M., & Rodríguez-Testal, J. F. (2020). The relationship with the voices as a dialogical experience: The role of self-focused attention and dissociation. *Journal of Clinical Psychology*, 76(3), 549–558.

Perrin, P. B., Sutter, M. E., Trujillo, M. A., Henry, R. S., & Pugh, M., Jr. (2020). The minority strengths model: Development and initial path analytic validation in racially/ethnically diverse LGBTQ individuals. *Journal of Clinical Psychology*, 76, 118–136.

Perrine, C. G., Pickens, C. M., Boehmer, T. K., King, B. A., Jones, C. M., DeSisto, C. L., . . . Lung Injury Response Epidemiology/Surveillance Group. (2019). Characteristics of a multistate outbreak of lung injury associated with e-cigarette use, or vaping—United States, 2019. *Morbidity and Mortality Weekly Report*, 68(39), 860–864.

Perry, J. C. (2001). Dependent personality disorder. In G. O. Gabbard (Ed.), *Treatment of psychiatric disorders* (pp. 2353–2368). Washington, DC: American Psychiatric Press.

Perugi, G., Hantouche, E., & Vannucchi, G. (2017). Diagnosis and treatment of cyclothymia: The "primacy" of temperament. *Current Neuropharmacology*, 15(3), 372–379.

Pescosolido, B. A., & Manago, B. (2019). Evolving public views on the likelihood of violence from people with mental illness: Stigma and its consequences. *Health Affairs*, 38, 1735–1743.

Pescosolido, B. A., Martin, J. K., Long, S., Medina, T. R., Phelan, J. C., & Link, B. G. (2010). "A disease like any other"? A decade of change in public reactions to schizophrenia, depression, and alcohol dependence. *American Journal of Psychiatry*, 167, 1321–1330.

Petersen, L., Sørensen, T. I. A., Andersen, P. K., Mortensen, P. B., & Hawton, K. (2013). Genetic and familial environmental effects on suicide—An adoption study of siblings. *PLOS One*, 8(10), e77973. https://doi.org/10.1371/journal.pone.0077973

Peterson, C., & Seligman, M. (2005). *Character strengths and virtue: A handbook and classification*. New York: Oxford University Press.

Pettigrew, J. A., & Novick, A. M. (2021). Hypoactive sexual desire disorder in women: Physiology, assessment, diagnosis, and treatment. *Journal of Midwifery & Women's Health*, 66(6), 740–748. https://doi.org/10.1111/jmwh.13283

Phillips, A., & Daniluk, J. C. (2004). Beyond "survivor": How childhood sexual abuse informs the identity of adult women at the end of the therapeutic process. *Journal of Counseling and Development*, 82, 177–184.

Phillips, K. A. (2005). *The broken mirror: Understanding and treating body dysmorphic disorder* (2nd ed., revised). New York: Oxford University Press.

Phillips, K. A., Hart, A. S., Simpson, H. B., & Stein, D. J. (2014). Delusional versus nondelusional body dysmorphic disorder: Recommendations for DSM-5. *CNS Spectrums*, 19(1), 10–20.

Phillips, N. (2018). Aurora theater shooter's psychiatric reports unsealed by 2015 trial judge. https://www.denverpost.com/2018/07/03/james-holmes-psychiatric-reports-unsealed/

Phillips, S. P., King, N., Michaelson, V., & Pickett, W. (2019). Sex, drugs, risk and resilience: Analysis of data from the Canadian Health Behaviour in School-aged Children (HBSC) study. *European Journal of Public Health*, 29(1), 38–43.

Phipps, S. (2011). Positive psychology and war: An oxymoron. *American Psychologist, 66*, 641–642.

Physiopedia. (2019). Migraine headache case study. https://www.physio-pedia.com/index.php?title=Migraine_Headache_Case_Study&oldid=215891

Piazza-Gardner, A. K., & Barry, A. E. (2013). Appropriate terminology for the alcohol, eating, and physical activity relationship. *Journal of American College Health, 61*, 311–313.

Piccirillo, M. L., Beck, E. D., & Rodebaugh, T. L. (2019). A clinician's primer for idiographic research: Considerations and recommendations. *Behavior Therapy, 50*, 938–951.

Pike, K. M., & Dunne, P. E. (2015). The rise of eating disorders in Asia: A review. *Journal of Eating Disorders, 3*, 33. https://doi.org/10.1186/s40337-015-0070-2

Pillai, V., Cheng, P., Kalmbach, D. A., Roehrs, T., Roth, T., & Drake, C. L. (2016). Prevalence and predictors of prescription sleep aid use among individuals with DSM-5 insomnia: The role of hyperarousal. *Sleep, 39*, 825–832.

Pinedo, M. (2020). The impact of deportation policies on the substance using behaviors of US-citizen Latinos. *The International Journal on Drug Policy, 75*, 102605. https://doi.org/10.1016/j.drugpo.2019.11.013

Piotrowski, C. (2015). Clinical instruction on projective techniques in the USA: A review of academic training settings 1995–2014. *Journal of Projective Psychology and Mental Health, 22*, 83–92.

Piper, M. E., Cook, J. W., Schlam, T. R., Jorenby, D. E., & Baker, T. B. (2010). Anxiety diagnoses in smokers seeking cessation treatment: Relations with tobacco dependence, withdrawal, outcome and response to treatment. *Addiction, 106*, 418–427.

Plante, T. G. (2013). *Abnormal psychology across the ages*. Santa Barbara, CA: Praeger.

Plate, R. C., Jones, C., Zhao, S., Flum, M. W., Steinberg, J., Daley, G., . . . Waller, R. (2023). "But not the music": Psychopathic traits and difficulties recognising and resonating with the emotion in music. *Cognition & Emotion, 37*(4), 748–762. https://doi.org/10.1080/02699931.2023.2205105

Plateau, C. R., Bone, S., Lanning, E., & Meyer, C. (2018). Monitoring eating and activity: Links with disordered eating, compulsive exercise, and general well-being among young adults. *The International Journal of Eating Disorders, 51*(11), 1270–1276.

Platt, J. R. (2011). Lions vs. cattle: Taste aversion could solve African predator problem. https://blogs.scientificamerican.com/extinction-countdown/lions-vs-cattle-taste-aversion/

Pliszka, S. R. (2019). Is there long-term benefit from stimulant treatment for ADHD? *The American Journal of Psychiatry, 176*(9), 685–686.

Poeppl, T. B., Eickhoff, S. B., Fox, P. T., Laird, A. R., Rupprecht, R., Langguth, B., & Bzdok, D. (2015). Connectivity and functional profiling of abnormal brain structures in pedophilia. *Human Brain Mapping, 36*, 2374–2386.

Polak, K., Kelpin, S., & Terplan, M. (2019). Screening for substance use in pregnancy and the newborn. *Seminars in Fetal and Neonatal Medicine, 24*(2), 90–94.

Polanco-Roman, L., Anglin, D. M., Miranda, R., & Jeglic, E. L. (2019). Racial/ethnic discrimination and suicidal ideation in emerging adults: The role of traumatic stress and depressive symptoms varies by gender not race/ethnicity. *Journal of Youth and Adolescence, 48*(10), 2023–2037.

Polanco-Roman, L., Danies, A., & Anglin, D. M. (2016). Racial discrimination as race-based trauma, coping strategies, and dissociative symptoms among emerging adults. *Psychological Trauma: Theory, Research, Practice and Policy, 8*(5), 609–617.

Pollack, A. (2015). Viagra for women is backed by an F.D.A. panel. http://www.nytimes.com/2015/06/05/business/panel-backs-a-drug-to-increase-womens-sex-drive.html

Pols, M. (2015). Becoming myself. *People, 84*, 74–77.

Pompoli, A., Furukawa, T. A., Efthimiou, O., Imai, H., Tajika, A., & Salanti, G. (2018). Dismantling cognitive-behaviour therapy for panic disorder: A systematic review and component network meta-analysis. *Psychological Medicine, 48*(12), 1945–1953.

Pompoli, A., Furukawa, T. A., Imai, H., Tajika, A., Efthimiou, O., & Salanti, G. (2016). Psychological therapies for panic disorder with or without agoraphobia in adults: A network meta-analysis. *The Cochrane Database of Systematic Reviews, 4*(4), CD011004. https://doi.org/10.1002/14651858.CD011004.pub2

Pontillo, M., Tata, M. C., Averna, R., Demaria, F., Gargiullo, P., Guerrera, S., . . . Vicari S. (2019). Peer victimization and onset of social anxiety disorder in children and adolescents. *Brain Science.* https://www.ncbi.nlm.nih.gov/pmc/articles/PMC6627045/

Pope, H. G., Jr., & Hudson, J. I. (2007). "Repressed memory" challenge. http://www.butterfliesandwheels.com/printer_friendly.php?num5177

Pope, H. G., Jr., Poliakoff, M. B., Parker, M. P., Boynes, M., & Hudson, J. I. (2009). Response to R. E. Goldsmith, R. E. Cheit, & M. E. Wood, "Evidence of dissociative amnesia in science and literature: Culture-bound approaches to trauma." *Journal of Trauma and Dissociation, 10*, 254–257.

Porter, J. (2012). Stress, high school, tics and secondary stress response. http://www.stressstop.com/blog/read-entry.php?eid542

Portnoff, L., McClintock, C., Lau, E., Choi, S., & Miller, L. (2017). Spirituality cuts in half the relative risk for depression: Findings from the United States, China, and India. *Spirituality in Clinical Practice, 4*(1), 22–31.

Posar, A., & Visconti, P. (2019). Long-term outcome of autism spectrum disorder. *Turk Pediatri Arsivi, 54*(4), 207–212.

Posner, J., Hellerstein, D. J., Gat, I., Mechling, A., Klahr, K., Wang, Z., . . . Peterson, B. S. (2013). Antidepressants normalize the default mode network in patients with dysthymia. *JAMA Psychiatry, 70*(4), 373–382.

Post, R. M., Altshuler, L. L., Kupka, R., McElroy, S. L., Frye, M. A., Rowe, M., . . . Nolen, W. A. (2017). More childhood onset bipolar disorder in the United States than Canada or Europe: Implications for treatment and prevention. *Neuroscience and Biobehavioral Reviews*, 74(Pt A), 204–213.

Potter, R., Patterson, B. W., Elbert, D. L., Ovod, V., Kasten, T., Sigurdson, W., . . . Bateman, R. J. (2013). Increased in vivo amyloid-b42 production, exchange, and loss in presenilin mutation carriers. *Science Translational Medicine, 5,* 189ra77. https://doi.org/10.1126/scitranslmed.3005615

Poulin, C., Shiner, B., Thompson, P., Vepstas, L., Young-Xu, Y., Goertzel, B., . . . McAllister, T. (2014). Predicting the risk of suicide by analyzing the text of clinical notes. *PLOS One, 9*(1), e85733. https://doi.org/10.1371/journal.pone.0085733

Pourkalbassi, D., Patel, P., & Espinosa, P. S. (2019). Conversion disorder: The brain's way of dealing with psychological conflicts. Case report of a patient with non-epileptic seizures. *Cureus, 11*(1), e3902. https://doi.org/10.7759/cureus.3902

Pozza, A., & Dèttore, D. (2020). Modular cognitive-behavioral therapy for affective symptoms in young individuals at ultra-high risk of first episode of psychosis: Randomized controlled trial. *Journal of Clinical Psychology, 76*(3), 392–405.

Prefit, A. B., Cândea, D. M., & Szentagotai-Tătar, A. (2019). Emotion regulation across eating pathology: A meta-analysis. *Appetite, 143,* 104438. https://doi.org/10.1016/j.appet.2019.104438

Price, A. J., Collado-Torres, L., Ivanov, N. A., Xia, W., Burke, E. E., Shin, J. H., . . . Jaffe, A. E. (2019). Divergent neuronal DNA methylation patterns across human cortical development reveal critical periods and a unique role of CpH methylation. *Genome Biology, 20*(1), 196. https://doi.org/10.1186/s13059-019-1805-1

Price, J. H., & Khubchandani, J. (2019). The changing characteristics of African-American adolescent suicides, 2001–2017. *Journal of Community Health, 44*(4), 756–763.

Price, M. N., & Green, A. E. (2023). Association of gender identity acceptance with fewer suicide attempts among transgender and nonbinary youth. *Transgender Health, 8*(1), 56–63.

Prisciandaro, J. J., Mellick, W., Mitaro, E., & Tolliver, B. K. (2019). An evaluation of the impact of co-occurring anxiety and substance use disorder on bipolar disorder illness outcomes in STEP-BD. *Journal of Affective Disorders, 246,* 794–799.

Proudfoot, J., Doran, J., Manicavasagar, V., & Parker, G. (2010). The precipitants of manic/hypomanic episodes in the context of bipolar disorder: A review. *Journal of Affective Disorders, 133,* 381–387.

Puhl, R. M., Peterson, J. L., & Luedicke, J. (2013). Weight-based victimization: Bullying experiences of weight loss treatment-seeking youth. *Pediatrics, 131,* e1–e9.

Pulcu, E., Lythe, K., Elliott, R., Green, S., Moll, J., Deakin, J. F., & Zahn, R. (2014). Increased amygdala response to shame in remitted major depressive disorder. *PLOS One, 9,* e86900. https://doi.org/10.1371/journal.pone.0086900

Pull, C. B. (2013). Too few or too many? Reactions to removing versus retaining specific personality disorders in DSM-5. *Current Opinion in Psychiatry, 26,* 73–78.

Purse, M. (2013). Brief reactive psychosis—An inside story. http://bipolar.about.com/od/interviews/a/brief-reactive-psychosis-experience.htm

Purty, A., Nestadt, G., Samuels, J. F., & Viswanath, B. (2019). Genetics of obsessive-compulsive disorder. *Indian Journal of Psychiatry, 61*(Suppl 1), S37–S42.

Qaseem, A., Owens, D. K., Etxeandia-Ikobaltzeta, I., Tufte, J., Cross, J. T., Jr., Wilt, T. J., . . . Yost, J. (2023). Nonpharmacologic and pharmacologic treatments of adults in the acute phase of major depressive disorder: A living clinical guideline from the American College of Physicians. *Annals of Internal Medicine, 176*(2), 239–252.

Quick, V. M., & Byrd-Bredbenner, C. (2014). Disordered eating, sociocultural media influencers, body image, and psychological factors among a racially/ethnically diverse population of college women. *Eating Behaviors, 15*(1), 37–41.

Quinn, S. O. (2012). Credibility, respectability, suggestibility, and spirit travel: Lurena Brackett and animal magnetism. *History of Psychology, 15,* 273–282.

Quiroz, Y. T., Zetterberg, H., Reiman, E. M., Chen, Y., Su, Y., Fox-Fuller, J. T., . . . Lopera, F. (2020). Plasma neurofilament light chain in the presenilin 1 E280A autosomal dominant Alzheimer's disease kindred: A cross-sectional and longitudinal cohort study. *The Lancet: Neurology, 19*(6), 513–521.

Quittkat, H. L., Hartmann, A. S., Düsing, R., Buhlmann, U., & Vocks, S. (2019). Body dissatisfaction, importance of appearance, and body appreciation in men and women over the lifespan. *Frontiers in Psychiatry, 10,* 864. https://doi.org/10.3389/fpsyt.2019.00864

Qureshi, I. A., & Mehler, M. F. (2014). Epigenetics of sleep and chronobiology. *Current Neurology and Neuroscience Reports, 14,* 432.

Rachman, S., Marks, I. M., & Hodgson, R. (1973). The treatment of obsessive compulsive neurotics by modeling and flooding in vivo. *Behaviour Research and Therapy, 11,* 463–471.

Radomsky, A. S., Alcolado, G. M., Abramowitz, J. S., Alonso, P., & Wing, W. (2014). Part 1—You can run but you can't hide: Intrusive thoughts on six continents. *Journal of Obsessive-Compulsive and Related Disorders, 3,* 269–279.

Radonic, E., Rados, M., Kalember, P., Bajs-Janovic, M., Folnegovic-Smalc, V., & Henigsberg, N. (2011). Comparison of hippocampal volumes in schizophrenia, schizoaffective and bipolar disorder. *Collegium Antropologicum, 35,* 249–252.

Radparvar, S. (2023). The clinical assessment and treatment of inhalant abuse. *Permanente*

Journal, 27(2), 99–109. https://doi.org/10.7812/TPP/22.164

Raine, A. (2018). Antisocial personality as a neurodevelopmental disorder. *Annual Review of Clinical Psychology, 14,* 259–289.

Rajanala, S., Maymone, M., & Vashi, N. A. (2018). Selfies—Living in the era of filtered photographs. *JAMA Facial Plastic Surgery, 20*(6), 443–444.

Ramachandraih, C. T., Subramanyam, N., Bar, K. J., Baker, G., & Yeragani, V. K. (2011). Antidepressants: From MAOIs to SSRIs and more. *Indian Journal of Psychiatry, 53,* 180–182.

Raman, R., Jarrett, R. T., Cull, M. J., Gracey, K., Shaffer, A. M., & Epstein, R. A. (2021). Psychopharmaceutical prescription monitoring for children in the child welfare system. *Psychiatric Services (Washington, DC), 72*(3), 295–301. https://doi.org/10.1176/appi.ps.202000077

Ramos, R. (1998). *An ethnographic study of Mexican American inhalant abusers in San Antonio.* Austin: Texas Commission on Alcohol and Drug Abuse. http://www.dshs.state.tx.us/sa/research/populations/Inhale98S.pdf

Rand Corporation. (2010). Invisible wounds: Mental health and cognitive care needs of America's returning veterans. http://www.rand.org/pubs/research_briefs/RB9336/index1.html

Rao, V., Handel, S., Vaishnavi, S., Keach, S., Robbins, B., Spiro, J., . . . Berlin, F. (2007). Psychiatric sequelae of traumatic brain injury: A case report. *American Journal of Psychiatry, 164,* 728–735.

Rastelli, M., Knauf, C., & Cani, P. D. (2018). Gut microbes and health: A focus on the mechanisms linking microbes, obesity, and related disorders. *Obesity (Silver Spring, MD), 26*(5), 792–800.

Rastrelli, G., Corona, G., & Maggi, M. (2018). Testosterone and sexual function in men. *Maturitas, 112,* 46–52. https://doi.org/10.1016/j.maturitas.2018.04.004

Rathbone, C. J., Moulin, C. J., & Conway, M. A. (2009). Autobiographical memory and amnesia: Using conceptual knowledge to ground the self. *Neurocase: The Neural Basis of Cognition, 15,* 405–418.

Rauch, S., Kim, H. M., Powell, C., Tuerk, P. W., Simon, N. M., Acierno, R., . . . Hoge, C. W. (2019). Efficacy of prolonged exposure therapy, sertraline hydrochloride, and their combination among combat veterans with posttraumatic stress disorder: A randomized clinical trial. *JAMA Psychiatry, 76*(2), 117–126.

Ravitz, P., Watson, P., Lawson, A., Constantino, M. J., Bernecker, S., Park, J., & Swartz, H. A. (2019). Interpersonal psychotherapy: A scoping review and historical perspective (1974–2017). *Harvard Review of Psychiatry, 27*(3), 165–180.

Read, J., Kirsch, I., & McGrath, L. (2019). Electroconvulsive therapy for depression: A review of the quality of ECT versus sham ECT trials and meta-analyses. *Ethical Human Psychology and Psychiatry, 21,* 64–103.

Read, J., & Mati, E. (2013). Erectile dysfunction and the Internet: Drug company manipulation of public and professional opinion. *Journal of Sex and Marital Therapy, 39,* 541–559.

Ream, M. A., & Lehwald, L. (2018). Neurologic consequences of preterm birth. *Current Neurology and Neuroscience Reports, 18*(8), 48. https://doi.org/10.1007/s11910-018-0862-2

Reardon S. (2023). US could soon approve MDMA therapy: Opening an era of psychedelic medicine. *Nature, 616*(7957), 428–430. https://doi.org/10.1038/d41586-023-01296-3

Rebhi, H., Damak, R., Cherif, W., Ellini, S., Cheour, M., & Ellouze, F. (2019). Impact of duration of untreated psychosis on quality of life and cognitive functions. *L'Encephale, 45*(1), 22–26.

Rector, N. A., Beck, A. T., & Stolar, N. (2005). The negative symptoms of schizophrenia: A cognitive perspective. *Canadian Journal of Psychiatry, 50,* 247–257.

Redden, S. A., Mueller, N. E., & Cougle, J. R. (2023). The impact of obsessive-compulsive personality disorder in perfectionism. *International Journal of Psychiatry in Clinical Practice, 27*(1), 18–24. https://doi.org/10.1080/13651501.2022.2069581

Redolfi, S., Arnulf, I., Pottier, M., Lajou, J., Koskas, I., Bradley, T. D., & Similowski, T. (2011). Attenuation of obstructive sleep apnea by compression stockings in subjects with venous insufficiency. *American Journal of Respiratory and Critical Care Medicine, 183,* A6161.

Redvers, N., & Blondin, B. (2020). Traditional Indigenous medicine in North America: A scoping review. *PLOS One, 15*(8), e0237531. https://doi.org/10.1371/journal.pone.0237531

Reed, I. (2007). Why Salem made sense: Culture, gender, and the Puritan persecution of Witchcraft, *Cultural Sociology, 1,* 209–234.

Rees, C. S., & Pritchard, R. (2015). Brief cognitive therapy for avoidant personality disorder. *Psychotherapy (Chicago), 52*(1), 45–55.

Reich, S. G., & Savitt, J. M. (2019). Parkinson's disease. *The Medical Clinics of North America, 103*(2), 337–350.

Reinders, A. A. T. S., Marquand, A. F., Schlumpf, Y. R., Chalavi, S., Vissia, E. M., Nijenhuis, E. R. S., . . . Veltman, D. J. (2019). Aiding the diagnosis of dissociative identity disorder: Pattern recognition study of brain biomarkers. *The British Journal of Psychiatry, 215*(3), 536–544.

Reinelt, E., Aldinger, M., Stopsack, M., Schwahn, C., John, U., Baumeister, S. E., . . . Barnow, S. (2014, January 10). High social support buffers the effects of 5-HTTLPR genotypes within social anxiety disorder. *European Archives of Psychiatry and Clinical Neuroscience, 264*(5), 433–439. https://doi.org/10.1007/s00406-013-0481-5

Reinhardt, M., Schlögl, M., Bonfiglio, S., Votruba, S. B., Krakoff, J., & Thearle, M. S. (2016). Lower core body temperature and greater body fat are components of a human thrifty phenotype. *International Journal of Obesity (2005), 40*(5), 754–760.

Reinhart, R. J. (2019). Fewer in U.S. continue to see vaccines as important. https://news.gallup.com/poll/276929/fewer-continue-vaccines-important.aspx

Reinhold, N., & Markowitsch, H. J. (2009). Retrograde episodic memory and emotion: A perspective from patients with dissociative amnesia. *Neuropsychologia, 47,* 2197–2206.

Reisner, S. L., Vetters, R., Leclerc, M., Zaslow, S., Wolfrum, S., Shumer, D., & Mimiaga, M. J. (2015). Mental health of transgender youth in care at an adolescent urban community health center: A matched retrospective cohort study. *Journal of Adolescent Health, 56,* 274–279.

Reist Gibbel, M., Regueiro, V., & Pargament, K. I. (2019). A spiritually integrated intervention for spiritual struggles among adults with mental illness: Results of an initial evaluation. *Spirituality in Clinical Practice, 6,* 240–255

Reitsma, L., Boelen, P. A., de Keijser, J., & Lenferink, L. I. M. (2023). Self-guided online treatment of disturbed grief, posttraumatic stress, and depression in adults bereaved during the COVID-19 pandemic: A randomized controlled trial. *Behaviour Research and Therapy, 163,* 104286. https://doi.org/10.1016/j.brat.2023.104286

Rembert, B. (2017). Clinical significance of psychotic-like experiences in children and adolescents. *Psychiatria Polska, 51,* 271–282.

Reséndiz-Hernández, J. M., & Falfán-Valencia, R. (2018). Genetic polymorphisms and their involvement in the regulation of the inflammatory response in asthma and COPD. *Advances in Clinical and Experimental Medicine, 27*(1), 125–133.

Ressler, K. J., & Rothbaum, B. O. (2012). Augmenting obsessive-compulsive disorder treatment: From brain to mind. *JAMA Psychiatry, 70,* 1129–1131.

Reynolds, G., Field, A. P., & Askew, C. (2014). Effect of vicarious fear learning on children's heart rate responses and attentional bias for novel animals. *Emotion, 14*(5), 995–1006. https://doi.org/10.1037/a0037225

Rhea, D. J., & Thatcher, W. G. (2013). Ethnicity, ethnic identity, self-esteem, and at-risk eating disordered behavior differences of urban adolescent females. *Eating Disorders, 21,* 223–237.

Rhee, S. H., Woodward, K., Corley, R. P., du Pont, A., Friedman, N. P., Hewitt, J. K., . . . Zahn-Waxler, C. (2021). The association between toddlerhood empathy deficits and antisocial personality disorder symptoms and psychopathy in adulthood. *Development and Psychopathology, 33*(1), 173–183. https://doi.org/10.1017

Rice, J. (2020). Why we must improve police responses to mental illness. https://www.nami.org/Blogs/NAMI-Blog/March-2020/Why-We-Must-Improve-Police-Responses-to-Mental-Illness

Richards, J. C., Alvarenga, M., & Hof, A. (2000). Serum lipids and their relationships with hostility and angry affect and behaviors in men. *Health Psychology, 19,* 393–398.

Richter, J., Brunner, R., Parzer, P., Resch, F., Stieltjes, B., & Henze, R. (2014). Reduced cortical and subcortical volumes in female adolescents with borderline personality disorder. *Psychiatry Research, 221*(3), 179–186.

Richter, P., & Ramos, R. T. (2018). Obsessive-compulsive disorder. *Continuum, 24,* 828–844.

Richwine, J. (2009). IQ and immigration policy. ProQuest Dissertations and Theses. https://gwern.net/doc/iq/ses/2009-richwine.pdf

Ricketts, E. J., Snorrason, Í., Kircanski, K., Alexander, J. R., Thamrin, H., Flessner, C. A., . . . Woods, D. W. (2018). A latent profile analysis of age of onset in pathological skin picking. *Comprehensive Psychiatry, 87,* 46–52.

Ridaura, V. K., Faith, J. J., Rey, F. E., Cheng, J., Duncan, A. E., Kau, A. L., . . . Gordon, J. I. (2013). Gut microbiota from twins discordant for obesity modulate metabolism in mice. *Science, 341,* 1241214.

Rideout, V., Fox, S., & Well Being Trust. (2018). Digital health practices, social media use, and mental well-being among teens and young adults in the U.S. *Articles, Abstracts, and Reports, 1093.* https://digitalcommons.psjhealth.org/publications/1093

Rides at the Door, M., & Shaw, S. (2023). The other side of the ACEs pyramid: A healing framework for Indigenous communities. *International Journal of Environmental Research and Public Health, 20*(5), 4108. https://doi.org/10.3390/ijerph20054108

Rieber, R. W. (2006). *The bifurcation of the self: The history and theory of dissociation and its disorders.* New York: Springer.

Rieder, J. K., Kleshchova, O., & Weierich, M. R. (2022). Estradiol, stress reactivity, and daily affective experiences in trauma-exposed women. *Psychological Trauma: Theory, Research, Practice and Policy, 14*(5), 738–746.

Rief, W., Barsky, A. J., Bingel, U., Doering, B. K., Schwarting, R., Wöhr, M., & Schweiger, U. (2016). Rethinking psychopharmacotherapy: The role of treatment context and brain plasticity in antidepressant and antipsychotic interventions. *Neuroscience and Biobehavioral Reviews, 60,* 51–64.

Rienecke, R. D., & Richmond, R. L. (2017). Psychopathology and expressed emotion in parents of patients with eating disorders: Relation to patient symptom severity. *Eating Disorders, 25*(4), 318–329.

Riley, M., Hernandez, A. K., & Kuznia, A. L. (2018). High blood pressure in children and adolescents. *American Family Physician, 98*(8), 486–494.

Rimmele, F., Müller, B., Becker-Hingst, N., Wegener, S., Rimmele, S., Kropp, P., & Jürgens, T. P. (2023). Medication adherence in patients with cluster headache and migraine: An online survey. *Scientific Reports, 13*(1), 4546. https://doi.org/10.1038/s41598-023-30854-y

Rink, L., Pagel, T., Franklin, J., & Baethge, C. (2016). Characteristics and heterogeneity of schizoaffective disorder compared with unipolar depression and schizophrenia— A systematic literature review and meta-analysis. *Journal of Affective Disorders, 191,* 8–14.

Ritchie, K., Norton, J., Mann, A., Carrière, I., & Ancelin, M. L. (2013). Late-onset agoraphobia: General population incidence and evidence for a clinical subtype. *American Journal of Psychiatry, 170,* 790–798.

Ritz, T., Meuret, A. E., & Simon, E. (2013). Cardiovascular activity in blood-injection-injury phobia during exposure: Evidence for diphasic response patterns? *Behaviour Research and Therapy, 51,* 460–468.

Roberts, A. L., Gilman, S. E., Breslau, J., Breslau, N., & Koenen, K. C. (2011). Race/ethnic differences in exposure to traumatic events, development of post-traumatic stress disorder, and treatment-seeking for post-traumatic stress disorder in the United States. *Psychological Medicine, 41*(1), 71–83.

Roberts, C. A., Quednow, B. B., Montgomery, C., & Parrott, A. C. (2018). MDMA and brain activity during neurocognitive performance: An overview of neuroimaging studies with abstinent "Ecstasy" users. *Neuroscience and Biobehavioral Reviews, 84,* 470–482.

Robertson, W. C., Jr. (2010). Tourette syndrome and other tic disorders. http://emedicine.medscape.com/article/1182258-overview

Robinson, D. G., Schooler, N. R., Marcy, P., Gibbons, R. D., Hendricks Brown, C., John, M., . . . Kane, J. M. (2022). Outcomes during and after early intervention services for first-episode psychosis: Results over 5 years from the RAISE-ETP Site-Randomized Trial. *Schizophrenia Bulletin, 48*(5), 1021–1031.

Robinson, E., Haynes, A., Sutin, A., & Daly, M. (2020). Self-perception of overweight and obesity: A review of mental and physical health outcomes. *Obesity Science and Practice, 6*(5), 552–561.

Robinson, T. E., Yager, L. M., Cogan, E. S., & Saunders, B. T. (2014). On the motivational properties of reward cues: Individual differences. *Neuropharmacology, 76*(Pt B), 450–459.

Rockwell, D. (2019). A presidential address: The state of humanistic psychology. *The Humanistic Psychologist, 47,* 329–334.

Rodda, A., & Estes, A. (2018). Beyond social skills: Supporting peer relationships and friendships for school-aged children with autism spectrum disorder. *Seminars in Speech and Language, 39*(2), 178–194.

Roder, V., Mueller, D. R., & Schmidt, S. J. (2011). Effectiveness of integrated psychological therapy (IPT) for schizophrenia patients: A research update. *Schizophrenia Bulletin, 37*(Suppl 2), S71–S79.

Rodgers, R. F., Lowy, A. S., Halperin, D. M., & Franko, D. L. (2016). A meta-analysis examining the influence of pro-eating disorder websites on body image and eating pathology. *European Eating Disorders Review, 24*(1), 3–8.

Rogers, C. R. (1959). A theory of therapy, personality, and interpersonal relationships, as developed in client-centered framework. In S. Koch (Ed.), *Psychology: A study of science* (Vol. 3, pp. 123–148). New York: McGraw-Hill.

Rogers, C. R. (1961). *On becoming a person.* Boston: Houghton Mifflin.

Rogers, M. L., & Joiner, T. E. (2019). Interactive effects of acute suicidal affective disturbance and pain persistence on suicide attempt frequency and lethality. *Crisis, 40,* 413–421.

Rogers, S. J., Estes, A., Lord, C., Munson, J., Rocha, M., Winter, J., . . . Talbott, M. (2019). A multisite randomized controlled two-phase trial of the early start Denver model compared to treatment as usual. *Journal of the American Academy of Child and Adolescent Psychiatry, 58*(9), 853–865.

Rohsenow, D. J., Monti, P. M., Martin, R. A., Michalec, E., & Abrams, D. B. (2000). Brief coping skills treatment for cocaine abuse: 12-month substance use outcomes. *Journal of Consulting and Clinical Psychology, 68,* 515–520.

Rojas Saffie, J. P., & Eyzaguirre Bäuerle, N. (2023). Etiology of gender incongruence and its levels of evidence: A scoping review protocol. *PLOS One, 18*(3), e0283011. https://doi.org/10.1371/journal.pone.0283011

Rollnick, S., Miller, W. R., & Butler, C. C. (2008). *Motivational interviewing in health care: Helping patients change behavior.* New York: Guilford Press.

Romero, N., Sanchez, A., & Vazquez, C. (2014). Memory biases in remitted depression: The role of negative cognitions at explicit and automatic processing levels. *Journal of Behavior Therapy and Experimental Psychiatry, 45,* 128–135.

Rondeaux, C. (2006). Can castration be a solution for sex offenders? http://www.washingtonpost.com/wp-yn/content/article/2006/07/04/AR2006070400960_pf.html

Rosenfarb, I. S., Bellack, A. S., & Aziz, N. (2006). Family interactions and the course of schizophrenia in African American and white patients. *Journal of Abnormal Psychology, 115,* 112–120.

Rosenhan, D. L. (1973). On being sane in insane places. *Science, 179,* 250–258.

Rosenström, T., Ystrom, E., Torvik, F. A., Czajkowski, N. O., Gillespie, N. A., Aggen, S. H., . . . Reichborn-Kjennerud, T. (2017). Genetic and environmental structure of DSM-IV criteria for antisocial personality disorder: A twin study. *Behavior Genetics, 47*(3), 265–277.

Rosenthal, D. G., Learned, N., Liu, Y., & Weitzman, M. (2013). Characteristics of fathers with depressive symptoms. *Maternal and Child Health Journal, 17,* 119–128.

Ross, K., Freeman, D., Dunn, G., & Garety, P. (2011). Can jumping to conclusion be reduced in people with delusions? An experimental investigation of a brief reasoning training module. *Schizophrenia Bulletin, 37,* 324–333.

Ross, M. W. (2014). Do research ethics need updating for the digital age? *Monitor on Psychology, 45.* https://www.apa.org/monitor/2014/10/research-ethics

Ross, R., Rand, D., & Pennycook, G. (2019). Beyond "fake news": The role of analytic thinking in the detection of inaccuracy and partisan bias in news headlines. https://psyarxiv.com/cgsx6/

Rossi, V., Galizia, R., Tripodi, F., Simonelli, C., Porpora, M. G.,

& Nimbi, F. M. (2022). Endometriosis and sexual functioning: How much do cognitive and psycho-emotional factors matter? *International Journal of Environmental Research and Public Health*, 19(9), 5319. https://doi.org/10.3390/ijerph19095319

Rossiter, K. (2018). My journey with anxiety and panic disorder. https://www.becomingyou.co.za/journey-anxiety-panic-disorder/

Rostad, W. L., Gittins-Stone, D., Huntington, C., Rizzo, C. J., Pearlman, D., & Orchowski, L. (2019). The association between exposure to violent pornography and teen dating violence in grade 10 high school students. *Archives of Sexual Behavior*, 48(7), 2137–2147.

Rothenberger, A., & Roessner, V. (2019). Psychopharmacotherapy of obsessive-compulsive symptoms within the framework of Tourette syndrome. *Current Neuropharmacology*, 17(8), 703–709.

Rothmore J. (2020). Antidepressant-induced sexual dysfunction. *The Medical Journal of Australia*, 212(7), 329–334. https://doi.org/10.5694/mja2.50522

Rowe, C., Deledalle, A., & Boudoukha, A. H. (2022). Psychiatric comorbidities of obsessive-compulsive disorder: A series of systematic reviews and meta-analyses. *Journal of Clinical Psychology*, 78(4), 469–484

Rowland, D. L., Castleman, J. M., Bacys, K. R., Csonka, B., & Hevesi, K. (2023). Do pornography use and masturbation play a role in erectile dysfunction and relationship satisfaction in men? *International Journal of Impotence Research*, 35(6), 548–557. https://doi.org/10.1038/s41443-022-00596-y

Roy-Byrne, P. P., Craske, M. G., & Stein, M. B. (2006). Panic disorder. *Lancet*, 368, 1023–1032.

Rozel, J. S., & Mulvey, E. P. (2017). The link between mental illness and firearm violence: Implications for social policy and clinical practice. *Annual Review of Clinical Psychology, 13*, 445–469.

Ruan, Y., Tang, J., Guo, X., Li, K., & Li, D. (2018). Dietary fat intake and risk of Alzheimer's disease and dementia: A meta-analysis of cohort studies. *Current Alzheimer Research*, 15(9), 869–876. https://doi.org/10.2174/1567205015666180427142350

Rubino, F., Puhl, R. M., Cummings, D. E., Eckel, R. H., Ryan, D. H., Mechanick, J. I., . . . Dixon, J. B. (2020). Joint international consensus statement for ending stigma of obesity. *Nature Medicine*, 26(4), 485–497.

Ruch, D. A., Sheftall, A. H., Schlagbaum, P., Rausch, J., Campo, J. V., & Bridge, J. A. (2019). Trends in suicide among youth aged 10 to 19 years in the United States, 1975 to 2016. *JAMA Network Open*, 2(5), e193886. https://doi.org/10.1001/jamanetworkopen.2019.3886

Rudd, M. D., Goulding, J., & Bryan, C. (2011, May). Student veterans: A national survey exploring psychological symptoms and suicide risk. Presentation at the Meetings of the American Psychological Association, Washington, DC.

Rude, M. (2022). These states still have laws banning sodomy in 2022. https://www.out.com/news/2022/7/12/these-states-still-have-laws-banning-sodomy-2022#rebelltitem1

Rudigera, J. A., & Winstead, B. A. (2013). Body talk and body-related co-rumination: Associations with body image, eating attitudes, and psychological adjustment. *Body Image*, 11, 462–471.

Rudovic, O., Lee, J., Dai, M., Schuller, B., & Picard, R. W. (2018). Personalized machine learning for robot perception of affect and engagement in autism therapy. *Science Robotics*, 3(19).

Ruiz, B. (2021). Why some experts and patients want to rename schizophrenia: Interview with Raquelle Mesholam-Gately and Matcheri Keshavan. https://www.madinamerica.com/2021/09/experts-patients-want-rename-schizophrenia-interview-matcheri-keshavan-raquelle-mesholam-gately/

Rumpf-Whitten, S. (2023). New Jersey student ends her life after months of bullying, video of school hallway beating circulates online. https://www.foxnews.com/us/new-jersey-student-ends-life-months-bullying-video-school-hallway-beating-circulates-online

Russell-Williams, J., Jaroudi, W., Perich, T., Hoscheidt, S., El Haj, M., & Moustafa, A. A. (2018). Mindfulness and meditation: Treating cognitive impairment and reducing stress in dementia. *Reviews in the Neurosciences*, 29(7), 791–804.

Ryan, S. M., & Ollendick, T. H. (2018). The interaction between child behavioral inhibition and parenting behaviors: Effects on internalizing and externalizing symptomology. *Clinical Child and Family Psychology Review*, 21(3), 320–339.

Ryder, A. G., Sun, J., Dere, J., & Fung, K. (2014). Personality disorders in Asians: Summary, and a call for cultural research. *Asian Journal of Psychiatry*, 7, 86–88.

Rynar, L., & Coccaro, E. F. (2018). Psychosocial impairment in DSM-5 intermittent explosive disorder. *Psychiatry Research*, 264, 91–95.

Sabbag, S., Prestia, D., Robertson, B., Ruiz, P., Durand, D., Strassnig, M., & Harvey, P. D. (2015). Absence of bias in clinician ratings of everyday functioning among African American, Hispanic and Caucasian patients with schizophrenia. *Psychiatry Research*, 229(1–2), 347–352.

Sabri, B., Simonet, M., & Campbell, J. C. (2018). Risk and protective factors of intimate partner violence among South Asian immigrant women and perceived need for services. *Cultural Diversity and Ethnic Minority Psychology*, 24(3), 442–452.

Sack, R. L., Auckley, D., Auger, R. R., Carskadon, M. A., Wright, K. P., Jr., & Vitiello, M. V. (2007). Circadian rhythm sleep disorders: Part I. Basic principles, shift work and jet lag. *Sleep*, 30, 1460–1483.

Sacktor, N. (2018). Changing clinical phenotypes of HIV-associated neurocognitive disorders. *Journal of Neurovirology*, 24(2), 141–145.

Sadeh, N., Miller, M. W., Wolf, E. J., & Harkness, K. L. (2015). Negative emotionality and disconstraint influence PTSD symptom course via exposure to new major adverse life events. *Journal of Anxiety Disorders, 31,* 20–27.

Safarinejad, M. R. (2006). Female sexual dysfunction in a population-based study in Iran: Prevalence and associated risk factors. *International Journal of Impotence Research, 18,* 382–395.

Sagalyn, D. (2012). Health experts question army report on psychological training. http://www.pbs.org/newshour/updates/military-jan-june12-csf_training_01-02

Saha, P., & Sen, N. (2019). Tauopathy: A common mechanism for neurodegeneration and brain aging. *Mechanisms of Ageing and Development, 178,* 72–79.

Saito, T., Toda, H., Inoue, T., Koga, M., Tanichi, M., Takeshita, S., . . . Yoshino, A. (2019). Relationship between the subtypes of child abuse and affective temperaments: Comparison of depression and bipolar disorder patients and healthy controls using the reclassified Child Abuse and Trauma Scale. *Journal of Affective Disorders, 257,* 396–403.

Sajatovic, M., Tatsuoka, C., Cassidy, K. A., Klein, P. J., Fuentes-Casiano, E., Cage, J., . . . Levin, J. B. (2018). A 6-month, prospective, randomized controlled trial of customized adherence enhancement versus bipolar-specific educational control in poorly adherent individuals with bipolar disorder. *The Journal of Clinical Psychiatry, 79*(6). https://doi.org/10.4088/JCP.17m12036

Saklofske, D. H., Hildebrand, D. K., & Gorsuch, R. L. (2000). Replication of the factor structure of the Wechsler Adult Intelligence Scale—Third edition with a Canadian sample. *Psychological Assessment, 12,* 436–439.

Saks, E. R. (2007). *The center cannot hold: My journey through madness.* New York: Hyperion.

Saks, E. R. (2013). Successful and schizophrenic. http://www.nytimes.com/2013/01/27/opinion/sunday/schizophrenic-not-stupid.html?_r50

Sakurada, K., Konta, T., Watanabe, M., Ishizawa, K., Ueno, Y., Yamashita, H., & Kayama, T. (2020). Associations of frequency of laughter with risk of all-cause mortality and cardiovascular disease incidence in a general population: Findings from the Yamagata Study. *Journal of Epidemiology, 30*(4), 188–193.

Salgado-Pineda, P., Caclin, A., Baeza, I., Junque, C., Bernardo, M., Blin, O., & Funlupt, P. (2007). Schizophrenia and the frontal cortex: Where does it fail? *Schizophrenia Research, 91,* 73–81.

Salk, R. H., Hyde, J. S., & Abramson, L. Y. (2017). Gender differences in depression in representative national samples: Meta-analyses of diagnoses and symptoms. *Psychological Bulletin, 143*(8), 783–822.

Salk, R. H., Petersen, J. L., Abramson, L. Y., & Hyde, J. S. (2016). The contemporary face of gender differences and similarities in depression throughout adolescence: Development and chronicity. *Journal of Affective Disorders, 205,* 28–35.

Sallinger, R. (2012). James Holmes saw three mental health professionals before shooting. http://www.alipac.us/f19/james-holmes-saw-three-mental-health-professionals-before-shooting-262890

Salmani, Z., Zargham-Boroujeni, A., Salehi, M., Killeen, T., & Merghati-Khoei, E. (2015). The existing therapeutic interventions for orgasmic disorders: Recommendations for culturally competent services, narrative review. *Iran Journal of Reproductive Medicine, 13,* 403–412.

Salvatore, G., Russo, B., Russo, M., Popolo, R., & Dimaggio, G. (2012). Metacognition-oriented therapy for psychosis: The case of a woman with delusional disorder and paranoid personality disorder. *Journal of Psychotherapy Integration, 22,* 314–329.

Salvatore, J. E., & Dick, D. M. (2018). Genetic influences on conduct disorder. *Neuroscience and Biobehavioral Reviews, 91,* 91–101.

Salvatore, P., Bhuvaneswar, C., Tohen, M., Khalsa, H. M., Maggini, C., & Baldessarini, R. J. (2014). Capgras' syndrome in first-episode psychotic disorders. *Psychopathology, 47*(4), 261–269.

Salvatore, T., Dodson, K. D., Hull, A., Harr, D., & Brown, J. (2018). Elder abuse as a risk factor for suicidal behavior in older adults. *The Forensic Mental Health Practitioner, 1,* 1–7.

Samarrai, F. (2013). New Center for Open Science designed to increase research transparency, provide free technologies for scientists. https://news.virginia.edu/content/new-center-open-science-designed-increase-research-transparency-provide-free-technologies

SAMHSA (2023). Results from the 2021 National Survey on Drug Use and Health: Graphics from the Key Findings Report. https://www.samhsa.gov/data/sites/default/files/reports/rpt39443/2021_NNR_figure_slides.pdf

Sami, M., Worker, A., Colizzi, M., Annibale, L., Das, D., Kelbrick, M., . . . Collaborators. (2020). Association of cannabis with glutamatergic levels in patients with early psychosis: Evidence for altered volume striatal glutamate relationships in patients with a history of cannabis use in early psychosis. *Translational Psychiatry, 10*(1), 111. https://doi.org/10.1038/s41398-020-0790-1

Sampedro-Piquero, P., Alvarez-Suarez, P., & Begega, A. (2018). Coping with stress during aging: The importance of a resilient brain. *Current Neuropharmacology, 16*(3), 284–296.

Sampson, M., Melnyk, B. M., & Hoying, J. (2020). The MINDBODYSTRONG intervention for new nurse residents: 6-month effects on mental health outcomes, healthy lifestyle behaviors, and job satisfaction. *Worldviews on Evidence-Based Nursing, 17*(1), 16–23.

Samuelson, K. W., Bartel, A., Valadez, R., & Jordan, J. T. (2017). PTSD symptoms and perception of cognitive problems: The roles of posttraumatic cognitions and trauma coping self-efficacy. *Psychological Trauma: Theory, Research, Practice, and Policy, 9*(5), 537–544.

San Francisco Women Against Rape. (n.d.) Facts and information. http://www.sfwar.org/facts.html

Sanchez, C. (2022). Billie Eilish on living with Tourette's syndrome: "It's part of me." https://www.harpersbazaar.com/celebrity/latest/a40091846/billie-eilish-tourette-syndrome/

Sanchez, O. (2019). Endless fear: Undocumented immigrants grapple with anxiety, depression under Trump. https://news.yahoo.com/endless-fear-undocumented-immigrants-grapple-170444635.html?.tsrc=jtc_news_index

Sandin, S., Lichtenstein, P., Kuja-Halkola, R., Larsson, H., Hultman, C. M., & Reichenberg, A. (2014). The familial risk of autism. *JAMA*, 311(17), 1770–1777.

Sansone, R. A., & Sansone, L. A. (2011). Personality pathology and its influence on eating disorders. *Innovations in Clinical Neuroscience*, 8, 14–18.

Sansone, R. A., & Sansone, L. A. (2015). Borderline personality in the medical setting. *The Primary Care Companion for CNS Disorders*, 17(3), 10.4088/PCC.14r01743.

Santa Maria, M. P., Hill, B. D., & Kline, J. (2019). Lead (Pb) neurotoxicology and cognition. *Applied Neuropsychology: Child*, 8(3), 272–293.

Santee, J., Barnes, K., Borja-Hart, N., Cheng, A. L., Draime, J., Edwards, A., . . . Sawkin, M. (2022). Correlation between pharmacy students' implicit bias scores, explicit bias scores, and responses to clinical cases. *American Journal of Pharmaceutical Education*, 86(1), 8587. https://doi.org/10.5688/ajpe8587

Santiago, P. N., Ursano, R. J., Gray, C. L., Pynoos, R. S., Spiegel, D., Lewis- Fernandez, R., . . . Fullerton, C. S. (2013). A systematic review of PTSD prevalence and trajectories in DSM-5 defined trauma exposed populations: Intentional and non-intentional traumatic events. *PLOS One*, 8(4), e59236. https://doi.org/10.1371/journal.pone.0059236

Santini, Z. I., Koyanagi, A., Tyrovolas, S., Mason, C., & Haro, J. M. (2015). The association between social relationships and depression: A systematic review. *Journal of Affective Disorders*, 175, 53–65.

Sanvisens, A., Hernández-Rubio, A., Zuluaga, P., Fuster, D., Papaseit, E., Galan, S., . . . Muga, R. (2021). Long-term outcomes of patients with cocaine use disorder: A 18-years addiction cohort study. *Frontiers in Pharmacology*, 12,

625610. https://doi.org/10.3389/fphar.2021.625610

Sarafidou, S. (2018). Life quality and the self: A person-centered case study of Alzheimer's disease. *Journal of Aging and Geriatric Psychiatry*, 2(2), 7–122.

Sarafrazi, N., Hughes, J. P., Borrud, L., Burt, V., & Paulose-Ram, R. (2014). *Perception of weight status in U.S. children and adolescents aged 8–15 years, 2005–2012.* NCHS data brief, no 158. Hyattsville, MD: National Center for Health Statistics.

Sateia, M. J., Buysse, D. J., Krystal, A. D., Neubauer, D. N., & Heald, J. L. (2017). Clinical practice guideline for the pharmacologic treatment of chronic insomnia in adults: An American Academy of Sleep Medicine Clinical practice guideline. *Journal of Clinical Sleep Medicine*, 13(2), 307–349.

Satir, V. (1967). A family of angels. In J. Haley & L. Hoffman (Eds.), *Techniques of family therapy* (pp. 99–113). New York: Basic Books.

Satow, R. (1979). Where has all the hysteria gone? *Psychoanalytic Review*, 66, 463–477.

Sattler, S., Sauer, C., Mehlkop, G., & Graeff, P. (2013). The rationale for consuming cognitive enhancement drugs in university students and teachers. *PLOS One*, 8, e68821. https://doi.org/10.1371/journal.pone.0068821

Sauer K. S., & Witthöft, M. (2022). Inhibitory learning versus habituation in an experimental exposure intervention for people with heightened health anxiety: Increase of distress tolerance as a joint mechanism of change? *Journal of Experimental Psychopathology*, 13(4). doi:10.1177/20438087221138716

Sauer-Zavala, S., Bentley, K. H., Steele, S. J., Tirpak, J. W., Ametaj, A. A., Nauphal, M., . . . Barlow, D. H. (2019). Treating depressive disorders with the unified protocol: A preliminary randomized evaluation. *Journal of Affective Disorders*, 264, 438–445.

Savage, M. (2020). How COVID-19 is changing women's lives. https://www.bbc.com/worklife/article/20200630-how-covid-19-is-changing-womens-lives

Savarese, M., & Di Perri, M. C. (2020). Excessive sleepiness in shift work disorder: A narrative review of the last 5 years. *Sleep and Breathing*, 24(1), 297–310.

Saw, A., Berenbaum, H., & Okazaki, S. (2013). Influences of personal standards and perceived parental expectations on worry for Asian American and White American college students. *Anxiety, Stress and Coping*, 26(2), 187–202.

Sawchuk, C. N., Roy-Byrne, P., Noonan, C., Craner, J. R., Goldberg, J., Manson, S., . . . AI-SUPERPFP Team. (2017). Panic attacks and panic disorder in the American Indian community. *Journal of Anxiety Disorders*, 48, 6–12.

Scarella, T. M., Boland, R. J., & Barsky, A. J. (2019). Illness anxiety disorder: Psychopathology, epidemiology, clinical characteristics, and treatment. *Psychosomatic Medicine*, 81(5), 398–407.

Schachter, S., & Latané, B. (1964). Crime, cognition, and the autonomic nervous system. *Nebraska Symposium on Motivation*, 12, 221–274.

Schaefer, L. M., Burke, N. L., Calogero, R. M., Menzel, J. E., Krawczyk, R., & Thompson, J. K. (2018). Self-objectification, body shame, and disordered eating: Testing a core mediational model of objectification theory among White, Black, and Hispanic women. *Body Image*, 24, 5–12.

Schaefer, L. M., Smith, K. E., Anderson, L. M., Cao, L., Crosby, R. D., Engel, S. G., . . . Wonderlich, S. A. (2020). The role of affect in the maintenance of binge-eating disorder: Evidence from an ecological momentary assessment study. *Journal of Abnormal Psychology*, 129(4), 387–396.

Schäfer, S. K., Sopp, M. R., Staginnus, M., Lass-Hennemann, J., & Michael, T. (2020). Correlates of mental health in occupations at risk for traumatization: A cross-sectional study. *BMC Psychiatry*, 20(1), 335. https://doi.org/10.1186/s12888-020-02704-y

Scheim, A. I., Baker, K. E., Restar, A. J., & Sell, R. L. (2022). Health and health care among transgender adults in the United States. *Annual Review of Public Health*, 43, 503–523.

Schepis, T. S., Teter, C. J., Simoni-Wastila, L., & McCabe, S. E. (2018). Prescription tranquilizer/sedative misuse prevalence and correlates across age cohorts in the US. *Addictive Behaviors, 87*, 24–32.

Schieve, L. A., Tian, L. H., Drews-Botsch, C., Windham, G. C., Newschaffer, C., Daniels, J. L., . . . Danielle Fallin, M. (2018). Autism spectrum disorder and birth spacing: Findings from the study to explore early development (SEED). *Autism Research, 11*(1), 81–94.

Schindler, S. E., Li, Y., Todd, K. W., Herries, E. M., Henson, R. L., Gray, J. D., . . . Dominantly Inherited Alzheimer Network. (2019). Emerging cerebrospinal fluid biomarkers in autosomal dominant Alzheimer's disease. *Alzheimer's and Dementia, 15*(5), 655–665.

Schlax, J., Wiltink, J., Beutel, M. E., Münzel, T., Pfeiffer, N., Wild, P., . . . Michal, M. (2020). Symptoms of depersonalization/derealization are independent risk factors for the development or persistence of psychological distress in the general population: Results from the Gutenberg Health Study. *Journal of Affective Disorders, 273*, 41–47.

Schmauk, F. J. (1970). Punishment, arousal, and avoidance learning. *Journal of Abnormal Psychology, 76*, 325–335.

Schmetze, A. D., & McGrath, R. (2014). Phencyclidine (PCP)-related psychiatric disorders. http://emedicine.medscape.com/article/290476-overview

Schmidt, U., Kaltwasser, S. F., & Wotjak, C. T. (2013). Biomarkers in posttraumatic stress disorder: Overview and implications for future research. *Disease Markers, 35*, 43–54.

Schneider, A., Huber, L., Lohse, J., Linde, K., Greissel, A., Sattel, H., . . . Hapfelmeier, A. (2023). Association between somatic symptom disorder and symptoms with daily life impairment after SARS-CoV-2 infection: Results from a population-based cross-sectional study. *Journal of Psychosomatic Research, 168*, 111230. https://doi.org/10.1016/j.jpsychores.2023.111230

Schnierle, J., Christian-Brathwaite, N., & Louisias, M. (2019). Implicit bias: What every pediatrician should know about the effect of bias on health and future directions. *Current Problems in Pediatric and Adolescent Health Care, 49*(2), 34–44.

Schoenbaum, M., Sutherland, J. M., Chappel, A., Azrin, S., Goldstein, A. B., Rupp, A., & Heinssen, R. K. (2017). Twelve-month health care use and mortality in commercially insured young people with incident psychosis in the United States. *Schizophrenia Bulletin, 43*(6), 1262–1272.

Schofield, P., Ashworth, M., & Jones, R. (2011). Ethnic isolation and psychosis: Re-examining the ethnic density effect. *Psychological Medicine, 41*, 1263–1269.

Scholten, W., Batelaan, N., & Van Balkom, A. (2020). Barriers to discontinuing antidepressants in patients with depressive and anxiety disorders: A review of the literature and clinical recommendations. *Therapeutic Advances in Psychopharmacology, 10*, 2045125320933404. https://doi.org/10.1177/2045125320933404

Schonfeldt-Lecuona, C., Connemann, B. J., Spitzer, M., & Herwig, U. (2003). Transcranial magnetic stimulation in the reversal of motor conversion disorder. *Psychotherapy and Psychosomatics, 72*, 286–290.

Schooler, D., & Daniels, E. A. (2014). "I am not a skinny toothpick and proud of it": Latina adolescents' ethnic identity and responses to mainstream media images. *Body Image, 11*, 11–18.

Schori, A., Jackowski, C., & Schön, C. A. (2022). How safe is BDSM? A literature review on fatal outcome in BDSM play. *International Journal of Legal Medicine, 136*(1), 287–295. https://doi.org/10.1007/s00414-021-02674-0

Schrader, C., & Ross, A. (2021). A review of PTSD and current treatment strategies. *Missouri Medicine, 118*(6), 546–551.

Schrader, H., Bøhmer, T., & Aasly, J. (2019). The incidence of diagnosis of Munchausen syndrome, other factitious disorders, and malingering. *Behavioural Neurology, 2019*, 3891809. https://doi.org/10.1155/2019/3891809

Schramm, E., Klein, D. N., Elsaesser, M., Furukawa, T. A., & Domschke, K. (2020). Review of dysthymia and persistent depressive disorder: History, correlates, and clinical implications. *The Lancet: Psychiatry, 7*(9), 801–812.

Schreiber, F. R. (1973). *Sybil.* Chicago: Regnery.

Schreier, A., Wolke, D., Thomas, K., Horwood, J., Hollis, C., Gunnell, D., . . . Harrison, G. (2009). Prospective study of peer victimization in childhood and psychotic symptoms in a nonclinical population at age 12 years. *Archives of General Psychiatry, 66*, 527–536.

Schrempft, S., van Jaarsveld, C., Fisher, A., Herle, M., Smith, A. D., Fildes, A., & Llewellyn, C. H. (2018). Variation in the heritability of child body mass index by obesogenic home environment. *JAMA Pediatrics, 172*(12), 1153–1160. https://doi.org/10.1001/jamapediatrics.2018.1508

Schroeder, A. R., Dehghan, M., Newman, T. B., Bentley, J. P., & Park, K. T. (2019). Association of opioid prescriptions from dental clinicians for US adolescents and young adults with subsequent opioid use and abuse. *JAMA Internal Medicine, 179*(2), 145–152.

Schroeder, K., Schuler, B. R., Kobulsky, J. M., & Sarwer, D. B. (2021). The association between adverse childhood experiences and childhood obesity: A systematic review. *Obesity Reviews: An Official Journal of the International Association for the Study of Obesity, 22*(7), e13204. https://doi.org/10.1111/obr.13204

Schroll, J. B., & Lauritsen, M. P. (2022). Premenstrual dysphoric disorder: A controversial new diagnosis. *Acta Obstetricia et Gynecologica Scandinavica, 101*(5), 482–483. https://doi.org/10.1111/aogs.14360

Schrut, A. (2005). A psychodynamic (non-Oedipal) and brain function hypothesis regarding a type of male sexual masochism. *Journal of the American Academy of*

Psychoanalysis and Dynamic Psychiatry, 33, 333–349.

Schuler, M. S., Tucker, J. S., Pedersen, E. R., & D'Amico, E. J. (2019). Relative influence of perceived peer and family substance use on adolescent alcohol, cigarette, and marijuana use across middle and high school. *Addictive Behaviors, 88,* 99–105.

Schulte, I. E., & Petermann, F. (2011). Familial risk factors for the development of somatoform symptoms and disorders in children and adolescents: A systematic review. *Child Psychiatry and Human Development, 42,* 569–583.

Schulte, M. H., Cousijn, J., den Uyl, T. E., Goudriaan, A. E., van den Brink, W., Veltman, D. J., . . . Wiers, R. W. (2014). Recovery of neurocognitive functions following sustained abstinence after substance dependence and implications for treatment. *Clinical Psychology Review, 34*(7), 531–550.

Schultze-Lutter, F., Nenadic, I., & Grant, P. (2019). Psychosis and schizophrenia-spectrum personality disorders require early detection on different symptom dimensions. *Frontiers in Psychiatry, 10,* 476. https://doi .org/10.3389/fpsyt.2019.00476

Schwartz-Mette, R. A., & Smith, R. L. (2018). When does co-rumination facilitate depression contagion in adolescent friendships? Investigating Intrapersonal and interpersonal factors. *Journal of Clinical Child and Adolescent Psychology, 47*(6), 912–924.

Schwasinger-Schmidt, T. E., & Macaluso, M. (2019). Other antidepressants. *Handbook of experimental pharmacology, 250,* 325–355.

Schweizer, T., Schmitz, J., Plempe, L., Sun, D., Becker-Asano, C., Leonhart, R., & Tuschen-Caffier, B. (2017). The impact of pre-existing anxiety on affective and cognitive processing of a virtual reality analogue trauma. *PLOS One, 12*(12), e0190360. https:// doi.org/10.1371/journal .pone.0190360

Sciberras, E., Mulraney, M., Silva, D., & Coghill, D. (2017). Prenatal risk factors and the etiology of ADHD—Review of existing evidence. *Current Psychiatry Reports,* 19(1), 1. https://doi.org/10.1007 /s11920-017-0753-2

Scoboria, A., Wade, K. A., Lindsay, D. S., Azad, T., Strange, D., Ost, J., & Hyman, I. E. (2017). A mega-analysis of memory reports from eight peer-reviewed false memory implantation studies. *Memory, 25*(2), 146–163.

Scripter, C. (2018). Headache: Tension-type headache. *FP Essentials, 473,* 17–20.

Scudellari, M. (2013, July 1). Worried sick. http://www.the-scientist.com /?articles.view/articleNo/36126 /title/Worried-Sick

Seabrook, R. C., McMahon, S., & O'Connor, J. (2018). A longitudinal study of interest and membership in a fraternity, rape myth acceptance, and proclivity to perpetrate sexual assault. *Journal of American College Health, 66,* 510–518.

Seaton, E. K., & Zeiders, K. H. (2020). Daily racial discrimination experiences, ethnic–racial identity, and diurnal cortisol patterns among Black adults. *Cultural Diversity and Ethnic Minority Psychology, 27*(1), 145–155. https://doi.org/10.1037 /cdp0000367

Seery, M. D., Holman, E. A., & Silver, R. C. (2010). Whatever does not kill us: Cumulative lifetime adversity, vulnerability, and resilience. *Journal of Personality and Social Psychology, 99,* 1025–1041.

Seftel, A. D., Rosen, R. C., Hayes, R. P., Althof, S., Goldfisher, E., Shen, W., & Sontag, A. (2014). Effect of once-daily tadalafil on confidence and perceived difficulty in performing sexual intercourse in men who were incomplete responders to as-needed PDE5 inhibitor treatment. *International Journal of Clinical Practice, 68,* 841–849.

Segal, Z. V., Dimidjian, S., Beck, A., Boggs, J. M., Vanderkruik, R., Metcalf, C. A., . . . Levy, J. (2020). Outcomes of online mindfulness-based cognitive therapy for patients with residual depressive symptoms: A randomized clinical trial. *JAMA Psychiatry, 77*(6), 1–11.

Sehatzadeh, S., Daskalakis, Z. J., Yap, B., Tu, H. A., Palimaka, S., Bowen, J. M., & O'Reilly, D. J. (2019). Unilateral and bilateral repetitive transcranial magnetic stimulation for treatment-resistant depression: A meta-analysis of randomized controlled trials over 2 decades. *Journal of Psychiatry and Neuroscience, 44*(3), 151–163.

Seidman, L. J., & Mirsky, A. F. (2017). Evolving notions of schizophrenia as a developmental neurocognitive disorder. *Journal of the International Neuropsychological Society, 23*(9–10), 881–892.

Seidman, L. J., Shapiro, D. I., Stone, W. S., Woodberry, K. A., Ronzio, A., Cornblatt, B. A., . . . Woods, S. W. (2016). Association of neurocognition with transition to psychosis: Baseline functioning in the second phase of the North American Prodrome Longitudinal Study. *JAMA Psychiatry, 73*(12), 1239–1248.

Seife, C. (2012). Is drug research trustworthy? The pharmaceutical industry funnels money to prominent scientists who are doing research that affects its products— And nobody can stop it. *Scientific American, 307,* 56–63.

Sekar, A., Bialas, A. R., de Rivera, H., Davis, A., Hammond, T. R., Kamitaki, N., . . . McCarroll, S. A. (2016). Schizophrenia risk from complex variation of complement component 4. *Nature, 530*(7589), 177–183.

Selby, E. A., & Joiner, T. E., Jr. (2013). Emotional cascades as prospective predictors of dysregulated behaviors in borderline personality disorder. *Personality Disorders, 4,* 168–174.

Seligman, M. E. P., & Csikszentmihalyi, M. (2000). Positive psychology: An introduction. *American Psychologist, 55,* 5–14.

Selkie, E., Adkins, V., Masters, E., Bajpai, A., & Shumer, D. (2020). Transgender adolescents' uses of social media for social support. *Journal of Adolescent Health, 66,* 275–280.

Sellbom, M. (2019). The MMPI-2-Restructured Form (MMPI-2-RF): Assessment of personality and psychopathology in the twenty-first century. *Annual*

Review of Clinical Psychology. https://doi.org/10.1146 /annurev-clinpsy-050718-095701

Sempértegui, G. A., Karreman, A., Arntz, A., & Bekker, M. H. (2013). Schema therapy for borderline personality disorder: A comprehensive review of its empirical foundations, effectiveness and implementation possibilities. *Clinical Psychology Review, 33,* 426–447.

Senova, S., Clair, A. H., Palfi, S., Yelnik, J., Domenech, P., & Mallet, L. (2019). Deep brain stimulation for refractory obsessive-compulsive disorder: Towards an individualized approach. *Frontiers in Psychiatry, 10,* 905. https://doi.org /10.3389/fpsyt.2019.00905

Senova, S., Rabu, C., Beaumont, S., Michel, V., Palfi, S., Mallet, L., & Domenech, P. (2019). Vagus nerve stimulation and depression. *Presse Medicale, 48*(12), 1507–1519.

Serra, G., Uchida, M., Battaglia, C., Casini, M. P., De Chiara, L., Biederman, J., . . . Wozniak, J. (2017). Pediatric mania: The controversy between euphoria and irritability. *Current Neuropharmacology, 15*(3), 386–393.

Serretti A. (2017). Genetics and pharmacogenetics of mood disorders. Genetyka i farmakogenetyka zaburzeń nastroju. *Psychiatria Polska, 51*(2), 197–203. https:// doi.org/10.12740/PP/68914

Seto, M. C. (2012). Is pedophilia a sexual orientation? *Archives of Sexual Behavior, 41,* 231–236.

Seto, M. C., & Lalumière, M. L. (2010). What is so special about male adolescent sexual offending? A review and test of explanations through meta-analysis. *Psychological Bulletin, 136,* 526–575.

Sevincer, A. T., & Oettingen, G. (2014). Alcohol myopia and goal commitment. *Frontiers in Psychology, 5,* 169. https://doi.org /10.3389/fpsyg.2014.00169

Shah, M., Adams-Huet, B., Rao, S., Snell, P., Quittner, C., & Garg, A. (2013). The effect of dietary counseling on nutrient intakes in gastric banding surgery patients. *Journal of Investigative Medicine, 61,* 1165–1172.

Shan, Z., Li, Y., Baden, M. Y., Bhupathiraju, S. N., Wang, D.

D., Sun, Q., . . . Hu, F. B. (2020). Association between healthy eating patterns and risk of cardiovascular disease. *JAMA Internal Medicine,* e202176. https://doi.org/10.1001 /jamainternmed.2020.2176

Shankman, S. A., Funkhouser, C. J., Klein, D. N., Davila, J., Lerner, D., & Hee, D. (2018). Reliability and validity of severity dimensions of psychopathology assessed using the Structured Clinical Interview for DSM-5 (SCID). *International Journal of Methods in Psychiatric Research, 27*(1). doi:10.1002 /mpr.1590

Shapero, B. G., Curley, E. E., Black, C. L., & Alloy, L. B. (2019). The interactive association of proximal life stress and cumulative HPA axis functioning with depressive symptoms. *Depression and Anxiety, 36*(11), 1089–1101.

Shapero, B. G., Stange, J. P., McArthur, B. A., Abramson, L. Y., & Alloy, L. B. (2019). Cognitive reappraisal attenuates the association between depressive symptoms and emotional response to stress during adolescence. *Cognition and Emotion, 33*(3), 524–535.

Shapero, B. G., Weiss, R. B., Burke, T. A., Boland, E. M., Abramson, L. Y., & Alloy, L. B. (2017). Kindling of life stress in bipolar disorder: Effects of early adversity. *Behavior Therapy, 48*(3), 322–334.

Shapiro, D. L., Ferguson, S., Hernandez, K., Kennedy, T., & Black, R. (2019). Ethnic adjustment abuses in forensic assessment of intellectual abilities. *Practice Innovations, 4,* 265–281.

Sharma, S., Powers, A., Bradley, B., & Ressler, K. J. (2016). Gene × environment determinants of stress- and anxiety-related disorders. *Annual Review of Psychology, 67,* 239–261.

Shaw, P., Eckstrand, K., Sharp, W., Blumenthal, J., Lerch, J. P., Greenstein, D., . . . Rapoport, J. L. (2007). Attention-deficit/hyperactivity disorder is characterized by a delay in cortical maturation. *Proceedings of the National Academy of Sciences, 104,* 19649–19654.

Sheffield, J. M., Karcher, N. R., & Barch, D. M. (2018). Cognitive deficits in psychotic disorders: A lifespan perspective.

Neuropsychology Review, 28(4), 509–533.

Shekriladze, I., Javakhishvili, N., & Tchanturia, K. (2019). Culture change and eating patterns: A study of Georgian women. *Frontiers in Psychiatry, 10,* 619. https://doi.org/10.3389 /fpsyt.2019.00619

Shelby, G. D., Shirkey, K. C., Sherman, A. L., Beck, J. E., Haman, K., Shears, A. R., . . . Walker, L. S. (2013). Functional abdominal pain in childhood and long-term vulnerability to anxiety disorders. *Pediatrics, 132,* 475–482.

Shi, C., Taylor, S., Witthöft, M., Du, X., Zhang, T., Lu, S., & Ren, Z. (2022). Attentional bias toward health-threat in health anxiety: A systematic review and three-level meta-analysis. *Psychological Medicine, 52*(4), 604–613.

Shi, J., Geng, J., Yan, R., Liu, X., Chen, Y., Zhu, R., . . . Lu, Q. (2018). Differentiation of transformed bipolar disorder from unipolar depression by resting-state functional connectivity within reward circuit. *Frontiers in Psychology, 9,* 2586. https://doi .org/10.3389/fpsyg.2018.02586

Shiban, Y., Pauli, P., & Mühlberger, A. (2013). Effect of multiple context exposure on renewal in spider phobia. *Behaviour Research and Therapy, 51,* 68–74.

Shim, I. H., Woo, Y. S., Kim, M. D., & Bahk, W. M. (2017). Antidepressants and mood stabilizers: Novel research avenues and clinical insights for bipolar depression. *International Journal of Molecular Sciences, 18*(11), 2406. https://doi.org/10.3390 /ijms18112406

Shively, S. B., Horkayne-Szakaly, I., Jones, R. V., Kelly, J. P., Armstrong, R. C., & Perl, D. P. (2016). Characterisation of interface astroglial scarring in the human brain after blast exposure: A post-mortem case series. *The Lancet: Neurology, 15*(9), 944–953.

Shneidman, E. S. (1998). *The suicidal mind.* New York: Oxford University Press.

Shokri-Kojori, E., Wang, G. J., Wiers, C. E., Demiral, S. B., Guo, M., Kim, S. W., . . . Volkow, N. D. (2018). β-Amyloid accumulation in the human brain after one night of sleep deprivation. *Proceedings of the National Academy of Sciences of the United States of America, 115*(17), 4483–4488.

Short, N. A., Stentz, L., Raines, A. M., Boffa, J. W., & Schmidt, N. B. (2019). Intervening on thwarted belongingness and perceived burdensomeness to reduce suicidality among veterans: Subanalyses from a randomized controlled trial. *Behavior Therapy, 50,* 886–897.

Shrivastava, A., Shah, N., Johnston, M., Stitt, L., & Thakar, M. (2010). Predictors of long-term outcome of first-episode schizophrenia: A ten-year follow-up study. *Indian Journal of Psychiatry, 52,* 320–326.

Sibitz, I., Unger, A., Woppmann, A., Zidek, T., & Amering, M. (2011). Stigma resistance in patients with schizophrenia. *Schizophrenia Bulletin, 37,* 316–323.

Sibolt, G., Curtze, S., Melkas, S., Pohjasvaara, T., Kaste, M., Karhunen, P. J., . . . Erkinjuntti, T. (2013). Post-stroke depression and depression-executive dysfunction syndrome are associated with recurrence of ischemic stroke. *Cerebrovascular Diseases, 36,* 336–343.

Sibrava, N. J., Beard, C., Bjornsson, A. S., Moitra, E., Weisberg, R. B., & Keller, M. B. (2013). Two-year course of generalized anxiety disorder, social anxiety disorder, and panic disorder in a longitudinal sample of African American adults. *Journal of Consulting and Clinical Psychology, 81,* 1052–1062.

Sibrava, N. J., Bjornsson, A. S., Pérez Benítez, A., Moitra, E., Weisberg, R. B., & Keller, M. B. (2019). Posttraumatic stress disorder in African American and Latinx adults: Clinical course and the role of racial and ethnic discrimination. *The American Psychologist, 74*(1), 101–116.

Sicras-Mainar, A., Maurino, J., Ruiz-Beato, E., & Navarro-Artieda, R. (2014). Prevalence of metabolic syndrome according to the presence of negative symptoms in patients with schizophrenia. *Neuropsychiatric Disease and Treatment, 11,* 51–57.

Siebert, D. C., & Wilke, D. J. (2007). High-risk drinking among young adults: The influence of race and college enrollment. *American Journal of Drug and Alcohol Abuse, 33,* 843–850.

Siegel, M. (1979). Privacy, ethics, and confidentiality. *Professional Psychology, 10,* 249–258.

Siemaszko, C. (2019). A "public relations nightmare": Boy band star accuses ex-girlfriend of Munchausen by proxy. https://www.nbcnews.com/news/us-news/public-relations-nightmare-boy-band-star-accuses-ex-girlfriend-munchausen-n1001121

Sierk, A., Daniels, J. K., Manthey, A., Kok, J. G., Leemans, A., Gaebler, M., . . . Walter, H. (2018). White matter network alterations in patients with depersonalization/derealization disorder. *Journal of Psychiatry and Neuroscience, 43*(5), 347–357.

Sierra, M. (2012). *Depersonalization: A new look at a neglected syndrome.* New York: Cambridge University Press.

Sieswerda, S., & Arntz, A. (2007). Successful psychotherapy reduces hypervigilance in borderline personality disorder. *Behavioral and Cognitive Psychotherapy, 35,* 387–402.

Sikich, L., Kolevzon, A., King, B. H., McDougle, C. J., Sanders, K. B., Kim, S. J., . . . Veenstra-VanderWeele, J. (2021). Intranasal oxytocin in children and adolescents with autism spectrum disorder. *New England Journal of Medicine, 385*(16), 1462–1473.

Silberstein, J., & Harvey, P. D. (2019). Cognition, social cognition, and self-assessment in schizophrenia: Prediction of different elements of everyday functional outcomes. *CNS Spectrums, 24*(1), 88–93.

Silveira, É., Jr., & Kauer-Sant'Anna, M. (2015). Rumination in bipolar disorder: A systematic review. *Revista Brasileira de Psiquiatria, 37*(3), 256–263.

Silver, J., Simons, A., & Craun, S. (2018). *A study of the pre-attack behaviors of active shooters in the United States between 2000–2013.* Washington, DC: Federal Bureau of Investigation, U.S. Department of Justice.

Sim, L. A., Sadowski, C. M., Whiteside, S. P., & Wells, L. A. (2004). Family-based therapy for adolescents with anorexia nervosa. *Mayo Clinic Proceedings, 79,* 1305–1308.

Simiola, V., Neilson, E. C., Thompson, R., & Cook, J. M. (2015). Preferences for trauma treatment: A systematic review of the empirical literature. *Psychological Trauma: Theory, Research, Practice and Policy, 7*(6), 516–524.

Simmons, A. M. (2002, January 13). Eating disorders on rise for South African blacks. *Los Angeles Times,* p. A3.

Simone, M., Telke, S., Anderson, L. M., Eisenberg, M., & Neumark-Sztainer, D. (2022). Ethnic/racial and gender differences in disordered eating behavior prevalence trajectories among women and men from adolescence into adulthood. *Social Science & Medicine (1982), 294,* 114720. https://doi.org/10.1016/j.socscimed.2022.114720

Simons, T. (2014). Local bowler finds renewed energy with silver cross sleep apnea treatment. http://joliet.patch.com/groups/silver-cross-health/p/local-bowler-finds-renewed-energy-with-silver-cross-sleep-apnea-treatment

Simpson, H. B., van den Heuvel, O. A., Miguel, E. C., Reddy, Y., Stein, D. J., Lewis-Fernández, R., . . . Wall, M. (2020). Toward identifying reproducible brain signatures of obsessive-compulsive profiles: Rationale and methods for a new global initiative. *BMC Psychiatry, 20*(1), 68. https://doi.org/10.1186/s12888-020-2439-2

Sin, J., Henderson, C., Cornelius, V., Chen, T., Elkes, J., Woodham, L. A., . . . Gillard, S. (2020). COPe-support—A multicomponent digital intervention for family carers for people affected by psychosis: Study protocol for a randomized controlled trial. *BMC Psychiatry, 20*(1), 129. https://doi.org/10.1186/s12888-020-02528-w

Singer, H. S. (2005). Tourette's syndrome: From behaviour to biology. *Lancet Neurology, 4*(3), 149–159.

Singh, N. N. (2022). Neuro case challenge: A 35-year-old with angry, aggressive outbursts, memory loss, and insomnia. https://reference.medscape.com /viewarticle/888807_2

Sinha-Deb, K., Sarkar, S., Sood, M., & Khandelwall, S. K. (2013). Wires in the body: A case of factitious disorder. *Indian Journal of Psychological Medicine, 35,* 209–221.

Siroosbakht, S., Rezakhaniha, S., & Rezakhaniha, B. (2019). Which of available selective serotonin reuptake inhibitors (SSRIs) is more effective in treatment of premature ejaculation? A randomized clinical trial. *International Journal of the Brazilian Society of Urology, 45*(6), 1209–1215.

Sisti, D., Mann, J. J., & Oquendo, M. A. (2020). Toward a distinct mental disorder-suicidal behavior. *JAMA Psychiatry, 77,* 671–672.

Skeen, S., Laurenzi, C. A., Gordon, S. L., du Toit, S., Tomlinson, M., Dua, T., . . . Melendez-Torres, G. J. (2019). Adolescent mental health program components and behavior risk reduction: A meta-analysis. *Pediatrics, 144*(2), e20183488. https://doi.org /10.1542/peds.2018-3488

Skeie-Larsen, M., Stave, R., Grønli, J., Bjorvatn, B., Wilhelmsen-Langeland, A., Zandi, A., & Pallesen, S. (2022). The effects of pharmacological treatment of nightmares: A systematic literature review and meta-analysis of placebo-controlled, randomized clinical trials. *International Journal of Environmental Research and Public Health, 20*(1), 777. https://doi .org/10.3390/ijerph20010777

Skelton, M., Khokhar, W. A., & Thacker, S. P. (2015). Treatments for delusional disorder. *Schizophrenia Bulletin, 41*(5), 1010–1012.

Skewes, M. C., & Blume, A. W. (2019). Understanding the link between racial trauma and substance use among American Indians. *The American Psychologist, 74*(1), 88–100.

Skewes, M. C., Hallum-Montes, R., Gardner, S. A., Blume, A.

W., Ricker, A., & FireMoon, P. (2019). Partnering with native communities to develop a culturally grounded intervention for substance use disorder. *American Journal of Community Psychology, 64*(1-2), 72–82.

Skinner, A. C., Ravanbakht, S. N., Skelton, J. A., Perrin, E. M., & Armstrong, S. C. (2018). Prevalence of obesity and severe obesity in US children, 1999–2016. *Pediatrics, 141*(3), e20173459. https:// doi.org/10.1542/peds.2017-3459

Skinner, B. F. (1990). Can psychology be a science of mind? *American Psychologist, 45,* 1206–1210.

Skinner, M. D., Lahmek, P., Pham, H., & Aubin, H. J. (2014). Disulfiram efficacy in the treatment of alcohol dependence: A meta-analysis. *PLOS One, 9,* e87366. https://doi.org/10.1371/journal .pone.0087366

Skoy, E. T., Eukel, H. N., Frenzel, J. E., Werremeyer, A., & McDaniel, B. (2016). Use of an auditory hallucination simulation to increase student pharmacist empathy for patients with mental illness. *American Journal of Pharmaceutical Education, 80*(8), 142. https://doi .org/10.5688/ajpe808142

Slavich, G. M., Giletta, M., Helms, S. W., Hastings, P. D., Rudolph, K. D., Nock, M. K., & Prinstein, M. J. (2020). Interpersonal life stress, inflammation, and depression in adolescence: Testing social signal transduction theory of depression. *Depression and Anxiety, 37*(2), 179–193.

Sloan, E., Hall, K., Moulding, R., Bryce, S., Mildred, H., & Staiger, P. K. (2017). Emotion regulation as a transdiagnostic treatment construct across anxiety, depression, substance, eating and borderline personality disorders: A systematic review. *Clinical Psychology Review, 57,* 141–163.

Sloane, C., Burke, S. C., Cremeens, J., Vail-Smith, K., & Woolsey, C. (2010). Drunkorexia: Calorie restriction prior to alcohol consumption among college freshman. *Journal of Alcohol and Drug Education, 54*(2), 17–34.

Smallheer, B. A., Vollman, M., & Dietrich, M. S. (2018). Learned helplessness and depressive

symptoms following myocardial infarction. *Clinical Nursing Research, 27*(5), 597–616.

Smaragdi, A., Chavez, S., Lobaugh, N. J., Meyer, J. H., & Kolla, N. J. (2019). Differential levels of prefrontal cortex glutamate+glutamine in adults with antisocial personality disorder and bipolar disorder: A proton magnetic resonance spectroscopy study. *Progress in Neuro-Psychopharmacology and Biological Psychiatry, 93,* 250–255.

Smith, A. D., Refsum, H., Bottiglieri, T., Fenech, M., Hooshmand, B., McCaddon, A., . . . Obeid, R. (2018). Homocysteine and dementia: An International consensus statement. *Journal of Alzheimer's Disease: JAD, 62*(2), 561–570. https://doi.org/10.3233 /JAD-171042

Smith, A. D., Smith, S. M., de Jager, C. A., Whitbread, P., Johnston, C., Agacinski, G., . . . Refsum, H. (2010). Homocysteine- lowering by B vitamins slows the rate of accelerated brain atrophy in mild cognitive impairment: A randomized controlled trial. *PLOS One, 5*(9), e12244. https://doi.org/10 .1371/journal.pone.0012244

Smith, A. R., Zuromski, K. L., & Dodd, D. R. (2018). Eating disorders and suicidality: What we know, what we don't know, and suggestions for future research. *Current Opinion in Psychology, 22,* 63–67.

Smith, C. S. (2003, September 27). Son's wish to die, and mother's help, stir French debate. *New York Times,* pp. A1, A4.

Smith, G. C., Clarke, D. M., Handrinos, D., Dunsis, A., & McKenzie, D. P. (2000). Consultation-liaison psychiatrists' management of somatoform disorders. *Psychosomatics, 41,* 481–489.

Smith, M. R. (2013). 50 years later, Kennedy's vision for mental health not realized. http://seattletimes.com/htm l/nationworld/2022091710_ mentalhealthxml.html

Smith, M., Segal, J., & Robinson, L. (2013). Suicide prevention. http:// www.helpguide.org/mental /suicide_prevention.htm

Smith, P. N., Cukrowicz, K. C., Poindexter, E. K., Hobson, V., & Cohen, L. M. (2010). The acquired capability for suicide: A comparison of suicide attempters, suicide ideators, and non-suicidal controls. *Depression and Anxiety*, 27, 871–877.

Snell-Rood, C., & Carpenter-Song, E. (2018). Depression in a depressed area: Deservingness, mental illness, and treatment in the contemporary rural U.S. *Social Science & Medicine (1982)*, 219, 78–86.

Snow, K. (2015). Jacob's journey: Life as a transgender 5-year-old. https://www.nbcnews.com /storyline/transgender-kids/jacob -s-journey-life-transgender-5-year -old-n345131

So, J. K. (2008). Somatization as a cultural idiom of distress: Rethinking mind and body in a multicultural society. *Counselling Psychology Quarterly*, 21, 167–174.

Soares, C. N. (2019). Depression and menopause: An update on current knowledge and clinical management for this critical window. *The Medical Clinics of North America*, 103(4), 651–667.

Soidla, K., & Akkermann, K. (2020). Perfectionism and impulsivity based risk profiles in eating disorders. *The International Journal of Eating Disorders*, 53(7), 1108–1119. https://doi.org/10 .1002/eat.23285

Sokol, Y., Levin, C., Linzer, M., Rosensweig, C., Hubner, S., Gromatsky, M., . . . Goodman, M. (2022). Theoretical model of recovery following a suicidal episode (COURAGE): Scoping review and narrative synthesis. *BJPsych Open*, 8(6), e200.

Sola, C. L., Chopra, A., & Rastogi, A. (2010). Sedative, hypnotic, anxiolytic use disorders. http:// emedicine.medscape.com /article/290585-overview

Solé, E., Garriga, M., Valentí, M., & Vieta, E. (2017). Mixed features in bipolar disorder. *CNS Spectrums*, 22(2), 134–140.

Soler, J., Arias, B., Moya, J., Ibáñez, M. I., Ortet, G., Fañanás, L., & Fatjó-Vilas, M. (2019). The interaction between the ZNF804A gene and cannabis use on the risk of psychosis in a non-clinical sample. *Progress in Neuro-psychopharmacology and Biological Psychiatry*, 89, 174–180.

Sollman, M. J., Ranseen, J. D., & Berry, D. T. R. (2010). Detection of feigned ADHD in college students. *Psychological Assessment*, 22, 325–335.

Solomon, M., Iosif, A. M., Reinhardt, V. P., Libero, L. E., Nordahl, C. W., Ozonoff, S., . . . Amaral, D. G. (2018). What will my child's future hold? Phenotypes of intellectual development in 2-8-year-olds with autism spectrum disorder. *Autism Research*, 11(1), 121–132.

Solovitch, S. (2014). Conspiracy of silence. When the psychiatrist has bp. http://www.bphope.com/Item .aspx/102/conspiracy-of-silence -when-the-psychiatrist-has-bp

Sommer, I. E., Brand, B. A., Gangadin, S., Tanskanen, A., Tiihonen, J., & Taipale, H. (2023). Women with schizophrenia-spectrum disorders after menopause: A vulnerable group for relapse. *Schizophrenia Bulletin*, 49(1), 136–143.

Sommers-Flanagan, J., & Shaw, S. L. (2017). Suicide risk assessment: What psychologists should know. *Professional Psychology: Research and Practice*, 48(2), 98–106.

Song, T. J., Lee, M. J., Choi, Y. J., Kim, B. K., Chung, P. W., Park, J., . . . Cho, S. J. (2019). Differences in characteristics and comorbidity of cluster headache according to the presence of migraine. *Journal of Clinical Neurology (Seoul, Korea)*, 15(3), 334–338. https:// doi.org/10.3988/jcn.2019.15.3.334

Songco, A., Hudson, J. L., & Fox, E. (2020). A cognitive model of pathological worry in children and adolescents: A systematic review. *Clinical Child and Family Psychology Review*, 23, 229–249.

Soreff, S., & McInnes, L. A. (2014). Bipolar affective disorder. http:// emedicine.medscape.com /article/286342-overview

Sørensen, H. J., Mortensen, E. L., Schiffman, J., Reinisch, J. M., Maeda, J., & Mednick, S. A. (2010). Early developmental milestones and risk of schizophrenia: A 45-year follow-up of the Copenhagen Perinatal Cohort. *Schizophrenia Research*, 118, 41–47.

Sørensen, K. D., Wilberg, T., Berthelsen, E., & Råbu, M. (2019). Lived experience of treatment for avoidant personality disorder: Searching for courage to be. *Frontiers in Psychology*, 10, 2879.

Sorkin, A., Weinshall, D., & Peled, A. (2008). The distortion of reality perception in schizophrenia patients, as measured in virtual reality. *Studies in Health Technology and Informatics*, 132, 475–480.

Sosoo, E. E., Bernard, D. L., & Neblett, E. W. (2020). The influence of internalized racism on the relationship between discrimination and anxiety. *Cultural Diversity and Ethnic Minority Psychology*, 26, 570–580.

Sousa Filho, D., Kanomata, E. Y., Feldman, R. J., & Maluf Neto, A. (2017). Munchausen syndrome and Munchausen syndrome by proxy: A narrative review. *Einstein (Sao Paulo, Brazil)*, 15(4), 516–521.

Sousa, G. S., Santos, M., Silva, A., Perrelli, J., & Sougey, E. B. (2017). Suicide in childhood: A literature review. *Ciência & Saúde Coletiva*, 22, 3099–3110.

Southward, M. W., & Cheavens, J. S. (2020). Quality or quantity? A multistudy analysis of emotion regulation skills deficits associated with borderline personality disorder. *Personality Disorders: Theory, Research, and Treatment*, 11(1), 24–35.

Soutullo, C., & Figueroa-Quintana, A. (2013). When do you prescribe antidepressants to depressed children? *Current Psychiatry Reports*, 15, 366. https://doi.org/10.1007 /s11920-013-0366-3

Spanos, N. P. (1978). Witchcraft in histories of psychiatry: A critical analysis and an alternative conceptualization. *Psychological Bulletin*, 85, 417–439.

Spanos, N. P. (1994). Multiple identity enactments and multiple personality disorder: A sociocognitive perspective. *Psychological Bulletin*, 116, 143–165.

Spence, S. H., Donovan, C. L., March, S., Gamble, A., Anderson, R., Prosser, S., . . . Kenardy, J.

(2008). Online CBT in the treatment of child and adolescent anxiety disorders: Issues in the development of BRAVE–ONLINE and two case illustrations. *Behavioural and Cognitive Psychotherapy*, 36, 411–430.

Spencer-Thomas, S. (2018). "Man therapy": Engaging men in their mental health. https://www.irmi.com/articles/expert-commentary/man-therapy-engaging-men-in-their-mental-health

Spielmans, G. I., Jureidini, J., Healy, D., & Purssey, R. (2013). Inappropriate data and measures lead to questionable conclusions. *JAMA Psychiatry*, 70, 121–123.

Spielmans, G. I., Spence-Sing, T., & Parry, P. (2020). Duty to warn: Antidepressant black box suicidality warning is empirically justified. *Frontiers in Psychiatry*, 11, 18. https://doi.org/10.3389/fpsyt.2020.00018

Spinhoven, P., van Hemert, A. M., & Penninx, B. W. (2018). Repetitive negative thinking as a predictor of depression and anxiety: A longitudinal cohort study. *Journal of Affective Disorders*, 241, 216–225.

Spira, A. P., Gamaldo, A. A., An, Y., Wu, M. N., Simonsick, E. M., Bilgel, M., . . . Resnick, S. M. (2013). Self-reported sleep and b-amyloid deposition in community-dwelling older adults. *JAMA Neurology*, 70, 1537–1543.

Spitzer, R. L., Gibbon, M., Skodol, A. E., Williams, J. B., & First, M. B. (Eds.). (1994). *DSM-IV: Casebook* (pp. 121–122). Washington, DC: American Psychiatric Publishing.

Sprayregen, M. (2023). Here are all the anti-trans bills that have become law in 2023. https://www.lgbtqnation.com/2023/03/here-are-all-the-anti-trans-bills-that-have-become-law-in-2023/

Sproch, L. E., & Anderson, K. P. (2018). A novel in-home relapse prevention treatment for anorexia nervosa. *Clinical Case Studies*, 17, 499–514.

St. Louis, E. K., & Boeve, B. F. (2017). REM sleep behavior disorder: Diagnosis, clinical implications, and future directions. *Mayo Clinic Proceedings*, 92(11), 1723–1736.

Stabouli, S., Erdine, S., Suurorg, L., Jankauskienė, A., & Lurbe, E. (2021). Obesity and eating disorders in children and adolescents: The bidirectional link. *Nutrients*, 13(12), 4321. https://doi.org/10.3390/nu13124321

Stahl, E. A., Breen, G., Forstner, A. J., McQuillin, A., Ripke, S., Trubetskoy, V., . . . Bipolar Disorder Working Group of the Psychiatric Genomics Consortium. (2019). Genome-wide association study identifies 30 loci associated with bipolar disorder. *Nature Genetics*, 51(5), 793–803.

Stallman, H. M., Kohler, M., & White, J. (2018). Medication induced sleepwalking: A systematic review. *Sleep Medicine Reviews*, 37, 105–113.

Stanciu, C. N., Penders, T. M., & Rouse, E. M. (2016). Recreational use of dextromethorphan, "robotripping"—A brief review. *American Journal on Addictions*, 25(5), 374–377.

Stanford, F. C., Tauqeer, Z., & Kyle, T. K. (2018). Media and its influence on obesity. *Current Obesity Reports*, 7(2), 186–192. https://doi.org/10.1007/s13679-018-0304-0

Starcevic, V., & Janca, A. (2018). Pharmacotherapy of borderline personality disorder: Replacing confusion with prudent pragmatism. *Current Opinion in Psychiatry*, 31(1), 69–73.

Stargell, N. A., Kress, V. E., Paylo, M. J., & Zins, A. (2016). Excoriation disorder: Assessment, diagnosis and treatment. *The Professional Counselor*, 6, 50–60.

Stark, J. (2004, July 25). Twin sisters, a singular affliction. *Bellingham Herald*, p. A1.

Stefanidis, E. (2006). Being rational. *Schizophrenia Bulletin*, 32, 422–423.

Stehman, C. R., Testo, Z., Gershaw, R. S., & Kellogg, A. R. (2019). Burnout, drop out, suicide: Physician loss in emergency medicine, part I. *Western Journal of Emergency Medicine*, 20, 485–494.

Stein, A., Craske, M. G., Lehtonen, A., Harvey, A., Savage-McGlynn, E., Davies, B., . . . Counsell, N. (2012). Maternal cognitions and mother–infant interaction in postnatal depression and generalized anxiety disorder. *Journal of Abnormal Psychology*, 121, 795–809.

Stein, G. L., Castro-Schilo, L., Cavanaugh, A. M., Mejia, Y., Christophe, N. K., & Robins, R. (2019). When discrimination hurts: The longitudinal impact of increases in peer discrimination on anxiety and depressive symptoms in Mexican-origin youth. *Journal of Youth and Adolescence*, 48(5), 864–875.

Steinberg, J. S., Arshad, A., Kowalski, M., Kukar, A., Suma, V., Vloka, M., . . . Rozanski, A. (2004). Increased incidence of life-threatening ventricular arrhythmias in implantable defibrillator patients after the World Trade Center attack. *Journal of the American College of Cardiology*, 44, 1261–1264.

Steiner, T. J., Stovner, L. J., Jensen, R., Uluduz, D., Katsarava, Z., & Lifting the Burden: The Global Campaign against Headache. (2020). Migraine remains second among the world's causes of disability, and first among young women: Findings from GBD2019. *The Journal of Headache and Pain*, 21(1), 137. https://doi.org/10.1186/s10194-020-01208-0

Steinhausen, H. C., & Weber, S. (2009). The outcome of bulimia nervosa: Findings from one-quarter century of research. *American Journal of Psychiatry*, 166, 1331–1341.

Stemper, B. D., Shah, A. S., Harezlak, J., Rowson, S., Mihalik, J. P., Duma, S. M., . . . CARE Consortium Investigators. (2019). Comparison of head impact exposure between concussed football athletes and matched controls: Evidence for a possible second mechanism of sport-related concussion. *Annals of Biomedical Engineering*, 47(10), 2057–2072.

Stephenson, K. R., & Meston, C. M. (2016). Heterosexual women's causal attributions regarding impairment in sexual function: Factor structure and associations with well-being. *Archives of Sexual Behavior*, 45(8), 1989–2001.

Stepp, S., Chung, T., & King, K. M. (2021). Substance use and sexual minority status: Examining the mediating roles of stress and emotion dysregulation in young adult women. *Clinical Psychological Science, 9*(6), 1095–1114.

Stern, R. A., Adler, C. H., Chen, K., Navitsky, M., Luo, J., Dodick, D. W., . . . Reiman, E. M. (2019). Tau positron-emission tomography in former National Football League players. *New England Journal of Medicine, 380*(18), 1716–1725.

Stetka, B. S., Christoph, U., & Correll, M. D. (2013, May 21). A guide to DSM-5. *Medscape.* http://www.medscape.com/viewarticle/803884_1

Stettin, G. (2020). *America's state of mind U.S. trends in medication use for depression, anxiety and insomnia.* https://www.express-scripts.com/corporate/americas-state-of-mind-report

Stevens, M., King, D. L., Dorstyn, D., & Delfabbro, P. H. (2019). Cognitive-behavioral therapy for Internet gaming disorder: A systematic review and meta-analysis. *Clinical Psychology and Psychotherapy, 26*(2), 191–203.

Stevenson-Hoare, J., Heslegrave, A., Leonenko, G., Fathalla, D., Bellou, E., Luckcuck, L., . . . Escott-Price, V. (2023, February 13). Plasma biomarkers and genetics in the diagnosis and prediction of Alzheimer's disease. *Brain, 146*(2), 690–699. https://doi.org/10.1093/brain/awac128.

Stewart, J. G., Shields, G. S., Esposito, E. C., Cosby, E. A., Allen, N. B., Slavich, G. M., & Auerbach, R. P. (2019). Life stress and suicide in adolescents. *Journal of Abnormal Child Psychology, 47*(10), 1707–1722.

Stice, E., Gau, J. M., Rohde, P., & Shaw, H. (2017). Risk factors that predict future onset of each DSM-5 eating disorder: Predictive specificity in high-risk adolescent females. *Journal of Abnormal Psychology, 126*(1), 38–51.

Stice, E., Marti, C. N., & Rohde, P. (2013). Prevalence, incidence, impairment, and course of the proposed DSM-5 eating disorder diagnoses in an 8-year prospective community study of young women. *Journal of Abnormal Psychology, 122*(2), 445–457.

Stice, E., Marti, C. N., Shaw, H., & Jaconis, M. (2009). An 8-year longitudinal study of the natural history of threshold, subthreshold, and partial eating disorders from a community sample of adolescents. *Journal of Abnormal Psychology, 118,* 587–597.

Stiles, B. L., & Clark, R. E. (2011). BDSM: A subcultural analysis of sacrifices and delights. *Deviant Behavior, 32,* 158–189.

Stilo, S. A., & Murray, R. M. (2019). Non-genetic factors in schizophrenia. *Current Psychiatry Reports, 21*(10), 100. https://doi.org/10.1007/s11920-019-1091-3

Stone, D. M., Holland, K. M., Bartholow, B., Crosby, A. E., Davis, S., & Wilkins, N. (2017). Preventing suicide: A technical package of policies, programs, and practices. Atlanta: National Center for Injury Prevention and Control, Centers for Disease Control and Prevention.

Stone, D. M., Mack, K. A., & Qualters, J. (2023). Notes from the field: Recent changes in suicide rates, by race and ethnicity and age group: United States, 2021. *MMWR: Morbidity and Mortality Weekly Report, 72,* 160–162.

Stone, D. M., Simon, T. R., Fowler, K. A., Kegler, S. R., Yuan, K., Holland, K. M., . . . Crosby, A. E. (2018). Vital signs: Trends in state suicide rates—United States, 1999–2016 and circumstances contributing to suicide—27 states, 2015. *Morbidity and Mortality Weekly Report, 67,* 617–624.

Stoner, R., Chow, M. L., Boyle, M. P., Sunkin, S. M., Mouton, P. R., Roy, S., . . . Courchesne, E. (2014). Patches of disorganization in the neocortex of children with autism. *New England Journal of Medicine, 370,* 1209–1219.

Storebø, O. J., Stoffers-Winterling, J. M., Völlm, B. A., Kongerslev, M. T., Mattivi, J. T., Jørgensen, M. S., . . . Simonsen, E. (2020). Psychological therapies for people with borderline personality disorder. *Cochrane Database of Systematic Reviews, 5*(5), CD012955. https://doi.org/10.1002/14651858.CD012955.pub2

Stossel, S. (2014). Surviving anxiety. http://www.theatlantic.com/magazine/archive/2014/01/surviving_anxiety/355741

St-Pierre-Delorme, M.-E., Lalonde, M. P., Perreault, V., Koszegi, N., & O'Connor, K. (2011). Inference-based therapy for compulsive hoarding: A clinical case study. *Clinical Case Studies, 10,* 291–303.

Strain, J. J. (2018). The psychobiology of stress, depression, adjustment disorders and resilience. *The World Journal of Biological Psychiatry, 19*(Suppl 1), S14–S20.

Strain, J. J. (2019). The adjustment disorder diagnosis, its importance to liaison psychiatry, and its psychobiology. *International Journal of Environmental Research and Public Health, 16*(23), 4645. https://doi.org/10.3390/ijerph16234645

Straub, R. H., & Cutolo, M. (2018). Psychoneuroimmunology—Developments in stress research. *Wiener Medizinische Wochenschrift (1946), 168*(3–4), 76–84.

Straube, A., & Andreou, A. (2019). Primary headaches during lifespan. *The Journal of Headache and Pain, 20*(1), 35. https://doi.org/10.1186/s10194-019-0985-0

Strauss, A. Y., Kivity, Y., & Huppert, J. D. (2019). Emotion regulation strategies in cognitive behavioral therapy for panic disorder. *Behavior Therapy, 50*(3), 659–671.

Strauss, G. P., Harrow, M., Grossman, L. S., & Rosen, C. (2010). Periods of recovery in deficit syndrome schizophrenia: A 20-year multi-follow-up longitudinal study. *Schizophrenia Bulletin, 36*(4), 788–799.

Strawn, J. R., Welge, J. A., Wehry, A. M., Keeshin, B., & Rynn, M. A. (2015). Efficacy and tolerability of antidepressants in pediatric anxiety disorders: A systematic review and meta-analysis. *Depression and Anxiety, 32,* 149–157. https://doi.org/10.1002/da.22329

Strobel, C., Quadflieg, N., Voderholzer, U., Naab, S., & Fichter, M. M. (2018). Short- and long-term outcome of males treated for anorexia nervosa: A review of the literature. *Eating and Weight Disorders, 23*(5), 541–552.

Stroebel, S. S., O'Keefe, S. L., Beard, K. W., Kuo, S. Y., Swindell, S. V., & Kommor, M. J. (2012). Father-daughter incest: Data from an anonymous computerized survey. *Journal of Child Sexual Abuse, 21*(2), 176–199.

Stroebel, S. S., O'Keefe, S. L., Beard, K. W., Kuo, S. Y., Swindell, S., & Stroupe, W. (2013a). Brother-sister incest: Data from anonymous computer-assisted self interviews. *Journal of Child Sexual Abuse, 22*, 255–276.

Stroebel, S. S., O'Keefe, S. L., Griffee, K., Kuo, S. Y., Beard, K. W., & Kommor, M. J. (2013b). Sister-sister incest: Data from an anonymous computerized survey. *Journal of Child Sexual Abuse, 22*, 695–719.

Ströhle, A., Gensichen, J., & Domschke, K. (2018). The diagnosis and treatment of anxiety disorders. *Deutsches Arzteblatt International, 155*(37), 611–620.

Strong, Y. N., Cao, D. Y., Zhou, J., Guenther, M. A., Anderson, D. J., Kaye, A. D., . . . Urits, I. (2023). Koro syndrome: Epidemiology, psychiatric and physical risk factors, clinical presentation, diagnosis, and treatment options. *Health Psychology Research, 11*, 70165. https://doi.org/10.52965/001c.70165

Stroup, T. S., & Gray, N. (2018). Management of common adverse effects of antipsychotic medications. *World Psychiatry, 17*(3), 341–356.

Stubbe, D. E. (2019). Engaging youths for accurate risk assessment in the context of school shootings. *Focus, 17*, 387–390.

Su, Y., & Zheng, L. (2023). Stability and change in asexuality: Relationship between sexual/romantic attraction and sexual desire. *Journal of Sex Research, 60*(2), 231–241.

Su, Z., Mackert, M., Li, X., Han, J. K., Cook, B., & Wyeth, B. (2020). "Study natural" without drugs: An exploratory study of theory-guided and tailored health campaign interventions to prevent nonmedical use of prescription stimulants in college students. *International Journal of Environmental Research and Public Health, 17*(12), 4421. https://doi.org/10.3390/ijerph17124421

Substance Abuse and Mental Health Services Administration (SAMHSA). (2012). *National strategy for suicide prevention 2012: How you can play a role in preventing suicide.* Washington, DC: Substance Abuse and Mental Health Services Administration.

Substance Abuse and Mental Health Services Administration (SAMHSA). (2015). *A journey toward help and hope: Your handbook for recovery after a suicide attempt.* HHS Publication No. SMA-15-4419. Rockville, MD: Center for Mental Health Services, Substance Abuse and Mental Health Services Administration.

Substance Abuse and Mental Health Services Administration (SAMHSA). (2019). *Key substance use and mental health indicators in the United States: Results from the 2018 National Survey on Drug Use and Health.* Rockville, MD: Center for Behavioral Health Statistics and Quality, Substance Abuse and Mental Health Services Administration. https://www.samhsa.gov/data/sites/default/files/cbhsq-reports/NSDUHNationalFindings Report2018/NSDUHNational FindingsReport2018.htm#suicidal

Substance Abuse and Mental Health Services Administration (SAMHSA). (2022). *Key substance use and mental health indicators in the United States: Results from the 2021 National Survey on Drug Use and Health* (HHS Publication No. PEP22-07-01-005, NSDUH Series H-57). Center for Behavioral Health Statistics and Quality, Substance Abuse and Mental Health Services Administration. https://www.samhsa.gov/data/report/2021-nsduh-annual-national-report

Substance Abuse and Mental Health Services Administration (SAMHSA). (2023a). *2021 National Survey on Drug Use and Health.* https://www.samhsa.gov/data/sites/default/files/2022-12/2021NSDUHFFRHighlights092722.pdf

Substance Abuse and Mental Health Services Administration (SAMHSA). (2023b). Results from the 2021 National Survey on Drug Use and Health: Graphics from the key findings report. https://www.samhsa.gov/data/sites/default/files/reports/rpt39443/2021_NNR_figure_slides.pdf

Sudhakar, V., & Richardson, R. M. (2019). Gene therapy for neurodegenerative diseases. *Neurotherapeutics, 16*(1), 166–175.

Sue, D., & Sue, D. M. (2008). *Foundations of counseling and psychotherapy: Evidence-based practices for a diverse society.* Hoboken, NJ: John Wiley & Sons.

Sue, D. W., Sue, D., Neville, H. A., & Smith, L. (2022). *Counseling the culturally diverse* (9th ed.). Hoboken, NJ: John Wiley & Sons.

Sugawara, H., Tsutsumi, T., Inada, K., Ishigooka, J., Hashimoto, M., Takebayashi, M., & Nishimura, K. (2019). Association between anxious distress in a major depressive episode and bipolarity. *Neuropsychiatric Disease and Treatment, 15*, 267–270.

Sugg, N. (2015). Intimate partner violence: Prevalence, health consequences, and intervention. *The Medical Clinics of North America, 99*(3), 629–649.

Suglia, S. F., Solnick, S., & Hemenway, D. (2013). Soft drinks consumption is associated with behavior problems in 5-year-olds. *Journal of Pediatrics, 163*, 1323–1328.

Suh, B., & Luthar, S. S. (2020). Parental aggravation may tell more about a child's mental/behavioral health than adverse childhood experiences: Using the 2016 National Survey of Children's Health. *Child Abuse and Neglect, 101*, 104330. https://doi.org/10.1016/j.chiabu.2019.104330

Sultan, R. S., Correll, C. U., Schoenbaum, M., King, M., Walkup, J. T., & Olfson, M. (2018). National patterns of commonly prescribed psychotropic medications to young people. *Journal of Child and Adolescent Psychopharmacology, 28*(3), 158–165.

Sultan, R. S., Wang, S., Crystal, S., & Olfson, M. (2019). Antipsychotic treatment among youths with attention-deficit/hyperactivity disorder. *JAMA Network Open, 2*(7), e197850. https://doi.org/10.1001/jamanetworkopen.2019.7850

Sun, M., Rith-Najarian, L. R., Williamson, T. J., & Chorpita, B. F. (2019). Treatment features associated with youth cognitive behavioral therapy follow-up effects for internalizing disorders: A meta-analysis. *Journal of Clinical Child and Adolescent Psychology*, 48(Suppl 1), S269–S283.

Sundstrom, E. (2004). First person account: The clogs. *Schizophrenia Bulletin*, 30, 191–192.

Suominen, K., Mantere, O., Valtonen, H., Arvilommi, P., Leppämäki, S., & Isometsä, E. (2009). Gender differences in bipolar disorder type I and II. *Acta Psychiatrica Scandanavica*, 120, 464–473.

Surgeon General's Advisory. (2023). Our epidemic of loneliness and isolation. https://www.hhs.gov/sites/default/files/surgeon-general-social-connection-advisory.pdf

Svob, C., Wickramaratne, P. J., Reich, L., Zhao, R., Talati, A., Gameroff, M. J., . . . Weissman, M. M. (2018). Association of parent and offspring religiosity with offspring suicide ideation and attempts. *JAMA Psychiatry*, 75(10), 1062–1070.

Swan, A. J., Kendall, P. C., Olino, T., Ginsburg, G., Keeton, C., Compton, S., . . . Albano, A. M. (2018). Results from the Child/Adolescent Anxiety Multimodal Longitudinal Study (CAMELS): Functional outcomes. *Journal of Consulting and Clinical Psychology*, 86(9), 738–750.

Swanson, S. A., & Colman, I. (2013). Association between exposure to suicide and suicidality outcomes in youth. *Canadian Medical Association Journal*, 185, 870–877.

Swartz, M. S., Bhattacharya, S., Robertson, A. G., & Swanson, J. W. (2017). Involuntary outpatient commitment and the elusive pursuit of violence prevention: A view from the United States. *Canadian Journal of Psychiatry*, 62, 102–108.

Swendsen, J., Burstein, M., Case, B., Conway, K. P., Dierker, L., He, J., & Merikangas, K. R. (2012). Use and abuse of alcohol and illicit drugs in US adolescents: Results of the National Comorbidity Survey—Adolescent supplement. *Archives of General Psychiatry*, 69, 390–398.

Szaflarski, M., Klepinger, D. H., & Cubbins, L. A. (2019). Alcohol use/abuse and help-seeking among U.S. adults: The role of racial-ethnic origin and foreign-born status. *Journal of Ethnicity in Substance Abuse*, 18(2), 183–210.

Szasz, T. S. (1987). Justifying coercion through theology and therapy. In J. K. Zeig (Ed.), *The evolution of psychotherapy* (pp. 158–174). New York: Brunner/Mazel.

Szuhany, K. L., Malgaroli, M., Miron, C. D., & Simon, N. M. (2021). Prolonged grief disorder: Course, diagnosis, assessment, and treatment. *Focus*, 19(2), 161–172. https://doi.org/10.1176/appi.focus.20200052

Taghizadeh, N., Eslaminejad, A., & Raoufy, M. R. (2019). Protective effect of heart rate variability biofeedback on stress-induced lung function impairment in asthma. *Respiratory Physiology and Neurobiology*, 262, 49–56.

Takaesu, Y. (2018). Circadian rhythm in bipolar disorder: A review of the literature. *Psychiatry and Clinical Neurosciences*, 72(9), 673–682.

Takahashi, T., Tsunoda, M., Miyashita, M., Ogihara, T., Okada, Y., Hagiwara, T., . . . Amano, N. (2011). Comparison of diagnostic names of mental illnesses in medical documents before and after the adoption of a new Japanese translation of "schizophrenia." *Psychiatry and Clinical Neurosciences*, 65, 89–94.

Takayanagi, Y., Sasabayashi, D., Takahashi, T., Furuichi, A., Kido, M., Nishikawa, Y., . . . Suzuki, M. (2020). Reduced cortical thickness in schizophrenia and schizotypal disorder. *Schizophrenia Bulletin*, 46(2), 387–394.

Takeuchi, H., Suzuki, T., Remington, G., Bies, R. R., Abe, T., Graff-Guerrero, A., . . . Uchida, H. (2012). Effects of risperidone and olanzapine dose reduction on cognitive function in stable patients with schizophrenia: An open-label, randomized, controlled, pilot study. *Schizophrenia Bulletin*, 39, 993–998.

Takeuchi, J. (2000). Treatment of a biracial child with schizophreniform disorder: Cultural formulation. *Cultural Diversity and Ethnic Minority Psychology*, 6, 93–101.

Talarowska, M. (2020). Epigenetic mechanisms in the neurodevelopmental theory of depression. *Depression Research and Treatment*, 2020, 6357873. https://doi.org/10.1155/2020/6357873

Talavage, T. M., Nauman, E. A., Breedlove, E. L., Yoruk, U., Dye, A. E., Morigaki, K., . . . Leverenz, L. J. (2014). Functionally-detected cognitive impairment in high school football players without clinically-diagnosed concussion. *Journal of Neurotrauma*, 31, 327–338.

Tanaka, T., Yamamoto, T., & Haruno, M. (2017). Brain response patterns to economic inequity predict present and future depression indices. *Nature Human Behaviour*, 1(10), 748–756.

Tariq, S., & Barber, P. A. (2018). Dementia risk and prevention by targeting modifiable vascular risk factors. *Journal of Neurochemistry*, 144(5), 565–581.

Tarr, P. (2018). Homelessness and mental illness: A challenge to our society. https://www.bbrfoundation.org/sites/default/files/pdfs/bb_magazine-september2018.pdf

Tatu, L., Aybek, S., & Bogousslavsky, J. (2018). Munchausen syndrome and the wide spectrum of factitious disorders. *Frontiers of Neurology and Neuroscience*, 42, 81–86.

Tatulian, S. A. (2022). Challenges and hopes for Alzheimer's disease. *Drug Discovery Today*, 27(4), 1027–1043. https://doi.org/10.1016/j.drudis.2022.01.016

Taylor, C. A., Bell, J. M., Breiding, M. J., & Xu, L. (2017). Traumatic brain injury-related emergency department visits, hospitalizations, and deaths: United States, 2007 and 2013. *Morbidity and Mortality Weekly Report: Surveillance Summaries (Washington, DC: 2002)*, 66(9), 1–16. https://doi.org/10.15585/mmwr.ss6609a1

Taylor, C. T., Pearlstein, S. L., Kakaria, S., Lyubomirsky, S., & Stein, M. B. (2020). Enhancing social connectedness in anxiety and depression through amplification of positivity: Preliminary treatment outcomes and process of change. *Cognitive Therapy and Research*, 44(4), 788–800.

Taylor, K. N., Harper, S., & Chadwick, P. (2009). Impact of mindfulness on cognition and affect in voice hearing: Evidence from two case studies. *Behavioural and Cognitive Psychotherapy*, 37, 397–402.

Tedeschi, R. G., & McNally, R. J. (2011). Can we facilitate posttraumatic growth in combat veterans? *American Psychologist*, 66, 19–24.

Terman, L. M., & Merrill, M. A. (1960). *Stanford-Binet intelligence scale*. Boston: Houghton Mifflin.

Testai, F. D., Gorelick, P. B., Aparicio, H. J., Filbey, F. M., Gonzalez, R., Gottesman, R. F., . . . Song, S. Y. (2022). Use of marijuana: Effect on brain health. A scientific statement from the American Heart Association. *Stroke*, 53(4), e176–e187. https://doi.org/10.1161/STR.0000000000000396

Tetteh-Quarshie, S., & Risher, M. L. (2023). Adolescent brain maturation and the neuropathological effects of binge drinking: A critical review. *Frontiers in Neuroscience*, 16, 1040049. https://doi.org/10.3389/fnins.2022.1040049

Thaker, V. V., Osganian, S. K., deFerranti, S. D., Sonneville, K. R., Cheng, J. K., Feldman, H. A., & Richmond, T. K. (2020). Psychosocial, behavioral and clinical correlates of children with overweight and obesity. *BMC Pediatrics*, 20(1), 291. https://doi.org/10.1186/s12887-020-02145-2

The Lancet Neurology. (2010). Dispelling the stigma of Huntington's disease. *The Lancet Neurology*, 9, 751. https://doi.org/10.1016/S1474-4422(10)70170-8

Thippaiah, S. M., George, V., Birur, B., & Pandurangi, A. (2018). A case of concomitant pseudocyesis and Couvade syndrome variant. *Psychopharmacology Bulletin*, 48(3), 29–32.

Thom, A., Sartory, G., & Johren, P. (2000). Comparison between one-session psychological treatment and benzodiazepine in dental phobia. *Journal of Consulting and Clinical Psychology*, 68, 378–387.

Thomas, L. (2019). Diagnostic criteria for orthorexia. https://www.news-medical.net/health/Diagnostic-Criteria-for-Orthorexia.aspx

Thomas, P. (1995). Thought disorder or communication disorder: Linguistic science provides a new approach. *British Journal of Psychiatry*, 166, 287–290.

Thompson, J., Stansfeld, J. L., Cooper, R. E., Morant, N., Crellin, N. E., & Moncrieff, J. (2020). Experiences of taking neuroleptic medication and impacts on symptoms, sense of self and agency: A systematic review and thematic synthesis of qualitative data. *Social Psychiatry and Psychiatric Epidemiology*, 55(2), 151–164.

Thompson, M., & Gibbs, N. (2012, July 23). Why can't the army win the war on suicide? *Time*, pp. 23–31.

Thompson, P. M., Vidal, C., Giedd, J. N., Gochman, P., Blumenthal, J., Nicolson, R., . . . Rapoport, J. L. (2001). Mapping adolescent brain change reveals dynamic wave of accelerated gray matter loss in very early-onset schizophrenia. *Proceedings of the National Academy of Sciences*, 98, 11650–11655.

Thorgaard, M. V., Frostholm, L., Walker, L., Jensen, J. S., Morina, B., Lindegaard, H., . . . Rask, C. U. (2017). Health anxiety by proxy in women with severe health anxiety: A case control study. *Journal of Anxiety Disorders*, 52, 8–14.

Thorndike, R. L., Hagen, E. P., & Sattler, J. M. (1986). *The Stanford-Binet intelligence scale: Guide for administration and scoring* (3rd ed.). Chicago: Riverside.

Thurston, R. C., & Kubzansky, L. D. (2009). Women, loneliness, and incident coronary heart disease. *Psychosomatic Medicine*, 71, 836–842.

Thurston, R. C., Chang, Y., Matthews, K. A., von Känel, R., & Koenen, K. (2019). Association of sexual harassment and sexual assault with midlife women's mental and physical health. *JAMA Internal Medicine*, 179(1), 48–53.

Thylstrup, B., & Hesse, M. (2009). "I am not complaining"—Ambivalence construct in schizoid personality disorder. *American Journal of Psychotherapy*, 63, 147–167.

Thylstrup, B., Schrøder, S., Fridell, M., & Hesse, M. (2017). Did you get any help? A post-hoc secondary analysis of a randomized controlled trial of psychoeducation for patients with antisocial personality disorder in outpatient substance abuse treatment programs. *BMC Psychiatry*, 17(1), 7. https://doi.org/10.1186/s12888-016-1165-2

Tierney, J. (1988, July 3). Research finds lower-level workers bear brunt of work- place stress. *Seattle Post Intelligencer*, pp. K1–K3.

Tindle, H. A., Chang, Y.-F., Kuller, L. H., Manson, J. E., Robinson, J. G., Rosal, M. C., . . . Matthews, K. A. (2009). Optimism, cynical hostility, and incident coronary heart disease and mortality in the Women's Health Initiative. *Circulation*, 120, 656–662.

Titus-Lay, E., Eid, T. J., Kreys, T. J., Chu, B., & Malhotra, A. (2020). Trichotillomania associated with a 25-hydroxy vitamin D deficiency: A case report. *The Mental Health Clinician*, 10(1), 38–43.

Tobin, J. J., & Friedman, J. (1983). Spirits, shamans, and nightmare death: Survivor stress in a Hmong refugee. *American Journal of Orthopsychiatry*, 53, 439–448.

Todd, C. L. (2018). Compulsive sexual behavior is now recognized as a disorder, but it isn't the same as sex addiction. https://www.msn.com/en-us/health/sexualhealth/compulsive-sexual-behavior-is-now-recognized-as-a-disorder-but-it-isn%e2%80%99t-the-same-as-sex-addiction/ar-BBL9rGM?li=BBnba9O

Toledo, F., Dubé, J. J., Goodpaster, B. H., Stefanovic-Racic, M., Coen, P. M., & DeLany, J. P. (2018). Mitochondrial respiration is associated with lower energy expenditure and lower aerobic capacity in African American women. *Obesity*, 26(5), 903–909.

Tolin, D. F., Frost, R. O., Steketee, G., & Muroff, J. (2015). Cognitive behavioral therapy for hoarding disorder: A meta-analysis. *Depression and Anxiety*, 32(3), 158–166.

Tolin, D. F., Hallion, L. S., Wootton, B. M., Levy, H. C., Billingsley, A. L., Das, A., . . . Stevens, M. C. (2018). Subjective cognitive function in hoarding disorder. *Psychiatry Research*, 265, 215–220.

Tomita, K. K., Testa, R. J., & Balsam, K. F. (2019). Gender-affirming medical interventions and mental health in transgender adults. *Psychology of Sexual Orientation and Gender Diversity*, 6, 182–193.

Tomiyama, A. J. (2019). Stress and obesity. *Annual Review of Psychology*, 70, 703–718.

Tomiyama, A. J., Hunger, J. M., Nguyen-Cuu, J., & Wells, C. (2016). Misclassification of cardiometabolic health when using body mass index categories in NHANES 2005–2012. *International Journal of Obesity (2005)*, 40(5), 883–886.

Torgerson, T., Khojasteh, J., & Vassar, M. (2020). Public awareness for a sexual assault hotline following a *Grey's Anatomy* episode. *JAMA Internal Medicine*, 180, 456–458.

Torres-Ferrús, M., Ursitti, F., Alpuente, A., Brunello, F., Chiappino, D., de Vries, T., . . . School of Advanced Studies of European Headache Federation (EHF-SAS) (2020). From transformation to chronification of migraine: Pathophysiological and clinical aspects. *The Journal of Headache and Pain*, 21(1), 42. https://doi.org/10.1186/s10194-020-01111-8

Tozzi, L., Farrell, C., Booij, L., Doolin, K., Nemoda, Z., Szyf, M., . . . Frodl, T. (2018). Epigenetic changes of FKBP5 as a link connecting genetic and environmental risk factors with structural and functional brain changes in major depression. *Neuropsychopharmacology*, 43(5), 1138–1145.

Trefan, L., Houston, R., Pearson, G., Edwards, R., Hyde, P., Maconochie, I., . . . Kemp, A. (2016). Epidemiology of children with head injury: A national overview. *Archives of Disease in Childhood*, 101(6), 527–532.

Treichel, J. (2011). Ignoring cultural factors can compromise therapy. http://psychnews.psychiatryonline.org/newsarticle.aspx?articleid5115860

Trevor Project. (2019). The Trevor Project research brief: Data on transgender youth. https://www.thetrevorproject.org/wp-content/uploads/2019/02/The-Trevor-Project-Research-Brief-February-2019.pdf

Trimble, M. (2019). WHO: Anti-vaccine movement a top threat in 2019. https://www.usnews.com/news/national-news/articles/2019-01-16/who-names-vaccine-hesitancy-as-top-world-threat-in-2019

Tron, G. (2019). Where is Trisha Meili, the Central Park jogger, now? https://www.oxygen.com/martinis-murder/where-is-trisha-meili-the-central-park-jogger-now

Truesdell, J. (2020). Munchausen by proxy moms: These mothers harmed their children to gain sympathy for themselves. https://people.com/crime/munchausen-moms-gallery-harmed-children-sympathy/?

Tse, S., Tsoi, E. W., Hamilton, B., O'Hagan, M., Shepherd, G., Slade, M., . . . Petrakis, M. (2016). Uses of strength-based interventions for people with serious mental illness: A critical review. *International Journal of Social Psychiatry*, 62, 281–291.

Tsiachristas, A., Thomas, T., Leal, J., & Lennox, B. R. (2016). Economic impact of early intervention in psychosis services: Results from a longitudinal retrospective controlled study in England. *BMJ Open*, 6(10), e012611. https://doi.org/10.1136/bmjopen-2016-012611

Tsoulis-Reay, A. (2016). What it's like to be a celibate pedophile. http://nymag.com/scienceofus/2016/08/what-its-like-to-be-a-celibate-pedophile.html

Tucker, C. (2012). New research aimed at mental health: U.S. veterans struggle with pain, stigma of post-traumatic stress. *Nations Health*, 42, 1–12.

Tunks, E. R., Weir, R., & Crook, J. (2008). Epidemiologic perspective on chronic pain treatment. *Canadian Journal of Psychiatry*, 53, 235–242.

Turban, J. L., King, D., Carswell, J. M., & Keuroghlian, A. S. (2020). Pubertal suppression for transgender youth and risk of suicidal ideation. *Pediatrics*, 145(2), e20191725. https://doi.org/10.1542/peds.2019-1725

Turner, E. H., Matthews, A. M., Linardatos, E., Tell, R. A., & Rosenthal, R. (2008). Selective publication of antidepressant trials and its influence on apparent efficacy. *New England Journal of Medicine*, 358, 252–257.

Turner, S., Mota, N., Bolton, J., & Sareen, J. (2018). Self-medication with alcohol or drugs for mood and anxiety disorders: A narrative review of the epidemiological literature. *Depression and Anxiety*, 35(9), 851–860.

Turnwald, B. P., Goyer, J. P., Boles, D. Z., Silder, A., Delp, S. L., & Crum, A. J. (2019). Learning one's genetic risk changes physiology independent of actual genetic risk. *Nature Human Behaviour*, 3(1), 48–56.

Turtle, L., & Robertson, M. M. (2008). Tics, twitches, tales: The experiences of Gilles de la Tourette's syndrome. *American Journal of Orthopsychiatry*, 78, 449–455.

Turton, R., Chami, R., & Treasure, J. (2017). Emotional eating, binge eating and animal models of binge-type eating disorders. *Current Obesity Reports*, 6(2), 217–228.

Twenge, J. M., Sherman, R. A., & Wells, B. E. (2016). Changes in American adults' reported same-sex sexual experiences and attitudes, 1973–2014. *Archives of Sexual Behavior*, 45, 1713–1730.

Twohig, M. P., & Levin, M. E. (2017). Acceptance and Commitment Therapy as a treatment for anxiety and depression: A review. *The Psychiatric Clinics of North America*, 40(4), 751–770.

Tynan, W. D. (2008). Oppositional defiant disorder. http://emedicine.medscape.com/article/918095-print

Tynan, W. D. (2010). Conduct disorder. http://emedicine.medscape.com/article/918213-print

Tyson, P., Law, C., Reed, S., Johnsey, E., Aruna, O., & Hall, S. (2016). Preventing suicide and self-harm. *Crisis*, 37(5), 353–360.

U.S. Census Bureau. (2018). 1-year American Community Survey estimates. https://www.governing.com/gov-data/census/state-minority-population-data-estimates.html

U.S. Department of Health & Human Services (DHHS). (2021). Child abuse and neglect fatalities 2019: Statistics and interventions. https://www.childwelfare.gov/pubpdfs/fatality.pdf

U.S. Department of Justice. (2012). An updated definition of rape. https://www.justice.gov/opa/blog/updated-definition-rape

U. S. Department of Veterans Affairs. (2022). National veteran suicide prevention annual report. https://www.mentalhealth.va.gov/docs/data-sheets/2022/2022-National-Veteran-Suicide-Prevention-Annual-Report-FINAL-508.pdf

U.S. Environmental Protection Agency (EPA). (2023). America's children and the environment. https://www.epa.gov/americaschildrenenvironment

U.S. Food and Drug Administration (FDA). (2007). Anti-depressant use in children, adolescents, and adults. http://www.fda.gov/NewsEvents/Newsroom/PressAnnouncements/2007/ucm108905.htm

U.S. Food and Drug Administration (FDA). (2019). FDA approves new treatment for hypoactive sexual desire disorder in premenopausal women. https://www.fda.gov/news-events/press-announcements/fda-approves-new-treatment-hypoactive-sexual-desire-disorder-premenopausal-women

U.S. Government Accountability Office. (2017, July 20). Aviation security: TSA does not have valid evidence supporting most of the revised behavioral indicators used in its behavior detection activities. Washington, DC: GAO-17-608R.

Ucok, A. (2007). Other people stigmatize . . . But, what about us? Attitudes of mental health professionals towards patients with schizophrenia. Archives of Neuropsychiatry, 44, 108–116.

Udo, T., Bitley, S., & Grilo, C. M. (2019). Suicide attempts in US adults with lifetime DSM-5 eating disorders. BMC Medicine, 17(1), 120. https://doi.org/10.1186/s12916-019-1352-3

Ueda, K., & Black, K. J. (2021). A comprehensive review of tic disorders in children. Journal of Clinical Medicine, 10(11), 2479. https://doi.org/10.3390/jcm10112479

Ulatowska, J., & Sawicka, M. (2017). Recovered memories in clinical practice—A research review. Psychiatria Polska, 51(4), 609–618.

Ungar, M., & Liebenberg, L. (2013). Ethnocultural factors, resilience, and school engagement. School Psychology International, 34, 514–526.

United Nations. (2019). The United Nations sustainable goals report. https://unstats.un.org/sdgs/report/2019/goal-01/

United Nations. (2020). Policy brief: The impact of COVID-19 on women. https://www.unwomen.org/en/digital-library/publications/2020/04/policy-brief-the-impact-of-covid-19-on-women

United Nations Office on Drugs and Crime. (2020). World drug report. New York: United Nations. https://www.unodc.org/unodc/press/releases/2020/June/media-advisory---global-launch-of-the-2020-world-drug-report.html

Urban, C., Arias, S. A., Segal, D. L., Camargo, C. A., Jr., Boudreaux, E. D., Miller, I., & Betz, M. E. (2020). Emergency department patients with suicide risk: Differences in care by acute alcohol use. General Hospital Psychiatry, 63, 83–88.

Usher, L. V., DaWalt, L. S., Hong, J., Greenberg, J. S., & Mailick, M. R. (2020). Trajectories of change in the behavioral and health phenotype of adolescents and adults with fragile X syndrome and intellectual disability: Longitudinal trends over a decade. Journal of Autism and Developmental Disorders, 50(8), 2779–2792.

Vachon-Presseau, E., Berger, S. E., Abdullah, T. B., Huang, L., Cecchi, G. A., Griffith, J. W., . . . Apkarian, A. V. (2018). Brain and psychological determinants of placebo pill response in chronic pain patients. Nature Communications, 9(1), 3397. https://doi.org/10.1038/s41467-018-05859-1

Vahid, B., & Marik, P. E. (2007, September suppl). Severe emphysema associated with cocaine smoking: A case study. Journal of Respiratory Diseases, pp. 12–20.

Vaknin, S. (2012). The borderline patient—A case study. http://www.healthyplace.com/personality-disorders/malignant-self-love/borderline-patient-a-case-study

Valentine, S. E., & Shipherd, J. C. (2018). A systematic review of social stress and mental health among transgender and gender non-conforming people in the United States. Clinical Psychology Review, 66, 24–38.

Valotassiou, V., Malamitsi, J., Papatriantafyllou, J., Dardiotis, E., Tsougos, I., Psimadas, D., . . . Georgoulias, P. (2018). SPECT and PET imaging in Alzheimer's disease. Annals of Nuclear Medicine, 32(9), 583–593.

van Anders, S. M. (2012). Testosterone and sexual desire in healthy women and men. Archives of Sexual Behavior, 41, 1471–1484.

van den Heuvel, O. A., Boedhoe, P., Bertolin, S., Bruin, W. B., Francks, C., Ivanov, I., . . . ENIGMA-OCD Working Group. (2020). An overview of the first 5 years of the ENIGMA Obsessive-Compulsive Disorder Working Group: The power of worldwide collaboration. Human Brain Mapping. https://doi.org/10.1002/hbm.24972

Van der Feltz-Cornelis, C. M., Allen, S. F., & Van Eck van der Sluijs, J. F. (2020). Childhood sexual abuse predicts treatment outcome in conversion disorder/functional neurological disorder: An observational longitudinal study. Brain and Behavior, 10(3), e01558.

van der Gaag, M., Stant, A. D., Wolters, K. J. K., Burkens, E., & Wiersma, D. (2011). Cognitive behavioral therapy for persistent and recurrent psychosis in people with schizophrenia-spectrum disorder: Cost-effectiveness analysis. British Journal of Psychiatry, 198, 59–65.

van der Put, C. E., Assink, M., Gubbels, J., & Boekhout van Solinge, N. F. (2018). Identifying effective components of child maltreatment interventions: A meta-analysis. Clinical Child and Family Psychology Review, 21(2), 171–202.

van der Valk, E. S., Savas, M., & van Rossum, E. (2018). Stress and obesity: Are there more susceptible individuals? Current Obesity Reports, 7(2), 193–203.

van der Werf, M., Thewissen, V., Dominguez, M. D., Lieb, R., Wittchen, H., & Van Os, J.

(2011). Adolescent development of psychosis as an outcome of hearing impairment: A 10-year longitudinal study. *Psychological Medicine, 41*, 477–485.

Van Diest, I. (2019). Interoception, conditioning, and fear: The panic threesome. *Psychophysiology, 56*(8), e13421. https://doi.org/10.1111/psyp.13421

Van Heeringen, C., & Marusic, A. (2003). Understanding the suicidal brain. *British Journal of Psychiatry, 183*, 282–284.

Van Houtem, C. M., Laine, M. L., Boomsma, D. I., Ligthart, L., van Wijk, A. J., & De Jongh, A. (2013). A review and meta-analysis of the heritability of specific phobia subtypes and corresponding fears. *Journal of Anxiety Disorders, 27*(4), 379–388.

Van Lierde, E., Goubert, L., Vervoort, T., Hughes, G., & Van den Bussche, E. (2020). Learning to fear pain after observing another's pain: An experimental study in schoolchildren. *European Journal of Pain, 24*, 791–806.

Van Noppen, B., & Steketee, G. (2009). Testing a conceptual model of patient and family predictors of obsessive compulsive disorder (OCD) symptoms. *Behaviour Research and Therapy, 47*, 18–25.

Van Orden, K., & Deming, C. (2018). Late-life suicide prevention strategies: Current status and future directions. *Current Opinion in Psychology, 22*, 79–83.

Van Rheenen, T. E., Cropley, V., Zalesky, A., Bousman, C., Wells, R., Bruggemann, J., . . . Pantelis, C. (2018). Widespread volumetric reductions in schizophrenia and schizoaffective patients displaying compromised cognitive abilities. *Schizophrenia Bulletin, 44*(3), 560–574.

van Strien, T. (2018). Causes of emotional eating and matched treatment of obesity. *Current Diabetes Reports, 18*(6), 35. https://doi.org/10.1007/s11892-018-1000-x

van Strien, T., Snoek, H. M., van der Zwaluw, C. S., & Engels, R. C. (2010). Parental control and the dopamine D2 receptor gene (DRD2) interaction on emotional eating in adolescence. *Appetite, 54*, 255–261.

Vanden Brook, T. (2019). Shanahan calls for reforms as military sexual assaults rise by 38%; highest for young women. https://www.usatoday.com/story/news/politics/2019/05/02/military-sexual-assaults-climb-2016-2018-pentagon-army-navy-marines-alcohol/3625405002/

Vandentorren, S., Pirard, P., Sanna, A., Aubert, L., Motreff, Y., Dantchev, N., . . . Baubet, T. (2018). Healthcare provision and the psychological, somatic and social impact on people involved in the terror attacks in January 2015 in Paris: Cohort study. *The British Journal of Psychiatry, 212*(4), 207–214.

Vander Zanden, C. M., & Chi, E. Y. (2020). Passive immunotherapies targeting amyloid beta and tau oligomers in Alzheimer's disease. *Journal of Pharmaceutical Sciences, 109*(1), 68–73.

VandeVrede, L., Boxer, A. L., & Polydoro, M. (2020). Targeting tau: Clinical trials and novel therapeutic approaches. *Neuroscience Letters, 731*, 134919. https://doi.org/10.1016/j.neulet.2020.134919

Vanltallie, T. B. (2019). Traumatic brain injury (TBI) in collision sports: Possible mechanisms of transformation into chronic traumatic encephalopathy (CTE). *Metabolism: Clinical and Experimental, 100S*, 153943. https://doi.org/10.1016/j.metabol.2019.07.007

Vater, A., Ritter, K., Strunz, S., Ronningstam, E. F., Renneberg, B., & Roepke, S. (2014, February 10). Stability of narcissistic personality disorder: Tracking categorical and dimensional rating systems over a two-year period. *Personality Disorders: Theory, Research, and Treatment, 5*, 305–313.

Vatne, M., & Naden, D. (2016). Crucial resources to strengthen the desire to live: Experiences of suicidal patients. *Nursing Ethics, 23*(3), 294–307.

Vaucher, J., Keating, B. J., Lasserre, A. M., Gan, W., Lyall, D. M., Ward, J., . . . Holmes, M. V. (2018). Cannabis use and risk of schizophrenia: A Mendelian randomization study. *Molecular Psychiatry, 23*(5), 1287–1292.

Vega, H., Cole, K., & Hill, K. (2019). Interventions for children with reactive attachment disorder. *Nursing, 49*(6), 50–55.

Veling, W., Selten, J.-P., Mackenbach, J. P., & Hoek, H. W. (2007). Symptoms at first contact for psychotic disorder: Comparison between native Dutch and ethnic minorities. *Schizophrenia Research, 95*, 30–38.

Ventriglio, A., Bhat, P. S., Torales, J., & Bhugra, D. (2019). Sexuality in the 21st century: Leather or rubber? Fetishism explained. *Medical Journal, Armed Forces India, 75*(2), 121–124. https://doi.org/10.1016/j.mjafi.2018.09.009

Ventus, D., Gunst, A., Arver, S., Dhejne, C., Öberg, K. G., Zamore-Söderström, E., . . . Jern, P. (2019). Vibrator-assisted start–stop exercises improve premature ejaculation symptoms: A randomized controlled trial. *Archives of Sexual Behavior.* https://doi.org.ezproxy.library.wwu.edu/10.1007/s10508-019-01520-0

Verboom, C. E., Sentse, M., Sijtsema, J. J., Nolen, W. A., Ormel, J., & Penninx, B. W. (2011). Explaining heterogeneity in disability with major depressive disorder: Effects of personal and environmental characteristics. *Journal of Affective Disorders, 132*, 71–81.

Verma, P. K., Walia, T. S., Chaudhury, S., & Srivastava, S. (2019). Family psychoeducation with caregivers of schizophrenia patients: Impact on perceived quality of life. *Industrial Psychiatry Journal, 28*(1), 19–23.

Versey, H. S. (2017). Caregiving and women's health: Toward an intersectional approach. *Women's Health Issues, 27*(2), 117–120.

Veterans Administration. (2016). VA conducts nation's largest analysis of veteran suicide. https://www.va.gov/opa/pressrel/pressrelease.cfm?id=2801

Veterans Administration. (2019). 2019 national veteran suicide prevention annual report. https://www.mentalhealth.va.gov/docs/data-sheets/2019/2019_National_Veteran_Suicide_Prevention_Annual_Report_508.pdf

Veterans Administration (2022). *National Veteran Suicide Prevention Annual Report. 2022.* https://www.mentalhealth.va.gov/docs/data-sheets/2022/2022-National-Veteran-Suicide-Prevention-Annual-Report-FINAL-508.pdf

Vetter, N. C., Backhausen, L. L., Buse, J., Roessner, V., & Smolka, M. N. (2020). Altered brain morphology in boys with attention deficit hyperactivity disorder with and without comorbid conduct disorder/oppositional defiant disorder. *Human Brain Mapping, 41*(4), 973–983.

Viding, E., & McCrory, E. J. (2018). Understanding the development of psychopathy: Progress and challenges. *Psychological Medicine, 48*(4), 566–577.

Vieta, E., Salagre, E., Grande, I., Carvalho, A. F., Fernandes, B. S., Berk, M., . . . Suppes, T. (2018). Early intervention in bipolar disorder. *The American Journal of Psychiatry, 175*(5), 411–426.

Vijay, A., Becker, J. E., & Ross, J. S. (2018). Patterns and predictors of off-label prescription of psychiatric drugs. *PLOS One, 13*(7), e0198363. https://doi.org/10.1371/journal.pone.0198363

Villagonzalo, K. A., Dodd, S., Ng, F., Mihaly, S., Langbein, A., & Berk, M. (2011). The relationship between substance use and posttraumatic stress disorder in a methadone maintenance treatment program. *Comprehensive Psychiatry, 52*, 562–566.

Vinciguerra, F., Graziano, M., Hagnäs, M., Frittitta, L., & Tumminia, A. (2020). Influence of the Mediterranean and ketogenic diets on cognitive status and decline: A narrative review. *Nutrients, 12*(4), 1019. https://doi.org/10.3390/nu12041019

Viskovich, S., & Pakenham, K. I. (2019). Randomized controlled trial of a web-based Acceptance and Commitment Therapy (ACT) program to promote mental health in university students. *Journal of Clinical Psychology, 76*(6), 929–951. https://doi.org/10.1002/jclp.22848.

Vogt, D., Vaughn, R., Glickman, M. E., Schultz, M., Drainoni, M.-L., Elwy, R., . . . Eisen, S. (2011). Gender differences in combat-related stressors and their association with post-deployment mental health in a nationally representative sample of U.S. OEF/OIF veterans. *Journal of Abnormal Psychology, 120*, 797–806.

Volbrecht, M. M., & Goldsmith, H. H. (2010). Early temperamental and family predictors of shyness and anxiety. *Developmental Psychology, 46*, 1192–1205.

Volkert, J., Gablonski, T. C., & Rabung, S. (2018). Prevalence of personality disorders in the general adult population in Western countries: Systematic review and meta-analysis. *The British Journal of Psychiatry, 213*(6), 709–715.

Volkow, N. D., Wang, G. J., Tomasi, D., & Baler, R. D. (2013). Obesity and addiction: Neurobiological overlaps. *Obesity Reviews, 14*, 2–18.

Volkow, N. D., Wise, R. A., & Baler, R. (2017). The dopamine motive system: Implications for drug and food addiction. *Nature Reviews: Neuroscience, 18*(12), 741–752.

Volpe, K. D., & Kean, S. (2023). More support and critique of AAP Guidelines for Childhood Obesity. https://www.clinicaladvisor.com/home/topics/obesity-information-center/support-critique-aap-guideline-children-obesity/

von Lojewski, A., & Abraham, S. (2014). Personality factors and eating disorders: Self-uncertainty. *Eating Behaviors, 15*, 106–109.

Voss, A., Bogdanski, M., Langohr, B., Albrecht, R., & Sandbothe, M. (2020). Mindfulness-based student training leads to a reduction in physiological evaluated stress. *Frontiers in Psychology, 11*, 645. https://doi.org/10.3389/fpsyg.2020.00645

Voss, R. M., & Das, J. M. (2020). *Mental status exam.* Treasure Island, FL: StatPearls.

Vowels, L. M., Vowels, M. J., & Mark, K. P. (2021). Uncovering the most important factors for predicting sexual desire using explainable machine learning. *The Journal of Sexual Medicine, 18*(7), 1198–1216.

Vowles, K. E., Sowden, G., Hickman, J., & Ashworth, J. (2019). An analysis of within-treatment change trajectories in valued activity in relation to treatment outcomes following interdisciplinary acceptance and commitment therapy for adults with chronic pain. *Behaviour Research and Therapy, 115*, 46–54.

Vu, M., Li, J., Haardörfer, R., Windle, M., & Berg, C. J. (2019). Mental health and substance use among women and men at the intersections of identities and experiences of discrimination: Insights from the intersectionality framework. *BMC Public Health, 19*(1), 108. https://doi.org/10.1186/s12889-019-6430-0

Wacker, E. C., & Dolbin-MacNab, M. L. (2020). Feminist-informed protective factors for subthreshold eating disorders. *Qualitative Health Research, 30*(10), 1546–1560. https://doi.org/10.1177/1049732320921832

Waddell, J. T., Elam, K. K., & Chassin, L. (2022). Multidimensional impulsive personality traits mediate the effect of parent substance use disorder on adolescent alcohol and cannabis use. *Journal of Youth and Adolescence, 51*(2), 348–360. https://doi.org/10.1007/s10964-021-01556-3

Wadden, T. A., Tronieri, J. S., & Butryn, M. L. (2020). Lifestyle modification approaches for the treatment of obesity in adults. *American Psychologist, 75*(2), 235–251.

Wagner, B., Hofmann, L., & Grafiadeli, R. (2021). The relationship between guilt, depression, prolonged grief, and posttraumatic stress symptoms after suicide bereavement. *Journal of Clinical Psychology, 77*(11), 2545–2558.

Wagner-Skacel, J., Bengesser, S., Dalkner, N., Mörkl, S., Painold, A., Hamm, C., . . . Reininghaus, E. Z. (2020). Personality structure and attachment in bipolar disorder. *Frontiers in Psychiatry, 11*, 410. https://doi.org/10.3389/fpsyt.2020.00410

Wahlbeck, K., Cresswell-Smith, J., Haaramo, P., & Parkkonen, J. (2017). Interventions to mitigate the effects of poverty and inequality on mental health. *Social Psychiatry and Psychiatric Epidemiology, 52*(5), 505–514.

Wainwright, L. D., Glentworth, D., Haddock, G., Bentley, R., & Lobban, F. (2014). What do relatives experience when supporting someone in early psychosis? *Psychology and Psychotherapy: Theory, Research, and Practice*. https://doi.org/10.1111/papt.12024

Waldorf, M., Vocks, S., Düsing, R., Bauer, A., & Cordes, M. (2019). Body-oriented gaze behaviors in men with muscle dysmorphia diagnoses. *Journal of Abnormal Psychology, 128*(2), 140–150.

Walfish, S., Barnett, J. E., Marlyere, K., & Zielke, R. (2010). "Doc, there's something I have to tell you": Patient disclosure to their psychotherapist of unprosecuted murder and other violence. *Ethics and Behavior, 20*, 311–323.

Walker, D. D., Stephens, R. S., Towe, S., Banes, K., & Roffman, R. (2015). Maintenance check-ups following treatment for cannabis dependence. *Journal of Substance Abuse Treatment, 56*, 11–15.

Walker, J. R., & Furer, P. (2008). Interoceptive exposure in the treatment of health anxiety and hypochondriasis. *Journal of Cognitive Psychotherapy, 22*, 367–380.

Walker, R. L., Talavera, D. C., Nomamiukor, F., Madubata, I. J., Alfano, C., & Vujanovic, A. A. (2019). Sleep-related problems and suicide behavior and ideation among black and white trauma-exposed psychiatric inpatients. *Comprehensive Psychiatry, 91*, 22–28.

Walker, W. H., II, & Borniger, J. C. (2019). Molecular mechanisms of cancer-induced sleep disruption. *International Journal of Molecular Sciences, 20*(11), 2780. https://doi.org/10.3390/ijms20112780

Walkup, J. (1995). A clinically based rule of thumb for classifying delusions. *Schizophrenia Bulletin, 21*, 323–331.

Wallace, E. R., & Gach, J. (2008). *History of psychiatry and medical psychology with an epilogue on psychiatry and the mind-body relation*. New York: Springer.

Walsh, J. L., Senn, T. E., & Carey, M. P. (2013). Longitudinal associations between health behaviors and mental health in low-income adults. *Translational Behavioral Medicine, 3*, 104–113.

Walters, E. R., & Lesk, V. E. (2015). Time of day and caffeine influence some neuropsychological tests in the elderly. *Psychological Assessment, 27*, 161–168.

Wallis, C. (2022). The pandemic has created a 'zoom boom' in remote psychotherapy. Retrieved from https://www.scientificamerican.com/article/the-pandemic-has-created-a-zoom-boom-in-remote-psychotherapy/

Walther, S., Stegmayer, K., Wilson, J. E., & Heckers, S. (2019). Structure and neural mechanisms of catatonia. *The Lancet: Psychiatry, 6*(7), 610–619.

Walton, E., Bernardoni, F., Batury, V. L., Bahnsen, K., Larivière, S., Abbate-Daga, G., . . . Ehrlich, S. (2022). Brain structure in acutely underweight and partially weight-restored individuals with anorexia nervosa: A coordinated analysis by the ENIGMA Eating Disorders Working Group. *Biological Psychiatry, 92*(9), 730–738. https://doi.org/10.1016/j.biopsych.2022.04.022

Walton, M. T., Cantor, J. M., & Lykins, A. D. (2015). An online assessment of personality, psychological, and sexuality trait variables associated with self-reported hypersexual behavior. *Archives of Sexual Behavior, 46*(3), 721–733.

Wan, Y., Chen, R., Ma, S., McFeeters, D., Sun, Y., Hao, J., & Tao, F. (2019). Associations of adverse childhood experiences and social support with self-injurious behaviour and suicidality in adolescents. *The British Journal of Psychiatry, 214*, 146–152.

Wang, C., & Holtzman, D. M. (2020). Bidirectional relationship between sleep and Alzheimer's disease: Role of amyloid, tau, and other factors. *Neuropsychopharmacology, 45*(1), 104–120.

Wang, J., Lloyd-Evans, B., Giacco, D., Forsyth, R., Nebo, C., Mann, F., & Johnson, S. (2017). Social isolation in mental health: A conceptual and methodological review. *Social Psychiatry and Psychiatric Epidemiology, 52*(12), 1451–1461.

Wang, Q., Wall, C. A., Barney, E. C., Bradshaw, J. L., Macari, S. L., Chawarska, K., & Shic, F. (2020). Promoting social attention in 3-year-olds with ASD through gaze-contingent eye tracking. *Autism Research, 13*(1), 61–73.

Wang, Y. (2016). After years of alleged bullying, an Ohio teen killed herself. Is her school district responsible? http://www.msn.com/en-us/news/us/after-years-of-alleged-bullying-an-ohio-teen-killed-herself-is-her-school-district-responsible/ar-BBtmrtC

Wang, Y., Zuo, C., Xu, Q., Hao, L., & Zhang, Y. (2020). Attention-deficit/hyperactivity disorder is characterized by a delay in subcortical maturation. *Progress in Neuropsychopharmacology and Biological Psychiatry, 104*, 110044. https://doi.org/10.1016/j.pnpbp.2020.110044

Wang, Z., Xu, F., Ye, Q., Tse, L. A., Xue, H., Tan, Z., . . . Wang, Y. (2018). Childhood obesity prevention through a community-based cluster randomized controlled physical activity intervention among schools in China: The health legacy project of the 2nd World Summer Youth Olympic Games (YOG-Obesity study). *International Journal of Obesity (2005), 42*, 625–633.

Ward, A. R., Sibley, M. H., Musser, E. D., Campez, M., Bubnik-Harrison, M. G., Meinzer, M. C., & Yeguez, C. E. (2019). Relational impairments, sluggish cognitive tempo, and severe inattention are associated with elevated self-rated depressive symptoms in adolescents with ADHD. *Attention Deficit and Hyperactivity Disorders, 11*(3), 289–298.

Warren, M., Beck, S., & Delgado, D. (2019). The state of obesity: Better policies for a healthier America 2019. https://www.tfah.org/wp-content/uploads/2019/09/2019Obesity ReportFINAL-1.pdf

Washington Post. (2012). *Washington Post*–Kaiser Family Foundation poll of Black women in America. http://www.washingtonpost.com/wp-srv/special/nation/black-women-in-america

Watkins, E. R., Taylor, R. S., Byng, R., Baeyens, C., Read, R., Pearson, K., & Watson, L. (2012). Guided self-help concreteness training as an intervention for major depression in primary care: A phase II randomized controlled trial. *Psychological Medicine, 42,* 1359–1371.

Watson, A. C., & Compton, M. T. (2019). What research on crisis intervention teams tells us and what we need to ask. *Journal of the American Academy of Psychiatry and Law, 47,* 422–426.

Watson, E. (2019). Is rebirthing therapy safe and effective? https://www.healthline.com/health/rebirthing

Watson, H. J., Yilmaz, Z., Thornton, L. M., Hübel, C., Coleman, J., Gaspar, H. A., . . . Bulik, C. M. (2019). Genome-wide association study identifies eight risk loci and implicates metabo-psychiatric origins for anorexia nervosa. *Nature Genetics, 51*(8), 1207–1214.

Watson, J. B., & Rayner, R. (1920). Conditioned emotional reactions. *Journal of Experimental Psychology, 3,* 1–14.

Watson, N. F., Harden, K. P., Buchwald, D., Vitiello, M. V., Pack, A. I., Strachan, E., & Goldberg, J. (2014). Sleep duration and depressive symptoms: A gene-environment interaction. *Sleep, 37,* 351–358.

Wauthia, E., Lefebvre, L., Huet, K., Blekic, W., El Bouragui, K., & Rossignol, M. (2019). Examining the hierarchical influences of the Big-Five dimensions and anxiety sensitivity on anxiety symptoms in children. *Frontiers in Psychology, 10,* 1185. https://doi.org/10.3389/fpsyg.2019.01185

WCPO Staff. (2016). Emilie Olsen case: Allstate goes to court so it won't have to pay insurance claim. https://www.wcpo.com/news/local-news/hamilton-county/fairfield/emilie-olsen-case-allstate-goes-to-court-so-it-wont-have-to-pay-insurance-claim

Weber, S. R. (2020). Use of mixed amphetamine salts in a patient with depersonalization/derealization disorder. *Innovations in Clinical Neuroscience, 17*(1–3), 45–48.

Wechsler, D. (1981). *Wechsler adult intelligence scale.* New York: Harcourt, Brace, Jovanovich.

Weersing, V. R., Jeffreys, M., Do, M. T., Schwartz, K. T., & Bolano, C. (2017). Evidence base update of psychosocial treatments for child and adolescent depression. *Journal*

of Clinical Child and Adolescent Psychology, 46(1), 11–43.

Weierstall, R., & Giebel, G. (2016). The sadomasochism checklist: A tool for the assessment of sadomasochistic behavior. *Archives of Sexual Behavior, 46*(3), 735–745.

Weinberger, A. H., Smith, P. H., Allen, S. S., Cosgrove, K. P., Saladin, M. E., Gray, K. M., . . . McKee, S. A. (2015). Systematic and meta-analytic review of research examining the impact of menstrual cycle phase and ovarian hormones on smoking and cessation. *Nicotine and Tobacco Research, 17*(4), 407–421.

Weiner, S. (2019). Finding my purpose after schizophrenia. https://www.nami.org/Blogs/NAMI-Blog/June-2019/Finding-My-Purpose-After-Psychosis?

Weir, K (2018, Nov). The ascent of digital therapies. *Monitor on Psychology, 49,* 80.

Weiser, M., Levi, L., Zamora, D., Biegon, A., SanGiovanni, J. P., Davidson, M., . . . Davis, J. M. (2019). Effect of adjunctive estradiol on schizophrenia among women of childbearing age: A randomized clinical trial. *JAMA Psychiatry, 76*(10), 1009–1017. https://doi.org/10.1001/jamapsychiatry.2019.1842

Weissenberger, S., Ptacek, R., Klicperova-Baker, M., Erman, A., Schonova, K., Raboch, J., & Goetz, M. (2017). ADHD, lifestyles and comorbidities: A call for an holistic perspective—From medical to societal intervening factors. *Frontiers in Psychology, 8,* 454. https://doi.org/10.3389/fpsyg.2017.00454

Weller, J., & Budson, A. (2018). Current understanding of Alzheimer's disease diagnosis and treatment. *F1000Research, 7,* F1000 Faculty Rev-1161. https://doi.org/10.12688/f1000research.14506.1

Wells, A. (2005). The metacognitive model of GAD: Assessment of meta-worry and relationship with DSM-IV generalized anxiety disorder. *Cognitive Therapy and Research, 29,* 107–121.

Wells, A. (2009). *Metacognitive therapy for anxiety and depression.* New York: Guilford Press.

West, M. L., & Sharif, S. (2023). Cannabis and psychosis. *Child and Adolescent Psychiatric Clinics of North America, 32*(1), 69–83.

Westefeld, J. S. (2018). Suicide prevention and psychology: A call to action. *Professional Psychology: Research and Practice, 50,* 1–10.

Westen, D., Defife, J. A., Bradley, B., & Hilsenroth, M. J. (2010). Prototype personality diagnosis in clinical practice: A viable alternative to DSM-5 and ICD-11. *Professional Psychology: Research and Practice, 41,* 482–487.

Westheimer, R. K., & Lopater, S. (2005). *Human sexuality: A psychosocial perspective.* Baltimore, MD: Lippincott Williams & Wilkins.

Westphal, M., & Bonanno, G. A. (2007). Posttraumatic growth and resilience to trauma: Different sides of the same coin or different coins? *Applied Psychology: An International Review, 56,* 417–427.

Wetzler, S., Hackmann, C., Peryer, G., Clayman, K., Friedman, D., Saffran, K., . . . Pike, K. M. (2020). A framework to conceptualize personal recovery from eating disorders: A systematic review and qualitative meta-synthesis of perspectives from individuals with lived experience. *The International Journal of Eating Disorders, 53*(8), 1188–1203. https://doi.org/10.1002/eat.23260

Whealin, J. M., Ciro, D., Dasaro, C. R., Udasin, I. G., Crane, M., Moline, J. M., Harrison, D. J., Luft, B. J., Todd, A. C., Feder, A., & Pietrzak, R. H. (2022). Race/ethnic differences in prevalence and correlates of posttraumatic stress disorder in World Trade Center responders: Results from a population-based, health monitoring cohort. *Psychological Trauma: Theory, Research, Practice and Policy, 14*(2), 199–208.

Whealin, J. M., Pitts, B., Tsai, J., Rivera, C., Fogle, B. M., Southwick, S. M., & Pietrzak, R. H. (2020). Dynamic interplay between PTSD symptoms and posttraumatic growth in older military veterans. *Journal of Affective Disorders, 269,* 185–191.

Wheaton, M. G., Berman, N. C., Fabricant, L. E., & Abramowitz, J. S. (2013). Differences in obsessive-compulsive symptoms and obsessive beliefs: A comparison between African Americans, Asian Americans, Latino Americans, and European Americans. *Cognitive Behaviour Therapy*, 42(1), 9–20. https://doi.org/10.1080

White, E. K., & Warren, C. S. (2013). Body checking and avoidance in ethnically diverse female college students. *Body Image*, 11, 583–590.

White, K. S., Craft, J. M., & Gervino, E. V. (2010). Anxiety and hypervigilance to cardiopulmonary sensations in non-cardiac chest pain patients with and without psychiatric disorders. *Behaviour Research and Therapy*, 48, 394–401.

White, L., McDermott, J., Degnan, K., Henderson, H., & Fox, N. (2011). Behavioral inhibition and anxiety: The moderating roles of inhibitory control and attention shifting. *Journal of Abnormal Child Psychology*, 39, 735–747.

Whitman, I. R., Agarwal, V., Nah, G., Dukes, J. W., Vittinghoff, E., Dewland, T. A., & Marcus, G. M. (2017). Alcohol abuse and cardiac disease. *Journal of the American College of Cardiology*, 69(1), 13–24.

Whitmer, D. A., & Woods, D. L. (2013). Analysis of the cost effectiveness of a suicide barrier on the Golden Gate Bridge. *Crisis*, 34, 98–106.

Wichniak, A., Wierzbicka, A., Walęcka, M., & Jernajczyk, W. (2017). Effects of antidepressants on sleep. *Current Psychiatry Reports*, 19(9), 63. https://doi.org/10.1007/s11920-017-0816-4

Wick, M. R., & Keel, P. K. (2020). Posting edited photos of the self: Increasing eating disorder risk or harmless behavior? *The International Journal of Eating Disorders*, 53(6), 864–872. https://doi.org/10.1002/eat.23263

Wickramasekera, I. (1976). Aversive behavior rehearsal for sexual exhibitionism. *Behavior Therapy*, 7(2), 167–176.

Wickwire, E. M., Shaya, F. T., & Scharf, S. M. (2016). Health economics of insomnia treatments: The return on investment for a good night's sleep. *Sleep Medicine Reviews*, 30, 72–82.

Widiger, T. A., & Crego, C. (2019). The bipolarity of normal and abnormal personality structure: Implications for assessment. *Psychological Assessment*, 31(4), 420–431.

Wiepjes, C. M., Nota, N. M., de Blok, C., Klaver, M., de Vries, A., Wensing-Kruger, S. A., . . . den Heijer, M. (2018). The Amsterdam Cohort of Gender Dysphoria Study (1972–2015): Trends in prevalence, treatment, and regrets. *Journal of Sexual Medicine*, 15, 582–590.

Wierenga, C. E., Bischoff-Grethe, A., Melrose, A. J., Irvine, Z., Torres, L., Bailer, U. F., . . . Kaye, W. H. (2015). Hunger does not motivate reward in women remitted from anorexia nervosa. *Biological Psychiatry*, 77(7), 642–652. https://doi.org/10.1016/j.biopsych.2014.09.024

Wiersma, D., Nienhuis, F. J., Sloof, C. J., & Giel, R. (1998). Natural course of schizophrenic disorders: A fifteen-year follow-up of a Dutch incidence cohort. *Schizophrenia Bulletin*, 24, 75–85.

Wilbur, D. Q. (2019). He once tried to kill President Reagan. Now John Hinckley says he's "happy as a clam." https://www.latimes.com/nation/la-na-pol-hinckley-living-in-freedom-20190326-story.html

Wilding, J. P. H., Batterham, R. L., Davies, M., Van Gaal, L. F., Kandler, K., Konakli, K., . . . STEP 1 Study Group. (2022). Weight regain and cardiometabolic effects after withdrawal of semaglutide: The step 1 trial extension. *Diabetes, Obesity & Metabolism*, 24(8), 1553–1564. https://doi.org/10.1111/dom.14725

Wilhelm, S., Phillips, K. A., Didie, E., Buhlmann, U., Greenberg, J. L., Fama, J. M., . . . Steketee, G. (2014). Modular cognitive-behavioral therapy for body dysmorphic disorder: A randomized controlled trial. *Behavior Therapy*, 45(3), 314–327.

Wilhelm, S., Phillips, K. A., Greenberg, J. L., O'Keefe, S. M., Hoeppner, S. S., Keshaviah, A., . . . Schoenfeld, D. A. (2019). Efficacy and posttreatment effects of therapist-delivered cognitive behavioral therapy vs supportive psychotherapy for adults with body dysmorphic disorder: A randomized clinical trial. *JAMA Psychiatry*, 76(4), 363–373.

Williams, A., & McInnis, M. G. (2019). Sex differences in the incidence of antidepressant-induced mania (AIM) in bipolar disorders. *Neuropsychopharmacology*, 44(1), 224–225.

Williams, D. R., & Cooper, L. A. (2019). Reducing racial inequities in health: Using what we already know to take action. *International Journal of Environmental Research and Public Health*, 16(4), 606. https://doi.org/10.3390/ijerph16040606

Williams, D. R., Lawrence, J. A., & Davis, B. A. (2019). Racism and health: Evidence and needed research. *Annual Review of Public Health*, 40, 105–125.

Williams, K., Elliott, R., McKie, S., Zahn, R., Barnhofer, T., & Anderson, I. M. (2020). Changes in the neural correlates of self-blame following mindfulness-based cognitive therapy in remitted depressed participants. *Psychiatry Research: Neuroimaging*, 304. https://doi.org/10.1016/j.pscychresns.2020.111152

Williams, M. T. (2020). The OCD-racism connection and its impact on people of color. https://www.psychologytoday.com/us/blog/culturally-speaking/202009/the-ocd-racism-connection-and-impact-people-color

Williams, S. S. (2016). The terrorist inside my husband's brain. *Neurology*, 87, 1308–1311.

Wilson, N., Kariisa, M., Seth, P., Smith, H., 4th, & Davis, N. L. (2020). Drug and opioid-involved overdose deaths—United States, 2017–2018. *Morbidity and Mortality Weekly Report*, 69(11), 290–297.

Wiśniowiecka-Kowalnik, B., & Nowakowska, B. A. (2019). Genetics and epigenetics of autism spectrum disorder—Current evidence in the field. *Journal of Applied Genetics*, 60(1), 37–47.

Winsper, C., Bilgin, A., Thompson, A., Marwaha, S., Chanen, A. M., Singh, S. P., . . . Furtado, V. (2020). The prevalence of personality disorders in the community: A global systematic review and meta-analysis. *The British Journal of Psychiatry, 216*(2), 69–78.

Winter, J. (2013). Police warned Navy about gunman's mental instability 6 weeks ago, report says. http://www.foxnews.com/us/2013/09/18/navy-yard-shooter-heard-voices-through-walls-thought-people-sending-vibrations/#ixzz2fFS8OFbo

Witkiewitz, K., Wilson, A. D., Pearson, M. R., Montes, K. S., Kirouac, M., Roos, C. R., . . . Maisto, S. A. (2019). Profiles of recovery from alcohol use disorder at three years following treatment: Can the definition of recovery be extended to include high functioning heavy drinkers? *Addiction (Abingdon, England), 114*(1), 69–80.

Wittchen, H.-U., & Hoyer, J. (2001). Generalized anxiety disorder: Nature and course. *Journal of Clinical Psychiatry, 62,* 15–21.

Wittstein, I. S., Thiemann, D. R., Lima, J. A. C., Baughman, K. L., Schulman, S. P., Gerstenblith, G., . . . Champion, H. C. (2005). Neurohumoral features of myocardial stunning due to sudden emotional stress. *New England Journal of Medicine, 352,* 539–548.

Wolff, J., Frazier, E. A., Esposito-Smythers, C., Burke, T., Sloan, E., & Spirito, A. (2013). Cognitive and social factors associated with NSSI and suicide attempts in psychiatrically hospitalized adolescents. *Journal of Abnormal Child Psychology, 41,* 1005–1013.

Wollschlaeger, B. (2007). The science of addiction: From neurobiology to treatment. *Journal of the American Medical Association, 298,* 809–810.

Wolpe, J. (1958). *Psychotherapy by reciprocal inhibition.* Stanford, CA: Stanford University Press.

Wolpe, J. (1973). *The practice of behavior therapy.* New York: Pergamon.

Wolraich, M. L., Chan, E., Froehlich, T., Lynch, R. L., Bax, A., Redwine, S. T., . . . Hagan, J. F., Jr. (2019). ADHD diagnosis and treatment guidelines: A historical perspective. *Pediatrics, 144*(4),

e20191682. https://doi.org/10.1542/peds.2019-1682

Won, C., Mahmoudi, M., Qin, L., Purvis, T., Mathur, A., & Mohsenin, V. (2014). The impact of gender on timeliness of narcolepsy diagnosis. *Journal of Clinical Sleep Medicine, 15,* 89–95.

Won, E., & Kim, Y. K. (2017). An oldie but goodie: Lithium in the treatment of bipolar disorder through neuroprotective and neurotrophic mechanisms. *International Journal of Molecular Sciences, 18*(12), 2679. https://doi.org/10.3390/ijms18122679

Wong, C., Meaburn, E. L., Ronald, A., Price, T. S., Jeffries, A. R., Schalkwyk, L. C., . . . Mill, J. (2014). Methylomic analysis of monozygotic twins discordant for autism spectrum disorder and related behavioural traits. *Molecular Psychiatry, 19*(4), 495–503.

Wong, C., Smith, R. G., Hannon, E., Ramaswami, G., Parikshak, N. N., Assary, E., . . . Mill, J. (2019). Genome-wide DNA methylation profiling identifies convergent molecular signatures associated with idiopathic and syndromic autism in post-mortem human brain tissue. *Human Molecular Genetics, 28*(13), 2201–2211.

Woo, J. S., Brotto, L. A., & Gorzalka, B. B. (2012). The relationship between sex guilt and sexual desire in a community sample of Chinese and Euro-Canadian women. *Journal of Sex Research, 49,* 290–298.

Wood, M. D., Capone, C., Laforge, R., Erickson, D. J., & Brand, N. H. (2007). Brief motivational intervention and alcohol expectancy challenge with heavy drinking college students: A randomized factorial study. *Addictive Behaviors, 32,* 2509–2528.

Woods, D. W., & Houghton, D. C. (2014). Diagnosis, evaluation, and management of trichotillomania. *The Psychiatric Clinics of North America, 37*(3), 301–317.

Woods, J. M., & Nashat, M. (2012). Psychoanalysis and the Rorschach. *Rorschachiana, 33,* 95–99.

World Health Organization (WHO). (2011). Mental retardation: From knowledge to action. http://www.searo.who.int/en/Section1174

/Section1199/Section1567/Section1825_8090.htm

World Health Organization (WHO). (2016). Headache disorders. https://www.who.int/en/news-room/fact-sheets/detail/headache-disorders

World Health Organization (WHO). (2020a). Depression. https://www.who.int/news-room/fact-sheets/detail/depression

World Health Organization (WHO). (2020b). Gender disparities in mental health. https://www.who.int/mental_health/prevention/genderwomen/en/

World Health Organization (WHO). (2021). *Suicide.* https://www.who.int/news-room/fact-sheets/detail/suicide

World Health Organization (WHO). (2023a). Dementia. https://www.who.int/news-room/fact-sheets/detail/dementia

World Health Organization (WHO). (2023b). Obesity and overweight. https://www.who.int/en/news-room/fact-sheets/detail/obesity-and-overweight

World Health Organization (WHO). (2023c). Tobacco. https://www.who.int/news-room/fact-sheets/detail/tobacco

Woud, M. L., Zhang, X. C., Becker, E. S., McNally, R. J., & Margraf, J. (2014). Don't panic: Interpretation bias is predictive of new onsets of panic disorder. *Journal of Anxiety Disorders, 28*(1), 83–87.

Wozney, L., Huguet, A., Bennett, K., Radomski, A. D., Hartling, L., Dyson, M., . . . Newton, A. S. (2017). How do ehealth programs for adolescents with depression work? A realist review of persuasive system design components in internet-based psychological therapies. *Journal of Medical Internet Research, 19*(8), e266. https://doi.org/10.2196/jmir.7573

Wright, A. G., Pincus, A. L., & Lenzenweger, M. F. (2013). A parallel process growth model of avoidant personality disorder symptoms and personality traits. *Personality Disorders, 4,* 230–238.

Wright, C., Beattie, S., Galper, D., Church, A., Bufka, L., Brabender, V., & Smith, B. (2017). Assessment practices of professional psychologists: Results of a national survey. *Professional Psychology: Research and Practice, 48,* 73–78.

Wright, J. H., Owen, J., Eells, T. D., Antle, B., Bishop, L. B., Girdler, R., . . . Ali, S. (2022). Effect of computer-assisted cognitive behavior therapy vs usual care on depression among adults in primary care: A randomized clinical trial. *JAMA Network Open, 5*(2), e2146716. https://doi.org/10.1001 /jamanetworkopen.2021.46716

Wu, L. T., Payne, E. H., Roseman, K., Kingsbury, C., Case, A., Nelson, C., & Lindblad, R. (2019). Clinical workflow and substance use screening, brief intervention, and referral to treatment data in the electronic health records: A National Drug Abuse Treatment Clinical Trials Network Study. *EGEMS (Washington, DC), 7*(1), 35. https:// doi.org/10.5334/egems.293

Wu, Q. E., Zhou, A. M., Han, Y. P., Liu, Y. M., Yang, Y., Wang, X. M., & Shi, X. (2019). Poststroke depression and risk of recurrent stroke: A meta-analysis of prospective studies. *Medicine, 98*(42), e17235. https://doi.org/10.1097 /MD.0000000000017235

Wunderink, L., Nieboer, R. M., Wiersma, D., Sytema, S., & Nienhuis, F. J. (2013). Recovery in remitted first-episode psychosis at 7 years of follow-up of an early dose reduction/discontinuation or maintenance treatment strategy: Long-term follow-up of a 2-year randomized clinical trial. *JAMA Psychiatry, 70,* 913–920.

Wurtele, S. K., Simons, D. A., & Moreno, T. (2014). Sexual interest in children among an online sample of men and women: Prevalence and correlates. *Sexual Abuse, 26,* 546–568.

Xavier, M. J., Roman, S. D., Aitken, R. J., & Nixon, B. (2019). Transgenerational inheritance: How impacts to the epigenetic and genetic information of parents affect offspring health. *Human Reproduction Update, 25*(5), 518–540.

Xu, G., Snetselaar, L. G., Jing, J., Liu, B., Strathearn, L., & Bao, W. (2018). Association of food allergy and other allergic conditions with autism spectrum disorder in children. *JAMA Network Open, 1*(2),

e180279. https://doi.org/10.1001 /jamanetworkopen.2018.0279

Xu, G., Strathearn, L., Liu, B., O'Brien, M., Kopelman, T. G., Zhu, J., . . . Bao, W. (2019). Prevalence and treatment patterns of autism spectrum disorder in the United States, 2016. *JAMA Pediatrics, 173*(2), 153–159.

Xu, Y., Schneider, F., Heimberg, R. G., Princisvalle, K., Liebowitz, M. R., Wang, S., & Blanco, C. (2012). Gender differences in social anxiety disorder: Results from the national epidemiologic sample on alcohol and related conditions. *Journal of Anxiety Disorders, 26,* 12–19.

Yadegar, M., Guo, S., Ricketts, E. J., & Zinner, S. H. (2019). Assessment and management of tic disorders in pediatric primary care settings. *Current Developmental Disorders Reports, 6*(3), 159–172.

Yalçın, İ., Boysan, M., Eşkisu, M., & Çam, Z. (2022). Health anxiety model of cyberchondria, fears, obsessions, sleep quality, and negative affect during COVID-19. *Current Psychology (New Brunswick, NJ),* 1–18. Advance online publication. https://doi.org/10.1007 /s12144-022-02987-2

Yalom, I. D. (2005). *The theory and practice of group psychotherapy.* New York: Basic Books.

Yamagata, A. S. , Brietzke, E., Rosenblat, J. D., Kakar, R., & McIntyre, R. S. (2017). Medical comorbidity in bipolar disorder: The link with metabolic-inflammatory systems. *Journal of Affective Disorders, 211,* 99–106.

Yanek, L. R., Kral, B. G., Moy, T. F., Vaidya, D., Lazo, M., Becker, L. C., & Becker, D. M. (2013, June 28). Effect of positive well-being on incidence of symptomatic coronary artery disease. *American Journal of Cardiology, 112,* 1120–1125.

Yang, A. C., & Tsai, S. J. (2017). New targets for schizophrenia treatment beyond the dopamine hypothesis. *International Journal of Molecular Sciences, 18*(8), 1689. https://doi.org/10.3390 /ijms18081689

Yang, J., Millman, L. S. M., David, A. S., & Hunter, E. C. M. (2023). The prevalence of

depersonalization-derealization disorder: A systematic review. *Journal of Trauma & Dissociation, 24*(1), 8–41.

Yang, X., Daches, S., George, C. J., Kiss, E., Kapornai, K., Baji, I., & Kovacs, M. (2019). Autonomic correlates of lifetime suicidal thoughts and behaviors among adolescents with a history of depression. *Psychophysiology, 56*(8), e13378. https://doi .org/10.1111/psyp.13378

Yao, J., Lv, D., & Chen, W. (2018). Multiple myeloma, misdiagnosed as somatic symptom disorder: A case report. *Frontiers in Psychiatry, 9,* 557. https://doi.org /10.3389/fpsyt.2018.00557

Yap, M., Cardamone-Breen, M. C., Rapee, R. M., Lawrence, K. A., Mackinnon, A. J., Mahtani, S., & Jorm, A. F. (2019). Medium-term effects of a tailored web-based parenting intervention to reduce adolescent risk of depression and anxiety: 12-month findings from a randomized controlled trial. *Journal of Medical Internet Research, 21*(8), e13628. https:// doi.org/10.2196/13628

Yaroslavsky, I., Allard, E. S., & Sanchez-Lopez, A. (2019). Can't look away: Attention control deficits predict rumination, depression symptoms and depressive affect in daily life. *Journal of Affective Disorders, 245,* 1061–1069.

Yasgur, B. S. (2023). Clinicians are talking: Euthanasia for mental illness. Right or wrong? https:// www.medscape.com/view article/995146?form=fpf

Yasumura, A., Omori, M., Fukuda, A., Takahashi, J., Yasumura, Y., Nakagawa, E., . . . Inagaki, M. (2019). Age-related differences in frontal lobe function in children with ADHD. *Brain and Development, 41*(7), 577–586.

Yates, G. P., & Feldman, M. D. (2016). Factitious disorder: A systematic review of 455 cases in the professional literature. *General Hospital Psychiatry, 41,* 20–28.

Yates, G., & Bass, C. (2017). The perpetrators of medical child abuse (Munchausen syndrome by proxy)—A systematic review of 796 cases. *Child Abuse and Neglect, 72,* 45–53.

Yates, W. R. (2014). Anxiety disorders. http://emedicine.medscape.com/article/286227-clinical

Yatham, L. N., Kennedy, S. H., Parikh, S. V., Schaffer, A., Bond, D. J., Frey, B. N., . . . Berk, M. (2018). Canadian Network for Mood and Anxiety Treatments (CANMAT) and International Society for Bipolar Disorders (ISBD) 2018 guidelines for the management of patients with bipolar disorder. *Bipolar Disorders*, *20*(2), 97–170.

Yatham, S., Sivathasan, S., Yoon, R., da Silva, T. L., & Ravindran, A. V. (2018). Depression, anxiety, and post-traumatic stress disorder among youth in low and middle income countries: A review of prevalence and treatment interventions. *Asian Journal of Psychiatry*, *38*, 78–91.

Yee, C. S., Hawken, E. R., Baldessarini, R. J., & Vázquez, G. H. (2019). Maintenance pharmacological treatment of juvenile bipolar disorder: Review and meta-analyses. *International Journal of Neuropsychopharmacology*, *22*(8), 531–540.

Yeung, A. S., Brandt, A. S., O'Neill, M. A., Chen, J. A., Trinh, N. T., & Stern, T. A. (2019). Capacity assessment and involuntary commitment in psychiatric and medical settings: Clinical, legal, and cultural considerations. *The Primary Care Companion for CNS Disorders*, *21*(3), 19f02472. https://doi.org/10.4088/PCC.19f02472

Yeung, A., & Deguang, H. (2002). Somatoform disorders. *Western Journal of Medicine*, *176*.

Yeung, N. C., Lu, Q., Wong, C. C., & Huynh, H. C. (2016). The roles of needs satisfaction, cognitive appraisals, and coping strategies in promoting posttraumatic growth: A stress and coping perspective. *Psychological Trauma: Theory, Research, Practice and Policy*, *8*(3), 284–292.

Y-Hassan, S., & Tornvall, P. (2018). Epidemiology, pathogenesis, and management of takotsubo syndrome. *Clinical Autonomic Research*, *28*(1), 53–65.

Yiend, J., Allen, P., Lopez, N. D., Falkenberg, I., Tseng, H. H., &

McGuire, P. (2019). Negative interpretation biases precede the onset of psychosis. *Behavior Therapy*, *50*(4), 718–731.

Yong, S. J., Tong, T., Chew, J., & Lim, W. L. (2020). Antidepressive mechanisms of probiotics and their therapeutic potential. *Frontiers in Neuroscience*, *13*, 1361. https://doi.org/10.3389/fnins.2019.01361

Yoon, S., Shi, Y., Yoon, D., Pei, F., Schoppe-Sullivan, S., & Snyder, S. M. (2020). Child maltreatment, fathers, and adolescent alcohol and marijuana use trajectories. *Substance Use & Misuse*, *55*(5), 721–733. https://doi.org/10.1080/10826084.2019.1701033

You, Z., Song, J., Wu, C., Qin, P., & Zhou, Z. (2014). Effects of life satisfaction and psychache on risk for suicidal behaviour: A cross-sectional study based on data from Chinese undergraduates. *BMJ Open*, *4*(3), e004096. https://doi.org/10.1136/bmjopen-2013-004096

Young, S., Hollingdale, J., Absoud, M., Bolton, P., Branney, P., Colley, W., . . . Woodhouse, E. (2020). Guidance for identification and treatment of individuals with attention deficit/hyperactivity disorder and autism spectrum disorder based upon expert consensus. *BMC Medicine*, *18*(1), 146. https://doi.org/10.1186/s12916-020-01585-y

Younger, J. (2015). My life with orthorexia. https://www.yahoo.com/beauty/my-life-with-orthorexia-118873503443.html

Youssef, N. A. (2022). Potential societal and cultural implications of transgenerational epigenetic methylation of trauma and PTSD: Pathology or resilience? *The Yale Journal of Biology and Medicine*, *95*(1), 171–174.

Yu, K. Y., Pope, S. C., & Perez, M. (2019). Clinical treatment and practice recommendations for disordered eating in Asian Americans. *Professional Psychology: Research and Practice*, *50*, 279–287.

Yuan, S., Wu, H., Wu, Y., Xu, H., Yu, J., Zhong, Y., . . . Wang, C. (2022). Neural effects of cognitive behavioral therapy in psychiatric disorders: A systematic review

and activation likelihood estimation meta-analysis. *Frontiers in Psychology*, *13*, 853804. https://doi.org/10.3389/fpsyg.2022.853804

Yueh, B. (2020). The threshold of clinical significance. *JAMA Otolaryngology Head and Neck Surgery*, *146*, 98–100.

Zablotsky, B., Black, L. I., Maenner, M. J., Schieve, L. A., Danielson, M. L., Bitsko, R. H., . . . Boyle, C. A. (2019). Prevalence and trends of developmental disabilities among children in the United States: 2009–2017. *Pediatrics*, *144*(4), e20190811. https://doi.org/10.1542/peds.2019-0811

Zablotsky, B., & Terlizzi, E. P. (2020). *Mental health treatment among children aged 5–17 years: United States, 2019*. NCHS Data Brief, no 381. Hyattsville, MD: National Center for Health Statistics.

Zaboski, B. A., 2nd, Merritt, O. A., Schrack, A. P., Gayle, C., Gonzalez, M., Guerrero, L. A., . . . Mathews, C. A. (2019). Hoarding: A meta-analysis of age of onset. *Depression and Anxiety*, *36*(6), 552–564.

Zachar, P., First, M. B., & Kendler, K. S. (2020). The DSM-5 proposal for attenuated psychosis syndrome: A history. *Psychological Medicine*, *50*(6), 920–926.

Zaffar, W., & Arshad, T. (2020). The relationship between social comparison and submissive behaviors in people with social anxiety: Paranoid social cognition as the mediator. *PsyCh Journal*. https://doi.org/10.1002/pchj.352

Zago, S., Piacquadio, E., Monaro, M., Orrù, G., Sampaolo, E., Difonzo, T., . . . Heinzl, E. (2019). The detection of malingered amnesia: An approach involving multiple strategies in a mock crime. *Frontiers in Psychiatry*, *10*, 424. https://doi.org/10.3389/fpsyt.2019.00424

Zaman, R., Hankir, A., & Jemni, M. (2019). Lifestyle factors and mental health. *Psychiatria Danubina*, *31*(Suppl 3), 217–220.

Zanarini, M. C., Parachini, E. A., Frankenburg, F. R., & Holman, J. B. (2003). Sexual relationship difficulties among borderline patients and Axis II comparison subjects. *Journal of Nervous and Mental Disease, 191,* 479–482.

Zanatta, D. P., Rondinoni, C., Salmon, C. E. G., & Del Ben, C. M. (2019). Brain alterations in first episode depressive disorder and resting state fMRI: A systematic review. *Psychology and Neuroscience, 12*(4), 407–429.

Zaninotto, P., & Steptoe, A. (2019). Association between subjective well-being and living longer without disability or illness. *JAMA Network Open, 2*(7), e196870. https://doi.org/10.1001/jamanetworkopen.2019.6870

Zapolski, T. C., Garcia, C. A., Jarjoura, G. R., Lau, K. S., & Aalsma, M. C. (2016). Examining the influence of ethnic/racial socialization on aggressive behaviors among juvenile offenders. *Journal of Juvenile Justice, 5*(1), 65–79.

Zeanah, C. H., Egger, H. L., Smyke, A. T., Nelson, C. A., Fox, N. A., Marshall, P. J., & Guthrie, D. (2009). Institutional rearing and psychiatric disorders in Romanian preschool children. *American Journal of Psychiatry, 166,* 777–785.

Zehra, A., Burns, J., Liu, C. K., Manza, P., Wiers, C. E., Volkow, N. D., & Wang, G. J. (2018). Cannabis addiction and the brain: A review. *Journal of Neuroimmune Pharmacology, 13*(4), 438–452.

Zeidan, J., Fombonne, E., Scorah, J., Ibrahim, A., Durkin, M. S., Saxena, S., . . . Elsabbagh, M. (2022). Global prevalence of autism: A systematic review update. *Autism Research: Official Journal of the International Society for Autism Research, 15*(5), 778–790.

Zeiders, K. H., Landor, A. M., Flores, M., & Brown, A. (2018). Microaggressions and diurnal cortisol: Examining within-person associations among African-American and Latino young adults. *Journal of Adolescent Health, 63*(4), 482–488.

Zeiders, K. H., Umaña-Taylor, A. J., & Derlan, C. L. (2013). Trajectories of depressive symptoms and self-esteem in Latino youths: Examining the role of gender and perceived discrimination. *Developmental Psychology, 49,* 951–963.

Zelviene, P., & Kazlauskas, E. (2018). Adjustment disorder: Current perspectives. *Neuropsychiatric Disease and Treatment, 14,* 375–381.

Zerdzinski, M. (2008). Olfactory obsessions—Individual cases or one of the symptoms of obsessive-compulsive disorder? An analysis of 2 clinical cases. *Archives of Psychiatry and Psychotherapy, 3,* 23–27.

Zhang, B., Weuve, J., Langa, K. M., D'Souza, J., Szpiro, A., Faul, J., . . . Adar, S. D. (2023). Comparison of particulate air pollution from different emission sources and incident dementia in the US. *JAMA Internal Medicine, 183*(10), 1080–1089. https://doi.org/10.1001/jamainternmed.2023.3300

Zhang, F., Niu, L., Liu, X., Liu, Y., Li, S., Yu, H., & Le, W. (2020). Rapid eye movement sleep behavior disorder and neurodegenerative diseases: An update. *Aging and Disease, 11*(2), 315–326.

Zhang, H., Watson-Singleton, N. N., Pollard, S. E., Pittman, D. M., Lamis, D. A., Fischer, N. L., . . . Kaslow, N. J. (2019). Self-criticism and depressive symptoms: Mediating role of self-compassion. *Omega, 80*(2), 202–223.

Zhang, J. P., Robinson, D., Yu, J., Gallego, J., Fleischhacker, W. W., Kahn, R. S., . . . Lencz, T. (2019). Schizophrenia polygenic risk score as a predictor of antipsychotic efficacy in first-episode psychosis. *American Journal of Psychiatry, 176*(1), 21–28.

Zhang, L., Hu, X., Lu, L., Li, B., Hu, X., Bu, X., . . . Huang, X. (2020). Anatomic alterations across amygdala subnuclei in medication-free patients with obsessive-compulsive disorder. *Journal of Psychiatry and Neuroscience, 45*(3), 334–343.

Zhang, L., Opmeer, E. M., van der Meer, L., Aleman, A., Ćurčić-Blake, B., & Ruhé, H. G. (2018). Altered frontal-amygdala effective connectivity during effortful emotion regulation in bipolar disorder. *Bipolar Disorders, 20*(4), 349–358.

Zhao, D., Post, W. S., Blasco-Colmenares, E., Cheng, A., Zhang, Y., Deo, R., . . . Guallar, E. (2019). Racial differences in sudden cardiac death. *Circulation, 139*(14), 1688–1697.

Zhao, J. L., Cross, N., Yao, C. W., Carrier, J., Postuma, R. B., Gosselin, N., . . . Dang-Vu, T. T. (2022). Insomnia disorder increases the risk of subjective memory decline in middle-aged and older adults: A longitudinal analysis of the Canadian Longitudinal Study on Aging. *Sleep, 45*(11), zsac176. https://doi.org/10.1093/sleep/zsac176

Zhao, Y., Zhu, R., Xiao, T., & Liu, X. (2020). Genetic variants in migraine: A field synopsis and systematic re-analysis of meta-analyses. *The Journal of Headache and Pain, 21*(1), 13. https://doi.org/10.1186/s10194-020-01087-5

Zheng, H., Gao, T., Zheng, Q. H., Lu, L. Y., Hou, T. H., Zhang, S. S., . . . Li, Y. (2022). Acupuncture for patients with chronic tension-type headache: A randomized controlled trial. *Neurology.* Advance online publication. https://doi.org/10.1212/WNL.0000000000200670

Zheng, J., Zheng, D., Su, T., & Cheng, J. (2018). Sudden unexplained nocturnal death syndrome: The hundred years' enigma. *Journal of the American Heart Association, 7*(5), e007837. https://doi.org/10.1161/JAHA.117.007837

Zhou, S., Banawa, R., & Oh, H. (2021). The mental health impact of COVID-19: Racial and ethnic discrimination against Asian American and Pacific Islanders. *Frontiers in Psychiatry, 12,* 708426. https://doi.org/10.3389/fpsyt.2021.708426

Zickgraf, H. F., & Barrada, J. R. (2022). Orthorexia nervosa vs. healthy orthorexia: Relationships with disordered eating, eating behavior, and healthy lifestyle choices. *Eating and Weight Disorders, 27*(4), 1313–1325. https://doi.org/10.1007/s40519-021-01263-9

Zimmerman, M., Martinez, J. A., Attiullah, N., Friedman, M., Toba, C., Boerescu, D. A., & Rahgeb, M. (2012). Why do some depressed outpatients who are in remission according to the Hamilton

Depression Rating Scale not consider themselves to be in remission? *Journal of Clinical Psychiatry, 73,* 790–795.

Zito, J. M., Burcu, M., Ibe, A., Safer, D. J., & Magder, L. S. (2013). Antipsychotic use by Medicaid-insured youths: Impact of eligibility and psychiatric diagnosis across a decade. *Psychiatric Services, 64,* 223–229.

Zubair, U., Khan, M. K., & Albashari, M. (2023). Link between excessive social media use and psychiatric disorders. *Annals of Medicine and Surgery (2012), 85*(4), 875–878. https://doi.org/10.1097/MS9.0000000 000000112

Zucker, K. J., & Cohen-Ketteris, P. T. (2008). Gender identity disorder in children and adolescents. In D. Rowland & L. Incrocci (Eds.), *Handbook of sexual and gender identity disorders* (pp. 376–422). Hoboken, NJ: Wiley.

Zulfarina, M. S., Syarifah-Noratiqah, S. B., Nazrun, S. A., Sharif, R., & Naina-Mohamed, I. (2019). Pharmacological therapy in panic disorder: Current guidelines and novel drugs discovery for treatment-resistant patient. *Clinical Psychopharmacology and Neuroscience, 17*(2), 145–154.

Zvolensky, M. J., Garey, L., Allan, N. P., Farris, S. G., Raines, A. M., Smits, J., . . . Schmidt, N. B. (2018). Effects of anxiety sensitivity reduction on smoking abstinence: An analysis from a panic prevention program. *Journal of Consulting and Clinical Psychology, 86*(5), 474–485.

Zvolensky, M. J., Kauffman, B. Y., Bogiaizian, D., Viana, A. G., Bakhshaie, J., & Peraza, N. (2019). Worry among Latinx college students: Relations to anxious arousal, social anxiety, general depression, and insomnia. *Journal of American College Health,* 1–8. https://doi.org/10.1080/07448481 .2019.1686004

Zvolensky, M. J., Kauffman, B. Y., Shepherd, J. M., Viana, A. G., Bogiaizian, D., Rogers, A. H., . . . Peraza, N. (2020). Pain-related anxiety among Latinx college students: Relations to body vigilance, worry, anxious arousal, and general depression. *Journal of Racial and Ethnic Health Disparities, 7*(3), 498–507.

Zwaigenbaum, L., Brian, J. A., & Ip, A. (2019). Early detection for autism spectrum disorder in young children. *Paediatrics and Child Health, 24*(7), 424–443.

Name Index

Subject Index

Assisted suicide, 345
Asthma, 218–220, 219f
Asthmatic bronchiole, 219f
Astrapophobia, 157t
Asymptomatic relatives, 136
Ataque de nervios, 245
Atherosclerosis, 213, 213f, 411, 490
Ativan, 164, 402
Attachment disorders, 606–609
Attention-deficit/hyperactivity disorder (ADHD), 621–626
  biological dimension, 623–624
  characteristics, 622t
  defined, 622
  etiology, 623–624
  psychological, social, socio-cultural dimensions, 624
  treatment, 625–626
Attenuated psychosis syndrome, 444
Attributional style, 283
Atypical antidepressants, 290
Atypical antipsychotics, 53, 459
Auditory hallucination, 438–440
Aura, 217
Aurora, Colorado shooting (2012), 654, 657, 674
Autism spectrum disorder (ASD), 626–635
  Asperger's syndrome, 631
  biological influences, 631–633
  continuum of symptoms, 629t
  defined, 626
  early warning signs, 630t
  etiology, 631–633
  intervention/treatment, 634–635
  symptoms, 627–631
Autistic savant, 629
Autogynephilia, 546
Autonomic nervous system (ANS), 46
Autosomal-dominant Alzheimer's disease, 496
Aversive behavior rehearsal, 552
Avoidance, 202
Avoidant personality disorder, 566t, 578–579
Avolition, 442
Axon, 47

B
Bacteria, 380
Barbiturates, 402
Base rate, 124–125
Bath salts (MPDV), 410, 450

BDD. *See* Body dysmorphic disorder (BDD)
BDI-II. *See* Beck Depression Inventory-II (BDI-II)
Beck Depression Inventory-II (BDI-II), 93–94
Beck's six types of faulty thinking, 282t
BED. *See* Binge-eating disorder (BED)
Bedlam, 20
Behavior
  ASMC, 366
  cultural influences on, 12–13
  describing, 5
  explaining, 5–6
  hypersexual, 521
  modifying, 7–8
  operant, 60
  predicting, 6–7
  self-destructive, 573
  sexual, 520–522
  socio-political influences on, 12–13
  voluntary, 60, 61
Behavioral activation therapy, 294–295
Behavioral factors, 106
Behavioral inhibition, 152
Behavioral models
  behavioral therapies, 62
  classical conditioning paradigm, 59–60
  criticisms of, 62
  observational learning paradigm, 61
  operant conditioning paradigm, 60–61
Behavioral symptoms
  depression, 270
  hypomania/mania, 271–272
Behavioral therapies, 62
  depressive disorders, 294–295
  obsessive-compulsive (OCD) and related disorders, 186–187
Behavioral treatments, 186–187, 294–297
Behavioral undercontrol, 414
Behavioral variation, 10f
Behaviorism, 23
Bell Curve, The (Herrnstein/Murray), 95–96
Bender-Gestalt Visual-Motor Test, 96, 96f
Benzodiazepines, 53, 164, 402, 512
Beta-amyloid plaques, 496
Beta-blockers, 164

Binge drinking, 397
Binge eating, 357–359
Binge-eating disorder (BED), 359–361
  associated characteristics, 360
  course and outcomes, 360–361
  physical complications, 360
  treatment, 375
Binge-eating/purging anorexia nervosa type, 355–356
Biochemical treatment
  panic disorders, 170–171
  phobias, 164
Biofeedback training, 225–226
Biological challenge tests, 137
Biological dimension
  antisocial personality disorder (APD), 583–585, 583f
  anxiety disorders, 149–152
  attention-deficit/hyperactivity disorder (ADHD), 623–624
  bipolar disorders, 302–304
  conduct disorder, 617–618
  depressive disorders, 277–280
  dissociative disorders, 255–256
  eating disorders, 371–373
  gender dysphoria, 538–541
  generalized anxiety disorder (GAD), 172–173
  obesity, 378–380
  obsessive-compulsive (OCD) and related disorders, 182–184
  overview, 44
  phobias, 159–160
  psychophysiological disorders, 220–222
  resilience model, 44f
  schizophrenia, 446–451
  sexual dysfunctions, 529–530
  somatic symptom and related disorders, 240–242
  substance-use disorders, 417–419
  suicide, 328–330
  trauma-related disorders, 204–206, 204f
Biological factors, 105
  biology-based treatment techniques, 52–55. *See also* Biology-based treatment techniques
  epigenetics, 51–52
  genetics/heredity, 50–52
  human brain, 45–47. *See also* Brain
  neuroplasticity, 50
Biological influences, 43

anxiety, trauma, and stressor-related disorders, 606–610
ASD. *See* Autism spectrum disorder (ASD)
attachment disorders, 606–609
child abuse and neglect, 607
conduct disorder (CD), 615t, 616–617
contemporary trends/future directions, 641–642
defined, 604
DMDD, 611
Down syndrome, 636
dyslexia/dyscalculia, 639
externalizing disorders, 613–620
fetal alcohol syndrome (FAS), 638
fragile X syndrome, 636
intellectual disability (ID), 620t, 635–639
intermittent explosive disorder (IED), 614–615, 615t
internalizing disorders, 606–613
learning disorder, 620t, 639–641
mood disorders, 610–613
neurodevelopmental disorders. *See* Neurodevelopmental disorders
nonsuicidal self-injury (NSSI), 609–610
oppositional defiant disorder (ODD), 614, 615t
pediatric bipolar disorder (PBD), 612–613, 612t
PTSD, 609
selective mutism, 606
separation anxiety disorder, 606
tic disorder, 620–622, 620t
Tourette's disorder, 621
Children
obesity, 378
pedophilic disorder, 548–550
psychopathology. *See* Child
sexual abuse, 124
suicide, 321–324
China, collectivity *vs.* individuality, 74
Chlorpromazine, 29, 53, 459
Cholesterol, 491
Chronic motor or vocal tic disorder, 621
Chronic traumatic encephalopathy (CTE), 488–490
Cialis, 533, 534t
Cigarette smoking, 406

Circadian-related treatments, 290
Circadian rhythms, 280, 508
Circadian rhythm sleep disorder, 508
Civil commitment, 6, 657–662
assessing dangerousness, 659–661
criteria for, 658–659
defined, 657
procedures in, 661
protection against involuntary commitment, 662
Classical conditioning, 59–60, 59f
Classical conditioning perspective, 161
Classification and labeling, 109
"Cleanup" enzymes, 398
Clinical interview, 88, 91
Clinical psychologist, 96
Clinical research, 117–142
analogue studies, 131–132
base rates, 124–125
biological research strategies, 135–138. *See also* Biological research
case study, 132–133, 133–134
characteristics of, 122–126
contemporary trends/future directions, 139–141
correlational studies, 129–131, 136
epidemiological research, 139
ethical considerations, 129
experiments, 126–129
field studies, 132
hypothesis, 119
increased appreciation for, 31
internal validity, 121–122, 127
levels of evidence, 121t
operational definitions, 123–124
placebo group, 128
reliability of measures/observations, 124
scientific method, 119
single-participant studies, 132–135
statistical significance, 125–126
theory, 119
validity of measures/observations, 124
Clinical Trials Network, 429
Club drugs, 411
Cluster A personality disorders
paranoid personality disorder, 567–568

schizoid personality disorder, 566t, 568
schizotypal personality disorder, 566, 569–570
Cluster B personality disorders
antisocial personality disorder (APD), 566t, 570–572
borderline personality disorder (BPD), 566t, 572–575
histrionic personality disorder, 566t, 576
narcissistic personality disorder, 566t, 577–578
Cluster C personality disorders
avoidant personality disorder, 566t, 578–579
dependent personality disorder, 566t, 580–581
obsessive-compulsive personality disorder (OCPD), 566t, 581–582
Cluster headaches, 216–218, 216f, 218
Cocaine, 404
Cocaine addiction, 404
Cocaine use, 417
Coffee drinking, 329
Cognitive-behavioral models, 63–66
criticisms of, 65
Ellis's A-B-C theory of personal, 63
phobias, 162
somatic symptom and related disorders, 242–243
therapeutic approaches, 65
Cognitive-behavioral therapy (CBT), 64–65
binge-eating disorder, 375
borderline personality disorder, 574
bulimia nervosa, 374
depressive disorders, 295–296
generalized anxiety disorder (GAD), 173
neurocognitive disorders, 503–504
panic disorders, 171–172
phobias, 164–167
psychophysiological disorders, 226
schizophrenia, 462–464
sleep disorders, 511
suicide, 343–344
trauma-related disorders, 210–211
Cognitive impairment tests, 96
Cognitive model, 65

Mindfulness-based stress reduction, 65
    psychophysiological disorders, and, 226
Mind That Found Itself, A (Beers), 21
Minnesota Multiphasic PersonalityInventory (MMPI), 93–94
Minnesota Multiphasic Personality Inventory-3 (MMPI-3), 93–94
Minor tranquilizers, 52, 53
Mixed features, 301
MMPI. *See* Minnesota Multiphasic Personality Inventory (MMPI)
MMPI-3. *See* Minnesota Multiphasic Personality Inventory (MMPI-3)
M'Naghten rule, 652
Mobile apps, 32
Model, 38, 39
Modeling, 61
Modeling agencies, 374
Modeling therapy, 165, 167
Models of abnormal behavior multipath. *See also* Multipath model
Moderate drinking, 397
Monoamine oxidase inhibitors (MAOIs), 53, 164, 290
Monophobia, 157t
Monozygotic (MZ) twins, 136
Mood, 268
Mood disorders, 364, 610–613
Mood stabilizers, 53
Mood symptoms, 272–273
Moral, ethical and legal issues surrounding suicide, 346–348
Moral treatment movement, 20–21
Morgellons disease, 469
Motivational enhancement therapy, 421
Motor tics, 621
MRI. *See* Magnetic resonance imaging (MRI)
Multicultural counseling, 76
Multicultural model, 74, 76–77
Multicultural perspective, 76
Multicultural psychology
    cultural and ethnic bias, in diagnosis, 26
    cultural values and influences, 25
    social conditioning, 24–25
    sociopolitical influences, 25
Multipath model, 40–44
    antisocial personality disorder, 583f

anxiety disorders, 150f
conduct disorder, 617f
depressive disorders, 278f
dissociative disorders, 256f
eating disorders, 364f
generalized anxiety disorder (GAD), 173f
neurocognitive disorders, 485f
obesity, 379f
obsessive-compulsive (OCD) and related disorders, 182f
panic disorders, 168f
phobias, 161
post-traumatic stress disorder (PTSD), 205f
psychophysiological disorders, 220f
schizophrenia, 446f
sexual dysfunctions, 530f
somatic symptom and related disorders, 241f
substance-use disorders, 413f
suicide, 329f
Multiple-baseline study, 134, 134f
Munchausen syndrome, 239
Munchausen syndrome by proxy. *See* Factitious disorder imposed on another
Muscle dysmorphia, 180–181
Muse (alprostadil), 534t
MXE. *See* Methoxetamine (MXE)
Myelin, 48
Myelination, 48
Mysophobia, 157t
MZ twins. *See* Monozygotic (MZ) twins

N

Nalmefene, 422
Naltrexone, 422
NAMI. *See* National Alliance of Mental Illness (NAMI)
Narcissistic personality disorder, 110, 566t, 577–578
Narcolepsy, 507–508
Narcotics Anonymous, 419
National Alliance of Mental Illness (NAMI), 15
National Committee for Mental Hygiene, 21
Native Indians, and suicide, 335–336
Natural catastrophes, 203
Naturalistic observations, 89
Navy Yard shooting, 435
NEBA. *See* Neuropsychiatric EEG-Based Assessment Aid (NEBA) system

Negative affectivity, 592, 596t
Negative alternations in mood or cognition, 202
Negative appraisal, 153
Negative emotional stage, 222
Negative hallucination, 438–440
Negative information perspective, 162
Negative reinforcement, 61
Negative symptoms of schizophrenia, 442
Negative thinking patterns, 283–284
Neural circuits, 47
Neural stem cells, 50
Neurocognitive disorders, 101t, 478–505
    Alzheimer's disease, and, 494–497. *See also* Alzheimer's disease (AD)
    biological treatment, 503
    cognitive/behavioral treatment, 503–504
    defined, 478
    delirium, 482–483
    dementia with Lewy bodies (DLB), 497–499
    environmental support, and, 504–505
    etiology of, 483–502
    event causes of, 484t
    frontotemporal lobar degeneration (FTLD), and, 499
    genetic testing, 501
    head injury, 487
    HIV infection, and, 501–502
    Huntington's disease (HD), and, 500–501
    lifestyle changes, and, 504
    major neurocognitive disorder, 479–480
    mild neurocognitive disorder, 481–482
    multipath model of, 485f
    normal aging *vs.* disorder symptoms, 481t
    Parkinson's disease (PD), and, 499–500
    rehabilitation services, 502–503
    substance abuse, and, 493
    traumatic brain injury (TBI), 485–490. *See also* Traumatic brain injury (TBI)
    treatment of, 502–505
    types of, 478–483
    vascular, 490–493